a LANGE medi

MW00759242

CURRENT
Diagnosis & Treatment
Emergency Medicine

SEVENTH EDITION

Edited by

C. Keith Stone, MD
Professor and Chair
Department of Emergency Medicine
Texas A&M University Health Science Center
College of Medicine
Scott & White Healthcare
Temple, Texas

Roger L. Humphries, MD
Associate Professor and Chair
Department of Emergency Medicine
University of Kentucky College of Medicine
Lexington, Kentucky

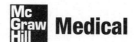 **Medical**

New York   Chicago   San Francisco   Lisbon   London   Madrid   Mexico City
Milan   New Delhi   San Juan   Seoul   Singapore   Sydney   Toronto

CURRENT Diagnosis & Treatment: Emergency Medicine, Seventh Edition

2 3 4 5 6 7 8 9 0 DOC/DOC 15 14 13 12

ISBN 978-0-07-170107-5
MHID 0-07-170107-9
ISSN 0894-2293

Notice

Medicine is an ever-changing science. As new research and clinical experience broaden our knowledge, changes in treatment and drug therapy are required. The authors and the publisher of this work have checked with sources believed to be reliable in their efforts to provide information that is complete and generally in accord with the standards accepted at the time of publication. However, in view of the possibility of human error or changes in medical sciences, neither the authors nor the publisher nor any other party who has been involved in the preparation or publication of this work warrants that the information contained herein is in every respect accurate or complete, and they disclaim all responsibility for any errors or omissions or for the results obtained from use of the information contained in this work. Readers are encouraged to confirm the information contained herein with other sources. For example and in particular, readers are advised to check the product information sheet included in the package of each drug they plan to administer to be certain that the information contained in this work is accurate and that changes have not been made in the recommended dose or in the contraindications for administration. This recommendation is of particular importance in connection with new or infrequently used drugs.

This book was set in Minion by Thomson Digital.
The editors were Anne M. Sydor and Peter J. Boyle.
The production supervisor was Sherri Souffrance.
Project management was provided by Anand Kumar, Thomson Digital.
The art manager was Armen Ovsepyan.
The designer was Alan Barnett; the cover art director is Anthony Landi.
RR Donnelley was printer and binder.

This book is printed on acid-free paper.

I dedicate this edition to my late father. I learned so much from you that has shaped both my personal and professional life. Your greatest strength ultimately led to your untimely passing from this earth. Even in death, you have given me one more valuable lesson to learn as I live my life.

C. Keith Stone

Contents

Authors

Brian Adkins, MD
Assistant Professor, Department of Emergency Medicine, University of Kentucky College of Medicine, Lexington, Kentucky
Genitourinary Trauma

Thomas W. Allen, DO, MPH
Department of Emergency Medicine, University of Oklahoma School of Community Medicine, Tulsa, Oklahoma
Disaster Medicine

Zachary E. Armstrong, MD
Resident, Department of Emergency Medicine, University of Louisville, Louisville, Kentucky
Gastrointestinal Bleeding

Shah Ashfaq, BS
University of Kentucky College of Medicine, Lexington, Kentucky
Pediatric Emergencies

Kavon Azadi, MD
Resident, Department of Emergency Medicine, University of Oklahoma, Tulsa, Oklahoma
Dermatologic Emergencies

Douglas J. Borys, PharmD
Adjunct Associate Professor, Department of Central Texas Poison Center, Irma Lerma Rangel College of Pharmacy, Texas A&M University Health Science Center, Kingsville, Texas
Poisoning

Rebecca C. Bowers, MD, FACEP
Assistant Professor, Department of Emergency Medicine, University of Kentucky, Lexington, Kentucky
Disorders Due to Physical & Environmental Agents

Jonathan C. Brantley, MD
Chief Resident, Department of Emergency Medicine, University of Kentucky, Lexington, Kentucky
Legal Aspects of Emergency Care

Eric J. Brown, MD, MS
Chief Resident, Department of Emergency Medicine, University of Oklahoma College of Medicine, Tulsa, Oklahoma
Psychiatric Emergencies

Boyd Burns, DO, FACEP, FAAEM
Assistant Professor, Department of Emergency Medicine, University of Oklahoma School of Community Medicine, Tulsa, Oklahoma
Dermatologic Emergencies

Craig Carter, DO
Associate Professor, Department of Emergency Medicine, University of Kentucky College of Medicine, Lexington, Kentucky
Pediatric Emergencies

Royce Coleman, MD
Department of Emergency Medicine, University of Louisville, Louisville, Kentucky
Orthopedic Emergencies

Christopher Colvin, MD
Assistant Professor, Department of Emergency Medicine, Scott & White Memorial Hospital, Temple, Texas
Procedural Sedation & Analgesia

Justin Coomes, MD
Resident, Department of Emergency Medicine, University of Louisville, Louisville, Kentucky
Abdominal Pain

Kimrey J. Daniel, MD
Resident, Department of Emergency Medicine, Scott & White Memorial Hospital, Temple, Texas
Prehospital Emergency Services; Eye Emergencies

Daniel F. Danzl, MD
Professor and Chair, Department of Emergency Medicine, University of Louisville, Louisville, Kentucky
Metabolic & Endocrine Emergencies

Elizabeth Davis, MD
Assistant Professor, Department of Emergency Medicine, University of Kentucky, Lexington, Kentucky
Gastrointestinal Emergencies

Sameer Desai, MD
Assistant Professor, Department of Emergency Medicine, University of Kentucky, Lexington, Kentucky
Cardiac Emergencies

Colby Dorroh, MD
Resident, Department of Emergency Medicine, University of Louisville, Louisville, Kentucky
Emergency Procedures

Dorian Drigalla, MD, FACEP
Assistant Professor, Department of Emergency Medicine,
College of Medicine, Texas A&M University Health
Science Center, Scott & White Memorial Hospital
and Clinic, Temple, Texas
Burns & Smoke Inhalation

Charles A. Eckerline, Jr, MD, FACEP
Associate Professor, Department of Emergency Medicine,
University of Kentucky Medical Center,
Lexington, Kentucky
Legal Aspects of Emergency Care

Bill Ewen, MD
Assistant Clinical Professor, International EM Fellow,
Division of Emergency Medicine,
University of Texas Southwestern Medical Center,
Dallas, Texas
Hand Trauma

S. Derrick Fowler, MD
Resident Physician, Department of Emergency Medicine,
University of Kentucky, Lexington, Kentucky
Vertebral Column & Spinal Cord Trauma

David A. Fritz, MD, FACEP
Assistant Professor, Department of Emergency Medicine,
Scott & White Memorial Hospital, Temple, Texas
Emergency Bedside Ultrasound; Vascular Emergencies

Jennifer Gemmill, MD
Resident Physician, Department of Emergency Medicine,
Scott & White Memorial Hospital, Temple, Texas
Burns & Smoke Inhalation

Eric C. Goshorn, MD
University of Louisville, Louisville, Kentucky
Basic & Advanced Cardiac Life Support

Robert D. Greenberg, MD, FACEP
Assistant Professor, Department of Emergency Medicine,
College of Medicine, Texas A&M University Health
Science Center, Temple, Texas
Eye Emergencies

Marshall Hall, MD
Chief Resident, Department of Emergency Medicine,
University of Kentucky, Lexington, Kentucky
Maxillofacial & Neck Trauma

Raymond G. Hart, MD, MPH
Assistant Clinical Professor, Department of Emergency
Medicine, University of Louisville School of Medicine,
Louisville, Kentucky
Hand Trauma

Joseph Heidenriech, MD
Assistant Professor, Department of Emergency Medicine,
College of Medicine, Texas A&M Health Science Center,
Scott & White Memorial Hospital, Temple, Texas
Cardiac Arrhrthmias; Genitourinary Emergencies

Martin R. Huecker, MD
Chief Resident, Department of Emergency Medicine,
University of Louisville, Louisville, Kentucky
Chest Pain; Metabolic & Endocrine Emergencies

Roger L. Humphries, MD
Associate Professor and Chair,
Department of Emergency Medicine,
University of Kentucky College of Medicine,
Lexington, Kentucky
Head Injuries

Jon Jaffe, MD
Assistant Professor, Department of Emergency Medicine,
College of Medicine, Texas A&M University Health
Science Center, Temple, Texas
Infectious Disease Emergencies

Jonathan Jones, MD
Attending Physician, Department of Emergency Medicine,
Bay Medical Center, Panama City, Florida
Chest Trauma

Thomas R. Jones, MD, MDiv, FAAEM
Associate Professor, Department of Emergency, College of
Medicine, Texas A&M University Health Science Center,
Scott & White Memorial Hospital, Temple, Texas
Approach to the Emergency Department Patient; Wound Care

Andrew Juergens, MD
Resident, Department of Emergency Medicine, Scott &
White Memorial Hospital, Temple, Texas
Syncope

Justin A. Kan, MD
Resident, Department of Emergency Medicine, University
of Louisville, Louisville, Kentucky
Basic & Advanced Cardiac Life Support

Justin Knowles, MD
Assistant Professor, Department of Emergency Medicine,
  University of Kentucky, Lexington, Kentucky
Compromised Airway

Julia Martin, MD, FACEP
Associate Professor, Department of Emergency Medicine,
  University of Kentucky, Lexington, Kentucky
The Multiply Injured Patient

Dylan B. Medley, MD
Resident, Department of Emergency Medicine,
  Scott & White Memorial Hospital, Temple, Texas
Coma

Daniel E. Melville, MD
Assistant Professor, Department of Family and
  Community Medicine, University of Kentucky,
  Lexington, Kentucky
Abdominal Trauma

Sonya C. Melville, MD
Assistant Professor, Department of Emergency Medicine,
  University of Kentucky, Lexington, Kentucky
Abdominal Trauma

David L. Morgan, MD
Professor, Department of Emergency Medicine, Texas A&M
  University Health Science Center, Temple, Texas
*Nuclear, Biologic, & Chemical Agents, Weapons of Mass
  Destruction; Poinsoning*

James E. Morris, MD, MPH
Assistant Professor, Department of Emergency Medicine,
  College of Medicine, Texas A&M University Health
  Science Center, Temple, Texas
Coma; Fluid, Electrolyte, & Acid–Base Emergencies

M. Virginia Mustain, MD
Assistant Professor, Department of Emergency Medicine,
  University of Kentucky, Lexington, Kentucky
Disorders Due to Physical & Environmental Agents

Daniel J. O'Brien, MD, FACEP, FAAEM
Associate Professor, Emergency Medicine, Department of
  Emergency Medicine, University of Louisville School of
  Medicine, Louisiville, Kentucky
Chest Pain

Christopher Ortiz, MD
Resident, Department of Emergency Medicine,
  Scott & White Memorial Hospital, Temple, Texas
*Nuclear, Biologic, & Chemical Agents; Weapons of
  Mass Destruction*

William Randall Partin, MD, FACEP, FAAEM
Associate Clinical Professor, Department of Dept.
  of Emergency Medicine, School of Medicine,
  University of Louisville, Louisville, Kentucky
Emergency Procedures

Melissa Platt, MD
Assistant Professor, Department of Emergency Medicine,
  University of Louisville, Louisville, Kentucky
Abdomial Pain; Obstetric & Gynecologic Emergencies & Rape

Kimberly J. Powers, MD
Resident, Department of Emergency Medicine,
  University of Kentucky, Lexington, Kentucky
Gastrointestinal Emergencies

Timothy G. Price, MD, FACEP, FAAEM
Associate Professor, Department of Emergency Medicine,
  University of Louisville, Louisville, Kentucky
Gastrointestinal Bleeding

Allison Rains, MD
Assistant Professor, Department of Emergency Medicine,
  University of Kentucky, Lexington, Kentucky
Compromised Airway

Taylor Ratcliff, MD
Resident, Department of Emergency Medicine, Scott &
  White Memorial Hospital, Temple, Texas
Infectious Disease Emergencies

Alison Reiland, MD
Resident, Department of Emergency Medicine, University
  of Louisville, Louisville, Kentucky
Orthopedic Emergencies

Jason Seamon, DO, MHS, FACEP, FAAEM
Program Director & Assistant Professor, Department of
  Emergency Medicine, University of Kentucky, Lexington,
  Kentucky
*Arthritis & Back Pain; Vertebral Column & Spinal Cord
  Trauma*

Alicia A. Shirakbari, MD
Assistant Professor, Department of Emergency Medicine,
  University of Kentucky Medical Center, Lexington,
  Kentucky
Maxillofacial & Neck Trauma

David A. Smith, MD
Assistant Professor, Department of Emergency Medicine,
  Texas A&M University Health Science Center, College of
  Medicine, Scott & White Healthcare, Temple, Texas
Pulmonary Emergencies

Timothy C. Stallard, MD
Associate Professor, Department of Emergency Medicine, Texas A&M University Health Sciences Center, Temple, Texas
Emergency Disorders of the Ear, Nose, Sinuses, Oropharynx, & Mouth

Gregory A. Starr, MD
Department of Emergency Medicine, University of Oklahoma School of Community Medicine, Tulsa, Oklahoma
Disaster Medicine

Seth Stearley, MD
Assistant Professor, Department of Emergency Medicine, University of Kentucky, Lexington, Kentucky
Chest Trauma

Maria Stephan, MD
Associate Professor, Department of Emergency Medicine, University of Kentucky, Lexington, Kentucky
Pediatric Emergencies

Charles E. Stewart, MD, EMDM
Department of Emergency Medicine, University of Oklahoma School of Community Medicine, Tulsa, Oklahoma
Disaster Medicine

C. Keith Stone, MD
Professor and Chair, Department of Emergency Medicine, Texas A&M University Health Science Center, College of Medicine, Scott & White Healthcare, Temple, Texas
Respiratory Distress; Syncope; Seizures; Headache; Neurologic Emergencies

Margaret Strecker-McGraw, MD, FACEP
Assistant Professor, Department of Emergency Medicine, Division of Prehospital Medicine, Scott & White Memorial Hospital, Texas A&M University Health Science Center, Temple, Texas
Prehospital Emergency Services; Syncope; Hematologic Emergencies

Ryan Tucker, MD
Resident, Department of Emergency Medicine, University of Louisville School of Medicine, Louisville, Kentucky
Obstetric & Gynecologic Emergencies & Rape

Salvator J. Vicario, MD
Associate Professor of Emergency Medicine, Department of Emergecy Medicine, University of Louisville School of Medicine, Louisville, Kentucky
Basic & Advanced Cardiac Life Support

Lori Whelan, MD
Assistant Professor, Department of Emergency Medicine, University of Oklahoma, Tulsa, Oklahoma
Psychiatric Emergencies

Mark Andrew Wilson, MD
Resident Physician, Department of Emergency Medicine, Scott & White Memorial Hospital, Temple, Texas
Hematologic Emergencies

Ryan P. Woods, MD
Department of Emergency Medicine, University of Kentucky Medical Center, Lexington, Kentucky
Arthritis & Back Pain

William F. Young, Jr. MD
Associate Professor, Department of Emergency Medicine, University of Kentucky, Lexington, Kentucky
Shock

Preface

Current Emergency Diagnosis & Treatment, seventh edition, is designed to present concise, easy-to-read, practical information on the diagnosis and treatment of a wide spectrum of conditions that present to the emergency department. The chapters emphasize the immediate management of life-threatening problems and then present the evaluation and treatment of specific disorders. We trust that this text will aid all practitioners of emergency medicine in providing care to their patients.

OUTSTANDING FEATURES

In keeping with the tradition of the *Current* series, CEDT strives to provide the reader with a broad-based text written in a clear and succinct manner. Our goal is to provide practicing emergency physicians quick access to accurate and useful information that will aid in their everyday practice of emergency medicine.

Because this text focuses on the practical aspects of emergency care, there is little discussion of the basic science or pathophysiology of disease processes. In addition, discussion of management restricts the material presented to treatments routinely provided in the ED.

INTENDED AUDIENCE

CEDT will be useful to all practitioners of emergency medicine, including physicians, residents, medical students, as well as physician extenders. It will also provide valuable information for emergency nurses and prehospital care providers.

ORGANIZATION

This edition retains the priority-based and problem-oriented organization of previous editions. Chapters in Section I, "Special Aspects of Emergency Medicine," are written in a non-structured free text format. Chapters in Section II, "Management of Common Emergency Problems," are presented in a problem-based format. Life-threatening disorders are discussed first followed by a presentation of specific disorders. This chapter format is carried out in the remainder of the book in both Section III "Traumatic Emergencies" and Section IV "Non-trauma emergencies."

SPECIAL TO THIS EDITION

- A new chapter on bedside ultrasound
- A new chapter on procedural sedation
- A new section on pandemic flu
- Updates of all chapters

ACKNOWLEDGMENTS

We would like to thank the staff at McGraw-Hill, Anne Sydor, Peter Boyle, and Jennifer Orlando for their patience and support throughout the preparation of the manuscript. In addition, we again would like to thank our families, Gail and Chase; Kris, Maddie, and Jack, for their love and indulgence to allow us to dedicate the hours needed to work on this edition.

C. Keith Stone, MD
Roger L. Humphries, MD
May 2011

Approach to the Emergency Department Patient

T. Russell Jones, MD, Mdiv

What Is Emergency Medicine?	Principles of Emergency Medicine
Unique Aspects of Emergency Medicine Practice	Conclusion

WHAT IS EMERGENCY MEDICINE?

An emergency is commonly defined as any condition perceived by the prudent layperson—or someone on his or her behalf—as requiring immediate medical or surgical evaluation and treatment. On the basis of this definition, the American College of Emergency Physicians states that the practice of emergency medicine has the primary mission of evaluating, managing, and providing treatment to these patients with unexpected injury and illness.

So what does an emergency physician (EP) do? He or she routinely provides care and makes medical treatment decisions based on real-time evaluation of a patient's history; physical findings; and many diagnostic studies, including multiple imaging modalities, laboratory tests, and electrocardiograms. The EP needs an amalgam of skills to treat a wide variety of injuries and illnesses, ranging from the diagnosis of an upper respiratory infection or dermatologic condition to resuscitation and stabilization of the multiple trauma patient. Furthermore, these physicians must be able to practice emergency medicine on patients of all ages. It has been said that EPs are masters and mistresses of negotiation, creativity, and disposition. Clinical emergency medicine may be practiced in emergency departments (EDs), both rural and urban; urgent care clinics; and other settings such as at mass gathering incidents, through emergency medical services (EMS), and in hazardous material and bioterrorism situations.

Emergency medicine serves as the US health care safety net. It provides valuable clinical and administrative services to the health care delivery system, including care for the indigent and others who lack access to health care, and has evolved as the most visible and vital component of a patchwork of health care providers and facilities. EDs have become the routine, and often the only, source of care for many of the uninsured, thereby acting as a critical safety net for our fragmented health care delivery system.

Finally, EDs are the only element of the health care system whose function has been delineated by federal law. Initially authorized in 1986, the Emergency Medical Treatment and Active Labor Act mandates that all EDs provide screening, stabilization, and appropriate transfer to *all* patients with *any* medical condition. Emergency medicine is often the last resort for many patients and frequently the access point for competent, comprehensive, and efficient medical care.

UNIQUE ASPECTS OF EMERGENCY MEDICINE PRACTICE

An EP faces numerous challenges. The first and most distinctive challenge is that of limited time. Time constraints occur because of the severity and acuity of the illness and also because of the ever-present worry that someone else will need the physician's attention. The second challenge for the EP is that he or she needs to quickly assess and make therapeutic decisions on the basis of limited information. The EP may also be providing medical control for patients in the prehospital environment. In addition, the EP also will need to determine what care was given prior to arrival and what impact the intervention made. History may be provided from bystanders or EMS providers and given to the physician second hand.

The EP has a different mindset than other specialties. The main concern of the EP is not necessarily the diagnosis, but a process of thinking aimed at ruling in or out serious pathology that is life- or limb-threatening. The classic model of history taking followed by a physical examination and then diagnostic testing must often be compressed and conducted simultaneously when time is of the essence and the patient's life is threatened.

The evaluation of patients should proceed in a parallel fashion rather than the time-honored serial method. The mindset that patients must be triaged and registered in the waiting room when there are beds available must be abandoned. Patients should be taken straight away to any available room where the physician and nurse assess the patient and get the history while the patient is simultaneously having an intravenous line with blood work drawn and registration occurring in the room. The single intervention of in-room registration can decrease the length of stay of the patient by an average of 15 minutes.

The ED is a unique environment in that hospital EDs are required by federal law to evaluate patients without regard to ability to pay. In 2005, there were an estimated 45–48 million Americans without health insurance. This puts financial strains on both hospitals and physicians. In addition, patients with nonurgent health problems use the ED for a variety of reasons. Studies have found that the majority of patients were not aware of other places to go for their care. When an ED reaches 140% of its capacity, the number of patients leaving without being seen will increase. This leads to patient dissatisfaction and an increased risk of litigation, not to mention the potential that the patient is leaving with a potential life threat that has not been identified.

Because of a number of factors, it may be difficult to get on-call physicians to care for patients seen in the ED. In a recent study conducted in California, it was found that the lack of insurance had a negative impact on the availability to obtain specialty physician assistance. The seven specialties noted to have the greatest difficulty in obtaining specialty consultations were plastic surgery, ENT, dentistry, psychiatry, neurosurgery, ophthalmology, and orthopedics. This was found despite the medical staff bylaws that required on-call ED coverage. It is up to the EP to be the patient advocate, even when that means holding patients in the department until they can get the care they need or the appropriate laboratory or specialty evaluation to let them safely go home.

It is imperative that the EP be informed about the resources that are available to the patients after discharge. It is a simple matter to send patients to see a physician that they already have a relationship with. It may not be such an easy matter for the uninsured or indigent patient. Various clinics in the community can assist patients with needs such as prenatal care or those with diabetes or HIV. In addition, the physician must inquire about domestic violence and elderly abuse and remain vigilant about the potential of child abuse.

EPs work in an environment in which patients die. Despite the circumstances surrounding the patient's death,

the EP needs to get answers to a myriad of questions: Why the person died, will the illness have an impact on survivors, does the illness put health care workers and society at risk, should an autopsy be performed for medical or legal reasons, and does the family desire organ donation? In interacting with survivors, the EP should avoid clichés that can be misleading and let the survivors know that the patient has died, in whatever language is appropriate. The EP needs to be on guard for the occasional violent reaction by survivors, so doors need to be open and security may need to be in close proximity. It behooves EPs to find positive ways to take care of themselves and the ED staff from emotionally traumatic events through techniques such as stress debriefing or counseling.

PRINCIPLES OF EMERGENCY MEDICINE

It is often said that ED patients "don't read the textbook," meaning that their presentations do not fit nicely into specific textbook diagnoses or classical presentations of illness. However, a cornerstone of an EP's practice is the recognition of patterns in a patient's presentation; therefore, the prudent physician must be a detective and scientist to muddle through the muck of vague signs and symptoms to find the pattern.

The principles of emergency medicine are simply questions that must be answered to provide effective care to patients who have entrusted EPs with their care. The questions are not to be used as a cookbook approach to the management of these often complex medical and psychosocial issues but are to be used as a simple method to guide the prudent EP through the quagmire of clinical emergency medicine.

A. Is the Patient About to Die?

Obviously, this is the first and most important question to answer. Every patient's presentation is quickly prioritized to one of the following acuities:

1. Critical—Patient has symptoms consistent with a life-threatening illness or injury with a high probability of death if immediate intervention is not begun.

2. Emergent—Patient has symptoms of illness or injury that may progress in severity if treatment is not begun quickly.

3. Nonurgent—Patient has symptoms that have a low probability of progression to a more serious condition.

Look for *symptoms* of a life-threatening emergency, not a specific disease entity. Anticipate impending life-threatening emergencies in the apparently stable patient.

B. What Steps Must Be Undertaken to Stabilize the Patient?

Act quickly to stabilize the critically ill or injured patient. Focus on the primary survey (airway, breathing, circulation, and neurologic deficits), and make necessary interventions as each issue is identified. Do not delay necessary primary interventions while awaiting completion of ancillary testing.

C. What Are the Most Potential Serious Causes of the Patient's Presentation?

Thinking of the worst-case scenario, develop a mental list of the most deadly causes of the patient's presentation by asking, "What will kill this patient the fastest?" Once the list has been developed, the vital signs, history, physical examination, and ancillary assessments should identify or confirm those causes highest on the list.

D. Could There Be Multiple Causes of the Patient's Presentation?

In addition to constant reevaluation and reprioritization of the differential diagnosis, continually ask, "Is this all there is?" For example, is the new-onset seizure and hypoglycemia in an older diabetic patient from intentional or accidental medication overdose or perhaps worsening renal insufficiency? Is the near-syncope and abdominal pain in an apparently intoxicated college coed from a ruptured ectopic pregnancy or perhaps a ruptured spleen secondary to undisclosed physical abuse by her boyfriend? Frequent reassessment and thoughtful inquiry as to the multiple possibilities responsible for each patient's condition is imperative.

E. Can a Treatment Assist in the Diagnosis in an Otherwise Undifferentiated Illness?

Often, in emergency medicine, treatment response foretells a diagnosis. A case in point is the unconscious patient with no available collateral history. The patient's response to empiric administration of naloxone will include or exclude narcotic overdose as a contributor to the obtundation. Referred to as the "diagnostic–therapeutic" concept, it underscores the emergency medicine philosophy that an established diagnosis is not a prerequisite to initiating appropriate treatment. Pitfalls can exist. For example, sublingual nitroglycerin and so-called GI cocktails can relieve symptoms of chest pain resulting from the same cause.

F. Is a Diagnosis Mandatory or Even Possible?

After the emergency issues have been addressed, the patient and EP are often left with an undifferentiated symptom complex. This frequently elicits an uncomfortable response by nonemergency medicine trained physicians. The EP should become accustomed to and comfortable with the notion of determining the disposition for nonemergency patients—having treated their symptoms and excluding emergency conditions—without a specific diagnosis.

G. Does This Patient Need to Be Admitted to the Hospital?

Having appropriately answered the preceding questions, make the bottom-line disposition decision. Once assessments and treatments are under way, decide whether an emergency condition exists. Consider other subtleties. Does the patient have timely, accessible follow-up? How far away from a medical facility does the patient live? Are unresolved abuse or self-care issues involved? Are you, as the EP, comfortable discharging the patient?

H. IF the Patient Is Not Being Admitted, is the Disposition Safe and Adequate for the Patient?

More frequently than not, patients are discharged home from the ED. However, many patients do not receive a specific diagnosis, and some symptoms may persist. Recommend appropriate follow-up, and provide written discharge instructions. Instruct the patient when to return for further evaluation should symptoms change or worsen. Provide the patient with information regarding treatment and diagnosis as well. In patients who choose to leave against medical advice, the EP must make it clear that there are no hard feelings and the patient is welcome to return at any time.

CONCLUSION

Emergency medicine has seen a tremendous growth and increase in awareness of the unique aspects of the profession. It remains a challenging and fulfilling experience for many physicians and an appealing choice of specialties for medical students. As emergency medicine matures as a specialty, its importance as the US health care safety net and its integral status as front-line medicine will continue to expand and grow.

American College of Emergency Physicians: Definition of emergency medicine, as approved by the ACEP Board of Directors, April 2001. Available at: www.acep.org/practres.aspx?id=29164.

Gorelick MH et al: Effect of in-room registration on emergency department length of stay. Ann Emerg Med 2005;45:128 [PMID: 15671967].

Leap E: Because We're So Good. Emerg Med News 2010;32(3):7.

Northington W et al: Use of an emergency department by nonurgent patients. Am J Emerg Med 2005;23:131. [PMID: 15765330].

Polevoi S et al: Factors associated with patients who leave without being seen. Acad Emerg Med 2005;12:232 [PMID: 15741586].

Rudkin S et al: The state of ED on-call coverage in California. Am J Emerg Med 2004;22:575 [PMID: 15666264].

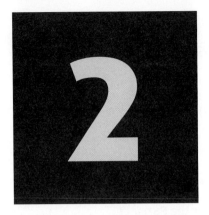

Prehospital Emergency Services

Margaret Strecker-McGraw, MD, FACEP

Kimrey J. Daniel, MD

Development of modern prehospital emergency medical services (EMS) stems primarily from lessons learned from providing medical care to soldiers in military conflicts and from government mandates.

In the 1960s, the President's Committee for Traffic Safety recognized the need to address health, transportation, and medical care in order to reduce fatalities and injuries on our nation's roadways.

In 1966, the National Academy of Science published a report entitled *Accidental Death and Disability: The Neglected Disease of Modern Society*. It described deficiencies in prehospital care regarding ambulance systems and the hazardous conditions of emergency care provision. The issues raised in this survey compounded with public outcry prompted the drafting of federal legislation, the Highway Safety Act of 1966. The legislation was intended to help states develop programs to improve emergency care. It required each state to have a highway safety program that complied with uniform federal standards including emergency services. Initial National Highway Transportation Safety Administration (NHTSA) efforts were focused on improving the education of prehospital personnel. Funding was provided to develop state emergency services offices. International activity around the same time included Professor Frank Pantridge (1916–2004) and colleagues demonstrating improvement in patient outcomes by outfitting cardiac defibrillators on ambulances in Belfast, Ireland.

The first national conference on EMS resulted in the development of a curriculum, certification process, and national registry for EMS personnel. In the 1970s, EMS systems were established by the Department of Transportation (DOT)–NHTSA in selected areas around the country to provide standardized ambulance services. As prehospital services expanded, so did the role of the EMS provider.

COMPONENTS OF AN EMERGENCY MEDICAL SERVICES SYSTEM

Public law 93-154: Emergency Medical Services System Act of 1973 identified the following essential components of an EMS system:

1. Communications
2. Training
3. Manpower
4. Mutual aid
5. Transportation
6. Accessibility
7. Facilities
8. Critical care units
9. Transfer of care
10. Consumer participation

11. Public education
12. Public safety agencies
13. Standard medical records
14. Independent review and evaluation
15. Disaster linkage

Unfortunately, this neglected two other essentials: medical direction and system financing.

Multiple changes have occurred over the ensuing years, and each component of the EMS system has gone through many stages of development. Federal financing has virtually been abolished by the Consolidated Omnibus Budget Reconciliation Act, which has shifted the burden on state and local agencies. In 1988, the Statewide EMS Technical Assessment Program was established by NHTSA and defined elements necessary to all EMS systems.

Communications

Communications are a critical part of prehospital emergency care. From universal access for the public to the EMS system, to adequate radio space for providers to communicate with each other in spite of disaster, communications are the lifeblood of EMS.

The 911 universal access system provides entry into the emergency system. The Wireless Communications and Public Safety Act of 1999 was enacted with the goal of implementing 911 as the universal access to emergency services. Enhanced 911 allows automatic reporting of number and location of the caller. Wireless enhanced 911 will soon provide the same automatic reporting from wireless phones. The FCC also regulates 911 services for satellite services, text telephone devices, and voice over Internet protocol devices.

A 911 call connects the caller with an emergency medical dispatcher (EMD), who then coordinates with other public agencies, for example, fire and police, and then prioritizes and dispatches resources available to the scene.

EMDs are trained to assign determinants that direct the level of response, that is, lights and sirens, and number of providers. They also give callers prearrival instructions for comfort and lifesaving interventions until prehospital personnel arrive on the scene.

Currently, EMS communications are changing from wide band to narrow band frequencies. Previously, prehospital providers used VHF or UHF 25-kHz bandwidths, but beginning in 2011, the FCC will no longer approve applications for these bandwidths. Nonfederal emergency providers that use frequencies below 512 MHz are required to transition to 12.5-kHz bandwidth by January 1, 2013. The goal of this change is to free up and streamline existing bandwidths, with a transition at some unspecified time in the future to a 6.25-kHz bandwidth.

Additionally, the FCC has designated the upper half of the 700-MHz public safety band for nationwide interoperable (real-time communication between different public safety groups) communications, to be administered at the state level. Most 700- and 800-MHz systems are trunked, meaning channels are shared among a group of users.

Federal goals for EMS communications include: demonstration of response-level communications within 1 hour for routine events involving multiple jurisdictions and agencies by 2010, by 2011 same for non-UASI jurisdictions, and by 2013 all jurisdictions' response level within 3 hours of significant event (as outlined in the National Emergency Communications Plan).

Transportation

Since 1966, requirements for vehicles used to provide emergency medical care have become standardized. Care is also provided in rotor- and fixed-wing aircraft. Many EMS services are fire based, and first responder vehicles include fire trucks and nonambulance trucks and automobiles. Bike EMS providers patrol civic events, and providers on motorcycles are a critical part of the system in Europe.

EMS vehicles may be equipped for basic life support (BLS), advanced life support (ALS), or specialty care depending on the need and availability (eg, specialized transport systems and vehicles for neonates, patients on ECMO, and intensive care transports).

Facilities

EMS systems typically include hospitals with a variety of treatment capabilities. These may include any number and mix of local community hospitals with limited services, moderate-sized facilities with more advanced capabilities, and tertiary care facilities with capabilities to provide all levels of care. Hospital facilities are also frequently classified according to their relationship to EMS in addition to their ability to provide definitive care.

1. *Base station hospitals*: Physicians or specially trained personnel, generally paramedics or nurses, with physician backup provide EMS units with online medical supervision during treatment and transport. In many EMS systems, the base station hospital may also be the one most capable of providing definitive care.

2. *Receiving hospitals*: Receiving hospitals are facilities within the EMS's geographic service area to which patients may be transported. The receiving hospital may be selected according to its proximity; capabilities; and patient, family, or physician preference.

In general, patients should be transported to the nearest facility capable of treating them, but since not all hospitals have equal capabilities they are sometimes bypassed. Bypass is driven by the EMS system generally by local or regional protocol that directs and allows transport directly to specialized facilities, for example, burn centers, trauma centers, or cardiac care centers rather than stopping at the closest facility. Diversion is a request by a hospital for an EMS provider to not bring a patient to them due to lack of capacity or capability.

The Joint Commission on Accreditation of Healthcare Organizations has categorized hospitals into four levels of acute care based on availability of physicians, nurses, allied health personnel, and other hospital resources. This ranges from a level 1 that is a comprehensive facility to a level 4 that is a triage and lifesaving aid station. Hospitals may also be categorized by the type and level of specialty care they can provide. The most well-known system is the American College of Surgeons Verification of Trauma Centers:

Level 1: A full-service trauma center that provides comprehensive care with immediate availability of services and a commitment to research and education.

Level 2: Similar to a level 1 center in ability to provide most clinical care, but does not necessarily include a commitment to education or research.

Level 3: Provides initial stabilization and lifesaving care prior to transfer to a higher-level facility if necessary.

▶ Training and Human Resources

EMS providers are trained in accordance with regional, state, and federal standards.

A. First Responders

First responders include law enforcement, rescue squad members, firefighters, or volunteer EMS personnel. This level of training requires approximately 40 hours of didactic and clinical training in basic first aid and cardiopulmonary resuscitation (CPR).

At the most basic provider level, providers are known as emergency medical responder (EMR), formerly known as emergency care attendants (ECAs)—training includes basic lifesaving interventions, and providing assistance to higher level of skill providers before and during transport.

B. Emergency Medical Technicians

The National Registry of Emergency Medical Technicians currently recognizes three levels of training: EMT-A (basic), EMT-I (intermediate), and EMT-P (paramedic). Each level requires specific training as defined by state protocol.

1. EMT-A—Basic EMTs constitute the essential workforce of EMS systems throughout the United States. Most state laws require at least one certified EMT onboard ambulance vehicles that transport patients.

The basic EMT course requires at least 81 hours of training standardized by the DOT. Basic classes frequently exceed this minimum by up to 140 hours. Students learn basic principles of patient care, how to identify signs and symptoms central to patient assessment and diagnosis, and how to provide treatment in specific emergencies. The use of automated external defibrillators (AEDs) is also now standard curriculum for EMTs in most regions. Optional modules for EMTs include advanced airway management, intravenous access, and assisting patients with self-administration of medications. Additionally, some states allow administration of medications, including epinephrine in anaphylaxis, albuterol in asthma, and aspirin in suspected cardiac chest pain.

2. EMT-I—Advanced Emergency Care Technician, also known as EMT-I, is trained to provide a level of advanced care in areas that are underserved by paramedics. The scope of practice has evolved since 1990 to incorporate many advanced cardiac life support procedures, including cardiac monitoring, treatment of arrhythmias, defibrillation, and advanced airway management with either endotracheal intubation or an alternative airway.

3. EMT-P—Advanced EMTs (paramedics) receive over 1000 hours of training in ALS techniques. Their skills include the basic EMT procedures as well as intravenous cannulations, invasive airway management, recognition and treatment of cardiac dysrhythmias, defibrillation, and the use of specific emergency medications. In addition to extensive classroom training, EMT-P personnel also complete clinical training and a field internship with experienced paramedic teams.

▶ Special Qualifications

Additional training is available at all levels for specific care settings. A Winter Emergency Care course has been developed by the National Ski Patrol to address special situations that occur in ski areas. Similarly, there are Wilderness modules at all levels of training that provide additional training for care provided in a remote setting with anticipated long evacuations and transportation.

EMT-tactical courses train EMTs and paramedics to deliver care so they may support or be a part of law enforcement, for example, SWAT, team. Finally, paramedic–critical-care training enables the advanced provider to provide care to critically injured or ill patients who are being transferred from one facility to another.

The air and surface transport nurse is generally a registered nurse with or without additional paramedic training. He or she usually serves on helicopters and fixed-wing and specialty care transports. Other personnel who provide care on specialty teams, especially pediatric and neonatal transports, include respiratory therapists and nurse practitioners.

Physician team members are more frequent outside of the United States. Within the United States, they are generally found only on rotor or fixed-wing transports.

▶ Resource Management

Each state must have central control of EMS resources to ensure all patients have equal access to acceptable emergency care. State EMS agencies are typically responsible for allocating funds to local systems, implementing legislation regarding the prehospital practice of medicine, licensing and certification of field providers and personnel, enforcing regulations, and appointing advisory councils.

At the municipal and regional level, the EMS agency is responsible for managing the local systems resources, developing operational protocol, and establishing standards and guidelines. Local agencies develop policies consistent with the state requirements, implement a quality assurance or quality improvement program to ensure that the patient's best interest is served, and develop mutual aid agreements. Mutual aid agreements ensure a continuum of care during multiple casualty incidents and can be between departments, municipalities, or states. The agreements should provide for situations that may overwhelm local or regional resources.

Local agencies are typically composed of community representatives, including emergency physicians, EMS providers, firefighters, police, and local citizens. EMS providers may function in a variety of ways. They may be a part of a municipal fire department or independent as in the "third service" model, with fire and police being the first and second services provided. Providers may also be independent businesses with municipal contracts or community, usually volunteer, based.

Responses

Many possible combinations of prehospital services exist with the variables of BLS versus ALS, volunteer versus paid, governmentally run versus independent with or without first responders or a tiered response. There may even be a mixture of providers to serve the emergency and nonemergency transport needs of a community. No one system is ideal, and all have advantages and disadvantages.

Medical Direction

Prehospital care by EMS personnel is a delegated medical practice. EMS systems must retain a physician who is legally responsible for clinical and patient care aspects of the system. The medical director, in conjunction with local and state entities, develops and oversees training programs and clinical protocols and authorizes EMS personnel under his or her direction. He or she participates in personnel and equipment selection, directs the quality improvement and quality assurance programs, provides direct input into patient care, and is a liaison between the EMS system and other health care agencies. The medical director is the ultimate authority for all medical direction.

Medical direction may be described as online or offline. Online medical communication provides EMTs with clinical consultation in the field via telephone or radio communication with a physician at a base station. Offline medical communication is a function of the EMS organization. Nonphysician prehospital personnel operate under standing orders and treatment protocols developed by a physician medical director that are appropriate for the provider's level of training. These protocols determine the type and level of care administered at the emergency site. Physicians who provide online medical supervision of paramedics from base hospitals may permit paramedics to deviate from established protocols or to provide treatment not specifically covered in standing orders as long as prehospital providers do not deviate from their given scope of practice. The medical director assumes authority for offline medical direction via policies, procedures, standing orders, and field protocols.

Protocols and standing orders are instruments developed and approved by the medical director to instruct and guide prehospital personnel. As every system is different in its composition, geographic coverage, and capabilities, there is no ideal set of protocols or standing orders that can be applied broadly. The breadth and depth of the protocols are most dependent on the system's ability to monitor the care given.

Field supervision and direct observation of care by the medical director, known to many as grassroots medical direction, is the most effective means to manage and oversee the care provided. This is commonly practiced in larger communities that can afford full-time medical direction. Unfortunately, EMS medical direction has been poorly valued and many times is undercompensated or uncompensated and as a result is inconsistent.

Trauma Systems

Each state should develop a system of specialized care for trauma patients, including acute care trauma centers and rehabilitation programs. It must also develop systems for assigning and transporting patients to those facilities.

Regulation, Policy, and Quality Improvement

EMS organizations are administered by the states. Currently, there is no federal agency that oversees EMS. Each state must have laws, regulations, policies, and procedures that govern its EMS system. The individual state is also required to provide leadership to local jurisdictions and is responsible for education and data collection. These agencies may supply medical protocols, or otherwise establish scope of practice, and oversee communication systems. States coordinate disaster response and planning. In addition, each state and system must have a quality improvement system in place for continuing evaluation and upgrading of its EMS system.

Current discussion centers on moving EMS under the umbrella of Homeland Security from its current place under the NTHSA. Placing EMS under this umbrella will facilitate its interaction with other divisions, and place EMS in line for federal funding. Resistance to the idea comes from fire department–associated systems and organizations.

▶ Public Education and Information

EMS systems provide for education of the public not only to recognize an emergency but also how to access the EMS system and initiate BLS. Classes in CPR, AED operation, and control of bleeding are offered to encourage bystanders to take an active role in providing emergency care prior to the arrival of trained personnel.

EMS DELIVERY DURING NATURAL DISASTERS AND TERRORIST ATTACKS

Over the past decade, a multitude of natural and manmade disasters have illuminated the deficiencies in EMS coordination and administration during such disasters. In order to facilitate communication and coordination of EMS during these events, the National Incident Management System (NIMS) was created to improve preparation, coordination, and incident management in disaster situations. NIMS was designed to allow federal, state, and local governments to work together to "prepare for, respond to, and recover from" domestic disasters, regardless of how large or small. Its goal is to provide both flexibility and standardization in delivery of emergency care during disasters. This includes coordinating diverse groups and ensuring adequate communication between them.

Other entities have come into being since the World Trade Center attacks in 2001. The Emergency Care Coordination Center within the Department of Health and Human Services was created to facilitate coordination between levels and types of EMS at a federal level.

FUTURE OF EMS

In 2007, the NHSTA, which currently oversees the EMS system, convened to reevaluate where EMS is now, and where it is headed. Renewed focus on research, collecting data, evidenced-based medicine, increasing standardization, and, eventually, reciprocal state licensure and national licensure is on the agenda as EMS heads into the 21st century.

EMS is a relatively new field, with potential for growth and expansion. Federal mandates for research and education will encourage evidence-based practice to become the accepted norm for providers. Improved technology and education such as transmission of field EKGs will allow EMS to provide cutting edge care as first responders. Prehospital providers will coordinate disaster care with local, state, and federal agencies, and continue to improve in this area through hard-won experience and constant review and evaluation.

700 MHz Public Safety Spectrum: http//www.fcc.gov/pshs/public-safety-spectrum/700-MHz/, Washington, DC. Accessed April 30, 2010.

Brice J, Alson RL: Emergency preparedness in North Carolina: Leading the way. N C Med J 2007;68:276–278 [PMID: 17694850].

Department of Homeland Security: National Emergency Communications Plan. http://www.dhs.gov/xlibrary/assets/national_emergency_communications_plan.pdf, Washington DC, July 2008. Accessed April 30, 2010.

Developing and Maintaining State, Territorial, Tribal and Local Government Emergency Plans. http://www.fema.gov/pdf/about/divisions/npd/cpg_101_layout.pdf, Washington, DC, 2009. Accessed May 4, 2010.

Emergency Medical Services Outcome Evaluation DOT HS 809 603, July 2003.

Erich J: Big Investments, Big Payoff. In EMS: Emergency Medical Services Magazine. August 2008. Vol. 37(8):114.

Federal EMS: A Lesson Learned From Katrina. http://www.emsresponder.com/web/online/EMSRespondercom-Columns/Federal-EMS—A-Lesson-Learned-From-Katrina/20$1958, October 2005. Accessed April 30, 2010.

Hurricane Katrina: EMAC Team Operational Lessons Learned. http//www.jems.com/news_and_articles/articles/Hurricane_Katrina_EMAC_Team_Operational.html, February 16, 2006. Accessed April 30, 2010.

In a Moment's Notice: Surge Capacity for Terrorist Bombings Challenges and Proposed Solutions. U.S. Department of Health and Human Services, Centers for Disease Control and Prevention, National Center for Injury Prevention and Control, Division of Injury Response, Atlanta, Georgia, April 2007.

Institute of Medicine: Quality Through Collaboration: The Future of Rural Health. The National Academies Press, 2005.

Institute of Medicine: Future of Emergency Care Series: Emergency Medical Services at the Crossroads. National Academies Press 1st ed. May 9, 2007.

Mackenzie EJ, Carlini AR: Configurations of EMS systems: A pilot study. US Department of Transportation, NHTSA, March 2008.

Mass Casualty Information for Emergency Medical Services (EMS) Providers: http://emergency.cdc.gov/masscasualties/ems.asp, Atlanta, GA. Accessed April 30, 2010.

McGinnis L: Rural and Frontier Emergency Medical Services: Agenda for the Future. National Rural Health Association, 2004.

McGinnis KK: The future of emergency medical services communications systems: Time for a change. N C Med J 2007;68: 283–285 [PMID 17694852].

National Rural Health Association Issue Paper: Recruitment and Retention of a Quality Health Workforce in Rural Areas. A Series of Policy Papers on the Rural Health Careers Pipeline. Number 14: Issues of Preserving Rural Professional Quality of Life, May 2006.

PSWN Program: Information Brief. Fire and EMS Communications Interoperability. http://www.safecomprogram.gov/NR/rdonlyres/7305F51F-B70B-4C6A-B80C-352486ADE3E2/0/fireems_summary.pdf, Washington, DC. Accessed April 30, 2010.

Rural EMS Committee: Strategic Plan. http//www.nasemso.org/Projects/RuralEMS/documents/StrategicPlan200804.pdf, Fall Church, VA, 2008. Accessed April 30, 2010.

Rural Issues Committee Annual Report/2009 Workplan/Budget Request: http//www.nasemso.org/Projects/RuralEMS/documents/2008Report.pdf, Fall Church, VA, 2008. Accessed April 30, 2010.

Strom KJ, Eyerman J: Interagency Coordination: Lessons Learned from the 2005 London Train Bombings. http://www.ojp.usdoj.gov/nij/journals/261/coordination.htm, Washington, DC, 2008. Accessed April 30, 2010.

The White House: The Federal Response to Hurricane Katrina: Lessons Learned. http://georgewbush-whitehouse.archives.gov/reports/katrina-lessons-learned/appendix-e.html, Washington, DC, 2006. Accessed April 30, 2010.

Understanding FCC Narrowbanding Requirements: http//www.ojp.usdoj.gov/nij/topics/technology/communication/fcc-narrowbanding.htm, Washington, DC, 2008. Accessed April 30, 2010.

What is the National Incident Management System: http//www.nimsonline.com/what-is-the-national-incident-management-system.html, 2010. Accessed April 30, 2010.

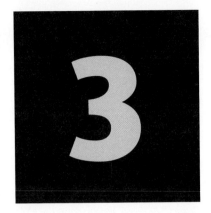

Nuclear, Biologic, & Chemical Agents; Weapons of Mass Destruction

David L. Morgan, MD

Christopher Ortiz, MD

Nuclear Weapons
Biologic Weapons
   Bacterial Agents
   Viral Agents
   Biologic Toxins

Chemical Weapons
   Nerve Agents
   Pulmonary Agents
   Vesicants
   Cyanide Agents
   Chemical Decontamination

For centuries, military forces have utilized nonconventional weapons using various chemical and biologic agents. During World War I, powerful chemical weapons were developed that affected hundreds of thousands of soldiers. Nuclear weapons were first created during World War II with devastating results. Today, thousands of these nuclear, biologic, and chemical weapons of mass destruction are stored in facilities throughout the world. An accident at any of these facilities could result in a large number of civilian casualties. In addition, many terrorist organizations are now actively attempting to purchase, steal, or develop such weapons for their use. As with most mass casualty situations, emergency physicians will be at the forefront of patient care. This chapter attempts to provide specific information regarding the management of nuclear, biologic, and chemical weapons injuries.

▼ NUCLEAR WEAPONS

A terrorist attack utilizing a nuclear weapon would most likely involve the detonation of a nuclear bomb or the detonation of a conventional explosive that also dispersed radioactive material (so-called dirty bomb).

▶ General Considerations

The detonation of a nuclear weapon results in a much larger blast area and much hotter fireball than that produced by conventional explosives. If victims survive the blast trauma and thermal burns, they are at risk for radiation injuries. There are four types of radioactive particles that may cause damage when they interact with body tissue:

1. *Alpha particles* are large particles that are stopped by the epidermis and cause no significant external damage. Internal contamination, from the inhalation or ingestion of contaminated particles, may cause local tissue injury.
2. *Beta particles* are small particles that can penetrate the superficial skin and cause mild-burn-type injuries.
3. *Gamma rays* are high-energy particles that can enter tissues easily and cause significant damage to multiple body systems.
4. *Neutrons* are large particles that are typically produced only during nuclear detonation. Like gamma rays, they cause significant tissue injury.

The effect that radiation will have on the body depends on the type of radiation, the amount of exposure, and the body system involved. Tissues that display higher rates of cellular mitosis, such as the gastrointestinal and hematopoietic systems, are more severely affected. At very high radiation doses, neurovascular effects will also be seen. Radiation injury may cause either abnormal cell function or cell death.

▶ Clinical Findings

A. Symptoms and Signs

The symptoms and signs of radiation exposure occur in three phases: prodromal, latent, and symptomatic.

1. Prodromal phase—Patients will develop nonspecific symptoms of nausea, vomiting, weakness, and fatigue. Symptoms generally last no longer than 24–48 hours. With higher radiation exposures, symptoms will occur earlier and last longer.

2. Latent period—The latent period duration depends on the dose of radiation and the body system involved (neurologic, several hours; gastrointestinal, 1–7 days; hematopoietic, 2–6 weeks).

3. Symptomatic phase—Symptoms will depend largely on the body system affected, which will depend on the radiation dose. At doses of 0.7–4 Gy, the hematopoietic system will begin to manifest signs and symptoms of bone marrow suppression. Because of their long life span, erythrocytes are less severely affected than are the myeloid and platelet cell lines. Neutropenia and thrombocytopenia may be significant and lead to infectious and hemorrhagic complications. At doses of 6–8 Gy, gastrointestinal symptoms develop. Nausea, vomiting, diarrhea (bloody), and severe fluid and electrolyte imbalances will occur. The neurovascular system becomes affected at doses of 20–40 Gy. Symptoms include headache, mental status changes, hypotension, focal neurologic changes, convulsions, and coma. Exposures in this range are uniformly fatal.

B. Laboratory and X-Ray Findings

Obtain a complete blood count with differential for all patients sustaining a radiation injury. Although symptomatic bone marrow suppression may not be evident for some weeks, a drop of the absolute lymphocyte count of 50% at 24–48 hours is indicative of significant exposure. Monitor electrolytes in patients with gastrointestinal symptoms.

▶ Treatment

In the absence of aggressive medical therapy, the LD_{50} (the dose of radiation that will kill 50% of those exposed) is approximately 3.5 Gy. Aggressive medical care affords improved survival. Treat all life-threatening injuries associated with blast or thermal effects according to standard advanced trauma life support protocols. Perform surgical procedures early to avoid the electrolyte and hematopoietic effects that will occur. Clean wounds extensively and close them as soon as possible to prevent infection. Treat nausea and vomiting with standard antiemetic medications (prochlorperazine, promethazine, ondansetron). Treat fluid and electrolyte abnormalities with appropriate replacement.

Anemia and thrombocytopenia can be treated with transfusion therapy. Leukopenia may be treated with hematopoietic growth factors such as sargramostim and filgrastim. In some instances, bone marrow transplantation may be utilized. Follow neutropenic precautions at absolute neutrophil counts below 500. Some authors recommend prophylactic antibiotics at counts below 100. Use broad-spectrum antibiotics to treat infections. Infection is the most common cause of death in radiation patients.

▶ Decontamination

Remove all contaminated clothing. Change contaminated dressings and splints. Thoroughly clean the patient's skin with soap and water or a 0.5% hypochlorite solution. Hair should be washed and in some instances removed. Eyes may be washed with large amounts of water or sterile saline. All contaminated materials should be bagged if possible and sent for proper disposal.

▶ Disposition

Patients who have been decontaminated and have only mild transient symptoms can be safely discharged. Because of the variable and lengthy latent period involved with this disorder, early admission is not indicated. Patients should be closely monitored and admitted when warranted.

Bushberg JT, Kroger LA, Hartman MB, Leidholdt EM Jr, Miller KL, Derlet R, Wraa C: Nuclear/radiological terrorism: Emergency department management of radiation casualties. J Emerg Med 2007;32:71–85 [PMID: 17239736].

Coleman CN, Hrdina C, Bader JL, Norwood A, Hayhurst R, Forsha J, Yeskey K, Knebel A: Medical response to a radiologic/nuclear event: integrated plan from the Office of the Assistant Secretary for Preparedness and Response, Department of Health and Human Services. Ann Emerg Med 2009;53:213–222 [PMID: 18387707].

▼ BIOLOGIC WEAPONS

Many agents may be used as biologic weapons. The most likely pathogens are presented here. Biologic agents can be classified as bacterial agents, viral agents, and biologic toxins. A high index of suspicion will be required in order to identify patients who have experienced a biologic attack. A large number of patients with severe febrile illnesses will be the most likely clue. Keep in mind that the attack most likely occurs by aerosol release of infectious material several days prior to patient presentation.

BACTERIAL AGENTS

See Table 3–1.

Table 3–1. Clinical Findings and Treatment of Bacterial Biologic Agent Infection.[a]

Agent	Syndrome	Incubation	Symptoms		Treatment[a]	
			Early	Late	First-line	Prophylaxis
Anthrax (*Bacillus anthracis*; gram-positive, sporulating)	Inhalational	1–7 d	Fever, chills, nausea and vomiting, headache, cough, dyspnea, chest pain, abdominal pain	High fever, diaphoresis, cyanosis, hypotension, lymphadenopathy, shock, death (within 3 d of late symptom onset)	Ciprofloxacin, 400 mg IV q 12 h, or doxycycline, 200 mg IV, and then 100 mg IV q 12 h. Without use of vaccine, treat for 60 days; with use of vaccine, treat for 30 days. As patient improves, may begin oral therapy	Ciprofloxacin, 500 mg PO b.i.d. × 1 wk, or doxycycline, 100 mg PO b.i.d. × 4 wk and begin vaccine
	Gastrointestinal (upper)		Oral or esophageal ulcer	Regional lymphadenopathy, sepsis		
	Gastrointestinal (lower)		Nausea and vomiting, diarrhea (bloody)	Acute abdomen, sepsis		
	Cutaneous	2 d	Pruritic papule → ulcer → vesicle → painless eschar	Regional lymphadenopathy, occasional sepsis (1–2 wk after onset)		
Plague (*Yersinia pestis*; gram-negative bacillus)	Bubonic	1–7 d	Fever, chills, malaise, lymphadenopathy	Necrotic lymphadenitis (1–10 cm) called a bubo, possible sepsis	Streptomycin, 30 mg/kg/d IM divided b.i.d. 10–14 d, or gentamicin, 5 mg/kg IV × 10–14 d	Doxycycline, 100 mg PO b.i.d. × 7 d, or ciprofloxacin, 500 mg PO b.i.d. × 7 d
	Septicemia (can be primary or secondary)		Fever, chills, dyspnea, hypotension, purpura	Gangrene of nose and extremities, disseminated intravascular coagulation, death		
	Pneumonic	1–6 d	Fever, chills, productive cough, dyspnea, hypoxia, nausea and vomiting	Sepsis		
Tularemia (*Francisella tularensis*; aerobic, gram-negative coccobacilli)	Ulceroglandular	Patients with any type may present with fever, chills, headache, myalgia, malaise, maculopapular rash; all types can spread hematogenously	Papule (inoculation site) → pustule → tender ulcer (yellow exudates, black base), painful regional lymphadenopathy		Streptomycin, 10 mg/kg/d IM divided b.i.d. × 10 d, or gentamicin, 5 mg/kg IV × 10 d	Doxycycline, 100 mg PO b.i.d. × 14 d, or ciprofloxacin, 500 mg PO b.i.d. × 14 d

Table 3–1. Clinical Findings and Treatment of Bacterial Biologic Agent Infection.[a] *(Continued)*

Agent	Syndrome	Incubation	Symptoms		Treatment[a]	
			Early	Late	First-Line	Prophylaxis
	Glandular			Same as above except without ulcer		
	Occuloglandular			Painful conjunctivitis, lymphadenopathy, ulcerations on palpebral conjunctiva		
	Oropharyngeal			Exudative pharyngotonsillitis, lymphadenopathy		
	Pneumonic			Pharyngitis, bronchiolitis, hilar lymphadenopathy, pneumonia, pulmonary failure, death		
	Typhoidal			Sepsis		
Brucellosis (pleomorphic gram-negative coccobacilli)		1–3 wk	Fever, chills, malaise, myalgias	May afflict a variety of organs or organ systems	Rifampin, 600 mg/d PO, plus doxycycline, 200 mg/d PO × 6 wk	Same as treatment course, but may be shortened to 3 wk
Q fever (*Coxiella burnetii*)	Can be acute or indolent in its course	5–30 d	Fever, chills, headache, malaise, myalgia, anorexia	May afflict a variety of organs or organ systems. Endocarditis and gastrointestinal symptoms are common	Tetracycline, 500 mg PO q 6 h × 5–7 d, or doxycycline, 100 mg PO b.i.d. × 5–7 d	Same as treatment course
Glanders and melioidosis (*Burkholderia* spp; gram-negative bacillus)	Localized	1–2 wk	Wound contamination, cellulitis, lymphadenopathy lymphangitis	Sepsis can result with all modes of infection; death from sepsis occurs in 7–10 d	Local disease: amoxicillin-clavulanate, 60 mg/kg/d divided t.i.d. × 60 d. Severe disease: ceftazidime, 120 mg/kg/d divided t.i.d., plus trimethoprim-sulfamethoxazole, 8 mg/kg/d divided q.i.d. × 2 wk, followed by prolonged oral therapy	Trimethoprim-sulfamethoxazole (160/800 mg) PO b.i.d. × 14 d
	Pulmonary		Fever, chills, cough, dyspnea			
	Septicemic		Fever, chills, malaise, abscesses, headache, pustular rash			

[a]Alternatives to the regimens given here may be used.

1. Anthrax

Bacillus anthracis is a gram-positive, sporulating rod. Anthrax infection occurs naturally after contact with contaminated animals or contaminated animal products. A biologic attack would likely involve the aerosol release of anthrax spores. Clinically, the disease occurs in three forms: inhalational, gastrointestinal, and cutaneous.

▶ Clinical Findings

A. Symptoms and Signs

1. Inhalational anthrax—Inhalational anthrax is the form of disease most likely expected after a terrorist attack. After spores are inhaled, an incubation period occurs, usually lasting 1–7 days. However, incubation periods of up to 60 days have been observed. Initially, nonspecific symptoms of fever, cough, headache, chills, vomiting, dyspnea, chest pain, abdominal pain, and weakness occur. This stage may last from a few hours to a few days. Following these non-specific symptoms, a transient period of improvement may be seen. When the second stage of disease is reached, high fever, diaphoresis, cyanosis, hypotension, lymphadenopathy, shock, and death will occur. Often, death will occur within hours once the second stage is reached. The average time from onset of symptoms to death is 3 days. Once the initial symptoms of inhalational anthrax develop, the overall mortality rate may be as high as 95%. Early diagnosis of anthrax infection and rapid initiation of therapy may improve survival.

2. Gastrointestinal anthrax—Gastrointestinal anthrax occurs when spores are ingested into the digestive tract. Two forms of the disease occur: oropharyngeal and abdominal. Oropharyngeal disease occurs when spores are deposited in the upper gastrointestinal tract. An oral or esophageal ulcer develops followed by regional lymphadenopathy and eventual sepsis. In abdominal anthrax, the spores are deposited in the lower gastrointestinal tract. Symptoms include nausea, vomiting, bloody diarrhea, and the development of an acute abdomen with sepsis. Mortality rates for gastrointestinal anthrax are in excess of 50%.

3. Cutaneous anthrax—Cutaneous anthrax is the most common naturally occurring form of the disease. It occurs when spores come in contact with open skin lesions. This usually occurs on the arms, hands, and face. Following exposure, a small, often pruritic, papule will develop. Eventually, this papule will turn into a small ulcer over 2 days, then progress to a small vesicle, and ultimately to a painless black eschar with surrounding edema. Then, over a period of 1–2 weeks, the eschar will dry and fall off. Regional lymphadenitis or lymphadenopathy may also occur. In some case, secondary sepsis may develop. Without treatment, cutaneous anthrax has a mortality rate of 20%; however, the mortality rate drops to 1% with treatment.

4. Anthrax meningitis—Anthrax meningitis can occur as a complication of any other form of anthrax. Symptoms include headache and meningismus. Anthrax meningitis carries a mortality rate of nearly 100%.

B. Laboratory and X-Ray Findings

Multiple laboratory studies can be used to identify anthrax. In fulminant cases, the organism may be seen on routine Gram stain. Blood cultures, wound cultures, and nasal cultures may be obtained. Given the lack of an infiltrate, sputum cultures are rarely useful. Often *Bacillus* spp. are thought to be the contaminant; therefore, notify laboratory personnel of possible anthrax. Confirmatory enzyme-linked immunoassay (ELISA) and polymerase chain reaction (PCR) tests are available at some national reference laboratories. Patients with inhalational anthrax will display a wide mediastinum on chest x-ray without infiltrate.

▶ Treatment and Prophylaxis

Because anthrax has a rapid and fulminant course, do not delay treatment while awaiting confirmatory tests. Delaying empiric treatment for even hours may significantly increase mortality.

A. Antibiotics

Most naturally occurring strains of anthrax are sensitive to penicillin. Some strains, however, are penicillin resistant. Weapons-grade anthrax is likely to be penicillin resistant. As a result, the first-line therapy is now ciprofloxacin; doxycycline is an acceptable alternative (see Table 3–1). Treatment should continue for 60 days. If cultures were obtained, later sensitivity testing may direct antibiotic use.

B. Supportive Care

Patients may require intensive medical support such as airway management, hemodynamic support, and various measures to manage multisystem organ failure.

C. Prophylaxis

Individuals thought to be at high risk for anthrax exposure should receive treatment as though infection has occurred. Later, laboratory analysis may allow discontinuation of therapy. An anthrax vaccination is available and requires injections at 0, 2, and 4 weeks, followed by injections at 6, 12, and 18 months. An annual booster is also required. If a combination of vaccination and antibiotics is used during treatment, the course of antibiotics may be shortened to 30 days.

▶ Infection Control

No data indicate that anthrax is spread via person-to-person contact. Use standard precautions during patient care activities (Table 3–2).

Table 3–2. Levels of Protection Required During Patient Care Activities.

Protection Level	Required Equipment
Standard precautions	Universal precautions; hand washing; protective gloves; gown, mask, eye protection, if splash risk exists
Droplet precautions	Same as standard precautions, except add surgical or Hepa filter mask
Airborne precautions	Same as standard precautions, except add negative pressure room, strict isolation; Hepa filter mask required

2. Plague

Yersinia pestis is a nonmotile, gram-negative bacillus. Plague occurs naturally after the bite of an infected arthropod vector. Biologic attack would most likely involve the aerosolized release of *Y. pestis*. Plague occurs in three clinical forms: bubonic plague, septicemic plague, and pneumonic plague.

▶ Clinical Findings

A. Symptoms and Signs

1. Bubonic plague—Bubonic plague is the most common naturally occurring form of the disease. Infection begins with the bite of a contaminated flea. A latent period then occurs and may last up to 1 week, followed by fevers, chills, and weakness. Eventually, the organism will migrate to the regional lymph nodes where it causes destruction and necrosis. A swollen and tender lymph node called a bubo will develop, which ranges from 1 to 10 cm. Some patients may develop secondary sepsis. Without treatment, bubonic plague has an estimated mortality rate of 50%; however, with antibiotic therapy the mortality rate falls to 10%.

2. Septicemic plague—Septicemic plague may occur either as a complication of other forms of plague or as a primary entity. Symptoms include fever, dyspnea, hypotension, and purpuric skin lesions. Gangrene of the nose and extremities may occur, hence the name "black death." Complications of disseminated intravascular coagulation may also be evident. Without treatment, septicemic plague has an estimated mortality rate of 100%; however, with antibiotic therapy the mortality rate falls to 40%.

3. Pneumonic plague—Pneumonic plague may occur either as a complication of other forms of plague or as a primary entity. It is the most likely form of the disease to result from a terrorist attack. A latent period of 1–6 days following exposure is likely. Patients will then develop signs and symptoms of severe pulmonary infection including fever, cough, dyspnea, hypoxia, and sputum production. Gastrointestinal symptoms of nausea, vomiting, and diarrhea may also occur.

Pneumonic plague has an estimated mortality rate of 100% if antibiotic therapy is not begun within 24 hours.

B. Laboratory and X-Ray Findings

Y. pestis can be identified by several different staining techniques, including routine Gram, Wright, Giemsa, and Wayson stains. Blood cultures, sputum cultures, and cultures of lymph node aspirates may be useful. Specialized rapid confirmatory tests are available at some laboratories. In patients with pneumonic plague, chest x-ray will display a patchy or confluent infiltrate.

▶ Treatment and Prophylaxis

Plague has a rapid disease progression, and any delay in empiric treatment will cause significant increases in mortality.

A. Antibiotics

Streptomycin or gentamicin is the drug of choice for the treatment of plague (see Table 3–1). Alternative antibiotics include doxycycline, ciprofloxacin, and chloramphenicol.

B. Supportive Care

Patients may require intensive medical support such as airway management, hemodynamic support, and other measures to manage multisystem organ failure.

C. Prophylaxis

Patients in a community experiencing a pneumonic plague epidemic should receive antibiotic therapy if they develop a cough or a fever above 38.5°C (101.2°F). Any person who has been in close contact with an individual with plague should receive a 7-day course of antibiotics.

▶ Infection Control

Pneumonic plague can be spread from person to person by aerosol droplets. Use droplet precautions, and either the patient or the caregivers should wear masks (see Table 3–2). Once the patient has received 48 hours of antibiotics and has improved clinically, standard precautions may be used.

3. Tularemia

Francisella tularensis is a nonmotile, aerobic, gram-negative coccobacillus. Two strains of tularemia are known to exist. *F. tularensis* biovar tularensis is considered highly virulent, whereas *F. tularensis* biovar palaearctiais more benign. Tularemia occurs naturally after the bite of an infected arthropod vector or after exposure to contaminated animal products. Biologic attack would most likely involve the release of aerosolized *F. tularensis*. Tularemia displays multiple clinical forms including ulceroglandular, glandular, oculoglandular, oropharyngeal, pneumonic, and typhoidal forms. The form of disease depends on the site and type of inoculation.

▶ Clinical Findings

A. Symptoms and Signs

Patients with any form of tularemia may present with the abrupt onset of fever, chills, headache, malaise, and myalgias. Often a maculopapular rash is seen.

1. Ulceroglandular tularemia—Ulceroglandular tularemia usually occurs after handling infected animals or after the bite of an infected arthropod vector. At the inoculation site, a papule will form that will eventually become a pustule and then a tender ulcer. The ulcer may have a yellow exudate and will slowly develop a black base. Regional lymph nodes will become swollen and painful.

2. Glandular tularemia—Glandular tularemia displays signs and symptoms similar to ulceroglandular tularemia, except that no ulcer formation is noted.

3. Oculoglandular tularemia—After ocular inoculation, a painful conjunctivitis will develop with regional lymphadenopathy. Lymphadenopathy may involve the cervical, submandibular, or preauricular chains. In some cases, ulcerations occur on the palpebral conjunctiva.

4. Oropharyngeal tularemia—After inoculation of the pharynx, an exudative pharyngotonsillitis will develop with cervical lymphadenopathy.

5. Pneumonic tularemia—Pneumonic tularemia occurs after inhalation of *F. tularensis* or following secondary spread from other infectious foci. A terrorist attack will most likely cause this form of disease. The findings of pulmonary involvement are variable and include pharyngitis, bronchiolitis, hilar lymphadenitis, and pneumonia. Early in the course of disease, systemic symptoms may predominate over pulmonary symptoms. In some cases, however, pulmonary disease progresses rapidly to pneumonia, pulmonary failure, and death.

6. Typhoidal tularemia—In this form of tularemia, systemic signs and symptoms of disease are present without a clear infectious site. Signs and symptoms include fever, chills, headache, malaise, and myalgias.

Any form of tularemia may be complicated by hematogenous spread leading to pneumonia, meningitis, or sepsis. The overall mortality rates for untreated tularemia range from 10% to 30%; however, with antibiotic therapy, mortality rates drop to less than 1%.

B. Laboratory and X-Ray Findings

F. tularensis requires special growth media. Notify laboratory personnel of a possible tularemia specimen so that proper plating can be performed. Cultures may be obtained from sputum, pharyngeal, or blood specimens. Specialized ELISA and PCR confirmatory tests are also available at some reference laboratories. In the case of pneumonic tularemia, chest x-ray may demonstrate peribronchial infiltrates, bronchopneumonia, or pleural effusions.

▶ Treatment and Prophylaxis

A. Antibiotics

Streptomycin and gentamicin are considered the drugs of choice for the treatment of tularemia (see Table 3–1). Ciprofloxacin has also displayed efficacy against tularemia. Second-line agents such as tetracycline and chloramphenicol may be used, but these agents are associated with higher rates of treatment failure. A 10-day course of antibiotics should be used. For second-line agents, a 14-day course should be used.

B. Supportive Care

Rarely, patients may require intensive medical support such as airway management, hemodynamic support, and other measures to manage multisystem organ failure.

C. Prophylaxis

Some data suggest that a 14-day course of antibiotics begun during the incubation period may prevent disease. Antibiotic choices are the same as for treatment. A live attenuated vaccine for tularemia also exists and is often used for at-risk laboratory workers. Vaccination decreases the rate of inhalational tularemia but does not confer complete protection. Given tularemia's short incubation period, and the incomplete protection of the vaccine, postexposure vaccination is not recommended.

▶ Infection Control

Significant person-to-person transmission of tularemia does not occur. Standard precautions are sufficient during patient care activities (see Table 3–2).

4. Brucellosis

Brucellae are small aerobic, gram-negative, pleomorphic coccobacilli. Many *Brucella* spp. occur naturally; however, only four species are infectious to humans. Each species typically infects a particular host organism, and human infection follows contact with contaminated animal material. The *Brucella* spp. that are infectious to humans are *B. melitensis* (found in goats), *B. suis* (found in swine), *B. abortus* (found in cattle), and *B. canis* (found in dogs). *B. suis* has been weaponized in the past.

▶ Clinical Findings

A. Symptoms and Signs

The symptoms and signs of brucellosis are similar whether infection is contracted via oral, inhalational, or percutaneous routes. The usual incubation period following infection is

1–3 weeks. Because *Brucella* spp. infection can involve multiple body systems, a wide range of clinical findings is typical. Nonspecific symptoms are common and include fever, chills, malaise, and myalgias. Osteoarticular involvement may manifest as joint infections or vertebral osteomyelitis. Respiratory symptoms include cough, dyspnea, and pleuritic chest pain. Cardiovascular complications are numerous and include endocarditis, myocarditis, pericarditis, and mycotic aneurysms. Gastrointestinal symptoms include nausea, vomiting, diarrhea, and hepatitis. Multiple types of genitourinary infections can also occur. Neurologic involvement may cause meningitis, encephalitis, cerebral abscesses, cranial nerve abnormalities, or Guillain–Barré syndrome. Patients may also develop anemia, thrombocytopenia, or neutropenia. Central nervous system and cardiac involvement, although infrequent, account for most fatalities. *Brucella* spp. are not known for their lethality, and infection has an estimated mortality rate of less than 2%. Its interest as a biologic weapon stems from the prolonged disease course and significant morbidity.

B. Laboratory and X-Ray Findings

Brucella spp. will grow on standard culture media. Because of their slow growth, cultures may need to be maintained for at least 6 weeks. Specialized biphasic culture techniques may improve isolation. A more common diagnostic modality is a serum tube agglutination test. ELISA and PCR studies are available at some reference laboratories. If vertebral involvement is suspected, spinal x-rays, magnetic resonance imaging, computed tomography scanning, or bone scintigraphy may be helpful.

▶ Treatment and Prophylaxis

A. Antibiotics

Because of the high rate of treatment failure, single-drug therapy is not recommended. A prolonged course of multiple antibiotics is now considered to be the standard of care. The most common regimen involves the use of rifampin and doxycycline given for a 6-week period (see Table 3–1). Other antibiotics that have displayed efficacy against *Brucella* spp. include gentamicin, streptomycin, trimethoprim–sulfamethoxazole, and ofloxacin. In patients with serious infections, a three-drug parenteral regimen is the norm.

B. Supportive Care

Rarely, patients may require intensive medical support such as airway management, hemodynamic support, and other measures to manage multisystem organ failure.

C. Prophylaxis

No human vaccine against *Brucella* spp. currently exists. Some physicians recommend a 3- to 6-week course of antibiotics following a high-risk exposure such as a biologic attack.

▶ Infection Control

Person-to-person spread of brucellosis is thought to be uncommon. Standard precautions are sufficient during patient care activities (see Table 3–2).

5. Q Fever

Q fever is caused by a rickettsial organism known as *Coxiella burnetii*. *C. burnetii* has a worldwide distribution and occurs naturally in many domesticated animals (dogs, cats, sheep, goats, cattle). The organism is shed in feces, urine, milk, and placental material. Much like anthrax, *C. burnetii* produces a sporelike form. Humans become infected by inhaling contaminated aerosols.

▶ Clinical Findings

A. Symptoms and Signs

After infection, a typical incubation period ranges from 5 to 30 days. The symptoms and signs of Q fever are nonspecific and may occur acutely or have an indolent course. Typical symptoms and signs include fever, chills, malaise, myalgias, headache, and anorexia. If cough occurs, it tends to occur late in the disease process and may or may not be associated with pneumonia. Various cardiac manifestations may occur and include endocarditis, myocarditis, and pericarditis. Gastrointestinal findings are common and include nausea, vomiting, diarrhea, and hepatitis. A nonspecific maculopapular rash may develop. Although not as common, various neurologic symptoms may also occur.

In some patients, Q fever may become a chronic condition. Chronic Q fever is typically manifested as endocarditis and tends to affect previously diseased cardiac valves. Although Q fever can be debilitating, it is usually not fatal. Mortality rates are generally less than 2.5%.

B. Laboratory and X-Ray Findings

C. burnetii is difficult to grow in culture and sputum analysis is equally futile. Several serologic tests are available and include indirect fluorescent antibody staining, ELISA, and complement fixation. These tests often must be conducted at specialized reference laboratories. Elevated liver enzymes are also common in *C. burnetii* infection.

▶ Treatment and Prophylaxis

A. Antibiotics

Most cases of *C. burnetii* infection will resolve without antibiotic therapy. Regardless, antibiotics are recommended because treatment will lower the rate of complications. A 7-day course of either doxycycline or tetracycline is usually sufficient (see Table 3–1). Fluoroquinolones are an acceptable alternative.

B. Supportive Care

Rarely, patients may require intensive medical support such as airway management, hemodynamic support, and other measures to manage multisystem organ failure.

C. Prophylaxis

Prophylactic antibiotics should be started 8–12 days after initial exposure. Antibiotics are ineffective if started sooner. A 7-day course of either doxycycline or tetracycline is usually sufficient. Fluoroquinolones are an acceptable alternative. An investigational vaccine exists but is not yet available to the general public.

▶ Infection Control

Person-to-person spread of the disease is unlikely. Standard precautions are sufficient while engaging in patient care activities (see Table 3–2).

VIRAL AGENTS

1. Smallpox

Smallpox is a disease caused by the variola virus, which is a DNA virus of the genus *Orthopoxvirus*. It occurs in two strains: the more severe variola major and a milder form, variola minor. Smallpox was essentially eradicated worldwide by an aggressive treatment and vaccination campaign conducted by the World Health Organization. The last naturally occurring case was in Somalia in 1977. Two stockpiles of the virus remain, one in the Centers for Disease Control and Prevention in Atlanta and the other in the Institute of Virus Preparations in Moscow.

▶ Clinical Findings

A. Symptoms and Signs

Disease begins with inhalation of the variola virus. After an initial exposure, a 7- to 17-day incubation period begins, during which the virus replicates in the lymph nodes, bone marrow, and spleen. A secondary viremia then develops leading to high fever, malaise, headache, backache, and in some cases delirium. After approximately 2 days, a characteristic rash will develop. The rash begins on the extremities and moves to the trunk. The palms and soles are not spared. The rash follows a typical progression beginning as macules, then papules, and eventually becoming pustular. Eventually, lesions will form scabs that separate, leaving small scars. The rash appears similar to chickenpox, except that all the lesions in smallpox will be in similar stages of development. In unvaccinated individuals, mortality rates associated with variola major are approximately 30%. Variola minor has a similar progression to variola major, but toxicity and rash are not as severe. In unvaccinated individuals, the mortality rates associated with variola minor

are approximately 1%. In 10% of cases, a variant form of rash will develop. A hemorrhagic rash displaying petechiae and frank skin hemorrhage may occur. This variant of smallpox carries a mortality rate of nearly 100%. Likewise, a malignant form exists in which the pustules remain soft and velvety to the touch.

B. Laboratory and X-Ray Findings

Analysis of pustular fluid will yield virus particles. All samples should be sealed in two airtight containers. Variola can easily be recognized via electron microscopy. The virus itself can be grown in cell cultures or on chorioallantoic egg membranes. Further characterization of strains can be accomplished via biologic assays. PCR analysis is available at some reference laboratories.

▶ Treatment and Prophylaxis

A. Specific Therapy

Currently there is no specific therapy for smallpox other than supportive care. Many investigational drugs are currently under study. Strict patient isolation, preferably at home, should be used. Any person having close contact with infected patients should be either quarantined or monitored for signs of infection. Antibiotics may be used if secondary bacterial infection occurs.

B. Prophylaxis

Smallpox vaccination is very effective at preventing the disease and gives immunity for 5–10 years. Universal smallpox immunization of the general population was discontinued over 30 years ago when smallpox was eradicated. Because of the risk of possible terrorist attack, there has recently been a preemptive initiation of smallpox vaccination for selected health care workers. However, the smallpox vaccine has several rare complications. Postvaccinal encephalitis occurs in approximately 1 in 300,000 vaccinations and is fatal in 25% of patients. Immunocompromised patients who are vaccinated may develop a condition known as progressive vaccinia, which is often fatal. In this condition, the initial inoculation site failed to heal, became necrotic, and necrosis spread to adjacent tissues. In some patients with eczema, a postvaccination condition known as eczema vaccinatum may occur. Here, vaccinial lesions occur in areas previously involved with eczema. Fortunately, the eruptions are usually self-limited. In some patients, a secondary generalized vaccinia could develop. In others, inadvertent autoinoculation of eyes, mouth, or other areas may occur. Many of these complications are treated with vaccinia immune globulin. Data indicate that vaccination within 4 days of smallpox exposure may lessen subsequent illness. Cidofovir has also displayed some efficacy in preventing smallpox infection if given within 48 hours. However, cidofovir is not more effective than the vaccine and is associated with significant renal toxicity.

▶ Infection Control

Smallpox is highly infectious. Infection is spread by aerosol droplets. It is generally thought that each index case will subsequently infect 10–20 secondary individuals. The period of infectivity begins with the onset of rash and ends when all scabs separate. Use airborne precautions during patient care activities (see Table 3–2). Any material in contact with patients should be either autoclaved or washed in a bleach solution.

2. Hemorrhagic Fever

Viral hemorrhagic fever represents a clinical syndrome caused by several RNA viruses. These viruses exist in four different families: the Arenaviridae, the Filoviridae, the Flaviviridae, and the Bunyaviridae. Numerous viruses in each family may cause slightly different forms of hemorrhagic fever. The different forms of hemorrhagic fever are often named by their geographic origin (Table 3–3). Human infection occurs after contact with infected animals or infected arthropod vectors. Many of these viruses are also highly infectious in the aerosol form. This characteristic makes these viruses potential biologic weapons.

▶ Clinical Findings

A. Symptoms and Signs

Several clinical aspects of hemorrhagic fever are unique to the individual forms (Table 3–3). Many symptoms and signs, however, are common to all types of hemorrhagic fever. Alterations in the vascular bed and increased vascular permeability lead to the dominant features of this disease. Early symptoms and signs include fever, conjunctival injection, mild hypotension, prostration, facial flushing, vomiting, diarrhea, and petechial hemorrhages. Eventually some patients may develop shock and mucous membrane hemorrhage. In some instances, evidence of hepatic, pulmonary, and neurologic involvement will be present. Secondary bacterial infection is also common.

B. Laboratory and X-Ray Findings

A number of nonspecific laboratory abnormalities may be seen, including leukopenia, thrombocytopenia, proteinuria, hematuria, and elevated liver enzymes. Definitive diagnosis is possible with various rapid enzyme immunoassays and with viral culture.

▶ Treatment and Prophylaxis

A. Specific Therapy

Ribavirin is a nucleoside analog that has been shown to improve mortality in some forms of hemorrhagic fever. Dosing is as follows: 30 mg/kg IV as an initial dose, followed by 16 mg/kg IV every 6 hours for 4 days, and then 8 mg/kg IV every 8 hours for 6 days. Ribavirin is usually most effective if begun within 7 days. Unfortunately, ribavirin is thought

Table 3–3. Specific Forms of Hemorrhagic Fever and Typical Findings Seen With Each Form.

Disease Form	Specific Features
Arenaviridae	
Argentine hemorrhagic fever	Progression or frank hemorrhage
Bolivian hemorrhagic fever	Progression or frank hemorrhage
Venezuelan hemorrhagic fever	Progression or frank hemorrhage
Lassa fever	Severe peripheral edema, hearing loss in survivors
Bunyaviridae	
Congo–Crimean hemorrhagic fever	Hepatitis, jaundice, severe hemorrhage
Rift Valley fever	Hepatitis, jaundice, retinitis
Filoviridae	
Ebola and Marburg forms	Hepatitis, jaundice
Flaviviridae	
Dengue fever	Pulmonary involvement
Yellow fever	Hepatitis, jaundice, pulmonary involvement

to be ineffective against the filoviruses and the flaviviruses. Convalescent plasma containing neutralizing antibodies is also effective in some cases.

B. Supportive Care

Intravenous lines and other invasive procedures should be limited. Use fluid resuscitation with caution. Because of increases in vascular permeability, peripheral edema and pulmonary edema are frequent complications of volume replacement. If frank disseminated intravascular coagulopathy develops, consider heparin therapy.

C. Prophylaxis

A vaccine against yellow fever is currently available. Many other investigational vaccines exist but are not currently available to the general public. Protocols also exist for the use of ribavirin in high-risk exposures.

▶ Infection Control

The causal agents of hemorrhagic fever are highly infectious. Use caution when using sharps or when coming into contact with the body fluids of the patients. Some forms are spread via aerosol, and patients with significant cough should be placed under airborne precautions. All laboratory specimens should be double sealed in airtight containers.

3. Viral Encephalitis

Much like viral hemorrhagic fever, viral encephalitis represents a clinical syndrome caused by numerous viruses. Of the pathogens that cause viral encephalitis, members of the family Togaviridae are thought to have the potential as biologic weapons. The family Togaviridae includes the eastern equine encephalitis (EEE) virus, western equine encephalitis (WEE) virus, and Venezuelan equine encephalitis (VEE) virus. VEE virus has been weaponized in the past. In nature, these viruses are spread by infected arthropod vectors and they infect humans as well as equines. They are also infectious in aerosol form, hence their utility as biologic weapons.

▶ Clinical Findings

A. Symptoms and Signs

Nearly all forms of infection will cause nonspecific symptoms and signs of fever, chills, malaise, myalgias, sore throat, vomiting, and headache. A large number of associated equine deaths may lead one to suspect equine encephalitis. The degree to which encephalitis develops depends on the pathogen involved. Although nearly all cases of VEE are symptomatic, encephalitis occurs in less than 5% of cases. If encephalitis does develop, and the patient recovers, residual neurologic sequelae usually do not occur. Without encephalitis, VEE has an expected mortality rate of less than 1%. Although uncommon, if encephalitis develops, the mortality rate increases to approximately 20%. In contrast, EEE tends to progress to neurologic involvement. Encephalitis is usually severe and residual neurologic findings are common. With EEE, mortality rates range from 50% to 75%. WEE displays an intermediate degree of severity, with an overall estimated mortality rate of approximately 10%. If encephalitis develops, confusion, obtundation, seizures, ataxia, cranial nerve palsies, and coma may occur.

B. Laboratory and X-Ray Findings

Although nonspecific, leukopenia and lymphopenia are common. In cases of encephalitis, cerebral spinal fluid analysis will display a lymphocytic pleocytosis. A number of serologic studies such as ELISA, complement fixation, and hemagglutination inhibition may aid diagnosis. Although time consuming, the gold standard test for VEE involves viral isolation following inoculation of cell cultures of suckling mice. Additional specialized tests may be available only at regional reference laboratories.

▶ Treatment and Prophylaxis

A. Specific Therapy

Unfortunately, no specific treatment for equine encephalitis exists. Supportive care is all that can be offered. Headache may be treated with typical analgesics. Seizures are treated with typical anticonvulsant medications.

B. Supportive Care

Patients may require intensive medical support such as airway management, hemodynamic support, and other measures to manage multisystem organ failure.

C. Prophylaxis

An investigational vaccine against VEE virus exists. It does not provide protection against all strains of VEE virus, and some patients will not display an effective antibody response. In 20% of the patients receiving the vaccine, fever, malaise, and myalgias may develop.

▶ Infection Control

Infection is not spread by person-to-person contact. Standard precautions are sufficient during patient care activities. To limit the spread of disease, patient exposure to arthropod vectors should be prevented.

BIOLOGIC TOXINS

See Table 3–4.

1. Botulinum Toxin

Botulism is caused by a protein toxin produced by *Clostridium botulinum*. *C. botulinum* is a gram-positive, spore-forming, obligate anaerobe found naturally in the soil. Many authorities consider botulinum toxin to be among the most potent naturally occurring poisons. The toxin occurs in seven antigenic types, designated types A–G. Once absorbed, toxin will bind to motor neurons and prevent the release of acetylcholine, causing a flaccid muscle paralysis. Natural infection occurs in three forms: wound botulism, foodborne botulism, and intestinal botulism. Wound botulism occurs after *C. botulinum* contaminates an open wound, subsequently producing toxin. Foodborne botulism occurs after ingesting food already contaminated by the toxin. Intestinal botulism, typically seen in infants, occurs after ingesting food contaminated by *C. botulinum*, which in turn produces toxin. Although not occurring naturally, botulism can also be caused by inhalation of the toxin. This is the form of botulism that will likely occur following biologic attack. Contamination of food or water supplies also represents a possible terrorist threat. Food contamination, however, is unlikely to induce the large numbers of affected persons that would be seen following aerosol exposure. Water contamination would be difficult because current purification techniques are effective in neutralizing botulinum toxin.

▶ Clinical Findings

A. Symptoms and Signs

After initial exposure, an incubation period ranging from 12 to 80 hours will occur. The duration of the incubation

Table 3–4. Clinical Findings Associated with Biologic Toxins.

Biologic Toxin	Latent Period	Route	Early Symptoms	Late Symptoms
Botulism (*Clostridium botulinum*)	12–80 h	Gastrointestinal	Nausea, vomiting, diarrhea	Both forms: lower muscle group paralysis, respiratory failure
		Inhalational	Flaccid paralysis of bulbar musculature (ptosis, diplopic, dysphagia, dysarthria, dysphonia, mydriasis)	
Ricin (extract from castor bean)	4–8 h	Gastrointestinal	Nausea and vomiting, hematemesis, bloody diarrhea, melena, visceral organ necrosis	Circulatory collapse
		Inhalational	Fever, chills, cough, chest pain, dyspnea	Bronchitis, pneumonia, acute respiratory distress syndrome, respiratory failure
T-2 mycotoxins (produced from fungi)		Cutaneous	Pain, erythema, blister, necrosis, ocular irritation, rhinorrhea, oral pain	All forms: weakness, dizziness, ataxia, and bone marrow suppression
		Gastrointestinal	Abdominal pain, nausea and vomiting, diarrhea (bloody)	
		Inhalational	Chest pain, cough, dyspnea	
Staphylococcal entero-toxin B (staphylococcal bacteria)	4–10 h	Ingestion	All forms: fever, chills, headache, myalgia	Nausea and vomiting, diarrhea (bloody)
	3–12 h	Inhalation		Chest pain, cough dyspnea, respiratory failure

period depends on the type and amount of exposure. After the incubation period, a flaccid symmetric muscle paralysis will affect the bulbar musculature. Patients often display ptosis, diplopia, dysphagia, dysarthria, and dysphonia. Dilated, poorly reactive pupils are common. Eventually the paralysis will extend to the lower muscle groups, leading to paralysis. Airway compromise is common and patients may lose respiratory function.

If foodborne exposure is involved, gastrointestinal symptoms such as nausea, vomiting, and diarrhea may occur. Botulism does not cause altered sensorium, sensory changes, or fever.

B. Laboratory and X-Ray Findings

A mouse bioassay is the definitive test for botulism. Specimens for evaluation may be obtained from suspected food, blood, gastric contents, or possibly stool. This type of diagnostic testing is not widely available, and specimens may need to be sent to specialized laboratories. In addition to laboratory studies, electromyograms may display patterns consistent with botulism.

▶ Treatment and Prophylaxis

A. Specific Therapy

A botulinum antitoxin can be obtained from many state health departments or from the Centers for Disease Control and Prevention. Antitoxin therapy is most effective when given early in the disease course. It acts by binding free toxin but will not restore nerve terminals that have already been compromised. The civilian antitoxin is effective in neutralizing the three most common types of botulinum toxin found to affect humans (types A, B, and E). If other forms of toxin are utilized, an investigational heptavalent antitoxin may be available from the military. The military antitoxin is effective against all types of toxin (types A–G). Because some patients may develop allergic reactions to the antitoxin, a test dose is recommended.

B. Supportive Care

Patients may require intensive medical support such as airway management and ventilator support. Parenteral or tube feedings may be required. Treat secondary bacterial infections with antibiotics. Avoid clindamycin and amino-glycoside antibiotics because they may worsen neurologic blockade.

C. Prophylaxis

Some evidence suggests that initiation of antitoxin prior to the onset of symptoms may prevent disease. Unfortunately, large amounts of the antitoxin are not available. A more prudent course of action would be to institute antitoxin therapy at the first signs of illness.

▶ Infection Control

Person-to-person transmission of botulism does not occur. Standard precautions are sufficient during patient care activities (see Table 3–2). If food is suspected of being contaminated, thorough cooking will neutralize the toxin.

2. Ricin

Ricin is a polypeptide toxin that causes cell death by inhibiting protein synthesis. It occurs naturally as a component of the castor bean from the castor plant, *Ricinus communis*. Accidental ricin toxicity has occurred following ingestion of castor beans. Although ricin is less toxic than many other potential biologic agents, it is inexpensive, easy to produce, and can be aerosolized. These characteristics make it a potential biologic weapon. Ricin may be delivered by parenteral injection, ingestion, or inhalation. Ingestion and inhalation are the likely modes of biologic attack.

▶ Clinical Findings

A. Symptoms and Signs

The signs and symptoms of ricin intoxication depend on the type and amount of exposure. Parenteral exposure causes necrosis of local tissues and regional lymph nodes. As the toxin spreads, visceral organs become involved, manifested as a moderate to severe gastroenteritis. Parenteral exposure is an unlikely means of biologic attack. If ricin is ingested, symptoms of gastrointestinal exposure will occur and may include nausea, vomiting, hematemesis, bloody diarrhea, melena, or visceral organ necrosis. If death occurs following parenteral or gastrointestinal exposure, it is usually secondary to circulatory collapse.

The most likely means of biologic attack involve aerosol exposure. Inhalation of ricin is manifested by direct pulmonary toxicity. Between 4 and 8 hours after exposure, the patient may develop fever, cough, chest pain, and dyspnea. Findings consistent with an aerosol exposure include bronchitis, bronchiolitis, interstitial pneumonia, and acute respiratory distress syndrome. If death occurs, it is usually secondary to respiratory failure and generally will occur within 36–72 hours.

B. Laboratory and X-Ray Findings

Various laboratory tests, including ELISA, PCR, and immunohistochemical staining, may aid in the diagnosis of ricin toxicity. In the event of pulmonary involvement, chest x-ray may display bilateral infiltrates or noncardiogenic pulmonary edema.

▶ Treatment and Prophylaxis

The treatment of ricin toxicity depends largely on the mode of exposure.

A. Parenteral Exposure

With parenteral exposure, treatment is largely supportive.

B. Gastrointestinal Exposure

The treatment of gastrointestinal exposure primarily involves the elimination of toxin. This can be accomplished by vigorous gastric lavage and by the use of cathartics such as magnesium citrate or whole bowel irrigation. Activated charcoal may be considered. Correct electrolyte abnormalities and maintain adequate volume status. Treat secondary bacterial infections with appropriate antibiotics.

C. Pulmonary Exposure

With pulmonary exposure, treatment involves providing adequate ventilatory support. Patients may require oxygen, intubation, and ventilator management. Treat secondary bacterial infections with appropriate antibiotics.

D. Prophylaxis

Ricin vaccines are under development.

▶ Infection Control

Ricin intoxication is not spread by person-to-person contact. Standard precautions are sufficient during patient care activities (see Table 3–2).

3. T-2 Mycotoxins

Like penicillin, mycotoxins are a diverse group of compounds produced by fungi for environmental protection. These compounds are frequently toxic to many animal species including humans. The T-2 mycotoxins are a particular group of compounds produced by fungi of the genus *Fusarium*. Although the actions of the T-2 mycotoxins are not completely understood, they are known to inhibit DNA and protein synthesis. They are most toxic to rapidly dividing cell lines.

Many properties of these compounds make them attractive as biologic weapons. Specifically, they are resistant to destruction by ultraviolet radiation and are heat stabile. T-2 mycotoxins confer toxicity after ingestion, inhalation, or dermal exposure. Unlike most other biologic agents, they can be absorbed directly through the skin.

Clinical Findings

A. Symptoms and Signs

With T-2 mycotoxin exposure, contamination via dermal, gastrointestinal, and pulmonary routes may occur simultaneously. The earliest symptoms and signs may begin within minutes to hours. Dermal exposure may manifest as skin pain, erythema, blistering, and skin necrosis. Toxin exposure to the eyes and upper airway may cause ocular pain, redness, tearing, sneezing, rhinorrhea, oral pain, blood-tinged mucus, and epistaxis. Patients with pulmonary involvement will display chest pain, cough, and dyspnea. Signs and symptoms of gastrointestinal toxicity include abdominal pain, nausea, vomiting, and a bloody diarrhea. With systemic toxicity, patients may develop weakness, dizziness, and ataxia. Similar to radiation exposure, these toxins may also cause bone marrow suppression resulting in thrombocytopenia and neutropenia.

B. Laboratory and X-Ray Findings

Two primary forms of laboratory testing may be used to identify T-2 mycotoxins. First, antigen detection can be performed on urine samples. The metabolites of the T-2 mycotoxins are eliminated primarily in the urine and feces. These metabolites are detectable in the urine up to 1 month after exposure. Second, mass spectrometric evaluation can be conducted on various body fluids. Appropriate samples include nasal secretions, pulmonary secretions, urine, blood, and stomach contents.

Treatment and Prophylaxis

A. Specific Therapy

The treatment of T-2 mycotoxin poisoning is essentially supportive care. Remove all contaminated clothing and wash the patient's skin with large amounts of soap and water. Treat dermal burns with standard therapy. Treat secondary bacterial infections with appropriate antibiotics. Ocular involvement requires irrigation with water or sterile saline. Activated charcoal may aid in gastrointestinal decontamination. Patients with pulmonary involvement may require advanced respiratory techniques such as intubation or ventilatory support.

B. Prophylaxis

Vaccines against the T-2 mycotoxins are under study. The early use of soap and water may prevent skin toxicity.

Infection Control

The T-2 mycotoxins are dispersed as an oily liquid. Contact with this liquid may cause cross-contamination. Therefore, remove all contaminated clothing and wash the patient's skin with soap and water. Standard precautions are sufficient during patient care activities (see Table 3–2).

4. Staphylococcal Enterotoxin B

Staphylococcal aureus produces a number of exotoxins that produce disease in humans. One such exotoxin, staphylococcal enterotoxin B (SEB), is a causal agent of the gastrointestinal symptoms seen in staphylococcal food poisoning. It is a heat-stabile toxin that belongs to a group of compounds known as super antigens. These compounds have the ability to activate certain cells in the immune system, causing a severe inflammatory response. This response causes injury to various host tissues. Aside from injury caused by SEB in natural infections, it can be aerosolized, making it a potential biologic weapon. Biologic attack could involve deliberate contamination of foodstuffs, although a more likely scenario would involve an aerosol release.

Clinical Findings

A. Symptoms and Signs

After exposure to SEB, a variable incubation period occurs, ranging from 4 to 10 hours for gastrointestinal exposure and from 3 to 12 hours for inhalational exposure. Regardless of the type of exposure, nonspecific symptoms and signs will develop and include fever, chills, headache, malaise, and myalgias. If the exposure occurred via the gastrointestinal route, then patients will also develop nausea, vomiting, and diarrhea. Conversely, if the exposure occurred via an inhalational route, the patient will also develop chest pain, cough, and dyspnea. Death is rare but in severe cases may occur from respiratory failure. Patients generally recover from symptoms after 1–2 weeks.

B. Laboratory and X-Ray Findings

The presence of SEB can be confirmed by identifying specific antigens via ELISA testing. Obtain serum and urine samples. Urine samples are more productive because toxin tends to accumulate in the urine. In the case of aerosol exposure, respiratory and nasal swabs may also demonstrate toxin if samples are obtained within 1 day of exposure. With inhalational exposure, the chest x-ray is usually normal but in severe cases may demonstrate pulmonary edema.

Treatment and Prophylaxis

A. Specific Therapy

The treatment of SEB exposure is largely supportive. Correct electrolyte abnormalities and maintain volume status. If pulmonary edema develops, patients may benefit from diuretic therapy and in some cases may require intubation and ventilatory support. Steroids may be given to lessen the inflammatory response, but this approach is controversial. Treat secondary bacterial infections with appropriate antibiotics.

B. Prophylaxis

Vaccines against SEB are under study.

▶ Infection Control

Person-to-person transmission of toxin is not a hazard. Standard precautions are sufficient during patient care activities (see Table 3–2).

Bioterrorism Agents/Diseases: http://emergency.cdc.gov/agent/agentlist.asp, Atlanta, GA. Accessed on May 4, 2010.

Gilsdorf JR, Zilinskas RA: New considerations in infectious disease outbreaks: The threat of genetically modified microbes. Clin Infect Dis 2005;40:1160–1165 [PMID: 15791517].

Kman NE, Nelson RN: Infectious agents of bioterrorism: A review for emergency physicians. Emerg Med Clin North Am 2008;26:517–547 [PMID: 18406986].

Paterson RR: Fungi and fungal toxins as weapons. Mycol Res 2006;110:1003–1010 [PMID: 16908123].

Reichert E, Clase A, Bacetty A, Larsen J: Alphavirus antiviral drug development: scientific gap analysis and prospective research areas. Biosecur Bioterror 2009;7:413–427 [PMID: 20028250].

▼ CHEMICAL WEAPONS

Like radiation and biologic agents, many chemicals can be developed into weapons of mass destruction (Table 3–5). Chemical weapons are particularly attractive to rogue governments and terrorist organizations because of their low cost, stability, and ease of production. In fact, a chemical nerve agent was already used by a terrorist organization. Aum Shinrikyo released sarin in the Tokyo subway in 1995. Chemical agents can be delivered as liquids, vapors, or components of explosive devices. They are generally categorized as nerve agents, pulmonary agents, vesicants, and cyanide agents.

NERVE AGENTS

The nerve agents are a diverse group of compounds that were first developed by the Germans prior to World War II. GA (tabun) was the first nerve agent produced, followed by several others including GB (sarin), GD (soman), GF, and VX. Each of these agents has different physical characteristics, of which volatility is the most critical. These agents are classified as organophosphates and induce toxicity by binding to and inhibiting various forms of the acetylcholine esterase enzyme. This causes increased levels of acetylcholine, leading to hyperstimulation of both central and peripheral muscarinic and nicotinic receptors. Toxicity can occur either from skin contact or from inhalation of vapor.

▶ Clinical Findings

A. Symptoms and Signs

1. Latent period—When nerve agent exposure occurs as a vapor, there is generally no significant latent period and symptoms will develop within minutes. Likewise, the clinical effects of vapor exposure do not tend to progress over time. In contrast, liquid contamination may have a significant

Table 3–5. Clinical Findings Associated with Chemical Agents.

Chemical Agents	Latent Period	Early Findings	Late Findings
Nerve agents	Vapor: none Liquid: up to 18 h	Rhinorrhea, salivation, sweating, increased pulmonary secretions, fasciculations, mood swings, difficulty concentrating	Weakness, paralysis, vomiting, diarrhea, increased urination, seizures, coma, apnea
Lung agents (phosgene)	0–24 h	Mucous membrane irritation, rhinorrhea, cough, dyspnea, chest pain	Pulmonary edema, hypotension, laryngeal spasm
Vesicants			
Sulfur mustard	2–48 h	Ocular pain, conjunctivitis, photophobia, blepharospasm, erythema, burning blister formation, mucous membrane damage, cough, nausea, vomiting, diarrhea	Corneal clouding, dyspnea, mental status changes, seizures, pulmonary edema, respiratory failure, bone marrow suppression
Lewisite	No latency	Similar to sulfur agents, but it also directly affects vascular permeability and causes third spacing and more systemic effects	
Cyanide	None	Tachycardia, hypertension, tachypnea, anxiety, mental status changes	"Cherry red" appearance to skin, coma, seizures, cardiac arrest

latent period depending on the amount of skin exposure. With small exposures, latent periods of up to 18 hours may be seen. Further, with liquid contact, symptoms and signs may progress over a period of time.

2. Clinical syndromes—The findings that will develop following nerve agent poisoning depend on the amount and type of exposure. As the degree of exposure increases, so does the severity of symptoms. The general clinical syndromes of nerve agent toxicity are as follows:

(A) CENTRAL NERVOUS SYSTEM—The effects on the central nervous system may range from mild to severe depending on the degree of exposure. Mild symptoms and signs include mood swings, difficulty concentrating, poor judgment, and sleep disturbances. With more significant exposures, coma, convulsions, and apnea may occur.

(B) PERIPHERAL NICOTINIC STIMULATION—The symptoms and signs of peripheral nicotinic receptor stimulation are manifest primarily as alterations in skeletal muscle functioning. The degree of involvement depends on the degree of exposure. Initially muscle fasciculations or weakness will occur and may eventually progress to paralysis.

(C) PERIPHERAL MUSCARINIC STIMULATION—The symptoms and signs of peripheral muscarinic receptor stimulation are manifest primarily as increased exocrine gland and smooth muscle activity. Typical symptoms and signs of exocrine gland stimulation include rhinorrhea, salivation, sweating, increased gastrointestinal secretions, and increased pulmonary secretions. Increased pulmonary secretions may be severe enough to compromise the patient's airway. Increased smooth muscle activity will cause vomiting, diarrhea, increased urination, and abdominal pain.

B. Laboratory and X-Ray Findings

Acetylcholine esterase exists in various tissues within the body. Two important subpopulations of acetylcholine esterase are the plasma cholinesterase and the erythrocyte cholinesterase. Decreased activity within either population may indicate nerve agent exposure. Of the two forms, the erythrocyte cholinesterase is the more sensitive indicator of exposure.

▶ Treatment

A. Specific Therapy

The treatment of nerve agent toxicity involves the use of three primary medications. The first, atropine, is an anticholinergic medication used to counteract the hyperstimulation of peripheral muscarinic receptors. Atropine (1–2 mg IV; if no effect, double dose every 5 minutes until secretions dry) should generally be given until secretions begin to dry. Atropine will not prevent central nervous system or nicotinic toxicity. In contrast, pralidoxime chloride (2-PAM), 1–2 g IV given over 15–30 minutes, ameliorates nicotinic toxicity

by breaking the bond formed between the nerve agent and the esterase enzyme. The nerve agent–esterase bond may be broken as long as the compound has not aged, a process by which the bond becomes irreversible. For most of the nerve agents, the aging process is not clinically significant. One notable exception is GD (soman), which ages after only 2 minutes and is refractory to 2-PAM therapy. Finally, a common complication of severe intoxication is seizure activity. Seizures may be treated with benzodiazepines.

B. Supportive Care

Patients may require intensive medical support such as airway management and ventilatory support. Frequent suctioning of secretions may also be required.

▶ Decontamination

For more specific information on decontamination, see the section "Chemical Decontamination."

PULMONARY AGENTS

Many different chemicals can be classified as pulmonary or lung agents. All have a similar mechanism of toxicity, producing delayed onset of pulmonary edema. Of these agents, carbonyl chloride (phosgene) has been the most studied. Because phosgene is the prototypical lung agent, most of the discussion here relates to phosgene; however, the principles of management can be applied to all lung agents. As a military agent, phosgene was first used during World War I and today can be found in numerous industrial applications. Because of its high volatility, phosgene forms a gas readily, often with the faint scent of freshly cut hay. It is not absorbed through the skin, but when inhaled, it causes toxicity. After inhalation, phosgene is deposited in the peripheral airways, where it undergoes acetylation reactions. Subsequent damage to the alveolar-capillary membrane will occur, resulting in pulmonary edema. Phosgene may also interact with mucous membranes, causing local irritation.

▶ Clinical Findings

A. Symptoms and Signs

As noted previously, the primary effect of phosgene involves lung toxicity, although with some exposures, patients may have transient irritation to the eyes, nose, and mouth. In some cases, rhinorrhea and oral secretions may be significant. Patients may also complain of mild chest discomfort and cough secondary to bronchial irritation. In significant exposures, early death may occur secondary to laryngeal spasm. Despite these early effects, most of the toxicity of phosgene exposure is delayed. After inhalation, a variable latent period of up to 24 hours will ensue. The length of the latent period depends on the dose of phosgene delivered and will be shorter with higher exposures. Eventually the patient may develop symptoms and signs consistent with pulmonary edema, including dyspnea, hypoxia, chest pain, and cough. In some cases, pulmonary edema may be severe enough to cause hypotension. The degree to which each patient is affected depends on the severity of exposure. In severe exposures, death may occur.

B. Laboratory and X-Ray Findings

No clinical test exists for the diagnosis of phosgene exposure. Appropriate studies such as arterial blood gas measurements and chest x-ray should be used to manage pulmonary edema. Hemoconcentration secondary to pulmonary edema may also be evident.

▶ Treatment
A. Bed Rest

Any activity, even walking, may increase the severity of pulmonary edema. As a result, discourage patients from any physical activity.

B. Upper Respiratory Symptoms

In some cases, upper airway secretions may be significant. Nasal, oral, or bronchial secretions should be suctioned, if needed. If bronchospasm develops, it may be treated with intravenous steroids and inhaled bronchodilators. Treat secondary bacterial infections with appropriate antibiotics.

C. Lower Airway Symptoms

If pulmonary edema develops, it should be managed with standard medical interventions including supplemental oxygen, intubation, and ventilator management. Positive end-expiratory pressure is a useful ventilator adjunct. Treat secondary bacterial infection with antibiotics.

D. Hypotension

Secondary hypotension may develop in the event of severe pulmonary edema. Treatment of hypotension is problematic, given the increased permeability of the alveolar-capillary membrane. Supplemental crystalloid or colloid solutions can be used but they may worsen pulmonary edema. Vasopressor agents such as dopamine may also be used.

▶ Decontamination

No specific decontamination is required except removing the patient from the phosgene gas.

VESICANTS

Vesicants are a group of related compounds known to cause skin lesions, primarily blisters. Despite their predilection for skin involvement, multiple systemic effects are also seen.

Although multiple agents may be used as vesicants, sulfur mustard and lewisite are the most common.

1. Sulfur Mustard

Sulfur mustard (mustard) was first used as a chemical weapon during World War I. Mustard is a lipophilic compound that is readily absorbed through intact skin. It causes significant dermal toxicity and after systemic absorption will affect various body systems. Exposure can occur after contact with mustard vapor or liquid. At different ambient temperatures, mustard may exist in either form. It displays a characteristic odor of garlic or mustard, hence its name. The exact mechanism of mustard toxicity is not known but appears to involve DNA alkylation. Mustard also displays mild cholinergic activity. After systemic absorption, cell lines undergoing active mitosis are affected the most.

▶ Clinical Findings
A. Symptoms and Signs

The symptoms and signs of mustard toxicity depend on the dose and mechanism of exposure. Unfortunately, initial mustard exposure is not symptomatic, and the patient may be unaware of contamination. Given the initial lack of symptoms, patients may not decontaminate, thus increasing toxicity. Depending on the dose, the latent period after exposure may range from 2 to 48 hours. In mild exposures, patients may display only mild dermal injury; in severe exposures, death may occur within hours. The specific symptoms and signs of mustard toxicity depend on the body areas exposed and the degree of systemic absorption. As noted, the skin is typically affected and will display areas of erythema, burning, and blister formation. The blisters may become large and express a clear to straw-colored fluid. The fluid does not contain mustard agent.

The eyes are one of the organs most sensitive to mustard exposure and may develop symptoms and signs first. Following ocular exposure, ocular pain, photophobia, conjunctivitis, and blepharospasm may occur. The superficial layers of the cornea may be denuded, leading to corneal clouding with visual changes.

With injury to the respiratory tree, patients may develop oronasal burning, rhinorrhea, sore throat, or epistaxis. In more severe exposures, findings of cough, dyspnea, mucous membrane necrosis, airway muscular damage, pulmonary edema, and respiratory failure may be seen. Symptoms and signs of gastrointestinal exposure may result either from the direct toxicity of mustard exposure or from mustard's cholinergic affects. Nausea, vomiting, diarrhea, and constipation are common findings.

Severe mustard exposure may also affect the central nervous system; mental status changes and seizure activity are the most common findings. Given mustard's interference with DNA activity, delayed findings of bone marrow suppression may also occur.

B. Laboratory and X-Ray Findings

With exposure to mustard, an early leukocytosis is typical. If bone marrow suppression develops, later findings of anemia, leukopenia, and thrombocytopenia may be seen. If wound or pulmonary secretions become more purulent, a secondary bacterial infection should be suspected and Gram stain and culture obtained. Gastrointestinal symptoms may require electrolyte monitoring. The primary metabolite of mustard agent thiodiglycol may be detected in the urine in contaminated patients. Such specialized testing usually can be conducted only at reference or military laboratories. In the event of pulmonary involvement, chest x-ray may demonstrate a focal or diffuse pneumonitis and occasionally pulmonary edema.

▶ Treatment

A. Decontamination

The most critical aspect in the treatment of mustard toxicity is removal of the chemical agent. This is problematic given the initial lack of symptoms. Even delayed decontamination, however, may lessen subsequent toxicity. Washing contaminated areas with either large amounts of soapy water or 0.5% hypochlorite solution is the preferred method of decontamination. For more specific information on decontamination, see the section "Chemical Decontamination."

B. Specific Therapy

With skin injuries, leave small blisters intact and unroof larger lesions. Clean unroofed areas frequently and cover them with antibiotic cream (Polysporin, silver sulfadiazine). Treat other irritated areas of skin with systemic analgesics or topical lotions. With ocular exposure, use topical antibiotics to prevent secondary bacterial infections. Topical anticholinergics may prevent the discomfort of ciliary spasm. With pulmonary involvement, treat associated cough with typical antitussive medications. Treat episodes of bronchospasm with systemic steroids and inhaled bronchodilators. Treat secondary bacterial infection with appropriate antibiotics. Supplemental oxygen, intubation, or ventilator management may be required in some patients. Typical gastrointestinal antispasmodics may ameliorate the symptoms of gastrointestinal exposure. Bone marrow transplant, growth factor utilization, and factor replacement are alternatives for the treatment of bone marrow suppression.

▶ Decontamination

As noted above, toxin can be removed by washing contaminated surfaces with large amounts of soapy water or 0.5% hypochlorite solution. For more specific information on decontamination, see the section "Chemical Decontamination."

2. Lewisite

Much like sulfur mustard, exposure to lewisite causes injury to contaminated body surfaces and may lead to systemic symptoms. Unlike mustard, however, lewisite exposure causes symptoms and signs without a significant latent period. Lewisite is a volatile agent with the odor of geraniums. Its exact mechanism of action is unknown, but it is thought that the arsenic component of lewisite may inhibit various enzymes.

▶ Clinical Findings

A. Symptoms and Signs

As noted above, the symptoms and signs of lewisite exposure begin without a significant latent period. Even though findings of exposure begin early, it may take several hours for symptoms to fully develop. The severity of clinical findings depends on the degree and method of exposure. Shortly after skin exposure, an area of dead skin will develop that will subsequently blister. These lesions may take up to 18 hours to fully develop. Skin necrosis may also be evident. Symptoms and signs of ocular exposure are similar to those associated with mustard toxicity and include conjunctivitis, iritis, edema, ocular pain, and corneal injury. If pulmonary toxicity develops, findings of cough, dyspnea, and pulmonary edema may occur. Lewisite causes increases in vascular permeability that may lead to third spacing of fluid with subsequent hypotension. In some cases, gastrointestinal, renal, and liver involvement may be seen.

B. Laboratory and X-Ray Findings

No specific test for lewisite exposure is currently available.

▶ Treatment

A. Decontamination

As with mustard exposure, the cornerstone of treatment involves early decontamination. Compared with mustard exposure, decontamination is usually more successful with lewisite exposure, given the early onset of symptoms. Standard washing with soap and water or 0.5% hypochlorite solution is sufficient.

B. Supportive Care

Patients may require intensive medical support such as airway management, hemodynamic support, and various measures to manage multisystem organ failure.

C. Specific Therapy

British antilewisite (dimercaprol), 2–3 mg/kg every 4 hours, is a compound that can be given IM to decrease the effects of lewisite exposure.

CYANIDE AGENTS

Cyanide has a high affinity for trivalent iron compounds and will bond to the cytochrome a3 complex within the mitochondria. The cytochrome a3–cyanide bond effectively blocks aerobic cellular respiration, and anaerobic metabolism ensues. Cyanide exposure most often occurs naturally after inhalation of smoke from burning synthetic materials. In a biologic attack, cyanide exposure would likely follow an aerosol release. Cyanide gas is known to exhibit the scent of bitter almonds.

▶ Clinical Findings

A. Symptoms and Signs

After inhalation of cyanide gas, the cytochrome a3 enzyme is effectively blocked. Because cells can no longer utilize oxygen, they will convert to anaerobic metabolism, leading to a lactic acidosis. This inability to utilize oxygen effectively smothers the patient. Tachycardia, hypertension, and tachypnea will be seen initially. As symptoms and signs progress, anxiety, mental status changes, coma, seizures, cardiac arrest, and death will occur. Because cyanide does not alter oxygen–hemoglobin saturation, cyanosis will not develop. In fact, the inability to utilize oxygen increases the venous oxygen saturation, leading to a cherry red appearance to the skin. It generally takes 6–8 minutes for death to occur following cyanide exposure.

B. Laboratory and X-Ray Findings

An elevated blood cyanide concentration confirms the diagnosis. Given the short time interval to death, such testing is not useful in the acute setting but may later confirm the diagnosis. Two rapid tests, an elevated venous blood oxygen saturation and an increased lactic acid level, are characteristic of cyanide poisoning.

▶ Treatment

A. Specific Therapy

In addition to cyanide's affinity for certain iron compounds, it also has a high affinity for sulfhydryl groups and for the methemoglobin complex. These two characteristics are the basis of the cyanide antidote kit. The kit contains three components: amyl nitrite (used if no vascular access is available), sodium nitrite, and sodium thiosulfate. First, the patient is given a nitrite compound (inhalation of an amyl nitrate ampule or sodium nitrite), which will cause the formation of methemoglobin. The dose of sodium nitrite is based on the patient's weight and hemoglobin concentration although 300 mg IV is the usual dose for nonanemic adults. Given the high affinity of methemoglobin for cyanide, it will preferentially bind the compound and help to remove it from the cytochrome a3 complex. Second, the patient is given sodium thiosulfate (typically 12.5 g IV for an adult), which interacts

with cyanide, forming thiocyanate. Thiocyanate is then excreted in the urine.

Recently, hydroxocobalamin (a form of vitamin B$_{12}$) was approved to treat cyanide poisoning. A 5-mg IV injection will bind circulating and cellular cyanide molecules to form cyanocobalamin that is then excreted in the urine within a few minutes. A second 5-mg dose can be given if necessary.

B. Supportive Measures

Severe lactic acidosis may be treated with bicarbonate administration. Seizures may be treated with benzodiazepines. In many cases, patients require intubation and ventilator support.

▶ Decontamination

The only effective mode of decontamination involves removing the patient from the cyanide gas.

CHEMICAL DECONTAMINATION

Because of the risk of cross-contamination to health care workers, the need for patient decontamination should be emphasized. All patients suspected of experiencing a chemical weapons attack should be decontaminated as soon as possible. Optimally, patient decontamination should be conducted in the field. Often this is not practical and a decontamination station should be established in a secure location adjacent to the health care facility. All persons conducting decontamination duties should be provided adequate protective clothing and should receive specialized training.

Decontamination involves physical removal and chemical deactivation of toxin. Remove all clothing, jewelry, dressings, and splints. Wash the patient with copious amounts of soap and water. Avoid vigorous scrubbing because this may facilitate toxin absorption. After physical removal of toxin, any remaining toxin can be chemically deactivated. This may take some time and thus is considered secondary to physical removal of toxin. The most common neutralizing solution is 0.5% hypochlorite solution, which detoxifies many chemical agents via oxidation reactions. Hypochlorite solution should not be used to decontaminate open peritoneal wounds, open chest wounds, exposed neural tissue, or ocular tissue. Irrigate these areas with copious amounts of normal saline. All contaminated materials should be bagged and sent for proper disposal.

Hall AH, Saiers J, Baud F: Which cyanide antidote? Crit Rev Toxicol 2009;39:541–552 [PMID: 19650716].

Jokanović M: Current understanding of the mechanisms involved in metabolic detoxification of warfare nerve agents. Toxicol Lett 2009;1881:1–10 [PMID: 19433263].

Wattana M, Bey T: Mustard gas or sulfur mustard: an old chemical agent as a new terrorist threat. Prehosp Disaster Med 2009; 241:19–29 [PMID: 19557954].

Disaster Medicine

Gregory A. Starr, MD

Thomas W. Allen, DO, MPH

Charles E. Stewart, MD, EMDM

OVERVIEW OF DISASTER MEDICINE

More than 4 million people worldwide have lost their lives and hundreds of millions have suffered due to natural and man-made disasters during the past 30 years. The dollars lost in damages and reconstruction costs are staggering. Hundreds of billions have gone to rebuild the infrastructure and to replace the personal property damaged or lost as a result of these disasters. Ongoing assistance may be required many years after the disasters to sustain and reconstruct the lives of those affected.

Disaster medicine and prevention is a system of study and medical practice encompassing the disciplines of emergency medicine and public health. The multidisciplinary nature of disaster planning and response has traditionally resulted in various definitions of disasters and events that cause mass casualties. Some commonality in terminology has evolved in the organizational aspects of emergency medical disaster response:

Austere medicine: Medicine practiced on-location without the amenities provided by an organized medical system. Austere medicine is often practiced in temporary shelters, with quite limited equipment. The goal is to provide temporary "fixes" to restore functionality or save life.

Disaster: Any event that overwhelms the emergency medical system resources available at a given time in a given jurisdiction. This may be a city/county, a region, a state, or even a country.

Incident Command System (ICS) and Incident Management System (IMS): Initially used by the military and fire departments. ICS has evolved over the past two decades into the current disaster management tools of choice for disaster command, operations, planning, logistics, and finance from the federal to local level.

Multiple (or Mass) Casualty Incident (MCI): Any event that causes a large number of individuals to become ill or injured. Sometimes called **Multiple Victim Incident (MVI).**

Medical disaster: Any event that causes a large number of individuals to become ill or injured and overwhelms the medical system resources available at a given time in a given jurisdiction.

Mutual aid: Agreements between neighboring communities to provide support and assistance in the event of a disaster.

National Response Framework (NRF): This is the current evolution of the US government national response plan. The ability for augmenting flexibility continues to be the driving force for the current version of the NRF. National or federal framework for coordinating the population and infrastructure of our nation including federal, state, local, tribal, and private sector resources in the event of a disaster.

Mitigation: Critical foundation in the effort to reduce the loss of life and property from natural and/or man-made disasters by avoiding or lessening the impact of a disaster and providing value to the public by creating safer communities. Mitigation seeks to fix the cycle of disaster damage, reconstruction, and repeated damage. These activities or actions, in most cases, will have a long-term sustained effect.

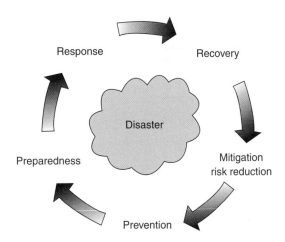

▲ **Figure 4-1.** The disaster life cycle.

public warnings and protection modalities to be implemented such as sheltering and evacuations to occur long before the inciting event occurs.

IMPACT OR EMERGENCY PHASE

This is the event. This phase may be relatively short or prolonged. The magnitude of damage, prioritization, and identification of injured and required resources is determined. Planning and preemptive actions will have the greatest effect on mitigation of the impact phase.

RESCUE PHASE

This phase represents the response to the emergency, the period where immediate time-sensitive action will save lives.

RECOVERY PHASE

This phase consists of all of the components required to return a population to a functioning society. The duration of this phase is variable and may last weeks to years.

▼ DISASTER CYCLE

Disasters follow a pattern of development and have a distinguishable life cycle of various durations. This sequence of events has been termed the disaster life cycle (Figure 4–1). Disaster planning, response, and research may be simplified by using the disaster cycle as a model for complex events. Five phases supplement the disaster life cycle.

INTERDISASTER PHASE

The interdisaster period is where there is a sequence of events that lead to the occurrence of a disaster. Evaluation of local hazards that may lead to a disaster or augment the destructive effects of a disaster is paramount to risk assessment strategies.

WARNING PHASE

The warning phase develops next and marks the time during which a particular event is likely to occur. Historically, weather and seismic prediction models have allowed for

▼ CATEGORIES OF DISASTER AND MASS CASUALTY EVENTS

Disasters are generally thought of in terms of being natural or man-made. Technically, however, all disasters are man-made. A palm tree felled by a hurricane is a natural event caused by a natural hazard. When the society builds a high-rise hotel on the same shore and the hurricane destroys the hotel, it is the same natural event, but because men built the hotel knowing the risks entailed in this location, it is now potentially a disaster.

Specific types of disasters produce different patterns and numbers of injuries and have different effects on the social and physical environment. It is important to be familiar with these disaster categories in terms of scope, scale, and historical impact.

EARTHQUAKES

An earthquake is the most likely large-scale event in the United States. Earthquake intensity is commonly measured by the Richter scale, a logarithmic scale that measures the intensity of seismic waves. An earthquake of 2.0 magnitude is barely felt, whereas an 8.0-magnitude event is greatly destructive. There have been six major earthquakes greater than 8.0 on the Richter scale in the history of the United States. An earthquake of a given magnitude may produce varying amounts of destruction, depending on a complex interaction of many factors, including the type of ground underlying a structure, the degree of ground failure (eg, landslide, soil failures), and the construction quality of overlying structures.

Injuries are most often due to structural collapse, the degree of which will also depend heavily on local structural engineering standards. Illness also occurs as a result of disruption of existing community infrastructure (eg, food supply, power, sanitation, ongoing support for persons with chronic disease). Predictably, the patterns of injury seen among casualties include severe orthopedic, neurologic, and thoracic crush injuries, lacerations, tetanus and dysentery infections, environmental exposure, and exacerbations of chronic medical problems.

Current problematic areas for earthquake activity include the Enriquillo fault line in the Caribbean in which lies Haiti and the New Madrid fault of the mid-eastern United States.

TROPICAL CYCLONES (HURRICANES, TYPHOONS, AND TROPICAL CYCLONES)

Tropical cyclones (hurricanes in the United States and Atlantic, typhoons in the eastern Pacific, tropical cyclones elsewhere) are a circulating mass of clouds, rain, and wind around a clear central area of extreme low barometric pressure. They occur most commonly in the late summer months.

The intensity of tropical cyclones is rated on a 5-point scale. For hurricanes approaching the United States, this information is available from the National Weather Service, which can also provide information about a storm's probable path. Damage is due to high winds, which can exceed 150 mph, storm surges, tornadoes, and inland flooding. Of these four, inland flooding causes more property damage and loss of life.

Casualties may be caused by trauma from flying debris or structural collapse; by drowning; by famine related to damaged agriculture and food distribution systems; by disease related to loss of power, water, and sanitation; and

occasionally by violence related to loss of public safety. Casualties may be significantly reduced by early warning systems and evacuation efforts.

TORNADOES AND SEVERE STORMS

Annually in the United States, tornadoes and severe thunderstorms are the most common cause of death due to natural disasters. Approximately 100,000 severe storms (eg, involving thunder, high winds, and hail) occur each year in the United States, including 1000 tornadoes. Most commonly affected are the states in "tornado alley," the area between the Rocky Mountains and Appalachian Mountains. No state is completely free of the risk of tornado. Tornadoes usually occur during the summer months and during late afternoons. Only about 3–4% of all tornadoes produce injury, and most deaths occur in a small number of highly destructive events. Casualties are related to trauma from structural collapse, flying debris, or being knocked to the ground or thrown. Head injuries, crush injuries, fractures, contusions, and lacerations are common.

As with all disasters, secondary illness and injury may occur, although tornadoes most commonly tend to produce random, isolated groups of casualties wherever they touch down, rather than diffuse area-wide casualties and destruction to community infrastructure. Multitornado storms such as occurred in Moore, Oklahoma, during 1999 can cause widespread damage. Casualty mitigation through early warning and evacuation is hard to manage because tornadoes are difficult to predict and the time frame for evacuation or protective cover is brief.

FLOODS

Floods can be divided into riverine floods, hurricane (storm) flooding, flash floods, and tsunamis. Riverine floods are typically seasonal and result from excessive rains or snow melts that lead to rivers overflowing their banks in a floodplain area. Flash floods occur in areas where rainfall produces surface water that exceeds the runoff or absorptive capacity of the soil. Storm flooding as a result of hurricanes is covered above. Tsunamis are caused by earthquakes or volcanic eruptions at sea. Rarely, flooding can be caused by failure of a dike or dam, usually due to heavy rains.

In the United States, the number of deaths each year from floods is small and sporadic. Property damage can be considerable, as are secondary effects on crops, sanitation, and vector-borne infections. When casualties occur, they are usually due to drowning. Mitigation (eg, through watershed engineering projects and limiting development on floodplains) and early warning are the most effective means of reducing deaths.

Tsunamis or tidal waves occur during sudden geologic events occurring at sea, such as earthquakes and volcanic eruptions. The tsunami will be worse if the epicenter of the seismic event resides in relatively shallower water. The giant

Phases of a pandemic

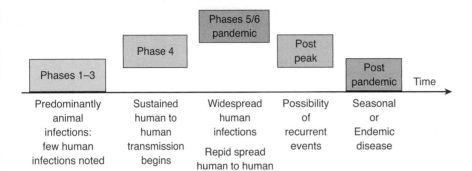

▲ **Figure 4–2.** Phases of pandemic flu.

wave of water may travel from the epicenter at hundreds of miles per hour. The onset is often heralded by a sudden ebb of water that exposes the seafloor and is followed in minutes by a wall of water that may rise to 100 ft. Massive damage occurs to the shore and structures; casualties are due to drowning. Mitigation through early warning is the most effective means of reducing casualties. Sea walls and locating structures on high ground can provide some additional relief.

VOLCANOES

Volcanoes are channels of molten rock (magma) from deep in the earth that vent to the surface in one of several forms. They may cause eruptions of molten rock (lava) or spew ash and debris. Volcanoes tend to be localized to the boundaries of tectonic plates (eg, the Pacific Rim). Injury is most commonly due to falling debris, collapse of structures under the weight of ash, being buried in mudslides or lava flows, or toxic effects of gases (eg, carbon dioxide, hydrogen sulfide). Effects on agriculture and property can be extensive. In many cases, early warning, although imprecise, can allow evacuation and mitigate casualties.

WINTER STORMS

A winter storm can range from a moderate snow over a few hours to blizzard conditions with blinding wind-driven snow that lasts several days. Some winter storms may be large enough to affect several states, while others may affect only a single community. Many winter storms are accompanied by sustained low temperatures and heavy winds.

Frostbite and hypothermia are of main concerns with trapped motorists, homeless people, and those trapped at home, without utilities or other services. Incorrect venting of heating devices and/or generators is a major cause of carbon monoxide poisoning during disasters. Fires are common with use of inappropriate alternative heating devices. Of course, trapped without heat or proper clothing, people

may suffer hypothermia or cold injuries. Property damage may occur due to pipeline freezing with subsequent building flooding, structural overload with snow and/or ice, and falling tree limbs or trunks. Automobile accidents are common.

PANDEMICS AND PLAGUES

A disease epidemic occurs when there are more cases of that disease than normal. A pandemic is a worldwide epidemic of a disease. A pandemic may occur when a disease appears against which the population has little or no immunity. With the increase in worldwide transport and urbanization and crowded conditions in some countries, epidemics due to a new disease or novel organism are more likely to occur around the world. The World Health Organization has defined six phases of a pandemic to provide a global framework to aid countries in preparedness and response planning for a possible pandemic (Figure 4–2). Pandemics can be either mild or severe in the illness and death they cause, and the severity of a pandemic can change over the course of that pandemic. Examples of pandemics and plagues are listed in Table 4–1.

MAN-MADE DISASTERS (SEE ALSO CHAPTER 2)

▶ Bioterrorism

Agents such as anthrax, plague, and smallpox may be used as biologic weapons. This may differ little from epidemics and plagues, but is caused by the deliberate efforts of man.

▶ Chemical Emergencies and Industrial Accidents

Agents such as ricin, chlorine, and nerve agents can be used as weapons or may be the result of release of chemical agents from industrial sources. Industrial accidents that cause large-scale disasters most commonly result in the release of

Table 4–1. Selected Pandemics and Plagues Throughout History.

Event	Years
Black Death (probably bubonic plague)	1300s
Typhus	1501-1587
Influenza	1732-1733, 1775-1776, 1857-1859, 1889-1892
Cholera	1816-1826, 1829-1851, 1852-1860, 1863-1875, 1899-1923
Bubonic plague	1855
Spanish flu (avian flu)	1918-1920
El Tor (*Vibrio cholerae*)	1960s
HIV/AIDS	1980s to present
Swine flu (H1N1)	2009-2010

a hazardous material. The most notorious occurred in 1984 in Bhopal, India, where a release of methyl isocyanate killed more than 2000 and injured up to 200,000.

Injuries vary depending on the nature of the agent. Asphyxia, respiratory distress, skin and eye irritations, neurologic abnormalities, or teratogenic effects may occur. In addition, explosive effects are not uncommon in industrial accidents.

Radiation Emergencies

Release of radiation from dirty bombs, nuclear blasts, or reactor accidents can be associated with major disasters. In nuclear accidents, injuries are due to the immediate blast effects, exposure to toxic chemicals used at reactor sites (eg, sulfuric acid, chlorine, ammonia), and radiation exposure. Aside from the atomic explosions in Japan in World War II, few deaths have resulted from nuclear disasters, although several significant incidents have occurred. The most deadly was the 1986 Chernobyl reactor explosion in the former Soviet Union, in which 27 people died and 135,000 were evacuated, many of whom were exposed to high radiation levels. The Chernobyl radiation release is considered the worst nuclear power plant accident in history. Over 400 times more radioactive material was released from the power plant explosion than the atomic bomb that was dropped on Hiroshima.

Mass Casualties

Explosions, blasts, and injuries causing mass casualties may be industrial, agricultural (grain elevators), or terrorism. The patterns of injury include direct blast injuries, fragment wounds, injuries sustained by the force of the blast, and injuries from the chemical products of the explosive.

Fires

Collectively, fires produce approximately 5000 deaths and 300,000 injuries each year in the United States, although the number has been on a steady decline since the 1950s. Under the right conditions, hot gases can produce winds that collect in a rotating cyclone (called a fire storm). Most deaths are due to asphyxiation from carbon monoxide and other toxic gases and due to burns. When exits are blocked, casualties from both fire and inhalation of toxic gases and crowd-related injuries may occur.

Transportation Accidents

Transportation accidents are the most common incidents producing multiple casualties in the United States. Airplane crashes produce a high ratio of fatalities to total injuries; highway accidents have the opposite characteristic. Railway accidents may produce significant injuries if passengers are involved and also have resulted in release of hazardous materials. Ship and ferry accidents are often complicated by adverse weather conditions.

Transportation accidents are the prototypical geographically localized multicasualty events practiced in most communities' disaster drills. They are realistically apt to occur, and they lend themselves to management within the jurisdiction and structure of local emergency medical services (EMS). The patterns of injury are well known to most emergency workers and consist of fractures, contusions, lacerations, and head and thoracoabdominal blunt injury.

Structural Collapse and Explosions

Structural failure of a building or man-made structure can be precipitated by natural forces (eg, earthquake) or may occur unexpectedly (eg, the Hyatt skywalk collapse in Kansas City, 1981; 113 dead and 200 injured). However, most such events in the United States have been limited in scope and have not produced many casualties. Injuries are predictable and consist of head injuries, fractures, lacerations, and blunt thoracoabdominal injuries.

Acts of Terrorism

Historically, acts of violence in the civilian arena are usually limited to a small number of casualties. Explosives are by far the most common modality used in modern terrorist attacks. Given the September 11, 2001, attack on the World Trade Center, the prior bombing there in the parking structure, the bombing of the Murrah Federal Building in Oklahoma City in 1995, the sarin gas attack in Tokyo, and the 2001 anthrax scare, it is obvious that acts of terrorism can strike close to home and affect a hospital's ability to properly care for a large influx of patients.

The 2001 anthrax scare in the United States and known world stockpiles and instability of biologic and chemical warfare programs around the world have demonstrated that bioterrorism is a very real threat. Hospital surveillance requires a high level of suspicion. A bioterrorism event that goes unrecognized or may be dismissed as a natural epidemic may compromise hospital staff and patients not associated with the disaster. Establishing an effective response requires hospital, local, state, and federal cooperation and training. An effective response should include the following four steps: detection and diagnosis, declaration of need, defense, and drug therapy.

OPERATIONAL ISSUES IN DISASTERS

CATEGORIZATION OF DISASTERS

Disasters may be more effectively categorized from an operational perspective. It can be argued that no disaster will fit neatly into any category whether operational, response based, or descriptive. Currently, we employ an operational "all-hazards" approach that creates a system to analyze, plan, and respond to a multitude of synchronous and asynchronous disasters.

▶ Open

An open disaster occurs in a widespread area where the location and number of casualties is often unknown. Many open disasters are natural in origin such as an earthquake, hurricane, or tornado. (It could be easily argued that Chernobyl and Bhopal were man-made open disasters.) The control of patient flow and ultimate disposition of patients becomes challenging. Open disasters often have substantial degradation of the medical system from the disaster. Open events may produce casualties for several days.

▶ Closed

A closed disaster occurs in a geographically confined area often with little or no warning. Terrorism events, structural failures, chemical plant explosions, and transportation accidents typically comprise this category of disaster. (Arguably, a tornado would fit this definition.) Frequently, the number of casualties and their names may be known to authorities, such as in an aircraft accident.

The first units to respond may be overwhelmed, but a robust emergency medical system can often cope with the relatively limited response. Ingress and egress of response units may be problematic due to the geographic proximity of the event. Hospitals close to the disaster are usually overwhelmed with sudden surges of patients occurring without warning, but substantial degradation of the overall medical system does not usually occur. Local infrastructures remain intact and resources are not usually overwhelmed.

Lessons learned from terrorism and MCIs such as the Oklahoma City bombing gave Incident Commanders (ICs) of more recent disasters training and tools to limit inflow of responders and minimize patient surges at health care facilities by transporting to the most appropriate levels of care and hospitals providing staging and treatment areas outside the emergency departments of their hospitals.

▶ Finite

A finite disaster by definition has a measurable endpoint. A tornado, terrorism event, solitary aircraft accident, or large traffic accident is typical of a finite disaster. Casualties occurring after the event are minimal and not usually as a result of the original disaster. Initial patient surges to health care facilities will peak within 2 hours. Subsequently, there will be very little, if any, further patient presentations. Often damage will be extensive, but the causative event will have terminated. Attention is concentrated on rescue and recovery.

This may be a relatively artificial distinction. In many disasters due to natural hazards, the endpoint of the natural event such as a tornado or hurricane may be quite easily measured. The number of injuries sustained during rebuilding may be ongoing for many months.

▶ Ongoing

In the ongoing disaster casualties continue to occur after the initial event and after the initial emergency response. Initial emergency resources are exhausted at an unusually fast rate. Mutual aid at the national and international levels is common.

Examples of such ongoing disasters include influenza pandemics, tsunamis and floods, and complex humanitarian emergencies such as sustained armed conflicts where a country or region is so poor or underdeveloped that it is completely unable to create a sustained response to a disaster. Ongoing disasters have components of both open and finite disasters. As with an open event, the ICS structure is maintained. However, efforts must be very flexible, and long-range vision and contingency planning is necessary for the successful management of the ongoing type of disasters. Resource requirements will exceed those of the finite event, and affected individuals will continue to grow and overwhelm resources. Difficult decisions regarding rationing of care become evident as the ability to care for critically ill patients who require surgery or cardiopulmonary support becomes impossible.

OPERATIONAL ISSUES

▶ Geographic Effect

Casualties capable of self-transport will usually travel to the closest health care facility. This can also be compounded by EMS personnel doing the same in the interest of critical care patient rapid transport and the desire for a rapid turnaround time in order to return to the scene to further assist in the response. Techniques have been developed to mitigate this effect. For example, the Israeli technique of "far-first" transport of wounded has decreased the load on hospitals closer to the incident.

▶ Interval Wave Phenomenon

Casualties frequently arrive to the hospital in two waves after a disaster. The first wave occurs within 30–60 minutes of a disaster. This includes all survivors who have self-transported or used local or family transportation from the scene to the hospital. This was seen in the World Trade Center attack and Oklahoma City bombing. The first patients arrived at the emergency department within 15 minutes of the disaster, but the highest flow occurred between 60 and 90 minutes.

The second wave begins to arrive within 1–3 hours of impact and comprises those who have been extricated and transported and those transported by formal emergency services. Patients transported by EMS have a much higher acuity and admission rate than for all other forms of transport. Adhering to strict triage principles, creation of hospital staging areas, and good EMS communication during an event will mitigate these effects.

▶ Communications Failure

Communications is often found to be the earliest breakdown in a disaster. A failure in communication is a failure in response. In a disaster, it may not be clear which communication modalities are functional and what facilities and resources are "online."

Whether it is destruction of trunked lines, power failure, collapse of antenna towers, or simple overload of cellular communications, emergency planners should count on disruption of communications. Lessons learned and concurrent reviews of ongoing and past disasters stress planning for contingencies based on interoperability, simplicity, redundancy, and in extreme cases more rudimentary forms of communication.

Communications between different agencies and hospitals often use different terminology, frequencies, and equipment. This must be mitigated in preplanning with joint frequencies, terminology, and compatible equipment. Amateur radio operators, HAMS, often provide appropriate continuing communication with reliable, simple, and easily maintained equipment. Whenever communication between agencies during a disaster is ongoing, clear simple language must be utilized.

▶ Samaritan Effect

Most disasters result in an outpouring by the lay public, including voluntary medical personnel. While well meaning, these volunteers may arrive without basic protective equipment, food, water, or medical supplies and tools. This was noted in hurricane Katrina. This may cause a logistical challenge to coordinating disaster relief services. While these individuals' intentions are indeed altruistic, most lack the proper training in these environments and may ultimately become causalities and further impede rescue efforts. If individuals wish to respond to a disaster, they become significantly more effective as part of an organized team coordinated by the IC. With training, coordination, equipment, supplies, and logistical support, the volunteer medical provider can truly make a difference.

In addition to these altruistic but untrained individuals, miscreants and poseurs may also respond, identifying themselves as medical, psychiatric, or social work professionals. Local precredentialing of providers at multiple hospitals within a municipality can provide a ready source of professionals if damage occurs to one hospital within the municipality. The federal program, Emergency System for Advance Registration of Volunteer Health Professionals (ESAR-VHP), established in 2006, can provide four levels of credentials for volunteers who cross state lines:

- Level 1: Verified active hospital practice
- Level 2: Verified active clinical practice (nonhospital)
- Level 3: Verified state licensure or certification (in good standing)
- Level 4: Verified education or experience (no verification of licensure or clinical practice)

▶ Disaster Supply Issues

In the first 24 hours of a disaster, the availability of pre-event stockpiles of supplies and equipment will be the main determinant of the effectiveness and success of the response. This is often known as the "come as you are effect." Despite lay public wishes and media pronouncements, the logistics tail remains relatively constant.

Simply put, it takes a significant amount of time for even an on-call unit to be paged, gather together, draw/ready equipment in stores, and then deploy to another location. Travel to the disaster site may be marred by road hazards, fires, fuel supply problems, weather, and even destroyed bridges or tunnels. The state government may be able to supply additional help and supplies within 2–24 hours depending on proximity and effect of the disaster on the supply and equipment storage facilities, road conditions, resource availability, and scope of the disaster. Federal units and supplies often take an additional 12–96 hours depending on where the resources are based. Austere conditions including weather, warfare, and unstable governments will affect supply delivery systems.

There are multiple strategies for aid delivery to disaster victims. Supply management through preparation from lessons learned and natural courses of prior events combined with contingency plans for multiple disasters in a single area will maximize the logistical aspects and utilization strategies of supply management.

▼ DISASTER PREPAREDNESS IN THE UNITED STATES

Recent terrorism such as New York City in 9/11, London, Madrid, and Mumbai has substantially changed disaster planning in this country and throughout the world. Federal, state, and local governments as well as voluntary disaster relief organizations, the private sector, and international sources have organized a national disaster response framework for providing assistance following a major disaster or emergency. Within this framework, the federal government can provide personnel, equipment, supplies, facilities, and managerial, technical, and advisory services in support of state and local disaster assistance efforts. Various federal statutory authorities and policies establish the basis for providing these resources.

US NATIONAL RESPONSE FRAMEWORK

The NRF is a scalable, flexible, and adaptable system to address a major disaster or emergency as defined under the Stafford Act (Table 4–2). This framework establishes a process and structure for the systematic, coordinated, and effective delivery of federal assistance to address the consequences of any major disaster or emergency in the United States. This includes a natural catastrophe; fire, flood, or explosion regardless of cause; or any other occasion or instance for which the President of the United States determines that federal assistance is needed to supplement state and local efforts and capabilities. Any reference to a disaster, major disaster, or emergency generally means a Presidentially declared major disaster or emergency under the Stafford Act. Under the Stafford Act, the Federal Emergency Management

Table 4–2. Emergency Support Functions (ESF) Outlined in the National Response Framework.

ESF 1: Transportation
ESF 2: Communications
ESF 3: Public Works and Engineering
ESF 4: Firefighting
ESF 5: Information and Planning
ESF 6: Mass Care (this may involve medical providers)
ESF 7: Resource Support
ESF 8: Health (this is usually medical providers)
ESF 9: Search and Rescue
ESF 10: Hazardous Materials
ESF 11: Food & Water
ESF 12: Energy
ESF 13: Military Support
ESF 14: Public Information
ESF 15: Volunteers & Donations
ESF 16: Law Enforcement
ESF 17: Animal Protection & Agriculture
ESF 18: Business Industry & Economic Stabilization

Agency (FEMA) from the Department of Homeland Security serves as the primary coordinating agency for disaster response and recovery activities. Initial tasks include notification, activation, mobilization, deployment, staffing, and facility setup. The NRF outlines the following:

- Lead agencies for each support function for planning and coordination of that support function;

- The array of federal response, recovery, and mitigation resources available to augment local and regional resources;

- The types of federal response assistance most likely to be needed in a specific disaster process;

- The methodology for implementing and managing specific incidents and subsequent federal mitigation programs and support/technical services;

- A focus for interagency and intergovernmental emergency preparedness, planning, training, exercising, coordination, and information exchange;

- The development of detailed supplemental plans and procedures to implement federal response and recovery activities rapidly and efficiently;

- The responses to the consequences of terrorism, in accordance with Presidential Decision Directives that set forth US counterterrorism policies.

The Department of Homeland Security processes a Governor's request for disaster assistance, coordinates federal operations under a disaster declaration, and appoints a Federal Coordinating Officer (FCO) for each declared state. In continuing operations, the Department of Homeland Security provides support for logistics management; communications and information technology; financial management; community relations, congressional affairs, public information, and other outreach; and information collection, analysis, and dissemination (Figure 4–3).

The Terrorism Incident Annex creates a unified response to a terrorism incident involving two or more of the following plans: the FRP, the Federal Bureau of Investigation (FBI) Weapons of Mass Destruction (WMD) Incident Contingency Plan, and the Department of Health and Human Services (HHS) Health and Medical Services Support Plan for the Federal Response to Acts of Chemical/Biological Terrorism.

NATIONAL INCIDENT MANAGEMENT SYSTEM

While the NRF delineates our nation's responsibilities for the responses to a disaster, the National Incident Management System (NIMS) establishes and defines a systematic approach to managing disasters from the national to local level. Homeland Security Presidential Directive (HSPD)-5, Management of Domestic Incidents, directed the development and administration of the NIMS. The intent is for NIMS to be flexible for any disaster, yet standardized in organization and function regardless of the breadth of the disaster. Inherent to

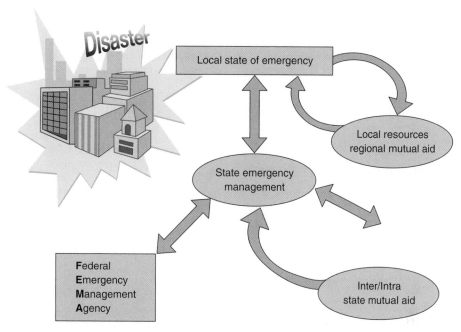

▲ **Figure 4–3.** Disaster response coordination.

the need for flexibility, there is ongoing refinement of NIMS to incorporate best practices and lessons learned from recent incidents. The current focus is on eliminating redundancy, defining the dichotomy between NIMS and the ICS, expansion of the planning, training of communities, and coordination of mutual aid. In addition, the roles of the private sector, nongovernmental organizations (NGO), and elected and appointed officials have been further defined.

The NIMS components include preparedness, communications and information management, and resource management. The NIMS and the NRF predicate that all incidents should typically be managed at the local level first. Implicit to this premise is that communities adequately prepare by activities conducted on an ongoing basis in advance of any potential disaster. Preparedness involves a unified approach. Development of multidisciplinary city, county, and statewide councils of representatives from emergency operations, fire, EMS, police, medical providers, and hospitals in turn standardizes protocols, engages in training exercises, determines supply and equipment needs, and evaluates and revises to develop best practices.

NIMS addresses issues concerning communication mismatch or the "Babel Effect" by requiring the development of emergency and incident communications and information systems that specifically require interoperability and redundancy.

Interagency resource management can be challenging as stockpiling supplies and pharmaceuticals may lead to overburdening of any of the involved entities. NIMS enables a process to acquire, mobilize, inventory, and reimburse supplies and equipment. It guides components critical to the acquisition and certification of equipment that will perform to certain standards.

NIMS mandates the use of national standards to ensure emergency personnel possess the knowledge, skills, and experience necessary to execute incident management and emergency response. Many of these emergency supplies will be designated as "dual use" in order to maximize "in-place" supply levels and ensure that additional training for use of this equipment is ongoing.

INCIDENT COMMAND SYSTEM

The NIMS components provide a framework to facilitate effective management during incident response. The ICS provides standardization of the broad spectrum of activities and organizations providing emergency management during an incident response. Local emergency management personnel within a single jurisdiction manage most incidents. Incidents that rapidly expand geographically or technically may require significant resources and operational support that are not available or where local resources will be rapidly consumed early in the disaster cycle. A single incident that covers a large geographic area will need to coordinate multiple local emergency incident and management systems. ICS provides a flexible mechanism for management of incidents where additional resources are required to complex incidents with national implications.

Acts of biologic, chemical, radiological, and nuclear terrorism may present unique challenges for the traditional ICS structure. Incidents that are not site specific, are geographically dispersed, or evolve over longer periods of time will require extraordinary coordination among all participants, including federal, state, tribal, and local governments, as well as NGOs and the private sector.

The ICS is based on 14 proven management principles that contribute to the strength and efficiency of the overall system.

▶ Common Terminology

The ICS terminology allows diverse incident management and support organizations to work together across a wide variety of incident command and management scenarios. There exists a uniform terminology as it relates to the naming of functional units that operate under ICS since common names for emergency resources including personnel, facilities, and major equipment and supply items enhance interoperability.

▶ Modular Organization

The ICS organizational structure develops in a modular fashion based on the size, complexity, and the unique hazard created by the incident. As the disaster becomes more complex or expands geographically, the organization expands from the top down as functional responsibilities are delegated.

▶ Management by Objectives

The ICS management objectives are communicated throughout the entire ICS organization and include specific and measurable procedures for accomplishment of incident management milestones during a disaster.

▶ Incident Action Planning

Every incident must have an action plan. An Incident Action Plan (IAP) provides means of communicating the overall incident objectives. The format is based on the requirements of the incident and the decision of the IC or Unified Command (UC). Initially, a formal IAP does not capture response operations but relies on the experience and direction of the IC. In the event an incident is projected to extend beyond one operational period, becomes more complex, or involves a UC, preparing a written IAP will become inherent to maintaining effective and safe operations.

▶ Manageable Span of Control

Span of control is defined as the number of subordinates a manager can safely and effectively manage in a stressful situation, and has been clearly delineated by the military under combat stresses. Span of control is the key to adequately supervise and control subordinates, to supply and equipment management, or to maintain the functionality of designated facilities from the IC or UC. The type of incident and distances between personnel and resources are just some of the factors that will influence span-of-control considerations.

▶ Incident Facilities and Locations

Operational support facilities are established at various points from incident. The IC will direct the identification and location of facilities based on the requirements of the situation and nature of disaster. Designated facilities include incident command posts, bases, camps, staging areas, mass casualty triage areas, and point-of-distribution sites.

▶ Comprehensive Resource Management

An accurate, real-time inventory of the supply chain and resources is a critical component to managing personnel, strike teams, equipment, supplies, and facilities available for assignment or allocation.

▶ Integrated Communications

Incident communications are facilitated by linking the operational and support units of the ICS. Communication equipment, systems, and protocols should follow ICS Form 205 to achieve integrated voice and data communications.

▶ Establishment and Transfer of Command

The command function must be clearly established from the beginning of incident operations. Command requirements at the incident may be ongoing several hours or even days into an event. The agency with primary jurisdictional authority over the incident designates the individual at the scene responsible for establishing command. In complex events there may not be an apparent primary authority and the designation of the IC may be brought about by extensive deliberations and negotiations in a process termed Joint Command. Command is transferred from individual to individual by a process that includes a briefing that captures all essential information for continuing safe and effective operations.

▶ Chain of Command and Unity of Command

Chain of command is the orderly line of authority within the ranks of an organization. All individuals have a designated supervisor to whom they report at the scene of the incident. Incident managers must be able to direct the actions of all personnel under their supervision in unity and in succession of the chain of command.

Unified Command

UC allows agencies with different functional authorities and responsibilities to work together effectively without affecting individual agency authority and operations.

Accountability

Accountability at all levels and within individual functional areas during incident operations is necessary to insure task success and completion. Completion of the milestones involved with incident action planning, command designation, unity of command, span of control, and resource tracking are the principles of accountability required for successful incident management.

Dispatch/Deployment

Resources should respond only when tasked or when dispatched by an appropriate authority through established resource management systems. This decreases the problems of spontaneous deployment by avoiding overburdening the recipient agency and compounding accountability challenges to the local ICS.

Information and Intelligence Management

The key action items for the scene commander to implement on designation results from information obtained from all aspects of disaster cycle. Accurate information gathering can help with mitigation of the disaster events, including resource logistics, media handling, disbursement of civilian emergency information, and simultaneous disaster surveillance.

PREHOSPITAL DISASTER PLANNING

The evolution of the modern EMS continues be a testament to our nation's ability to develop the most successful approaches to casualty mitigation and resolution of disasters in the austere environment. The most critical tasks in a disaster include identification of the disaster, situational awareness, triage, and transporting to an appropriate facility.

Disaster identification may involve both prevention and surveillance. EMS plays a fundamental role in local disaster planning and education within the communities they serve. EMS interaction with all levels of governmental and nongovernmental agencies that provide the safety and health care infrastructure to communities provides a unique opportunity to cross political and territorial issues. This allows the EMS leaders to initiate community education programs and coordinated disaster training. EMS knowledge of infrastructure and geography optimizes planning for ingress, egress, staging areas, casualty collection points, and command posts.

EMS personnel should be educated in the implementation of ICS in a disaster response. Equipment, supplies, training, and protocols used in a disaster must be the same that are used during day-to-day operations to ensure familiarity and operability in severely stressful situations. Multiple military training programs have validated that in times of stress, the provider will first respond within the training provided. Scene organization is crucial to manage outside agency and Samaritan relief efforts. Plans must be practiced, reviewed, and updated to reflect lessons learned from recent disasters and training scenarios. Executive exercises and tabletop exercises must be transformed into live multiagency training exercises on a regular basis to ensure that all levels of provider have been trained in needed techniques in the disaster.

SCENE ORGANIZATION AND MEDICAL COMMAND

EMS providers, police, and firefighters are typically the scene's first responders in a disaster. Crucial immediate lifesaving measures are instituted by these providers. Their forward position allows for frontline scene assessment and will at least initially shape the nature of the response team's reaction plan. First responders should conduct a scene report following the "Situation Report" (SITREP). This is an organized report that the provider transmits over the radio to his or her superiors, which always includes, but is not limited to, who, what, when, where, and why. It may be presented in many formats, depending on the units involved, but it is always the best assessment of the most senior person present of the situation. It should include:

- Situation/safety—Evaluates and classifies type of disaster and risks to responders.

- Estimated number of casualties—Rapid determination of sick and not sick.

- Resources available—Immediate determination of the type and availability of resources.

- Resources needed at the scene and potential hospital involvement.

These responders then need to establish a medical command (MC) and start triage. The MC within the ICS is responsible for all operations regarding triage, casualty stabilization, treatment, and transportation of casualties to definitive treatment facilities. The medical commander is not the IC, but serves to coordinate the medical response and serves as an advisor to the IC. Typical staff officers needed at scene include:

Staging officer—The staging officer commands all local and mutual aid resources and identifies the areas for resource staging. The staging site should be close to the triage areas. Immediate danger zones such as the direction of expanding fires and secondary and tertiary incendiary devices must be considered in the development of triage, casualty collection points, and staging sites.

Transportation officer—The transportation officer allocates casualties to ambulances and commandeered vehicles, tracks patient movements from treatment areas to hospitals, and works with the communications officer to notify facilities of incoming casualties.

Triage officer (TO)—The job of the TO is to prioritize treatment and evacuate casualties but not to provide any treatment. In many communities, a Medical Emergency Response Center (MERC) is a clearinghouse of information for disaster logistics and the local and regional facilities that will be responding to a disaster. The MERC may also be a coordinator to supply medical providers to facilities that have capacity but are short of providers. This was seen during tropical storm Allison as Texas Medical Center physicians were cross-credentialed to suburban Houston hospitals to perform surgeries and care for critical care patients. The MERC may be located in a city or county EOC or it may be within a particular hospital as the jurisdiction dictates.

SCENE TRIAGE

Triage is a process of sorting patients and classifying them by categories in terms of relative urgency. The objective in triage is to benefit the most number with the available resources. In disasters patients whose injuries are so severe that their survival is unlikely are given a low triage priority.

This paradigm is often difficult for physicians and nurses to accept. Typically, the responsibility for the TO is delegated to a senior EMS leader or senior physician with medical and disaster experience. Junior physicians are not typically designated as the TO as they will more often than not attempt to intervene rather than sort casualties.

Detailed patient assessment information is difficult to document in the field during a disaster. Triage tags that are simple and visual have been devised that can be attached to the patient. These tags often have substantial shortcomings and can be altered by patients. Few disasters have documented triage tag use during the disaster unless the EMS units practice with them on a regular basis. This may be due to unfamiliarity with the tag, or lack of field supplies of tags. The senior author has used colored indelible markers to similar effect in several local disasters.

Patients can be rapidly assessed and categorized using the Simple Triage and Rapid Treatment (START) plan. START utilizes heart rate, respiratory rate, and mental status to categorize patients into the four-level methodology. A similar system has been proposed by the AMA based on response to vocal commands followed by examination of the patient.

▶ Triage Categories

The most effective triage systems are simple and require no complex scoring methodology. A four-level system is commonly used in the United States:

1. **Immediate (I—red):** Patients have life-threatening injuries that probably are survivable with immediate treatment. Examples are tension pneumothorax, respiratory distress, major external hemorrhage, and airway injuries. Ideally, with limited resources, the only patients categorized as red will be those who would benefit from immediate short-duration treatment, and then could be retriaged as yellow.

2. **Delayed (II—yellow):** Patients require definitive treatment, but no immediate threat to life exists. Patients can wait for treatment without jeopardy. Examples include minor extremity fractures, laceration with hemorrhage controlled, and burns over less than 25% of body surface area.

3. **Minimal (III—green):** Patients have minimal injuries, are ambulatory, and can self-treat or seek alternative medical attention independently. Examples include minor lacerations, contusions, and abrasions.

4. **Expectant (0—black):** Patients have lethal injuries and will usually die despite treatment. Examples include devastating head injuries, major third-degree burns over most of the body, and destruction of vital organs. Retriage of this group may be done as resources become available.

POSTDEPLOYMENT PHASE

The postdeployment phase involves the transition and standing down of equipment and personnel, recovery and replacement of equipment and supplies, debriefing, and analysis of all personnel and agencies involved. Process improvement or "lessons learned" are ideally placed in a central database.

▼ HOSPITAL AND EMERGENCY DEPARTMENT DISASTER MANAGEMENT

The term disaster may have a slightly different meaning to a hospital than to the community. Although a community MCI may overwhelm local EMS resources and require the activation of a community disaster plan, much of the response and resource requirement may relate to public safety needs, victim rescue, or hazard suppression, with relatively few casualties requiring hospitalization. In addition, the distribution of victims among several area hospitals may lessen the impact on a single institution, as will the existence of special destination criteria (eg, burns, trauma, and pediatrics). However, internal problems at a hospital, such as utility failure, minor fires, and broken sewer lines, may require the evacuation of the hospital or shut down critical services (eg, x-ray, laboratory), causing bottlenecks or patient-flow problems. Even unexpected staffing problems coupled with a higher-than-normal emergency department census can be a minor "disaster" within a facility from time to time. As a result, hospitals should have well-tested plans to provide special organization and management during such times. These plans should include the possibility that the hospital itself may be damaged or the site of the disaster, such as in a hurricane, earthquake, or tornado.

PLANNING AND DRILLING

Community disasters large enough to require activation of a hospital's disaster plan are rare. Therefore, it is usually only through disaster drills that health care workers can gain experience with in-hospital disaster management. This is usually a committee or task force effort, and it should prominently involve input from emergency physicians and nurses in the hospital as well as from representatives of administration, plant services, security, and the like.

The Joint Commission on Accreditation of Healthcare Organizations mandates that member hospitals have an emergency management plan, which is implemented at least twice a year in the form of drills or in response to an actual event (JCAHO Standard EC-420). Community involvement is required in at least one of these exercises. Disaster plans are commonly classified qualitatively in terms of the type of incident (eg, external or internal).

MOBILIZATION OF DISASTER RESOURCES WITHIN THE HOSPITAL

▶ Personnel

Additional personnel resources, such as doctors, nurses, orderlies, and registration clerks, should be quickly mobilized and sent to the emergency department where incoming patients may soon arrive. Special support areas, such as radiology, the blood bank, clinical laboratories, operating and recovery rooms, and central supply, may also need additional staff.

▶ Supplies

Disaster cache medical supplies, registration packets, stretchers, blood products, and the like should be delivered immediately to the emergency department.

▶ Space

The emergency department should be surveyed quickly and patients with non-life-threatening complaints should be moved to another area or if possible discharged to open up treatment rooms for incoming victims. The operating and recovery rooms should be placed on standby and elective cases postponed. The intensive care units should review existing patients to identify those who can be moved to the wards. Opening a separate clinic area for minor complaints may be helpful.

TRIAGE AND RETRIAGE FOR INCOMING VICTIMS

An experienced physician or nurse should perform triage for arriving casualties at the door and direct them to resuscitation (or operating) areas, treatment rooms, or waiting areas, using principles similar to those outlined earlier (ie, immediate, delayed, minimal, expectant levels). The staff must realize that triage is fluid and that patients may need recategorization as disease processes unfold and trauma responses occur.

Use of the triage tags or other information supplied by field paramedics is important, not only to learn about the victim's prehospital course but also to chart information until a formal medical record can be established.

PROVISION OF TREATMENT

After emergency lifesaving treatment, such as airway control, has been provided, the emphasis is on providing definitive treatment rapidly for those who need it immediately and are likely to survive as a result. (Do the most good for the most people.) Unlike in the field, care need not be austere, but priority ranking is important and minor treatments may be delayed. Surgical resuscitation may be best handled in the operating room, because it tends to tie up personnel, space, and equipment in the emergency department.

COMMAND AND COMMUNICATIONS ORGANIZATION

It is important to rapidly establish an in-hospital Emergency Operations Center capable of communicating with each of the departments, coordinating logistics, and assessing resource and capacity needs. The Hospital Emergency Incident Command Structure, which evolved from the ICS model, is a management tool that the medical community has adopted for this purpose. It enables hospitals to communicate with differing agencies using a common language, provides a clear chain of command, and is a flexible plan, much as ICS has helped the prehospital provider.

MEDIA RELATIONS

A press area should be set aside and a media liaison and hospital spokesperson designated to keep the public informed of events. Accurate victim counts as well as names of victims are of intense interest to concerned relatives. The spokesperson should be well informed, articulate, and able to communicate a coherent message to the public and the media.

PLANT SERVICES

An assessment of the structural integrity of the facility is critical in many disasters with involvement of the hospital. Problems should be communicated to the local ambulance dispatch center and/or MERC so that additional victims may be diverted elsewhere if damage to sections of the hospital degrades the care available.

SPECIALTY MANAGEMENT OF HAZARDOUS MATERIALS AND RADIATION

Variations in the basic plan are required for different types of incidents and disasters. An important variation occurs when a hazardous or radioactive substance is involved. Although sizable casualties of this type are rare in the United States, they may occur, particularly along transportation routes.

▼ THE OVERWHELMED MEDICAL SYSTEM

America has not faced a situation where the medical community has been completely overwhelmed since the Civil War! Due to budget constraints, just-in-time logistics, and staffing, we have little surge capacity. In disaster medicine planning, it is very easy to come up with situations where regional medical care systems would be overwhelmed. This could include hurricanes such as Katrina, widespread acts of terrorism, large tornadoes such as Moore, Oklahoma, in 1999, or a major earthquake in the New Madrid fault. Dual use and surge strategies are cutting-edge paradigm shifts, which maximize survival, minimize morbidity, and optimize resource management.

During such a disaster, local and potentially regional resources will become overwhelmed. Hospitals must maintain and even expand their ability to provide critical care to patients during a disaster. In any of these scenarios, degradation of medical care provided to the public will occur. Even though the facilities are overwhelmed, there will continue to be a need to provide adequate and interval care that is sufficient for the diseases that the public presents with. This is a divergence from what is traditionally expected: the standard of care. This revised disaster standard could be termed a "sufficiency" of medical care designed to meet necessary health care needs for survival. With proper prior planning, this degradation will be graceful and will continue to provide a "sufficiency" of medical care to the vast majority.

SURGE CAPACITY

A surge hospital or facility serves as an alternate facility that can be used to provide sufficient medical care when a primary medical facility is destroyed, contaminated, or overwhelmed. The facilities may be abruptly acquired in situations that require "in-place" strategies because of local impact of the disaster or preplanned locations in anticipation of large casualties or refugees to a particular site, such as an inland location in a hurricane scenario.

Implicit to this is planning for expanding the treatment of the less critically or urgently ill to other areas of the hospital medical center or to offsite facilities that can help meet this requirement for "sufficiency" of care. Lower-acuity patients and treatment areas are created within the alternate areas or facilities. The designated area within the facility may be a patient treatment area with the medical center or hospital such as a day surgery or endoscopy suite that will retain the standard of care and relative licensing requirements for a medical facility, but serve as an ad hoc intensive care unit with staff that understand the monitoring equipment and are trained in its use.

A surge facility may also be an abandoned retail store or even a veterinary facility. Clearly, these facilities may not meet the credentialing criteria for a human medical facility. Plans for alterations in accepted standards of care must be discussed with state and local health departments well in advance. The concept of sufficiency of need encompasses such facilities. During the evacuations for Hurricane Rita, this planning allowed St. Joseph's Hospital to stay at 80% capacity and able to do all services that required hospital-level intensity of service—births, operations, and acute myocardial infarctions.

DUAL USE EQUIPMENT

The concept of dual use ensures supplies and equipment that are used on a daily bases are identical to those earmarked for a disaster. This allows practitioners to use additional supplied equipment with a confident and competent response to emergencies and disasters. The US military has a long history of utilizing such systems.

Mobile ICUs, radiographic scanners, operating rooms, and emergency departments that meet US medical facility standards can be kept safe in remote locations or can be used as semipermanent additions to existing facilities to augment surge requirements as these facilities link to and extend the capabilities to existing facilities. For example, additional CT scanners are often shared among rural hospitals. Similar facilities have been constructed for ICU beds, operating suites, and even emergency departments. Use of these facilities that can be transferred by commercial tractor-trailer drivers to a parking lot in a disaster area can rapidly augment medical care in the region. In the event of a disaster, the strike team can deploy fully certified equipment that is used on a daily basis.

American Federation of Medical Boards: Responding in Times of Need: Katrina and Beyond. http://www.fsmb.org/pdf/PUB_Responding_In_Times_of_Need.pdf, 2006. Accessed April 1, 2010.

Aylwin CJ, Koenig TC, Brennan NW et al: Reduction in critical mortality in urban mass casualty incidents: Analysis of triage, surge, and resource use after the London bombings on July 7, 2005. Lancet 2006;368:2219–2225.

Birnbaum M, Sundnes KO: Health disaster management: Guidelines for evaluation and research in the "Utstein style". Chapter 3: Overview and concepts. Prehosp Disaster Med 2002;17:31–55.

Carlton PK: Medical Response and Reconstruction—Sheltering. Paper presented at Gimme Shelter, 2010, Tulsa, OK.

Chandler R, Feinber S: Failure in communication = failure in response: Continuity of operations planning goes beyond business as usual. 9-1-1 Magazine 2007;(March):60–62.

Cushman JG, Pachter HL, Beaton HL: Two New York City hospitals' surgical response to the September 11, 2001, terrorist attack in New York City. J Trauma 2003;54:147–155.

Dale W: An outbreak of carbon monoxide poisoning after a major ice storm in Maine. J Emerg Med 2000;18:87–93.

Frykberg ER: Principles of mass casualty management following terrorist disasters. Ann Surg 2004;239:319–321.

Gomez AM, Dominguez CJ, Pedrueza CL, Calvente RR, Lillo VM, Canas JM: Management and analysis of out-of-hospital health-related responses to simultaneous railway explosions in Madrid, Spain. Eur J Emerg Med 2007;14:247–255.

Marples DR: The Chernobyl disaster: Its effect on Belarus and Ukraine. In Mitchell JK (editor): *The Long Road to Recovery: Community Responses to Industrial Disaster*. United Nations University Press, 1996:183–231.

Noji EK, Sivertson KT: Injury prevention in natural disasters: A theoretical framework. Disasters 1987;11:290–296.

Shrivastava P: Long-term recovery from the Bhopal crisis. In Mitchell JK (editor). *The Long Road to Recovery: Community Responses to Industrial Disaster*. United Nations University Press, 1996:121–147.

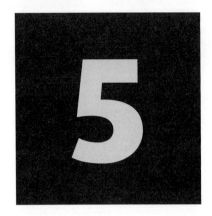

Legal Aspects of Emergency Care

Charles A. Eckerline, Jr., MD, FACEP

Jonathan C. Brantley, MD

Medical malpractice lawsuits and medicolegal issues are a major concern for physicians and health care institutions. Most physicians expect to become involved in some manner in litigation alleging physician negligence. There are nearly 125,000 active lawsuits in the United States alleging physician malpractice on any given day. To put this number in perspective, consider that there are only 69,000 students currently enrolled in US medical schools. The physician named in a suit, however, may not always be a target defendant. In some circumstances, physicians who have provided treatment to a patient suing another physician may be subpoenaed to testify in court. Physicians may also become involved in litigation by agreeing to present medical opinion.

The filing of a malpractice action is likely to generate a great deal of emotional stress for the defendant physician. This chapter discusses medicolegal problem areas in the emergency department (ED) and suggests ways in which the emergency medicine physician can avoid malpractice litigation.

The true extent of the ED malpractice problem is unknown, partly because EDs and emergency physicians are insured by many different insurance companies that have not pooled their claim information and partly because many claims involve events that occurred not only in the ED but also in other parts of the hospital. It is clear, however, that disputes have increased attention to risk management; the number of ED malpractice claims and the size of malpractice judgments are increasing.

The net effect of malpractice suits has been to make emergency physicians, like physicians in general, practice so-called defensive medicine. Modern EDs provide mainly episodic care in a high-pressure environment that affords little time for leisurely contemplation and consultation when the diagnosis or best course of treatment is in doubt. In addition, prompt follow-up or consultation is often impossible to provide. These conditions mandate obtaining more supportive laboratory or radiographic studies than might be obtained otherwise (defensive medicine).

This chapter is intended to provide the practitioner with an overview of relevant medicolegal aspects of emergency medicine. The outcome of a particular malpractice case depends on its particular facts. Furthermore, both statutory and case law may vary considerably in different jurisdictions. For all these reasons, this chapter is not offered as legal advice.

GENERAL LEGAL PRINCIPLES

CRIMINAL VERSUS CIVIL LAW

There are two major types of law in the United States: criminal and civil. In a criminal lawsuit, the state or federal government sues an individual for actions considered to be against public interest, such as theft, murder, or rape. Such suits are intended to protect the public by apprehending and punishing the offender in a particular case and by deterring others from similar harmful conduct. Punishments range from fines to incarceration or even death in some jurisdictions. Given the relative severity of the punishment, the prosecution must prove its case beyond a reasonable doubt, a heavier evidentiary burden than in civil cases.

Civil cases typically involve a dispute between two or more persons or parties, in which the suing party (the plaintiff) seeks redress or compensation for an injury arising from the alleged wrongdoing of the defendant. Such cases may involve contract disputes, property disputes, or torts. A civil suit seeks to resolve the dispute and, if necessary, compensate the plaintiff, usually with money damages. Civil cases are concerned less with punishment than with compensation to the injured party. The suing party must prove his or her case by a preponderance of the evidence. Medical malpractice is a civil cause of action, a subset of tort law known as professional negligence.

NEGLIGENCE

Negligence, broadly defined, is the failure to do something that a reasonable person similarly situated would do, or doing something that a reasonable person similarly situated would not do. Negligence is a basic concept of tort law and courts have long used it to remedy damages caused by such imprudent behavior. It is also the predominant (but not sole) theory of liability in medical malpractice actions. To recover against a negligent physician, a plaintiff patient must prove each of the following four elements: (1) a duty of care, (2) a breach of that duty, (3) proximate cause, and (4) damages. Thus, succinctly stated, negligence in the medical malpractice setting is the breach of a duty of care proximately causing damages.

▶ Duty of Care

The duty of care is a physician's obligation to provide treatment according to an accepted standard of care. This obligation usually exists in the context of a physician–patient relationship but can extend beyond it in some circumstances. The physician–patient relationship clearly arises when a patient requests treatment and the physician agrees to provide it. However, creation of this relationship does not necessarily require mutual assent. An unconscious patient presenting to the ED is presumed to request care and the physician assessing such a patient is bound by a duty of

care. The Emergency Medical Treatment and Active Labor Act (EMTALA) requires ED physicians to assess and stabilize patients coming to the ED before transferring or discharging them. Such an assessment presumably creates the requisite physician–patient relationship. As intimated above, courts often extend this duty of care outside the immediate physician–patient relationship to include foreseeable third parties at risk for foreseeable harm. A more detailed discussion of EMTALA is included later in this chapter.

▶ Breach of Duty

When caring for a patient, a physician is obligated to provide treatment with the knowledge, skill, and care ordinarily used by reasonably well-qualified physicians practicing in similar circumstances. In some jurisdictions, these similar circumstances include the peculiarities of the locality in which the physician practices. This locality rule was developed to protect the rural practitioner who was sometimes deemed to have less access to the amenities of urban practices or education centers. However, the locality rule is being replaced by a national standard of care in recognition of improved information exchange, ease of transportation, and the more widespread use of sophisticated equipment and technology.

Establishing the standard of care in a given case requires the testimony of medical experts in most circumstances, unless the breach alleged is sufficiently egregious to be self-evident to the lay jury member—for example, amputating the wrong limb or leaving surgical implements in the operative field. A physician specializing in a given field will be held to the standard of other specialists in the same field, rather than to the standard of nonspecialists.

▶ Proximate Cause

In order to recover in a malpractice lawsuit, the plaintiff must prove that the defendant's negligence more likely than not caused the injury sustained. The connection between the negligent act or omission and the injury must be reasonably foreseeable and probable in a natural course of events rather than speculative or merely possible. Courts have approached the concept of proximate cause in a number ways. The "but for" rule states that the defendant's conduct is a cause of the event if the event would not have occurred without it, that is, the event would not have occurred but for the defendant's conduct. For example, but for the physician negligently transfusing an Rh-negative woman with Rh-positive blood, the woman's unborn child would not have suffered hemolytic disease of the newborn and its complications. When it is foreseeable that two or more causes could result in the event, such as when a negligent act aggravates an underlying disease process, proximate cause may be found when the act in question is a substantial factor in bringing about the event.

This brief discussion of proximate cause only hints at the complexity of the issue, which is often much easier to state than to apply. The jury is charged with the responsibility of determining whether proximate cause exists and, as a practical matter, will find proximate cause if the conduct is of such closeness and significance to the event that imposition of legal liability is warranted.

▶ Damages

Damages are awarded as compensation for loss or injury suffered as a proximate result of negligent conduct. A plaintiff may recover compensatory damages for disability or disfigurement, pain and suffering, the expense of past and future medical treatment and services, lost earnings, the loss of the services of a spouse, funeral expenses, and other expenses. In some states, punitive damages may also be awarded if the defendant acted with malicious intent or with reckless disregard for the consequences of his or her actions, that is, with willful or wanton misconduct. The jury determines the amount of damages awarded. This determination is afforded great weight by reviewing courts and will be amended only if it is clear from the evidence that the jury was moved by sympathy or prejudice in reaching its decision.

STATUTE OF LIMITATIONS

The statute of limitations is a law that specifies the time within which a lawsuit must be initiated. In other words, any person who feels that he or she may have a claim against another person must file that claim before the time period specified in the statute of limitations runs out. Failure to do so forever bars the claim. Despite its appearance, this law is not intended to shield the wrongdoer. Rather, its purpose is to promote timely filing of claims and thus to allow the defendant to prepare an adequate defense while memories are fresh, witnesses are available, and material facts are accessible.

The length of time varies for different causes of action, but the time frame for negligence actions (and, hence, most medical malpractice actions) is 2 years in most states. The time period typically begins to run once the aggrieved person knows or reasonably should know that a claim exists, not simply once the offense has occurred. However, most limitations statutes also include a longer, maximum time measured from the occurrence of the offense, known as the statute of repose. Both time periods will be extended if the offending party fraudulently conceals the negligent conduct or intentionally misleads the aggrieved party. Finally, of special note, most statutes of limitations do not begin to run against a minor until he or she reaches the age of majority. The age of majority varies from 18 to 21 years.

RES IPSA LOQUITUR

The plaintiff in a medical malpractice case has the burden of proving each of the elements of the cause of action and, in order to carry that burden, normally must present direct factual evidence showing that the defendant acted negligently. However, in those instances where the injury would not have occurred in the absence of negligence, such as when a patient emerges from an abdominal surgery with a shoulder injury, the plaintiff may invoke the doctrine of *res ipsa loquitur*, which translated literally means "the thing speaks for itself."

Under this doctrine, which arose in response to medical professionals' notorious unwillingness to testify against one another, the defendant's negligence may be inferred from circumstantial evidence alone when direct evidence of the cause of injury is primarily within the knowledge or control of the defendant. To invoke this doctrine, the plaintiff must demonstrate that (1) the injury is of the kind that ordinarily does not occur in the absence of negligence, (2) the injury was caused by an agency or instrumentality within the exclusive control of the defendant, and (3) the patient did nothing to contribute to the injury. The legal effect of successfully invoking this doctrine is to create an inference of a breach of the standard of care and to shift to the defendant the burden of proving that no breach occurred. In essence, it makes the defendant speak when he or she would prefer to remain silent and about things it would be extremely difficult or impossible for the plaintiff to discover. The burden of proof shifts to the defendant only with relation to the breach of the standard of care. The plaintiff still retains the burden of proof with relation to the other elements of the cause of action. Although this doctrine is typically mentioned as a way to avoid the use of expert testimony to establish negligence, as a practical matter, expert testimony is still usually required to show that the injury would not have occurred in the absence of negligence.

LIABILITY FOR THE ACTS OF OTHERS: VICARIOUS LIABILITY

Normally, a person is liable only for his or her own negligent conduct. However, according to the principles of vicarious liability, a physician or hospital may be liable for the negligent conduct of employees or agents. This doctrine was developed in the realm of employment, and a number of justifications for its use have been offered. The employer, it is deemed, has general control over the employment situation and must bear the responsibility for this supervisory control. The employer selects and trains his or her employees and should therefore pay for their negligence just as he or she profits from their efforts. The employer is better able to absorb losses and to distribute them to the public through increased prices, rates, or insurance. Essentially, these justifications describe a public policy to deliberately allocate risk. The losses caused by the torts of employees that are sure to occur in the conduct of the employer's enterprise are placed on the enterprise itself, as a required cost of doing business.

Within the employment relationship, *respondeat superior* (Latin for "let the master answer") confers legal liability on the employer for the actions of the employee. A hospital or a physician may therefore be found liable for the negligence of an employed office worker, physician's assistant, or nurse. Similarly, a medical partnership may be held liable for the negligent acts of one of its partners, each of whom is an agent of the partnership. Liability is conferred, however, only if the agent or employee committed the negligent act within the scope of his or her employment. An employer will not be held liable for the intentionally wrongful acts of employees, such as sexual assault while at work, because such acts are not considered to be in furtherance of the business enterprise.

Traditionally, hospitals were not held liable for the negligence of physicians working in the hospital as independent contractors, such as physicians with admitting privileges. In this instance, the hospital was not deemed to have sufficient control over the actions of the physician to justify application of vicarious liability principles. In recent years, however, there has been an emerging trend to hold the hospital liable for the actions of independent contractor physicians who provide hospital-based services integral to the business enterprise of the hospital. The negligence of independent contractor physicians working in fields such as emergency medicine, radiology, and anesthesiology has been attributed to the hospitals where they work under the doctrine of apparent agency. Courts have reasoned that if the hospital holds itself out to the public as providing a given service and enters into a contractual relationship with physicians to provide this service, and the public looks to the hospital for this service without regard to the identity of the particular physician providing care, the hospital should be vicariously liable as an employer.

DUTY TO PROVIDE EMERGENCY CARE

At one time, US common law did not require a physician or hospital to provide medical treatment to all who sought it. Thus, private, and some public, hospitals could refuse emergency care to a patient if the treatment would result in no compensation to the hospital.

A series of abuses of the privilege not to provide emergency care and the transfers of patients to hospitals that would accept those persons unable to pay caused mounting concern over the practice of so-called patient dumping. This concern resulted in landmark legislation that has had a huge impact on the practice of emergency medicine.

Congress enacted EMTALA as part of the Consolidated Omnibus Reconciliation Act of 1985. EMTALA applies to emergency care provided to all patients presenting to hospitals that have a Medicare contract and receive third-party payment from Medicare or Medicaid. It requires that anyone presenting to an ED requesting an examination be provided with an appropriate medical screening examination, sufficient to determine whether an emergency medical condition exists. This includes the use of appropriate ancillary services.

If no emergency medical condition is found, the duty to patients under EMTALA ends, although any alleged failure to provide appropriate care could still result in a malpractice claim. If an emergency medical condition is discovered, EMTALA requires stabilizing treatment for any emergency medical condition or labor. EMTALA restricts the transfer of patients with emergency medical conditions or women in active labor until the condition has been stabilized unless the benefits of transfer outweigh the risks.

A receiving hospital may not refuse an appropriate transfer. For hospitals with specialized capabilities such as burn units, trauma centers, or neonatal intensive care units, transfers cannot be refused unless the receiving facility does not have the capacity to care for the patient. Hospitals that receive inappropriate transfers are required to report suspected EMTALA violations within 72 hours. The law provides for civil monetary penalties and revocation of a hospital's Medicare certification for violations. In addition, civil suits may be filed in state or federal court, bypassing any peer review or arbitration system established in some states as part of the tort reform.

EMTALA began as well-intentioned effort to address the problem of patient dumping. It has expanded far beyond its original intent to apply to psychiatric patients and even patients who have not yet arrived in the ED. This has placed an additional burden on emergency physicians as well as hospitals that transfer or receive transferred patients.

Hospitals have an interest in educating their medical staff about EMTALA. Emergency physicians are often most knowledgeable about these issues and are looked to for leadership. The responsibilities of emergency care are so important that any hospital that does not have a qualified emergency physician on duty might find itself unable to discharge its full legal duty to the public under the law.

GOOD SAMARITAN LAWS

Good Samaritans are statutes enacted in each state to protect health care professionals who render aid at the scene of an emergency from civil liability. These statutes are intended to encourage assistance in emergency situations by providing an affirmative defense to suits arising from the event. Statutes vary somewhat in terms of whom they protect, ranging from physicians to all individuals. The statutes generally require that the person rendering aid act reasonably, in good faith, without compensation, and without gross negligence or harmful intent.

Good Samaritan statutes have provided protection to physicians who were not officially on call but who responded to an ED case. Several jurisdictions have applied good Samaritan statutes to staff physicians called to an emergency in a hospital room. Good Samaritan protection does not apply to emergency medicine physicians seeing patients in the ED or to emergency medical services personnel in the field in the course of their employment. Good Samaritan statutes also do not create an affirmative duty to render aid.

▼ COMMON LEGAL PROBLEMS IN THE ED

CONSENT

▶ General Principles Relating to Consent

Consent, as a legal doctrine, arose out of cases alleging battery by a physician. In these cases, a surgeon performing a surgery for which consent had not been obtained was likened to nonconsensual touching, which is the definition of the tort of battery. Thus, it was immaterial that the patient needed the surgery, that the surgeon had performed the surgery well, or even that the patient would have consented if he or she had been asked. Infringing on the patient's right to decide what would be done with his or her body was the essential wrongdoing. The right to be free from nonconsensual touching is fundamental in US civil and criminal law, in that battery is actionable in both arenas. These cases established that right in medical contexts as well.

Subsequent case law has extended this doctrine from simple consent, agreeing to a procedure despite no discussion of risks or alternative treatments, to the modern concept of informed consent, which requires physicians to give patients adequate information about proposed treatments.

▶ Doctrine of Informed Consent

Under the modern doctrine of informed consent, a physician should discuss with the patient the following elements: the patient's diagnosis, the nature and purpose of the proposed treatment, the risks and expected outcomes of the proposed treatment, alternative treatments and their risks, and the consequences of no treatment.

In order to successfully sue for lack of informed consent, a plaintiff must prove that (1) the physician failed to obtain full and informed consent and (2) this failure proximately caused the injury, that is, the patient would not have consented to the procedure had the material risks been disclosed. Regarding the first element, most jurisdictions follow a physician-oriented standard of disclosure. Under this standard, a physician is required to disclose what a reasonable medical practitioner of the same school in the same or similar circumstances would disclose. However, a number of jurisdictions, including New Jersey and Pennsylvania, follow a patient-oriented standard of disclosure. Under this standard, a physician is required to disclose the information that a reasonable person in the patient's situation would consider important in choosing a course of treatment. Reasonable people can disagree about which standard is more appropriate. The physician-oriented standard is sometimes derided as allowing the medical community to specify its own scope of disclosure, which may be out of touch with the needs of the individual patient. By contrast, detractors of the patient-oriented standard point out that it is too prone to misuse by sympathetic juries in cases where inevitably the undisclosed, unusual complication has occurred.

In order to prove the causation element, most jurisdictions require that the plaintiff prove that a reasonable person in the patient's situation would not have consented to the proposed treatment had adequate information been given.

▶ Exceptions to Consent Requirements

Several exceptions to informed consent–disclosure requirements have been consistently recognized throughout the United States. In medical emergencies, when the patient is unconscious or unable to communicate, or when there is no time to obtain informed consent, the physician may provide treatment under the theory of implied consent. In this circumstance, the law presumes that the compelling need for treatment outweighs the need to obtain informed consent. When a patient receives recurrent medical care and thus has prior knowledge of the nature of the ongoing treatment, as well as the material risks and alternatives, then the physician generally need not make duplicative disclosures in order to obtain informed consent. However, if the patient's condition or other circumstances change, the physician should apprise the patient of this change and renew the consent previously obtained.

A patient may expressly waive the right to informed consent by stating that he or she does not wish to be informed about certain information pertaining to the course of treatment. When this occurs, the physician should inquire why the patient does not wish to be informed and should document these reasons in the medical record. If the patient knowingly and intelligently waives this right, and has reasonable justifications for doing so, then nondisclosure will be defensible in court.

The final exception to consent requirements is known as the doctrine of therapeutic privilege. It arises in situations in which the patient is so anxious or fragile that full disclosure might cause serious emotional or physical harm. Circumstances justifying use of this doctrine are exceptionally rare, and physicians asserting this privilege must carefully document their decision making in the medical record. A physician's concern that the patient might forego recommended treatment if adequately apprised of its risks is not a sufficient reason to invoke this doctrine.

▶ Authority to Give Consent

Informed consent obtained after adequate disclosure by the treating physician will be meaningful only if the patient has the authority to give consent. Under US law, all adults are presumed to be competent to make decisions about their treatment and thus to have the authority to give or withhold consent. However, a physician should question this presumption of competence when the patient's mental capacity is altered due to physical or mental illness, intoxication, or diminished consciousness due to injury or other causes.

Competence, broadly defined, is the ability to make decisions. The word competence, however, has many legal and medical connotations, so in general it is better to use the term capacity when discussing a patient's ability to understand and make decisions with regard to medical situations that confront patients. Most patients have the capacity to understand their medical condition and the proposed treatments in a general way and can appreciate the consequences of accepting or refusing the proposed treatment. If a patient lacks the requisite mental capacity to make informed decisions, the physician should seek consent from a qualified surrogate decision-maker. If the patient has previously been determined to lack this capacity, he or she will likely have an appointed guardian with the responsibility to make medical decisions. If the patient has an advance directive such as a durable power of attorney or a living will, this document will identify the surrogate decision-maker. If no such documentation exists, most states have enacted statutes that identify a hierarchy of family members who can give or withhold consent for a patient who becomes incompetent acutely. Given the circumstances in most EDs, when treating a patient who lacks the capacity to receive informed consent, a physician should always involve a patient's closest family members in the decision-making process. Further, a physician should carefully document in the medical record evidence justifying the determination of a patient's lack of capacity and his or her attempts to obtain consent from a qualified surrogate decision-maker.

Intoxicated Patients

Intoxicated patients are frequent ED patients and present a special risk to the ED physicians. Their altered mental status may mask serious injuries that are too easily attributed to their intoxication, and the treating physician must exercise a heightened suspicion while evaluating such patients for injuries. Depending on the degree of their intoxication, patients may be so altered that they may not possess the capacity to consent to or refuse treatment. In this situation an emergency physician is required to obtain consent from a qualified surrogate decision-maker, as discussed above. In general, the emergency physician should assume that an intoxicated patient does not have the capacity to consent and that the patient may have a serious injury or illness, and should therefore perform a complete medical screening evaluation. A liberal restraint policy may be necessary to allow for proper evaluation. However, once the patient demonstrates mental capacity and there is no apparent life threat, the physician has no legal right to detain the patient any longer, regardless of whether the patient's blood alcohol level is at or below the state legal limit for intoxication.

Police Custody

Patients who have been arrested and are on their way to jail, or persons already in jail, are often brought to the ED for evaluation and possibly treatment. Impending or actual incarceration does not alter their rights concerning consent for treatment. Sufficient consent for examination and treatment must be obtained.

Minors

In general, a minor does not have legal competence, and the consent of a minor's parent or legal guardian must be obtained before treatment can be rendered. Of course, several exceptions exist. In a medical emergency, consent will be implied by law. Most states allow an emancipated minor to consent to his or her medical care. An emancipated minor is a minor who is or has been married, who lives alone and is financially independent, or who has children of his or her own. Most states also allow minors to give consent for treatment of specific conditions such as pregnancy, sexually transmitted diseases, or chemical dependency. Consent laws vary considerably from state to state, and emergency physicians should become familiar with their own states' consent laws.

Patient Refusal to Consent

Any competent adult patient may refuse to consent to a proposed treatment, even if that treatment is necessary to save the patient's life. The guiding principle being observed is patient autonomy: all competent patients have the right to decide what will be done with their bodies.

If a patient decides to leave the ED without treatment and against medical advice, the risks of doing so should be explained and the patient should be asked to sign a form releasing the hospital and ED staff from liability. If the patient refuses to sign this form, this fact and the circumstances of the patient's departure should be documented in the medical record.

If a patient is incompetent, he or she does not have the right to refuse treatment because such a patient is not deemed to have the capacity to make an informed decision. In this circumstance, the physician has an obligation to protect the patient, restrain the patient if necessary, and render appropriate care. This delicate balancing of patient autonomy and physician authority requires a sort of cost–benefit analysis on the physician's part in each case. An intoxicated patient refusing to consent to suturing of a small laceration might be afforded greater autonomy than a previously healthy person who refuses treatment of an acute myocardial infarction. Although a physician faced with the second scenario cannot simply override a competent patient's wishes, the physician should investigate more fully the patient's understanding of his or her condition, the proposed treatment, and the likely consequences of the decision.

With these principles in mind, a few special cases should be noted. A psychiatric patient should be evaluated to determine if he or she is a threat to self or others. If so, the patient should be held for further psychiatric evaluation and therapy. However, the psychotic state itself does not necessarily render the patient incompetent. A psychiatric patient's right to refuse psychotropic medications has generally been upheld by the courts. If available, the safest alternative for the emergency physician is to consult a psychiatrist to conduct this evaluation.

Narcotics users who present to the ED in respiratory arrest and receive naloxone may become intensely uncomfortable due to the effects of narcotic reversal and acute withdrawal. They may desire to leave the ED to seek more narcotics. However, naloxone has a shorter half-life than heroin and other narcotics, and the patient remains at significant risk for recurrent respiratory arrest. At a minimum, such patients should be held in the ED for at least one half-life of naloxone.

ED personnel should use reasonable therapeutic restraint to evaluate and provide treatment to violent patients, because there is a correlation between violence and acute organic brain syndrome. If restraining such a patient places the staff at risk of harm, the patient should be allowed to "escape" and the police should be notified that the patient may be a threat to self or others. Circumstances of the incident should be carefully documented in the medical record.

The right of Jehovah's Witness patients to refuse receiving blood products is a troublesome area for physicians. Courts have generally upheld this right for competent adults, but a number of exceptions exist, depending on whether the state can demonstrate a compelling or overriding interest for authorizing the transfusion. Transfusions have been authorized when the patient has dependents or is pregnant or when there is a reasonable doubt about the strength of the patient's convictions. Courts typically do not allow a Jehovah's Witness parent to refuse treatment for a minor. The safest course of action for a physician facing this dilemma is to contact hospital staff or legal counsel for guidance.

Finally, although parents' decisions about their child's care are typically respected, they should not be allowed to place the child at risk of serious harm. Courts have repeatedly held, under the doctrine of *parens patriae* (the state's paternalistic interest in children), that a parent does not have the right to refuse lifesaving treatment for a child, even on religious grounds. If faced with such a situation, the physician should contact hospital counsel and take temporary protective custody of the child based on child neglect. The physician may be hesitant to take custody of the child, but it should not be for fear of liability; the physician is protected from civil and criminal liability under child abuse and neglect statutes. In the past 30 years, no case has been reported in which a parent has successfully sued a physician for providing nonnegligent care to a child without parental consent.

▶ Consent for Blood Alcohol Samples

Many states have enacted statutes regarding driving under the influence; these statutes define intoxication on the basis of blood alcohol concentration. They typically specify that a person arrested under the statute is deemed to have consented to blood tests for the purpose of determining the blood alcohol level. If the patient does not allow medical personnel to obtain the sample, such refusal may result in summary suspension of the patient's driver's license. These statutes usually provide physicians with civil liability protection for use of the results of these samples in legal proceedings. In some states, this implied consent extends only to the testing of urine and breath samples but not to blood samples. The provisions of these statutes vary from state to state, and emergency physicians should become familiar with the laws of the states in which they practice.

PSYCHIATRIC EMERGENCIES

Patients with psychiatric disorders or altered mental status for other reasons (ie, drugs, alcohol, organic dysfunction) are often unable to test and evaluate external reality and may experience delusions, hallucinations, and personality disintegration (see also Chapter 49). Such patients present special legal hazards with regard to the legal principles of assault and battery as well as false imprisonment. The key question in deciding when and to what degree physical restraint can be used on a patient with mental illness is whether the patient is likely to cause self-harm or harm to others. The ED staff may use appropriate and reasonable efforts, including the use of restraints, to protect the patient from self-harm and from harming others. If the staff fails to use necessary, reasonable restraints, it risks incurring liability to innocent third parties injured by the patient and may incur liability to the patient if the patient causes self-harm. By contrast, unnecessary or excessive force may result in liability for injuries sustained by the patient. What constitutes excessive force depends on the circumstances of each case.

Hospitals are required to have specific restraint policies and forms. ED staff must be familiar with these policies and document their compliance on the appropriate forms. The ED record should contain an objective and thorough documentation of the patient's behavior and mental status, the physician's reason for restraints, and the method and duration of restraint.

The problem may be complicated when an alert and apparently competent patient protests against being held in the ED for further assessment and demands to leave before his or her evaluation is complete. The ED staff may be held liable for false imprisonment if such a patient is later determined not to be a danger to self or others. Actions for false imprisonment may arise when a person is unlawfully deprived of personal liberty by another person without giving consent and is aware of such deprivation, and when no defense of privilege applies. Although the potential for liability exists in such cases, the incidence of claims is low.

Conversely, ED staff may face liability for failure to hold and further assess a mentally unstable person if the patient is released and then causes self-harm or harms others. Physicians who discharged psychiatric patients who subsequently committed suicide have been found liable for wrongful death of these patients in lawsuits brought by the patients' survivors, if the juries concluded that the decisions to discharge their patients were made in a negligent manner. This scenario exposes the ED staff to a greater risk of litigation than the risk of false imprisonment.

Maintaining the patient in the ED for a reasonable period of time for examination and evaluation by a psychiatric health professional may be the most prudent course of action. If a psychiatrist or other mental health professional is not available, the ED physician must decide whether to discharge the patient or start procedures for involuntary commitment to a psychiatric facility. Laws vary greatly with regard to emergency involuntary commitments. The ED staff should be familiar with the laws in their local jurisdiction. As a general principle, the decision to restrain a mentally ill patient for a thorough evaluation is more easily defended than the decision to allow a potentially dangerous patient to be discharged. The key is thorough documentation.

ABANDONMENT

Abandonment is the unilateral termination of the physician–patient relationship by the physician without the patient's consent and without giving the patient sufficient opportunity to secure the services of another competent physician. Although much ED care is episodic in nature and does not involve follow-up treatment, the ED physician and staff still have a responsibility to provide appropriate discharge instructions.

ED physicians may be liable for negligent disposition of the patient if they do not give follow-up care instructions appropriate for the patient's condition. This principle also requires the translation of follow-up instructions for patients who do not read English, if the ED is in an area where it would be reasonable to require the presence of translating personnel in the ED. The area of follow-up instructions is also one of concern to the Joint Commission. When frequently required in an emergency care area, a means of communications should be available in the language of the predominant population groups served by the ED.

▶ Follow-Up Care

EDs are designed to provide episodic care for emergency problems. Patients discharged from the ED frequently require referral for follow-up care. Because of a shortage of primary care physicians and certain specialists, and frequently a lack of financial resources by ED patients, arranging appropriate follow-up care can be difficult. Generally, the ED physician should refer the discharged patient to a physician available from the on-call list. When follow-up becomes unavailable for whatever reason, the patient should be instructed to return to the ED.

▶ Instruction Sheets

Discharge instruction sheets should be provided to every ED patient and should be signed by the patient or guardian. The instruction sheets should be as specific as possible

and appropriate for the discharge diagnosis. The patient's signatures on the instruction sheet should certify that he or she has received the form and has been given oral instructions as indicated on the sheet. A copy of the signed instruction sheet should be retained in the patient's medical record.

▶ Telephone Consultation

Patients may also allege abandonment or negligence via telephone consultation. An example is the patient who is discharged from the ED, experiences a reoccurrence of symptoms, calls the ED, and is told not to worry about it until morning. If the patient's condition worsens, or if the patient receives any advice subsequently deemed to be inappropriate, the ED staff may be liable for negligence and abandonment. As a general rule, although it is reasonable to answer basic questions, the ED staff should not provide diagnoses or treatment to patients over the telephone.

REPORTABLE EVENTS

All governments have statutes and administrative regulations that require reporting of certain events by ED physicians and staff. Reportable events include child or elder abuse, rape, gunshot and stab wounds, assaults, or other suspicious injuries; certain communicable disease including most sexually transmitted diseases, hepatitis, tuberculosis, and HIV infection; animal bites; and the receipt of patients who are dead on arrival (DOA). Emergency physicians and staff should know which events are reportable and the procedure for reporting them in the area in which they practice, because these rules vary by state and county.

▶ Child Abuse

All US jurisdictions and many other countries have regulations or statutes requiring the reporting of actual or suspected child abuse. Some of the statutes allow the reporter to exercise discretion in deciding whether to report, whereas others require reporting of all cases under penalty of fine or imprisonment.

Many states' reporting statutes grant immunity from civil liability (eg, immunity from charges of slander) to the reporting party. These immunity provisions were intended to make the public (including physicians and nurses) more inclined to report suspected child abuse cases by eliminating the fear of being sued by the parents. In some states, immunity for reporting and for participating in subsequent judicial proceedings is provided without any express qualification. Other states provide immunity for actions taken "in good faith" or "without malice." Generally, no immunity provision will protect ED staff members who broadcast to third parties with no official status or right to know that the parents are child abusers.

In states lacking statutes granting immunity, the emergency physician and, more important, the child victim will be better off if suspicion of child abuse is reported to the appropriate agency. Failure to report a reasonably suspected case of child abuse may result in criminal penalties for failure to report according to state law and may also result in civil liability for negligence in failing to report.

Sexual Assault

All states have procedures for handling sexual assault investigations. ED staff must recognize that rape is a legal conclusion and not a medical diagnosis.

Protocols for management of rape victims are given in Chapter 38.

Gunshot and Stab Wounds

Most jurisdictions require that injuries from acts of violence, such as gunshot and stab wounds, or any alleged assaults be reported to the appropriate reporting agency. Reports of violent wounds of any sort should generally be reported to the local police.

Communicable Diseases

Public health laws generally require the reporting of certain communicable diseases, including sexually transmitted infections, HIV infection, infectious encephalitis, food poisoning, hepatitis, meningococcal infections, plague, bioterrorism, anthrax, and many others. Both documented and suspected cases should be reported. Lists of reportable diseases vary by locale and should be reviewed by the emergency physician.

In general, although all medical personnel who are aware of the patient's diagnosis (including the attending physician, nurses, and laboratory personnel) are obligated to report cases of communicable disease, the hospital should develop a specific mechanism to ensure compliance with local laws. Reporting in the United States is generally accomplished by means of a short written form (the Confidential Morbidity Report card). With certain virulent diseases (eg, plague, botulism, anthrax), reporting by telephone or e-mail may be required for obvious reasons. In most states, failure to report is a misdemeanor punishable by fines or brief imprisonment. The physician who fails to notify the health department when he or she diagnoses a reportable event faces a risk of license revocation or civil suit if secondary cases or other damages result from the failure to report. The need of the health department to know of these conditions transcends the absolute confidentiality of the physician–patient relationship. The physician should discuss with the patient the need for reporting to preserve their therapeutic relationship.

Individuals other than those in the health department may be notified of the patient's diagnosis directly by the physician if there is an immediate risk to the patient's health. This notification may also be made by the health department. However, individuals not at immediate risk of contracting infection from the patient (this usually includes employers, fellow employees, landlords, and casual acquaintances) should not be informed of the patient's diagnosis by the physician. To do so could leave the physician at risk of civil liability for breach of confidentiality. The patient about whom such information is disclosed may bring a lawsuit alleging wrongful disclosure of private information. Also, the physician risks liability for defamation, which is defined broadly as that which tends to injure the plaintiff's reputation or to diminish the esteem or respect in which the plaintiff is held.

Animal Bites

Reporting laws in the United States usually require that the emergency physician and staff report an animal bite to the appropriate local health official within a specified number of hours after the bite has occurred. Such reporting is an obvious safeguard to protect the public from vicious animals and from the spread of animal-borne infections, especially rabies.

See Chapter 30 for management of bites.

Epilepsy

In many states, epilepsy and other neurologic impairments, especially those resulting in episodic loss of consciousness, are reportable to the agency responsible for motor vehicle licensing. The time period after a seizure during which a patient may not drive varies widely among the states but is usually a period of at least 3–6 months without a recurrent seizure. It is also important to provide appropriate discharge instructions to patients so that they will avoid potentially dangerous activities.

Dead on Arrival

All states in the United States require that receipt of a body DOA at the ED be reported to the coroner or medical examiner for possible investigation and for assessment of the need for postmortem examination. In such cases, the emergency physician and staff should do nothing to the corpse that would interfere with the gathering of evidence by the coroner or medical examiner. For example, the ED staff should not attempt to obtain blood and tissue for laboratory studies; all specimens in such cases should be obtained by the coroner or medical examiner. Similarly, the corpse should not be used to practice cardiopulmonary resuscitation, endotracheal intubation, or other procedures.

THE MEDICAL RECORD

The importance of medical records cannot be overstated. The medical record is both a legal document and a means of recording the cause of a patient's illness. It is subject to review by hospital administration, the medical staff including consulting or subsequent treating physicians, third-party payers, state and national accreditation agencies, patients, and occasionally attorneys.

Medical records serve many purposes, including the following:

- Recording information important to patient care now and in the future;
- Delineating level of care for billing;
- Providing medicolegal documentation to support compliance with the standard of care.

When crucial facts such as vital signs or the results of specific examinations were not recorded in the patient's medical records, courts and juries may conclude that they were not done. Although the medical record is a summary of the patient's visit rather than a verbatim account of everything that transpired, it behooves the emergency physician and staff to document carefully with specific attention to pertinent negatives and positives for the particular presenting complaint. Invariably, should an unfavorable outcome or litigation occur, the physician would wish he or she had provided better documentation of care.

The Joint Commission requires that a medical record be established and maintained for every ED patient. The record must contain the following elements:

- Patient identification
- Time and means of arrival
- Appropriate vital signs
- Documentation of pertinent history and physical findings
- Emergency care given prior to patient arrival
- Diagnostic and therapeutic orders
- Clinical observations, including the results of treatment
- Reports of procedures, tests, and results
- Conclusions reached on completion of examination and treatment
- Diagnostic impression
- Final disposition
- Patient condition on discharge or transfer
- Documentation of discharge instructions

Other important items include the following:

- List of allergies
- Current medication
- Possibility of pregnancy, if germane
- Tetanus immunization history, if germane
- Name of patient's private physician
- Documentation of prescriptions given to the patient
- Patient's signature acknowledging receipt and understanding of discharge instructions
- Documentation of a medical screening examination
- Documentation of leaving against medical advice

The information contained in the patient's medical record is confidential and should not be disclosed to the police, press, or other parties without the patient's written consent. Exceptions arise when the patient's medical record is sought by a valid subpoena or court order. The emergency physician can be forced to release confidential information by a court order requiring such release.

Medical records of patients seen in the ED because of drug or alcohol abuse must be handled with particular attention to confidentiality to avoid litigation for defamation. All descriptions of the patient's clinical condition must be stated in an objective manner. Extraneous subjective remarks betraying the physician's or nurse's attitudes about the patient have no place in the medical record.

EMERGENCY PHYSICIAN AND MEDICAL STAFF INTERACTION

The practice of hospital-based emergency medicine involves constant interaction with many members of the medical staff as well as the hospital administration and governing body. The emergency physicians practice in something of a fish bowl, where their clinical skills are under constant prospective and retrospective scrutiny by the entire medical staff. As a result, emergency physicians and other staff must work in a highly charged professional environment.

A potential problem for the ED is created when a patient is instructed by a medical staff physician to go to the ED for treatment and the physician then either fails to meet the patient and keep the appointment or fails to notify the ED staff of the patient's imminent arrival. The emergency physician must decide whether to exercise clinical control over the patient and institute diagnosis and treatment. If the patient is a nonemergency patient and wishes to be seen only by the private physician, there is no difficulty for the ED staff. However, when the patient's clinical problem requires immediate attention, the emergency physician may be sued for negligence if necessary emergency care is not given despite the wishes of the private physician. As a general rule, when in doubt, it is better to err on the side of treatment, assuming that the patient has consented to treatment in the first place. An effort should be made to contact the private physician under these circumstances, but administrative considerations should never interfere with appropriate patient care.

Another difficulty for the emergency physician is dealing with medical staff physicians' requests that the emergency physician write admission orders for patients admitted through the ED. The responsibility for writing admission orders should rest with the medical staff physician to whose service the patient has been admitted. Having the emergency physician write admission orders as a convenience for the medical staff still occurs at many hospitals, but it is a policy that should be discouraged. It blurs the transfer-of-care responsibility, exposes the emergency physician to unnecessary liability, and may delay prompt examination by the admitting physician.

Once a patient has been admitted through the ED, hospital bylaws usually specify how soon the patient must be seen by the admitting physician. If the patient's condition is serious, the patient should be seen as soon as possible after admission. All admitted patients should be seen within a reasonable time depending on their clinical condition. To ensure that this happens, the emergency physician should accurately convey the patient's clinical condition to the admitting physician. If uncertainty exists, the admitting physician should be asked to examine the patient.

Another area of potential conflict between the hospital staff and the emergency physician is the area of on-call specialty consultation. EMTALA requires hospitals to provide a list of on-call physicians who will respond to requests from emergency physicians for specialty consults and follow-up care. If emergency specialty consultation is requested and the on-call specialist fails to respond, the emergency physician may transfer the patient by certifying that the benefit of transfer outweighs the risks. Care must be taken to document requests for on-call consultation in a timely, accurate, and objective manner.

Problems such as these involving the ED and medical staff are of a delicate political nature. The ED and medical staff must keep lines of communication open so that these difficult areas can be discussed dispassionately. If this open communication does not exist, the inevitable result is strained personal and professional relations, which can cause a lowered standard of patient care and create a climate of confusion that engenders litigation.

EXPERT WITNESS

Emergency medicine physicians may be asked to provide expert witness testimony in medical malpractice cases. Regardless of how one feels about the current legal process for resolving malpractice suits, fair, accurate, and impartial opinions by emergency physicians familiar with the standard of care are essential. Serving as an expert witness can be an intimidating experience. If opposing counsel is unable to rebut the opposing expert's opinions, they often attempt to discredit the expert.

The American College of Emergency Physicians has issued expert witness guidelines for the specialty of emergency medicine (policy stated September 1995), stated as follows:

Expert witnesses are called on to assess the standard of care for emergency physicians in matters of alleged medical malpractice and peer review. Expert witnesses in the specialty of emergency medicine should meet the following criteria:

- *Be certified by a recognized certifying body in emergency medicine;*

- *Be in the active clinical practice of emergency medicine for three years immediately before the date of the incident;*

- *Be currently licensed in a state, territory, or area constituting legal jurisdiction of the United States as a doctor of medicine or osteopathic medicine;*

- *Abide by the following guidelines for an expert witness:*

  - *The expert witness should possess current experience and ongoing knowledge in the area in which he or she is asked to testify.*

  - *The expert witness should be willing to submit the transcripts of depositions and testimony to peer review.*

  - *Pursuant to Opinion 9.07 of the Current Opinions of the American Medical Association's Council on Ethical and Judicial Affairs, the expert witness should not testify on a contingency-fee basis or offer expert witness services on a contingency-fee basis through an agent, representative, or other third party.*

  - *The expert witness should not provide expert medical testimony that is false or without medical foundation. The key to this process is a thorough review of available and appropriate medical records and literature concerning the case being examined. The expert's opinion after this process is completed should reflect the state of medical knowledge at the time of the incident.*

  - *The expert witness should review the medical facts in a thorough, fair, and impartial manner and should not exclude any relevant information to create a view favoring the plaintiff or the defendant.*

  - *Expert witnesses are chosen on the basis of their experience in the area in which they are providing testimony and not solely on the basis of offices or positions held in medical specialty societies, unless such positions are material to the witness' expertise. Emergency physicians should not engage in advertising or solicit employment as expert witness where such advertising or solicitation contains representations about the physician's qualifications, experience, or background that are false or deceptive.*

In 2003, the American College of Emergency Physicians announced the availability of an "Expert Witness Re-Affirmation Statement" that can be used by members testifying in physician liability cases.

The statement was developed by ACEP's Professional Liability Task Force in response to members' concerns about untruthful and unethical testimony. The statement was modeled after a similar document utilized by the American College of Obstetricians and Gynecologists.

The ACEP statement calls for an expert witness to affirm that he or she has relevant expertise and will provide true and impartial testimony based on generally accepted standards. ACEP members who testify as expert witnesses are professionally obligated to adhere to the principles enunciated in the reaffirmation.

When joining the College, members agree to abide by ACEP's Code of Ethics for Emergency Physicians. That document includes a policy on expert witness testimony. The reaffirmation confirms their willingness to abide by that policy.

When providing expert witness testimony, ACEP recommends that members sign a copy of the reaffirmation statement *and present it to an attorney who can introduce it in direct examination of the member and in direct or cross-examination of other witnesses designated as experts.*

The statement is available at http://www.acep.org/download.cfm?resource=1024.

NATIONAL PRACTITIONER DATA BANK

The Health Care Quality Improvement Act (HCQIA) was passed by Congress in 1986 and called for the establishment of the National Practitioner Data Bank for Advice Information on Physicians and Other Health Care Providers (NPDB). Its purpose is to collect data on medical malpractice payments. All medical malpractice payments must be reported to the NPDB. What effect HCQIA and the NPDB will have on health care and the availability of insurance is yet to be determined.

HARVESTING OF ORGANS FOR TRANSPLANTATION

Emergency physicians can be expected to be confronted with the issue of organ or tissue donation. Hospitals should have specific policies in place that address the issue and emergency staff should be familiar with them. Most states have statutes that require notification of the organ donation association in the event of any death that meets criteria for possible organ or tissue donation.

HEALTH CARE REFORM

It is possible that future legislation would include some type of tort reform, as a means of cost containment, but that has not been part of the bills under current consideration. Fear of liability clearly drives physicians to order extra medical treatments or diagnostic tests to avoid liability. The true cost of defensive medicine continues to be hotly debated, but the US Department of Health and Human Services estimate that these unnecessary expenditures add between $60 and $108 billion to the total cost of health care each year. Given the limited resources to pay the enormous costs associated with health care, it would seem to reason that any meaningful comprehensive health care reform initiatives will need to include tort reform as well.

American College of Emergency Physicians Policy Statement: Expert Witness Guidelines for the Specialty of Emergency Medicine. American College of Emergency Physicians, Policy #400114, Approved August 2000.

American College of Emergency Physicians: The National Report Card on the State of Emergency Medicine. 2009 ed. http://www.emreportcard.org/uploadedFiles/ACEP-ReportCard-10-22-08.pdf.pdf.

American Medical Association Website: www.ama-assn.org/ama1/pub/upload/mm/399/mlr tp.pdf.

Bitterman RA: Medicolegal and risk management. In Marx JA et al (editors): *Rosen's Emergency Medicine Concepts and Clinical Practice*. 5th ed. Mosby, 2002.

Freedman DL: National Practitioner Data Bank. ED Legal Lett 1999;10(8).

Henry GL, Sullivan DJ: *Emergency Medicine Risk Management*. 2nd ed. American College of Emergency Physicians, 1997.

Huber JR: Foresight American College of Emergency Physicians, *EMTALA—New Developments in the Regulatory Guidelines and an Update of Recent Court Opinions*. Issue 48, June 2000.

Magauran BG: Risk management for the emergency physician: Competency and decision making capacity, informed consent and refusal of care against medical advice. Emerg Med Clin North Am 2009;27:605–614.

Keeton WP: *Prosser and Keeton on Torts*. 5th ed. West, 1999.

LeBlang TR, Basanta WE, Kane RJ: *The Law of Medical Practice in Illinois*. 2nd ed. Lawyers Cooperative Publishing, 1997.

Peth HA: The Emergency Medical Treatment and Active Labor Act: Guidelines for compliance. Emerg Med Clin North Am 2004;22:225–240.

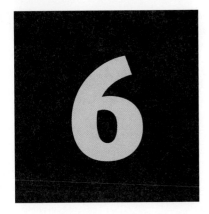

Emergency Bedside Ultrasound

David A. Fritz, MD, FACEP

EMERGENCY BEDSIDE ULTRASOUND BASICS

MACHINE CHARACTERISTICS FOR BEDSIDE USE

Deciding on the type of ultrasound machine to obtain for your emergency department depends on balancing the cost versus the features desired on the machine.

Early portable ultrasound units had the advantages of low cost and user-friendly interfaces with limited adjustment options. Small viewing screens were problematic, and multiple probes could not be used simultaneously. Image quality was reduced but battery power and rapid power-up allowed immediate imaging.

Traditional, larger ultrasound machines commonly used by radiologists are designed for the radiology suite, where patients are brought to the machine. There are obvious disadvantages in bringing these to the patient bedside in a crowded emergency department, and many have a prolonged power-up period causing a delay in image acquisition. The cost of these machines is also prohibitive in most emergency departments.

Ultrasound machines designed specifically for bedside applications are now available. Small physical profiles, digital storage, fast power-up, multiple probe ports, and high-quality images are made possible by technological advances. Basic features ideal for the emergency department setting are listed in Table 6–1.

▶ Probes

There are three main types of ultrasound probes or transducers: curved, linear, and phased array (Figure 6–1). Curved probes are used for abdominal and obstetric imaging. Linear probes are used for soft tissue and small parts imaging. Phased array probes use computer control to "bend" the ultrasound beam from a flat, small footprint to a wider pie-shaped wedge distally. This is usually called the "cardiac" probe but is also excellent to image between ribs and is often used for abdominal imaging.

Many ultrasound probes allow for use of variable frequencies. Curved array probes used for abdominal imaging, for example, may have settings from 2.5 to 5 MHz. Soft tissue probes and intracavitary/transvaginal probes may allow for settings above 7 MHz. There is an inverse relationship between the resolution of a probe and its penetration.

Most emergency departments will require a minimum of three probes, depending on the types of ultrasound examinations and procedures anticipated (Table 6–2): one for abdominal imaging, one for high-resolution shallow imaging, and an intracavitary probe. While more probes would seem beneficial, the probes make up a large portion of the cost of the system and expenditures for extra or specialty probes are unlikely to be justified.

▶ ED Physician Training

The American Medical Association's (AMA) policy on ultrasound states that specialty societies should determine

Table 6–1. Characteristics of an Ideal Bedside Ultrasound Machine.

Low cost
High-quality images
Portability
Durability
Small physical profile
Quick power-up
Internal power supply (battery)
Multiple probe ports (minimum 3)
Digital storage and image transfer
Movie/clip capable
Color Doppler
Easy to clean/disinfect

Table 6–2. Type of Ultrasound Probes Used for Examinations and Procedures.

Examination/Procedure	Probe Type
FAST exam	Curved array 2.5–5.5 MHz or phased array 2.5–5.5 MHz
Enhanced FAST exam	Curved array 2.5–5.5 MHz or phased array 2.5–5.5 MHz *plus* linear small parts probe 5–10 MHz
Aorta, gallbladder	Curved array 2.5–5.5 MHz or phased array 2.5–5.5 MHz
Cardiac	Phased array 2.5–5.5 MHz or curved array 2.5–5.5 MHz
Transabdominal OB	Curved array 2.5–5.5 MHz or phased array 2.5–5.5 MHz
Transvaginal OB	Curved array intracavitary probe
Peritonsillar abscess	Curved array intracavitary probe
Central line guidance	Linear small parts probe 5–10 MHz
Foreign body	Linear small parts probe 5–10 MHz

what constitutes proficiency for their members, and recommends that hospital medical staff base credentialing on those specialty guidelines. The American College of Emergency Physicians (ACEP) policy agrees with the AMA policy and adds that emergency physicians "should possess appropriate training and hands-on experience to perform and interpret limited bedside ultrasound imaging." The Accreditation Council for Graduate Medicine Education (ACGME) considers ultrasound a key procedural competency for emergency medicine residents.

There is currently no universally accepted certification process for bedside ultrasound. ACEP's guidelines for basic competency recommend 150 proctored examinations performed during emergency medicine residency plus scheduled didactic sessions, or a 16- to 24-hour course with combined didactic and hands-on training for a practice-based pathway.

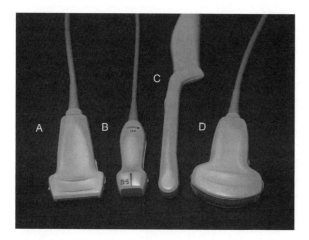

▲ **Figure 6–1.** Common ultrasound probes. **A:** Linear small parts probe (soft tissue probe). **B:** Phased array. **C:** Intracavitary curved array. **D:** Curved array.

Some emergency physicians have obtained certification from the American Registry for Diagnostic Medical Sonography. This requires either a continuous, 12-month training program in clinical sonography (eg, ultrasound fellowship) or documentation of ultrasound training in residency and the performance of 800 ultrasound examinations, and passage of a two-part written examination.

There are proponents for a standardized certification process for ultrasound in emergency medicine, and others who believe that emergency ultrasound is simply a technological extension of the physical examination, the use of which should not be limited. Supporters of the last can point to use of the EKG, slit lamp, and fiber optics as examples of "specialty" tools adopted by emergency physician to facilitate patient care.

▶ Physics of Ultrasound

Ultrasound is a mechanical wave propagated through a medium at frequency above 20,000 Hz. Diagnostic ultrasound generally uses frequencies from 2.5 to 10.5 MHz. The ultrasound waves are generated by the application of electrical current to piezoelectric crystals in the ultrasound transducer (probe). The wave then propagates through tissue, reflecting a portion of the energy back to the probe at each change in tissue density, until all of the energy in the wave is lost through reflection, refraction, or absorption. The reflected waves again contact the piezoelectric crystals that generate a small electric current that is analyzed by a computer processor. The data are then translated onto the display screen.

The amount of ultrasound energy reflected depends on the differences in density (and "stiffness" or *bulk modulus*) at each tissue interface. Great differences in density, such as between bone and tissue or air and tissue, cause virtually all of the ultrasound wave to be reflected back to the probe. This prevents ultrasound imaging beneath lung tissue, gas-filled bowel, or bone.

The depth to which ultrasound will penetrate depends on the frequency. The higher the frequency, the better the resolution but the distance from the skin you can image is reduced. Lower-frequency probes are used for deep abdominal imaging while higher-frequency probes are used to give high-resolution images of shallow structures.

▶ ALARA Principle

The concept of using the lowest power setting possible to obtain a diagnostic image arose from the use of plain radiography and was extended to ultrasound. Early machines sometimes had both diagnostic and therapeutic capabilities; the therapeutic settings could deliver high energy levels that could potentially cause tissue damage. ALARA is an acronym for "As Low As Reasonably Achievable," and it reminds the sonographer to set power levels (when adjustable) to the lowest level that allows proper imaging. There have been no substantiated reports of fetal injury or tissue damage with the use of modern diagnostic ultrasound.

▶ Ultrasound Artifacts

Ultrasound can produce artifacts that may both aid and hinder interpretation of images. The recognition of artifact will help prevent misinterpretation of findings.

▶ Acoustic Enhancement

An ultrasound wave loses energy or attenuates as it passes through tissue; this is due mostly to reflection as interfaces between tissues of different density are encountered. When there are no differences in density, such as when imaging through collections of urine, blood, or other homogenous fluid, no energy is reflected. This allows more energy to arrive at the structures beneath the fluid and to reflect back to the probe. Structures underlying fluid collections will appear to be brighter (more echogenic) than other structures at the same depth (Figure 6–2).

▶ Reverberation Artifact

Brightly reflective (echogenic) structures may cause reverberation artifact (also known as comet-tail or ring-down artifact). This results from ultrasound energy bouncing from the probe to a highly reflective structure, back to the probe and so on, causing the appearance of a "comet tail" trailing down away from the echogenic structure. This often occurs beneath metallic foreign bodies and air pockets (Figure 6–3).

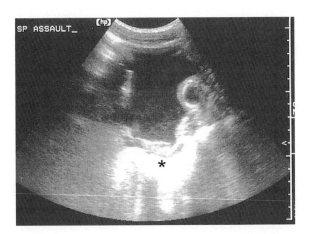

▲ **Figure 6–2.** Acoustic enhancement. Note the bright area of acoustic enhancement (*) below the black fluid collection, in this case intraperitoneal blood.

▶ Edge Shadow

As ultrasound waves strike a curved structure, some of that energy is reflected (or refracted, or both) away from the probe. As the angle increases, more energy is reflected away until a critical angle is reached where no part of the wave returns to the probe. This results in an apparent "shadow" at the edges of curved structures such as vessels imaged in short axis, gallbladder in short axis, etc. It is particularly important to recognize edge shadow (or "critical angle") artifact to prevent confusion with true shadowing structures such as gallstones or foreign bodies (Figure 6–4).

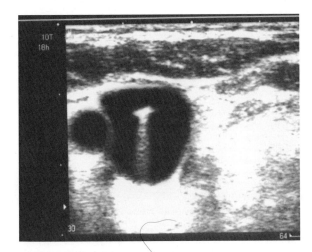

▲ **Figure 6–3.** Reverberation artifact. The brightly reflective tip of a needle within the internal jugular causing a ring-down or comet-tail artifact.

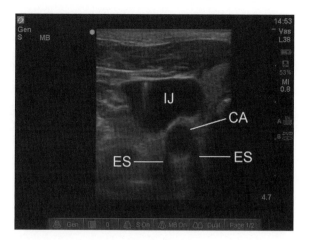

▲ **Figure 6–4.** Edge shadow artifact. The carotid artery (CA) demonstrates two edge shadow (ES) artifacts on either side. This occurs when ultrasound waves strike the vessel wall at a critical angle, deflecting the waves away from the probe.

Knobology

The term "knobology" simply refers to the various adjustments and settings available on a particular ultrasound machine. An emergency physician working in an unfamiliar department should familiarize himself or herself with the control functions before the shift. Some machines will have slide potentiometers (also known as "time gain compensators") that adjust the gain (brightness) at various depths while compact machines often have automatic adjustments.

At a minimum, the physician should know the position and function of the power switch, freeze, save and print controls, frequency selection toggle, and the caliper/calculation button. Every machine will have different options, so refer to your technical manual or the clinical/technical representative for your brand's capabilities. Table 6–3 describes the function of common ultrasound machine controls and functions.

GENERAL IMAGING CONSIDERATIONS

Probe Direction

Ultrasound probes have a marker, either a printed dot or a raised ridge, on one side of the probe to establish probe direction. This marker will correspond to an icon on the display screen that is usually found at the top left corner (but can be reversed or inverted). By convention, the probe marker is positioned generally to the patient's right or cephalad while imaging. This convention aids review of static images; for example, a long-axis image of the abdominal aorta will always show the proximal portion to the left of the

Table 6–3. Description of Common Ultrasound Controls and Function.

Calculations	Used in conjunction with calipers. Calculations available generally depend on the probe being used and the type of exam; obstetric settings might allow for calculating fetal heart rate
Calipers	This control places one or more icons on the screen that can be moved to measure objects or select points in tracings for calculations
Color Doppler	Color Doppler assigns two colors to represent flow toward or away from the probe. Often used to determine blood flow in a vessel or structure
Depth	Depth controls the depth of field on your screen; the depth is usually measured in centimeters to the right of the monitor screen
Doppler	Used to determine the velocity of flow through a vessel
Dynamic range	Dynamic range determines how many shades of gray will be displayed between black and white. In practice, lower numbers increase contrast while higher numbers visualize subtle differences in tissue. The range available is typically 30–70 dB
Freeze	The freeze button "freezes" the image on the screen to allow saving, printing, or measurements
Harmonic imaging	Also called tissue harmonics, this function allows the incorporation of harmonic waves generated by the original ultrasound wave to allow better resolution at lower frequencies. Also tends to improve contrast
M-mode	"Motion" mode. A line is positioned vertically across the display; when activated, the image within the line is scrolled across the screen. Useful for calculation of fetal heart rate and measuring cardiac structures
On/off	Turns machine on/off
Power	Power is the amount of ultrasound energy sent from the probe. If this control is present, set as low as possible to achieve satisfactory images

screen. Organs should be imaged in long and short axes relative to the organ itself, but the probe marker should be kept generally to the right and/or facing cephalad.

Axes of Movement

The three axes of movement of the ultrasound probe are similar to those of an airplane: pitch, roll, and yaw. Inexperienced sonographers should move the probe in one axis at a time while attempting to image structures to avoid confusion. It is preferable to hold the probe in the dominant hand while standing to the patient's right side facing the head.

Conducting Gel

Ultrasound requires the use of a conducting gel to eliminate air between the probe and skin. Ultrasonic medium gel is preferred but in a pinch any clear gel or in fact water or blood can be used. Sterile gel is available for ultrasound-guided procedures.

Brightness Control

The brightness level of the screen should be set so that fluid and vessels appear black on the display screen. The frequency should be adjusted so that the highest resolution is achieved while providing adequate depth penetration.

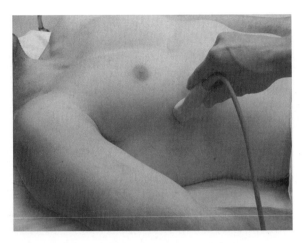

▲ **Figure 6–5.** Morison's pouch probe placement. The probe is placed between the 8th and 11th ribs parallel to the ribs on the mid- or anterior axillary line. The probe marker is directed toward the right shoulder.

▼ PRIMARY INDICATIONS

THE FAST EXAM

The Focused Assessment with Sonography for Trauma (FAST) examination is a multiview examination of the intra-abdominal space and heart. The goals of the FAST exam are to identify free intraperitoneal fluid or pericardial effusion. Originally designed to assess traumatic injuries, the FAST is also a useful tool for the rapid assessment of any hemodynamically unstable patient.

Four basic views comprise the FAST examination: Morison's pouch (right upper quadrant), cardiac, splenorenal (left upper quadrant), and bladder (pelvic).

Morison's Pouch View

The right upper quadrant view (a.k.a. Morison's pouch view or perihepatic view) is sensitive for the detection of free fluid and is generally the first ultrasound image learned by emergency physicians. The right upper quadrant view visualizes the right lobe of the liver, the right kidney, and the potential space that lies between them known as Morison's pouch. Detection of intraperitoneal fluid after trauma strongly indicates significant intra-abdominal injury, and in the unstable patient is a recognized indication for immediate exploratory laparotomy. The actual visualization of solid organ injuries, that is, splenic or hepatic lacerations, is unusual with ultrasound.

sTo obtain the Morison's pouch view, the probe is placed between the right 8th and 11th ribs on the mid- or anterior axillary line (Figure 6–5). Some sonographers recommend the probe be held coronal to the body but this allows interference by rib shadows; holding the probe parallel to the ribs with the probe marker pointing to the posterior axilla allows an unobstructed view. The probe is adjusted so that the right

kidney is visualized (Figure 6–6). The presence of a black (anechoic) stripe between the liver and kidney indicates free intraperitoneal fluid (Figure 6–7). Care should be taken to image the subdiaphragmatic area cephalad to the liver as well. The white outline of the kidney is Gerota's fascia; fluid between this and the kidney is not intraperitoneal and indicates renal hematoma, renal cysts, or other pathology.

Blood initially appears black on ultrasound; as it coagulates, the image "lightens" and can appear similar to tissue but the stippled appearance of renal and hepatic parenchyma is more homogenous than mixed blood and clot. As with any

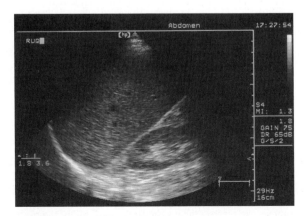

▲ **Figure 6–6.** Normal Morison's pouch view. The right lobe of the liver is at the top left of the image; the right kidney is at bottom right. The bright line between the two is Gerota's fascia.

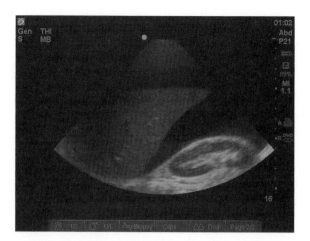

▲ **Figure 6–7.** Positive Morison's pouch view. Note the black fluid between the liver and the bright Gerota's fascia around the right kidney.

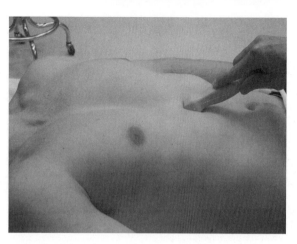

▲ **Figure 6–8.** Subxyphoid cardiac view. The probe is placed below the xyphoid process and directed under the sternum. The angle of the probe will vary but is generally quite shallow.

ultrasound view, the probe should be "panned" through the area of interest to allow the detection of subtle abnormalities. Representative views should be saved for the medical record and quality improvement review.

▶ Cardiac View

The cardiac view is a rapid, one-view examination of the heart specifically used to detect pericardial effusion. In the context of the FAST examination, the cardiac view is generally not meant to evaluate ejection fraction, wall motion abnormalities, etc.

The subxyphoid view is the most commonly used cardiac view. The probe is placed under the xyphoid process almost horizontal with the floor and aimed directly under or slightly left of the sternum; the probe marker should face the patient's right side (Figure 6–8). The probe should be adjusted so that the right and left ventricles are visualized in long axis (Figure 6–9). The display screen should show a portion of the liver at the top, followed in order by the right ventricle, intraventricular septum, and the left ventricle. A black stripe surrounding the myocardium indicates a pericardial effusion (Figure 6–10). Tiny amounts of fluid are normal in the pericardial space but these should not be visualized on ultrasound in nondependent areas. Any fluid seen in the nondependent pericardial space should be considered pathologic; however, an effusion should not always be attributed to trauma and clinical correlation is required, particularly in patients with chronic renal failure. Cardiac tamponade is a clinical syndrome; when evidence of right heart collapse during diastole is present on ultrasound, it is referred to as "imminent tamponade."

If difficulty is encountered identifying the heart, the patient should be asked to inspire fully and hold; the ventilated patient may be placed on an inspiratory pause. This will often bring the heart into the field of view. Ensure also that the depth of field is adequate to image the entire heart.

An alternate cardiac view is the left parasternal approach. This can be useful in the morbidly obese patient or in patients with significant abdominal tenderness in whom the subxyphoid view is impractical. The probe is placed just to the left of the sternum at about the fifth intercostal space

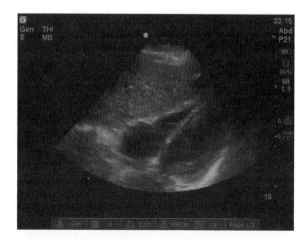

▲ **Figure 6–9.** Subxyphoid cardiac view. From the top of the image are seen liver, right ventricle, septum, and left ventricle.

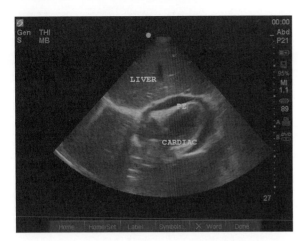

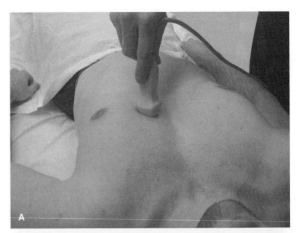

▲ **Figure 6–10.** Pericardial effusion. This subxyphoid cardiac view shows a rim of hypoechoic (black) fluid around the heart. This was a contained aortic rupture after a motor vehicle accident.

with the probe marker to the patient's right (Figure 6–11A). When the heart is visualized, the probe marker can be rotated cephalad, aiming toward the right shoulder to obtain a long-axis view (Figure 6–11B). The probe marker can be directed alternately toward the left shoulder to obtain a short-axis view (Figure 6–11C).

▶ Splenorenal View

The left upper quadrant view (a.k.a. splenorenal view or perisplenic view) is the most difficult FAST exam view for many beginning sonographers. While the probe placement is similar to the Morison's pouch view, the spleen lies more posterior than the Morison's pouch view's corresponding right hepatic lobe. The probe should be placed between the left 8th and 11th ribs at the mid- or posterior axillary line. The probe marker should be directed toward the posterior shoulder so that the probe lies parallel to the ribs. If the spleen cannot be visualized, the probe should be moved cephalad to next intercostal space (Figure 6–12).

The normal splenorenal view appears similar to the Morison's pouch view (Figure 6–13). The diaphragm, if visualized, should be seen on the left side of the display screen. The spleen should appear to the left and above the kidney. Free intraperitoneal fluid can be found on any side of the spleen; the entire region should be imaged to rule out subtle fluid collections. Fluid often collects cephalad to the spleen, just beneath the diaphragm. Blood or ascites will appear as a black or anechoic area (Figure 6–14).

Note that both Morison's pouch view and the splenorenal view can be used to image pleural effusions during the FAST examination. If an anechoic area is noted above the

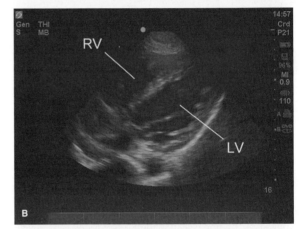

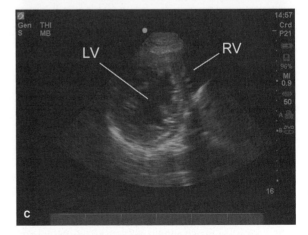

▲ **Figure 6–11. A:** Left parasternal cardiac view. The probe is placed just left of the sternum with the probe marker toward the right shoulder for a long-axis view (**B**) and toward the left shoulder for a short-axis view (**C**).

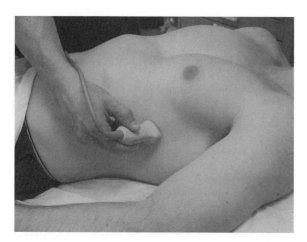

▲ **Figure 6–12.** Splenorenal probe placement. The probe is positioned in the left upper quadrant more posteriorly than the corresponding Morison's pouch view. The probe is parallel to the ribs with the probe marker facing the posterior left shoulder.

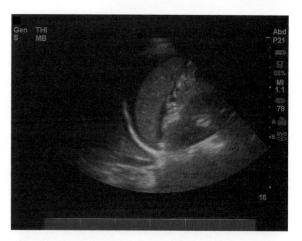

▲ **Figure 6–14.** Positive splenorenal view. A black rim of blood surrounds the spleen at left. Note the curved diaphragm at the lower left of the image.

diaphragm in either view, confirm by moving the probe to a different position, preferably above the diaphragm. The diaphragm can act as a strong reflector of ultrasound waves (a "specular" or mirrorlike reflector), and this can cause the pleural space to appear dark (Figure 6–15).

▶ **Bladder View**

The bladder or pelvic view is the simplest to obtain of all the FAST examination views. The probe is placed immediately cephalad to the pubic bone in the midline with the probe marker facing the head for a long-axis view (Figure 6–16A) or a short bladder view can be obtained with the probe marker to the patient's right (Figure 6–16B).

Free fluid will appear as an anechoic collection cephalad (to the left on the display screen) or posterior to the bladder (Figure 6–17). In a female, free fluid will collect cephalad or between the uterus and rectum—the Pouch of Douglas.

The bladder view may be difficult to obtain in patients with an empty bladder or after Foley catheter placement. Careful technique will allow the fluid-filled balloon of the Foley to be imaged. Free fluid can often still be visualized despite Foley placement. If a fluid collection is found on the long-axis bladder view, observe it for a time to ensure there is no encircling peristalsis that would indicate fluid within the bowel.

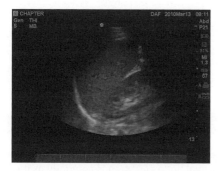

▲ **Figure 6–13.** Normal splenorenal view. In this view the spleen is at top left and the left kidney is at bottom right. Note the similarity to Morison's pouch view.

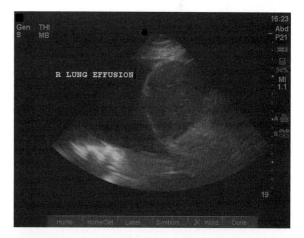

▲ **Figure 6–15.** Pleural effusion. This image was captured during a FAST exam. The liver is shown adjacent to the diaphragm. The black fluid on the left of the image is a hemothorax.

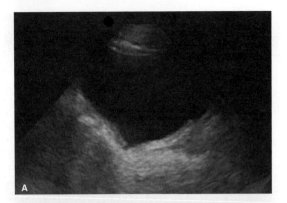

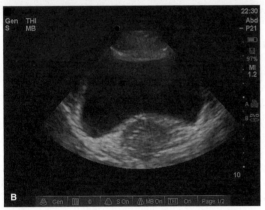

▲ **Figure 6–16.** Bladder long-axis view. **A:** In the long-axis view the normal bladder appears triangular in shape. **B:** When viewed in short axis, the normal bladder appears square. The circular structure below the bladder is the prostate gland.

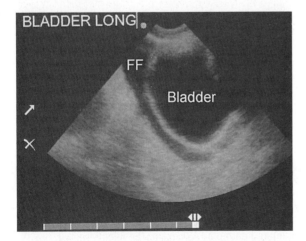

▲ **Figure 6–17.** Positive bladder view. In this view free fluid can be seen to the left of the bladder.

ABDOMINAL AORTA

The ruptured or rapidly expanding abdominal aortic aneurysm (AAA) is a true medical emergency. These patients are often hemodynamically unstable or become unstable during diagnostic imaging. The rapid diagnosis of an AAA with bedside ultrasound allows the clinician to mobilize necessary resources quickly and alerts team members to the seriousness of the situation.

▶ Imaging the Aorta

The abdominal probe is used to image the aorta in most patients. The depth control should be adjusted to ensure the anterior aspect of the vertebral bodies can be visualized. When using a probe with variable frequencies, choose the lowest frequency available to provide maximum penetration. These adjustments can be changed once the aorta is visualized to maximize image quality.

Place the probe in the midline of the anterior abdomen just below the xyphoid process with the probe marker facing the patient's head. The aorta and the inferior vena cava (IVC) run side by side at this level and must be differentiated. Pan slowly from the patient's right to left until first the IVC and then the aorta are visualized in long axis. Proximally the abdominal aorta runs deep to and following the contour of the posterior liver; it will angle toward the anterior abdomen until leveling off at the level of the renal arteries (Figure 6–18). The aorta tends to have more brightly reflective, thicker walls and often has a corrugated appearance while the IVC has smooth, thinner walls. The aorta may be highly calcified in older patients and patients with atherosclerotic disease. The celiac trunk arises from the

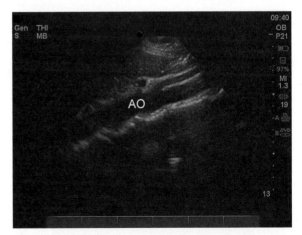

▲ **Figure 6–18.** Long-axis view of the proximal aorta. The proximal aorta (AO) trends anteriorly as it courses distally. The liver edge is seen above the aorta and the superior mesenteric artery can be seen arising from and running parallel to the proximal aorta.

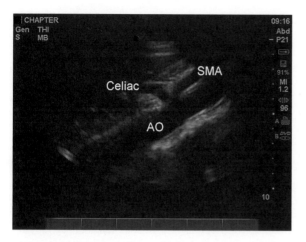

▲ **Figure 6–19.** Celiac trunk and the superior mesenteric artery. This long-axis view of the proximal aorta (AO) demonstrates the origins of the celiac trunk and superior mesenteric artery (SMA).

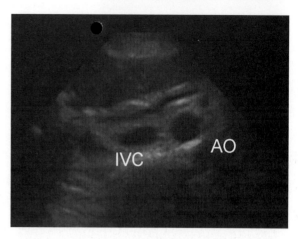

▲ **Figure 6–20.** Inferior vena cava and aorta, short-axis view. A proximal short-axis view of the abdominal aorta (AO) also reveals the inferior vena cava (IVC). The anterior aspect of a thoracic vertebral body is seen just below these two vessels.

aorta anteriorly at this level; just caudad to this the superior mesenteric artery arises anteriorly and extends in a caudad and anterior direction. These vessels allow confirmation that the aorta, not the IVC, is being imaged (Figure 6–19). If it is unclear which vessel is being imaged, turn the probe marker to the patient's right to obtain a short-axis view of both vessels. In this view the IVC lies to the patient's right, or to the left of the aorta on the display screen. The IVC will often appear oval or flat in short axis, compared to the circular appearance of the aorta (Figure 6–20). When the aorta has been confirmed, save images in both long and short axes; the short-axis image should include measurements of the aorta horizontally and vertically.

If the aorta cannot be satisfactorily visualized, move the probe slightly left or right of midline. Gas from the duodenum can obscure underlying structures. Placing gentle downward pressure on the probe can displace the gas and improve the image. Alternately the patient can be asked to inspire deeply and hold; this brings the liver edge down over the proximal aorta where it acts as an "acoustic window," allowing ultrasound waves to pass unobstructed to the deeper structures.

Once the proximal aorta has been imaged, bring the probe caudally down the midline until it rests approximately halfway between the xyphoid process and umbilicus. With the probe marker once again facing the patient's head, visualize the aorta in long axis and pan left and right to confirm the relative position of the IVC. At this level the aorta should appear almost horizontal (Figure 6–21). This view captures the majority of aneurysms as it images the infrarenal aorta. Images of the midabdominal aorta should be saved in long and short axes and the short-axis image measured as above.

Ultrasound imaging of the distal abdominal aorta is accomplished by moving the probe down the midline of the

anterior abdomen until just cephalad to the umbilicus, with the probe marker cephalad. At this level the aorta angles deeply posterior and bifurcates into the common iliac arteries; the IVC is no longer visible. The long-axis view is obtained first, and then the probe marker is turned to the patient's right and images of the bifurcation are recorded (Figure 6–22).

The caliber of the aorta should decrease as it extends caudally; strictly speaking, any lack of tapering is considered aneurysmal. Most authorities suggest that an increase in normal caliber of greater than 50% or 3 cm constitutes an AAA (Figure 6–23). A major pitfall in ultrasound imaging

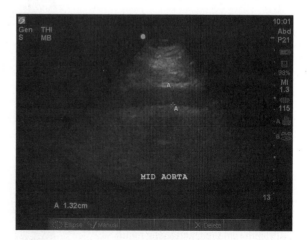

▲ **Figure 6–21.** Abdominal aorta, middle portion. The middle abdominal aorta is imaged in long axis. At this level it should appear horizontal.

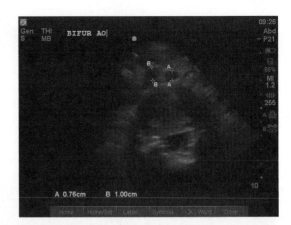

▲ **Figure 6–22.** Abdominal aorta bifurcation. In this short-axis view, the left (**A**) and right (**B**) common iliac arteries are measured.

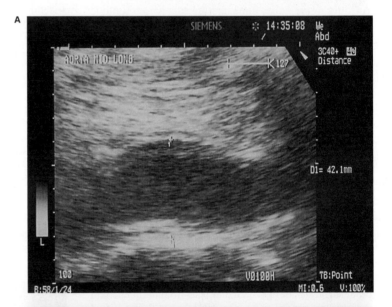

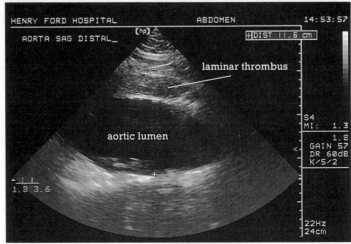

▲ **Figure 6–23.** Abdominal aortic aneurysm. **A:** This small infrarenal abdominal aortic aneurysm was asymptomatic. **B:** This patient presented with abdominal pain and was found to have a massive abdominal aortic aneurysm with laminar thrombus on bedside ultrasound.

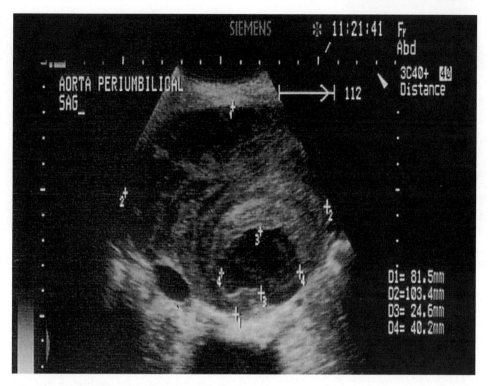

▲ **Figure 6–24.** Laminar thrombus. This short-axis view of a large abdominal aortic aneurysm demonstrates concentric rings of laminar thrombus that have formed within the aneurysm. Compare the size of the aneurysm to the caliber of the inferior vena cava, seen at the lower left of the aneurysm.

of the aorta is failure to recognize the common presence of laminar thrombus within the aneurysm. This thrombus may have a lumen of apparently normal caliber; if the lumen is measured instead of the walls of the aneurysm, the aorta may be mistakenly considered normal (Figure 6–24). Elderly patients will often have a tortuous aorta; if the aorta is not measured in true short axis, the dimensions will be artificially increased.

BILIARY SYSTEM

Imaging the biliary system can be technically challenging for the beginner sonographer. With practice and by following a few basic steps, the success rate is greatly improved.

▶ Biliary Imaging

The gallbladder can be imaged from a subcostal or intercostal approach. The most common technique is to place the probe under the xyphoid process with the probe marker facing cephalad, and then sliding the entire probe laterally along the inferior costal margin until the gallbladder is visualized. The presence of tenderness when the gallbladder is imaged and pressure directly exerted on the gallbladder is the "sonographic Murphy sign" and correlates with cholecystitis.

The intercostal technique is performed by placing the probe between the ribs 7 cm lateral to the xyphoid process. This usually places the probe directly over the gallbladder. A variant of the intercostal method is to place the probe in the anterior axillary line at or just below nipple level and aim sharply medial. The probe should be adjusted to parallel the ribs.

When the gallbladder is recognized, the probe should be finely adjusted to allow a long-axis view of the fundus, neck, interlobar fissure, and portal vein (Figure 6–25). This view should appear as an "exclamation point" with the portal vein being the point. Note that the portal vein has brightly reflective walls, where the hepatic veins and vena cava have thin walls that are poorly echogenic.

The gallbladder wall should be measured at its thinnest point on the anterior wall. Typically this is done with the gallbladder visualized in short axis (Figure 6–26). The upper limit of normal for thickness is 3 mm. Thickening can be due to cholecystitis but may also be due to contraction (recent food ingestion), congestive heart failure, cirrhosis, malnutrition, or other hypoproteinemic states.

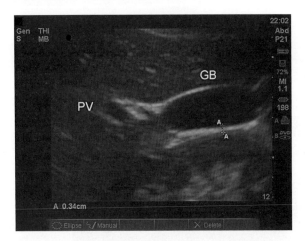

▲ **Figure 6–25.** Long-axis gallbladder. The gallbladder (GB) is imaged in long axis. As the gallbladder tapers down to the neck, the interlobar fissure is seen leading to the portal vein (PV).

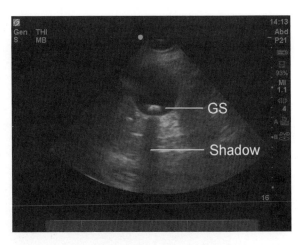

▲ **Figure 6–27.** Gallstones. In this short-axis view of the gallbladder, a single, brightly reflective gallstone (GS) rests at the dependent portion.

Gallstones are the most common intraluminal abnormality observed by ultrasound. They appear as mobile, highly reflective shadowing structures. They range from sandlike to golf-ball sized (Figure 6–27). Because tumors and polyps could be confused for gallstones, patient positioning should be changed during imaging to document mobility. A simple way to do this is to have the patient roll from a supine position to a left side down position. Gallstones lodged in the neck of the gallbladder will not be mobile. When stones completely fill the gallbladder, only the anterior wall and the anterior aspect of the stones will be visible with a strong shadow posteriorly; this is known as the wall echo shadow (WES) sign.

Gallbladder sludge is seen as a gravity-dependent layer of material within the gallbladder but not as dark or hypoechoic as the bile itself, which should be homogenous and black (Figure 6–28).

The common bile duct is imaged by first imaging the gallbladder in long axis so that the portal vein is visible as the point in the "exclamation point." Center the image on the portal vein and rotate the probe until the portal vein is seen in short axis with two smaller vessels seen anteriorly;

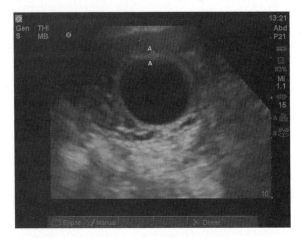

▲ **Figure 6–26.** Measuring gallbladder wall thickness. The gallbladder wall is measured at the anterior surface in short axis. Care must be taken to ensure the image is not oblique as this will exaggerate wall thickness.

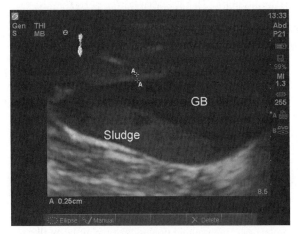

▲ **Figure 6–28.** Gallbladder sludge. A long-axis view of the gallbladder (GB) showing a layer of sludge. Note the sludge is much less reflective than a typical gallstone.

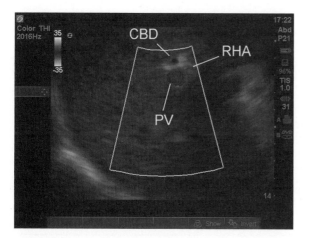

▲ **Figure 6–29.** Short-axis common bile duct. The portal vein (PV) is imaged in short axis with the right hepatic artery (RHA) and the common bile duct (CBD) seen anteriorly. Color flow Doppler is used to differentiate the bile duct (no flow) from the artery (red flow).

this is the "Mickey Mouse sign" with the right ear being the right hepatic artery and the left being the common bile duct (Figure 6–29). The common duct should be imaged in long axis as it continues distally and medially (Figure 6–30). The upper limit of normal for the common bile duct is 6 mm; dilation can be normal after cholecystectomy or with advanced age.

FIRST-TRIMESTER PREGNANCY

Emergency physician–performed ultrasound of the patient with first-trimester pregnancy reduces length of stay by hours and allows the clinician to diagnose time-dependent pathology such as ruptured ectopic pregnancy. Special attention must be given to patient comfort and privacy during these examinations, and a female chaperone should always be present.

The goal of first-trimester ultrasound for emergency medicine patients is to demonstrate the presence of a viable intrauterine pregnancy (IUP). The absence of an IUP in the patient with a positive pregnancy test should imply the presence of an ectopic pregnancy and is an indication for "formal" sonographic investigation by a radiologist or obstetric consultation.

Both transabdominal and transvaginal ultrasound may be used in the evaluation of the first-trimester pregnancy. The transabdominal technique identifies critical structures later in the first trimester than transvaginal ultrasound and may require a full urinary bladder. Most first-trimester emergency patients with abdominal pain and/or vaginal bleeding will require a pelvic examination as part of their workup; performing a transvaginal ultrasound in conjunction with this eliminates the need to duplicate patient preparation and may in fact eliminate the need for pregnancy testing if a viable IUP is demonstrated by ultrasound.

If a transabdominal technique is used, the abdominal probe is placed on the lower abdomen in the midline above the pubic bone with the probe marker cephalad. This is identical to the longitudinal bladder examination used in the FAST examination. The uterus is visualized in the long axis and the gestational sac identified (Figure 6–31).

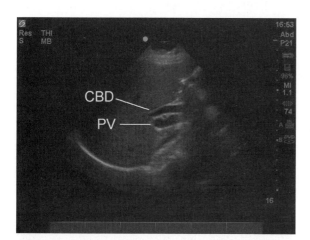

▲ **Figure 6–30.** Common bile duct. The common bile duct (CBD) is imaged in long axis just anterior to the portal vein (PV). This common bile duct is markedly dilated; this degree of dilation is often referred to as the "double barrel" sign.

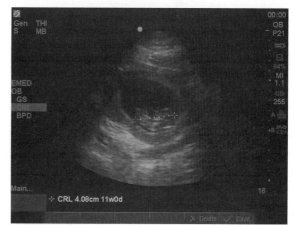

▲ **Figure 6–31.** Transabdominal obstetric ultrasound. This intrauterine pregnancy is about 11 weeks' gestational age based on crown–rump length measurements. The probe is placed just above the pubic bone with the probe marker to the patient's right.

The uterus should be imaged in its entirety in this axis. The probe marker should then be turned to the patient's right and the uterus reimaged in this plane. It is critical to ensure that there is at least 0.5 cm of myometrium between the outer wall of the uterus and the decidual reaction surrounding the gestational sac in all planes to avoid missing an interstitial pregnancy. Imaging may be improved if the patient's urinary bladder is allowed to fill; in some patients the transabdominal approach will not allow satisfactory images.

The transvaginal technique of first-trimester ultrasound allows better imaging of structures and earlier detection of IUP. The probe is prepared by placing ultrasound gel on the probe and covering with a protective barrier. Probe covers are relatively inexpensive but if unavailable a condom or even a clean glove may be used. A very small amount of lubricant, not ultrasound gel, may be placed on the protective barrier prior to insertion. The probe is inserted through the introitus under visual guidance with the probe marker anterior. Ideally the probe tip will rest in the anterior fornix on the anterior aspect of the cervix. This view should allow a longitudinal view of the cervix and uterus. Ensure the endometrial stripe is visualized from the cervix to the uterine fundus (Figure 6–32). Pan through the uterus from right to left to image the entire organ, saving representative images. After imaging in this plane, turn the probe marker to the patient's right to obtain coronal views. The bilateral adnexae should be imaged and representative views of the ovaries obtained.

If the patient has a positive pregnancy test and vaginal bleeding and/or abdominal pain, sonographic demonstration

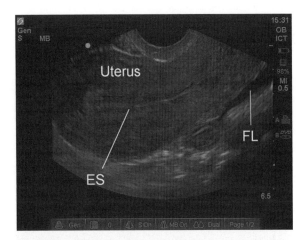

▲ **Figure 6-32.** Transvaginal uterine ultrasound. The uterus is imaged in long axis using a transvaginal technique. The endometrial stripe (ES) is seen at the center of the uterus. There is a normal, physiologic amount of free fluid (FL) in the cul-de-sac in this nonpregnant patient.

Table 6-4. Ultrasound Findings of Intrauterine Pregnancy.

Finding	Gestational Age (wk)	Comment
Intradecidual sign	4-5	Does not signify IUP
Gestational sac	5	May be ectopic
Double decidual ring	5	Only present in 50% of IUPs
Yolk sac	5-6	Identifies IUP
Fetal pole	6	Identifies IUP
Fetal heart rate	6	Identifies IUP
Limb buds	8	Identifies IUP

of an IUP should be made. If no IUP is seen on transvaginal ultrasound, a quantitative serum human chorionic gonadotropin (hCG) level should be obtained. If the hCG level is below 2000 mIU/mL (or your institution's discriminatory level), a reasonable option in the stable patient is to obtain a repeat hCG 48 hours later. If the level is above 2000 mIU/mL, formal imaging or obstetric consultation is indicated.

IUP can be reliably identified by 5 weeks using the transvaginal approach. Unless an intrauterine fetus with a heart beat is identified, at least one other "hard" sign of IUP must be demonstrated (Table 6–4). An IUP should be visualized on ultrasound when the hCG level is 2000 mIU/mL or higher.

▶ Intradecidual Sign

The intradecidual sign is an insensitive and nonspecific indicator of early pregnancy. It cannot be used to determine the presence of an IUP. It consists of a 2- to 4-mm fluid collection to one side of the endometrial stripe (Figure 6–33).

▶ Gestational Sac

The gestational sac is a midline fluid collection (Figure 6–34). The presence of an isolated gestational sac not containing a yolk sac or fetal pole and not surrounded by a double decidual sign (see below) cannot be used to establish the diagnosis of IUP.

▶ Double Decidual Sign

After implantation, a decidual reaction occurs around the developing embryo. Sonographically two layers may be visible, the decidua capsularis around the gestational sac and an eccentric ring around this, the decidua parietalis. This is known as the double decidual sac sign or double decidual ring (Figure 6–35). The double decidual sign is only visible

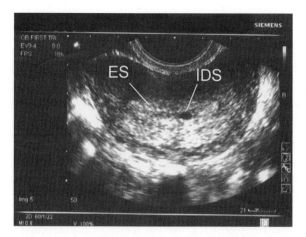

▲ **Figure 6–33.** Intradecidual sign. The intradecidual sign (IDS) may be seen in early gestation but is not a reliable indicator of intrauterine pregnancy. Note the small fluid collection just off the endometrial stripe (ES).

sonographically in about half of early pregnancies. Use caution when diagnosing an IUP based on this finding.

▶ **Yolk Sac**

The yolk sac is the first reliable indicator of IUP for the beginning sonographer. It is a thin-walled spherical structure found within the gestational sac (Figure 6–36).

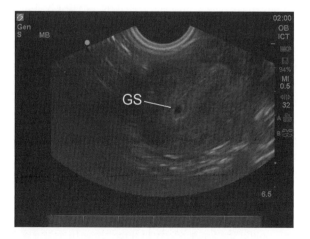

▲ **Figure 6–34.** Gestational sac. The uterus is seen in long axis with a gestational sac (GS) within the endometrial stripe. This may be an early intrauterine pregnancy or may represent a pseudogestational sac with an ectopic pregnancy.

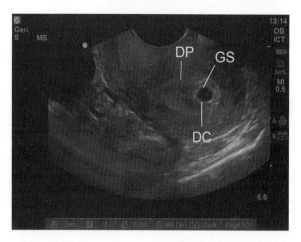

▲ **Figure 6–35.** Double decidual sign. The double decidual sign comprises two rings surrounding the gestational sac (GS): the decidua capsularis (DC) and the decidua parietalis (DP).

▶ **Fetal Pole**

The fetal pole is first visible on transvaginal ultrasound at about 6 weeks. It is usually found adjacent to the yolk sac, and by the time it is 5 mm, a fetal heart beat can be detected (Figure 6–37).

▶ **Fetal Heart Rate**

Fetal heart movement can be detected at about 6 weeks by transvaginal ultrasound, or when the hCG level is approximately 10,000 mIU/mL. Use M-mode ("motion" mode) to

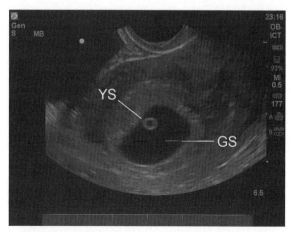

▲ **Figure 6–36.** Yolk sac. The yolk sac (YS) is a brightly reflective, thin-walled circular structure found within the gestational sac (GS).

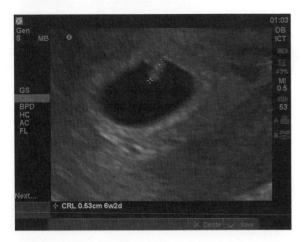

▲ **Figure 6–37.** Fetal pole. The fetal pole is detectible at about 6 weeks' gestation. In this image the yolk sac is out of plane and cannot be seen.

determine fetal heart rate (Figure 6–38). The average fetal heart rate is 110 beats per minute (bpm) at 6 weeks and will gradually increase to 170 bpm by week 8 before slowing to 160 bpm by week 14. Fetal heart rates lower than 100 are strongly associated with fetal demise.

▶ Diagnosing Ectopic Pregnancy

Ultimately the diagnosis of ectopic pregnancy requires the combination of laboratory, clinical, and ultrasound findings.

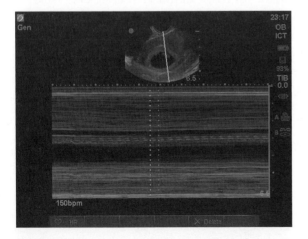

▲ **Figure 6–38.** M-mode heart rate determination. In this typical split screen M-mode display, the fetal heart rate is shown graphically at the bottom of the screen. Calipers are used to mark heart beats for measurement.

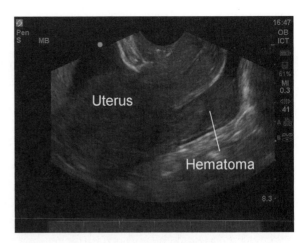

▲ **Figure 6–39.** Ectopic pregnancy. This hemodynamically unstable patient had a history of bilateral tubal ligation and a positive pregnancy test. No IUP is seen, and a hematoma is seen in the pouch of Douglas beneath the uterus.

For the emergency physician, the absence of hard signs of an IUP on ultrasound plus a quantitative hCG level above 1000 mIU/mL should trigger Ob/gyn consultation or formal ultrasound imaging to further investigate the possibility of an ectopic pregnancy. In stable patients with minimal symptoms, it may be reasonable to arrange repeat hCG testing in 48 hours; doubling of the level within 48 hours suggests early IUP.

The only ultrasound finding of ectopic pregnancy may be large amounts of free fluid in the pelvis (Figure 6–39). In some cases of ectopic pregnancy, fluid (blood) may be found in Morison's pouch.

ULTRASOUND-GUIDED PROCEDURES

Ultrasound allows direct visualization of anatomic structures during invasive procedures. This improves the success rate of the procedure and reduces complications.

▶ Foreign Body Removal

While some foreign bodies such as glass and metal are easily visualized with x-rays, others such as wood, plastic, thorns, etc, usually are not. Ultrasound allows visualization of the foreign body during the removal procedure and avoids radiation. The clinician may determine the position of the foreign body in three dimensions and discover its relationship to critical structures such as arteries and nerves.

The soft tissue probe is a high-resolution linear transducer that is ideal for the removal of foreign bodies. A sterile probe cover should be used and the machine adjusted

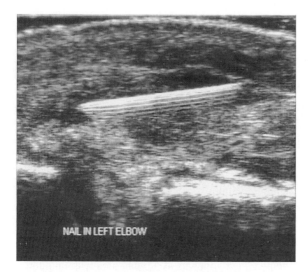

▲ Figure 6–40. Foreign body. This foreign body could not be located despite clear visualization on plain radiographs. Bedside ultrasound was used to locate and remove the finishing nail.

for the highest resolution possible. This limits ultrasound penetration but most foreign bodies will be found relatively superficial. The expected image will depend on the composition of the foreign body. Shadows and ring-down artifact will aid in identifying foreign bodies (Figure 6–40). If working alone, the clinician should mark the position of the foreign body with one hand while guiding forceps with the other.

If a foreign body is obscured by air within a tunneled skin defect, sterile saline may be poured into the cavity to allow visualization. If a foreign body is suspected in a hand or foot, the distal extremity can be submerged in water or saline for better ultrasound visualization.

▶ Thoracentesis and Paracentesis

The ability to mark pleural or peritoneal fluid during the procedure virtually eliminates the possibility of accidentally penetrating vital structures. Using the soft tissue probe with a sterile cover, the needle can be visualized entering the fluid collection. Alternately the safest needle insertion site can be marked on the skin after ultrasound confirmation and the procedure performed in the traditional method.

▶ Pericardiocentesis

The emergency pericardiocentesis is performed in critically ill patients with clinical signs and symptoms of cardiac tamponade. The use of ultrasound to assist in this procedure not only confirms the diagnosis but allows rapid localization of the pericardial effusion for drainage.

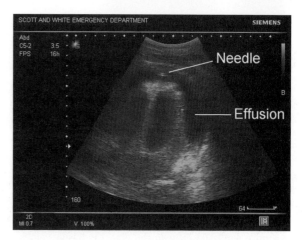

▲ Figure 6–41. Ultrasound-guided pericardiocentesis. Ultrasound of a patient during pericardiocentesis. The needle tip can be seen within the pericardial effusion.

The ultrasound probe is placed at the fifth costal interspace on the left of the sternum. The probe can be moved up or down a rib until the effusion is clearly visualized. The needle attached to a syringe is inserted beside the probe and visualized as it passes through the ribs into the effusion (Figure 6–41). When fluid from the effusion is aspirated, the syringe is removed and a wire is fed through the needle. A drainage catheter is then placed using standard Seldinger technique.

▶ Peripheral Access

Ultrasound-guided peripheral access can be performed anywhere a peripheral vessel is available. The soft tissue probe is used to locate the vessel and then guide the needle into the vessel under direct visualization. One specific vessel that is often overlooked by emergency physicians is the basilic vein, a large vein (5- to 6-mm diameter) located in the medial aspect of the mid-upper extremity.

The vessel is located by placing the probe at 90 degrees to the long axis of the mid-upper arm. Multiple vessels will be seen; placing gentle pressure on the probe will cause the basilic vein to collapse while the arteries remain circular. The probe is then turned to visualize the basilic vein in long axis. A 2.5- to 3-in angiocath needle is directed to the vessel under direct visualization. When the vessel is entered, the catheter is advanced, the needle removed, and the catheter secured in place (Figure 6–42).

▶ Central Venous Access

Ultrasound can be used to facilitate any central catheter placement including femoral, subclavian, or internal jugular but is most useful for the internal jugular. Research has found a significant reduction in procedure failure rate

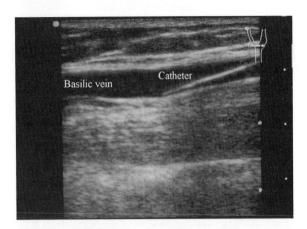

▲ **Figure 6–42.** Basilic vein catheter. The basilic vein is shown in long axis with catheter in place.

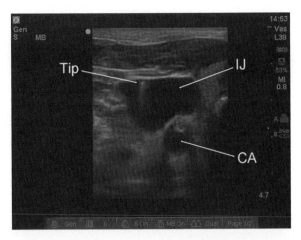

▲ **Figure 6–43.** Needle tip in internal jugular vein. The needle tip (TIP) appears as a bright area with ring-down artifact within the internal jugular vein (IJ). The carotid artery (CA) is visualized.

using ultrasound compared to traditional techniques. The soft tissue probe covered with a sterile sheath is placed on the anterior neck at the junction of the sternal head of the sternocleidomastoid and the clavicle with the probe marker to the patient's right using the clinician's non-dominant hand. The proceduralist should be standing at the head of the bed facing the patient's feet. The internal jugular and common carotid are visualized in short axis, and the vein is confirmed by placing gentle downward pressure on the probe that should collapse the vein but leave the carotid distended and circular. When the vessels are confirmed, the anticipated needle track is anesthetized under ultrasound guidance. The needle tip is then directed into the internal jugular lumen under direct visualization (Figure 6–43). An image should be saved at this point for documentation. Once dark red blood is aspirated, the ultrasound probe may be set aside and the procedure proceeds in the usual fashion.

It is useful to place the probe parallel to the vessel to confirm in long axis the catheter's track through the skin and into the internal jugular; it is possible to place the needle through the internal jugular and into the carotid artery.

▶ Ultrasound-Guided Abscess Drainage

Ultrasound is useful to evaluate presumed cellulitis and may change the management in many patients. Research has demonstrated that almost half of patients initially thought to have uncomplicated cellulitis were found to have an abscess requiring drainage when evaluated with ultrasound. While obvious abscesses do not require ultrasound guidance, most patients with cellulitis will benefit from ultrasound imaging.

A soft tissue probe with a protective cover should be used to scan the entire area over and surrounding cellulitic skin. An abscess will appear as a hypoechoic fluid collection or a

heteroechogenic collection with fluid of varying brightness on ultrasound (Figure 6–44). Using a skin marking pen can facilitate the procedure or the abscess can be drained under direct visualization.

American Medical Association Policy H-230.960: Privileging for Ultrasound Imaging. Res. 802, I-99; Reaffirmed: Sub. Res. 108, A-00.

American College of Emergency Physicians Policy: The Use of Ultrasound Imaging by Emergency Physicians. Approved by ACEP Board of Directors, June 2001.

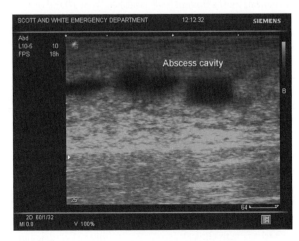

▲ **Figure 6–44.** Abscess cavity. The abscess should be scanned in two planes to ensure other abscess cavities are not missed.

American College of Emergency Physicians: American College of Emergency Physicians. ACEP Emergency Ultrasound Guidelines—2001. Ann Emerg Med 2001;38:470–481 [PMID: 11574810].

American College of Emergency Physicians: Emergency Ultrasound Guidelines. http://www.acep.org/workarea/down-loadasset.aspx?id=32878, Irving, TX, 2008. Accessed February 9, 2010.

American Registry for Diagnostic Medical Sonography: RDMS—Registered Diagnostic Medical Sonographer. http://www.ardms.org/default.asp?ContentID=63, Rockville, MD. Accessed February 9, 2010.

Accreditation Council for Graduate Medical Education: Emergency Medicine Guidelines. http://www.acgme.org/acWebsite/RRC_110/110_guidelines.asp, Chicago, IL. Accessed February 9, 2010.

Doubilet PM, Benson CB, Chow JS: Long-term prognosis of pregnancies complicated by slow embryonic heart rates in the early first trimester. J Ultrasound Med 1999;18:537–541 [PMID: 10447078].

Hind D, Calvert N, McWilliams R et al: Ultrasonic locating devices for central venous cannulation: Meta-analysis. BMJ 2003;327:361 [PMID: 12919984].

Rozycki GS, Shackford SR: Ultrasound, what every trauma surgeon should know. J Trauma 1996;40:1–4 [PMID: 8576968].

Shih CH: Effect of emergency physician-performed pelvic sonography on length of stay in the emergency department. Ann Emerg Med 1997;29:348–351 [PMID: 9055773].

Tezuka N, Sato S, Kanasugi H et al: Embryonic heart rates: Development in early first trimester and clinical evaluation. Gynecol Obstet Invest 1991;32:210–212 [PMID: 1778511].

Turkuer I, Atilla R, Topacoglu H et al: Do we really need plain and soft-tissue radiographies to detect radiolucent foreign bodies in the ED? Am J Emerg Med 2006;24:763–768 [PMID: 17098094].

Tayal VS, Hasan N, Norton HJ et al: The effect of soft-tissue ultrasound on the management of cellulitis in the emergency department. Acad Emerg Med 2006;13:384–388 [PMID: 16531602].

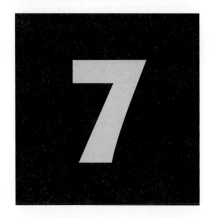

Emergency Procedures

William Randall Partin, MD, FACEP, FAAEM
Colby Dorroh, MD[1]

GENERAL INSTRUCTIONS FOR SKIN PREPARATION AND STERILE TECHNIQUE

▶ Skin Preparation

There are two types of skin preparation: skin cleansing and skin sterilization.

A. Skin Cleansing

Cleansing of the skin is sufficient for routine injections (subcutaneous, intramuscular, intravenous) and for simple venipuncture but not for venipuncture performed to draw blood for culture or to permit insertion of an indwelling device.

Skin cleansing is generally performed by swabbing the skin for a few seconds with a swab saturated with alcohol (70%) or organic iodine (eg, povidone–iodine or equivalent). To reduce the pain of venipuncture, the disinfectant should be allowed to dry on the skin before the skin is punctured. *Note*: This procedure merely cleans the skin; it does not sterilize it.

B. Skin Sterilization

Skin sterilization should be performed before all procedures that involve puncturing or cutting the skin, with the exception of routine venipuncture and simple injections. This procedure eliminates superficial skin bacterial, leaving only a few organisms deep in hair follicles or sweat glands. Skin sterilization may be omitted if the delay involved would jeopardize the patients' life (eg, thoracostomy for tension pneumothorax).

[1]This chapter is a revision of the chapter by David Knighton, MD, FACS, Richard M. Locksley, MD, & John Mills, MD, from the 4th edition.

A variety of techniques can be used to achieve skin sterilization:

1. Scrub the skin vigorously with copious amounts of 70% alcohol for 2 minutes or

2. Use a sterile 10×10 cm^2 (4×4 inch^2) gauze pad, and apply 2% iodine tincture to the area and allow the iodine to dry. Then remove it, using 70% alcohol on a sterile pad, because iodine may cause skin burns or

3. Apply an organic iodine disinfectant (eg, povidone–iodine or poloxamer–iodine) twice, allowing each application to dry. These particular disinfectants need not be removed before the procedure is started.

The following guidelines should be observed in all cases:

- Sterilize a much larger area of skin than is required for the procedure.

- Apply the disinfectant starting at the site of the procedure and extending outward in concentrically larger circles.

- Use sterile gloves to apply the disinfectant.

▶ Sterile Technique

It is virtually impossible to achieve sterile technique at the bedside in the emergency department comparable to that obtainable in an operating room; however, following the guidelines outlined below decreases the risk of infection. Good lighting is helpful for maintaining sterile technique and is essential for performing procedures successfully.

1. Wash hands thoroughly, preferably with antiseptic soap, before performing any procedure.

2. Have all necessary equipment assembled and opened at the bedside, so that once sterile gloves have been donned, only sterile instruments and equipment will be touched. Alternatively, an assistant can open packaged sterile supplies.

3. Put on sterile gloves.

4. Sterilize the skin as described above.

5. Enlarge the sterile field by surrounding the sterile skin with sterile drapes made of cloth or paper. These may come with a window in them which is used to isolate the area of sterile skin selected for the procedure.

6. Make sure that catheters, needles, stopcocks, and the like cannot roll off the drape onto the floor, perhaps at a critical moment.

7. When performing complicated procedures that require stricter sterile conditions (eg, insertion of a central venous catheter), wear a surgical cap, mask, and gown in addition to the sterile gloves.

▼ UPPER EXTREMITY VENIPUNCTURE

▶ Indications

Venipuncture is performed to obtain a sample of venous blood for laboratory testing.

▶ Contraindications

Contraindications to venipuncture are as follows:

- Cellulitis over the proposed site
- Phlebitis
- Venous obstruction
- Lymphangitis of the extremity
- Administration of intravenous fluid distal to the proposed site.

▶ Personnel Required

One person can perform venipuncture unaided.

▶ Equipment and Supplies Required

- Materials for skin cleansing (or skin sterilization, if blood culture is to be performed).

- Syringe of adequate size (10–50 mL) for the amount of blood needed or Vacutainer tubes and appropriate Vacutainer syringe hub (Vacutainer equipment consists of a needle with a point at each end, evacuated glass tubes with rubber stoppers, and a plastic barrel. Blood is forced into the evacuated tube when the needle connects the tube with the vein).

- Needle (21 gauge) for the syringe or a Vacutainer needle with an automatic valve or rubber cuff to stop blood flow while tubes are being changed. If a large amount of blood is to be drawn, it is advisable to use an 18-gauge needle. Use smaller-gauge needles or scalp vein needles for infants and children.

- Tourniquet.

- Receptacle tubes for blood for the desired laboratory tests.

- Gauze squares, 5×5 cm^2 (2×2 inch^2).

- Adhesive dressing.

▶ Positioning of the Patient

The upper extremity is the site most commonly used to draw venous blood. The patient should be in a comfortable position, with the upper extremity resting on a solid object. If the patient is in bed, the supine position is best, with the arm resting on the mattress close to the patient's side. The ambulatory patient should be sitting with the arm on a table or support at a comfortable height for the operator.

▶ Procedure

1. Assemble all necessary equipment and position as described above.

2. Apply the tourniquet above the antecubital fossa in a manner that will allow quick removal with one hand. The tourniquet should be tight enough to occlude venous return but not so tight as to cause arterial obstruction or patient discomfort. It should be removed before the extremity turns purple.

3. Locate an appropriate vein. Have the patient open and close the fist of the selected arm to help pump blood from the muscle compartment of the arm into the superficial venous circulation.

   a. *Antecubital veins:* The superficial basilic and cephalic veins course just under the skin on the volar side of the forearm. They run along the medial and lateral edge of the antecubital fossa at the elbow crease. In slender or muscular people, these veins often stand out and are easy to enter. If one of these veins is accessible, use it. In obese people, those who have had multiple venipunctures, and intravenous drug abusers, finding a patent antecubital vein (or any other vein) may be difficult.

   Palpate the antecubital fossa with the tip of the index finger and feel for the buoyant resilience of a distended vein. Be careful to differentiate the firm cord of a tendon or a thrombosed vein from the resiliency of a patent vessel. When the veins are not visible, they must be located by feel. Even a small vein deep in the subcutaneous tissue may be detected on the basis of its resilient feel.

   b. *Arm veins:* If a patient's antecubital vein cannot be found, examine the forearm on both the volar and the dorsal surfaces. Look for the faint bluish color of a vein under the skin, or better yet, feel for a vein with the tip of the index finger.

   c. *Hand veins:* If no vein is found on the forearm, proceed to the dorsal surface of the hand and use one of the superficial veins on the hand. These veins are small, collapse easily, and are usually inadequate for drawing a large amount of blood. If large amounts of blood are needed, it is often better to go to another anatomic site such as the femoral vein than to persist in trying to draw large quantities of blood from a small hand vein. By the time an adequate amount has been obtained, it usually clots in the syringe and another venipuncture then becomes necessary.

   Do not give up after one examination of the arm. Carefully palpate the arm two or three times if necessary. A vein suitable for venipuncture may be obscured (eg, by hair) and may therefore be missed on initial examination. Occasionally, slapping repeatedly over the vein with the pads of the

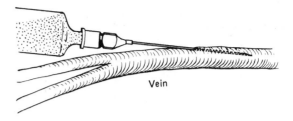

▲ **Figure 7–1.** Technique of percutaneous venipuncture. The needle should be inserted into the lumen of the vein at an angle of about 10–20°, and the bevel should be facing up. (Reproduced, with permission, from Krupp MA et al: *Physician's Handbook,* 21st ed. Lange, 1985.)

first and second fingers will help to distend a faint vein, or the patient can dangle the arm over the side of the bed to achieve the same result. Do not thrust blindly at a bluish mark on the patient's arm without first palpating the area to confirm that a patent vein is underneath.

4. Prepare the skin. Skin cleansing is adequate unless blood is being obtained for culture, in which case the skin must be sterilized (see Skin Preparation, above).

5. Grasp the syringe or Vacutainer in the dominant hand while palpating the vein with the index finger of the other hand. Exert traction on the vein by pulling distally (toward the operator) on the skin next to the puncture site. Align the needle with the course of the vein and make sure that the bevel is facing up. With a quick but smooth motion, push the needle through the skin at an angle of about 10–20° (Figure 7–1). Then carefully advance the needle into the lumen of the vein with a smooth motion.

6. When the vein has been properly penetrated, blood will flow back into the needle when the Vacutainer tube is pushed onto the needle.

7. If venous blood is not obtained on the first attempt, reassess the course of the vein. Try palpating the vein proximal to the needle site. Withdraw the needle to just below the skin and attempt a second venipuncture.

8. If a Vacutainer system is being used, simply fill all of the tubes required.

9. Draw enough blood to give accurate laboratory test results; clotted or hemolyzed specimens will give misleading information.

10. When enough blood has been obtained, remove the tourniquet, and then withdraw the needle quickly and smoothly. Have the patient immediately apply firm direct pressure on a 5 × 5 cm² (2 × 2 inch²) piece of gauze over the site for 3–5 minutes. If the site is antecubital,

flex the arm to stop the bleeding. Elevating the arm will speed hemostasis.

11. Gently mix each tube thoroughly if anticoagulant or preservative is present in the tube. At the patient's bedside, label the tubes with the patient's name, date of birth, and date of sample, and place any specimens on ice as required.

12. It is often helpful to put an adhesive dressing on the venipuncture site to absorb any blood that might ooze out.

INSERTION OF A PERIPHERAL INTRAVENOUS CATHETER

Catheter-clad needles (eg, Angiocath) are the standard used millions of times per year for easy access to the vascular system.

Indications

Peripheral venous catheterization with a catheter-clad needle is performed to gain peripheral venous access.

Contraindications

Contraindications to peripheral venous catheterization with a catheter-clad needle are as follows:

- Phlebitis of the extremity.
- Cellulitis over the projected site of insertion.
- Potential or existing lymphedema or venous occlusive edema of the extremity.
- Traumatic injury proximal to insertion site (eg, fracture).

Personnel Required

One person can insert a catheter-clad needle unaided.

Equipment and Supplies Required

- Materials for skin cleansing.
- Tourniquet.
- Precut tape to secure the catheter in place.
- Plastic-coated absorbent pad to place under the patient's arm.
- Catheter-clad needle (eg, Angiocath) of sufficient size for the rate and type of fluid to be infused, but smaller than the cannulated vein. For administration of electrolyte or glucose solutions at rates of less than 200 mL/h, a 20-gauge catheter is usually sufficient. For infusion of blood or colloid solutions or rapid infusion of electrolyte solutions (200–1000 mL/h), an 18-gauge catheter is mandatory and a 16-gauge is preferred. In patients with

multiple trauma, who may require large volumes of blood and electrolyte solutions, at least one, but preferably two large bore (16 or 14-gauge) catheters are indicated.

- Usually 1 L bag of fluid for intravenous administration, with proper connecting tubing. The equipment should be flushed and fully assembled ready for use.

Positioning of the Patient

Place peripheral intravenous catheters in the upper extremity if possible. Occasionally, a lower extremity intravenous catheter is necessary when all veins in the upper extremity are inaccessible and insertion of a central venous catheter is not practical. Intravenous catheters in the lower extremity are associated with a much higher incidence of infection and thrombosis than are those inserted in the upper extremity especially in patients with peripheral vascular disease or diabetes.

The patient should be in a comfortable supine or sitting position, with the extremity to be used resting on a firm surface.

Procedure

1. Connect a bag of fluid with the tubing, fill the connecting tubing with intravenous fluid, and make sure that all air is flushed from the tubing.

2. Apply the tourniquet above the antecubital fossa and secure it so that it can be quickly removed with one hand.

3. Have the patient open and close the fist to help distend the superficial veins with blood. If veins are difficult to identify, having the patient hang the arm below the level of the heart or wrapping the arm in a warm moist towel may be helpful.

4. Select an appropriate vein. The site at which two veins join is an excellent choice, because the vein is immobilized best in such a location. Possible sites include the radial aspect of the forearm just proximal to the wrist ("intern's vein"), the volar aspect of the forearm distal to the antecubital fossa on the ulnar side, and the dorsum of the hand. In slender people, these veins usually distend without difficulty; however, some individuals have deeply buried veins that can be found only by careful palpation. Remember that a vein does not have to be visualized in order to be successfully catheterized. Gently tapping over the vein may help to distend it and make identification and catheterization easier. If the vein lies deep in the subcutaneous tissue, make a mental picture of its course and branches by means of systematic palpation up and down the vein.

5. Inspect the catheter to make sure that it slides easily off the needle and that both the catheter and the needle are smooth.

6. Cleanse the skin around the insertion site.

7. Grasp the needle directly with the dominant hand. Insert the needle through the skin at an angle of about 10–20°, either on top of or next to the vein (see Figure 7–1).

8. Pull the skin taut distal to the venipuncture site and insert the needle and catheter into the vein. When the lumen of the vein is entered, blood flows back into the hub of the angiocath.

9. Make sure that both the needle and the catheter are in the lumen of the vein. Blood may flow back when only the needle is in the vein and the catheter tip is against the wall of the vessel and has not actually entered the vessel lumen. In this position, the catheter cannot be advanced over the needle into the vein. To avoid this complication, advance the needle and catheter into the vein about 4–6 mm (⅛–¼ inch) after blood initially returns. Check to be sure that blood continues to return when the needle and catheter are in this position.

10. Slide the catheter off the needle (Figure 7–2A). Hold the needle steady by its hub in one hand at an angle of 10–20° to the vein while gripping the hub of the catheter with the other hand, and gently push the catheter forward off the needle. Advance the catheter up to its hub while keeping the needle firmly in place. With practice, advancing the catheter and withdrawing the needle can be accomplished in one smooth motion. Be sure not to pull out both the catheter and needle at the same time. To reduce the incidence of needle sticks, most IV catheters in use today have a spring-loaded mechanism that allows the needle to be safely and rapidly withdrawn into the proximal housing of the catheter device. To avoid uncontrolled blood loss from the open catheter, occlude the vein proximal to the end of the catheter by applying direct pressure before pulling the needle out of the catheter.

11. *Note*: Occasionally, the catheter will encounter a valve in the vein that prevents complete advancement of the catheter. If this occurs, hold the catheter hub in place, remove the tourniquet, and connect the intravenous tubing to the catheter. Running intravenous fluid into the vein often opens the valve and allows complete insertion of the catheter.

12. Remove the tourniquet.

13. Attach the intravenous tubing to the catheter and check the flow. A properly located catheter should allow rapid

A
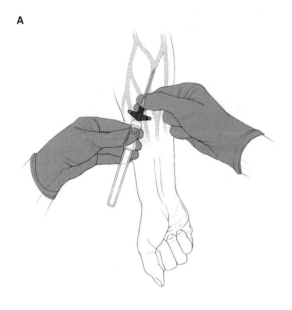

B
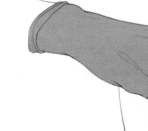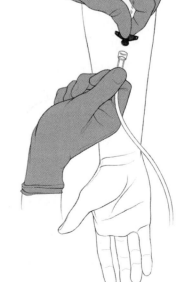

▲ **Figure 7–2. A:** Technique of removing the needle from the catheter-clad needle. **B:** Connecting the intravenous tubing.

influx of fluid. If flow is slow or there is no flow at all, withdraw the catheter a few millimeters and watch for change in the rate of flow. Occasionally, a branch vein or valve obstructs flow and moving the catheter will be all that is required to achieve good flow.

14. Occasionally, the catheter is pushed through the opposite wall of the vein, causing swelling and pain at the insertion site as the intravenous fluid dissects the subcutaneous tissues. In this case, withdraw the catheter and needle completely and try a second venipuncture in another vein or in the same vein proximal to the first insertion site. (Allow enough time for the first venipuncture to clot, or leave the catheter in place to occlude the venipuncture site until the more proximal catheter is inserted, and then withdraw the unused catheter.)

15. Secure the catheter in place with tape as shown in Figure 7–2B. Do not apply tape completely around the arm; it can act as a tourniquet and lead to distal edema. It is helpful to write the catheter gauge and date of insertion on the tape.

EXTERNAL JUGULAR VEIN CATHETERIZATION

▶ Indications

External jugular vein catheterization is performed to gain peripheral or central venous access when sites other than the external jugular vein (eg, internal jugular or subclavian vein) are inaccessible or if catheterization of those sites is contraindicated (eg, coagulopathy).

▶ Contraindications

Contraindications to external jugular vein catheterization are as follows:

- Agitated, uncooperative patient (relative contraindication).
- Cellulitis at the insertion site.
- Previous neck surgery (the position of the vein may be distorted or it may have been ligated or removed).

▶ Personnel Required

One person can perform simple external jugular vein catheterization unaided, although an assistant is helpful. Insertion of a central venous catheter through the external jugular vein by means of a J wire requires an assistant.

▶ Equipment and Supplies Required

A. Peripheral Venous Access

- Materials for skin sterilization.

- Catheter-clad needle (eg, Angiocath), 16–18 gauge.
- Container of intravenous solution and connecting tubing.
- Precut tape for securing the catheter.
- Plastic-coated absorbent pad to place under the patient's head and neck.
- Tincture of benzoin, 5 mL.

B. Central Venous Access

- Materials for skin sterilization.
- Materials for sterile technique (cap, mask, gloves, and gown).
- Lidocaine, 1%, with 10-mL syringe and 25-gauge needle.
- Sterile syringes with normal saline for flushing intravenous catheters and tubing.
- Most adults will need a 16–18-gauge catheter-clad needle. Make sure the needles and catheters are of the proper size and construction to accept and slip over the J wire.
- J wire (flexible angiography wire) 35.5-cm (14-inch) long, about 0.089 cm $\frac{1}{32}$ inch diameter, and with a curvature that has a radius of about 3 mm ($\frac{1}{8}$ inch).
- Silk skin suture (size 3-0) on a cutting needle.
- Needle holder.
- Straight scissors.
- IV bag and connecting tubing. All equipment must be flushed and fully assembled ready for use.
- Gauze squares, 10×10 cm^2 (4×4 inch^2).
- Plastic-coated absorbent pad to place under the patient's head and neck.
- Sterile drapes.
- Tincture of benzoin, 5 mL.

▶ Positioning of the Patient

The patient should be placed in the Trendelenburg position (20–30°), with the head turned 90° away from the side of insertion. Place the plastic-coated absorbent pad under the patient's head and neck.

▶ Anatomy Review

The external jugular vein courses from behind the angle of the jaw across to the sternocleidomastoid muscle and superficial to it to join the subclavian vein (Figure 7–3). The internal jugular vein and carotid artery lie deep to the external jugular vein and are separated from it by the sternocleidomastoid muscle.

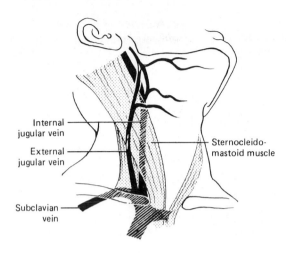

▲ **Figure 7–3.** Anatomic relationships of the external jugular vein. The external jugular vein originates at the level of the angle of the mandible in the parotid gland and it courses caudally and anteriorly across the sternocleidomastoid muscle. It enters the subclavian vein near the subclavian triangle.

▶ **Procedure**

A. Peripheral Venous Access

1. Assemble all necessary equipment, including the IV fluid and tubing, and make sure the tubing has been flushed to remove all air.

2. Position the patient.

3. Sterilize the skin around the area of insertion from the clavicle to the ear.

4. Have the patient take a deep breath and forcibly exhale against a closed glottis (Valsalva maneuver) to increase intrathoracic pressure and distend the external jugular vein with blood. It is sometimes helpful to have the patient put a thumb in his or her mouth and blow against it. If the patient is unable to cooperate, the vein may be distended by obstructing its outflow with a finger placed on the neck above the clavicle.

5. Make a mental note of the position and size of the vein.

6. Have the patient resume normal breathing as soon as the size and position of the vein have been determined.

7. Insert the catheter-clad needle into the vein halfway between the angle of the jaw and the clavicle. While the patient performs the Valsalva maneuver, apply traction cephalad on the vein and insert the catheter-clad needle into the vein lumen. Withdraw the needle, leaving the catheter in place. (See above for technique of catheterization using a catheter-clad needle.)

8. Connect the intravenous tubing to the catheter and start the intravenous infusion. To avoid air embolism, make sure that either the intrathoracic pressure is elevated (eg, by the Valsalva maneuver) or the hub of the needle is occluded with a thumb or finger.

9. Tape the tubing in place. When taping an intravenous line to the neck, it is helpful to use tincture of benzoin on both the patient's skin and the tubing. Tape the tubing up the side of the patient's neck and face superior to the ear, securing the line in several places with tape. Tightly secure all connections.

10. Short catheters inserted in the external jugular vein are difficult to secure because of the constant motion of the patient's neck. The catheter may become dislodged from the vein and cause infiltration of intravenous fluid into the soft tissues of the neck. Before administering blood or drugs through an external jugular catheter, check to see that there is free flow of fluid into the line, that the neck is not swollen, and that blood can reflux freely into the intravenous tube when the intravenous bag or bottle is lowered below the level of the patient.

B. Central Venous Access

1. Assemble all necessary equipment, including the container of intravenous fluid and tubing, and make sure the tubing has been flushed to remove all air.

2. Position the patient.

3. Sterilize the skin around the area of insertion from the clavicle to the ear.

4. Drape the area and observe sterile technique (don cap, mask, gloves, and gown).

5. Have the patient take a deep breath and forcibly exhale against a closed glottis (Valsalva maneuver).

6. Note the course of the vein, and then have the patient resume normal breathing.

7. Select an insertion point about 4 cm (1⅝ inch) above the clavicle and infiltrate the area with the 1% lidocaine with the 10-mL syringe and 25-gauge needle.

8. While keeping the vein distended (by Valsalva maneuver or occlusion of outflow with finger compression), insert the catheter-clad needle or the needle from a needle-clad catheter into the external jugular vein. If a catheter-clad needle is being used, remove the central needle at this point and cover the end of the catheter hub with a thumb to prevent aspiration of air.

9. Make sure the needle or catheter is properly placed in the vein by observing the return of blood through the catheter. Inject 5 mL of sterile saline or run intravenous fluid through the line to establish its patency.

10. Insert the J wire through the needle or catheter, curved end first; guide the wire around the bends in the course of the external jugular vein–subclavian vein junction

into the intrathoracic portion of the subclavian vein–superior vena cava system.

11. Secure the wire at the skin with a clamp or a finger. Do not allow the wire to slip all the way into the vein. If a catheter-clad needle is being used, slide the catheter over the wire and into position in the intrathoracic portion of the venous system. If a needle-clad catheter is being used, remove the insertion needle, taking care to grasp the J wire firmly to keep it from slipping forward all the way into the vein. Slip the catheter over the J wire and be careful not to let the J wire slip all the way into the vein as the catheter is being advanced.

12. Holding the catheter in place, remove the J wire and cover the end of the catheter hub with a thumb until the setup can be tested for return of blood. Then start the intravenous infusion.

13. Secure the catheter in place with the silk suture run first through the skin and then wrapped around the catheter.

14. Take the patient out of the Trendelenburg position.

15. Obtain a portable chest X-ray immediately to confirm placement of the catheter.

16. Dress the insertion site with a folded sterile 10×10 cm^2 (4×4 inch^2) gauze pad and tape the pad in place.

17. Remember to tightly secure all connections to prevent air embolism.

INTERNAL JUGULAR VEIN CATHETERIZATION

The internal jugular vein is used for the insertion of central venous catheters. Pulmonary complications (hemothorax, pneumothorax) occur less commonly than with subclavian vein catheterization, but arterial injury (eg, to the carotid artery) is more common.

▶ Indications

Internal jugular vein catheterization is performed to gain venous access for monitoring of central venous pressure, mixed central venous oxygen saturation, insertion of a transvenous pacemaker, or administration of medications or intravenous fluids.

▶ Contraindications

Contraindications to internal jugular vein catheterization are as follows:

- Previous neck injury that might have ligated or scarred the internal jugular vein and thereby altered its anatomy.
- Superior vena cava occlusion.
- Acquired or iatrogenic bleeding disorder.
- Cellulitis over the proposed insertion site.

- Agitated, uncooperative patient (relative contraindication).
- Patient receiving cardiopulmonary resuscitation (CPR).

▶ Personnel Required

The operator performing internal jugular vein catheterization requires an assistant to help handle sterile materials and position the patient.

▶ Equipment and Supplies Required

A. Materials

- Materials for skin sterilization.
- Materials for sterile technique (cap, mask, gloves, gown, and large sterile drape).
- Lidocaine, 1%, with 10-mL syringe and 25- and 22-gauge needles.
- Intravenous fluid with all necessary tubing. All equipment should be flushed and fully assembled ready for use.

B. Prepackaged Sterile Central Venous Access Trays

Prepackaged sterile central venous access trays are commercially available. The following items are required:

- Drapes.
- Gauze sponges, 10×10 cm^2 (4×4 inch^2).
- Nylon or silk skin suture (size 3-0 or 4-0) on a cutting needle.
- Needle holder.
- Straight scissors.
- Plastic-coated absorbent pad to place beneath the patient's arm.
- Syringe, 3 mL, with 22-gauge, 6.5-cm (2½-inch) needle (for use as a probe).
- Central venous catheter and insertion set. Many kinds are commercially available; most consist of an introducing needle and radiopaque catheter, usually 30.5-cm (12-inch) long.

▶ Positioning of the Patient

Use a bed or gurney that can be placed in the Trendelenburg position and that has a removable headboard. The patient should be supine, with the head turned 90° away from the side selected for insertion. Place the patient in as steep a Trendelenburg position as possible in order to fully distend the internal jugular vein and also to create increased pressure inside the vein, thus decreasing the chances of air embolism during insertion.

▶ Anatomy Review

The internal jugular vein leaves the base of the skull and courses laterally and posteriorly to the carotid artery and the carotid sheath. It joins the subclavian vein at the thoracic outlet. The internal jugular vein runs medial to the upper portion of the sternocleidomastoid muscle, deep to the triangle formed by the two heads at the midportion of this muscle, and deep to its clavicular head (see Figure 7–3).

▶ Procedure

A. Middle (Triangle) Approach

See Figure 7–4.

1. Assemble and arrange all necessary equipment, including the container of intravenous fluid and intravenous tubing, and make sure the tubing has been flushed to remove all air.

2. Position the patient, as described above.

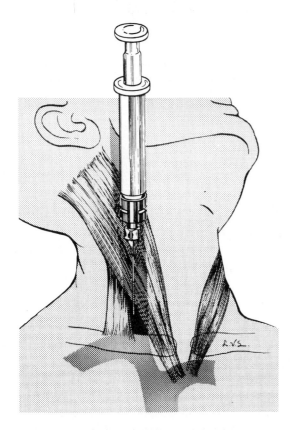

▲ **Figure 7–4.** Internal jugular vein catheterization—middle approach. (Reproduced, with permission, from Dunphy JE, Way LW (editors): *Current Surgical Diagnosis & Treatment,* 5th ed. Lange, 1981.)

3. Observe sterile technique (don cap, mask, gown, and gloves). Sterilize the skin around the area of insertion from the clavicle to the ear and drape the patient.

4. The sternocleidomastoid muscle will be clearly outlined when the patient lifts the head slightly. Make a mental picture of the triangle formed by the two heads of the muscle, which has its apex pointed cephalad and its base formed by the clavicle.

5. Palpate the carotid artery, and make a mental note of the course of the internal jugular vein, which runs lateral and deep to the artery.

6. Choose a point near the apex of the triangle formed by the sternocleidomastoid and anesthetize the skin with the 1% lidocaine with the 10-mL syringe and 25-gauge needle. Change to the 22-gauge needle and infiltrate a path through the subcutaneous tissue toward the internal jugular vein, directing the needle downward at an angle of 45° toward the ipsilateral nipple. Be careful when infiltrating the area to aspirate before injecting, so as to avoid injecting significant amounts of lidocaine into the vein. Omit this step if the patient is comatose.

7. Make a probe by placing the 22-gauge, 6.5-cm (2½-inch) needle on the 3-mL syringe.

8. Use this small-gauge needle as a probe to locate the internal jugular vein. Pierce the skin near the apex of the triangle formed by the sternocleidomastoid and direct the needle downward at a 30–45° angle toward the ipsilateral nipple. If the right hand is being used to guide the syringe and needle, palpate the carotid artery with the left hand to make sure that the needle is moving away from it. The needle should pierce the vein after advancing 2.5–4 cm (1–½ inch). If it does not, withdraw the needle until the point is just under the skin, reposition the needle in the subcutaneous tissue, and probe more medially, always keeping the left index finger on the carotid artery for reference. Once the needle has entered the internal jugular vein, dark venous blood should flow freely into the syringe. If the vein cannot be located after a few probing maneuvers, ask for assistance. *Caution:* Do not use the larger catheter insertion needle or a catheter-clad needle (eg, Angiocath) if the vein cannot be located with the probing needle. When the vein is located, withdraw the probing needle and remove it from the syringe.

9. Place the catheter insertion needle or catheter-clad needle on the syringe and follow the course of the probing needle to enter the internal jugular vein. Always recheck the landmarks and position of the carotid artery while inserting this large needle.

10. Maintain a slight vacuum in the attached syringe while inserting the larger needle. Once the needle has entered the vein, dark venous blood will flow freely into the syringe. While aspirating, rotate the needle 360° to make

sure that the bevel of the needle is completely within the vein; cessation of blood flow at any point indicates that the needle should be slowly advanced or withdrawn, because it is near one wall of the vein.

11. When it is clear that the needle is properly positioned in the lumen of the vein, disconnect the syringe, and immediately occlude the orifice of the needle to prevent air embolization during inspiration. Most central venous catheters are inserted using the Seldinger technique. This method involves the use of a flexible guide wire or J wire that is placed through the lumen of the needle. The needle is then removed while allowing the guide wire to remain in the lumen of the vein. A No. 11 scalpel blade is then used to make a small incision in the skin where the wire penetrates. Next, a semirigid dilator is advanced over the wire and into the lumen of the vein to create a tract for the more pliable catheter to follow. The dilator is removed continuing to keep the guide wire in place. Finally, the catheter is advanced over the wire and into the lumen of the vein and the guide wire is removed from the catheter leaving only the pliable catheter in place in the vein. An alternative is to place the dilator inside the catheter (most kits are designed to allow this) and then advance the dilator–catheter complex over the wire and into the vein lumen. This method permits dilation of the tract and insertion of the catheter simultaneously. After the dilator–catheter complex is advanced over the wire and into the vein lumen, the dilator and guide wire can then be removed leaving only the catheter behind in the lumen of the vein.

12. When the catheter is fully inserted, check again to be sure there is good return, attach the intravenous tubing, and start the fluid infusion. Anchor the catheter in place with the nylon or silk size 3-0 or 4-0 skin suture. Make sure that the catheter is well secured and tape it in place, using tincture of benzoin to help secure the tape to the skin and catheter. Tightly secure all connections. Cover the insertion site with a sterile 10×10 cm^2 (4×4 inch^2) gauze pad folded in half.

13. Take the patient out of the Trendelenburg position and obtain a chest X-ray immediately to check placement of the catheter and to detect possible pneumothorax.

B. Posterior Approach

See Figure 7–5.

1. (Steps 1–4 are the same as in the anterior approach.) Note the border where the posterior edge of the anterior belly of the sternocleidomastoid muscle meets the external jugular vein and anesthetize with the 1% lidocaine. Use a 25-gauge needle for superficial infiltration and a 22-gauge needle for deeper anesthesia.

2. Using a 22-gauge, 6.5-cm (2½-inch) needle attached to the 3-mL syringe as a probe, enter the skin just

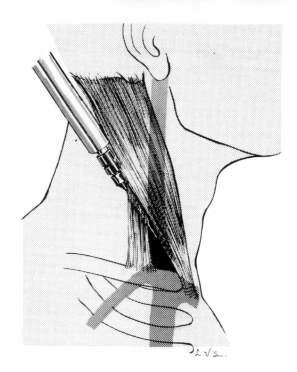

▲ **Figure 7–5.** Internal jugular vein catheterization—posterior approach. (Reproduced, with permission, from Dunphy JE, Way LW (editors): *Current Surgical Diagnosis & Treatment*, 5th ed. Lange, 1981.)

distal to the posterior edge of the sternocleidomastoid muscle about two-third of the way down, where the external jugular vein crosses the stern-ocleidomastoid muscle. Enter at a 45° angle to the vertical axis and 20° below the coronal plane. Direct the needle under the sternocleidomastoid muscle and toward the suprasternal notch. Pull back on the plunger as the needle is inserted. When the vein has been successfully entered, dark venous blood will flow back into the syringe. If the vein is not entered when the probing needle has been inserted its full length, withdraw the needle and try again.

3. When the vein has been located with the probing needle, withdraw this needle and insert the larger catheter insertion needle or catheter–needle combination. The needle should be attached to a syringe in which a slight vacuum is maintained.

4. When the vein has been successfully entered, dark venous blood will flow freely into the syringe.

5. Insert the catheter using the Seldinger technique, as described above.

The remaining steps are the same as in the anterior approach.

▼ INTERNAL JUGULAR VEIN CATHETERIZAION USING ULTRASOUND GUIDANCE

The practice of using ultrasound guidance for the placement of central venous catheters in the internal jugular vein is becoming more common. Several studies have shown that using ultrasound guidance for this procedure can lead to a significantly lower complication rate and an increased success rate, compared to the traditional anatomical approach. Ultrasound guidance may also offer additional benefit in patients whose anatomical landmarks are difficult to distinguish.

▶ Equipment and Supplies Required

In addition to the items needed for placement of an internal jugular vein catheter using the anatomic method, the following additional items will be needed:

- Ultrasound machine with high resolution (7–15 MHz) linear probe, also known as a vascular probe.
- Sterile ultrasound probe cover kit containing the following:
- Sterile probe cover
- Sterile rubber bands
- Sterile package of water-based gel
- Nonsterile bottle of water-based gel

▶ Procedure

1. As in the anatomical approach, assemble and arrange all necessary equipment, including the container of intravenous fluid and intravenous tubing, and make sure the tubing has been flushed to remove all air.

2. Position the ultrasound machine beside the patient with the screen facing the head of the bed. The screen should be easily seen from the position where you will be standing to perform the procedure.

3. Position the patient as described earlier.

4. Before sterilizing the field, visualize the internal jugular vein using the vascular ultrasound probe and the nonsterile bottle of water-based gel. Orient the probe in the transverse position, with the probe marker facing the patient's left shoulder. The marker on the probe should match the marker on the screen. To help identify which vessel is the vein, apply some mild pressure with the probe. The internal jugular vein will usually collapse with mild pressure from the probe, while the artery will stay patent under mild pressure. Scan up and down the vessel to confirm patency. Repeat the preliminary ultrasound examination on the patient's contralateral side for comparison. You may find that one side will provide easier access due to vessel patency, size, or anatomy.

5. Observe sterile technique (don cap, mask, gown, and gloves). Sterilize the skin around the area of insertion from the clavicle to the ear and drape the patient.

6. Once the area has been prepped and draped, you will need an assistant to help place the sterile cover over the ultrasound probe. First, place some of the sterile water-based gel down inside the end of the cover. Next, hold the probe cover with the opening facing up. Have an assistant lower the ultrasound probe into the cover. Grasp the probe in the cover and have the assistant pull the end of the cover over the probe cable. Secure the cover over the probe using the rubber bands. Apply sterile gel to the outside of the sterile probe cover.

7. Over the site of insertion anesthetize the skin with the 1% lidocaine with the 10-mL syringe and 25-gauge needle. Change to the 22-gauge needle and infiltrate a path through the subcutaneous tissue toward the internal jugular vein, directing the needle downward at an angle of 45° toward the ipsilateral nipple. Be careful when infiltrating the area to aspirate before injecting, so as to avoid injecting significant amounts of lidocaine into the vein. Omit this step if the patient is comatose.

8. Hold the probe over the insertion site to visualize the internal jugular vein. The probe should be positioned so that the vein is visible in the center of the ultrasound screen. Held in this position, the vein should be located under the center of the ultrasound probe.

9. Since visualization of the vein is made possible by the ultrasound, use of the smaller probing needle to locate the vein is typically not necessary.

10. While holding the probe over the insertion site with one hand, slowly insert the catheter insertion needle and syringe at a 40–60° angle from the plane of the neck, and approximately 1 cm back from the middle of the ultrasound probe (**picture 5**). Some may find it easier to have a gowned and gloved assistant hold the probe in position for you. Any time you advance the needle be sure to aspirate the syringe and have your eyes on the syringe as you advance. When applying pressure with the probing needle, you should be able to see soft tissue indent on the ultrasound screen. Use the tissue indentation to guide the direction of the needle. As you advance the needle further, eventually pressure applied to the needle will cause the vein to compress somewhat. Finally, the needle may come into view on the screen as it cannulates the vein. It is important to keep your eyes on the syringe and aspirate a vacuum any time you are advancing the needle so you will see the flash as soon as you enter the vessel. Concentrating solely on the ultrasound screen could cause you to miss the flash and penetrate through the vessel.

11. Once the needle has entered the vein, dark venous blood will flow freely into the syringe. While aspirating, rotate the needle 360° to make sure that the bevel of the needle is completely within the vein; cessation of blood flow

at any point indicates that the needle should be slowly advanced or withdrawn, because it is near one wall of the vein. Once the needle is in the vessel, the ultrasound probe may be set aside in the sterile field.

12. The remaining steps are the same as steps 11–13 in the Middle (Triangle) Approach.

SUBCLAVIAN VEIN CATHETERIZATION

Indications

Subclavian vein catheterization is performed to gain venous access for monitoring of central venous pressure, mixed central venous oxygen saturation, insertion of a transvenous pacemaker, or administration of medications or intravenous fluids.

Contraindications

Contraindications to subclavian vein catheterization are as follows:

- Edema or other manifestations of superior vena cava obstruction on the proposed side of insertion.
- Previous surgery or irradiation to the subclavicular area.
- Bleeding diathesis.
- Infection or cellulitis over the proposed insertion site.
- Pneumothorax on the contralateral site.
- Uncooperative patient.
- Patient receiving CPR.

Relative Contraindications

Relative contraindications to subclavian vein catheterization are as follows:

- Assisted ventilation with high end-expiratory pressures.
- Mastectomy on the proposed side of insertion.
- Severe hypovolemia (eg, hemorrhagic shock).
- Recently discontinued subclavian line in the same area.

Personnel Required

Two people are usually required to perform percutaneous subclavian vein catheterization. The operator inserts the catheter and an assistant opens sterile equipment and helps to position the patient.

Equipment and Supplies Required

A. Materials

- Materials for skin sterilization.
- Materials for sterile technique (cap, mask, gloves, gown, and large sterile drape).

- Lidocaine, 1%, with 10-mL syringe and 22- and 25-gauge needles.
- Intravenous fluid with connector tubing.
- Central venous catheter and insertion set. Many kinds are commercially available; most consist of an introducing needle and a radiopaque catheter, usually 30.5-cm (12-inch) long.
- Tincture of benzoin.
- Tape (including precut lengths).
- Standard bath towel.

B. Prepackaged Sterile Central Venous Access Trays

Prepackaged sterile central venous access trays are commercially available. The following items are required:

- Drapes.
- Gauze sponges, 10×10 cm^2 (4×4 inch^2).
- Nylon or silk suture (size 3-0 or 4-0) on a cutting needle.
- Needle holder.
- Straight scissors.
- Syringe, 3 mL, with 22-gauge, 6.5-cm (2½-inch) needle for use as a probe (optional).

Positioning of the Patient

Proper positioning of the patient is crucial to successful subclavian vein catheterization. Place the patient in the Trendelenburg position at an angle of 30°, with the patient's head at a comfortable height for the operator. This position fully distends the subclavian vein and creates positive pressure inside the vein when the catheter is inserted, thus preventing air embolism.

Place the rolled bath towel between the patient's scapulas to allow the shoulders to fall backward and flatten the clavicles. Both arms should be at the patient's sides.

Anatomy Review

The subclavian vein courses under the clavicle near the subclavian artery and the apex of the lung (Figure 7–6). The artery is superior and deep to the vein. With a percutaneous approach, the vein is entered before the artery can be accidentally punctured. Laterally, the artery and vein drop caudally to enter the axilla.

Procedure

1. Make sure that all equipment is close at hand and ready for use. Assemble the container of intravenous fluid and tubing and flush the tubing with fluid to remove all air.

2. Position the patient.

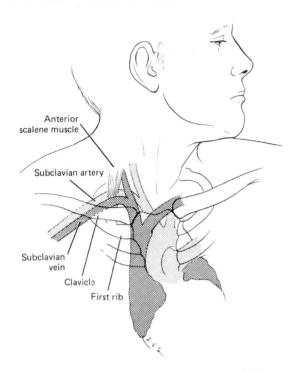

▲ **Figure 7–6.** Anatomic relationships of the subclavian vein.

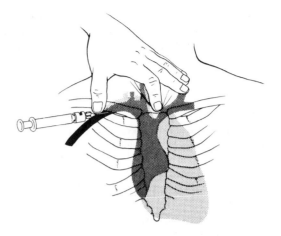

▲ **Figure 7–7.** Technique of subclavian vein catheterization. With the index finger in the suprasternal notch and the thumb marking the costoclavicular ligament, insert the needle just medial to the thumb.

3. Sterilize the skin over the insertion site from the lateral aspect of the clavicle to the ear to the suprasternal notch.

4. Unless the patient has a cervical spine injury, the head should be rotated away from the side of insertion, with the neck twisted as far as possible.

5. Observe sterile technique (don cap, mask, gloves, and gown).

6. Assemble the introducing needle and syringe and make sure that the catheter is close by and quickly available.

7. Drape the infraclavicular area.

8. Using the index finger, palpate inferior to the clavicle to find the costoclavicular ligament, which connects the clavicle and the first rib. This ligament lies where the clavicle bends posteriorly (about one-third the length of the clavicle from the suprasternal notch). Place the thumb between the clavicle and the first rib just lateral to this ligament and place the index finger in the suprasternal notch. The subclavian vein traverses the imaginary line connecting these two fingers (Figure 7–7).

9. Anesthetize the skin with the 1% lidocaine using the 10-mL syringe and the 25-gauge needle; then use the 22-gauge needle to anesthetize the subcutaneous tissue and the periosteum of the clavicle along the expected route of insertion (ie, the inferior border of the clavicle).

When anesthetizing, make sure that the needle is not in the vein (ie, that blood does not flow back when the plunger of the syringe is gently pulled back) before injecting lidocaine.

10. Reposition the index finger in the suprasternal notch and the thumb over the costoclavicular ligament. Place the catheter insertion needle or catheter-clad needle on the 3-mL syringe and insert the needle under the skin 3 cm (1¾₆ inch) caudal to the clavicle just medial to the thumb (see Figure 7–7). Insert the needle with the bevel facing up, so that its orientation can be maintained after it enters the vein. It may help to find the vein with a smaller needle (22-gauge, 6.5-cm [2½-inch] needle attached to a 3-mL syringe) before using the introducing needle.

11. Advance the needle at a 10–20° angle until it contacts the clavicle. Decrease the angle of the needle until the needle shaft is parallel to the patient's back and close to the correct alignment (pointing to the finger in the suprasternal notch). Push the needle slowly inferiorly along the clavicle until it reaches the inferior surface. Always keep the tip in contact with the clavicle and proceed slowly. When the inferior surface is reached, check the alignment of the needle with the suprasternal notch, and while pulling back on the plunger of the syringe, advance the needle toward the suprasternal notch, keeping the needle shaft parallel to the patient's back. When the needle enters the vein, venous blood will flow back into the syringe. If no blood flows out, slowly withdraw the needle while continuing to pull back on the plunger. Occasionally, blood will enter the syringe as the needle is being pulled out slowly.

12. If the first attempt fails, withdraw the needle completely and flush it with air to clean out any tissue from the needle lumen. This maneuver is important, because a second attempt at catheterization with an obstructed needle will also fail. Occasionally, directing the needle a little cephalad or a little deeper will locate the vein, but do not make misguided attempts in all directions, because of the danger of penetrating nearby structures such as the lung or the subclavian artery. Seek assistance if three or four attempts to locate the vein fail. If assistance is not obtainable, attempt catheterization on the other side (obtain a chest X-ray first to rule out pneumothorax) or insert an internal jugular venous catheter instead.

13. After the vein has been entered, rotate the needle so that the bevel faces caudally (toward the patient's feet) and make sure that there is free flow of blood. Occasionally, if the tip of the needle lies against the wall of the vein, blood will flow if the bevel is facing cephalad but not when the bevel is rotated. If this is the case, advance or withdraw the needle a short distance and check it again for blood flow.

14. When the needle is properly located in the lumen of the vein, hold it in place with the thumb and forefinger of one hand, remove the syringe, and immediately occlude the hub of the needle to prevent any air from entering the vein. (If a hypovolemic patient takes a deep breath just as the syringe is disconnected, air may be sucked into the vein, possibly causing air embolism.) If the needle is properly positioned, blood should flow freely from it.

15. The catheter can now be inserted using the Seldinger technique described earlier.

16. Evacuate the insertion syringe of all blood clots, attach it to the catheter hub, and withdraw some blood to make sure that the catheter is in the vein. The blood should flow freely. Remove the syringe. An assistant should then insert the intravenous tubing into the catheter hub and check for rapid flow.

17. Take the patient out of the Trendelenburg position.

18. Secure the catheter at the insertion site by placing the skin suture through the skin, tying it, and then looping it around the catheter three times and tying it again. Make sure that the lumen of the catheter is not constricted by the tie.

19. Cover the insertion site with a folded 10×10 cm^2 (4×4 inch^2) sterile gauze sponge and tape the sponge in place after applying tincture of benzoin to the skin to help secure the tape to the skin and the catheter.

20. Make sure that all connections are tight to prevent disconnection.

21. Obtain a chest X-ray immediately to check placement of the catheter and to detect possible pneumothorax.

▼ FEMORAL VEIN PHLEBOTOMY OR CATHETERIZATION

Femoral vein catheterization is an easy way to gain rapid access to the central venous system, for example, during CPR. Because infection is common at this site, the femoral vein should not be used for procedures requiring elective long-term venous access (eg, parenteral nutrition). Femoral vein phlebotomy is useful in patients in whom peripheral veins of the extremities are not palpable (eg, intravenous drug abusers). However, this route should not be used to obtain blood for culture.

▶ Indications

Femoral vein phlebotomy is used to obtain venous blood samples in patients in whom other sites cannot be used for venipuncture. Femoral vein catheterization is performed to gain central venous access.

▶ Contraindications

Contraindications to femoral vein phlebotomy or catheterization are as follows:

- Previous surgery in the groin.
- Prosthetic graft placement in the groin.
- Venous occlusive disease of the extremities.
- Acquired or congenital bleeding disorder.
- Cellulitis or burn over the proposed site of insertion.

▶ Personnel Required

One operator can perform femoral vein phlebotomy or catheterization unaided if the patient is cooperative, but it is helpful to have an assistant.

▶ Equipment and Supplies Required

A. Femoral Vein Phlebotomy

- Materials for skin cleansing.
- Syringe (20–30 mL) with 18- or 20-gauge needle.
- Gauze sponges, 5×5 cm^2 (2×2 inch^2).
- Specimen tubes for blood.
- Adhesive dressing.

B. Femoral Vein Catheterization

- Materials for skin sterilization.
- Materials for sterile technique (cap, mask, gloves, and gown).
- Lidocaine, 1%, with 10-mL syringe and 25-gauge needle.

- Catheter-clad needle (eg, Angiocath), 16–18-gauge and 12.5–20.5-cm (5–8-inch) long; or a central venous catheter kit.
- Container of intravenous infusion fluid with connecting tubing. All equipment should be flushed and fully assembled ready for use.
- Nylon or silk suture (size 3-0) on a cutting needle.
- Needle holder.
- Straight scissors.
- Drapes.
- Gauze sponges, 10×10 cm^2 (4×4 inch^2).
- Tape.

▶ Positioning of the Patient

The patient should be supine, with the leg externally rotated on the side selected for phlebotomy or catheterization.

▶ Anatomy Review

The femoral vein normally lies 1–2 cm (⅜–¾ inch) medial to the readily palpable femoral artery (Figure 7–8). In a patient without a palpable femoral pulse, the approximate position of the vein can be determined by dividing the distance from the anterior superior iliac spine to the pubic tubercle into three equal segments. The artery lies at the junction of the medial segment and the middle segment. The vein is about 1.5 cm (⅝ inch) medial to this point and to the artery.

▶ Procedure

A. Femoral Vein Phlebotomy

1. Cleanse the skin.
2. Locate the femoral artery with the nondominant hand.
3. Using the 20–30-mL syringe and the 18- or 22-gauge needle in the dominant hand, hold the needle at an angle of 90° to the long axis of the vein.
4. Insert the needle under the skin about 0.5 cm (³⁄₁₆ inch) medial to the artery and pull the plunger back gently to create a slight vacuum as the needle is advanced.
5. When the needle enters the vein, dark venous blood will flow back into the syringe. The blood should flow freely.
6. After obtaining the desired amount of blood, remove the needle quickly and apply direct pressure over the puncture site.
7. Fill the specimen tubes as described under Upper Extremity Venipuncture, above.

B. Femoral Vein Catheterization

1. Assemble all equipment and make sure that it is readily at hand.

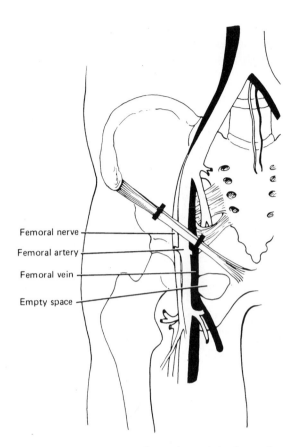

▲ **Figure 7–8.** Anatomic relationships of the femoral vein at the inguinal ligament.

Femoral nerve

Femoral artery

Femoral vein

Empty space

2. If necessary, shave the side of the groin chosen for insertion.
3. Observe sterile technique (don cap, mask, gloves, and gown).
4. Sterilize the skin around the groin and drape the area.
5. Locate the femoral artery. Infiltrate the skin 1.5 cm (⅝ inch) medial to the artery with the 1% lidocaine. Omit this step if the patient is comatose.
6. Using the catheter insertion needle attached to a syringe, insert the needle just under the skin and pull the plunger back gently to create a slight vacuum. Then advance the needle at an angle of 45° to the long axis of the vein; when the needle enters the vein, dark venous blood will flow back into the syringe. The blood should flow freely.
7. Advance the catheter into the vein. Once the catheter is in place, check to make certain that the blood flows freely. A central venous catheter could be inserted instead, using the Seldinger technique described earlier.

8. Obtain an X-ray immediately in order to check the position of the catheter.

9. If the femoral artery instead of the femoral vein is entered, brighter red blood will flow into the syringe under systemic arterial pressure. A patient in shock or cardiac arrest may have desaturated blood, with little arterial pressure, so that differentiation between arterial and venous puncture may be difficult. If the catheter is to be used solely for infusion of fluid or medication during emergency treatment (eg, CPR), temporary placement in the femoral artery is probably not harmful. If central venous access is required, withdraw the needle and catheter from the artery, maintain direct pressure over the area for 5 minutes, and then either try again on the same side or attempt catheterization on the opposite side.

▼ INTRAOSSEOUS INFUSION

▶ Indications

Intraosseous infusion (IO infusion) is an important vascular access route for both children and adults. It is performed when other techniques of venous cannulation have failed or would be too time consuming (eg, in the presence of cardiac arrest, trauma, shock). Complications are infrequent (0.6%) and consist mostly of osteomyelitis and infection in adjacent tissues.

▶ Site Selection

Several sites are suitable for infusion. In children the most commonly used site is the proximal tibia, just distal to the tibial tuberosity. Sites for IO line placement in adults include the proximal humerus, distal tibia, distal femur or sternum.

▶ Contraindications

Cutaneous infection or burn overlying the insertion site, previous attempt at IO placement in the extremity, fracture or major injury to the extremity proximal to the insertion site are contraindications.

▶ Personnel Required

One person can perform the procedure. An assistant is helpful.

▶ Equipment and Supplies Required

- Materials for skin sterilization.
- Lidocaine, 1%, with 5-mL syringe and 25-gauge needle.
- Sterile gloves.
- Short, large-bore bone marrow needle or 13–18-gauge Intraosseous infusion needles.

- 10-mL syringe.
- Intravenous infusion set, including sterile tubing and appropriate fluids for administration.
- Gauze sponges (eg, 10×10 cm^2 [4×4 inch^2]).
- Adhesive tape.

▶ Positioning of the Patient

The patient should be supine. If the proximal tibia is selected, the leg should be rotated slightly externally.

▶ Anatomy Review

The ideal insertion site on the tibia lies 1–2 cm distal to the tibial tuberosity on the anterior medial surface. On the femur it is 2–3 cm proximal to the lateral epicondyle in the midline.

▶ Procedure

1. Sterilize the skin.

2. Using sterile technique, locate the desired insertion site and infiltrate the skin with 1% lidocaine over a 2–3-cm area. Lidocaine should also be infiltrated along the anticipated course of insertion, down to and including the periosteum. For patients that are unconscious or obtunded, no local anesthetic is needed.

3. Using the bone marrow needle or intraosseous infusion needle, penetrate the skin perpendicularly. Advance the needle toward the bone at a 6° angle (directed away from the growth plate, caudal at the tibia, and rostral at the femur).

4. Use firm pressure to penetrate the cortex, employing a rotating or twisting motion. Upon entry into the marrow space, a sudden "give" will be felt. *Caution*: Errant placement of the needle can cause injury to the growth plate with resultant growth deformity.

5. Remove the trocar from the needle and attach a 10-mL syringe. Aspiration of blood and marrow contents confirms needle-tip placement in the marrow.

6. Connect a fluid-filled syringe or intravenous tubing to the needle and infuse under pressure.

7. Apply gauze 10×10 cm^2 (4×4 inch^2) sponges (cut midway) against the skin at the entry site, surrounding the needle. Occasionally, deep penetration of the needle through the bone cortex on the opposite side can occur, with delivery of infusion into surrounding tissue spaces. This can also occur if the needle becomes dislodged and withdrawn from its intramedullary position; tape the needle firmly in place. (Commercially available intraosseous infusion needles may have a lip to which tape can be attached or a screw mechanism, for securing the needle to the skin surface.)

▼ RADIAL ARTERY PUNCTURE: FOR BLOOD GAS AND pH ANALYSIS

▶ Indications

Indications for radial artery punctures are as follows:

- Need to obtain arterial blood for blood gas and pH determinations.
- Need to perform phlebotomy when other sites are inaccessible.

▶ Contraindications

Contraindications to radial artery puncture are as follows:

- Positive Allen test (see below), indicating that only one artery supplies the hand.
- Absence of palpable radial artery pulse.
- Cellulitis or other infection over the radial artery.
- Coagulation defects (relative contraindication).

▶ Personnel Required

One person can perform radial artery puncture unaided, but it is helpful to have an assistant to maintain pressure over the puncture site while the operator prepares the sample for transport to the laboratory.

▶ Equipment and Supplies Required

- Materials for skin cleansing.
- Lidocaine, 1%, with 5-mL syringe and 23–25-gauge, 1.5-cm (½-inch) needle.
- Heparinized syringe, 3–5 mL, preferably of glass or of siliconized plastic made especially for arterial blood sampling. To heparinize the syringe, aspirate 0.5 mL of heparin (100–1000 units/mL) into the syringe, hold the syringe upright, pull the plunger all the way out to the end, and then return all of the heparin to the original container. This procedure ensures that a small amount of heparin is in the tip of the syringe and needle hub that is adequate to heparinize the arterial blood gas sample but is not enough to affect the accuracy of blood gas determinations.
- Needle for arterial puncture, 23–25 gauge (depending on the size of the artery), 1.5-cm (½-inch) long.
- Ice for transport.

▶ Positioning of the Patient

The patient should be in a comfortable position, either supine or sitting. If respiratory difficulties require that the patient sit upright, the upper extremity selected should be extended on a stable surface such as a bedside table or on the side of the bed. The arm should be positioned with the volar side up.

▶ Anatomy Review

The radial artery runs along the lateral aspect of the volar forearm deep to the superficial fascia. The artery runs between the styloid process of the radius and the flexor carpi radialis tendon. The point of maximum pulsation of the radial artery can usually be palpated just proximal to the wrist.

▶ Allen Test

The Allen test should be performed to confirm the patency of the ulnar artery before any attempt is made to obtain a blood sample from the radial artery.

While the patient is elevating the arm and making a tight fist, occlude both radial and ulnar arterial flow with firm pressure over both the radial and the ulnar aspects of the volar forearm just proximal to the wrist. Allow a few minutes for the blood to drain from the hand and then lower the arm to waist level and have the patient open the hand. Release the pressure on the ulnar artery while keeping the radial artery occluded. Normal skin color should return to the ulnar side of the palm in 1–2 seconds, followed by quick restoration of normal color to the entire palm. A hand that remains white indicates either absence or occlusion of the ulnar artery, in which case radial artery puncture is contraindicated. Failure to perform this test may result in a gangrenous finger or loss of the hand from a spasm or clotting of the radial artery where there is no collateral flow through the ulnar artery.

▶ Procedure

1. Palpate the radial artery just proximal to the wrist and determine where the pulse is most prominent.

2. Locate the approximate position of the artery under the pad of the index finger by slowly rolling the finger from side to side. This maneuver causes the pulse to become alternately stronger and weaker and further helps to locate the relatively small artery.

3. Cleanse the skin over the proposed site of puncture.

4. Anesthetize the skin over the proposed site of puncture with 1% lidocaine using the 3–5-mL syringe and 23–25-gauge needle.

5. Using the index and middle fingers of the nondominant hand, identify again the point of maximal pulsation of the radial artery (Figure 7–9).

6. Attach the 23–25-gauge needle to the heparinized syringe, and holding the needle perpendicular to the arm, insert the needle into the skin in the anesthetized area. The smaller the needle, the less the risk of injury to the artery and the less painful the procedure to the patient.

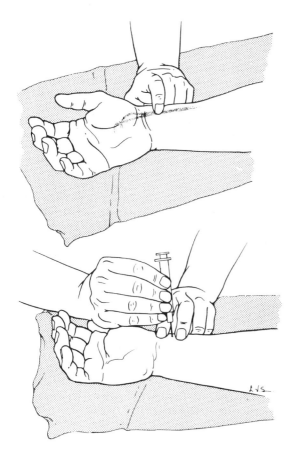

▲ **Figure 7–9.** Technique of radial artery puncture. The index and middle fingers are used to identify the point of maximum pulsation.

7. Guide the needle toward the point of maximum pulsation and watch for a sudden gush of arterial blood into the hub of the needle or the lower part of the syringe. Once the needle has entered the lumen of the radial artery, the force of arterial pulsation should fill the syringe if it is specially designed for arterial puncture (glass or siliconized plastic). If an ordinary plastic syringe is used, a small amount of suction may be required to obtain an adequate blood sample (only 1–2 mL of blood is required for blood gas and pH analysis).

8. If no blood is obtained with these maneuvers, it is possible that the needle has completely passed through the radial artery. Advance the needle until it meets the periosteum of the radius. Slowly withdraw the syringe and needle and look for the gush of arterial blood into the hub of the needle.

9. If this attempt is still unsuccessful, withdraw the needle to a position just under the skin, move it 1 mm (¹⁄₁₆ inch) to either side of the previous attempt, and try again.

Make at least three attempts before giving up and trying another site or seeking assistance.

10. Remove the needle from the artery with a smooth, swift motion and apply immediate direct pressure over the puncture site for 10 minutes. An assistant is helpful to apply pressure on the artery.

11. Evacuate all air bubbles from the sample by holding the syringe upright and allowing the bubbles to collect near the needle hub. Gently tapping the syringe with the end of a finger will help dislodge bubbles from the walls of the syringe. Once all of the air has been confined to the tip of the syringe, evacuate it by pushing on the plunger. Then, cap the needle with a rubber stopper, label the tube with the patient's name and number, and place the sample on ice for transport to the laboratory.

12. Return in 15 minutes and check for adequate per-fusion of the hand and for possible hematoma formation in the patient's wrist.

DIRECT LARYNGOSCOPY, OROTRACHEAL INTUBATION, AND NASOTRACHEAL INTUBATION

Please see Chapter 8 for a complete discussion of airway management.

▶ Indications

A. Orotracheal Intubation

Indications for orotracheal intubation area as follows:

- Inadequate oxygenation (eg, decreased arterial Po_2) that is not corrected by supplemental oxygen supplied by mask or nasal cannula.

- Inadequate ventilation (increased arterial Pco_2).

- Need to control and remove pulmonary secretions (bronchial toilet).

- Need to provide airway protection in an obtunded patient or a patient with a depressed gag reflex.

- Need to perform urgent or emergency diagnostic studies in a multiple injured or intoxicated patient or in an uncooperative patient with head injury.

B. Nasotracheal Intubation

Nasotracheal intubation is used less frequently than orotracheal intubation. It is mainly used when access to the trachea through the oropharynx is difficult and emergency cricothyrotomy is not indicated. The advantages of nasotracheal intubation are greater comfort for the patient and greater ease in communicating with the intubated patient through lip reading. Disadvantages include need for a smaller airway, which results in increased airway resistance; need for a more skilled operator, because the tube is usually inserted without direct vision; possible bleeding caused by passage of the nasotracheal tube through the nasopharynx; and sinusitis that may result owing to obstruction of the ostia of the sinuses.

▶ Contraindications

The following are only relative contraindications to tracheal intubation:

- Severe airway trauma or obstruction that does not permit safe passage of an endotracheal tube. Emergency cricothyrotomy is indicated in such cases.

- Cervical spine injury is no longer considered a contraindication to intubation. Rapid sequence induction followed by orotracheal intubation optimizes intubating conditions and with careful maintenance of in-line cervical immobilization has not been shown to lead to iatrogenic cervical spinal cord injury.

- Nasotracheal intubation is still performed by those with significant experience with the technique but is contraindicated in the apneic patient.

▶ Personnel Required

One person can perform direct laryngoscopy or tracheal intubation unaided in nontrauma patients. An assistant is required to maintain cervical spine immobilization for any patient who has a history of blunt trauma and requires intubation.

▶ Equipment and Supplies Required

- Self-refilling bag-valve-mask combination (eg, Ambu bag) or bag-valve unit (Ayres bag), connector, tubing, end-tidal CO_2 ($ETCO_2$) detector, and oxygen source. Assemble all items before attempting intubation.

- Laryngoscope with curved and straight blades of a size appropriate for the patient.

- Endotracheal tubes of several different sizes (Table 7–1). Low-pressure, high-flow cuffed balloons are preferred. Tracheal tubes used in nasotracheal intubation should be smaller than those used for orotracheal intubation.

- Oral and nasal airways.

- Tincture of benzoin and precut tape.

- Introducer (stylets or Magill forceps).

- Suction apparatus (tonsil tip and catheter suction).

- Syringe, 10 mL, to inflate the cuff.

- Mucosal anesthetics and astringents (eg, 1% lidocaine jelly and phenylephrine nasal spray).

- Water-soluble sterile lubricant.

Table 7–1. Guidelines for Endotracheal Tube Selection.

Age	Orotracheal Tube[a]	Nasotracheal Tube
Premature	2.0	Not applicable
Term	2.5	Not applicable
3–18 months	3–4	Not applicable
1½–3 years	4–5	Not applicable
3–5 years	5–6	5
5–7 years	6–6.5	5–6
8–14 years	7–8	6–7
Over 14 years		
Female	7–8	7
Male	7–9	7–8

[a]Inside diameter in millimeters.

▶ Positioning of the Patient

Unless contraindicated as in the trauma patient, the sniffing position—patient supine, with the neck extended, the occiput elevated, and the head tilted backward—permits visualization of the glottis and vocal cords and allows passage of the endotracheal tube. A towel rolled under the head usually makes it easier for the patient to maintain this position.

In infants younger than 1 month, the head and neck should be in a neutral position.

▶ Procedure

A. Mask Ventilation

Oxygen is delivered with a face mask at a rate of 10–15 L/min.

1. Select the proper-sized mask; it should cover the mouth and nose and fit snugly against the cheeks.

2. Place the nontrauma patient in the sniffing position.

3. Place the mask over the patient's mouth and nose with the right hand.

4. With the left hand, place the small and ring fingers under the patient's mandible and lift up to open the airway. Grasp the mask with the thumb and index finger and press it to the patient's face while lifting the mandible with the ring and small fingers.

5. Compress the bag with the right hand.

6. The chest should rise with each breath and airflow should be unimpeded. If not, reposition the mask and try again. Occasionally, insertion of an oral or nasal airway facilitates ventilation by mask. Because of the lack of support for the lips, elderly edentulous patients may be especially hard to ventilate using a mask.

B. Topical Anesthesia

Anesthetize the mucosa of the nose, oropharynx, and upper airway with cocaine, 4%, or lidocaine, 2%, if time permits and the patient is awake.

C. Direct Laryngoscopy

1. Place the patient in the sniffing position.

2. Check the laryngoscope and blade for proper fit and make sure that the light works.

3. Make sure that all materials are assembled and close at hand.

4. Curved blade technique: (1) Open the patient's mouth with the right hand and remove any dentures. (2) Grasp the laryngoscope in the left hand (Figure 7–10). (3) Spread the patient's lips and insert the blade between the teeth, being careful not to traumatize the teeth. (4) Pass the blade to the right of the tongue and advance the blade into the hypopharynx, pushing the tongue to the left and placing the tip of the blade into the vallecula. (5) Lift the laryngoscope upward and forward, without changing the angle of the blade, to expose the vocal cords.

5. Straight blade technique: Follow the steps outlined for curved blade technique, but advance the blade down the hypopharynx, and lift the epiglottis with the tip of the blade to expose the vocal cords. The tip of the laryngoscope blade fits below the epiglottis, which is no longer visible with the blade in position.

D. Orotracheal Intubation

1. Select the proper-sized tube (see Table 7–1). Most adult men take an endotracheal tube that has an inside diameter of 8–9 mm. Most adult women take an endotracheal tube that has 7–8-mm internal diameter. For children, a general rule is that the external diameter of the tube is equal to the diameter of the child's fifth digit fingernail. The formula ¼ age + 4 = endotracheal tube size is also very helpful in determining the proper tube size in children older than 1 year.

2. With the 10-mL syringe, inflate the balloon with 5–8 mL of air. Make sure that the balloon is functional and intact.

3. Lubricate the end of the tube (optional).

4. Insert the stylet and bend the tube and stylet gently into a crescent shape so that the tip of the stylet is at least 1 cm (⅜ inch) proximal to the end of the orotracheal tube.

5. Be sure that the syringe and the bag-valve combination are within easy reach.

6. If the patient is already hypoxic, ventilate the patient with the bag-valve combination with 100% oxygen until the pulse oximetry saturation increases into the 90% range.

7. Open the patient's mouth, remove dentures, and suction secretions or vomitus from the mouth.

8. Visualize the glottis and vocal cords and, by direct laryngoscopy, gently pass the tube through the vocal cords into the trachea. Occasionally, having an assistant press posteriorly on the anterior neck at the level of the cricoid cartilage will often help to bring an anteriorly placed larynx into view and facilitate intubation. This is known as the Sellick maneuver; it also helps reduce reflux of gastric contents into the hypopharynx.

9. Gently pass the tube next to the laryngoscope blade, through the vocal cords, and far enough so that the balloon is just beyond the cords.

10. Withdraw the stylet and inflate the cuff.

11. Connect the bag-valve combination and $ETCO_2$ detector and begin ventilation with 100% oxygen.

12. Confirm the tube is properly positioned by several methods. $ETCO_2$ detector color change confirms endotracheal intubation in the patient with spontaneous circulation but the color may not change in patients who have had cardiac arrest. Next, it is important to use auscultation to confirm appropriate placement. First, listen over the stomach with a stethoscope while ventilating the patient. If sounds of airflow are heard or if distention of the stomach occurs, the tube is in the esophagus. If the esophagus has been intubated instead of the trachea, remove the tube, ventilate the patient with a mask, and try again.

    Next, listen to each side of the chest, including the axilla, to be sure that the breath sounds are equal. If the left chest has more distant breath sounds than the right chest, try withdrawing the tube 1–2 cm (⅜–¾ inch) and ventilating again. This maneuver helps to correct intubation of the right main-stem bronchus as a cause of unequal ventilation. Airway anatomy makes intubation of the right main-stem bronchus more likely than intubation of the left. When breath sounds are equal on both sides and the thorax rises equally on both sides with each inspiration, note the position of the tube (eg, mark the tube at the patient's mouth).

13. Secure the tube in place with tracheostomy ribbon or tape.

14. Obtain a chest X-ray immediately to check tube placement.

15. Obtain arterial blood gas measurements to assess the adequacy of ventilation.

E. Nasotracheal Intubation

1. (Steps 1–6 are the same as those for orotracheal intubation, except that no stylet is needed. The tube must be

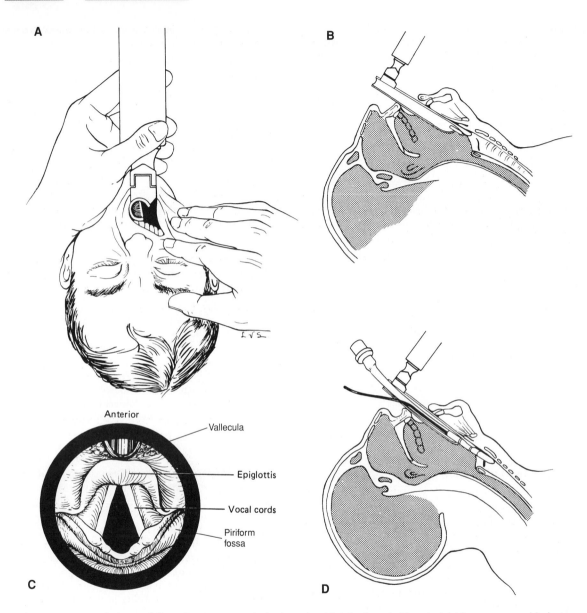

A

B

Anterior

Vallecula

Epiglottis

Vocal cords

Piriform fossa

C

D

▲ **Figure 7–10.** Technique of direct laryngoscopy and orotracheal intubation. **A:** The straight laryngoscope blade is passed behind the tongue and deep to the tip of the epiglottis. **B:** Lateral view showing straight laryngoscope blade deep to the tip of the epiglottis exposing glottic opening. **C:** View of glottis as seen through a laryngoscope with a curved blade. **D:** Insertion of endotracheal tube. (Parts A, B, and D reproduced, with permission, from Way LW (editor): *Current Surgical Diagnosis & Treatment*, 3rd ed. Lange, 1977. Part C reproduced, with permission, from Kempe CH, Silver HK, O'Brien D (editors): *Current Pediatric Diagnosis & Treatment*, 4th ed. Lange, 1976.)

checked and lubricated and all materials must be readily at hand.) Examine the patient's nose and determine if one nasal passage is larger than the other. If no difference is noted, use the left naris to better align the bevel of the endotracheal tube with the vocal cords. Insert the

lubricated nasotracheal tube in the external naris and pass it directly posteriorly until it meets the floor of the nasopharynx. The technique is similar to that used to pass a nasogastric tube (see Nasogastric Intubation, below).

2. Make sure that the natural bend in the tube (without the stylet in place) corresponds to the direction of passage, and with gentle, steady pressure, continue to advance the nasotracheal tube into the posterior pharynx. At this point, the tube may meet with obstruction. If the tube fails to pass into the posterior pharynx under gentle, steady pressure, withdraw the tube and attempt insertion in the opposite nostril.

3. Once the nasotracheal tube is in the pharynx, the patient's head may be flexed by lifting the occiput if no concern for cervical spine injury exists. This helps to guide the tube through the vocal cords anteriorly into the larynx. The patient may start to cough when the tube passes through the vocal cords.

4. If the patient is breathing spontaneously, listen at the external end of the tube. If the tube is properly positioned over the larynx, air should be heard coming in and out of the tube. If no air is heard, the tube has slipped posteriorly and is in the esophagus. Using the nonintubating hand, place the index finger and thumb on each side of the larynx. This allows for external palpation of the endotracheal tube if it deviates to either piriform fossa. Using the digits flanking the trachea, manually deviate the trachea toward the intubated nares to facilitate better alignment and allow for easier intubation.

5. When ventilation is heard, steady the patient's head in that position, and when inspiration begins, advance the tube into the trachea.

6. Once the tube is in the trachea, inflate the balloon and listen again to make sure that air is coming from the nasotracheal tube, and look at the tube to see the condensation of water vapor with exhalation.

7. Have an assistant steady the nasotracheal tube. Connect an air reservoir bag (eg, Ayers or Ambu bag) and $ETCO_2$ detector to the tube, ventilate the patient, and check for elevation of both sides of the chest on inspiration and the presence of breath sounds at each axilla in addition to color change on the $ETCO_2$ detector. As with orotracheal intubation, inadvertent intubation of the right main-stem bronchus (with poor ventilation of the left lung) occurs more commonly than intubation of the left bronchus.

8. When proper positioning of the tube in the trachea has been achieved, secure the tube in place with tracheostomy ribbon or tape. Make sure that there is no pressure on the external naris that might cause necrosis.

F. Removal of the Endotracheal Tube

1. Ventilate the patient with a bag-valve combination for 1–2 minutes with 100% oxygen.

2. Suction the patient's trachea, mouth, and hypopharynx before removing the tube.

3. Deflate the cuff by withdrawing all air with the 10-mL syringe.

4. Have the patient take a deep breath and remove the tube at the midpoint of expiration.

5. Suction the patient's mouth a second time to remove any remaining secretions.

6. Begin oxygen, 5 L/min, by mask.

NASOGASTRIC INTUBATION: FOR GASTRIC EVACUATION OR LAVAGE

▶ Indications

Indications for nasogastric intubation are as follows:

- Need to suppress vomiting caused by gastric distention or paralytic ileus.
- Need to perform gastric lavage (therapeutic or diagnostic).
- Need to perform gastric decompression.
- Need to perform gastric evacuation.

▶ Contraindications

Important contraindications to nasogastric intubation are as follows:

- Choanal atresia.
- Massive facial trauma or basilar skull fracture.
- Esophageal atresia or stricture.
- Ingestion of a caustic substance (eg, acid, lye), unless nasogastric intubation can be performed under direct vision.

Relative contraindications to nasogastric intubation are as follows:

- Recent gastric or esophageal surgery.
- Recent oropharyngeal or nasal surgery.
- Esophageal stricture.
- Esophageal burn.
- Zenker diverticulum.

▶ Personnel Required

One person can perform nasogastric intubation unaided, but an assistant is helpful.

▶ Equipment and Supplies Required

- Nasogastric tube of the proper diameter. There are two main types of tubes: straight suction tubes and sump suction tubes (with two lumens). The sump tube is less likely to be sucked against the stomach wall and become plugged. The only disadvantage is that because of the second air-inlet port, it has a slightly smaller lumen for suction than does a similarly sized straight suction tube. Most adults require a 16–18F sump tube. The limiting factor is the size of the naris. Children usually require a 10F nasogastric tube and infants an 8F tube. (Nasogastric size can be estimated by multiplying endotracheal tube size by 2.)

- Lubricant.
- Suction syringe with catheter tip.
- Connector (usually supplied with the nasogastric tube).
- Suction tube and suction device (wall suction, intermittent wall suction, or portable intermittent suction).
- Phenylephrine nasal spray, 0.5%, and benzocaine–tetracaine spray.
- Tincture of benzoin.
- Tape.

▶ Positioning of the Patient

The patient should be in a comfortable, supported sitting position. Unconscious patients should either be supine and flat or supine with the head slightly elevated. Children or unusually overreactive adults may be asked to sit on their hands as a reminder to keep them away from the nose and the tube as it is being passed into the stomach.

▶ Procedure

1. Explain exactly what the steps of the procedure will be and explain the need for the patient's help at certain points.

2. Determine the length of tubing necessary by measuring the distance between the ear and the umbilicus.

3. Lubricate the end of the tube with lubricant.

4. Apply 0.5% phenylephrine nasal spray to both nostrils to prevent epistaxis. If intractable gagging is a problem, benzocaine–tetracaine spray applied to the pharynx will help.

5. Insert the tube into the nostril at a 60–90° angle to the plane of the face and advance it straight back until it meets resistance (the patient usually signs when this happens).

6. Using the gentle pressure and pushing posteriorly and perpendicularly to the long axis of the head, advance the tip of the tube inferiorly and into the nasopharynx (Figure 7–11).

7. Have the patient take a small sip of water through the straw and hold it in the mouth without swallowing. Then have the patient swallow, and advance the tube into the esophagus simultaneously. If this maneuver is successful, the patient will gag. If it fails and the tube slips into the trachea, violent coughing will usually

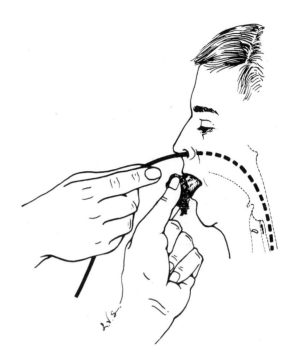

▲ **Figure 7-11.** Technique of nasogastric intubation.

ensue. Withdraw the tube into the oropharynx, and try again. The most important step is timing the advancement of the tube to coincide with the swallow. Patients with an altered sensorium sometimes tolerate tracheal intubation without any reflex coughing. The tube is improperly positioned if air exchange is heard.

8. When the tube is in the esophagus, advance it into the stomach. In adults, the tube is usually in the stomach when it is advanced to the next-to-the-last mark on the sump tube.

9. Once the nasogastric tube is in the stomach, withdraw some gastric fluid, and with a suction syringe inject air down the tube while listening over the left upper quadrant for the sound of air leaving the tube and bubbling in the stomach. If no sound is heard, reposition the tube and inject more air. If several attempts fail, check to make sure that the tube is not in the trachea or curled in the patient's mouth. Obtain a chest X-ray to check the position of the tube. Injecting a small amount of water-soluble contrast medium down the tube and visualizing its position with fluoroscopy or standard X-ray is the definitive confirmatory procedure. Never assume that the tube is in the correct position without performing some confirming maneuver. Nasogastric tubes have been left in the peripheral lung, cranial vault, extraesophageal mediastinum, and peritoneal cavity.

10. Apply tincture of benzoin to the nose before securing the tube to the nose with tape, and make sure that

the tube does not exert pressure on the external naris, which can result in pressure necrosis and sloughing of the naris.

▶ Special Problems

A. Intubated Patients

Inserting a nasogastric tube in an intubated patient can be difficult. Follow the steps outlined above, and remember to deflate the cuff of the endotracheal tube if the nasogastric tube becomes stuck in the upper esophagus. In an unresponsive intubated patient, it may occasionally be necessary to use Magill forceps and a laryngoscope to advance the tube into the esophagus under direct vision.

B. Comatose Patients

A comatose or obtunded patient cannot swallow at the right time to facilitate passage of the tube. The natural bend of the tube as it passes into the pharynx from the naris is anterior; the tube therefore tends to enter the trachea. Any one of the following maneuvers may be helpful (they should be performed in the order given here):

1. Flex the patient's head when passing the tube. Make sure the patient does not have a cervical spine injury if this is attempted in the emergency department.
2. After the tube passes into the hypopharynx, rotate the tube to direct the natural curve posteriorly and continue to advance it.
3. Pass the tube through the nostril and into the nasopharynx and insert a finger into the patient's mouth to manually guide the tube posteriorly into the esophagus.
4. Use a laryngoscope and Magill forceps to pass the tube into the esophagus under direct vision.

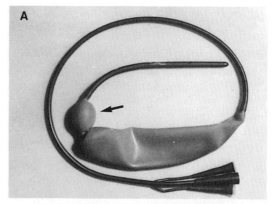

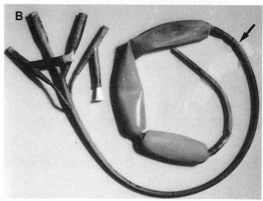

▲ **Figure 7–12.** Balloon tamponade for bleeding varices. **A:** The Sengstaken–Blakemore tube has a small gastric balloon (arrow) that can be inflated to 250 mL with air. **B:** The four-lumen Minnesota tube has a much larger gastric balloon that inflates to 450 mL and a series of aspirating ports (arrow) for removing secretions above the esophageal balloon.

▼ INSERTION OF SENGSTAKEN–BLAKEMORE OR MINNESOTA TUBE

Minnesota and Sengstaken–Blakemore tubes (Figure 7–12) are used to temporarily control hemorrhage from esophageal varices and the esophagogastric junction. The Sengstaken–Blakemore tube is a triple-lumen rubber tube with two balloons: One that is inflated in the lumen of the stomach and pressed against the esophagogastric junction and one that is inflated in the lumen of the esophagus to press directly against the varices. Two of the lumens are used to inflate the balloons; the third opens into a port on the distal tip of the tube and is used to irrigate and drain the stomach.

The Minnesota tube is currently preferable to the other tubes that are available. This tube has four lumens: two for filling the balloons, one that permits aspiration of gastric contents, and a fourth to aspirate the esophagus above the balloon. If a tube without an esophageal port is used (eg, a Sengstaken–Blakemore tube), a naso-gastric tube must be tied to the Sengstaken–Blakemore tube just above the esophageal balloon in order to remove secretions collecting there.

Effective use of the Sengstaken–Blakemore or Minnesota tube requires close attention to the pressure in each balloon and monitoring for continued bleeding from the esophagogastric varices (blood aspirated through the gastric aspiration port of the Sengstaken–Blakemore tube or above the esophageal balloon through a nasogastric tube or the esophageal port of the Minnesota tube). Proper insertion will also ensure that the gastric balloon is not inflated in the esophagus, which may lead to esophageal rupture.

With either tube, most patients require orotracheal or nasotracheal intubation first to protect the airway before balloon tamponade is attempted. Intubation must always be done in comatose patients.

Indications

Indications for insertion of a Sengstaken–Blakemore or Minnesota tube are as follows:

- Need to control massive upper gastrointestinal tract hemorrhage presumed to result from esophageal varices in a patient with hypovolemic shock.

- Need to control documented esophagovariceal hemorrhage in a patient with or without hemodynamic compromise.

Contraindications

Insertion of a Sengstaken–Blakemore or Minnesota tube is contraindicated in patients who have undergone previous gastroesophageal surgery.

Personnel Required

The operator will require an assistant.

Equipment and Supplies Required

- Sengstaken–Blakemore tube or Minnesota tube.
- No. 18 Salem sump tube if Sengstaken–Blakemore tube is used.
- Constant or intermittent wall or portable suction device.
- Mercury manometer or aneroid pressure gauge.
- Y connector.
- Rubber-clad clamps (3).
- Water-soluble lubricating jelly.
- Cocaine spray, 4%.
- Glass of water and a straw.
- Manometer-grade rubber tubing, 0.6–1 m (2–3 feet).
- Irrigating syringe (50 mL), water, basin.
- Football helmet with a face mask, if available.
- Sponge rubber to act as cuff around the tube.

Positioning of the Patient

The patient should be supine, with the head of the bed elevated 30–45° if possible. It is difficult to insert the tube with the patient in the Trendelenburg position.

Anatomy Review

Esophageal varices result from portal hypertension. When the distal esophageal veins become distended, they become susceptible to erosion and the overlying mucosa becomes thinner. Mechanical or chemical (reflux of gastric acid) irritation may rupture the varices, causing hemorrhage.

Procedure

1. Protect the airway. In stuporous patients or those with a diminished gag reflex, endotracheal intubation should be performed before passage of a Minnesota or Sengstaken–Blakemore tube.

2. Inflate the balloons to test for air leaks and lubricate the distal end of the tube and balloons.

3. Make sure that all necessary equipment is readily at hand.

4. Deflate the balloons completely.

5. Anesthetize the patient's nasal passages, pharynx, and hypopharynx with the 4% cocaine spray or benzocaine–tetracaine spray and wait for 2–3 minutes.

6. Pass the tube through one nostril with steady pressure until the tip of the tube is in the posterior pharynx.

7. Advance the tube into the esophagus as the patient swallows.

8. Advance the tube to at least the 50-cm mark. (In the typical adult, the tube should be in the stomach at this point.)

9. Fill the irrigating syringe with air and listen over the patient's stomach with a stethoscope while injecting air through the gastric aspiration port. If the tube is properly positioned, a gurgling sound will be heard in the stomach as air escapes from the tube. If no air is heard, withdraw the tube and insert it again. Do not inflate either balloon until the tube is known to be in the stomach.

10. When proper placement of the tube in the stomach has been confirmed, inflate the gastric balloon with air (250–275 mL for the Sengstaken–Blakemore tube; 450–500 mL for the Minnesota tube) and clamp the gastric balloon port with a rubber-clad clamp. If the patient develops substernal pain while the gastric balloon is being inflated, the balloon may be in the esophagus. Stop immediately, deflate the balloon, and push the tube farther into the stomach before attempting reinflation of the gastric balloon.

11. Pull back on the tube until resistance is felt, showing that tamponade of the gastroesophageal junction has been achieved. Secure the tube with a minimum of tension (about 0.45 kg [1 lb]) by taping a cuff of sponge rubber to the tube just distal to the patient's nostril.

12. Construct a pressure-reading mechanism by connecting the esophageal balloon port to a Y connector. Use part of the manometer-grade rubber tubing if needed. Connect the manometer or aneroid pressure gauge to one port of the Y connector and an inflating bulb of the 50-mL syringe to the other.

13. If inflation of the gastric balloon fails to stop the bleeding, inflate the esophageal balloon to 35–50 mm Hg of pressure, using manometer control. Use the lowest pressure possible that will control hemorrhage.

14. Aspirate through the gastric port of the tube and evacuate the stomach of all blood and water. Irrigate and aspirate the stomach, if necessary, to completely evacuate all contents.

15. Continue gastric lavage for 30 minutes and check for bright red blood. If bleeding continues, increase the esophageal balloon pressure by 5-mm Hg increments. Continue lavage to determine the exact pressure at which bleeding stops. Occlude the esophageal and gastric ports with a rubber-clad clamp proximal to the Y connector.

16. Record the pressures in the gastric and esophageal balloons, and transport the patient to an intensive care unit with one-on-one nursing.

17. Obtain a portable chest X-ray and abdominal film immediately to check for proper placement of the tube.

18. If a football helmet is available, secure the tube to the face mask instead of using pressure against the nostril to hold the tube in place.

19. If a Sengstaken–Blakemore tube is being used, pass a standard nasogastric Salem sump tube through the other nostril to evacuate all secretions that accumulate above the esophageal balloon. If a Minnesota tube is being used, attach the esophageal port to a suction device set to intermittent high suction.

20. If the patient is comatose and the tube cannot be passed through the nose, insert it through the mouth and guide it into the esophagus with a finger. An alternative is to use direct laryngoscopy and Magill forceps to guide the tube into the esophagus. Be careful not to puncture the balloon with the forceps.

21. Secure the tube as shown in Figure 7–13.

22. The pressure in both balloons should be checked every 30 minutes by releasing the rubber-clad clamps on the tube proximal to the Y connector while the tube used for inflation is occluded. This connects the balloon to the manometer for pressure measurement, and air leaks in the balloon can be quickly detected before bleeding recurs. Periodically irrigate and aspirate through the gastric port and through the esophageal port (Minnesota tube) or Salem sump tube (Sengstaken–Blakemore tube) to make sure that no gastric or esophageal bleeding goes undetected.

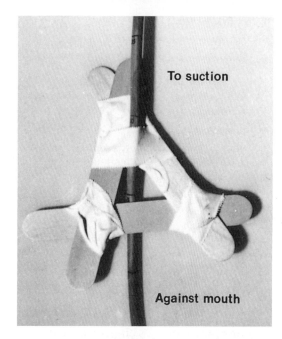

▲ **Figure 7–13.** Securing tamponade tube using crossed tongue blades. The insertion tube is secured to the corner of the mouth as shown. Foam or gauze may be placed between the triangle and the patient's mouth to prevent damage to gingival mucosa.

contraindications. The procedure should not be performed in children younger than 12 years. Transtracheal jet ventilation (TTJV, also known as needle cricothyrotomy) is the preferred method for this age group.

▶ Contraindications

Cricothyrotomy is contraindicated when any other less radical means of securing an airway is feasible.

▶ Personnel Required

One person can perform cricothyrotomy unaided, but an assistant is helpful.

▶ Equipment and Supplies Required

Because cricothyrotomy is almost always performed when speed is essential to save the patient's life, presterilized kits containing the required materials should be available in all hospital emergency departments. The following items are required:

- Materials for skin sterilization.
- Materials for sterile technique (cap, mask, gloves, and gown).

▼ CRICOTHYROTOMY

▶ Indications

Cricothyrotomy is performed when the airway must be secured or maintained and when attempts at orotracheal or nasotracheal intubation have failed. Transections or fracture of the trachea, larynx, or cricoid cartilage are

- Lidocaine, 1%, with 10-mL syringe and 25-gauge needle.
- Sponges, 10×10 cm^2 (4×4 inch^2).
- Drapes and rolled bath towel.
- No. 11 scalpel blade, mounted.
- Mosquito clamps (2).
- Kelly clamps (2).
- Self-retaining skin retractors.
- Low-pressure, high-flow orotracheal tube sized to the patient (usually a small [4–6-mm] tube is used to fit the small opening) or, if available, low-pressure cuffed tracheostomy tubes of various sizes.
- Syringe, 10 mL, to inflate the balloon on the orotracheal tube.
- Self-refilling bag-valve-mask combination (eg, Ambu bag) or bag-valve unit (eg, Ayres bag), connector, tubing, and oxygen source.
- Tincture of benzoin.
- Tape.

▶ Positioning of the Patient

The patient should be supine, with a rolled bath towel under the shoulders, and the neck hyperextended.

▶ Anatomy Review

The cricothyroid membrane (conus elasticus and cricothyroid ligament) lies between the thyroid cartilage superiorly and the cricoid cartilage inferiorly (Figure 7–14). The membrane is a poorly vascularized ligamentous structure that lies under the subcutaneous tissue between the laterally placed cricothyroid muscles.

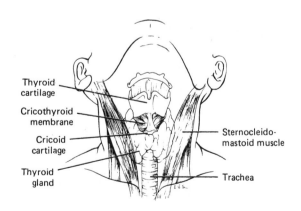

Thyroid cartilage
Cricothyroid membrane
Cricoid cartilage
Thyroid gland
Sternocleido-mastoid muscle
Trachea

▲ **Figure 7–14.** Anatomic relationships of cricothyroid membrane. (Reproduced, with permission, from Dunphy JE, Way LW (editors): *Current Surgical Diagnosis & Treatment*, 5th ed. Lange, 1981.)

▶ Procedure

1. Assemble all necessary equipment.
2. Position the patient.
3. Sterilize the skin of the neck from the chin to the sternal notch and laterally to the base of the neck, if time permits.
4. Observe sterile technique (don cap, mask, gloves, and gown) if time permits.
5. Check the endotracheal tube or tracheostomy tube for cuff leaks by inflating the tube with air from a syringe.
6. Identify the cricothyroid membrane. Using the 10-mL syringe with the 25-gauge needle, infiltrate the skin and underlying cricothyroid membrane with the 1% lidocaine in a line across the membrane while steadying the thyroid cartilage with the left hand. Omit this step if complete airway obstruction is present or if the patient is comatose.
7. Using the No. 11 blade, make a vertical incision in the skin overlying the cricothyroid membrane. Retract the skin with self-retaining retractors and relocate the cricothyroid membrane by palpation.
8. Make a horizontal incision through the cricothyroid membrane. Extend the incision in the cricothyroid membrane for approximately 1 cm on each side of the midline.
9. Using a mosquito or Kelly clamp in the left hand (with the point downward), insert the clamp into the incision and spread it. This maneuver alone is sufficient to provide an airway for a patient with supraglottic airway obstruction.
10. Grasp the endotracheal tube or tracheostomy tube with the right hand and insert the tube through the incision into the trachea, directing it caudally.
11. Connect the bag-valve unit to the tube and immediately ventilate the patient with 100% oxygen. Check for respiratory movement of the chest and the presence of bilaterally symmetric breath sounds.
12. Inflate the balloon just enough to stop any audible air leak during the inspiratory phase of positive-pressure ventilation.
13. Cut a 10×10 cm^2 (4×4 inch^2) gauze sponge halfway down the middle and wrap it around the tube. If an orotracheal tube is being used, fashion a necklace of adhesive tape, apply tincture of benzoin to the tube, and tape it in place. If a tracheostomy tube is being used, secure the wings of the tube by tying the tapes around the patient's neck, leaving enough slack so that an index finger can easily slide under the tape. Tying the tape too tightly can cause erosion of the skin and venous congestion above the tie, whereas tying it too loosely invites dislodging of the tube.
14. Suction the trachea.
15. Obtain a chest X-ray immediately to check the position of the tube.

▼ TRANSTRACHEAL JET VENTILATION

▶ Indications

Transtracheal jet ventilation is an alternative to cricothyrotomy in patients who require emergency assisted ventilation when conventional methods of endotracheal intubation are not possible.

▶ Contraindications

TTJV is contraindicated if conventional methods of endotracheal intubation can be successfully employed or if the proper equipment for TTJV is not available.

▶ Personnel Required

One person can perform the procedure unaided, although it is helpful to have an assistant to position the patient's head and handle equipment.

▶ Equipment and Supplies Required

- Materials for skin sterilization.
- Sterile gloves.
- Intravenous catheter, 12 or 14 gauge, or 13-gauge cannula designed specifically for TTJV that has lateral flanges to which tape may be attached.
- Bag-valve-mask set.
- 50-psi oxygen source.
- Demand valve device or Y adapter with connectors and tubing that connects to the 50-psi oxygen source.
- Adapter (eg, Luer-Lok) for connecting the demand valve outflow tubing to the catheter (Figure 7–15).
- Tape for securing catheter in place.
- Syringe, 3 mL.

▶ Positioning of the Patient

The patient is positioned supine with the head in the midline. It is helpful to have the neck slightly extended unless cervical spine injury is suspected.

▶ Anatomy Review

The cricothyroid membrane is a 1- to 1.5-cm membrane that lies inferior to the thyroid cartilage and superior to the cricoid cartilage. It can be located easily by palpating the protuberant midline portion of the thyroid cartilage ("Adams apple") and then moving the fingertip inferiorly 1.5 cm until it rests in a soft, flat depression between the thyroid cartilage and the cricoid cartilage. The examining fingertip will then be on the cricothyroid membrane.

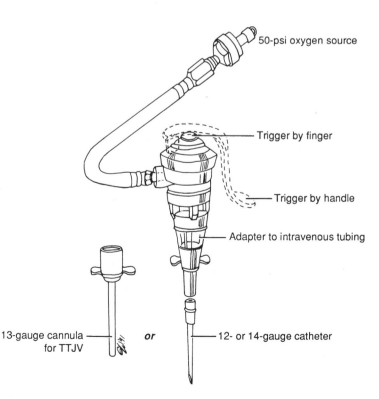

50-psi oxygen source

Trigger by finger

Trigger by handle

Adapter to intravenous tubing

13-gauge cannula for TTJV   *or*   12- or 14-gauge catheter

▲ **Figure 7–15.** 50-psi oxygen source is connected via a demand valve to the transtracheal jet ventilator.

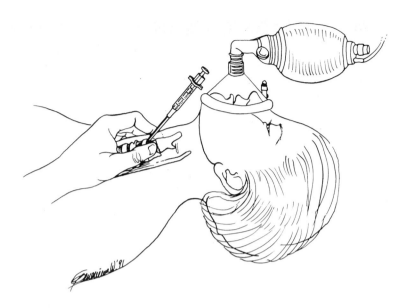

▲ **Figure 7–16.** Proper orientation for introducing transtracheal catheter. The trachea is stabilized with the hand.

▷ Procedure

1. Position the head as described above. Have an assistant hold the patient's head or use the tape across the forehead to prevent unexpected motion. If the patient requires assisted ventilation, provide it by a bag-valve-mask device.

2. Prepare the anterior surface of the neck with povidone-iodine.

3. Using sterile gloves, locate the cricothyroid membrane. It may be helpful to place the thumb and index finger of the nondominant hand on either side of the cricothyroid membrane to stabilize the trachea and anchor and stretch the skin slightly.

4. Connect the catheter or cannula to the 3-mL syringe. With the catheter or cannula and syringe in the dominant hand, pierce the skin and cricothyroid membrane at a 45° angle, directing the catheter tip inferiorly (Figure 7–16). When the catheter tip enters the tracheal lumen, a slight "give" will be felt. The patient may also cough when the catheter stimulates the tracheal wall. Traction in the syringe plunger during the entry will confirm lumen entry when air is withdrawn freely.

5. Slide the catheter sheath forward until it is snug against the skin, and then withdraw the needle.

6. Connect the inflow tubing on the demand valve or Y adapter to the 50-psi oxygen source and the outflow tubing to the catheter via the adapter. (*Note:* 50 psi may be obtained from a step-down regulator that supplies oxygen to a demand valve or from a venturi flow regulator opened wide to deliver 15 L/min.)

7. Begin ventilation at a rate of 20 breaths per minute, by pressing the button on the demand valve, or occluding the open port on the Y adapter, and inflating for 1 second, followed by a 2-second relaxation phase during which the patient will exhale passively through the oropharynx. Be prepared for secretions to be expelled during inflation as well as exhalation.

8. Tape the catheter firmly in place, with the hub of the catheter snug against the neck.

▽ THORACENTESIS

▷ Indications

Indications for thoracentesis are as follows:

- To relieve dyspnea or respiratory distress caused by accumulation of fluid in the pleural space.

- To obtain pleural fluid for diagnostic tests.

▷ Contraindications

Contraindications to thoracentesis are as follows:

- Severe coagulopathy (should be corrected before thoracentesis, unless severe respiratory failure is present, as determined by arterial blood gas analysis).

- Agitated, uncooperative patient (relative contraindication).

▷ Personnel Required

One person can perform thoracentesis unaided.

Equipment and Supplies Required

- Materials for skin sterilization.
- Materials for sterile technique (cap, mask, gloves, and gown).
- Lidocaine, 1%, with 5-mL syringe and 25- or 27-gauge needle.
- Sterile towels (4) or sterile paper drapes.
- Gauze sponges, 10×10 cm^2 (4×4 inch^2).
- Catheter-clad needle (eg, Angiocath), 16–18-gauge, 30.5-cm (12-inch) long; and 30-mL syringe to aid in insertion.
- Three-way stopcock.
- Luer-Lok syringe, 30 mL.
- °Sterile connecting tubing and empty intravenous bottle, or vacuum bottle specially designed for thoracentesis (if removal of more than a few hundred milliliters of fluid is anticipated). The connecting tube should not have a drip chamber.
- Collection vessels and culture media for laboratory analysis.

Positioning of the Patient

Thoracentesis is usually performed with the operator positioned behind the seated patient. Occasionally, thoracentesis must be performed in the lateral position when the patient cannot sit. For the posterior approach, the patient should be sitting on the edge of the bed or gurney with arms and trunk bent forward over a bedside stand and supported by the elbows or a pillow.

If the lateral approach must be used, have the patient lie at the edge of the bed on the affected side with the ipsilateral arm extended over the head. The midposterior line must be accessible for insertion of the needle. Elevating the head of the bed 30° is sometimes helpful.

Anatomy Review

Access to the pleural space is gained through the inter-costal spaces (Figure 7–17). Remember that nerves and blood vessels run on the underside of the rib and that the domes of the diaphragm are highest posteriorly, occasionally as high as the seventh intercostal space.

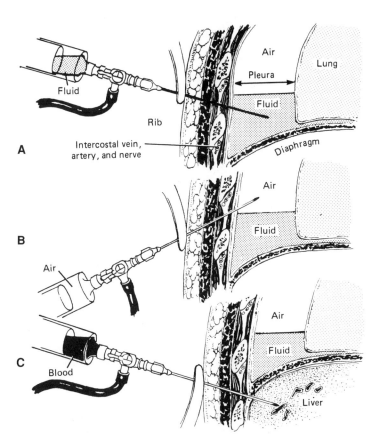

▲ **Figure 7–17.** Technique of thoracentesis using a regular steel needle (not catheter-clad). **A:** Successful tap, with fluid obtained. Note the position of the needle in relation to the intercostal neurovascular bundle, and the use of the clamp to steady the needle at skin level (do not use a clamp with a catheter-clad needle). **B:** Air is obtained if the position of the needle tip is too high (lung is punctured, or preexisting pneumothorax is entered, as in illustration). **C:** A bloody tap may result from excessively low position of the needle with puncture of the liver. (Reproduced, with permission, from Wilson JL (editor): *Handbook of Surgery*, 5th ed. Lange, 1973. Redrawn from GE Lindskog and AE Liebow.)

Procedure

Position the patient, and prepare all equipment.

A. Initial Preparation

1. If removing a large volume of fluid, assemble the connecting tubing and a collection vessel.

2. Observe sterile technique (don cap, mask, gloves, and gown) if time permits.

3. Arrange all of the equipment on a sterile field on a Mayo stand or bedside table.

4. Select the thoracentesis site by localizing the level of pleural fluid either by percussion (area of dullness) or ultrasonography. Insert the needle in the inter-costal space below the level of fluid in the midposterior line (posterior insertion) or the midaxillary line (lateral insertion).

5. Sterilize a wide area of skin around the proposed insertion site.

6. Drape the patient (this may be impossible if the patient is sitting).

7. Anesthetize the skin over the insertion site with the 1% lidocaine with a 25- or 27-gauge needle and 5-mL syringe. Then anesthetize the superior surface of the rib and the parietal pleura.

B. Catheter-Clad Needle (Eg, Angiocath) Insertion

1. Attach a 30-mL syringe to the catheter-clad needle and insert the needle through the skin over the rib selected. Advance the needle until it hits the rib.

2. Move the tip of the needle cephalad over the edge of the rib until it encounters the superior aspect of the rib.

3. Have the patient take a deep breath and hold it against a closed glottis.

4. Advance the needle over the superior surface of the rib and through the pleura into the pleural space. Maintain constant suction on the syringe so that the pleural fluid will enter the syringe instantly when the pleural space is entered. Apply controlled, gentle, steady pressure with both hands steadied on the patient's back to keep from suddenly spearing the lung. Do not use a Kelly clamp to grip a catheter-clad needle.

5. When the catheter has entered the pleural space, angle the needle caudally and push the catheter off the needle and into the base of the pleural space.

6. Occlude the lumen of the catheter and have the patient exhale and breathe normally.

7. Have the patient take a deep breath again and hold it; insert the 3-way stopcock into the catheter hub. Make

sure that the stopcock valve is set to occlude the catheter port. Have the patient resume normal breathing.

8. Connect the 30-mL Luer-Lock syringe to one port of the 3-way stopcock and (if needed) the intravenous tubing to the other.

9. Turn the stopcock valve to connect the syringe with the catheter and withdraw fluid from the pleural space. Then turn the stopcock so as to connect the syringe to the intravenous tubing and empty the syringe through the tubing into the intravenous bag or bottle. The first syringeful of fluid may be reserved for diagnostic tests.

10. Withdraw as much fluid as possible up to 1 L. In order to completely evacuate the pleural space, the patient may have to be rocked from side to side while fluid is being withdrawn.

11. At the termination of the procedure, the patient should take a deep breath and hold it while the catheter is quickly withdrawn. Cover the insertion site with a sterile occlusive dressing.

12. Obtain an upright portable chest X-ray to check for possible pneumothorax and residual fluid.

TUBE THORACOSTOMY: INSERTION OF A CHEST TUBE

Indications

Tube thoracostomy is performed in order to drain air or fluid from the pleural space.

Contraindications

There are no absolute contraindications to chest tube insertion. Usually, the patient is in distress and any relative contraindication (eg, coagulopathy) is superseded by the need to reinflate a compressed lung or drain fluid from the lungs.

Personnel Required

One operator can insert a chest tube alone; however, an assistant is helpful.

Equipment and Supplies Required

Most hospitals have sterile thoracostomy trays ready for use. If a tray is not available, assemble the following instruments and materials:

- Materials for skin sterilization.

- Materials for sterile technique (cap, mask, gloves, and gown).

- Lidocaine, 1%, with 10-mL syringe and 25- and 22-gauge needles.

- Sterile towels (4) or sterile paper drapes.
- Chest tube of the appropriate size and style to suit the clinical situation (see below).
- No. 11 surgical blade, mounted.
- Mayo clamp.
- Kelly clamp.
- Surgical silk suture (size 0) with large curved cutting needle.
- Needle holder.
- Petrolatum-impregnated gauze.
- Sterile gauze sponges, 10×10 cm^2 (4×4 inch^2).
- Plastic adhesive tape, 5-cm (2-inch) wide.
- Suction apparatus, 3-bottle, with water-seal, collection, and water-column sections (Figure 7–18). In the United States, this device is usually supplied as a unit with tall connectors and tubes included (eg, PleurEvac).
- Sterile Y connector (if two chest tubes are to be connected to the same suction apparatus).

▶ Positioning of the Patient

Tubes are usually inserted laterally when fluid, pus, or blood is drained, irrespective of whether air is also being removed. The patient should lie with the affected side up, and the ipsilateral arm extended over the head and grasping the top of the bed or the guardrail for security.

Rarely, chest tubes are inserted anteriorly to evacuate a pure pneumothorax. The patient should be supine, with the head raised about 10°. Position the bed or gurney at a comfortable height to prevent back strain for the operator.

▶ Anatomy Review

See Anatomy Review under Thoracentesis, above. Remember that the intercostal arteries and veins follow the inferior border of the rib.

▶ Procedure

1. Prepare all necessary equipment and arrange it on a sterile towel placed on a Mayo stand or bedside table.

2. Select the proper chest tube for insertion. In patients with trauma, insert the largest tube available (usually 36–40F). In patients without trauma, use a 26–32F chest tube, either straight or curved. In a patient with pure pneumothorax, a smaller chest tube (12–20F) is usually sufficient. A general rule is that a large tube effectively drains any substance from the pleural space and thus is preferred in emergencies, when the diagnosis may be unclear.

3. Assemble the suction apparatus according to the manufacturer's directions.

4. Connect the suction apparatus to a wall suction outlet and adjust the suction so that a steady stream of bubbles is produced in the water column.

5. Position the patient.

6. Determine the insertion site. Most tubes are inserted in the lateral thorax at the anterior axillary line, just lateral to the nipple. This places the tube in the fourth or fifth intercostal space, ensuring that it is above the dome of the diaphragm. Palpate the nearest rib and double-check the position; liver or spleen laceration can occur if the patient is not properly positioned.

7. Observing sterile technique, open the sterile instrument tray, arrange all necessary instruments, and make sure that everything is present.

8. Sterilize the skin over the insertion site and a wide area around it.

9. Again locate the rib for the insertion site and anesthetize the skin over the mid to inferior aspect of the rib with the 1% lidocaine with the 10-mL syringe and 25-gauge needle. Then anesthetize the surface of the rib and the tissue superior to it with the 22-gauge needle.

10. Drape the area around the insertion site.

11. Using the No. 11 blade, make a horizontal incision through the skin along the inferior aspect of the rib. The incision should be about 1½ times as wide as the tube selected. Incise the skin down to the subcutaneous tissue.

12. Use the Mayo clamp with the tips down as a dissector. Spread the tips to open tissue planes and create a tunnel aiming toward the superior aspect of the rib. Make sure the clamp stays next to the rib.

13. When the Mayo clamp is just over the superior edge of the rib, close the clamp and push it with steady pressure through the parietal pleura and into the chest. This maneuver requires more pressure that might be anticipated. Use steady, even, controlled pressure to provide control of the clamp after it has perforated the pleura. A lunging motion may cause a hole in the lung, heart, liver, or spleen.

    Once the clamp has penetrated the pleural space, air, fluid, blood, or pus may escape during expiration. Tension pneumothorax will whistle as air escapes under pressure, and the lung will collapse further during inspiration, because free air has access to the pleural space.

14. Widen the hole in the parietal pleura by spreading the Mayo clamp.

15. If a tube of large diameter is to be inserted, use the index finger to dilate the tract and hole in the pleura. This maneuver also ensures that entry has been made into the pleural space and not into a space inadvertently created between the parietal pleural and the chest wall.

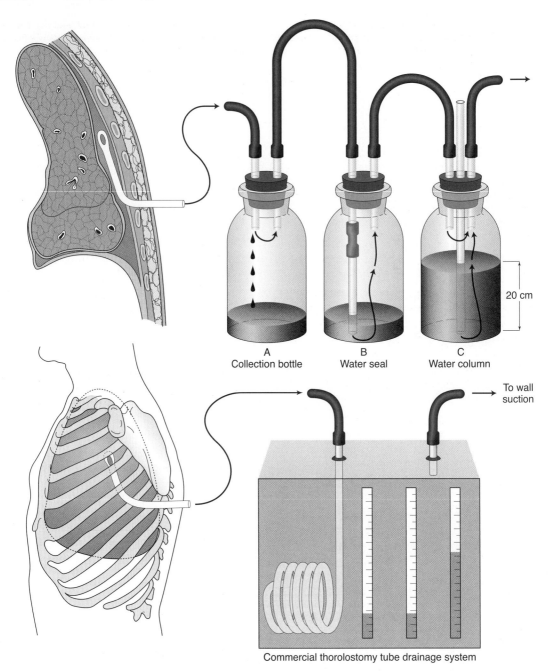

A
Collection bottle

B
Water seal

C
Water column

20 cm

To wall
suction

Commercial thorolostomy tube drainage system

▲ **Figure 7–18.** Diagram of tube thoracostomy and three-bottle suction apparatus. Bottle A is connected to the thoracostomy tube and collects pleural drainage for inspection and measurement of volume. Bottle B acts as a simple valve to prevent collapse of the lung if tubing distal to this point is opened to atmospheric pressure. Pulmonary air leak can be detected by the escape of bubbles from the submerged tube. Bottle C is a system for regulating the negative pressure delivered to the pleural space. Wall suction should be regulated to maintain continuous vigorous bubbling from the middle open tube in bottle C. The resulting negative pressure (in cm H_2O) is equal to the difference in the height of the fluid levels in bottles B and C. The Pleur-Evac system works in a similar manner. One end is attached to the chest tube and the other end is attached to suction. Each chamber of the Pleur-Evac is filled with sterile water to the level noted in the manufacturer's instructions. (Reproduced, with permission, from Dunphy JE, Way LW (editors): *Current Surgical Diagnosis & Treatment*, 5th ed. Lange, 1981.)

16. Grasp the end of the chest tube along the index finger and guide the tube down the tract into the pleural space, making sure that the last hole in the chest tube is within the pleural space. If a curved tube is being used, direct it inferiorly so that it lies along the base of the pleural space. A straight tube may be positioned inferiorly, laterally, or superiorly, depending on the clinical situation.

17. Connect the chest tube to the suction apparatus and make sure that the level in the water column varies with respiration. Usually, fluid, blood, or pus drains from the tube, a sign that the tube is properly positioned in the pleural space (unless the tube was inserted for pure pneumothorax). *Note*: If the tube has been inadvertently inserted between the parietal pleural and the chest wall, no fluid will drain from the tube and the level in the water column will not vary with respiration.

18. Sew the tube to the chest wall with the silk suture. Partially close the incision with a mattress stitch and use one throw of a square knot to close the skin around the tube. Then, wind both ends of the suture around the tube, starting at the bottom and working toward the top (as if lacing up a shoe). Tie the ends of the suture snugly around the top of the tube.

19. Wrap Xeroform or petrolatum-impregnated gauze around the tube to seal it to the skin. Cover the tube with two 10×10 cm^2 (4×4 inch^2) sterile gauze sponges, cut so that they fit around the tube. Tape the sponges and the tube in place. Tape connections of the chest tube to the suction tube and tape the chest tube to the patient's side below the insertion site.

20. Obtain a portable upright chest X-ray to check the position of the tube and to make sure that the lung is expanded and that all fluid has been evacuated.

▼ EMERGENCY THORACOTOMY

(See Chapter 24.) Emergency thoracotomy is performed to gain access to the heart and great vessels. It can occasionally be lifesaving, although controversy exists over the indications and the location where it should be performed. It should be performed only when the patient can be taken immediately afterward to the operating room.

▶ Indications

1. Traumatic cardiac arrest following penetrating chest trauma with signs of life in the prehospital setting (survival rate up to 40%).

2. Traumatic cardiac arrest following penetrating or blunt trauma with signs of life in the emergency department (exceedingly low survival rate for blunt trauma victims).

3. Cardiac tamponade with profound shock; patient is unresponsive to rapid volume expansion, is deteriorating, and is unlikely to survive until operation.

4. Blunt or penetrating trauma to the chest or abdomen with profound shock; patient is unresponsive to rapid volume expansion, is deteriorating, and is unlikely to survive until operation.

5. Massive chest or abdominal bleeding with profound shock; patient is unresponsive to rapid volume expansion, is deteriorating, and is unlikely to survive until operation.

▶ Contraindications

1. Traumatic cardiac arrest with no signs of life in the prehospital setting (survival rate virtually nil).

2. Appropriate operating facilities and personnel not immediately available.

3. Patient immediately responsive to volume expansion or decompression of tension pneumothorax.

▶ Personnel Required

One individual experienced in the technique is required to perform the procedure, another to maintain an airway and assist ventilation, and, ideally, a third to prepare and hand equipment to the operator. In most cases, patients have multiple, concomitant needs that are best met by a team.

▶ Equipment and Supplies Required

- Materials for skin sterilization.
- Sterile drapes.
- Scalpel with No. 10 blades.
- Rib spreaders.
- Vascular clamps.
- Nonvascular clamps.
- Suture scissors.
- Metzenbaum scissors (long).
- Needle holder (long).
- Suture (2-0 silk or comparable) on cutting needle.
- 10-in DeBakey tangential occlusion clamp.
- Suction catheter.
- Tissue forceps.
- Bone rongeur.
- Rib approximator.

▶ Positioning of the Patient

The patient should be supine. Place rolled sheet under the left scapula and lower ribs and elevate the left arm above the head to expose the left chest and axilla. The patient should be intubated and ventilated with positive pressure (manual bag-valve method or mechanical ventilator). Advance the endotracheal tube to selectively intubate the right main-stem bronchus. This allows the left lung to be manually collapsed, providing access to the heart. Remember to decrease tidal volumes by half and increase the respiratory rate to compensate for ventilation of a single lung.

▶ Anatomy Review

The favored approach to the heart in an emergency setting is through a left thoracotomy. The incision follows the rib interspace, with care taken to avoid the intercostal vessels that run beneath each rib. The internal mammary artery runs parallel to the lateral margin of the sternum and must be ligated should hemorrhage from this vessel occur.

▶ Procedure

1. Prepare the anterior thoracic surface generously on both sides with skin-sterilizing solution and cover it with sterile drapes to the extent that time allows.

2. Using the No. 10 scalpel blade, make a horizontal incision in the left fourth or fifth intercostal space, extending from the sternum to the posterior axillary line. It should be deep enough to expose the intercostal muscles and should follow the superior rib margin to avoid injury to the intercostal vascular bundle beneath the rib above. In women, make the incision beneath the breast.

3. With a scalpel or scissors, make a small opening through the intercostal muscles into the pleural space. Using Metzenbaum scissors, divide the intercostal muscles the entire length of the incision, remaining close to the superior margin of the rib. Ligate the internal mammary artery above and below. Using the scalpel or heavy scissors, cut through two sternocostal cartilages above the interspace.

4. Insert a rib spreader and spread the ribs as widely apart as possible. If necessary (eg, in penetrating trauma to the right chest), the incision may be extended across the sternum and into the right chest to increase exposure.

5. Inspect the heart. It will appear to be bluish if cardiac tamponade is present. To relieve tamponade or perform cardiac massage, open the pericardium. Pick up the anterior pericardium with forceps and incise it from apex to base, using Metzenbaum scissors. Be careful to avoid the left phrenic nerve, which courses longitudinally along the left lateral heart margin. Remove any clotted blood; suction excess blood as needed.

6. If observable cardiac contractions are inadequate, or if cardiac arrest has occurred, perform internal cardiac massage by gently compressing the heart with both hands. If ventricular fibrillation is present, a quivering motion will be observed. Perform defibrillation using the internal paddles, at an energy level of 5–50 J. If a myocardial laceration is present, it can be temporarily controlled with a fingertip or with a 3-0 polypropylene suture. Horizontal mattress sutures through Teflon pledgets will help prevent further laceration of the myocardium. Place sutures through the epicardium and myocardium only. Avoid the coronary arteries. Atrial wounds can be repaired with simple interrupted sutures.

7. Control massive bleeding from the lung or pulmonary vessels by crossclamping the hilum of the involved lung.

8. If the patient fails to respond rapidly to volume administration, or if intra-abdominal bleeding is suspected, incise the overlying pleural and crossclamp the aorta above the point where it enters the diaphragm. Be careful to avoid clamping the esophagus. As a temporary measure during internal cardiac massage, the aorta may be occluded with the index and long fingers placed behind the heart.

9. If resuscitation is successful, immediately transport the patient to the operating room for definitive care.

▼ PERICARDIOCENTESIS

Blind aspiration of the pericardium was formerly the only way to detect and treat a pericardial effusion. Complications of this technique included pneumothorax, myocardial or coronary artery laceration, and iatrogenic pericardial tamponade. Many emergency departments currently utilize bedside ultrasound to detect pericardial effusion. Ultrasound is quick, noninvasive, and can even provide guidance for pericardiocentesis in the symptomatic patient with pericardial effusion. Blind pericardiocentesis should be reserved for those situations in which a critically ill patient is suspected of having tamponade and no diagnostic tests are rapidly available to assist in the diagnosis or treatment.

▶ Indications

The following description of pericardiocentesis assumes that bedside emergency ultrasound or echocardiography are not rapidly available to evaluate and treat a suspected pericardial tamponade.

▶ Contraindications

In a patient who requires pericardiocentesis for decompensated or rapidly decompensating cardiac tamponade, there are no contraindications. In other patients, the following conditions are contraindications:

- Infection along the proposed course of pericardiocentesis.

- Bleeding diathesis (relative contraindication, especially if it can be corrected).

▶ Personnel Required

Three people are required to perform pericardiocentesis: the operator and an assistant to monitor the electrocardiograph and another physician besides the operator. A cardiothoracic surgeon should be available in case complications occur.

▶ Equipment and Supplies Required

Many hospitals have prepackaged sterile pericardiocentesis trays that contain many of the required items. If these are not available, the following instruments and materials are required:

- Materials for skin sterilization.

- Materials for sterile technique (cap, mask, gloves, and gown).

- Lidocaine, 1%, with 10-mL syringe and 25-gauge needle.

- Pericardiocentesis needle: 17-gauge, 12.5-cm (5-inch) thin-walled steel needle (usually a spinal needle) for aspiration. It is possible to use 16-gauge and even 14-gauge needles with plastic outer cannulas.

- Syringes: assorted sizes, including 50 mL (2), 30 mL (2), 10 mL (2), and 5 mL (1).

- No. 11 scalpel blade, mounted.

- Sterile conductive monitoring cable with alligator clamps at each end.

- Three-way stopcock.

- Silk suture (5-0) on a cutting needle.

- Straight clamp and needle holder.

- Needles: assorted sizes, including 25 gauge, 1.5 cm (⅝ inch) (1); 22 gauge, 2.5 cm (1 inch) (2); and 19 gauge, 4 cm (1½ inch) (5), for transferring specimens.

- Drapes.

- Sterile, capped, 15-mL specimen tubes (10).

- Heparin, to lightly heparinize cytologic specimen tubes.

- Specimen tubes, one purple-topped and three red-topped.

- Clean glass microscope slides.

- Microhematocrit centrifuge tubes with occlusive sealant.

- Ice bucket to hold cytologic specimens.

- Sterile dressing for entry and exit sites.

- CPR cart.

▶ Positioning of the Patient

The patient should be supine, and if time permits, the thorax should be elevated 30°. Optimize bed height and lighting for the operator.

▶ Procedure

A. Patient Preparation

Take the following steps, if time permits:

1. The patient should be in a bed where cardiac monitoring is available, preferably in a cardiac catheterization laboratory.

2. Position the patient, as described above.

3. Begin electrocardiographic monitoring with limb leads.

4. Gain secure intravenous access.

5. Give atropine, 0.6–1 mg intramuscularly or subcutaneously, before pericardiocentesis, because vagal responses during cardiac tamponade may be devastating.

6. Narcotics may be used as long as they do not depress consciousness or respiration.

7. Supplemental oxygen, 5–10 L/min, by mask or nasal cannula is advisable.

B. Observe Sterile Technique

1. Put on cap, mask, gloves, and gown.

2. Sterilize the skin in a wide area around the xiphoid process.

3. Drape the field widely with sterile towels if time permits.

C. Begin Pericardiocentesis

1. Locate the appropriate site to the right of and below the xiphoid process (Figure 7–19) and anesthetize the skin with the 1% lidocaine with the 10-mL syringe and 25-gauge needle. Switch to the 22-gauge needle and anesthetize the tissue beneath the xiphoid process along the track of the pericardiocentesis needle. Omit this step if the patient is comatose.

2. A small incision in the skin with the No. 11 scalpel blade may facilitate entry of the pericardiocentesis needle.

3. Attach the pericardiocentesis needle to a 30-mL syringe.

4. Perform pericardiocentesis. If this procedure is being done during active CPR, make sure that everything is ready beforehand, work rapidly, and stop CPR for only as long as necessary. Enter the selected site, just caudal and to the right of the xiphoid process, and direct the needle at an angle of 30–45° to the skin. Aim toward the patient's right shoulder. Advance the needle slowly and aspirate the fluid continuously. There is usually a

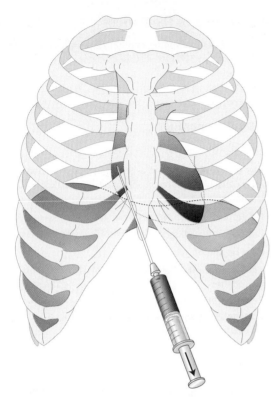

▲ **Figure 7–19.** Diagram of pericardiocentesis showing position of needle and anatomic relationships. (Reproduced, with permission, from Way LW (editor): *Current Surgical Diagnosis & Treatment*, 9th ed. Appleton & Lange, 1991.)

palpable feeling of resistance when the needle pierces the parietal pericardium.

If the attempt to penetrate the pericardium is unsuccessful and no fluid is aspirated, bring the needle back to the subcutaneous tissue and direct it more medially. Continue either until fluid is aspirated or until the needle hits the right side of the sternum, at which point it is safer to use fluoroscopic or echocardiographic guidance.

Pericardial aspiration by an anterior left inter-costal approach (usually the fourth left intercostal space just left of the sternum) is less satisfactory because it penetrates the pleural space and has a potential for laceration of the left anterior descending coronary artery or a branch of the internal mammary artery. This approach may be used as a last resort in a dying patient.

5. When fluid is aspirated and is flowing freely, the needle can be anchored at the chest wall with a surgical clamp to keep it from penetrating any farther. In cardiac tamponade due to pericardial hemorrhage, the fact that

pericardial blood does not clot (whereas intracardiac blood does) may be a helpful diagnostic clue.

6. Aspirate until the pericardium is dry by slowly withdrawing fluid. Secure any specimens that are required for diagnostic tests. In the presence of decompensated cardiac tamponade, removal of even a small amount of pericardial fluid should result in a dramatic improvement in the patient's hemodynamic status.

7. After aspiration is completed, withdraw the needle and gain hemostasis with pressure. A single suture may be required.

8. Cover the entry site with a sterile dressing.

▼ FOCUSED ASSESSMENT WITH SONOGRAPHY FOR TRAUMA

Focused assessment with sonography for trauma (FAST) is a rapid, noninvasive technique for determining the presence of intra-abdominal fluid (eg, blood or urine) in the trauma victim. It does not detect retroperitoneal fluid collections or hollow viscus injury such as bowel perforation. The FAST exam is a quick screening tool and should be performed immediately after the primary survey of the trauma victim.

▶ Indications

- Blunt thoracoabdominal trauma.
- Penetrating thoracoabdominal trauma.
- Suspected pericardial tamponade.
- Undetermined origin of hypotension in trauma patient.

▶ Contraindications

The FAST exam is contraindicated in the unstable trauma victim who requires immediate surgery.

▶ Personnel Required

One operator can perform a FAST exam unaided.

▶ Equipment and Supplies Required

- Ultrasound transmission gel (hypoallergenic).
- Ultrasound machine with 2.5–7-MHz transducer. Higher frequency allows for better resolution; however, a 3.5-MHz transducer is usually adequate for FAST exams performed on the adult trauma victim.
- An attached printer that allows images viewed to be transferred to photographic paper for documentation.

▶ Positioning of the Patient

The patient should be supine on a level surface. Reverse-Trendelenburg (head up) position increases the sensitivity in the suprapubic view while the Trendelenburg (head down) position increases sensitivity of the RUQ view.

Anatomy Review

FAST exams evaluate fluid collections in four anatomic locations. In the chest, the pericardial sac is viewed. In the abdomen, the Morison pouch in the right upper quadrant, the splenorenal recess in the left upper quadrant, and the pouch of Douglas in the suprapubic area are viewed. To optimally view the pelvis, a full bladder is required. When a Foley catheter is inserted before or during the FAST exam, remember to have the Foley drainage tubing clamped so as not to decompress the bladder. The distended bladder provides a good "acoustic window" to identify free fluid in the pelvis.

Procedure

1. Set up the ultrasound machine for FAST exams as instructed by the machine's manufacturer.
2. Enter the patient's name and medical record number using the machine's annotation keys.
3. Expose the patient's thoracoabdominal area and place ultrasound transmission gel in the following four locations: pericardial area, right upper quadrant, left upper quadrant, and suprapubic area (Figure 7–20).
4. Orient the transducer for sagittal sections of the body and place it in the subxiphoid region. This view identifies pericardial fluid collections.
5. Next, place the transducer on the right midaxillary region between the fourth and fifth ribs to view the Morison pouch. Keep the transducer in the intercostal space to avoid shadows created by the ribs.
6. Move the transducer, still in the sagittal plane, to the left posterior axillary line between the 9th and 11th ribs to view the splenorenal recess.
7. Finally, place the transducer, now oriented for the transverse view, about 4–5 cm superior to the pubic symphysis in the midline to view the pouch of Douglas.
8. Each view should be frozen on screen and printed. This documentation should be placed with the patient's medical record. Performing and interpreting FAST exams is not a difficult procedure, but it requires hands-on training, which should be undertaken by any emergency physician wishing to become prolific in its use.

Limitations

A FAST exam is helpful when the findings are positive; however, a negative study must be evaluated further (eg, with computed tomography [CT] scan, repeat evaluations, observation). A falsely negative FAST exam can result from several factors:

- Too little time has elapsed since the trauma for the blood to accumulate.

- Bleeding may be retroperitoneal and not visible on FAST exam.
- Solid organ injury with encapsulated bleeding is present.
- Hollow viscus injury is present.
- Inadequate volume of fluid. As little as 50 cc of fluid can be detected by some expert sonographers; however, it may take up to 250 cc of fluid to create an unequivocally positive FAST exam.

▼ ABDOMINAL PARACENTESIS

Indications

Indications for abdominal paracentesis are as follows:

- To determine the cause of ascites, including suspected intra-abdominal hemorrhage from trauma.
- To lower intra-abdominal pressure in tense ascites (rarely indicated in the emergency department).
- To obtain fluid for analysis and culture in patients with ascites who are thought to have an infection.

Contraindications

The following conditions are relative contraindications to abdominal paracentesis and most can be corrected or circumvented if paracentesis must be performed:

- Bleeding diathesis (coagulopathy or thrombocytopenia). Correct severe bleeding diathesis before performing paracentesis. Cautious paracentesis with a 22-gauge needle may be safely performed in patients with mild to moderate bleeding tendencies.
- Previous abdominal surgery.
- Severe bowel distention (correct with nasogastric suction and a rectal tube before performing paracentesis).

Personnel Required

One person can perform paracentesis unaided if the patient is cooperative. An assistant may be helpful if the patient is obese.

Equipment and Supplies Required

- Materials for skin sterilization.
- Materials for sterile technique (cap, mask, gloves, and gown).
- Lidocaine, 1%, with 10-mL syringe and 22- and 25-gauge needles.
- Needles in various sizes, including a longer 20- or 22-gauge spinal needle and a 19-gauge catheter-clad

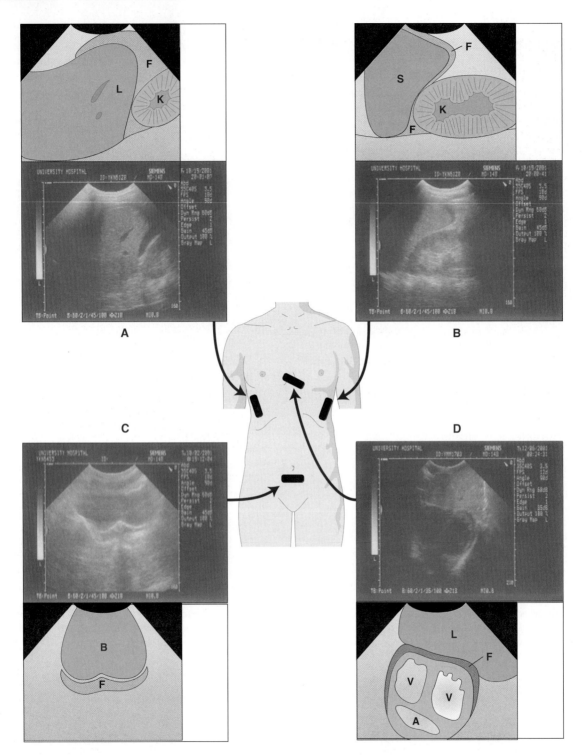

▲ **Figure 7–20.** Illustration of the four views for the FAST exam and where fluid would be seen in each view. A, atrium; B, bladder; F, fluid; K, kidney; L, liver; S, spleen; V, ventricle.

needle (eg, Angiocath). Use a 22-gauge, 4-cm (1½-inch) needle or spinal needle in patients with severe bleeding diathesis.

- Syringe, 50 mL.

- Drapes.

- Specimen tubes, both with and without anticoagulant, and a blood culture bottle.

- Ice bucket for cytology specimens.

- Gauze sponges, 10×10 cm^2 (4×4 inch^2).

- Topical antibacterial ointment.

- Tape and dressing material.

- Three-way stopcock, connector tubing, and 500-mL collection bottles (if therapeutic paracentesis is planned).

▶ Positioning of the Patient

Have the patient supine at the edge of the bed nearest the operator (right side of the bed for a right-handed operator), with the trunk elevated 45°. Allow 10 minutes for ascites to pool in the dependent portion of the abdomen and for air-filled bowel to float up away from the puncture site. Be sure the bladder has been emptied by voiding or catheterization.

The patient can be tipped 30° to either side if paracentesis of the lower quadrants is necessary.

▶ Procedure

1. Observe sterile technique (don cap, mask, gloves, and gown).

2. Sterilize the skin between the umbilicus and symphysis pubica and both lower quadrants.

3. Drape the field widely.

4. Using the 25-gauge needle, anesthetize the skin with the 1% lidocaine in the 10-mL syringe at the selected puncture site. The preferred site is on the poorly vascularized linea alba, about halfway between the symphysis pubica and the umbilicus (Figure 7–21). Change to the 22-gauge needle and anesthetize down to and including the peritoneum.

5. Attach the 19-gauge catheter-clad needle to a 50-mL syringe. In patients with severe coagulopathy and thrombocytopenia, use a 22-gauge needle. In markedly obese patients, use a 20-gauge spinal needle.

6. Puncture the skin. Keeping the needle perpendicular to the abdominal wall, maintain continuous negative suction in the syringe while slowly advancing the needle. In tense ascites, it may be useful to try Z-tracking the needle to minimize persistent leaking of ascitic fluid; that is, after penetrating the skin, move the needle and syringe 1–2 cm (⅜–¾ inch) before piercing the subcutaneous

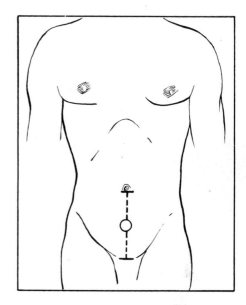

▲ **Figure 7–21.** Insertion site for abdominal paracentesis. (Reproduced, with permission, from Dunphy JE, Way LW (editors): *Current Surgical Diagnosis & Treatment*, 5th ed. Lange, 1981.)

tissue, but maintain the perpendicular approach. Repeat this maneuver at the level of the peritoneum, thus describing an oblique Z pattern through the various layers of tissue. In this manner, the track of the needle from the skin to the peritoneal space will not be a continuous line when the needle is removed.

7. The dense connective tissue of the peritoneum will yield a noticeable "pop" when pierced.

8. Fluid should flow freely into the syringe. To avoid bowel or visceral trauma, particularly in patients with bleeding tendencies, it is preferable to remove the steel needle, leaving the plastic catheter in place while specimens are collected. The patient can be safely moved into more dependent positions with the plastic catheter in place to facilitate draining of sufficient fluid for analysis. In most cases of diagnostic paracentesis, a single collection of 50 mL is adequate. At a minimum, fluid should be sent to the laboratory for cell count, tests for protein, cultures, and staining with Gram stain. For suspected neoplasia or for therapeutic relief of tense ascites, up to 1 L may be removed, although 750 mL is a more prudent upper limit in order to avoid adverse effects on intravascular volume. A 3-way stopcock can be used to minimize leakage while the operator is continually aspirating with a syringe. Alternatively, drainage can go directly into sterile 250–500-mL vacuum containers using connecting tubing.

9. After samples have been collected, remove the catheter or needle and apply firm pressure to the site for 5 minutes.

10. Apply topical antibacterial ointment and dress the site with a pressure dressing.

11. If leaking of ascitic fluid persists despite a pressure dressing, close the paracentesis tract with a mattress stitch.

PERITONEAL CATHETER INSERTION AND PERITONEAL LAVAGE

▶ Indications

Peritoneal lavage is performed to determine if intraperitoneal hemorrhage has occurred. With the proliferation of CT scanning and FAST exams, peritoneal lavage is used much less frequently; however, it continues to have a role in evaluation of the trauma victim when the victim is too unstable to be sent for CT scan or if ultrasound is inconclusive.

▶ Contraindications

Contraindications to peritoneal lavage are as follows:

- Previous intra-abdominal surgery of any kind.
- Pregnancy.
- Unstable patient who requires immediate surgery.

▶ Personnel Required

One operator and an assistant are required for peritoneal lavage using the percutaneous approach. Alternatively, one operator and two assistants are required for peritoneal lavage using the operative approach.

▶ Equipment and Supplies Required

Prepackaged trays with the necessary equipment are available commercially, or they can be made up by the hospital. The following items are required:

- Materials for skin sterilization.
- Materials for sterile technique (cap, mask, gloves, and gown).
- Sterile towels (4) or sterile paper drapes.
- Lidocaine, 1%, with 5-mL syringe and 25-gauge needle.
- No. 11 surgical blade, mounted.
- Peritoneal lavage catheter (11–18F) and introducing stylet.
- Sterile bag containing 1 L of lactated Ringer's injection or normal saline, with intravenous connector tubing.
- Nylon suture (size 4-0) on a cutting needle (percutaneous approach); chromic catgut (size 3-0) plus silk, nylon, or polypropylene sutures (size 3-0) (operative approach).

- Needle holder and straight scissors.
- Adhesive dressing.
- For operative technique only: Two Allis or Kocher clamps, one Kelly clamp, and two small right-angle retractors.

▶ Positioning of the Patient

The patient should be supine on a level surface. Examine the abdomen for scars; do not perform peritoneal lavage if abdominal surgery has been performed previously. If necessary, take diagnostic abdominal X-rays before performing peritoneal lavage (the procedure may produce artifacts on the X-ray [eg, ileus or intraperitoneal air]).

▶ Procedure

A. Preparatory Measures

1. Drain the bladder (by urination or catheterization, as required). Place nasogastric tube.

2. Position the patient and check to see that all equipment is at hand.

3. Sterilize the skin of the anterior abdominal wall from the umbilicus to the symphysis pubica.

4. Drape the operative site.

5. Observe sterile technique (don cap, mask, gloves, and gown).

6. Using the 1% lidocaine with the 5-mL syringe and 25-gauge needle, anesthetize the skin about 2 cm (¾ inch) caudal to the umbilicus in the midline. Then, directing the needle perpendicularly to the anterior abdominal wall, infiltrate the fascia (linea alba), preperitoneal space (between peritoneum and fascia), and parietal peritoneum. The needle will encounter resistance when it reaches the peritoneum.

B. Percutaneous Approach

1. Using the No. 11 blade, make a 0.5-cm (¼-inch) transverse incision through the skin and fascia to allow easy passage of the catheter and stylet.

2. Carefully insert the catheter and stylet into the anesthetized tract with gentle, steady, controlled pressure. (*Caution*: The abdominal aorta lies in the path of the catheter.) Control is best achieved by making sure that both hands are comfortably placed on the patient's abdomen and by advancing the catheter with steady pressure applied by the thumb and forefinger. Advance the catheter through the peritoneum and into the peritoneal cavity. There will be a definite give ("pop") as the catheter penetrates the peritoneum.

3. Once the catheter has penetrated the peritoneal cavity, slide it off the stylet and into the peritoneal cavity.

The catheter should slide easily. If any resistance is encountered, withdraw the catheter and stylet together, and attempt insertion again. Difficulty in advancing the catheter may indicate that the stylet has not entered the peritoneal cavity and that the catheter is being inserted into the space between the peritoneum and the fascia; alternatively, there may be adhesions in the peritoneal cavity that have fixed the intraperitoneal structures. Failure to make this important distinction may result in false-positive or false-negative findings or perforation of intraperitoneal structures.

C. Operative Approach

With this approach, a superficial laparotomy is performed to permit direct visualization of the peritoneum when the catheter is inserted. The advantage of this approach is that inadvertent insertion of the catheter into the preperitoneal space is unlikely to occur; however, more personnel are required to perform the procedure.

1. After the area has been anesthetized, use the No. 11 blade to make a 3-cm ($\frac{1}{16}$ inch) vertical incision in the midline about 1 cm ($\frac{3}{8}$ inch) inferior to the umbilicus.

2. Using the Kelly clamp, bluntly dissect through sub-cutaneous tissue to the fascia of the abdominal wall. Then incise the fascia for the length of the incision. Again using a Kelly clamp, spread the preperitoneal fat and expose the parietal peritoneum.

3. Using two Allis or Kocher clamps, grasp the peritoneum and lift it up to free it from any underlying visceral structures. (Grasp a bit of peritoneum with one clamp, grasp another bit with the second clamp about 1–2 cm [$\frac{3}{8}$–$\frac{3}{4}$ inch] away and release the first clamp. Repeat as needed. This method of alternately grasping and releasing the peritoneum separates it from underlying structures.)

4. Holding the peritoneum up between two clamps (Allis or Kocher), make a small stab wound through the peritoneum with a No. 11 scalpel blade.

5. Insert the catheter into the peritoneal cavity under direct vision.

D. Results

1. If blood does not return immediately, connect the intravenous tubing to the catheter and instill 1 L of sterile, warm Ringer's lactate or normal saline (Figure 7–22). Gently massage the abdomen to spread the fluid and roll the patient from side to side to make sure that the lavage fluid reaches all areas of the peritoneal cavity. Lower the intravenous bag to the floor. The fluid in the peritoneal cavity should flow out of the cavity and back into the bottle. Again, roll the patient from side to side to return as much fluid as possible to the bag.

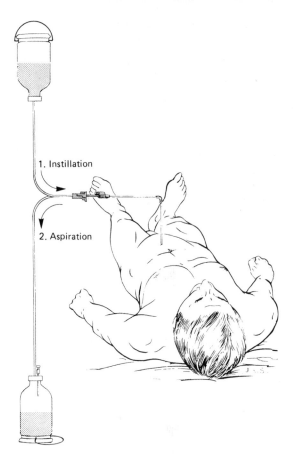

1. Instillation

2. Aspiration

▲ **Figure 7–22.** Technique of peritoneal lavage. (Reproduced, withpermission, from Dunphy JE, Way LW (editors): *Current Surgical Diagnosis & Treatment*, 5th ed. Lange, 1981.)

With either approach, gross blood may return after the catheter has been placed and the stylet has been removed. This finding signifies extensive intraperitoneal hemorrhage, and the patient should be prepared for surgery.

2. After as much of the fluid as possible has been removed from the peritoneal cavity (a reasonable return is 75–80% of the fluid instilled), remove the catheter and close the incision. Use the size 4-0 nylon skin suture if the percutaneous approach was used, and cover it with an adhesive dressing. To close the incision made for the operative approach, close the peritoneum with chromic catgut sutures; close the anterior abdominal fascia with interrupted silk, polypropylene, or nylon sutures; approximate the subcutaneous tissue with absorbable sutures; and close the skin.

If immediate laparotomy is necessary, leave the incision open and cover it with a sterile dressing that has been soaked in saline.

3. Make sure to record the amount of any excess fluid left in the patient's peritoneal cavity as fluid input on the fluid intake and output computation sheet.

▶ Interpretation

Significant intraperitoneal hemorrhage is indicated by grossly bloody lavage fluid or gross blood coming from the catheter. Lavage fluid with a hematocrit of 1% or higher also indicates significant intraperitoneal hemorrhage and suggests the need for laparotomy. Completely clear fluid indicates lack of significant intraperitoneal bleeding.

▼ INSERTION OF INDWELLING (FOLEY) URINARY CATHETER

▶ Indications

Indications for insertion of an indwelling urinary catheter are as follows:

- Diagnostic or therapeutic drainage of the urinary bladder.
- Need for a reliable and frequent assessment of urine output (eg, for treatment of shock).
- Need to perform retrograde cystography.

▶ Contraindications

The following are only relative contraindications to insertion of an indwelling urinary catheter:

- Previous urethral surgery.
- Suspected or known urethra trauma (free-floating prostate, blood issuing from urethra meatus). In this case, perform a urethrogram before urethral catheterization is attempted.

▶ Personnel Required

One person can insert an indwelling urinary catheter unaided. An assistant is helpful if the patient is uncooperative.

▶ Equipment and Supplies Required

Note: Most hospitals have disposable Foley insertion trays that contain most of the items listed below except for the catheter. It is important to check to see that the tray contains all of the needed materials and that the catheter, if it is supplied with the set, is of the proper size and desired material and has a balloon of the proper size.

- Foley catheter of the appropriate size, material, and contour (different catheters are discussed below).
- Urinary drainage bag and connecting tube.
- Sterile lubricant.
- Antiseptic solution and sterile cotton balls to sterilize the male urethral meatus and the female perineum.
- Sterile syringe, 5–10 mL, filled with enough sterile water to inflate the balloon on the catheter. The size of the balloon is usually printed on the catheter (usually 5 mL).
- Sterile gloves and drapes.

▶ Selecting a Catheter

The Foley catheter is used in almost all cases when an indwelling urinary catheter is required. It consists of a double-lumen rubber tube with a terminal retaining balloon. The larger channel is for drainage of urine and the smaller is for inflation of the balloon. Some indwelling catheters have a third lumen, for constant bladder irrigation. Foley catheters are of standard length (46 cm [18 inch]) but come in varying diameters that are numerically graded (French system), with the larger number indicating a larger diameter. Two sizes of balloon are commonly available: 5-mL balloons for routine catheterizations and 30-mL balloons for special situations. Most Foley catheters are made of rubber. Teflon or Silastic is sometimes used for long-term, indwelling catheters. (With the exception of the Coudé catheter, specialized shapes and contours are not discussed here, because they should be inserted by a urologist.)

- For routine, short-term catheterization in males or females, a 14F or 18F rubber catheter with a 5-mL balloon is satisfactory. Smaller sizes are required for children.
- Men with prostatic hypertrophy may require larger catheters (eg, 20–22F).

▶ Positioning of the Patient

A. Females

The patient should be in the lithotomy position. If she is comatose or under anesthesia, flex her knees and hips, and allow the legs to abduct. If the soles of the feet are pressed together, this position can easily be held by the patient without assistance.

B. Males

The patient should be supine.

▶ Anatomy Review

A. Females

The female urethra is short, and because there is no prostate gland, passage of a catheter is relatively easy. The only difficulty is locating the urethral meatus, which lies in the superior fornix of the vulva, above the vaginal opening and below the clitoris. It appears as a small dimple or slit in the midline.

B. Males

The urethra leaves the bladder at the trigone, passes through the prostate, and then runs the length of the penis to exit at the meatus at the tip of the glans.

▶ Procedure

A. Catheterization of Females

1. Assemble all necessary equipment.
2. Open the catheter tray and selected catheter and position them on a sterile field placed on a bedside table or stand so that all required materials are readily accessible.
3. Place a generous amount of lubricant on the sterile field.
4. Put on sterile gloves, and drape the perineal area.
5. Make sure that the catheter is open and the lubricating jelly is accessible.
6. Open the antiseptic packet and moisten the cotton swabs provided with antiseptic.
7. Be sure that the syringe is filled with enough sterile water to inflate the balloon being used.
8. Using the left hand (standing on the patient's right side), spread the labia and identify the superior fornix with the clitoris at the apex. Thoroughly cleanse the entire area with 4–5 swabs soaked in antiseptic. Clean the labia with front to back strokes with two successive swabs; then cleanse the urethral meatus with another two successive swabs.
9. The left hand continues to hold the labia spread apart from the rest of the procedure.
10. Make a loop in the Foley catheter for easier handling. Grasp the catheter with the right hand, coat the tip and proximal portion with lubricating jelly, and insert the catheter into the urethral meatus, which lies just below the clitoris. Advance the catheter until urine returns. Then advance it 4–5 cm (1⅝–2 inch) farther to make sure that the balloon is well within the bladder.
11. Inflate the balloon with the appropriate amount of sterile water (usually 5 mL; the balloon volume is usually printed on the catheter) and withdraw the catheter gently until the balloon is pulled snugly against the trigone (Figure 7–23).
12. Collect a small amount of urine in a sterile container for appropriate studies (urinalysis should be obtained routinely) and then connect the catheter to the urinary drainage bag.

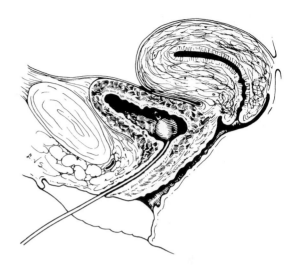

▲ Figure 7–23. Sagittal section of female bladder showing balloon of Foley catheter fitting snugly against the trigone.

13. Tape the Foley catheter and the urinary drainage tube to the upper thigh, leaving enough slack so that abduction of the legs will not put tension on the catheter.
14. *Note*: The most common mistake in catheterization of the female bladder is to miss the urethral meatus and inadvertently slip the catheter into the vagina. No urine will return. Leave the catheter in place in the vagina as a marker. Obtain a new, sterile catheter and try again. Remove the other catheter.

B. Catheterization of Males

1. (Steps 1–7 are the same as those described under Catheterization of Females, above.) Using the left hand (standing on the patient's right side), grasp the penis so that the shaft lies in the palm and the glans of the penis is free but secure. The penis should be held at a right angle to the abdomen. The left hand should remain in this position for the remainder of the procedure; it is no longer sterile. For uncircumcised patients, retract the foreskin over the glans.
2. Sterilize the glans and urethral meatus with 3–4 swabs dipped in antiseptic.
3. Put a single loop in the Foley catheter for easier handling, grasp the catheter in the right hand, and coat the tip of the catheter with lubricating jelly. It is often helpful to place some on the meatus as well.
4. Insert the catheter into the urethral meatus and advance it down the penile urethra to the base of the penis with successive, steady movements.

5. Advance the catheter through the membranous and prostatic urethra into the bladder.

6. Advance the catheter to the hilt (even if urine is obtained earlier) to ensure that the balloon is not inflated in the urethra. As soon as the catheter has been advanced to the hilt, release the penis to free both hands for inflation of the balloon.

7. Inflate the balloon with the proper amount of sterile water for its size (usually 5 mL) and withdraw the catheter until the balloon is pulled snugly against the trigone.

8. Obtain a specimen for appropriate tests (at a minimum, routine urinalysis should be performed). Connect the urinary drainage system bag to the catheter, and tape the catheter to the upper thigh, leaving sufficient slack so that movement of the leg will not pull on the catheter. If the patient is uncircumcised, remember to retract the foreskin back over the glans.

▶ Problem Solving

A. Males with Prostatic Enlargement or False Urethral Passages

Conventional technique usually fails in patients with significant prostatic hypertrophy or false urethral passage. Listed below are a few techniques that have proved successful in catheterizing these patients. *Caution*: Reasonable persistence in attempting catheterization is acceptable; however, there comes a time when further manipulations may rupture the urethra or create new false passages. If attempts using the guidelines outlined below are still unsuccessful, consult a urologist or insert a suprapubic catheter instead (see below).

1. Increase the size of the catheter—Large catheters are stiffer and provide more forceful dilatation of the prostatic urethra. The larger, blunt tip tends to follow the true urethra rather than following smaller false passages.

2. Lubricate the urethra—Fill a 30–50-mL sterile catheter-tipped syringe with the lubricating jelly and inject the jelly down the urethra with gentle pressure until no more can be injected. Then insert the catheter.

3. Inject lubricating jelly while the catheter is being passed—Fill the syringe as outlined above, insert the tip into the catheter, and fill the catheter with jelly. As the catheter is being passed, slowly inject more lubricant to ensure that the entire length of the catheter is lubricated and to help dilate the urethra just ahead of the catheter tip.

4. Use a Coudé catheter—A Coudé catheter has an upwardly deflected tip, which may navigate through a narrowed prostatic urethra more successfully than does a standard Foley catheter. The tip of the catheter should be directed anteriorly to facilitate passage through the prostatic urethra.

B. Traumatized Patients

Most patients with major trauma have a Foley catheter inserted during resuscitation. A rectal examination must be performed before a catheter is inserted in a male patient with major blunt trauma. Feel for the prostate and make sure that it is firmly attached to the surrounding tissues. A free-floating prostate or gross blood escaping from the urethra signifies urethral rupture until proved otherwise. In either case, Foley catheterization is contraindicated, and a suprapubic catheter should be inserted instead.

▼ PERCUTANEOUS SUPRAPUBIC CYSTOSTOMY

Suprapubic bladder cystostomy is a means of bypassing the urethra to provide drainage of the urinary bladder.

▶ Indications

Suprapubic bladder cystostomy is performed to provide bladder drainage when transurethral drainage is unsuccessful or contraindicated.

▶ Contraindications

Contraindications to suprapubic cystostomy are as follows:

• Nondistended, nonpalpable bladder.

• Carcinoma of the bladder, because percutaneous catheterization of the bladder might lead to seeding of the cancer along the track of the catheter.

• Gross hematuria, which would require a tube of large diameter to drain clots from the bladder.

• Recent cystostomy (the percutaneous technique might disrupt suture lines).

▶ Personnel Required

One person can perform percutaneous suprapubic cystostomy unaided, although an assistant may be helpful, particularly if the patient is uncooperative.

▶ Equipment and Supplies Required

Many prepackaged commercial kits are available for percutaneous suprapubic cystostomy. The following items are required:

• Materials for skin sterilization.

• Materials for sterile technique (cap, mask, gloves, and gown).

• Lidocaine, 1%, with 10-mL syringe and 25-gauge, 1-cm (½-inch) and 22-gauge, 4-cm (1½-inch) needles.

• Sterile towels (4) or sterile paper drapes.

• Razor.

- No. 11 scalpel blade, mounted.
- Catheter-clad needle (eg, Angiocath), 14 gauge, 30 cm (12 inch), or other commercially manufactured percutaneous suprapubic catheter set. A central venous catheter kit can also be used if no other equipment is available.
- Syringe, 50 mL.
- Closed urinary drainage system (sterile intravenous tubing and empty intravenous bag or bottle).
- Silk suture (size 3-0) on a curved cutting needle.
- Needle holder.
- Suture scissors.
- Antibacterial ointment.
- Sterile gauze sponges, 5 × 5 cm² (2 × 2 inch²), and tape.
- Rolled bath towel for placement under the patient's hips.

▶ **Positioning of the Patient**

The patient should be supine, with a rolled-up towel placed under the hips.

▶ **Anatomy Review**

The urinary bladder lies in the midline of the lower abdomen. When it is distended, its position can be detected by palpation or percussion.

▶ **Procedure**

1. Locate the distended bladder by palpation, percussion, or ultrasonography. If the bladder cannot be located, percutaneous suprapubic cystostomy should not be performed. If the bladder is not distended, it can usually be filled by oral or intravenous hydration.

2. Prepare the area just above the symphysis pubica by shaving the pubic hair and sterilizing the skin. Extend the sterile field with drapes.

3. Assemble all necessary equipment.

4. Observe sterile technique (don cap, mask, gloves, and gown).

5. Determine the insertion point by measuring cephalad 1–2 cm (⅜–¾ inch) from the superior edge of the symphysis pubica in the midline (Figure 7–24).

6. Using the 1% lidocaine with the 10-mL syringe and 25-gauge needle, anesthetize the skin at the point of insertion. Then switch to the 22-gauge needle to anesthetize the subcutaneous tissue and anterior wall of the bladder. If the position of the needle is correct, urine can be aspirated through the needle. Remove the needle.

7. Make a 0.5-cm (³⁄₁₆ inch) transverse incision in the skin over the anesthetized area with the No. 11 scalpel blade.

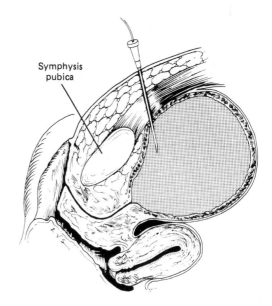

Symphysis pubica

▲ **Figure 7–24.** Suprapubic cystostomy. Sagittal section of distended bladder showing insertion site for catheter.

8. The technique for placing the catheter depends on the type of catheter used:

   a. *Catheter-clad needle:*

   (1) Attach a 50-mL syringe to the 14-gauge, 30-cm (12-inch) catheter-clad needle.

   (2) Insert the catheter unit through the skin incision.

   (3) Advance the catheter caudally at a 50–60° angle to the abdominal surface. Advance the catheter with a smooth, deliberate motion and steady the guiding hands on the patient's abdomen as necessary. A "give" is felt as the catheter and needle penetrate each successive layer of the fascia and bladder wall. Maintaining gentle suction with the syringe will cause aspiration of urine as soon as the bladder cavity has been entered.

   (4) Once the bladder has been entered, slip the catheter tip off the needle by holding the hub of the needle in the left hand and advancing the catheter with the right.

   (5) Advance the catheter about 6–8 cm (2⅜–3⅛ inch) to make sure that enough of it is within the bladder.

   (6) Attach the sterile intravenous tubing to the catheter hub. If no assistant is available, reattach the 50-mL syringe to the tubing to keep the system closed. Otherwise, have an assistant attach the end of the tubing to the empty

intravenous bag or bottle that is to receive the urine.

(7) Suture the catheter in place at the insertion site with the size 3-0 silk suture. Wind the ends of the suture around the catheter at least three times to make sure that it is secured to the abdominal wall.

(8) Apply antibacterial ointment to the insertion site, cover it with sterile 5×5 cm^2 (2×2 inch^2) gauze sponges, and tape the sponges in place.

(9) If not done earlier, attach the end of the tubing to the empty intravenous bag or bottle that is to receive the urine.

(10) Tape all connections.

b. *Central venous catheter kit*: Use the Seldinger technique, as previously discussed, to insert the catheter.

c. *Percutaneous suprapubic catheter*: Follow the manufacturer's instructions for use.

LUMBAR PUNCTURE

▶ Indications

Lumbar puncture is performed to obtain cerebrospinal fluid for diagnostic tests (eg, suspected meningitis, subarachnoid hemorrhage).

▶ Contraindications

Contraindications to lumbar puncture are as follows:

- Local infection of the lumbar area. Cervical or cisternal puncture should be performed instead.

- Suspected intracranial mass lesion (brain abscess, tumor, any posterior fossa lesion, subdural hematoma). Papilledema or focal cerebral defects (excluding ophthalmoplegia) suggest a mass lesion of the central nervous system. CT scan of the head should precede lumbar puncture in these circumstances.

- Bleeding diathesis (relative contraindication; should be corrected if time permits).

- Suspected spinal cord mass lesion (eg, epidural abscess, hematoma, or tumor). Myelography should be performed in consultation with a neurosurgeon to define the lower limit of the spinal block.

▶ Personnel Required

One person can perform lumbar puncture unaided if the patient is cooperative. An assistant can help with positioning of the patient, lighting, handling of samples, and the like, and is essential if the patient is uncooperative.

▶ Equipment and Supplies Required

Prepackaged sterile disposable lumbar puncture trays are commercially available. If the tray is to be assembled at the hospital, the following items are required:

- Materials for skin sterilization.

- Materials for sterile techniques (gloves and mask; cap and gown are optional).

- Spinal needles, 20 and 22 gauge (shorter, smaller-gauge needles are required for children).

- Manometer.

- Three-way stopcock.

- Cerebrospinal fluid collection tubes (5).

- Sponges, 10×10 cm^2 (4×4 inch^2).

- Lidocaine, 1%, with 5-mL syringe and 22- and 25-gauge needles.

- Sterile drapes.

- Adhesive dressing.

- Ice bucket for specimens that must be put on ice immediately.

▶ Positioning of the Patient

A. Lateral Decubitus

Place the patient in the lateral decubitus position lying on the edge of the bed and facing away from the operator. The patient should flex the lumbar spine as much as possible by assuming the fetal position (forehead bent toward knees and knees drawn up to abdomen). The patient's head should rest on a pillow, so that the entire craniospinal axis is parallel to the bed. Positioning is the most crucial aspect of successful lumbar puncture, and the three key elements of proper positioning are achieving maximal lumbar flexion (to open the intervertebral spaces), keeping the patient's spine parallel to the bed, and having the line of the patient's shoulders and pelvis perpendicular to the bed (to facilitate orientation of the needle track). Prevent pelvic rotation by keeping the patient's knees and ankles aligned. An assistant is useful to help the patient maintain the proper position.

B. Sitting

The patient sits facing away from the operator and bends over a bedside table to maximize lumbar flexion. This position is useful when cerebrospinal fluid pressure is low (eg, dehydration) or when the patient is obese. Cerebrospinal fluid pressure can be determined by having the patient lie in the decubitus position after the needle is in place.

After the patient has been properly positioned, raise the bed until the patient's lower lumbar spine is at the mid-chest level of the operator, who should be seated. Adjust the lighting for optimal effect.

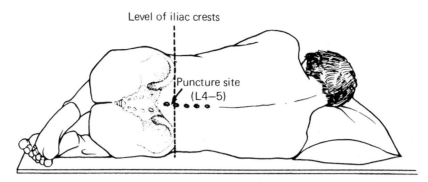

Level of iliac crests

Puncture site
(L4–5)

▲ **Figure 7-25.** Decubitus position for lumbar puncture. (Reproduced, with permission, from Krupp MA et al: *Physician's Handbook*, 21st ed. Lange, 1985.)

▶ Anatomy Review

Lumbar puncture should enter the subarachnoid space below the level of the conus medullaris, which extends to L1–L2 in most adults and L2–L3 in children. The L3–L4 interspace, the most commonly used site for lumbar puncture, is at the level of the posterior iliac crests (Figure 7–25). The L4–L5 interspace may be preferable, however, because a traumatic spinal tap at this level may leave cerebrospinal fluid obtained at the higher interspace uncontaminated with red blood cells (because of the caudal direction of flow of cerebrospinal fluid).

With the patient properly positioned, find the posterior iliac crest and palpate the spine at this level for the L3–L4 interspace. Other interspaces are counted from this landmark. The needle should enter the exact midpoint of the interspace between the spinous processes. Mark the point on the patient's skin with the end of a ballpoint pen or the indentation from a fingernail to facilitate locating the landmark after the skin has been sterilized.

It may be difficult to palpate the spinous processes in obese patients. Using the gluteal cleft to mark the mid-line, locate the sacral promontory, which is palpable even in obese patients. Move cephalad until the promontory ends, indicating the L5–S1 interspace; the L4–L5 interspace is then easily identified.

▶ Procedure

1. Observe sterile technique (don mask and gloves; cap and gown are optional).

2. Prepare all equipment. Assemble the manometer and stopcock (the channel from the spinal needle to the manometer should be open), open the specimen tubes, and draw up the 1% lidocaine into the 5-mL syringe with the 25-gauge needle.

3. Sterilize the skin in a wide field around the L2–L3 to L4–L5 interspaces.

4. Place a sterile drape under the patient that extends over the edge of the bed. Contamination of gloves may be avoided by folding the edge of the drape back over the gloves, pushing the edge beneath the patient's back, and carefully removing the gloved hands.

5. Place a second sterile drape over the topside of the patient, leaving only sterilized skin between the edges of the drapes. Although a drape with a center hole is preferred by some, it obscures the rest of the spine (a valuable landmark) and makes shifting to another interspace difficult.

6. Locate the puncture site and anesthetize the skin using the 1% lidocaine in the 5-mL syringe with the 25-gauge needle. Change to the 22-gauge needle before anesthetizing between the spinous processes. Be sure to apply vacuum to the syringe to make sure that the needle has not entered a blood vessel (blood in the syringe).

7. Hold the spinal needle between the index and middle fingers, with the thumb over the stylet. It may be held with two hands, if necessary, for stability. Avoid touching the tip and shaft of the needle, because starch granules from the gloves may be introduced into the subarachnoid space and can cause sterile arachnoiditis. The 20-gauge needle is better for transmitting pressure changes in cerebrospinal fluid, but the 22-gauge needle is adequate in most cases; smaller needles should be used in children.

8. Introduce the needle in the midline perpendicular to a line connecting the iliac crests, aiming about 30 degrees rostrally toward the umbilicus. Be sure the long axis of the needle is parallel to the bed and that the plane of the patient's back is perpendicular to the bed. In infants, the entry angle is nearer to the perpendicular, whereas in elderly patients, the angle may approach 45 degrees rostrally to pass beneath the osteophytic lipping of the spinous processes. The bevel of the needle should

be facing up (parallel to the spine) if the patient is in the lateral decubitus position, so that the fibers of the dura are split longitudinally.

9. Advance the needle slowly. There will be a "pop" as the needle passes through the ligamentum flavum and the spinal arachnoid membrane. Since the spinal venous plexus is anterior to the spinal canal, the chance of a traumatic spinal tap can be minimized by frequent checking of the position of the needle (withdraw the stylet).

10. If the needle hits bone deep in the penetration, withdraw to the ligamentum flavum and redirect the tip in a more caudal direction. (The needle will follow the same course unless it is drawn back through the ligamentum flavum.) Pain radiating to the leg or buttock is an obvious indication to direct the needle toward the midline and away from the involved side.

11. When cerebrospinal fluid begins to flow from the needle, discard the first few drops. Establish free flow of cerebrospinal fluid, rotating the bevel of the needle may be helpful. Do not aspirate cerebrospinal fluid unless it cannot be obtained by other means, because a nerve root may be trapped against the needle and injured. Replace the stylet halfway in the shaft of the needle to prevent leakage. If the patient is in a seated position and if cerebrospinal fluid pressures are to be obtained, have an assistant help the patient into the decubitus position, taking care not to move the needle.

12. Remove the stylet and attach the stopcock and the manometer to the needle.

13. If not already done, rotate the stopcock lever to open the channel between the needle and the manometer. Cerebrospinal fluid will rise into the manometer and the opening cerebrospinal fluid pressure can be measured. Normal pressure is between 780 and 180 mm H_2O. If pressure is elevated, make sure that the patient's position is not causing jugular or abdominal compression. Have the patient slowly relax and uncurl from the fetal position (if in the lateral decubitus position) and then inhale deeply. Cerebrospinal fluid pressure falls with inspiration and rises with expiration. Check pressure changes with the patient's head first flexed and then extended. To detect mass lesions in the spinal canal, look for a block to cerebrospinal fluid that is present only on either extension or flexion. Abnormally low pressures may be caused by dehydration.

14. Remove the manometer, and begin collecting samples of cerebrospinal fluid in the specimen tubes. This is most easily achieved by removing the 3-way stopcock and using the stylet to block flow between samples by replacing the stylet halfway in the shaft of the needle. Three tubes are routinely collected: Tube 1 (0.5–1 mL), tube 2 (2–3 mL), and tube 3 (2–4 mL) in adults (smaller amounts are collected in children). Frequently, however,

further information is desired, and more samples are collected in the extra tubes (see section on specimen collection, below). If in doubt, collect extra fluid in additional tubes.

15. Replace the manometer, and obtain a closing pressure if spinal subarachnoid block is suspected.

16. Remove the needle, and place a small adhesive bandage over the puncture site.

17. Draw venous blood for determination of glucose concentration. The ratio of blood glucose to cerebrospinal fluid glucose is helpful in the diagnosis of inflammatory disease.

18. Recommendations to have the patient lie supine after the procedure do not appear to affect the incidence of postdural puncture headache.

▶ Special Problems Encountered in Lumbar Puncture

A. Massive Obesity

If the patient is obese, landmarks are difficult to locate, and alternative methods for locating the L4–L5 interspace must be used (see Anatomy Review, above). Lumbar puncture with the patient sitting may be tried if attempts fail with the patient in the lateral decubitus position. The sitting position makes the midline easier to locate and increases lumbar flexion. A 12.5-cm (5-inch) needle may be required. The patient must be cooperative. Cerebrospinal fluid pressures are not measured in this position, but the patient may be carefully repositioned in the lateral decubitus position after the needle is in place to record cerebrospinal fluid pressures. If lumbar puncture in the sitting position is unsuccessful, a neurosurgeon can use the cervical approach (done at the bedside) or a neuroradiologist can attempt a fluoroscopically guided approach (performed in the radiology department).

B. Osteoarthritis

As the body ages, desiccation of the nucleus pulposus of the intervertebral disk occurs, with subsequent narrowing of the disk space. This change together with osteophytic "lipping" of the spinous process and calcification of the interspinous ligament and ligamentum flavum makes lumbar puncture difficult. A larger-gauge needle (eg, 18–19 gauge) facilitates passage through calcified posterior ligaments. It may occasionally be necessary to resort to an oblique approach performed by a radiologist using fluoroscopy.

C. Previous Lumbar Surgery

Lumbosacral spine films assist in defining the extent of surgery and fusion. If all of the posterior approaches are unavailable for lumbar puncture, obtain neurologic or neurosurgical consultation.

D. Inadvertent Arterial Puncture

If arterial blood is obtained during lumbar puncture, completely withdraw the needle. Obtain a fresh spinal needle for the next attempt, because clotted blood makes replacement of the stylet difficult and also contaminates the sample. If the patient has an underlying coagulopathy, it should be corrected and the patient should be observed for signs of compressive spinal epidural or subdural hematoma (Chapter 25).

E. High Opening Pressure

If high cerebrospinal pressures are unsuspected before lumbar puncture is performed, use the smallest needle possible. Collect the minimum amount of fluid necessary (usually that in the manometer is sufficient) and withdraw the needle. Watch the patient carefully for signs of impending herniation and treat accordingly. Obtain a closing cerebrospinal fluid pressure; remove only as much fluid as causes the initial pressure to drop by one-half. A rapid drop in cerebrospinal fluid pressure to low levels with removal of only a small amount of fluid may be an ominous sign indicating impending herniation. Obtain urgent neurosurgical consultation.

F. Hypotension

Cerebrospinal fluid pressure is proportionate to venous pressure and P_{CO_2}. Severe hypotension may decrease the volume of the subarachnoid space and make it difficult to penetrate. Slowly advance the needle, and each time the stylet is removed, attach a tuberculin syringe with a small air bubble in the hub, relying on the negative pressure in the epidural space to help define location (the bubble is sucked into the needle when the needle is in the epidural rather than the arachnoid space). Advancing the needle a few millimeters will place the tip within the subarachnoid space, permitting aspiration of cerebrospinal fluid.

The sitting position may be helpful in the patient with severe hypotension, provided that arterial blood pressure is sufficient to enable the patient to tolerate the upright position. The sitting position takes advantage of gravity to help raise cerebrospinal fluid pressure in the lumbar space.

G. Post-Lumbar Puncture Headache

Headache following lumbar puncture is unfortunately a relatively common complication of the procedure. It does not appear to be related to the duration that a patient remains supine after the procedure. Smaller, less traumatic (pencil point) needles may reduce the incidence. Medications such as oral or intravenous caffeine may be of benefit for headaches that continue despite bed rest. For persistent headaches, an epidural blood patch is usually effective in resolving the headache.

H. Blood in Cerebrospinal Fluid

Features that point to a traumatic spinal tap rather than to subarachnoid hemorrhage include (1) normal cerebrospinal fluid pressure, (2) absence of xanthochromia after centrifugation, (3) blood sample followed by clearer samples or bloodier samples, (4) white cell count proportionate to red cell count (700–1000 red blood cells per white blood cell; 1 mg/dL of protein per 1000 red blood cells), (5) changing red cell count in successive tubes, or (6) clot formation (rare). A repeat lumbar puncture at a higher interspace yields cerebrospinal fluid that is usually clear if the fluid was bloody owing to traumatic tap at a lower level. The presence or absence of crenated red cells is of no diagnostic value.

▶ Specimens

At a minimum, collect three tubes: Tube 1 (0.5–1 mL) for cell count, tube 2 (2–3 mL) for culture and Gram stain, and tube 3 for protein and glucose determinations and for chemistry studies (2–4 mL). Most authorities recommend another 0.5 mL for a VDRL (Venereal Disease Refererence Laboratory) study. There is no harm in collecting extra tubes, because a variety of other diagnostic tests may be indicated. If the specimen is bloody, perform comparison counts in tubes 1 and 3.

If subarachnoid hemorrhage is suspected, the supernatant in the tube should be examined for xanthochromia. Centrifuge 2–3 mL of cerebrospinal fluid at 1000 rpm for 5 minutes in a clinical centrifuge, and then examine the supernatant for the characteristic yellowish pigmentation of oxyhemoglobin and bilirubin. Xanthochromia does not appear until about 2–4 hours after hemorrhage, reaches a maximum around 6–48 hours, and may persist for 2–4 weeks (Table 7–2). Jaundice, hypercarotenemia, and elevated cerebrospinal fluid protein (> 150 mg/dL) may also cause xanthochromic spinal fluid. Xanthochromia does not occur in the supernatant after a traumatic spinal tap, because the bloody cerebrospinal fluid is not exposed to the enzyme in the subarachnoid space that converts hemoglobin to bilirubin.

Table 7–2. Pigmentation of the Cerebrospinal Fluid Following Hemorrhage.

	Appearance	Maximum	Disappearance
Oxyhemoglobin (pink)	½–4 hours	24–35 hours	7–10 days
Bilirubin (yellow)	8–12 hours	2–4 days	2–3 weeks

ARTHROCENTESIS: KNEE, SHOULDER, ELBOW, ANKLE, WRIST, HAND, AND FOOT JOINTS

The major peripheral joints can be aspirated safely in the emergency department. Aspiration of the hip and other joints of the axial skeleton usually requires the aid of specialists (orthopedic surgeons or rheumatologists) and the use of ancillary techniques (fluoroscopy and radionuclide scans); therefore, it is not discussed here.

► Indications

Indications for arthrocentesis are as follows:

- Need to obtain synovial fluid for diagnosis.
- Drainage of hemarthrosis when conservative management is unsuccessful.
- Instillation of local analgesic and anti-inflammatory agents into a joint.

► Contraindications

Contraindications to arthrocentesis are as follows:

- Soft tissue infection overlying proposed site of aspiration.
- Uncooperative patient (relative contraindication).
- Severe bleeding diathesis or anticoagulant therapy.

► Personnel Required

One person can perform arthrocentesis unaided if the patient is cooperative, although an assistant is helpful for handling samples and holding young children.

► Equipment and Supplies Required

- Materials for skin sterilization.
- Materials for sterile technique (mask and gloves; cap and gown are optional).
- Lidocaine, 1%, with 10-mL syringe and 22-gauge needle.
- Needles: 25 gauge, 1.5 cm (⅝ inch) (2); 22 gauge, 4 cm (1½ inch) (2); 20 gauge, 4 cm (1½ inch) (2); 27 gauge, 1.5 cm (½ inch) (1). Select a needle size appropriate to the joint to be aspirated.
- Syringes: 10 mL (2), 2 mL (2), 30 mL (1).
- Sterile gloves.
- Drapes.
- Gauze pads, 10×10 cm² (4×4 inch²) (2); 5×5 cm² (2×2 inch²) (2).
- Adhesive dressing.
- Sterile capped specimen tubes (2–3).

- Containers for synovial fluid: purple-topped or green-topped (EDTA or heparin anticoagulant, respectively, for cell count and differential and examination for crystals) (2); gray-topped (fluoride inhibitor for glucose) (1); red-topped (no anticoagulant) (3).
- Clean glass microscope slides and coverslips.

► Positioning of the Patient

See Procedure for Specific Joints, below.

► Procedure

1. Stabilize the joint to be aspirated. Identify landmarks and mark the entry point with a scratch or indentation on the skin.
2. Sterilize the skin in a wide field around the puncture site.
3. Assemble all necessary equipment.
4. Observe sterile technique (don mask and gloves; cap and gown are optional).
5. Anesthetize the skin with the 1% lidocaine with the 10-mL syringe and 22–27-gauge needle; continue down to the joint capsule.
6. Select an appropriate needle (usually 20 gauge for knee, shoulder, elbow, ankle, or wrist; 25 or 27 gauge for small hand joints) and syringe (10 mL for knee, shoulder, elbow, ankle, or wrist; 2 mL for hand joints). A large-bore needle (eg, 18 gauge) may be required for aspiration of pus in larger joints. Use the 30-mL syringe for large effusions.
7. Penetrate the skin at the selected site and cautiously advance the needle into the joint space; a "pop" will be felt when the needle passes through the synovium into the joint space. Aspirate continuously. Stop advancing the needle when joint fluid flows freely into the syringe.
8. Remove as much fluid as possible, but do not drain the joint dry if synovial biopsy is planned.
9. If joint fluid fails to flow freely, bring the needle all the way back to the subcutaneous tissue before redirecting it, in order to avoid joint trauma that might occur with deep probing.
10. After samples of fluid have been obtained, withdraw the needle and apply firm pressure over the site for 1–2 minutes.
11. Cover the site with an adhesive dressing.

► Procedure for Specific Joints

A. Knee

The joint space of the knee may be entered either medially or laterally (Figure 7–26). In either case, the leg should be fully

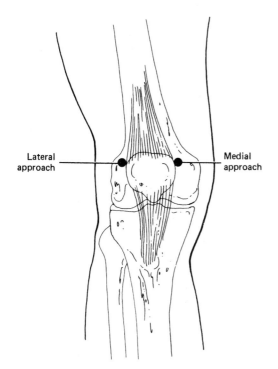

▲ **Figure 7–26.** Aspiration of the knee joint.
(Reproduced, with permission, from Way LW, ed. Current Surgical Diagnosis and Treatment, 11th ed. New York, NY: McGraw-Hill; 2003.)

extended, with the patient supine. Pressure on the opposite side of the joint will make the synovium bulge more prominently and assist in directing the needle.

From the lateral aspect, the entrance site is at the intersection of lines (extended from the upper and lateral margins of the patella). A 22-gauge, 4-cm (1½-inch) needle held parallel to the bed is directed medially and just deep to the patella and into the suprapatellar space. From the medial aspect, the needle is introduced anteromedially in the space between the patella and the medial condyle. The needle (held parallel to the bed) is advanced upward (toward the undersurface of the patella) and laterally, beneath the patella and into the joint space.

B. Shoulder

The shoulder joint can be aspirated from either an anterior or a posterior approach. The latter has the advantage of being out of the patient's line of vision.

For the posterior approach, the patient should sit in a chair and face backward (chest against the back of the chair). To open up the joint space and facilitate entry of the needle, the patient should put the arm of the site to be aspirated up against the chest and touch the opposite shoulder. This will adduct and internally rotate the arm. The head of the

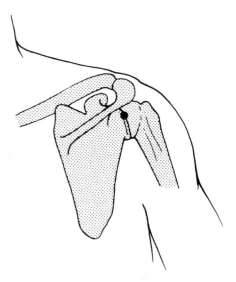

▲ **Figure 7–27.** Posterior approach to shoulder joint aspiration.

humerus is palpable posterolaterally. Use a 20- or 22-gauge, 4-cm (1½-inch) needle, and keep it parallel to the floor. Direct it about 30° medially into the joint space from a point just under the posteroinferior border of the acromion (Figure 7–27).

For the anterior approach, the patient should sit in a chair, facing forward, with the arm comfortably supported in the lap. Using a 20- or 22-gauge, 4-cm (1½ inch) needle, enter the joint space at a spot medial to the head of the humerus and just below the palpable tip of the coracoid process (Figure 7–28). Direct the needle slightly laterally and superiorly into the scapulohumeral joint space.

C. Elbow

Be certain to differentiate olecranon bursitis that does not involve the elbow joint from bulging synovium. Have the patient sit with the forearm supported from the elbow to the hand on a table, with the elbow joint in about 10–30° of flexion. With significant effusion, the bulging synovium should be evident laterally. Introduce the needle (usually a 20- or 22-gauge, 4-cm [1½-inch] needle) just below the lateral epicondyle and proximal to the olecranon process of the ulna (Figure 7–29). Advance the needle medially and slightly proximally into the joint space.

D. Ankle

Arthrocentesis of the ankle is more difficult than that of the other joints discussed here. The most common approach is anteromedial. Have the patient lie supine, with the knee extended and the foot slightly plantar-flexed. Identify the extensor hallucis longus tendon by

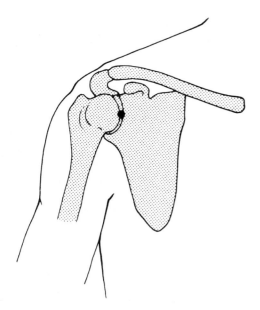

▲ **Figure 7–28.** Anterior approach to shoulder joint aspiration.

having the patient extend the great toe. Just anterior (1 cm [⅜ inch]) and inferior (1 cm [⅜ inch]) to the medial malleolus and lateral to the extensor tendon is a small depression. Introduce the needle in this depression and direct it toward the tibiotalar articulation (Figure 7–30). If swelling and pain are most severe on the side of the ankle, use a similar approach but from the anterolateral aspect of the joint. When subtalar disease is suspected (eg, pain on pronation and supination of the foot), the

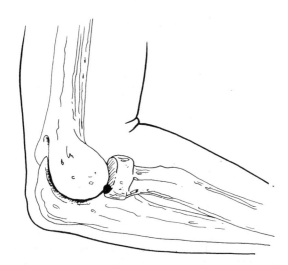

▲ **Figure 7–29.** Aspiration of the elbow joint.

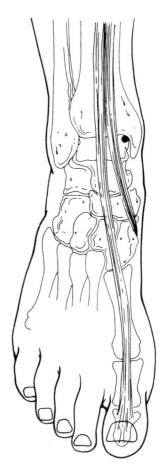

▲ **Figure 7–30.** Determination of the needle entry site for ankle joint aspiration. A small depression can be palpated about 1 cm (½ inch) anterior and inferior to the medial malleolus and lateral to the extensor hallucis longus.

needle is introduced more distally, at the talonavicular articulation. Although fluid is seldom obtained at the talonavicular joint, injection of anti-inflammatory agents may be readily accomplished.

E. Wrist

A bulging, inflamed joint space at the wrist can be entered dorsally at prominent areas of swelling; such areas are invariably found on the radial or ulnar aspects. Use a 20-or 22-gauge, 4-cm (1½-inch) needle.

For the radial (lateral) entry, position the hand with the palmar surface down and flex it over a rolled towel at the wrist. Aspirate the joint at the midpoint of the distal articulation of the radius, just medial to the extensor tendon of the thumb. The needle should be perpendicular to the skin during aspiration. The ulnar, or medial, approach is made in the middle of the palpable depression between the lateral aspect of the tip of the ulna and carpus. Position the hand as for a radial approach. Direct the needle ventrally toward the palmar surface and proximally into the joint space.

To administer corticosteroids into the carpal tunnel (to treat compression of the median nerve), place the needle between flexor creases of the wrist just lateral to the palmaris longus tendon (or medial to the flexor carpi radialis) and advance it distally until resistance to injection is minimal. (See Chapter 29 for details.)

F. Small Joints of the Hands and Feet

Systemic arthritides frequently involve the proximal and distal interphalangeal joints and the first metatarsophalangeal joint. Enter the joint in the midline just lateral to the extensor tendon on the dorsolateral aspect and gently work a 25- or 27-gauge needle into the joint space. A 2-mL syringe suffices for aspiration and is easier to handle than larger ones. Maintain a slight vacuum in the syringe so that any trauma to digital vessels will be recognized immediately (blood will appear in the syringe). Traction on the distal portion of the phalanx helps open the joint space, allowing easier access for the needle.

▶ Synovial Fluid Analysis

If minimal fluid is available, priorities must be established for processing the sample. If pyogenic arthritis is a diagnostic possibility, an appropriate approach would be to place one drop of fluid on a microscope slide for Gram stain, another into a hemacytometer for cell count, and the remainder of the sample for culture. If 10–20 mL or more of synovial fluid is obtained, complete synovianalysis can be performed, as outlined below; partial analysis is possible on even as little as 1 mL of fluid.

A. Physical Characteristics

1. Determine the total volume of fluid removed.

2. Assess color and clarity of fluid (normally a crystal-clear yellowish fluid through which print can be easily read).

3. Note viscosity by allowing a drop to fall from the needle. Normal joint fluid has high viscosity and easily forms a cord several inches long.

4. Perform the mucin clot test (Ropes test) by adding 1 mL of synovial fluid to diluted acetic acid (about 5%). Normally, the mucin in the fluid congeals within minutes, forming a gel (commonly called a clot) that remains firm for hours. In the case of infection or chronic inflammation, unstable gel forms, which is easily broken up by gentle agitation. Examine the gel again at 1 hour for friability; normal mucin gel should be unchanged after 1 hour.

B. Laboratory Studies

The choice of studies is guided by clinical circumstances. Gram stain and culture, cell count, and examination for crystal formation should always be performed when fluid from an acutely inflamed joint is being evaluated.

1. Cell count and differential—Place 2–10 mL of synovial fluid in a purple-topped (EDTA anticoagulant) or green-topped (heparin anticoagulant) tube for laboratory examination. If fluid is scanty, use 1–2 drops counterstained with methylene blue and perform a cell count in the emergency department with a hemacytometer. Normal synovial fluid contains fewer than 200 white cells per microliter, of which less than 25% are polymorphonuclear neutrophils.

2. Special stains—All joint fluid should be stained with Gram stain and examined by microscopy. Special stains for fungi and acid-fast bacilli should also be performed when chronic monarticular arthritis is being evaluated. These tests are specific but not sensitive for detection of fungal or mycobacterial arthritis.

3. Examination for crystals—Place a drop of synovial fluid on a clean glass microscope slide under a cover-slip. Examine the specimen immediately; if this is impossible, slow the evaporation of joint fluid by sealing the edges of the coverslip with nail polish or petrolatum. Crystals can be detected using light microscopy and tentatively identified on the basis of morphologic characteristics seen at ×400 magnification. Urate crystals are needle-shaped; calcium pyrophosphate crystals are more rhomboid-shaped; and cholesterol crystals are flat, with notched corners. Polarized light microscopy demonstrates the negative birefringence of urate crystals and the positive birefringence of calcium pyrophosphate. The presence of crystals both free in fluid and within leukocytes is pathognomonic of crystal-induced arthropathy. If the laboratory is doing the examination, collect 1–2 mL of fluid in a purple-topped (EDTA anticoagulant) or green-topped (heparin anticoagulant) tube.

4. Culture—Sterile, capped specimen tubes should be filled with 1–10 mL of fluid for bacterial cultures and, if indicated, mycobacterial and fungal cultures. In suspected gonococcal disease, chocolate agar should be inoculated with some of the fluid (in the emergency department if possible). When a potentially infected prosthetic joint is being evaluated, a jar of anaerobic transport media should also be inoculated.

5. Glucose determination—The glucose level of the synovial fluid can be used to determine the possibility a patient's symptoms are related to a septic joint. Place 0.5–1 mL of synovial fluid in a gray-topped (fluoride anticoagulant) tube. The sample must be compared with a simultaneously drawn blood sample. Blood glucose that is more than 40 mg/dL higher than synovial fluid glucose suggests infection.

6. Protein—Place 0.5–1 mL of synovial joint fluid in a red-topped (no anticoagulant) tube. Determine the total serum protein of a simultaneously drawn blood sample. Normal joint protein is about one-third that of serum.

7. Other studies—Less commonly indicated studies include cytology studies in possible pigmented villonodular synovitis or metastatic disease (5–10 mL in a lightly heparinized specimen tube); pH determinations (1–2 mL in a sealed heparinized syringe); complement levels; and tests for rheumatoid factor, antinuclear antibody, immunoglobulins, and various enzymes.

The presence of fat globules (often with blood) suggests intra-articular fracture.

INCISION AND DRAINAGE OF SUPERFICIAL ABSCESS

▶ Indications

A superficial abscess is incised in order to drain it.

▶ Contraindications

There are no contraindications to incision and drainage of a superficial abscess.

▶ Personnel Required

One person can usually incise and drain a superficial abscess unaided, although an assistant may be helpful to restrain an uncooperative patient.

▶ Equipment and Supplies Required

Many incision and drainage kits are commercially available. The following items are required:

- Materials for skin cleansing.
- Protective gown, mask, eye protection, and gloves.
- No. 11 surgical blade, mounted.
- Drapes.
- Curved Kelly and mosquito clamps.
- Forceps.
- Packing material, such as gauze strip packing.
- Sterile gauze sponges, 10×10 cm^2 (4×4 inch^2), and tape.
- Ethyl chloride skin-freezing solution (optional).
- Lidocaine, 1%, with 25-gauge needle and 5-mL syringe.
- Culture tube and slides.
- Sterile saline for irrigation.
- Irrigating syringe and basin.
- Needle, 18 gauge, with 5-mL syringe.
- Plastic-coated absorbent pad.

▶ Positioning of the Patient

The patient should be lying on a firm surface in a comfortable position, with the area to be drained in full view and firmly supported.

▶ Procedure

Anesthesia is the main difficulty in incision and drainage. Superficial abscesses suitable for drainage at the bedside are painful, and the patient should be assured that pain will decrease after the pressure is relieved and the pus is drained. Incising the skin and draining the pus are painful, however, and little relief can be obtained short of general or block anesthesia, both of which require an anesthesiologist and an operating room. Spraying the area with ethyl chloride to freeze the skin will prevent some but not all pain. Infiltrating the thick layer of skin over the pointing abscess with lidocaine is impossible, and injecting lidocaine into the abscess cavity is ineffective and may create more pain from increased pressure. Narcotic analgesics (eg, morphine, 2–10 mg intramuscularly or subcutaneously) may take the edge off the pain and relieve some of the patient's anxiety, but they will not provide total relief.

If an abscess is too large to be adequately drained at the bedside or if it appears that the patient may experience too much pain to be able to cooperate effectively, incision and drainage in the operating room is always an alternative.

A. Simple Abscess not Involving a Vital Structure

1. Assemble the necessary equipment and arrange it on a table or bedside stand.

2. Position the patient. Place the plastic-coated absorbent pad under the body part with the abscess to be drained.

3. Don sterile gloves and put on a gown, mask, and eye protection. Cleanse the skin over the area being drained. Drape the area, and have extra absorbent materials ready to catch any pus not absorbed by the drape.

4. If there is any doubt whether an abscess is actually present, take the 18-gauge needle and the 5-mL syringe and aspirate the suspected abscess at the point of maximum fluctuance. If no pus is found, reassess the clinical situation, and proceed with incision and draining if it is deemed appropriate.

5. If ethyl chloride or lidocaine is being used, it should be given at this time.

6. Using the No. 11 blade, open the abscess at the point of maximum fluctuance and allow the pus to drain under its own pressure. Using a quick, decisive motion minimizes the patient's discomfort. Collect the first portion of pus for Gram stain and culture and sensitivity testing.

7. After the pressure has been relieved, insert the Kelly or mosquito clamp and find the longest axis of the abscess. Point the curve of the clamp up at the farthest point from the central incision and determine the shortest possible length to be incised so that the abscess is completely drained. Incise the skin to that point, using swift upward motion of the No. 11 blade. If it is necessary to make a long incision to completely drain the abscess, infiltrate the skin in the most lateral aspect with lidocaine. Repeat the procedure in the opposite direction. Allow any further pus to drain. *Note*: It is important to obtain an opening in the abscess wide enough to allow complete drainage of all pus. If the abscess is not opened completely, complete drainage cannot occur, and resolution of the abscess will be delayed.

8. Using the clamp, break up any loculated pus in the cavity.

9. Irrigate the abscess with saline until all pus is removed.

10. Pack the abscess cavity with iodoform or plain gauze packing. Fill the cavity tightly enough to cause hemostasis but not so tightly that it causes pain.

11. Dress the area with the sterile 10×10 cm^2 (4×4 inch^2) sponge and tape. On the extremities or in areas where there is movement, consider dressing the site with an expanded bandage around the extremity.

12. Begin antimicrobial therapy, if indicated (eg, for facial abscesses, cellulitis). Remember to cover for community-acquired methicillin-resistant *Staphylococcus aureus* and consider trimethoprim/sulfamethoxazole unless a sulfa allergy exists.

13. Schedule a follow-up appointment in 1–2 days.

B. Incision and Drainage of Abscesses Over Special Areas

1. Face, head, and neck abscesses—The clinical situation in these anatomic areas must be carefully considered before incision and drainage is performed, because the large scar left by complete incision and drainage may be cosmetically unacceptable and because of the possibility of injuring vital structures beneath the skin. In small superficial abscesses on the face, drainage can be accomplished by making a small incision at the lower part of the abscess, removing all pus, and leaving a gauze wick in the incision to keep the wound from closing. Frequent irrigation will be needed during follow-up to keep the cavity clean and promote healing. Any abscess that is large or that might involve vital structures should be drained in the operating room by personnel experienced in this procedure.

2. Abscesses around joints—Make sure that the abscess does not involve the joint space. (Consult an orthopedic surgeon if there is any doubt.) If the abscess is superficial and does not involve the joint space, proceed with incision and drainage. Remember that splinting of the joint is necessary for adequate healing.

3. Abscesses around the anus—Differentiate pilonidal abscesses from perianal abscesses caused by anal fistulas. Perianal abscesses require surgical consultation and possibly drainage in the operating room.

4. Abscesses of the hands, wrists, ankles, and feet—The compact arrangement of many vital structures in the hand, wrist, ankle, and foot makes drainage of abscesses in these areas difficult to perform in the emergency department. It is recommended that any abscess around these structures be drained in the operating room by experienced personnel. Surgical consultation is advisable in all cases of abscesses in these areas.

▼ TRANSCUTANEOUS CARDIAC PACING

Transcutaneous cardiac pacing is a safe, rapid, noninvasive method of temporarily treating symptomatic bradyarrhythmias and asystole. Advances in technology have led to the development of defibrillators that are also capable of transcutaneous pacing. With these devices, transcutaneous pacing can be initiated in the prehospital setting or in the emergency department and is the procedure of choice in the treatment of asystole and bradycardic cardiac arrest.

▶ Indications

- Asystole.
- Symptomatic bradycardia (<40 beats/min) unresponsive to atropine.
- Overdrive pacing for tachyarrhythmias (atrial, ventricular, torsade de pointes) unresponsive to medical and electrical cardioversion.
- Transvenous pacing is difficult or contraindicated (eg, heart block in myocardial infarction treated with thrombolytic therapy).

▶ Complications

The main complications associated with transcutaneous pacing are pain and local skin erythema due to first-degree burns. With the newer devices, pain from cutaneous nerve and muscle stimulation is now reported as tolerable. The energy levels used for pacing have not been shown to produce any significant myocardial damage. Other persons coming into contact with the pacing impulses may experience mild tingling. The risk of inducing ventricular fibrillation during transcutaneous pacing is negligible.

▶ Personnel Required

One person can initiate transcutaneous pacing unaided.

▶ Equipment Required

- Transcutaneous pacing device, two pacing electrodes, and connecting cable.
- Optional electrodes and connecting cable for electrocardiographic monitoring are available with some models.

▶ Procedure

1. Place one pacing electrode over the left anterior chest. Place the other electrode posteriorly in the interscapular area. Attach the connecting cables as indicated on the labels.

2. If the pacing device is equipped for electrocardiographic monitoring, attach monitor leads to both shoulders and the left upper abdomen. *Note*: Standard electrocardiographic monitor results are usually uninterpretable owing to the strong pacing stimulus and movement artifact.

3. Set rate at 80 beats/min; select synchronous mode for bradycardia or asynchronous mode for asystole. (Depending on the model, rate and mode may be fixed and not operator-selected.) Turn on power; turn on pacing.

4. Begin at 70–80-mA current output.

5. Check for presence of a femoral pulse. Check the monitor for evidence of electrical capture (pacer spike before each QRS complex). If no pulse is detected, gradually increase the current output until pulse appears or highest current setting is reached. *Caution*: The carotid pulse is usually difficult to detect owing to muscle contractions. A Doppler stethoscope may be needed to ascertain the presence or absence of a pulse.

6. Reduce current output to the lowest setting associated with a palpable pulse and determine blood pressure.

7. If transcutaneous pacing is successful, interrupt pacing intermittently to check for return of spontaneous electrical activity. As soon as the patient is stable, if pacing is still needed, insert a transvenous pacemaker.

8. If transcutaneous pacing is unsuccessful and pacing is still required, attempt transvenous pacing.

Ortega F, Sekhar P, Song M, et al: Periferal intravenous cannulation. N Engl J Med 2008;359:e26.

Procedural Sedation and Analgesia

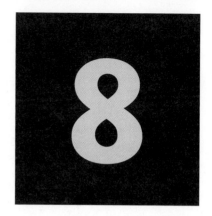

Christopher Colvin, MD

Procedural sedation and analgesia (PSA) has been proven safe and efficacious within the ED environment, and should be utilized when patients undergo painful procedures. The most important step beyond monitoring the patient involves extensive preparation, and at conclusion of the procedure, patients should return to their mental and physiologic baseline. In scenarios where the patient's severity of illness questions the applicability of ED sedation, one must judiciously review the risks and consider consultation with the anesthesiologist. Although the degrees of sedation can at times be ambiguous, observing the patient's progression and remaining vigilant for respiratory depression can diminish untoward effects and facilitate successful recovery and disposition.

BASICS OF PROCEDURAL SEDATION AND ANALGESIA

Sedation is often utilized to facilitate care in the ED. PSA has replaced the previous nomenclature of "conscious sedation." The American College of Emergency Physicians (ACEP) defines PSA as the "administration of sedatives or dissociative agents with or without analgesics to induce a state that allows the patient to tolerate unpleasant procedures while maintaining cardiorespiratory function. Procedural sedation and analgesia is intended to result in a depressed level of consciousness that allows the patient to maintain oxygenation and airway control independently."

The controversy over nonanesthesiologists providing PSA primarily involves this last statement. Patients can easily progress to each successive stage of sedation to the point of apnea and respiratory arrest. The practitioner's goal should be to avoid progressive unconsciousness and remain capable in managing their cardiopulmonary function when necessary. Despite concerns, the efficacy and safety of ED procedural sedations have been demonstrated in numerous studies, and PSA has become a core skill in emergency medicine training and practice.

LEVELS OF SEDATION

PSA is a spectrum involving light, moderate, deep, and general anesthesia levels necessitating the practitioner to be capable of recognizing the levels of sedation, and be prepared to rescue the next level of sedation if necessary. Some experts have proposed adding a separate category for dissociative anesthetics such as ketamine since its performance and side-effect profile differ a great deal from other forms of sedation. Each degree of sedation increases risk of cardiopulmonary instability with a likely need for aggressive intervention.

- **Minimal sedation (anxiolysis)**

  A drug-induced state during which patients respond normally to verbal commands. Although cognitive function and physical coordination may be impaired, airway reflexes, and ventilatory and cardiovascular functions are unaffected.

- **Moderate sedation/analgesia ("conscious sedation")**

  A drug-induced depression of consciousness during which patients respond purposefully to verbal commands, either alone or accompanied by light tactile stimulation. No interventions are required to maintain a patent airway, and spontaneous ventilation is adequate. Cardiovascular function is usually maintained.

- **Deep sedation/analgesia**

  A drug-induced depression of consciousness during which patients cannot be easily aroused but respond purposefully following repeated or painful stimulation. Reflex withdrawal from a painful stimulus is *not* considered a purposeful response. The ability to independently maintain ventilatory function may be impaired. Patients may require assistance in maintaining a patent airway, and spontaneous ventilation may be inadequate. Cardiovascular function is usually maintained.

- **General anesthesia**

  A drug-induced loss of consciousness during which patients are not arousable, even by painful stimulation. The ability to independently maintain ventilatory function is often impaired. Patients often require assistance in maintaining a patent airway, and positive pressure ventilation may be required because of depressed spontaneous ventilation or drug-induced depression of neuromuscular function. Cardiovascular function may be impaired.

ASSESSMENT

PSA is indicated for the anticipated need of pain relief, amnesia, and anxiolysis required for the patient's comfort. The sedative rugs, the dosage, depth, and duration of sedation must be considered prior to the initiation of the procedure. PSA requires a presedation assessment, sedation monitoring, and postsedation assessment prior to disposition. In the presedation assessment, history of prior anesthesia/sedation complications should be evaluated along with comorbid conditions and allergies. The American Society of Anesthesiologists (ASA) developed a physical status classification system. It describes patients' illness severity as categories I–VI (Table 8–1). Each category involves escalating degrees of progressive systemic disease, and is meant to be used for assessing the illness of the patient prior to surgery.

Patients scored as an ASA I–II can be reasonably sedated within the ED without elevating the risk of sequelae from underlying systemic pathology. Once the patient is deemed to be more ill (ie, ASA III–IV), it is often more appropriate to involve anesthesia within the parameters of elective or

Table 8–1. ASA Classification System.

ASA 1	A normal healthy patient
ASA 2	A patient with mild systemic disease
ASA 3	A patient with severe systemic disease
ASA 4	A patient with severe systemic disease that is a constant threat to life
ASA 5	A moribund patient who is not expected to survive without the operation
ASA 6	A declared brain-dead patient whose organs are being removed for donor purposes

non-life-threatening scenarios. ASA III classifications have been shown to be an independent risk factor for adverse outcomes in general anesthesia and pediatric sedation cases. Categories V and VI are usually not applicable within the ED setting. The downside to ASA classification is the inherent ambiguity of the definitions and the variable scoring between practitioners.

Patients should be screened for recent illnesses, hospitalizations, smoking, illicit drug use, GERD, CAD, HTN, cirrhosis, and other metabolic disorders as well. Pulmonary diseases such as asthma, cystic fibrosis, pulmonary fibrosis, tracheomalacia, and COPD could all potentially result in profound hypoxemia. Patient using supplemental oxygen at home would indicate an ASA class of III or IV requiring a critical review for the need of ED PSA. A history of GERD may predispose the patient to passive aspiration while sedated, and could result in laryngospasm or aspiration pneumonitis. A history of significant CAD or severe CHF would suggest a higher risk for myocardial events should hypoxemia or hypotension ensue. ED PSA would not be a satisfactory option for these patients.

Food and medication allergies should also be documented since egg and soy allergies would preclude the option to utilize propofol. Liver disease may indicate a decreased ability to metabolize barbiturates and benzodiazepenes, potentially prolonging sedation. Methohexital may induce seizure activity in patients with a history of a seizure disorder.

Airway assessment is integral in establishing an adequate sedation plan should aggressive maneuvers be necessary. Will the planned procedure involve occluding the airway (ie, oral laceration repairs, GI endoscopy)? Does the patient wear dentures, or have a large tongue, an overbite, or micrognathia? Patients with a Mallampati classification greater than III, inability to open the mouth more than 4 cm, a thyromental distance less than 6 cm, history of cervical spinal inflexibility, or history of previous difficult intubation all indicate a high risk for intubation failure. Should the patient be deemed at a high risk for airway failure, appropriate precautions should be implemented and the decision to abort the PSA should be entertained.

Airway adjuncts beyond direct laryngoscopy such as an intubating LMA, GlideScope, light wand, or fiberoptic scope should remain at the bedside. Supplemental oxygen may need to be delivered via non-rebreather (NRB) or nasal trumpet if the patient becomes unexpectedly obtunded. Above all else, protection of the patient's airway, and avoidance of respiratory depression, is tantamount to a successful sedation.

Hemodynamic stability must also be maintained. Many sedative agents and regimens result in vasodilatation, and once the patient develops a depressed level of consciousness, his or her sympathetic output may also decrease further potentiating bradycardia and decreased mean arterial pressure. Patients taking antihypertensive medications and those with dehydration or acute blood loss anemia should be volume resuscitated prior to PSA. Cardiac patients taking calcium channel blockers or beta-blockers have been shown to have a higher incidence of bradycardia and hypotension with PSA. Pressor agents such as norepinephrine, epinephrine, phenylephrine, dopamine, or ephedrine should be available in the event that fluid refractory shock takes place.

Patients should also be assessed for recent oral intake. Patients are at risk for aspiration of gastric contents when they reach deeper levels of sedation and lose their protective airway reflexes. Although small ED studies have shown no significant adverse outcomes with known oral intake prior to procedures, ASA guidelines recommend safety parameters of liquids requiring 2 hours and solids requiring 6 hours prior to a procedure.

Aspiration under general anesthesia has been estimated to have an incidence of 1:3420 with mortality in 1:125,109 cases with little data to suggest long-term sequelae. General anesthesia is at the extreme end of the sedation spectrum, and often mandates advanced airway manipulation; therefore, aspiration is much more likely. Although no study has demonstrated an elevated risk of aspiration for moderate to deep PSA in the ED, it is imperative to consider gastric contents and depth of sedation. Most authors have concluded that their sample sizes were often not large enough to detect statistically significant differences in study subjects. Patients presenting with a full stomach would benefit from observation and procedural delay for gastric emptying. Care should be taken to minimize the likelihood of aspiration, and precautions made to manage aspiration should it occur with wall suction, suction catheter, and additional personnel should the patient need to be log rolled into the lateral decubitus position.

MONITORING

Once the need for procedural sedation has been assessed, informed consent should be obtained from the patient. Patients should have mental status and function documented prior to and following the procedural initiation. Pediatric and adult patients alike should be placed on a cardiac monitor, pulse oximetry, blood pressure cuff, and, if available,

Table 8-2. Equipment for Procedural Sedation and Analgesia.

| High-flow oxygen |
| Non-rebreather mask |
| Ambu bag |
| Nasal trumpet |
| Advanced airway equipment |
| Cardiac monitor |
| Blood pressure monitor |
| Pulse oximetry/ETCO$_2$ |
| Reversal agents (ie, Narcan, flumazenil) ACLS medications |
| Defibrillator |
| Suction device with suction catheter |
| IV capabilities |

end-tidal CO_2 (ETCO$_2$). Studies have shown ETCO$_2$ to be more sensitive in detecting patients with respiratory depression than pulse oximetry, although there was no significant difference in outcome. Patients with deep sedation resulting in respiratory depression will show an increase in ETCO$_2$ greater than 10 mm Hg from baseline or a level above 50 mm Hg total before they demonstrate a decrease in oxygen saturation. Although the ETCO$_2$ does not differentiate the level of sedation, it can accurately detect respiratory depression.

While monitoring the patient's sedation course, heart rate, blood pressure, and oxygen saturations should be documented in serial timed intervals. Adverse events should be documented with additional descriptions of executed interventions. Standard reporting of adverse events includes apnea, oxygen saturation less than 90%, ETCO$_2$ > 50 mm Hg, bradycardia, hypotension, and emesis. Continuous cardiac monitoring is important to detect adverse rhythms, and can be helpful to determine pain response when the patient develops a sinus tachycardia. Additional tools that can often prove to be vital during sedations include ACLS medication access, advanced airway equipment, and supplemental oxygen via nasal cannula, NRB, or bag valve mask (BVM) (Table 8-2).

SEDATION SCALES

Multiple scales have been created and described for measuring patients' levels of comfort, agitation, and sedation in the ICU, OR, and ED environments. The scales provide practitioners a guide to determine depth of sedation, and need for smaller titrations, reversal, or additional medications. Most of the sedation scales include monitoring agitation that does not directly relate to elective procedural sedation in the ED.

The Ramsay Sedation Scale (RSS) has been utilized in studies on ED PSA to describe levels of sedation. It is a simple 6-score system with 1 being anxious or restless and 6 being no response to stimulus (Table 8-3). It has been validated for inter-rater reliability, and simplifies the PSA assessment.

Table 8–3. Ramsay Sedation Scale.

Score	Responsiveness
1	Patient is anxious and agitated or restless, or both
2	Patient is cooperative, oriented, and tranquil
3	Patient responds to commands only
4	Patient exhibits brisk response to light glabellar tap or loud auditory stimulus
5	Patient exhibits a sluggish response to light glabellar tap or loud auditory stimulus
6	Patient exhibits no response

The Richmond Agitation–Sedation Scale (RASS) is a 10-score system with 4+ (combative) to 1+ (restless) range for grading decreasing agitation, 0 for calmness, and −1 (drowsy) to −5 (unarousable) to quantify degree of responsiveness (Table 8–4). The RASS scale differentiates the varying degrees of agitation, whereas the RSS scale has only one category (1) for anxious, agitated, or restlessness. The RSS scale utilizes a physical stimulus (glabellar tap) to grade

Table 8–4. Richmond Agitation–Sedation Scale.

Score	Term	Description
+4	Combative	Overtly combative or violent; immediate danger to staff
+3	Very agitated	Pulls on or removes tube(s) or catheter(s) or has aggressive behavior toward staff
+2	Agitated	Frequent nonpurposeful movement or patient-ventilator dyssynchrony
+1	Restless	Anxious or apprehensive but movements not aggressive or vigorous
0	Alert and calm	
−1	Drowsy	Not fully alert, but has sustained (more than 10 seconds) awakening, with eye contact, to voice
−2	Light sedation	Briefly (less than 10 seconds) awakens with eye contact to voice
−3	Moderate sedation	Any movement (but no eye contact) to voice
−4	Deep sedation	No response to voice, but any movement to physical stimulation
−5	Unarousable	No response to voice or physical stimulation

responsiveness, but the RASS scale implements both verbal and physical stimuli to grade consciousness.

SEDATION CONCLUSION AND PATIENT DISPOSITION

Care should be taken toward the conclusion of the PSA to limit additional medication administration. Should the noxious stimuli cease (ie, distal radius fracture is reduced and splinted) shortly after the last dose, respiratory depression, hypotension, and bradycardia could likely ensue. Depending on the sedative regimen utilized, rapid degradation would mitigate these effects (ie, propofol, dexmedetomidine, etomidate). Longer-acting agents such as fentanyl and versed could create overt sedation 20–30 minutes beyond the last dose and completion of the ED procedure.

Patients should be capable of responding verbally once sedation has worn off, and once assessed they should return to the baseline mental status documented prior to the PSA. Postprocedural emesis can be common following agents such as ketamine, so complete return to baseline is recommended prior to administering oral intake. Studies suggest that a minimum post-PSA observation period of 30 minutes be exercised. Most adverse events such as hemodynamic instability and emesis should have been resolved by that time. Once the patient has successfully completed the post-PSA observation period, he or she may be safely discharged from the ED.

▼ AGENTS FOR PROCEDURAL SEDATION AND ANALGESIA

The ideal procedural agent for the ED acts quickly, creates excellent comfort for the patient, and resolves soon thereafter with little to no side effects. No sedative agent is perfect, but multiple agents exist to tailor to each patient encounter (Table 8–5). Analgesia can often be controlled with narcotics, but procedural sedation requires the addition of an amnestic to reach a steady state of comfort. Benzodiazepines are often included with narcotics to facilitate adequate sedation. Some agents such as ketamine can often serve as the sole agent in short procedures, whereas versed and fentanyl regimens remain the mainstay in numerous emergency departments. Propofol, although a strong agent for moderate to deep sedation, does not truly satisfy analgesic requirements; however, in multiple studies, it is often used solely for the entire PSA.

FENTANYL

Fentanyl is a strong synthetic opiate with potency nearly 100 times that of morphine. It lacks amnestic properties, so it is often used in combination with versed or propofol. The likelihood of respiratory depression increases greatly when fentanyl is administered with the aforementioned sedatives. It is renally excreted with a half-life of 3.5 hours. Dosing for

Table 8–5. Common Drugs for Procedural Sedation and Analgesia.

Drug	Dosage	Onset	Duration
Fentanyl	IV: 0.5–2 μg/kg	1–2 min	30–60 min
Ketamine	IV: 1–2 mg/kg	1–2 min	20–60 min
	IM: 3–5 mg/kg	5–10 min	60–120 min
Dexmedetomidine	IV: 1 μg/kg bolus over 10 min, and then a drip 0.5–0.75 μg/kg/h	10–15 min	2–3 min following discontinue
Versed	IV: 1–2.5 mg; titrate to effect	1–5 min	20–60 min
	IM: 0.1–0.15 mg/kg	10–15 min	60–120 min
Propofol	IV bolus over 1–2 min: 1 mg/kg, and then 0.5 mg/kg	30–60 s	2–5 min following discontinue
	IV drip: 5–50 μg/kg/min		
Etomidate	IV: 0.1–0.2 mg/kg	30–60 s	3–5 min
Methohexital	IV: 0.75–1.0 mg/kg, and then 0.5 mg/kg	30–60 s	5–7 min
Naloxone	IV: 0.4–2 mg	1–5 min	30–60 min
Flumazenil	IV: 0.2 mg; maximum dose of 3 mg	1–5 min	45–60 min

analgesia is 1–2 μg/kg IV, but is more optimal if administered as 0.5–1 μg/kg IV aliquots every 2–3 minutes. Time of onset is 1–2 minutes, with a duration of 30–45 minutes. Fentanyl does not induce histamine release, and is less likely to induce hypotension. It is also unlikely to cause a cross-reaction allergic response in patients with a known morphine allergy. Adverse effects include bradycardia, hypotension, increased intracranial pressure, and the potential for chest wall rigidity with large doses.

KETAMINE

Ketamine is a dissociative anesthetic that produces analgesic, amnestic, and sedative effects. It increases endogenous catecholamines by blocking the reuptake pathway facilitating sympathomimetic effects. It maintains protective airway reflexes, and can increase the heart rate and blood pressure as well as intracranial and intraocular pressures. Ketamine can also cause laryngospasm that may present as persistent coughing to complete occlusion with resultant hypoxemia. A recent history of viral upper respiratory infection, age < 3 months, parainfluenza infection with resultant subglottic narrowing (croup), and stimulation of the posterior pharynx (aggressive suctioning, endoscopy, bronchoscopy) has been demonstrated to increase the likelihood of laryngospasm.

The patient often demonstrates a persistent nystagmus with nonpurposeful movements, but he or she is unable to communicate. Prior to PSA initiation, it may be helpful to describe this phenomenon to friends or family in the room. Ketamine should be avoided in patients currently intoxicated with sympathomimetics such as cocaine or

methamphetamine, patients with head or ocular trauma, and patients with significant cardiovascular disease.

Drawbacks with ketamine use include the well-known emergence phenomena and postprocedural emesis. Benzodiazepenes have been shown to marginally decrease both effects. Ketamine dosing is 1–2 mg/kg IV with onset within 1–2 minutes, peak levels reached within 5 minutes, and total duration at 20–60 minutes. Ketamine is administered IM at 3–5 mg/kg with onset in 5–10 minutes, peak at 10–15 minutes, and duration 1–2 hours.

Ketamine is a sialagogue, and can produce an increase in tracheobronchial and salivary secretions. An anticholinergic such as atropine or glycopyrolate should be given to mitigate these effects. Glycopyrolate can be given IM/IV at 0.004 mg/kg (usual injection solution is 0.2 mg/mL). Atropine dosing should be 0.01 mg/kg IM/IV with a minimum dose of 0.1 mg, and maximum dose of 0.5 mg. Ketamine, versed, and atropine can be given within the same syringe.

DEXMEDETOMIDINE (PRECEDEX)

Precedex is a centrally acting 2-adrenergic agonist with sedating and analgesic effects. Although few studies have evaluated the use of dexmedetomidine for PSA in the ED setting, multiple studies have demonstrated the safety and efficacy of dexmedetomidine for PSA, surgical interventions, and ICU management. Dexmedetomidine has been utilized in pediatric and adult patients. Primary concerns with dexmedetomidine involve its ability to mitigate central sympathetic output. Patients can develop profound bradycardia, sinus arrest, heart block, and hypotension. Patients with a history of cardiovascular disease, heart block, or cardiomyopathy should not be administered dexmedetomidine for PSA. Anticholinergics are required to preempt adverse cardiac events. The standard regimen involves utilizing glycopyrolate at 0.2 mg IV prior to initiation of the PSA. Studies have shown this simple preventative measure significantly reduced episodes of bradycardia. The loading does for PSA is 1 mcg/kg bolus over 10 minutes followed by 0.5–0.75 mcg/kg/h. The loading does should not be shorter than 10 minutes in order to avoid bradycardia. Patients are capable of participating in painful procedures without developing respiratory depression, and once the PSA is completed, the agent is rapidly metabolized with a short recovery time. Patients should be continuously monitored while on dexmedetomidine, and a preprocedural ECG should be considered.

MIDAZOLAM (VERSED)

Midazolam is a benzodiazepine with sedating, anxiolytic, and amnestic effects, but no analgesic effects. It functions through GABA receptors resulting in an influx of chloride, and CNS depression occurs. It is often used in combination with a narcotic such as fentanyl, or a dissociative anesthetic such as ketamine. It is more rapid in onset than diazepam or lorazepam. Midazolam can be given PO, PR, IV, and IM, and atomized intranasally. It has been shown to diminish episodes of postprocedural emesis and emergence reactions with ketamine. Midazolam can cause hypotension and respiratory depression. PSA doses for adults should be titrated slowly with 1–2.5 mg IV doses at a time waiting 2–5 minutes between doses to assess response. Typical dosing regimen is 0.03–0.1 mg/kg IV. Pediatric patients should be dosed 0.05–0.1 mg/kg IV if age 6 months to 5 years, 0.025 mg to 0.05 mg/kg IV if 6–12 years of age, and 1–2.5 mg IV if aged 12–16 years. Patients who are administered narcotics simultaneously should have the midazolam dose decreased by 30% if under 60 years of age and 50% if over the age of 60. Alternate routes of midazolam and doses include:

- IM: 0.1–0.15 mg/kg
- Oral: 0.25–1 mg/kg
- Intranasal: 0.2–0.6 mg/kg
- Rectal: 0.25–0.5 mg/kg

Midazolam given IM will peak at 30 minutes with greater than 90% bioavailability. However, oral administration varies with peak onset depending on age (0.17–2.6 hours) with only 36% bioavailability. Elimination half-life IV is 3 hours in adults, and 2.9–4.5 hours in pediatric patients aged 6 months to 16 years. Median time of PSA with midazolam has been demonstrated to be 23 minutes versus 10 minutes for etomidate. Primary metabolism is hepatic with renal excretion highlighting the need to decrease dosages in patients with hepatic or renal disease. Pediatric patients requiring gentle anxiolysis for radiologic imaging can receive atomized intranasal midazolam to facilitate the study without the need for

parenteral administration. Midazolam is dosed at 1 mg/mL IV, and it is compatible with fentanyl.

PROPOFOL

Propofol is a nonopioid, nonbarbiturate, sedative hypnotic that is delivered via a lipid emulsion vehicle. Since the emulsion is composed of soy and egg products, patients with these food allergies should not receive this agent. Concentration is 10 mg/mL, and is given IV. Propofol for PSA is administered as a 1 mg/kg IV loading dose followed by 0.5 mg/kg IV maintenance dose, and is best given as 10–20 mg IV doses in adults over 1–2 minutes until desired level of sedation is attained. Propofol drips are initiated at 5–50 μg/kg/min and titrated to appropriate level of awareness for mechanical ventilation.

Propofol has no analgesic effects, and should be administered with a narcotic such as fentanyl if administered for mechanical ventilation. Risk for respiratory depression and apnea is increased if propofol is given in large, rapid boluses, and significantly more likely if given along with narcotics. It is often very difficult to correctly titrate the level of sedation with propofol, so it is imperative that continuous assessment of the patient's awareness be attained. Should a deeper level of sedation be achieved than warranted, discontinue the agent, observe, and execute rescue maneuvers as needed.

Propofol has the benefit of being rapidly metabolized following discontinuation of the PSA or drip, and this enables the practitioner to carefully observe the patient for a short period of time until resolution of sedation. Propofol is beneficial in emergent neurologic cases where serial examinations may be necessary to document progression, and it has been shown to decrease intracranial pressures. It also has been shown to have antiemetic and anticonvulsant properties. Long-term sequelae with propofol are not seen with short-term PSA doses, but include hyperlipidemia, pancreatitis, zinc deficiency, hepatomegaly, rhabdomyolysis, and propofol infusion syndrome. Short-term adverse effects include hypotension, hypoxemia, decreased cardiac output, respiratory depression, and apnea.

Ketamine and propofol combined or "ketofol" is a PSA regimen that has been utilized in the OR, and described in the anesthesia literature. The theory behind its benefits resides within the adverse event profiles of both drugs. Since ketamine can induce vomiting and emergence reactions following sedation, propofol can mitigate the events with its amnestic and antiemetic properties. Propofol can cause respiratory depression, apnea, hypotension, and depressed cardiac output, but when given with ketamine, there is a statistically significant decrease in respiratory depression, hypotension, and apnea. However, a study comparing propofol with fentanyl to propofol with ketamine demonstrated that nausea, vomiting, vertigo, and visual disturbances were much higher in the "ketofol" group suggesting that "ketofol" was a less than optimal regimen. The literature demonstrates that "ketofol" is fairly safe, and future comparative studies should consider evaluating the regimen against other common PSA strategies.

ETOMIDATE

Etomidate is a short-acting nonbarbiturate hypnotic with GABA-like effects. It has been studied exhaustively in induction of general anesthesia, rapid sequence intubation (RSI), and PSA. Typical dosing for RSI is 0.3 mg/kg, and dosing regimens for PSA are 0.1–0.2 mg/kg IV. The benefits include rapid onset of action, stable hemodynamic effects, and rapid metabolism.

Adverse events can include laryngospasm, hiccoughs, and myoclonus. Myoclonus can occur in upwards of 20–30% of cases that may make the procedure more difficult to complete (ie, shoulder reduction). No long-term sequelae are evidenced from the myoclonus, but the appearance may mimic seizure activity and may prompt an unnecessary workup. Etomidate has been shown to blunt response to the ACTH stimulation test suggesting an etiology for adrenal suppression. However, emergency department studies have not been able to demonstrate a statistically significant difference in outcome with hospitalized patients who received a single dose of etomidate for RSI. Although the adrenal suppressive effects typically last no longer than 6–8 hours, studies continue to debate this effect. Greater concern for adrenal suppression is found in patients receiving multiple doses or continuous infusions of etomidate.

METHOHEXITAL

Methohexital is an ultra-short-acting barbiturate used for anesthesia induction and PSA, and can be given IV, IM, and rectally. The dosing for PSA is 0.75–1.0 mg/kg IV, and can be redosed at 0.5 mg/kg IV every 2–5 minutes as needed. Pediatric patient dosing is 0.5–1.0 mg/kg IV. Its onset of action is 30 seconds with lasting clinical effect of 5–7 minutes. Although rapid progression of sedation can take place, airway protective mechanisms are functional. Similar to propofol, it is an amnestic with no analgesic effects. Methohexital can cause laryngospasm, hiccoughs, and if extravasated may result in tissue necrosis. It has also been shown to be a cardiac depressant that may result in hypotension.

▼ REVERSAL AGENTS

Rarely, one may need to administer reversal agents in the event that the patient has been deeply sedated to the state of general anesthesia. Although most agents are rapidly metabolized, and no additional medication is necessary, the midazolam and fentanyl regimen could last for 20–30 minutes. Narcan is more commonly given for opioid overdose, and flumazenil is indicated for benzodiazepine overdose. Although naloxone (Narcan) is relatively benign (symptoms

of withdrawal excluded), flumazenil can potentially be dangerous in patients dependent on benzodiazepenes, and precipitate a refractory seizure.

NALOXONE (NARCAN)

Naloxone is an opioid antagonist that competes directly with systemic narcotics. It binds all the opiate receptors, but appears to have a higher affinity for the mu receptor. Naloxone may be given through the endotracheal tube, IM, IV, IO, or subcutaneously. It is not recommended to administer Narcan via ET tube in newborn infants. Narcan is dosed at 0.4–2 mg IV for adults, and it is recommended to give smaller amounts for patients chronically on opioids in order to avoid overt withdrawal. Abrupt reversal in patients chronically administered narcotics may result in seizures, cardiac arrythmias, pulmonary edema, or profound agitation. Age-appropriate dosing is as follows:

- Newborns: 0.1 mg/kg IV/IM

- Pediatric < 5 years of age or < 20 kg: 0.1 mg/kg IV/IM/IO/SQ

- Pediatric > 5 years of age or > 20 kg: 2 mg IV/IM/IO/SQ

FLUMAZENIL

Flumazenil directly competes for the benzodiazepine binding site on the GABA receptor effectively reversing some aspects of the CNS depression (ie, respiratory depression). It does not facilitate the metabolism of benzodiazepenes, and resedation can occur once the flumazenil wears off. It is given IV, undergoes hepatic metabolism, and is excreted renally. The systemic half-life for adults is 40–70 minutes, and in pediatric patients it may range from 20 to 75 minutes. The initial dosing in adults is 0.2 mg IV over 30 seconds with additional doses of 0.3–0.5 mg given IV for a total maximum dose of 3 mg. Pediatric patients are dosed at 0.01 mg/kg up to 0.2 mg IV over 15 seconds. Repeat doses may be given in increments of 0.01 mg/kg up to a maximum dose of 0.05 mg/kg total or 1 mg total. Flumazenil can cause refractory seizures in patients on chronic benzodiazepenes, or patients with cyclic antidepressant overdoses. Should a patient develop seizure activity following flumazenil administration, benzodiazcpenes are unlikely to work despite large doses for competitive binding. Alternative adjuncts to mitigate the seizures include propofol or barbiturates.

Agrawal D, Manzi SF, Gupta R, Krauss B: Preprocedural fasting state and adverse events in children undergoing procedural sedation and analgesia in a pediatric emergency department. Ann Emerg Med 2003;42:636–646 [PMID: 14581915].

Arora S: Combining ketamine and propofol ("ketofol") for emergency department procedural sedation and analgesia: A review. West J Emerg Med 2008;8:20–23 [PMID: 19561698].

ASA Physical Status Classification System: http://www.asahq.org/clinical/physicalstatus.htm. Accessed July 16, 2010.

Bahn EL, Holt KR: Procedural sedation and analgesia: A review and new concepts. Emerg Med Clin North Am 2005;23: 503–517 [PMID: 15829394].

Bhana N, Goa KL, McClellan KJ: Dexmedetomidine. Drugs 2000;59(2):263–268 [PMID: 10730549].

Bhatt M, Kennedy RM, Osmond MH, Krauss B, McAllister JD, Ansermino JM, Evered LM, Roback MG, Consensus Panel on Sedation Research of Pediatric Emergency Research Canada (PERC), Pediatric Emergency Care Applied Research Network (PECARN): Consensus-based recommendations for standardizing terminology and reporting adverse events for emergency department procedural sedation and analgesia in children. Ann Emerg Med 2009;53:426–435 [PMID: 19026467].

Carrasco G: Instruments for monitoring intensive care unit sedation. Crit Care 2000;4:217–225 [PMID: 11094504].

Deitch K, Miner J, Chudnofsky CR, Dominici P, Latta D: Does end tidal CO_2 monitoring during emergency department procedural sedation and analgesia with propofol decrease the incidence of hypoxic events? A randomized, controlled trial. Ann Emerg Med 2010;55:258–264 [PMID: 19783324].

Di Liddo L, D'Angelo A, Nguyen B, Bailey B, Amre D, Stanciu C: Etomidate versus midazolam for procedural sedation in pediatric outpatients: A randomized controlled trial. Ann Emerg Med 2006;48:433–440 [PMID: 16997680].

Diaz-Guzman E, Mireles-Cabodevila E, Heresi GA, Bauer SR, Arroliga AC: A comparison of methohexital versus etomidate for endotracheal intubation of critically ill patients. Am J Crit Care 2010;19:48–54 [PMID: 20045848].

Godwin SA, Caro DA, Wolf SJ, Jagoda AS, Charles R, Marett BE, Moore J, American College of Emergency Physicians: Clinical policy: Procedural sedation and analgesia in the emergency department. Ann Emerg Med 2005;45:177–196 [PMID: 15671976].

Green SM, Krauss B: Barriers to propofol use in emergency medicine. Ann Emerg Med 2008;52:392–398 [PMID: 18295374].

Hohl CM, Sadatsafavi M, Nosyk B, Anis AH: Safety and clinical effectiveness of midazolam versus propofol for procedural sedation in the emergency department: A systematic review. Acad Emerg Med 2008;15:1–8 [PMID: 18211306].

Lee JS, Gonzalez ML, Chuang SK, Perrott DH: Comparison of methohexital and propofol use in ambulatory procedures in oral and maxillofacial surgery. J Oral Maxillofac Surg 2008;66:1996–2003 [PMID: 18848094].

McQueen A, Wright RO, Kido MM, Kaye E, Krauss B: Procedural sedation and analgesia outcomes in children after discharge from the emergency department: Ketamine versus fentanyl/midazolam. Ann Emerg Med 2009;54:191–197 [PMID: 19464072].

Meredith J, O'Keefe K, Galwankar S: Pediatric procedural sedation and analgesia. J Emerg Trauma Shock 2008;1:88–96 [PMID: 19561987].

Messenger DW, Murray HE, Dungey PE, van Vlymen J, Sivilotti ML: Subdissociative-dose ketamine versus fentanyl for analgesia during propofol procedural sedation: A randomized clinical trial. Acad Emerg Med 2008;15:877–886 [PMID: 18754820].

Miller M, Levy P, Patel M: Procedural sedation and analgesia in the emergency department: What are the risks? Emerg Med Clin North Am 2005;23:551–572 [PMID: 15829397].

Miner JR, Biros M, Krieg S, Johnson C, Heegaard W, Plummer D: Randomized clinical trial of propofol versus methohexital for procedural sedation during fracture and dislocation reduction in the emergency department. Acad Emerg Med 2003;10: 931–937 [PMID: 12957974].

Miner JR, Danahy M, Moch A, Biros M: Randomized clinical trial of etomidate versus propofol for procedural sedation in the emergency department. Ann Emerg Med 2007;49:15–22 [PMID: 16997421].

Miner JR, Heegaard W, Plummer D: End-tidal carbon dioxide monitoring during procedural sedation. Acad Emerg Med 2002;9:275–280 [PMID: 11927449].

Newman DH, Azer MM, Pitetti RD, Singh S: When is a patient safe for discharge after procedural sedation? The timing of adverse effect events in 1,367 pediatric procedural sedations. Ann Emerg Med 2003;42:627–635 [PMID: 14581914].

Riker RR, Shehabi Y, Bokesch PM, Ceraso D, Wisemandle W, Koura F, Whitten P, Margolis BD, Byrne DW, Ely EW, Rocha MG, SEDCOM (Safety and Efficacy of Dexmedetomidine Compared With Midazolam) Study Group: Dexmedetomidine vs midazolam for sedation of critically ill patients. JAMA 2009;301:489–499 [PMID: 19188334].

Roback MG, Wathen JE, Bajaj L, Bothner JP: Adverse events associated with procedural sedation and analgesia in a pediatric emergency department: A comparison of common parenteral drugs. Acad Emerg Med 2005;12:508–513 [PMID: 15930401].

Sessler CN: Sedation scales in the ICU. Chest 2004;126:1727–1730 [PMID: 15596665].

Sessler CN, Gosnell MS, Grap MJ, Brophy GM, O'Neal PV, Keane KA, Tesoro EP, Elswick RK: The Richmond agitation–sedation scale: Validity and reliability in adult intensive care unit patients. Am J Respir Crit Care Med 2002:166:1338–1344 [PMID: 12421743].

Vardy JM, Dignon N, Mukherjee N, Sami DM, Balachandran G, Taylor S: Audit of the safety and effectiveness of ketamine for procedural sedation in the emergency department. Emerg Med J 2008;25:579–582 [PMID: 18723707].

Willman EV, Andolfatto G: A prospective evaluation of "ketofol" (ketamine/propofol combination) for procedural sedation and analgesia in the emergency department. Ann Emerg Med 2007;49:23–30 [PMID: 17059854].

Zed PJ, Abu-Laban RB, Chan WW, Harrison DW: Efficacy, safety and patient satisfaction of propofol for procedural sedation and analgesia in the emergency department: A prospective study. Can J Emerg Med 2007;9:421–427 [PMID: 18072987].

Basic & Advanced Cardiac Life Support

Eric C. Goshorn, MD

Justin A. Kan, MD

Salvator J. Vicario, MD

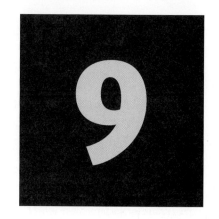

OVERVIEW OF CARDIAC ARREST

EPIDEMIOLOGY OF CARDIAC ARREST

Cardiac disease is the most common cause of death in the United States, with estimates ranging between 300,000 and 500,000 deaths annually. The American Heart Association (AHA) estimates that there are approximately 295,000 out-of-hospital cardiac arrests each year. As few as one fourth of these patients will have an attempted resuscitation. Only 3–8% of prehospital arrests will survive to discharge and have a reasonable functional recovery. Sudden cardiac death is often associated with an underlying history of coronary artery disease, which is seen in 80% of patients. Other causes include massive pulmonary embolism, renal failure, hypoglycemia, thyrotoxicosis, trauma, illicit drugs, and medications. The most common rhythms associated with cardiac arrest are ventricular arrhythmias (ventricular fibrillation [VF] and ventricular tachycardia [VT]). Asystole and pulseless electrical activity (PEA) are the next most common rhythms, at the time of first intervention.

DETERMINANTS OF CARDIAC ARREST SURVIVAL

The two most important factors for survival in the undifferentiated adult cardiac arrest victim are minimizing the elapsed time from patient collapse and the onset of effective cardiopulmonary resuscitation (CPR) and rapid defibrillation. Unfortunately, as many as 85% of arrests occur at home and not in a public place where there may be access to a defibrillator. Studies with patients in VF have demonstrated that for every minute that passes without intervention, the odds of survival decreases by 7–10% (decreased to 3–4% with effective CPR). Other factors related to a positive outcome include witnessed cardiac arrest and early use of advanced life support (ALS). Factors associated with poor prognosis include dyspnea as the presenting complaint, malignancy or sepsis as the underlying cause of cardiac arrest, coexistence of pneumonia, prolonged anoxia, presence of hypotension prior to cardiac arrest, and increasing age.

A patient who is not successfully resuscitated in the field is unlikely to be resuscitated in the emergency department. The risks of transporting a patient who remains in cardiac arrest after ALS procedures have been performed in the field may outweigh the likelihood of a successful resuscitation with good neurologic outcome. Medical directors should consider protocols to determine death and termination of resuscitative efforts in the field.

THE TEAM APPROACH TO CARDIAC ARREST

A resuscitation team has many pivotal participants in a cardiac arrest: the first responder, emergency medical service (EMS) personnel, the emergency department resuscitation team leader, emergency department resuscitation team members, and ancillary personnel. A successful resuscitation depends on a functional team. The responsibilities and expectations for each member must be identified prior to a resuscitation. Attempting to assign these roles after a resuscitation has already begun will simply add confusion to an already chaotic situation.

The composition of the resuscitation team is based largely on resource availability and institutional preferences. There must be a team leader who is responsible for the overall direction of the resuscitation. One member of the team is responsible for airway management. Another member will be necessary to provide support for this function, such as applying cricoid pressure, suctioning, or assisting in bag ventilation. Multiple team members may be required to provide chest compressions. The team leader must ensure that these providers do not become fatigued, by rotating the team members every 5 minutes. Vascular access must be obtained, and the team member performing this role can also administer medications. If a medication dispenser (eg, Pyxis) is being used, it is helpful to designate one person to manage it. Finally, it is helpful to have a recorder to record events, provide cues, track laboratory results, and communicate with areas outside of the resuscitation area. It is also important that the team leader control the number of people in the resuscitation area. Those individuals who are not part of the resuscitation may distract other members of the team.

Care providers are often trained as individuals, even though they most often respond as an integrated team. Utilization of team behaviors can minimize the number of errors, duplication of efforts, and loss of information that can occur during a resuscitation. Maintaining situational awareness is the key to being an essential team member. Reinforcing situational awareness in others emphasizes the team construct. Some mechanisms to enhance cross-monitoring include call outs and check backs. Call outs involve information that must be shared with the entire team (eg, calling out vital signs). Check backs are means to avoid order errors—the recipient of the order repeats the order verbatim, and then the orderer confirms that order verbatim. These techniques sustain dynamic situational awareness and allow for an organized, integrated team approach to comprehensive resuscitative care. Many universities and other institutions now have simulation

centers that can be utilized to more effectively train health care providers for resuscitations in realistic settings, both as individuals and in team settings.

FAMILY PRESENCE DURING RESUSCITATION

To allow family members to be present during a resuscitation or invasive procedure has been a subject of great debate. The majority of family members who have been surveyed indicate they would like to be present at the resuscitation. This is true for both adult and pediatric patient populations. The families often state that by being present they are able to provide emotional and spiritual support. The family's presence may also provide closure and facilitate grieving. Opponents of family presence argue that there may be disruption of code team functions and the event may cause lasting psychological damage to the witnessing family members. Neither of these concerns has been supported by the literature.

Eckstein M, Stratton SJ, Chan LS: Termination of resuscitative efforts for out-of-hospital cardiac arrests. Acad Emerg Med 2005;12(1):65–70 [PMID: 15635140].

Engdahl J et al: Time trends in long-term mortality after out-of-hospital cardiac arrest, 1980–1998, and predictors for death. Am Heart J 2003;145(5):826–833 [PMID: 12766739].

Halm MA: Family presence during resuscitation: A critical review of the literature. Am J Crit Care 2005;14(6):494–511 [PMID: 16249587].

Horsted TI et al: Outcome of out-of-hospital cardiac arrest—Why do physicians withhold resuscitation attempts? Resuscitation 2004;63(3):287–293 [PMID: 15582764].

Lloyd-Jones D, Adams RJ, Brown TM et al: Heart disease and stroke statistics—2010 update: A report from the American Heart Association. Circulation 2010;121(7):e46–e215 [PMID: 20019324].

Lund-Kordahl I, Olasveengen TM, Lorem T et al: Improving outcome after out-of-hospital cardiac arrest by strengthening weak links of the local chain of survival; quality of advanced life support and post-resuscitation care. Resuscitation 2010;81(4): 422–426 [PMID: 20122786].

Ornato JP, Perberdy MA: Prehospital and emergency department care to preserve neurologic function during and following cardiopulmonary resuscitation. Neurol Clin 2006;24(1):23–39 [PMID: 16443128].

Schuman SP, Hartmann TK, Geocadin RG: Intensive care after resuscitation from cardiac arrest: a focus on heart and brain injury. Neurol Clin 2006;24(1):41–59 [PMID: 16443129].

Spector PS: Diagnosis and management of sudden cardiac death. Heart 2005;91(3):408–413 [PMID: 15710742].

Wayne DB, Didwania A, Feinglass J et al: Simulation-based education improves quality of care during cardiac arrest team responses at an academic teaching hospital: A case–control study. Chest 2008;133(1):56–61 [PMID: 17573509].

Weng TI et al: Improving the rate of return of spontaneous circulation for out-of-hospital cardiac arrests with a formal, structured emergency resuscitation team. Resuscitation 2004;60(2):137–142 [PMID: 15036730].

▼ ADULT BASIC LIFE SUPPORT

THE CHAIN OF SURVIVAL

The AHA first proposed the phrase "the chain of survival" to describe the interrelated series of interventions that must be in place to maximize functional survival from sudden cardiac death. Any failure to implement a single link in the chain will lead to a decrease in survival. As depicted by the AHA, there are four links in the chain of survival: rapid access to medical care, early basic life support (BLS), early defibrillation, and early advanced cardiac life support (ACLS). Since that time, efforts have been made to expand this chain to include prevention prior to the event and secondary prevention of cardiac arrest. This includes lifestyle modifications (see below) and medical interventions such as statins for hypercholesterolemia, better control of diabetes, and the placement of implantable cardioverter defibrillators.

TECHNIQUES OF BASIC LIFE SUPPORT

▶ Early Prevention

As most cardiac arrests occur in the absence of trained medical personnel, it is imperative that we identify those patients at risk and decrease the likelihood of a cardiac event. Early prevention involves both primary prevention, including lifestyle modification (exercise and smoking cessation), and secondary prevention, including medical therapy. In addition, the patient and family should be educated on the signs and symptoms of chest pain related to cardiac ischemia. Patients with known cardiac disease should attempt to treat the pain with sublingual nitroglycerin. If, after taking the nitroglycerin, there is no relief, the patient should call the emergency number for his or her area. Patients without known disease should contact the emergency number if unremitting chest pain is present for more than 5 minutes. In the hospital setting, an early, organized response to chest pain, dyspnea, and abnormal vital signs can decrease the number of cardiac arrests.

▶ Early Access

As previously discussed, the need for immediate CPR and defibrillation following cardiac arrest cannot be overstated. On finding the unresponsive patient, a lone rescuer should immediately activate the EMS system and if available obtain an automated external defibrillator (AED). They should then provide adequate CPR. If two or more rescuers are present, CPR should be initiated immediately by one while the other activates EMS. As opposed to a lay provider, a lone health care worker may alter this sequence. If the event is likely asphyxial in origin, the provider may give five cycles of CPR before activating EMS. In the hospital setting, initiate the hospital's emergency response or "code" system. Early access

into the system is imperative to minimize the time delay until defibrillation.

▶ Early Basic Life Support

On finding an unresponsive patient and activating the EMS system, return to the patient to provide BLS until further help arrives. Assume a position alongside the patient's thorax so that rescue breathing and chest compressions can be done without repositioning one's body. Position the patient on a hard surface to allow for efficient chest compressions. Anticipate the arrival of a defibrillator, which is usually positioned on the left side, next to the patient's ear. Remember the importance of provider safety. If the provider is injured, it will obviously impair his or her ability to provide BLS and will add further strain to limited EMS resources.

▶ The ABCs (Airway, Breathing, and Circulation)

A. Airway

The first step of BLS is opening the patient's airway. This may be achieved using either the head tilt–chin lift or the jaw-thrust method. It is recommended that lay rescuers use the head tilt–chin lift method due to concern that the jaw thrust is more difficult to perform and may not be as effective in opening the airway. To perform the head tilt–chin lift, place one hand firmly on the patient's forehead and apply firm downward, backward pressure to tilt the head. Hook the fingers of the other hand under the bony part of the chin, lifting up the chin (Figure 9–1). If a health care provider is the rescuer and suspects C-spine injury, the jaw thrust is the method of choice to reduce movement of the neck. This maneuver is performed by using the index and middle fingers to grasp the angles of the mandible and lifting with both hands. The head is maintained in neutral position (Figure 9–2).

B. Breathing

After opening the patient's airway, breathing is assessed. This is done by leaning over the patient's open mouth and looking down at the chest for any rise or fall of breathing. Place an ear near the patient's mouth, listening for breathing or feeling the flow of air over the cheek. This should take no more than 10 seconds. In the absence of adequate breathing (agonal respirations are inadequate), perform mouth-to-mouth, mouth-to-mask, or bag–mask ventilation. Health care professionals should be familiar with all of these techniques. A mask with a one-way valve should be readily available in all health care settings to minimize the risk of contamination from the patient's oral secretions. A bag–mask should be available in all critical care areas and on crash carts.

1. Mouth to mouth—Maintain the airway by using the head tilt–chin lift method. Pinch the patient's nose shut.

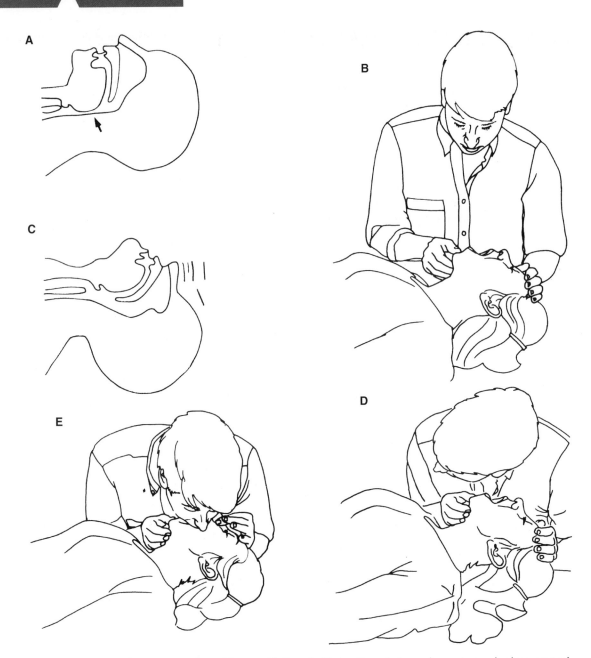

▲ **FIGURE 9–1.** Opening the airway and providing ventilation. **A:** Obstruction of airway by posterior displacement of tongue (arrow) in resting, supine position. **B** and **C:** Relief of lingual airway obstruction in supine position by forward displacement of mandible (head tilt–chin lift method). **D:** Rescuer checks for spontaneous breathing by listening and feeling for exhaled air while looking for chest movement. **E:** Mouth-to-mouth ventilation. While maintaining head tilt–chin lift, the rescuer uses his or her fingers to seal the victim's nose shut; rescuer takes a deep breath, seals mouth over victim's mouth, and exhales, watching for chest movement. Look, listen, and feel for passive exhalation.

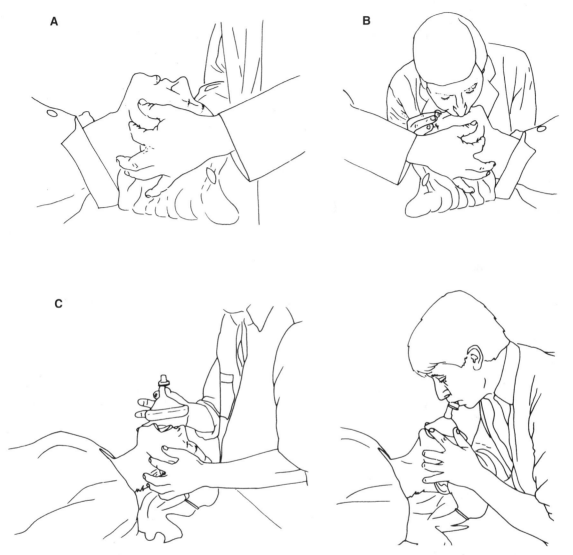

▲ **FIGURE 9–2.** Jaw-thrust maneuver. **A:** If C-spine injury is suspected, open airway by grasping and lifting angles of victim's lower jaw without tilting the head. **B** and **C:** Ventilation is best provided with the aid of a second rescuer or a pocket mask.

Seal your lips around the patient's mouth. Give two slow breaths over 2 seconds initially. There should be good chest rise and fall. If not, reposition the patient's airway and attempt to ventilate again. If there is still no movement of air, presume that the patient has a foreign body airway obstruction (FBAO) and attempt to clear it (see below).

2. Mouth to mask—A clear mask with or without a one-way valve (often called a pocket mask) can be used as an adjunct to mouth-to-mouth ventilation. Ventilations are provided in the same way as for mouth to mouth. It is often

easier and more effective for the inexperienced provider to adequately ventilate the patient with the pocket mask than with the bag–mask. When possible, the mask should be attached to supplemental oxygen. There are two techniques to achieve an effective seal with the mask.

A. CEPHALIC TECHNIQUE—Used when there is more than one provider. The provider ventilating the patient is positioned at the head of the bed. The mask is applied in one of the following two ways: with the thumbs and thenar eminences providing a seal, while the fingers are used to perform jaw thrust, or with the thumbs and index fingers providing a seal, while the remaining fingers provide a jaw thrust.

B. LATERAL TECHNIQUE—Used when there is only one provider, the lateral technique allows the provider to perform one-person CPR. With the provider at the patient's side, a head tilt–chin lift is applied. The hand closer to the top of the patient's head performs a head tilt while creating a seal on the upper part of the mask with index finger and thumb. The lower hand performs a chin lift with the fingers while creating a seal on the lower part of the mask with the thumb and thenar eminence.

3. Bag-mask ventilation—When two providers are available to manage the patient's airway, the mask is applied as with the cephalic technique of the pocket mask. Ventilations are then administered by the second provider squeezing the bag over 2 seconds and then releasing for 3 seconds. If only one provider is available for airway management, he or she must provide an adequate seal with one hand, using the index finger and thumb while providing a chin lift with the other three fingers. The other hand is used to squeeze the bag–mask. Optimizing the head tilt by positioning towels underneath the patient's shoulders may help, especially if the patient is obese. Ventilation can be improved by squeezing the bag against the provider's body. Whenever possible, use supplemental oxygen to provide up to a 100% concentration.

4. Cricoid pressure application—Cricoid pressure (Sellick maneuver) is the posterior displacement of the cricoid cartilage to close off the esophagus. This minimizes gastric insufflation associated with ventilation, as well as preventing reflux of gastric contents into the upper airway and lungs. This should be done only in the unconscious patient. The cricoid cartilage is found by first locating the thyroid cartilage with the index finger and then moving down the neck over the cricothyroid membrane. The first cartilage ring below the membrane is the cricoid cartilage. Moderate pressure (5–10 lb) is applied, pressing the cartilage with the thumb and index finger posteriorly toward the cervical spine.

C. Circulation

Circulation is assessed by palpation of the carotid pulse. The pulse is located in the groove lateral to the trachea. Check the pulse for no more than 10 seconds. If a pulse is present, rescue breathing can continue with one breath every 5–6 seconds. If a pulse is absent, start chest compressions. This is essential for providing blood flow during CPR. To perform chest compressions, identify the lower sternum in the center of the chest, between the nipples. The heel of the hand should be in this position, and place the second hand over the first so that they are overlapped and parallel. Compressions should depress the sternum 1.5–2.0 in, and then allow the chest to return to normal position. Chest

recoil allows venous return to the heart. Compressions are given at 100/min. The compression–ventilation ratio in adults should be 30:2, for both single rescuer and dual rescuer CPR. This results in minimal interruption of compressions and blood flow. Once a definitive airway is established, ventilations and compressions can be performed asynchronously.

▶ "Hands-Only" CPR

Recent recommendations published by the AHA recommend lay rescuers (non-health care providers) provide chest compression only CPR. This stems from research showing no survival advantage from ventilations during bystander-provided CPR compared to chest compressions only. Additionally, without interruptions to chest compressions, more blood flow is delivered to vital organs, and mouth-to-mouth resuscitation is thought to be one of the major psychological obstacles to would-be rescuers during a bystander-witnessed arrest.

FOREIGN BODY AIRWAY OBSTRUCTION

While uncommon, FBAO is a preventable cause of death. Identifying a patient with an FBAO may be as simple as recognizing the conscious patient with difficulty breathing, coughing, or the universal "I'm choking" sign, with fingers clutching around the throat, but it can be much more difficult to detect in the unconscious/altered level of consciousness patient. In the conscious patient, ask if he or she is choking. If the patient has a strong cough, is not cyanotic, does not have labored breathing or retractions, and can speak, then a partial obstruction with good air exchange exists. Observe the patient, but do not intervene initially. Allow the patient to attempt to clear the obstruction by himself or herself. If the patient has a weak cough, is cyanotic, has labored breathing, stridor, or has difficulty speaking, then a partial obstruction with poor air exchange exists. Prompt intervention is indicated. If the airway is obstructed completely, the patient is unable to speak or cough and may become cyanotic. Rapid intervention is essential.

The abdominal thrust (Heimlich maneuver) is used in the conscious choking patient. While standing behind the patient, position the fist with the thumb facing up over the umbilicus. Roll the fist so that the thumb is against the abdominal wall. Grasp the fist with the other hand. Apply sharp upward thrusts until the foreign body is cleared or the patient collapses and becomes unconscious. In the unconscious patient, position him or her on the floor. Perform a tongue–jaw lift by grasping the jaw and tongue with one hand and observe the airway. If a solid obstruction is visually identified, use the other hand to perform a finger sweep. Attempt to ventilate. If the first attempt does not succeed, reposition the airway and attempt to ventilate again. If the second attempt fails, perform the Heimlich maneuver by straddling the patient. Place the heel of one hand in the same location as that used for the standing abdominal thrust. Place the other hand over the top of the first. Provide five sharp upward thrusts. Repeat the sequence until the obstruction is relieved or alternative means of establishing the airway are available (eg, Magill forceps, surgical or needle cricothyroidotomy).

DEFIBRILLATION

Defibrillation is the intervention for the heart in pulseless VT and VF. When a critical level of energy reaches the myocardium, the ventricles become depolarized. This provides an opportunity for the sinoatrial node or another pacemaker to restore an organized perfusing rhythm. For this to occur, the provider must select the proper size paddles or self-adhesive pads, apply them in the correct position (Figure 9–3), use conductive gel, pregelled conductive pads, or saline-soaked gauze to minimize skin resistance, and apply 25 lb of pressure to the paddles. Increasing the energy selected will increase the energy delivered. Some studies now show benefit from 1 to 2 minutes of CPR prior to defibrillation. This recommendation has not yet been adopted into standard protocols; however, it may bear clinical consideration, especially while a defibrillator is being applied and charged.

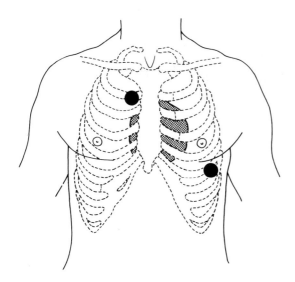

▲ **FIGURE 9–3.** Contact points for defibrillation electrodes (solid circles). Place one paddle electrode to the right of the sternum in the second or third interspace, and the other paddle should be at the cardiac apex. In children and thin adults, paddles may be placed directly over the heart in anteroposterior orientation.

The same techniques for defibrillation are used for synchronized cardioversion of tachydysrhythmias. The defibrillator must be placed in the synchronized mode. This is done by activating the SYNCH button on most defibrillators. This coordinates the shock so that it is not delivered during the relative refractory period (a shock during this period could result in VF). Most defibrillators will revert to an unsynchronized mode after delivering a synchronized shock. This allows for rapid defibrillation if VF occurs. For repeated synchronized cardioversion, the defibrillator must be resynchronized. A patient should be adequately sedated and receive analgesia prior to cardioversion, if circumstances permit.

▶ Defibrillation Waveforms

Waveforms indicate the flow of energy between the two paddles or pads of the defibrillator. A monophasic waveform travels in one direction, whereas a biphasic waveform travels initially in one direction and then reverses flow. Compared to monophasic waveforms, biphasic waveforms have the same rate of defibrillation, with less damage to the myocardium due to lower amounts of energy applied. Research indicates that the biphasic waveform is at least as effective as the monophasic waveform in terminating VF. Most defibrillators manufactured today use biphasic waveforms. Because lower-energy settings are used in biphasic defibrillators, the units are smaller and maintain a battery charge longer than monophasic models.

▶ Automated External Defibrillation

VF and pulseless VT are the most common dysrhythmias seen in cardiac arrest and may be successfully converted with defibrillation. However, in a matter of minutes this rhythm may degenerate into asystole, which is usually refractory to further interventions. It is thus imperative to deliver defibrillation as rapidly as possible. In an effort to improve the time of arrest till shock, the AHA has recommended the development of lay rescuer AED programs, with ideal sites in areas with large groups of people (ie, sporting events, airports, schools, and shopping malls). The AED is a computerized device that provides visual and often audible prompts to guide lay rescuers in safely defibrillating patients with sudden cardiac arrest. The device itself analyzes the patient's rhythm and determines if a shock is required. Several trials have shown a significant increase in survival to hospital discharge with a community AED program. This is true regardless of what type of first responder (emergency medical technician, firefighter, or police) used the AED.

Before applying the AED, the rescuer should initiate airway management and ventilations. If the patient has no pulse, an AED should be brought to the patient's side. If two rescuers are available, one can perform CPR while the AED is sought, but obtaining the AED is the critical action. The

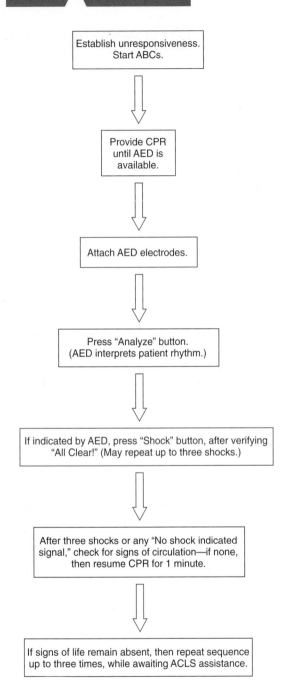

▲ **FIGURE 9–4.** Algorithm for usage of automated external defibrillator.

AED requires the rescuer to power on the device, apply the self-adhesive pads to the patient's chest, press the Analyze button, and, if an electrical shock is indicated, press the Shock button. The current algorithm for AED use is shown in Figure 9–4.

2005 American Heart Association guidelines for cardiopulmonary resuscitation and emergency cardiovascular care. Circulation 2005;112(24 Suppl):IV1–IV203 [PMID: 16314375].

Bobrow BJ, Ewy GA: Ventilation during resuscitation efforts for out-of-hospital primary cardiac arrest. Curr Opin Crit Care 2009;15(3):228–233 [PMID: 19469024].

Bradley SM, Gabriel EE, Aufderheide TP et al: Survival increases with CPR by emergency medical services before defibrillation of out-of-hospital ventricular fibrillation or ventricular tachycardia: observations from the Resuscitation Outcomes Consortium. Resuscitation 2010;81(2):155–162 [PMID: 19969407].

Bunch TJ, Hammill SC, White RD: Outcomes after ventricular fibrillation out-of-hospital cardiac arrest: Expanding the chain of survival. Mayo Clin Proc 2005;80(6):774–782 [PMID: 15945529].

Garza AG, Gratton MC, Salomone JA et al: Improved patient survival using a modified resuscitation protocol for out-of-hospital cardiac arrest. Circulation 2009;119(19):2597–2605 [PMID: 19414637].

Jacobs I et al: The chain of survival. Ann Emerg Med 2001;37 (4 Suppl):S5 [PMID: 11290965].

Nagao K: Chest compression-only cardiocerebral resuscitation. Curr Opin Crit Care 2009;15(3):189–197 [PMID: 19451816].

Ornato JP, Perberdy MA: Prehospital and emergency department care to preserve neurologic function during and following cardiopulmonary resuscitation. Neurol Clin 2006;24(1):23–39 [PMID: 16443128].

Sayre MR, Berg RA, Cave DM et al: Hands-only (compression-only) cardiopulmonary resuscitation: A call to action for bystander response to adults who experience out-of-hospital sudden cardiac arrest: A science advisory for the public from the American Heart Association Emergency Cardiovascular Care Committee. Circulation 2008;117;2162–2167 [PMID: 18378619].

▼ ADULT ADVANCED LIFE SUPPORT

If a patient does not respond to initial CPR and defibrillation, further interventions are required. And in cases where initial interventions are successful in restoring a perfusing rhythm, the patient may still require ALS (ie, airway, medications, and further evaluation) to optimize outcome.

ADVANCED AIRWAY MANAGEMENT

During a resuscitation, the risks and benefits of advanced airway management must be considered. To place a definitive airway requires time that may result in interruption of effective chest compressions. In addition, there is a risk of esophageal intubation that is highest in inexperienced providers. Once a definitive airway is in place, the risk of aspiration is significantly reduced and more effective ventilation can be performed. Current ACLS recommendations emphasize the use of effective bag valve mask ventilations rather than definitive airway placement during a resuscitation to minimize prolonged interruptions to effective chest compressions. Practice in most emergency departments still involves early placement of an advanced airway, as the skill level and training of most emergency room physicians will typically allow rapid, accurate insertion. Advanced airway techniques include endotracheal intubation, the use of the laryngeal mask airway, or the use of a double-lumen tube such as the esophageal–tracheal combitube or pharyngotracheal lumen airway.

Endotracheal intubation provides the best means of securing the airway; however, intubation should be attempted only by providers who are skilled in the procedure and who perform it at least 6–12 times per year. Placement of the tube should be confirmed by colorimetric end-tidal CO_2 detectors (although unreliable in prolonged cardiac arrest), esophageal detector devices, or capnography in addition to more traditional techniques. The details of endotracheal intubation are discussed in Chapters 7 and 10. When unable to secure an airway or to ventilate the patient using a bag–mask, the trained provider must perform a surgical or needle cricothyroidotomy.

VASCULAR ACCESS

While peripheral IVs are still commonly used for prehospital and in-hospital vascular access to deliver medications in resuscitations, intraosseous devices are becoming more prevalent in both EMS and emergency room practice that can provide more rapid and equally effective vascular access in the setting of arrest for drug and fluid delivery. Devices are available that use either powered or manual insertion techniques and can be inserted in a variety of sites in the adult patient. Central venous catheters may also be inserted in the hospital for more definitive access and central administration of medications.

SPECIFIC RHYTHMS

▶ Ventricular Fibrillation or Pulseless Ventricular Tachycardia

As mentioned previously, rapid defibrillation is essential in preventing progression of VF or pulseless VT to asystole. Recently, emphasis has been given to minimizing the interruption of CPR. In an unwitnessed arrest, it is now recommended that five cycles (2 minutes) of CPR be performed prior to defibrillation. It is felt that this will increase myocardial oxygen and energy substrates, increasing the likelihood of a restoration of spontaneous circulation (ROSC) to the myocardium following defibrillation. If the arrest was witnessed and a defibrillator is present, deliver the first shock immediately. The first shock is delivered at 360 or 200 J with a monophasic defibrillator or biphasic defibrillator, respectively. CPR is immediately resumed after the first shock.

Vasopressors (ie, epinephrine) may be given before or after the first shock, being careful not to interrupt CPR or defibrillation. Epinephrine is given at 0.5–1.0 mg IV every 3–5 minutes. Alternatively, a one-time dose of 40 U of vasopressin can replace the first or second dose of epinephrine. No further vasopressors may be given for 10 minutes after its administration. The pulse should only be checked if there is an organized rhythm on the monitor. Following the five cycles of CPR, a second shock should be performed if indicated. Again, 360 or 200 J with a monophasic defibrillator or biphasic defibrillator, respectively, is delivered. If VF or pulseless VT persists after two to three shocks, an antiarrhythmic (amiodarone or lidocaine) should be administered. Magnesium should be considered for torsades de pointes. The cycle of CPR, defibrillation, and vasopressors is continued until there is ROSC, a change in rhythm, or the resuscitation efforts are deemed futile.

▶ Pulseless Electrical Activity

PEA is the condition where there is an organized rhythm on the monitor in the absence of cardiac output. The key to successful resuscitation is identifying and treating the underlying cause. Determining the offending etiology can be facilitated by history, vital signs including temperature, electrocardiogram (ECG), blood gas analysis, electrolytes, and a focused physical examination. Initial interventions can be performed concurrently to address hypoxemia and hypovolemia. In addition to effective CPR, epinephrine (1 mg IV every 3–5 minutes) is given. As previously described, a onetime dose of vasopressin can replace the first or second dose of epinephrine. If the patient is bradycardic, atropine (1 mg IV) may be administered up to three times.

▶ Asystole

Asystole is usually a preterminal rhythm. As with PEA, the underlying causes must be addressed. Transcutaneous pacing may be considered early on, but it should be used only if the patient was witnessed entering asystole from a perfusing rhythm. Epinephrine (1 mg IV every 3–5 minutes) and atropine (1 mg IV every 3–5 minutes with a maximum of three doses) are administered. Vasopressin can replace the first or second dose of epinephrine as previously described. If an asystolic patient does not respond to ALS interventions in the field, resuscitation efforts may be terminated in the field without urgent transport.

▶ Tachydysrhythmia with a Pulse

If a patient has a tachydysrhythmia with evidence of poor perfusion (in which the tachydysrhythmia is the likely source), prompt cardioversion is indicated. Chest pain, dyspnea, altered level of consciousness, hypotension, and new-onset congestive heart failure are all indications of instability. Quickly perform synchronized cardioversion. Give the patient analgesic and sedative agents if circumstances permit.

In a hemodynamically stable patient with a tachydysrhythmia, clinical evaluation is needed to determine the source of the dysrhythmia. History and ECG are the two key diagnostic aids. The tachycardias are classified as narrow or wide complex. The most difficult differentiation is with the regular wide-complex tachycardias. The diagnostic dilemma is to decide whether the rhythm is supraventricular in origin with aberrant conduction or a true VT (Chapter 34). If the rhythm cannot be confirmed as supraventricular tachycardia (SVT), the patient should be presumed to have a VT, and appropriate treatment should be rendered. Treating a VT as an SVT can have disastrous results.

▶ Cardioversion

As mentioned above, the treatment for unstable tachycardia, which is not VF or pulseless VT, is synchronized cardioversion. Synchronization prevents the shock being delivered during the refractory period of the cardiac cycle, which may trigger VF. Escalate the dose of the second and subsequent shocks if ineffective. For unstable atrial flutter and other SVTs, the initial charge is 50–100 J. Escalate the dose of energy if ineffective. For unstable atrial fibrillation, the energy delivered is 100–200 J. And finally, for unstable VT with a pulse, the morphology and rate determine the energy delivered. If the VT is monomorphic, an initial charge of 100 J is delivered, and increased to 200, 300, and 360 J if ineffective. For polymorphic VT, treat in the same manner as VF.

▶ Bradycardia

As with tachydysrhythmia, a slow rhythm with signs of inadequate perfusion needs immediate intervention, regardless of the underlying pathology. A relative bradycardia with good perfusion may be observed while preparations are made to treat the underlying cause. Atropine (0.5–1.0 mg IV with up to 3 mg total) can be beneficial if parasympathetic tone is excessive. This is typically the case in depressed sinus node automaticity and in atrioventricular (AV) block secondary to acute myocardial infarction. Bradycardias secondary to degeneration of the conduction system (or disruption, as in a transplanted heart), or due to pharmacologic or metabolic causes, generally do not respond to atropine. Transcutaneous or transvenous pacing can be used as a bridge to a more permanent pacing mechanism. In addition, epinephrine or dopamine infusions may be required if the patient fails treatment with atropine or pacing.

PHARMACOLOGIC THERAPY

See Table 9–1.

▶ Vasoactive Agents

A. Epinephrine

Epinephrine is a mixed α- and β-agonist that has been shown to increase diastolic aortic blood pressure, coronary perfusion pressure, as well as cerebral blood flow. As such, it has been the mainstay of pharmacologic therapy in the pulseless patient, regardless of the underlying rhythm. The dose and frequency are described above. Epinephrine may be given through an endotracheal tube if IV access cannot be obtained. The endotracheal dose is 2.0–5.0 mg in 10 cm^3 of normal saline. High-dose epinephrine in adults is no longer recommended.

B. Vasopressin

Vasopressin (antidiuretic hormone) is an endogenous hormone that causes peripheral vasoconstriction, as well as vasoconstriction of the coronary, cerebral, and renal vasculature. Recent studies have indicated that vasopressin has no benefit over epinephrine in cardiac arrest. The dose and frequency are described in Table 9-1.

C. Dopamine

Dopamine is endogenous neurotransmitter that exhibits both α- and β-adrenergic effects, as well as dopaminergic effects that manifest in a dose-dependent fashion. Doses of greater than 20 μg/kg/min may have adverse effects on splanchnic perfusion and therefore should be avoided. Dopamine can also provoke tachydysrhythmias. If hypotension persists after optimization of filling pressures, dobutamine (as an inotropic agent) or norepinephrine (as a vasopressor) should be considered.

D. Norepinephrine

Norepinephrine is an adrenergic agent that affects α-receptors in the vasculature and β_1-receptors of the heart resulting in peripheral vasoconstriction and increased heart rate and contractility. It is used in states of severe shock and is recommended for management of hypotension when systolic pressures are less than 70 mm Hg. The starting infusion rate is 0.5–1.0 μg/min and titrated to effect, with a maximal infusion rate of 30 μg/min.

E. Dobutamine

Dobutamine is a synthetic catecholamine with potent β_1-agonist properties with little β_2- or α-adrenergic effects. As such, it can improve myocardial contractility and increase cardiac output. It is the initial agent of choice in patients with systolic blood pressure of 70–100 mm Hg. Paradoxically it can worsen hypotension in patients with inadequate preload. In addition, dobutamine can provoke tachyarrhythmias. It is run as an IV infusion of 2–20 mg/kg/min.

▶ Antidysrhythmics

A. Adenosine

Adenosine is an endogenous nucleoside that is a potent but short-lived AV nodal blocking agent. Along with vagal maneuvers, it is considered first-line therapy in paroxysmal

Table 9–1. Pharmacotherapy in Advanced Cardiac Life Support.[a]

Drug Name	Adult Dose	Pediatric Dose	Indications	Frequency	Effects
Epinephrine	1 mg IV OR 2–5 mg IV via ETT	0.01 mg/kg IV or 10 OR 0.1 mg/kg via ETT	Any pulseless rhythms	Every 3–5 min	Increases perfusion to myocardium and to brain by increasing peripheral vascular resistance
Vasopressin	40 units IV	Not indicated	VF, pulseless VT	Single dose, may be followed at 10 min by epinephrine	Increases peripheral vascular resistance
Amiodarone	For VF or pulseless VT: 300 mg IV push	For VF or pulseless VT: 5 mg/kg IV push	VF, pulseless VT, VT with a pulse, SVT	May use second dose of 150 mg for recurrent VF/VT. In children may be repeated in 5 mg/kg doses to a total of 15 mg/kg	Predominately class III antiarrhythmic, but has sodium, potassium channel, and α and β receptor blockade
Lidocaine	1.0–1.5 mg/kg IV push	Same	VF, pulseless VT, VT with a pulse	Second and subsequent doses of 0.75 mg/kg every 5 min to a total dose of 3 mg/kg	Class IB antiarrhythmic; suppresses ventricular automatically and electrical conduction
Magnesium	1–2 g IV slow push	25–50 mg/kg IV slow push	Torsade de pointes, known hypomagnesemia	Single dose	Can cause cutaneous flush, apnea, and hyporeflexia, if given too quickly
Procainamide	17 mg/kg IV slow bolus at maximum rate of 50 mg/min	15 mg/kg IV load; 3-6 mg/kg over 5 min, not to exceed 100 mg/dose	VT with a pulse	Continue infusion (4 mg/min) until QRS widening >50%, dysrhythmia terminated, onset of hypotension; or 17 mg/kg infused	Decreases myocardial excitability and conduction velocity
Atropine	Perfusing patients: 0.5 mg IV push q 5 min, to maximum of 3 mg Pulseless patients: 1.0 mg IV push q 5 min, to maximum of 3 mg	0.02 mg/kg: minimum dose of 0.1 mg	Bradycardia, asystole	May be repeated once up to maximum dose of 3 mg	Parasympatholytic, eliminates vagal tone
Adenosine	6 mg rapid IV push through proximal peripheral line; central line dose is one-half	0.1 mg/kg rapid IV push; maximum dose, 6 mg	SVT	If needed, second dose of 12 mg (pediatric, double initial dose up to 12 mg); third dose of 12–18 mg	Endogenous nucleoside causing brief asystole allowing dominant pacemaker to resume function
Diltiazem	0.25 mg/kg to a maximum dose of 20 mg IV push over 2 min	Same	SVT	Second dose of 0.35 mg/kg, maximum dose of 25 mg, at 15 min; after conversion, start diltiazem drip at 5–15 mg/h	Calcium channel blocker
Esmolol	500 μg/kg bolus over 1 min	100–500 μg/kg bolus over 1 min	SVT	May give another bolus if desired effect is not achieved; start drip 50 μg/kg/min	β-Blocker (short acting)
Atenolol	5 mg IV over 5 min	Not indicated	SVT, myocardial infarction	Repeat in 10 min, then give 50-mg oral load	β-Blocker (β_1 selective)

(continued)

Table 9–1. Pharmacotherapy in Advanced Cardiac Life Support.[a] *(Continued)*

Drug Name	Adult Dose	Pediatric Dose	Indications	Frequency	Effects
Metoprolol	5 mg IV push	Not indicated	SVT, myocardial infarction	Repeat twice at 5-min intervals, then give 50-mg oral load	β-Blocker (β_1 selective)
Dopamine	2-20 μg/kg/min	Same	Hypotension	Low doses are predominantly β; higher doses become predominantly α	Inotropic agent/vasopressor (combined α- and β-agonists)
Dobutamine	2-20 μg/kg/min	Same	Hypotension	Titrate to effect	Inotropic agent (β-agonist)
Norepinephrine	Start at 8-12 μg/min, then titrate to 2-4 μg/min for maintenance; maximum dose of 30 μg/min if hypotension unresponsive to lower doses	0.05-2 μg/kg/min	Hypotension	Titrate to effect	Vasopressor (predominately an α-agonist)
Phenylephrine	100-500 μg bolus IV	0.1-0.5 μg/kg/min	Hypotension	Every 5 min until desired effect, then continuous infusion of 40-180 μg/min	Vasopressor (pure α-agonist)

ETT, endotracheat tube; IO, intraosseoulsy; IV, intravenously; SVT, supraventricular tachycardia; VF, ventricular fibrillation; VT, ventricular tachycardia.
[a]Agents are listed from most effective (and most commonly used) to least.

supraventricular tachycardia (PSVT) secondary to a reentrant-type conduction defect. Adenosine should be considered only when a supraventricular rhythm is suspected. It should not be used as an aid in differentiating between PSVT with aberrant conduction and VT. It is associated with a prolonged sinus pause. The initial dose is 6 mg, given as a rapid bolus. If this fails to resolve PSVT, the dose is increased to 12 mg IV. If there is no response, this dose may be repeated in 1–2 minutes.

B. Amiodarone

Amiodarone is predominantly a class III antidysrhythmic (potassium channel blocker), but it also has some properties of class I (sodium channel blockade), class II (β-blockade), and class IV (calcium channel blockade) antidysrhythmics. This wide variety of effects makes amiodarone useful in treating both supraventricular and ventricular tachydysrhythmias. For VF and pulseless VT, the initial dose is 300 mg IV, which can be followed with a second dose of 150 mg if the arrhythmia persists. While amiodarone has been found to increase the rate of ROSC and prehospital survival from cardiac arrest, it has not been shown to increase survival to hospital discharge. Amiodarone is a

second-line agent for PSVT and can be used when adenosine fails to cardiovert.

C. Atropine

Atropine is an anticholinergic agent useful in the treatment of symptomatic bradycardias that are due to increased parasympathetic tone. It should not be used when infranodal pathology is suspected such as with second-degree Mobitz type II AV blocks. Atropine is indicated in the setting of asystole and bradycardic PEA. It is ineffective in the setting of previous heart transplant and may worsen ischemia during a myocardial infarction. Dosing is described in Table 9-1.

D. β-Adrenergic Blockers

β-Blockers (ie, atenolol, metoprolol, esmolol) are indicated for SVT for rate control in patients with preserved left ventricular function. Atenolol and metoprolol are β_1-blocking agents (cardioselective) available in both IV and oral formulations. Esmolol is a short-acting β_1-agent that must be given in a bolus and then maintained through a continuous infusion. This may be advantageous in patients who may respond negatively to β_2-blockade (eg, patients with chronic obstructive pulmonary disease). If an adequate response is not achieved after 5 minutes, the loading dose may be repeated and the infusion rate doubled.

E. Calcium Channel Blockers

Calcium channel blockers (ie, diltiazem and verapamil) are also indicated for rate control in SVT. They slow AV nodal conduction and prolong the AV nodal refractory period. Calcium channel blockers are contraindicated in atrial fibrillation or atrial flutter with rapid ventricular response when an accessory pathway such as Wolff–Parkinson–White syndrome exists, because it could lead to a life-threatening increase in the ventricular heart rate. Diltiazem is better tolerated in patients with impaired left ventricular function.

F. Lidocaine

Lidocaine is a class IB antidysrhythmic. It is commonly used for ventricular rhythms, both stable and unstable. Its use has largely been replaced by amiodarone. The initial dose in VF and pulseless VT is 1.0–1.5 mg/kg. Half of this dose may be repeated every 5–10 minutes, with a maximal total dose of 3 mg/kg. If successful in terminating the offending rhythm, a maintenance infusion of 3–5 mg/min may be administered.

G. Magnesium

Magnesium is indicated for patients who are known or suspected to have a low magnesium level, recurrent ventricular dysrhythmias, or for those with torsades de pointes.

H. Procainamide

Procainamide is a class IA antidysrhythmic, which is capable of suppressing both atrial and ventricular arrhythmias. It may be used in treatment of atrial fibrillation and atrial flutter (even in the presence of Wolff–Parkinson–White syndrome) in patients with preserved left ventricular function. In addition, procainamide may be used in SVT when vagal maneuvers and adenosine are ineffective. Its use should be avoided in patients with long QT intervals or when drugs that prolong the QT interval, such as amiodarone, have already been administered.

FIBRINOLYTIC THERAPY

Most cases of sudden cardiac death are secondary to an intravascular thrombosis, with the majority of these cases related to either an intracoronary thrombus or massive pulmonary embolus. The primary goal in treating these patients is restoring perfusion immediately. In the case of myocardial infarction, the two methods to restore coronary blood flow are fibrinolytic therapy and percutaneous coronary intervention (PCI). Multiple studies have found that in centers that can provide rapid PCI, there is improved outcome and a decreased rate of reocclusion when compared to fibrinolytic therapy. However, the presentation to PCI should occur within 90 minutes. Many facilities are unable to perform PCI, and transfer the patient to centers with catheterization capabilities. If the patient is unable to undergo PCI in the 90-minute period, fibrinolytic therapy should be initiated if not contraindicated. Ideally, if fibrinolytic therapy is to be initiated, it should occur within 30 minutes of the patient's presentation. Maximum benefit is seen in those patients who present within 3 hours from the onset of symptoms. Fibrinolytic administration by prehospital providers was studied in order to reduce time to administration. No improvement in outcomes was found. Fibrinolytic therapy is currently not recommended for administration by prehospital providers.

POSTRESUSCITATION STABILIZATION

Following successful ROSC after cardiac arrest, mortality is often associated with refractory cardiac damage, CNS injury, and sepsis. As described by the AHA, there are four objectives of postresuscitation stabilization after the patient has been transported to the emergency department: (1) optimize cardiopulmonary function and systemic perfusion, (2) identify the precipitating cause of the arrest, (3) prevent recurrence, and (4) begin measures to improve long-term survival and neurologic function.

Initial data gathering is directed to address the patient's history, underlying condition, and current physiologic status. The history may be obtained from family, friends, medical records, and prehospital care providers. Evaluate the patient's status by physical examination, laboratories, radiologic studies, and continuous hemodynamic monitoring. Routine postresuscitation studies include complete blood count, electrolytes (including glucose and magnesium), cardiac enzymes, toxicology, arterial blood gas, and a portable chest x-ray. Additional studies might include bedside echocardiography, pulmonary artery catheterization, heart catheterization, and computed tomography. Direct initial interventions are toward maintaining stable hemodynamic parameters, with the primary goal to restore adequate perfusion. Attach full monitoring equipment, if not done previously. Place a Foley catheter to monitor urine output.

Postresuscitation hypotension should be initially treated with small-volume (250–500 cm³) boluses of crystalloid solution. Pulmonary artery catheterization or central venous pressure monitoring may aid in determining the patient's fluid status. Consider other causes of hypotension, such as pneumothorax and pericardial tamponade. If bolus fluid therapy fails, add vasoactive (eg, norepinephrine) or inotropic (eg, dopamine) agents.

Hyperthermia increases the cerebral metabolic rate, which creates an imbalance between oxygen delivered and demanded. This can lead to anoxic cell death and initiate a subsequent systemic inflammatory response. Hypothermia, in contrast, can be beneficial to the patient. Studies using induced mild hypothermia (32–42°C or 89.6–93.2°F) have demonstrated increased survival to discharge and improved neurologic recovery. Many institutions have hypothermia protocols in place for postresuscitation patients.

Hyperglycemia is associated with worsening prognosis following global ischemia from cardiac arrest. Tight glucose control is felt to increase survival and reduce the incidence of developing infectious complications in the postresuscitation period.

TERMINATION OF RESUSCITATION

Ideally, termination of resuscitation efforts should occur when there is no further chance of survival or meaningful neurologic recovery. Efforts to resuscitate the victim should be stopped after 20–30 minutes of appropriate ACLS protocol, with no ROSC. In addition, bedside echocardiography can be used to evaluate for cardiac kinetic motion. Wall motion suggests the possibility that PEA has been inadequately resuscitated, whereas the absence of activity is associated with death.

One exception to the standard guidelines for termination of resuscitation is hypothermic cardiac arrest, which may occur from severe exposure or cold water drowning. Because of the protective effects of hypothermia, several cases of good neurologic recovery after prolonged resuscitation from hypothermic cardiac arrest have been documented. In general, continue resuscitation efforts until the patient has been rewarmed to a core temperature of 30–32°C (86–90°F).

2005 American Heart Association guidelines for cardiopulmonary resuscitation and emergency cardiovascular care. Circulation 2005;112(24 Suppl):IV1–IV203 [PMID: 16314375].

Abella BS et al: Induced hypothermia is underused after resuscitation from cardiac arrest: A current practice survey. Resuscitation 2005;64(2):181–186 [PMID: 15680527].

Aung T, Htay T: Vasopressin for cardiac arrest: a systematic review and meta-analysis. Arch Intern Med 2005;165(1):17–24 [PMID: 15642869].

Baker WF: Thrombolytic therapy: Current clinical Practice. Hematol Oncol Clin North Am 2005;19(1):147–181 [PMID: 15639112].

Eftestol T et al: Effects of cardiopulmonary resuscitation on predictors of ventricular fibrillation defibrillation success during out-of-hospital cardiac arrest. Circulation 2004;110(1):10–15 [PMID: 15210599].

El-Menyar AA: The resuscitation outcome: Revisit the story of the stony heart. Chest 2005;128(4):2835–2846 [PMID: 16236962].

Field JM, Soderberg ES: *ACLS Resource Text*. American Heart Association, 2007.

Hallstrom AP et al: Public Access Defibrillation Trial Investigators. Public-access defibrillation and survival after out-of-hospital cardiac arrest. NEJM 2004;351(7):637–646 [PMID: 15306665].

Neumar RW, Nolan JP, Adrie C, Aibiki M, Berg RA, Böttiger BW, Callaway C, Clark RS, Geocadin RG, Jauch EC, Kern KB, Laurent I, Longstreth WT Jr, Merchant RM, Morley P, Morrison LJ, Nadkarni V, Peberdy MA, Rivers EP, Rodriguez-Nunez A, Sellke FW, Spaulding C, Sunde K, Vanden Hoek T: Post-cardiac arrest syndrome: Epidemiology, pathophysiology, treatment, and prognostication. A consensus statement from the International Liaison Committee on Resuscitation. Circulation 2008;118(23):2452–2483 [PMID: 18948368].

Ngo AS, Oh JJ, Chen Y, Yong D, Ong ME: Intraosseous vascular access in adults using the EZ-IO in an emergency department. Int J Emerg Med 2009;2(3):155–160 [PMID: 20157465].

Ornato JP, Perberdy MA: Prehospital and emergency department care to preserve neurologic function during and following cardiopulmonary resuscitation. Neurol Clin 2006;24(1):23–39 [PMID: 16443128].

Salem P: Does the presence or absence of sonographically identified cardiac activity predict resuscitation outcomes of cardiac arrest patients? Am J Emerg Med 2005;23(4):459–462 [PMID: 16032611].

Shuster MN, Nolan J, Barnes TA: Airway and ventilation management. Cardiol Clin 2002;20(1):23–35 [PMID: 11845543].

Stadlbauer KH et al: Effects of thrombolysis during out-of-hospital cardiopulmonary resuscitation. Am J Cardiol 2006;97(1):305–308 [PMID: 16442386].

Sura A, Kelemen M: Early management of ST-segment elevation myocardial infarction. Cardiol Clin 2006;24(1):37–51 [PMID: 16326255].

▼ CARDIOPULMONARY RESUSCITATION IN INFANTS AND CHILDREN

Cardiac arrest in the pediatric population is most often secondary to respiratory arrest. In pediatric patients under 1 year of age, sudden infant death syndrome (SIDS) is the leading nontraumatic cause of death. Lesser causes include submersion injury, pulmonary disease, asphyxia, aspiration, and primary cardiac disease. The majority of these arrests are unwitnessed, with a subsequent delay in CPR and other intervention. As a result, the survival from cardiopulmonary arrest in the pediatric population is dismal, with few patients surviving till discharge from the hospital and the majority of those who do survive having significant neurologic sequelae.

The following terms apply to the pediatric patient:

- Newborn—first 24 hours of life, wherein the patient transitions from a fetal to a neonatal circulation
- Neonate—first 28 days of life
- Infant—first year of life
- Child—ages 1–8 years

For the purposes of BLS, an adult is someone older than 8 years. There can be significant overlap across the age lines in that it may be necessary to perform infant CPR on a toddler or adult chest compressions on a large child.

PEDIATRIC BASIC LIFE SUPPORT

Pediatric BLS uses the same basic techniques as adult BLS, but it is appropriately adapted for the anatomy and physiology of infants and children. The first significant difference between adult and pediatric BLS is the "phone fast" rather than "phone first" rule. Because the predominant cause of pediatric cardiac arrest is respiratory arrest, in the event that help cannot be obtained simultaneously with initiating CPR (ie, the lone rescuer situation), CPR should be performed for 2 minutes prior to interrupting to phone for help.

A. Airway

Opening the airway in a pediatric patient is similar to the procedure followed for adults. The head tilt–chin lift method is used for the patient not suspected of having trauma. The jaw thrust is used when C-spine injury secondary to trauma is a possibility. In the event of loss of consciousness secondary to FBAO, the rescuer may use the tongue–jaw lift to visualize the oropharynx and remove any foreign bodies. The jaw thrust is not recommended for the lay rescuer, as it is difficult to learn, and if not done correctly, does not properly open the airway.

B. Breathing

Ventilations are provided in a manner similar to adults. In infants, the mouth-to-mouth and nose technique can be used. The rescuer's mouth is placed over the infant's mouth and nose to create an effective seal. In children, mouth-to-mouth ventilation is performed as in adults. Mouth-to-nose ventilation is an alternative when the rescuer is unable to obtain an effective seal with the preferred technique. Ventilations should be delivered over 1.0–1.5 seconds. Initially, two ventilations should be delivered. An effective ventilation occurs when there is enough force and volume provided to make the chest rise. An appropriately sized bag–mask may be used by the trained provider (250-mL bag for neonates, 500-mL bag for infants and children). Supplemental oxygen should be used with the bag–mask when available. Cricoid pressure should be applied when giving a child rescue breaths prior to the insertion of an endotracheal tube.

C. Circulation

In the child, give 100 compressions per minute, with a compression–ventilation ratio of 30:2 in a lone rescuer scenario and 15:2 if there are two providers. In the neonate, this ratio is 3:1, with 90 compressions and 30 breaths performed per minute. In the infant, the preferred method for chest compressions is both hands encircling the chest with both thumbs providing compressions on the sternum (two-thumbs/encircling-hands technique). The alternative technique is using two fingers (either the index and middle finger or the middle and ring finger) from one hand to provide compressions. This technique may be more practical with a single rescuer. In children, the heel of one hand is used, but the technique is similar to the two-handed method used for adults. In all patients, the depth of compression is one third to one half the depth of the chest.

PEDIATRIC ADVANCED LIFE SUPPORT

Pediatric ALS is directed toward the same goals of ALS in the adult: ROSC with preserved neurologic function. Hence, much of the underlying theory and algorithms are similar. Several important differences are noted below. As with adults, preparation is crucial, and in emergency departments, a dedicated pediatric crash cart should be assembled. Accordingly, in the prehospital arena, it may be useful to have a dedicated pediatric bag or kit on hand. These carts and kits should have age-appropriate equipment and medications. A means of estimating approximate weight, vital signs, and drug doses should be used. The Broselow–Luten length-based tapes are an excellent example; however, given the prevalence of obesity in children in many practice environments, actual weight may be preferable for drug dosing to avoid underresuscitating the patient. If these guides are unavailable, the endotracheal tube size can be estimated in children over age 1 year as follows: tube size = (age in years/4) + 4. Endotracheal intubation provides another route to deliver some resuscitation medications (eg, lidocaine, epinephrine, atropine, and naloxone); however, drug absorption and efficacy by this route can be variable, and other routes are preferred.

The most common initial nonperfusing rhythm found in the pediatric population is asystole, with the incidence of other dysrhythmia increasing with the age of the patient population. The chance of ROSC increases in patients who present in VF or pulseless VT, which occurs in 5–15% of out-of-hospital cardiac arrests. Appropriate paddles are 4.5 cm for infants up to age 1 year or 10 kg, and adult paddles for all others. Paddle positioning may be either the same as for adults or anterior–posterior on the chest. Both positions are considered equally effective, as long as the pads do not touch. Using monophasic defibrillator, the initial energy setting for VF or pulseless VT is 2 J/kg at the beginning, followed by 4 J/kg. AEDs are recommended for 1–8 years of age. There is no literature supporting the use of AEDs in patients under 1 year of age. When using an AED on a child 1–8 years of age, use a pediatric attenuator system, which lowers the delivered energy to a dose suitable for children. Any identifiably treatable causes, such as a toxic ingestion, electrolyte abnormalities, or asthmatic exacerbations, should be addressed appropriately.

Vascular access in the pediatric patient in cardiac arrest should be achieved as rapidly as possible. The most rapid means of securing such access is through the use of an intraosseous catheter. The intraosseous needle can be placed in 30–60 seconds. It can be placed in any large bone containing marrow, although the proximal tibia is most recommended. High-dose epinephrine is no longer recommended and may be harmful, particularly in the setting of asphyxia.

2005 American Heart Association guidelines for cardiopulmonary resuscitation and emergency cardiovascular care. Circulation 2005;112(24 Suppl):IV1–IV203 [PMID: 16314375].

Bell MK, Lowe C: Push hard and push fast: The who, how, and why of pediatric advanced life support (PALS). Pediatr Emerg Med Pract 2009:(November):1–25.

Ralston MM, Haziniski MF, Zaritsky A et al (editors): *PALS Course Guide and PALS Provider Manual.* American Heart Association, 2007.

Topjian AA, Berg RA, Nadkarni VM: Pediatric cardiopulmonary resuscitation: Advances in science, techniques, and outcomes. Pediatrics 2008;122(5):1086–1098 [PMID: 18977991].

Topjian AA, Nadkarni VM, Berg RA: Cardiopulmonary resuscitation in children. Curr Opin Crit Care 2009;15(3):203–208 [PMID: 19469022].

Compromised Airway

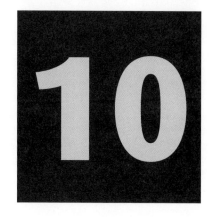

Justin Knowles, MD
Allison Rains, MD[1]

Immediate Management of the Compromised Airway	Bridging Devices for Ventilation in the Failed Airway
Principles of Intubation	Surgical Airways
Nonsurgical Devices and Techniques for Managing the Difficult Airway	Use of Drugs to Assist in Intubation
	Special Cases

IMMEDIATE MANAGEMENT OF THE COMPROMISED AIRWAY

Securing the airway and assuring adequate ventilation are the first priorities in the resuscitation of any acutely ill or injured patient. Without a patent airway and adequate gas exchange, other resuscitative measures will usually be futile. Thus, attention to the airway must precede or occur simultaneously with any other type of management. The exception is the initial defibrillation in cardiac arrest due to ventricular fibrillation, if it can be performed immediately. (See Figure 10–1.)

Assess the Airway

First, determine the patient's level of consciousness and note the presence of respirations and grade respiratory effort. In patients with known or suspected cervical spine (C-spine) injury, all assessments and maneuvers should be undertaken with the C-spine immobilized in a neutral position to prevent cord injury.

A. Apneic, Unconscious Patients

If the C-spine is not injured, place the head in the sniffing position with the chin lift maneuver to open the airway (Figure 10–2). For patients with potential C-spine injuries, a jaw-thrust maneuver should be used. Clear the airway of obstructions, using a rigid suction catheter to remove any blood, vomitus, or secretions from the oropharynx. Remove any large obstructing foreign bodies from the oropharynx manually or with Magill forceps (see Chapter 9).

If the patient remains apneic, assist ventilation using a bag–valve–mask device (eg, Ambu bag) or mouth-to-mouth breathing (see Chapter 9). If adequate personnel and equipment are available, immediately perform endotracheal intubation.

B. Patients with Respiratory Effort

Administer high-flow oxygen. Clear and position the airway as described above. Identify evidence of upper airway obstruction. Prolapse of the tongue and accumulation of secretions, blood, or vomitus are common causes of obstruction. Signs may include wheezing, sonorous respirations, stridor, cough, and dysphonia. Upper airway obstruction should be removed if present. Back blows or the Heimlich maneuver may clear the obstruction. If not, use suction or direct visualization and a Magill forceps or finger. Blind finger sweep is contraindicated. Obstructions that recur or persist require endotracheal intubation, either orotracheally or via cricothyroidotomy, tracheostomy, or percutaneous transtracheal jet ventilation (PTTJV) (see also Chapters 7, 9, and 50).

Evaluate the effectiveness of the patient's respiratory effort. Helpful signs include respiratory rate, tidal volume, accessory muscle use, level of consciousness, skin color, upper airway sounds, and auscultated lung sounds.

[1]This chapter is a revision of the chapter by Julia Nathan, MD, from the 4th edition.

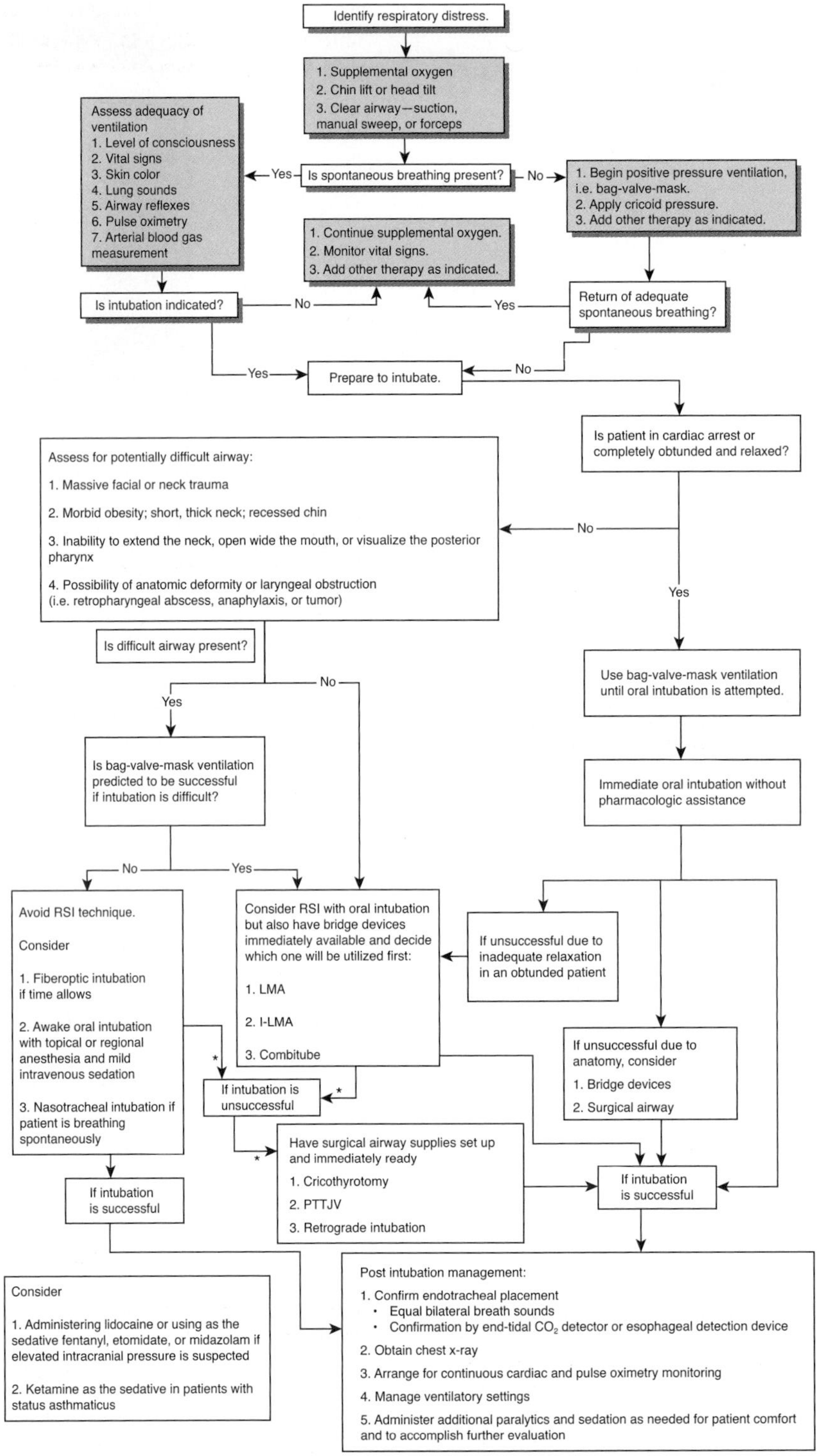

▲ **Figure 10–1.** Management of the compromised airway. I-LMA, intubating laryngeal mask airway; LMA, laryngeal mask airway; PTTJV, percutaneous transtracheal jet ventilation; RSI, rapid sequence induction.

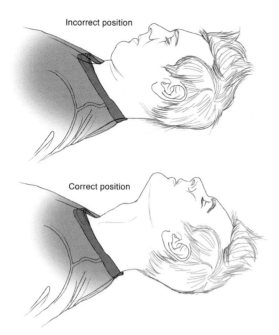

Incorrect position

Correct position

▲ **Figure 10–2.** In the sniffing position, the head is slightly extended and the neck is flexed on the shoulders. This aligns the axis of the airway with the mouth and pharynx, facilitating direct visualization of the cords during intubation. It is particularly important in young children and infants, in whom the larynx is considerably more anterior. A pad beneath the occiput improves flexion of the neck. This position cannot be used when there is cervical spine injury.

Further assessment may include pulse oximetry, arterial blood gas measurement, end-tidal CO_2 capnography, and chest radiography. If intubation is indicated (Table 10–1), continue high-flow oxygen and assist ventilation as needed. Assemble all items necessary for the appropriate method of intubation (Table 10–2). Check for equipment malfunction. If the patient is alert, inform him or her of your plan.

▶ Prepare for Intubation

A. High-Flow Oxygen

All patients with airway or ventilatory compromise require high-flow oxygen. Oxygen through a nasal cannula at flow rates up to 6 L/min provides a patient with 20–40% inspired oxygen concentration. A variety of masks are available that can accept oxygen flow rates of 5–15 L/min. Masks equipped with reservoirs and non-rebreathing valves can deliver oxygen concentrations close to 100% at flow rates of 10 L/min if an adequate seal can be maintained between the mask and face.

Table 10–1. Indications for Intubation.

Respiratory insufficiency
Apnea
Hypoxia
Hypoventilation
Airway obstruction
Foreign body
Fixed mass
Traumatic deformity
Continued bleeding, secretions, or emesis
Inability to protect airway
Altered mental status
Loss of normal airway reflexes
Need for hyperventilation
Head injury
Metabolic acidosis in critically ill or injured patient
Anticipated or impending airway compromise
Shock
Multiple trauma
Need for sedation or paralysis

Before attempting intubation, preoxygenate the patient with 100% oxygen for 5 minutes or have the patient perform eight vital capacity breaths. In a ventilating patient, this should provide 6–7 minutes of protection against hypoxia if the patient becomes apneic. Caution should be exercised because this time interval can be significantly shortened in an ill patient. In an apneic patient, preoxygenation with a bag–valve–mask unit provides 2–3 minutes of protection against hypoxia.

B. Suction

A rigid-tipped suction catheter should be available at all times to keep the airway clear of blood and secretions. The

Table 10–2. Essential Airway Management Equipment.

Oxygen
Nasal cannula
Non-rebreathing masks of various sizes
Suction—rigid pharyngeal, flexible
Oral and nasal airways—range of sizes
Bag-valve-mask units—adult and pediatric sizes
Water-soluble lubricant
Vasoconstrictive topicals
Anesthetic topicals (jelly and spray)
Laryngoscope handles
Laryngoscope blades—range of sizes (curved or straight based on operator preference)
Low-pressure cuff endotracheal tubes of varying sizes
Stylets
Intravenous access (advised)
End-tidal CO_2 detector or esophageal tube detector
Wire cutters

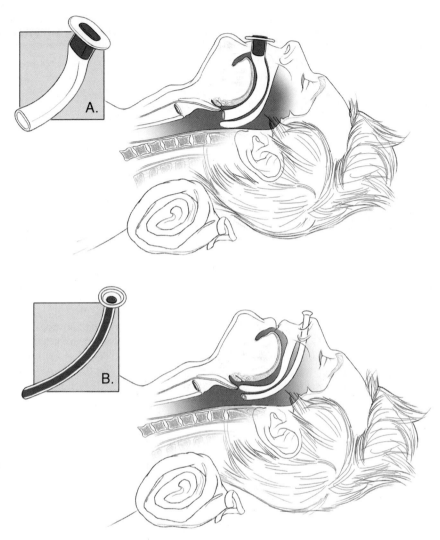

▲ **Figure 10–3.** Important basic airway devices to relieve upper airway obstruction from collapsed pharyngeal tissues. **A:** Oral airway. **B:** Nasal airway.

suction device should be set at 120 mm Hg. After intubation, suction the tracheobronchial tree with a sterile, flexible catheter as necessary.

C. Oral and Nasal Airways

When the jaw thrust or chin lift is ineffective in airway opening, a nasal or oral airway may support collapsed oropharyngeal tissues and permit adequate ventilation. A range of sizes should be readily available in all areas of the emergency department (Figure 10–3).

The oral airway should only be used in an obtunded patient. It may be inserted over a tongue blade or positioned upside down as it enters the mouth and rotated after the tongue is cleared. The former is preferred in pediatric patients as to prevent trauma to the soft palate. Positioned correctly, it retracts the tongue upward and anteriorly. Care must be taken not to push the tongue backward into the pharynx, worsening the obstruction. An oral airway that is too long could potentially displace the epiglottis over the larynx, resulting in complete obstruction.

The soft, rubber, noncuffed nasopharyngeal tube tends to be better tolerated in a semiobtunded patient. Lubricate the tube with anesthetic jelly before insertion. Insert it through the least obstructed nostril, advancing it posteriorly along the floor of the nostril until it bypasses the tongue. If it is too long, it may enter the esophagus, resulting in ineffective positive pressure ventilation and gastric distention. Epistaxis may occur during insertion, and suction should be available.

In patients with intact airway reflexes, placement of either device may cause emesis, gagging, or laryngospasm. During and after placement, head position should be maintained to optimize airway patency. Where indicated, spinal precautions must be maintained. Evaluate breath sounds after placement of either device to ensure that obstruction has not occurred. Care must be taken to avoid trauma during placement.

D. Positive Pressure Ventilation

Following airway opening, positive pressure ventilation may be used to preoxygenate a patient before intubation. Occasionally it may be the only form of ventilation available in an apneic patient when an airway cannot be secured. In general, however, it is not recommended for prolonged ventilation owing to gastric dilatation and technical difficulty.

The bag–valve–mask unit is the device most commonly used to provide positive pressure ventilation in the emergency department. The bag–valve–mask unit has a self-inflating reservoir that accepts 15-L/min oxygen flows. A non-rebreathing valve permits this reservoir air to enter through a separate port from air that is being expired. At these flow rates, inspired air will approach 100% oxygen, provided adequate seal is established. The self-filling bag permits use with spontaneously breathing patients. The unit can usually be attached to an endotracheal tube (ET) after intubation for manual bag-assisted tracheal ventilation.

The procedure for using the bag–valve–mask unit is described in Chapter 7. Use of this device is difficult in the hands of a single operator because effective bag–valve–mask ventilation depends on a tight seal between the mask and face. Often this requires two hands and a second operator to compress the bag. Many circumstances of anatomic variation, facial hair, or maxillofacial trauma make a tight seal impossible. During bag–valve–mask ventilation, proper head position must be maintained to preserve airway patency. Monitor the effectiveness of ventilation closely by frequent assessments of chest wall movement, lung sounds, and gastric dilatation.

The positive pressure generated by bag–valve–mask ventilation leads to gastric dilatation and abdominal distention. This results in decreased lung compliance and significant risk of emesis and aspiration. A clear mask is recommended to identify emesis. Suction equipment must be available. In patients with unprotected airways, cricoid pressure (the Sellick maneuver) is recommended (Figure 10–4). To perform the Sellick maneuver, apply firm, direct pressure on the circumferential cricoid cartilage. This will compress the esophagus posteriorly, decreasing gastric dilatation and reflux. If emesis occurs, release pressure on the cricoid to prevent esophageal rupture and aggressively suction the

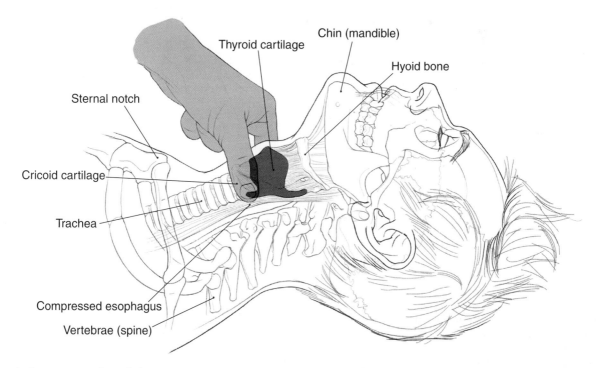

▲ **Figure 10–4.** The Sellick maneuver. Firm pressure on the cricoid cartilage compresses the esophagus, preventing aspiration of gastric contents when airway reflexes are absent.

hypopharynx. If bag–valve–mask ventilation must be prolonged for any reason, place a nasogastric tube to reduce gastric dilatation and its consequences. Because of operational difficulties and risks of aspiration, the bag–valve-mask is a temporizing measure under most circumstances. Patients who require bag-assisted ventilation should generally be intubated as soon as it can be accomplished safely and practically.

The mouth-to-mask technique is another method of providing positive pressure ventilation. This method may be easier for a single operator, because both hands can be used to seat the mask. Supplemental oxygen is provided via a port in the mask or via a nasal cannula worn by the operator.

E. Prehospital Airway Devices

Extraglottic devices can be used emergently, if no rapid sequence intubation (RSI) protocol exists or endotracheal intubation fails in the field. The esophageal tracheal Combitube (ETC) may even be potentially used as an ET if blind insertion results in tracheal placement, but this phenomenon is uncommon. Alternatively, the King LT airway is now becoming a popular device due to its ease of use and rapid deployment.

The ETC has found favor in prehospital and emergency department settings. It comprises two tubes that form a single double-lumen tube. A proximal balloon isolates the hypopharynx, whereas the distal balloon occludes the esophagus or the trachea, depending on its location. The tube is inserted blindly and is fairly stiff, so that it usually enters the esophagus. Tube 1 (larger tube) is closed distally with side holes for ventilation. Tube 2 (smaller tube) is open distally and gives a direct route to either the lungs or the stomach. Tube 1 is always ventilated first, when confirming placement of the tube. Advantages of the ETC include ease of placement, partial protection of the airway from aspiration, and lack of manipulation of the C-spine in the trauma patient.

The King LT airway is a single-lumen tube with two cuffs, but both are inflated simultaneously at a solitary site instead of the two required on an ETC. A ventilation port exists between the oropharyngeal and esophageal cuffs that provides ventilation toward the larynx. Insertion of King LT airway utilizes a similar technique as the ETC.

Esophageal tubes are contraindicated in semiobtunded patients, children, and patients less than 120 cm in height. Do not use them when there is known esophageal injury or ingestion of caustic substances. Complications are listed in Table 10–3. Because of reports of esophageal trauma, some authors recommend Gastrografin swallow or endoscopy after use of an esophageal obturator airway (EOA)-like device. Due to the established complication profile and the evolution of superior alternative devices, the use of esophageal tubes should be discouraged.

Patients intubated with an EOA in the field will need endotracheal intubation on arrival in the emergency

Table 10–3. Complications of Esophageal Airways.

Unrecognized endotracheal intubation
Incorrect positioning in pharynx
Inadequate mask or balloon seal
Esophageal or pharyngeal trauma due to placement, cardiopulmonary resuscitation, or retching
Tracheal compression due to incorrect balloon position
Balloon rupture or leakage
Anterior displacement of larynx
Emesis on removal
Gastric rupture

department. If an ETC or King LT airway is in place, it may be used temporarily for continued resuscitation, but a premium should be placed in establishing a cuffed, endotracheal intubation.

F. Cuffed Oropharyngeal Airway

The cuffed oropharyngeal airway is a modified oropharyngeal airway with a large distal inflatable cuff. It is inserted like a traditional oral airway, and the cuff is then inflated in the supraglottic space. This device is useful in resuscitation because of its ease of insertion and the low level of skill required to place it. The disadvantage of the device is that it has no distal balloon and gastric contents may be more easily aspirated as compared to the ETC.

Agro F et al: Associated techniques for tracheal intubation. Resuscitation 2000;47:343 [PMID: 11114469] (review of different techniques for establishing a patent airway).

Foley LJ et al: Managing the airway in the critically ill patient—Bridges to establish an emergency airway and alternate intubating techniques. Crit Care Clin 2000;16:429 [PMID: 10941582] (review of alternative airway management techniques).

Levitan RM et al: Airway management and direct laryngoscopy—A review and update. Crit Care Clin 2000;16:373 [PMID: 10941579] (review of airway management techniques).

Orebraugh SL: Difficult airway management in the emergency department. Emerg Med 2002;22:31 [PMID: 11809554] (review of techniques for managing the difficult airway).

Shuster M et al: Airway and ventilation management. Cardiol Clin 2002;20:23 [PMID: 11845543] (review of airway management techniques).

▼ PRINCIPLES OF INTUBATION

These principles of intubation management apply to all methods of airway management described in this chapter. Airway positioning, suction, and administration of 100% oxygen must precede any attempt at advanced airway control. Keep protective gear with the airway equipment, and use it routinely.

Table 10–4. Relative Contraindications for Orotracheal Intubation.

Mechanical obstruction in the hypopharynx or at the cords
Severe laryngeal/tracheal trauma
Unusual anatomic features
Presence of wiring due to jaw fracture

▶ Basic Orotracheal Intubation

Most patients can be intubated orally by direct laryngoscopic visualization of the cords. This is the method of choice, because the best assurance of correct tube placement is seeing the tube pass through the cords into the trachea. Please refer to Chapter 7 for complete discussion of basic laryngoscopy and orotracheal intubation technique.

When direct visualization is difficult (Table 10–4), various methods are available to improve visualization of the glottic opening. Backward, upward, rightward pressure (also known as the BURP maneuver) on the external larynx by an assistant to the intubator has been used with some success to increase the intubator's view of the glottic opening. An old technique that has resurfaced for use in the last few years, called external laryngeal manipulation (ELM), is probably even more successful at obtaining a better look at the glottis. This maneuver requires the intubator to use a bimanual technique for intubation. While attempting to visualize the glottis with the laryngoscope in the left hand, by traditional means, the intubator reaches around the anterior neck with the right hand and manipulates the external larynx in all directions while attempting to find a position in which the glottis can be better visualized. Once this position is noted, an assistant continues to hold the external laryngeal structures in this position while the intubator then passes the ET tube through the cords.

A head-elevated laryngoscopy position has also been found to be successful in increasing the view of the glottic opening. In patients who do not require C-spine immobilization, elevating the head so that the laryngeal structures are roughly level with anterior chest wall can also dramatically improve visualization of the glottic opening. This can be fairly easily accomplished with blankets, towels, or other material placed under the patient's head/neck, or by using the hand to help elevate the occiput. This maneuver is especially helpful in the obese patient with a large neck.

If the glottis is truly not visible after using these basic techniques, then other options are available. Blind intubation techniques, video laryngoscopy, fiberoptically assisted intubations, and surgical airways are all options in the difficult airway that cannot be intubated by direct means. These methods will be discussed in the next section.

▶ Universal Precautions

Airway management presents many opportunities for exposure to patient secretions. Wear adequate protective clothing, including a gown, gloves, mask, and either a face shield or goggles, any time the airway is manipulated. When the intubator's fingers are in the patient's mouth (eg, digital intubation, lighted stylet), care must be taken to prevent bite wounds. Place a bite block or dental prod before initiating intubation. Alternatively, place several layers of gauze between the intubator's hand and the patient's teeth. If the patient wears dentures, remove them before airway manipulation.

▶ Postintubation

After intubation, secure and assess the position of the ET by observing the chest wall for expansion. Auscultate both lung fields and the abdomen while ventilating. Inaudible lung sounds or the presence of abdominal sounds suggest esophageal placement. If breath sounds are louder on the right than on the left, suspect right mainstem intubation. Withdraw the tube 1–2 cm and auscultate again. Confirm the tube position by end-tidal CO_2 detector and chest x-ray.

Levitan R et al: Bimanual laryngoscopy: A videographic study of external laryngeal manipulation by novice intubators. Ann Emerg Med 2002;40:30 [PMID: 12085070] (study showing improved viewing of glottis using technique of ELM).

Levitan R et al: Head-elevated laryngoscopy position: Improving laryngeal exposure during laryngoscopy by increasing head elevation. Ann Emerg Med 2003;41:322 [PMID: 12605198] (study showing improved visualization of glottis using a head-elevated intubating position).

Levitan RM et al: Airway management and direct laryngoscopy—A review and update. Crit Care Clin 2000;16:373 [PMID: 10941579] (review of airway management techniques).

▼ NONSURGICAL DEVICES AND TECHNIQUES FOR MANAGING THE DIFFICULT AIRWAY

▶ Intubating Laryngeal Mask Airway

The laryngeal mask airway (LMA) is a device that has proven to be useful as an alternative for bag–valve–mask ventilation and as a rescue option in the difficult airway. The LMA is a semirigid tube with a distal inflatable balloon mask that is inserted blindly into the hypopharynx. The mask lies over the larynx and seals around the glottic opening. The LMA does not protect against aspiration. This device has been demonstrated to be easy to insert with limited prior training. The LMA is appropriate for use in adults and pediatrics, including neonates weighing more than 2 kg. The intubating LMA (I-LMA) is a modification of the LMA that has been developed to act as a conduit to allow blind passage of the ET through the glottis. The I-LMA has a metal handle attached to it that allows the user to stand at the head of a patient and manipulate it similarly to using laryngoscope handle in order to reposition the device and tube as needed.

▶ Lighted Stylet

Lighted stylet and light wand devices have been developed to aid in blind intubation. This method can be used when blood, secretions, or vomitus fill the hypopharynx. Because laryngoscopy need not be used, lighted stylets may be advantageous when the C-spine must remain immobilized. Blind intubation with a lighted stylet is most suitable for deeply comatose or apneic patients when there is little risk of stimulating protective reflexes or biting of the intubator's hand. Use a bite block or dental prod for protection. A lighted stylet can also be combined with direct laryngoscopy. Although there are no absolute contraindications to this technique, ambient lighting must be low to maximize its benefit. Obesity may diminish the intensity of transillumination. As for other blind techniques, avoid this method when direct laryngoscopy can be performed.

If necessary, one person can perform this technique unaided. These devices have a battery-powered light source at the top of a semiflexible stylet. A longer, floppy stylet is available for nasal intubations. The stylet is threaded into an ET. Aside from the lighted stylet, no special equipment is required.

Form the assembly of stylet and ET into a hook of slightly greater than 90°. The patient may be approached from the head if laryngoscopy is used. Otherwise, approach the patient from the right shoulder. While placing gentle traction on the tongue, pass the assembly into the mouth. When the epiglottis is reached, use a scooping or ladling motion to place the tip into the glottis. The appearance of transillumination at the neck indicates the position of the tube. Tracheal placement results in a bright, well-circumscribed area of transillumination at the cricothyroid membrane. The ET can then be advanced over the stylet into the trachea. Transillumination lateral to the midline indicates piriform sinus placement and need for repositioning. Esophageal placement causes little or no transillumination. The procedure is essentially the same for nasal intubation with a lighted stylet.

This procedure shares the same complications as other blind techniques: inadvertent malpositioning of the tube, hypoxia, and tissue damage.

▶ Video Laryngoscopes

Over the last few years, video laryngoscopes have been added to the airway armamentarium that many emergency physicians have ready to assist in challenging airway problems. The video laryngoscope, as its name implies, is a device with a video camera situated at the end of a curved blade that allows visualization of the anterior aspect of the hypopharynx and glottis. Because of the curve of the device, visualization of the glottis occurs without out alignment of the oropharyngeal and laryngotracheal axes that is required for successful intubation using conventional direct laryngoscopy. These devices utilize indirect laryngoscopy and can be particularly useful in difficult airway patients including those airways complicated by large body habitus or limited neck mobility. Many emergency physicians now preferentially turn to one of these airway management tools when managing difficult airway patients. Similar to the limitations discussed below with fiberoptic laryngoscopy, video laryngoscopes are centered around conditions that can obscure the lens of the device such as excessive oropharyngeal secretions or blood in the hypopharynx. Suctioning the airway prior to the intubation attempt may improve the chance of a successful intubation using video laryngosopes.

▶ Fiberoptic Intubation

Fiberoptic bronchoscopes may be used to locate the opening of the glottis when direct laryngoscopy cannot be used or is unsuccessful. The ET can then be advanced over the endoscope into the trachea. Although this procedure can be carried out without movement of the C-spine, it requires skill and practice. It can be performed either orally or nasally and oxygen can be insufflated during the procedure. It may be impossible when the hypopharynx is filled with blood or secretions. In addition, the equipment is expensive and easily damaged. Intubation via this method does require significant practice to become proficient.

▶ Gum Elastic Bougie

Gum elastic bougie was designed as a tracheal tube introducer. It is made of woven polyester with resin coating and is meant to be reused, although disposable ones are available. It is 60-cm long and 5 mm in diameter with an angled tip. When the glottis is impossible to visualize, this introducer can be angled under the epiglottis. If it passes into the trachea, a series of clicks will be palpable as it passes over the tracheal rings. Because of the diameter of the tube, it will no longer advance past 40 cm if in the airway. Once you are certain that it is in the airway, a tracheal tube from 6 to 8 mm may be passed over it into the trachea. The introducer is then removed. The bougie should not be used if one is completely unable to visualize the epiglottis.

▶ Nasotracheal Intubation

Please see Chapter 7 for description of method.

While this method of intubation is blind, it is relatively easy to perform in nonapneic patients. It is ideal in the patient who is awake and cannot undergo RSI or in those patients who have difficulty lying down secondary to severe shortness of breath (chronic obstructive pulmonary disease, congestive heart failure). It is contraindicated in the apneic patient and in those with severe facial trauma. This method has become less utilized in the recent years secondary to the use of RSI in most intubations. Prehospital providers occasionally still use it when RSI is not available to them.

▶ Retrograde Intubation

Retrograde intubation is indicated when oral or nasal intubation is contraindicated or technically impossible owing to anatomic, pathologic, or traumatic abnormalities. The advantages of this technique include maintenance of the C-spine in a neutral position and the benefits of any blind technique. In addition, it requires less skill than does fiberoptic intubation. Disadvantages include its time-consuming nature and the need to have the patient ventilating adequately throughout. This method is contraindicated when the airway is obstructed at or above the level of the cords. If the patient is unable to open the mouth, the retrograde wire must be passed out the nose for nasal intubation, which can be difficult and suboptimal in some settings.

Retrograde intubation can be performed by one operator, although an assistant is extremely helpful. Special equipment includes a needle of sufficient caliber to accept a guide wire and a wire approximately 70 cm in length. A small clamp or hemostat and Magill forceps are also useful. Local anesthetic is recommended.

The principle of retrograde intubation involves entering the trachea at the cricothyroid membrane with a guide wire that is threaded out the mouth or nose and used as a guide for blind oral or nasal intubation. After appropriate preparation of the neck, identify the cricothyroid membrane and surrounding landmarks. Pass a needle through the skin, and puncture the inferior third of the cricothyroid membrane with the needle directed about 30° caudad. Aspiration of air confirms tracheal placement. Rotate the needle to about 30° cephalad, and reaspirate to confirm tracheal position. Introduce the wire through the needle. As the wire is threaded through the needle, it often exits spontaneously through the mouth. Occasionally, however, it must be retrieved with fingers or forceps. When the wire is in hand at the lips or nares, the needle is removed. Fix the wire at the cricothyroid membrane with fingers or a small clamp. Thread the proximal end of the wire into the ET through the side hole (Murphy's eye). It should pass up through the lumen of the tube, exiting at its proximal end. Advance the lubricated tube along the wire until resistance is met, indicating that the tube is in the trachea, below the cords, pulled tight against the fixed wire. Release the wire at the skin and pull it out through the proximal end of the tube. Advance the tube to the appropriate position, and confirm placement in the usual manner.

Only a small number of cases of retrograde intubation have been described. Few serious complications have been reported.

Butler K et al: Management of the difficult airway: Alternative airway techniques and adjuncts. Emerg Med Clin North Am 2003;21:259 [PMID: 12793614] (a review of different methods both surgical and nonsurgical for managing the difficult airway).

Foley LJ et al: Managing the airway in the critically ill patient—Bridges to establish an emergency airway and alternate intubating techniques. Crit Care Clin 2000;16:429 [PMID: 10941582] (review of alternative airway management techniques).

Orebraugh SL: Difficult airway management in the emergency department. J Emerg Med 2002;22:31 [PMID: 11809554] (review of techniques for managing the difficult airway).

Pollack CV: The laryngeal mask airway—A comprehensive review for the emergency physician. J Emerg Med 2001;20:53 [PMID: 11165839] (review of the laryngeal mask airway indications, complications, and limitations).

Rodricks MB et al: Emergent airway management—Indications and methods in the face of confounding conditions. Crit Care Clin 2000;16:389 [PMID: 10941580] (review of management of the difficult airway, which includes review of current medications used in rapid-sequence protocols).

Shuster M et al: Airway and ventilation management. Cardiol Clin 2002;20:23 [PMID: 11845543] (review of airway management techniques).

▼ BRIDGING DEVICES FOR VENTILATION IN THE FAILED AIRWAY

In cases of patients who cannot be oxygenated or intubated, bridging devices provide the ability to ventilate a patient until a secure airway can be obtained that may help prevent the need for a surgical airway. These devices and methods of ventilation, while lifesaving in many situations, are not considered secure airways and do not prevent aspiration nor do they provide the best means of oxygenation and ventilation. A secure airway defined as a one in which a cuffed ET is situated below the cords must ultimately be obtained. Some of the following bridge devices may be successfully used between intubation attempts in the initially difficult airway to prevent dangerous episodes of hypoxia.

▶ Laryngeal Mask Airway

As stated in the section "Nonsurgical Devices and Techniques for Managing the Difficult Airway," the LMA is a very useful device that allows rapid insertion of a tube with which to ventilate through but provides minimal protection against aspiration. Please see previous section for description of use.

▶ Extraglottic Devices

As mentioned in previous sections, the ETC and King LT airway provide an excellent bridging device in hospital or prehospital failed airway situations. Please refer to the section "Prehospital Airway Devices" for description of use.

▶ Percutaneous Transtracheal Jet Ventilation

(See also Chapter 7.) PTTJV is an alternative technique for oxygenating a patient who cannot be intubated. It is unique in that positive pressure is generated by high-pressure oxygen delivered as an intermittent jet through high-pressure tubing and a percutaneously placed large-bore tracheal catheter. No bag reservoir or non-rebreathing valve is employed. PTTJV is less invasive than cricothyroidotomy and less time consuming than retrograde intubation (see above). It is relatively easily learned. With attention to detail, there are few complications. It can be used in awake or obtunded patients. Other advantages include presumed protection of the C-spine and possible expulsion of a pharyngeal foreign body by expired air. In the emergency department it is regarded as a temporizing measure while other methods of airway control can be established. Indications for PTTJV are the same as for cricothyroidotomy. PTTJV has been proven useful in the pediatric population.

Disadvantages include the need for either makeshift or commercially available special equipment. With prolonged use, retention of carbon dioxide may develop. Contraindications include anterior neck trauma, where high delivered pressures may lead to severe tissue disruption, and complete airway obstruction, where expired air cannot escape through the glottis. PTTJV shares the relative contraindications mentioned above for all invasive methods of airway control. Prior unsuccessful attempts at catheter placement may lead to air leak or subcutaneous emphysema after a second, successful attempt.

> Butler K et al: Management of the difficult airway: Alternative airway techniques and adjuncts. Emerg Med Clin North Am 2003;21:259 [PMID: 12793614] (a review of different methods both surgical and nonsurgical for managing the difficult airway).
>
> Orebraugh SL: Difficult airway management in the emergency department. J Emerg Med 2002;22:31 [PMID: 11809554] (review of techniques for managing the difficult airway).

▼ SURGICAL AIRWAYS

▶ Cricothyroidotomy

When there is complete upper airway obstruction or massive facial trauma that prohibits intubation from above, immediate access to the trachea can be obtained with cricothyroidotomy. In experienced hands, it is a rapid technique that maintains immobilization of the C-spine. It is a radical procedure with risk of significant short- and long-term negative outcomes. It is contraindicated whenever the airway can be secured by less invasive means. In children, cricothyroidotomy becomes technically more difficult as the landmarks become smaller. Patient age less than 10 years is a relative

contraindication for inexperienced practitioners. In children younger than 5 years, PTTJV or a tracheostomy is preferable if possible. Other relative contraindications include preexisting laryngeal disease, coagulopathy, anatomic deformities of the neck due to trauma or other causes, and lack of familiarity with the procedure. The equipment and technique for cricothyroidotomy are described in Chapter 7. Kits that use over-the-wire techniques, progressive dilatation, and trocar placement are available.

▶ Tracheostomy

Tracheostomy has little indication in emergency department management of the airway. Its only true indication is severe blunt trauma to the neck with fracture of the thyroid or cricoid cartilage, preventing access to the cricothyroid membrane. Tracheostomy is the preferred method of surgical airway management in the very small child when PTTJV is not possible. Because of the proximity of vascular, nerve, and visceral tissue, the risk of negative sequelae is high. A thorough knowledge of anatomy and careful surgical technique are critical to success. It should be performed only by surgeons experienced with the procedure.

> Bair AE, Panacek EA, Wisner DH, Bales R, Sakles JC. Cricothyrotomy: A 5-year experience at one institution. J Emerg Med 2003;24(2):151–156 [PMID: 12609644].

▼ USE OF DRUGS TO ASSIST IN INTUBATION

Some patients in the emergency department can be intubated without the use of pharmacologic intervention other than oxygen. However, when pharmacologic adjuncts are indicated, their use may dramatically reduce the difficulty of intubation and speed control of the airway. The patient's overall condition and the goal of intubation determine the choice of agent. Local, topical, or regional anesthesias are usually not considered options for an emergently compromised airway. For a semiobtunded or combative patient, use of neuromuscular blockade with sedation, usually in an RSI protocol, provides rapid control of the airway while protecting against aspiration of gastric contents.

Drugs that induce apnea must be used by or under the direct supervision of experienced clinicians prepared to obtain a surgical airway in the event of failed intubation. Equipment necessary for intubation and surgical airway must be prepared in advance and be available at the bedside before the patient is sedated or anesthetized.

▶ Rapid Sequence Intubation

A. General Considerations

Use of sedation alone to intubate a patient in the emergency department can be difficult and not without risk. Hypoventilation often occurs before the patient is adequately relaxed for intubation and prolonged bag–valve–mask ventilation may be required. Prolongation in airway control can delay other care and result in compromise of central nervous, cardiovascular, or pulmonary systems, further complicating the patient's postintubation course.

Every patient presenting with the need for an emergency airway should be approached as having a full stomach. These factors, combined with gastric distention due to bag–valve–mask ventilation, depressed airway reflexes, and the emetic effects of sedatives, raise the risk of aspiration.

The RSI protocol diminishes these difficulties in the awake patient who is agitated or who has altered mental status and requires oral intubation. A rapid-acting neuromuscular blocker is given to paralyze the patient. Though controversial, some protocols recommend a priming dose of a nondepolarizing neuromuscular blocker (such as vecuronium) to facilitate paralysis, reduce fasciculations, and limit elevations in intracranial pressure during laryngoscopy. Prior to administration of the paralytic, a short-acting sedative is added to decrease agitation and the noxious sensations associated with paralysis and intubation in awake or semiconscious patients. The patient is intubated immediately after paralysis. Further sedation and/or paralysis may then be necessary, as needed. During the short period when the patient is paralyzed and not intubated, the airway must be protected from aspiration with cricoid pressure.

The RSI protocol is generally unnecessary in a completely obtunded patient; however, if the patient has retained enough muscle tone to make intubation without paralytics difficult, RSI may facilitate a more rapid intubation. Because the RSI protocol will obscure the neurologic examination and physical manifestations of status epilepticus, only short-acting paralytics (such as succinylcholine) are recommended, or alternative plans to follow the neurologic condition of the patient must be made before inducing paralysis.

B. Equipment and Personnel Required

At least two individuals must be available to safely initiate the RSI protocol. Other than the drugs, no special equipment is required to induce neuromuscular blockade. Before giving any sedative or neuromuscular blocking agent, review the checklist in Table 10–5. The choice of sedative or anesthetic and neuromuscular blocking agent depends on the indication for intubation, patient condition, and user familiarity.

C. Procedure

Table 10–6 outlines the steps of the RSI protocol. The characteristics of the recommended drugs are mentioned in the section "Drugs Used During Intubation."

D. Additional Drugs

Several agents may be added to the RSI protocol under specific circumstances.

Table 10–5. Checklist for Initiation of RSI.

Baseline neurologic exam is completed
All materials for intubation are assembled
Materials for surgical airways are immediately available
Suction is working and available
Individuals have been designated as responsible for cricoid pressure cervical spine stabilization (in the setting of trauma)
The patient is preoxygenated

1. Atropine—Atropine, 0.01–0.02 mg/kg (minimum 0.1 mg to prevent reflex bradycardia) given immediately before the sedative, attenuates the vagal bradycardia associated with succinylcholine. Children, who tend to be more sensitive to the bradycardic and hypotensive effects of succinylcholine, benefit from pretreatment with atropine. Therefore, all children younger than 5 years should be pretreated with atropine before succinylcholine is administered. Pretreat adults with bradycardia and those receiving a second dose of succinylcholine.

2. Lidocaine—Lidocaine, 1.5 mg/kg given 1 minute before intubation, may attenuate elevations in intracranial pressure associated with succinylcholine and intubation. It may have some protective effect against laryngospasm and ventricular arrhythmias during intubation, as well.

3. Analgesics—If pain control is part of the management plan, a narcotic such as morphine sulfate (0.1 mg/kg),

Table 10–6. Rapid Sequence Intubation Protocol.

Preoxygenate with 100% oxygen (use bag-valve-mask ventilatory assistance only as needed)
Give rapid intravenous injection of sedative[a]
For trauma patients: maintain in-line cervical traction from induction and until cervical collar can be replaced after the endotracheal tube has been secured
Give rapid intravenous injection of succinylcholine,[b] 1-2 mg/kg (unless contraindicated)
Initiate cricoid pressure and stop bag-valve-mask ventilation
Observe for fasciculations followed by apnea
Immediately intubate on onset of apnea
Begin ventilation
Inflate endotracheal tube cuff and release cricoid pressure
Confirm tube position clinically to auscultate breath sounds; use end-tidal CO_2 detector
Secure tube
Provide additional sedation and paralysis as indicated

[a]Sedative drug choices: etomidate, 0.3 mg/kg; methohexital, 0.5–1 mg/kg; midazolam, 0.1-0.3 mg/kg; fentanyl, 1–5 mg/kg; ketamine, 1–2 mg/kg; thiopental, 1–4 mg/kg.
[b]Alternative neuromuscular blocker: vecuronium, 0.1-0.25 mg/kg; rocuronium, 0.6 mg/kg. (Use only when succinylcholine is contraindicated.)

fentanyl (1–2 μg/kg intravenously), or other analgesic should be added after intubation, because barbiturates have little analgesic effect and neuromuscular blockers have none.

▶ Drugs Used During Intubation

A. Succinylcholine

Succinylcholine is a depolarizing neuromuscular blocking agent.

1. Dose—1.0–1.5 mg/kg in adults, 1.5–2.0 mg/kg in children.

2. Onset—60 seconds to complete relaxation.

3. Duration—5–10 minutes.

4. Indications and advantages—

(a) Drug of choice for the RSI protocol under most circumstances owing to rapid onset, complete muscular relaxation, and short duration.

(b) Single dose in emergency department setting, usually well tolerated if appropriate precautions are taken (see below).

5. Contraindications—

(a) Risk factors for hyperkalemia (see Adverse Effects and Precautions, below).

(b) Hereditary pseudocholinesterase deficiency (1 in 2800 patients).

(c) Penetrating ocular trauma or glaucoma.

(d) Known family or personal history of malignant hyperthermia.

(e) Hypersensitivity to succinylcholine.

6. Adverse effects and precautions—

(a) Cardiovascular effects include bradycardia and hypotension, ventricular arrhythmias, and tachycardia or hypertension. Use with care in the setting of an irritable myocardium.

(b) Fasciculations (see above for sequelae).

(c) Hyperkalemia occurs in settings of subacute burns, subacute crush injuries, upper and lower motor neuron disease, and tetanus. Levels in excess of 9 mEq/L have been reported, and cardiac arrest may occur. Use may worsen hyperkalemia in renal failure patients.

(d) Pseudocholinesterase inhibition may occur in pregnancy, in renal or hepatic insufficiency, and with a variety of drugs.

(e) Malignant hyperthermia occurs in 1 in 50,000 patients.

(f) Histamine release may cause bronchospasm or anaphylactoid reaction.

(g) Intraocular pressure is elevated during fasciculations.

(h) Intracranial pressure may increase.

(i) Intragastric pressure may increase; use cricoid pressure until ET cuff is inflated.

(j) Always use sedation with alert patients; succinylcholine has no intrinsic analgesic or sedative effect.

B. Vecuronium

Vecuronium is a nondepolarizing neuromuscular blocking agent (NDNMB).

1. Dose—Standard dose is 0.1 mg/kg. To achieve rapid intubating conditions, 0.25 mg/kg may be used.

2. Onset—Dose dependent; standard doses achieve paralysis in 3–5 minutes, larger doses in 1–1.5 minutes.

3. Duration—Dose dependent; standard doses last 20–40 minutes and larger dose may prolong paralysis two to three times the usual duration.

4. Indications and advantages—

(a) One of the NDNMBs that can be used when succinylcholine is contraindicated.

(b) Relative short duration allows neurologic reevaluation and provides satisfactory paralysis for procedures such as computed tomography scan in an emergency setting.

(c) Minimal cardiovascular effects at usual doses.

(d) Reversible after partial recovery (evidence of head lift, respiratory effort, or muscle twitch response) with neostigmine, 0.04 mg/kg intravenously. Atropine, 0.02 mg/kg intravenously, must also be administered to prevent muscarinic side effects.

(e) Does not cause fasciculations or elevate intracranial pressure.

5. Contraindication—Known hypersensitivity to vecuronium.

6. Adverse effects and precautions—

(a) Reduce dosage in patients with myasthenia gravis to avoid prolonged blockade.

(b) Maintain cricoid pressure until inflation of ET cuff.

(c) Must use sedation or anesthesia in awake patients.

(d) Block is prolonged by aminoglycosides, lithium, quinidine, lidocaine, and propranolol and in hypermagnesemia, hyperkalemia, dehydration, hypothermia, and respiratory acidosis.

(e) Use during pregnancy only if clearly indicated.

C. Rocuronium

Rocuronium is a rapid-onset, short-acting NDNMB.

1. Dose—0.6 mg/kg.

2. Onset—1–2 minutes.

3. Duration—30 minutes.

4. Indications and advantages—Excellent choice for nondepolarizing neuromuscular blockade. Because of its rapid onset, rocuronium is a good alternative for use when succinylcholine is contraindicated.

5. Contraindication—Known hypersensitivity to rocuronium.

6. Adverse effects and precautions—

(a) Effects potentiated by electrolyte disturbances, neuromuscular diseases, and renal or hepatic failure.

(b) Use in pregnancy only if clearly indicated.

D. Pancuronium

Pancuronium is a longer-acting NDNMB.

1. Dose—0.05–0.2 mg/kg.

2. Onset—1–3 minutes.

3. Duration—Dose dependent, averaging 60–90 minutes.

4. Indications and advantages—

(a) Main use is prolonged blockade after intubation is complete.

(b) Does not promote bronchospasm.

(c) Reversible after partial recovery (see the section "Vecuronium").

(d) No elevated intracranial pressure or fasciculations.

5. Contraindications—

(a) Known hypersensitivity to pancuronium.

(b) Cardiovascular instability or history of congestive heart failure.

6. Adverse effects and precautions—

(a) History of myasthenia gravis (see the section "Vecuronium").

(b) Cardiovascular effects include increased heart rate, increased afterload, and ventricular arrhythmias. Use with caution in the setting of irritable myocardium.

(c) Blockade is prolonged by multiple drugs (see the section "Vecuronium").

(d) Duration profile is not optimal for use with the RSI protocol.

(e) Maintain cricoid pressure until inflation of ET cuff.

(f) Always use sedation or anesthesia in awake patients.

(g) Use in pregnancy only if clearly indicated.

E. Etomidate

Etomidate is a short-acting sedative-hypnotic.

1. Dose—0.3 mg/kg intravenously.

2. Onset—Within 1 minute.

3. Duration—3–5 minutes.

4. Indications and advantages—

(a) Alternative drug for sedation in RSI.

(b) Little to no cardiovascular side effects.

(c) Lowers intracranial and intraocular pressures.

5. Contraindication—Known hypersensitivity to etomidate.

6. Adverse effects and precautions—

(a) May cause hypotension in the hypovolemic patient.

(b) May cause apnea, laryngospasm, hiccups, and cough.

(c) May cause adrenal suppression with multiple doses.

(d) Local pain on injection.

(e) Skeletal muscle movements such as myoclonus.

(f) No recommendations for dosing in children younger than 10 years.

(g) May cause fetal malformation in pregnancy.

F. Midazolam

Midazolam is a short-acting benzodiazepine central nervous system depressant.

1. Dose—0.1–0.3 mg/kg.

2. Onset—Approximately 30 seconds, depending on rate of injection when given intravenously.

3. Duration—15–20 minutes.

4. Indications and advantages—

(a) Alternative induction agent for sedation in the RSI protocol (may have prolonged sedative effect).

(b) Minimal cardiovascular effects.

(c) May produce amnesia for several hours.

(d) Blunt intracranial pressure responses at high doses.

5. Contraindications—

(a) Known sensitivity to midazolam or benzodiazepines.

(b) Acute narrow-angle glaucoma.

6. Adverse effects and precautions—

(a) Respiratory depression or arrest.

(b) Cardiovascular effects usually minimal with bigeminy, premature ventricular contractions, and nodal rhythms.

(c) Laryngospasm and bronchospasm, cough, and hives.

(d) Local irritation at injection site.

(e) Nausea and vomiting.

(f) Potentiated by other central nervous system depressants; dose modifications recommended.

(g) Dose modifications recommended in patients with chronic obstructive pulmonary disease or congestive heart failure, in elderly patients, and in patients with renal failure.

(h) Possible increase in fetal malformations with pregnancy.

G. Fentanyl

Fentanyl is a short-acting narcotic anesthetic.

1. Dose—1–5 μg/kg intravenously.

2. Onset—60 seconds.

3. Duration—30–60 minutes.

4. Indications and advantages—

(a) Alternative drug for sedation in the RSI protocol (sedation may be prolonged with thiopental).

(b) Both analgesic and sedative effects.

(c) No histamine release.

(d) Blunts intracranial pressure response to intubation.

(e) Reversible with naloxone, 1–4 mg intravenously.

5. Contraindication—Known sensitivity to fentanyl.

6. Adverse effects and precautions—

(a) Respiratory depression and apnea. Respiratory depression may persist beyond analgesic and sedative effects.

(b) Muscle rigidity, which may occur with rapid injection of high doses.

(c) Rare bradycardia or cardiovascular depression.

(d) Nausea and vomiting.

(e) Effects potentiated by other central nervous system or respiratory depressants.

(f) Dose modifications recommended in patients with chronic obstructive pulmonary disease or congestive heart failure, in elderly patients, and in patients with renal failure.

(g) Possible increase in fetal malformations. Consider alternative drugs in pregnancy.

H. Ketamine

Ketamine is a dissociative anesthetic agent.

1. Dose—1–2 mg/kg.

2. Onset—60 seconds.

3. Duration—5–10 minutes.

4. Indications and advantages—

(a) Alternative drug for sedation and analgesia during the RSI protocol, particularly in hypotension.

(b) Sedative of choice in status asthmaticus patients because it may cause bronchodilation.

(c) Airway reflexes are usually maintained. Respiratory depression is usually minimal and transient.

(d) Myocardial depression is uncommon.

(e) Prominent analgesic effects.

5. Contraindications—

(a) Hypersensitivity to ketamine.

(b) Head injury.

(c) Severe hypertension.

6. Adverse effects and precautions—

(a) Elevated blood pressure and pulse rate are the most common cardiovascular effects. Hypotension, bradycardia, and arrhythmias have been reported. Use with caution if irritable myocardium is present or when hypertension would adversely affect patient course.

(b) Respiratory stimulation and maintained airway most common, but apnea, respiratory arrest, and laryngospasm also have been reported.

(c) Dysphoric emergence reactions.

(d) Nausea and vomiting.

(e) Local irritation at injection site.

(f) Increased intracranial pressure.

(g) Intraocular pressure may be increased.

(h) Muscle rigidity or myoclonus.

(i) Increased secretions. Consider pretreatment with atropine.

(j) Possible prolonged recovery when used concurrently with narcotics or barbiturates.

(k) Consider alternative drug in pregnancy and for patients younger than 2 months.

Rodricks MB et al: Emergent airway management—Indications and methods in the face of confounding conditions. Crit Care Clin 2000;16:389 [PMID: 10941580] (review of management of the difficult airway, which includes review of current medications used in rapid-sequence protocols).

Wadbrook PS: Advances in airway pharmacology—Emerging trends and evolving controversy. Emerg Med Clin North Am 2000;18:767 [PMID: 11130938] (review of drugs used for RSI protocol).

▼ SPECIAL CASES

▶ Management of the Pediatric Airway

Basic principles of airway management are similar for all age groups. However, anatomic and physiologic differences affect the emergency physician's equipment needs and management decisions when confronted with a pediatric airway emergency.

Table 10–7. Pediatric Vital Signs and Airway Equipment.

Age	Premature	Neonate	1 mo	6 mo	1 y	3 y	5 y	7 y	>10 y
Weight (kg)	1	2–3	4	7	10	12–14	16–18	20–26	>30
Heart rate	145	125	120	130	125	115	100	100	75
Respiratory rate	30–40	30–40	25–35		20–30		12–25		12–18
Endotracheal tube size (inner diameter in millimeter)	2.5–3.0	3	3.5	3.5	4	4.5	5–6	6–6.5	7
Length at teeth (cm)	8	10	12	12	16	16	18	20–22	
Laryngoscope blade size	0	0–1	1	1	1–2	1–2	2	2–3	3
				Straight				Curved	
Suction catheter size (F)	5	6	6–8	6–8	8	8–10	10	10–12	12

A. Unique Features

- In infants, the head is relatively larger in proportion to the body.
- The neck is more supple owing to a greater proportion of cartilaginous support tissue.
- The airway is smaller, resulting in increased resistance and susceptibility to obstruction due to edema, blood, or secretions.
- The mucosa is looser, permitting obstruction due to positioning and greater, faster distention from blood or edema.
- The adenoidal and tonsillar lymphatic tissues are larger and more friable than those of adults.
- The larynx is more cephalad and anterior.
- The epiglottis is larger and more floppy and protrudes into the airway more prominently.
- The narrowest portion of the airway in children younger than 5 years is the cricoid cartilage rather than the larynx, as in adults.
- The cricothyroid membrane is very small and does not lend itself to surgical manipulation.
- The carina branches symmetrically at 45°.
- The chest wall is thinner, and both airway and gastric sounds radiate easily, making auscultation less reliable.
- The chest wall is more pliable, and ventilation depends significantly on diaphragmatic movement.
- Oxygen consumption is 6–8 mL/kg/min in children, whereas adults usually consume about 3–4 mL/kg/min. Hypoxemia can occur more rapidly and is tolerated less well.
- Apnea occurs suddenly during a wide range of illnesses and injuries.
- Normal vital signs vary for different age groups (Table 10–7).

B. Equipment Required

All essential equipment (oxygen delivery systems, face masks, bag–valve–mask units, oral and nasal airways, laryngoscope blades, ETs, stylets, and suction devices) should be stocked in a variety of sizes to accommodate the anticipated population served by the facility (see Table 10–7). Oxygen should be humidified and warmed to prevent drying of secretions and subsequent airway obstruction. It has been classically taught that ETs for children younger than 8 years should be noncuffed to prevent damage to the cricoid ring. This notion has recently been challenged and many pediatric critical care specialists now routinely use modern high-volume, low-pressure cuffed ETs for intubation of all children. Correct tube size may be obtained from a table or gauged based on one of the following three methods:

1. The tube size should closely approximate the size of the child's small finger at the distal interphalangeal joint.
2. The tube size should closely approximate the size of the child's nares.
3. The tube size in millimeters is equal to (patient's age in years/4) + 4.

For patients younger than 4 years, a straight blade is preferred owing to the tendency of the epiglottis to protrude and cover the airway. In emergency departments where pediatric resuscitation is rare, precalculate the doses of commonly needed drugs, based on weights, and post them clearly in the resuscitation area or utilize length-based charts such as the Broselow–Luten tape.

C. Decision and Techniques

Evaluate for respiratory distress by assessing vital signs, skin signs, overall patient condition, use of accessory muscles, retractions, nasal flaring, and arterial blood gases or pulse oximetry. Since supplemental oxygen must be given and children often cannot tolerate a face mask, adequate oxygen supplementation can frequently be achieved by directing a stream of humidified 100% oxygen across the patient's face.

Airway positioning is essential. Alert patients will often choose the position of greatest airway patency and should not be forced to lie down. Infants and obtunded patients must be placed in the sniffing position (see Figure 10–2) unless C-spine injury is suspected or present. In this position, the neck is flexed slightly and the head is extended on the neck. The jaw thrust or chin lift is then used to lift the soft tissues out of the airway. Obstruction should be cleared.

Oral and nasal airways are less useful in children because they frequently stimulate laryngospasm or emesis when reflexes are intact. In addition, placement may traumatize the adenoidal or tonsillar soft tissues, resulting in significant bleeding, which can be difficult to control and may further complicate airway management.

In obtunded or paralyzed children, cricoid pressure should be used during positive pressure ventilation until intubation is confirmed. Bag–valve–mask ventilation is used initially for emergent oxygenation and ventilation in children because of the ease of attaining a seal and the smaller size of the chest cavity. Adequacy of ventilation is best assessed by observing chest wall motion, as auscultation is less reliable. Care should be taken to coordinate breaths with the bag–valve–mask unit with spontaneous ventilations, when present.

Definitive airway control involves oral endotracheal intubation. Blind nasal intubation is technically more difficult in children and is contraindicated in the emergency department. The increased adenoidal tissue is at risk for bleeding, and the anterior position of the larynx with the overlying epiglottis makes nasal tube placement more difficult. Until 5 years of age, children should be premedicated with atropine, 0.01–0.02 mg/kg (minimum 0.1 mg), to prevent bradycardia with intubation. Because auscultation can be unreliable, tube placement should be confirmed by a colorimetric end-tidal CO_2 detector, observation of chest wall movement, skin color, and radiographs.

Surgical airways in young children and infants are extremely difficult. They should be performed only as a last resort by surgeons with experience in pediatric head and neck surgery. There are high failure and complication rates. Most airways will be adequately managed by bag–valve–mask or oral intubation techniques.

D. Epiglottitis and Croup

These illnesses may cause severe airway edema and sudden obstruction. Diagnosis is based on clinical features and, when necessary, anteroposterior and lateral neck soft tissue views.

1. Croup—Croup progresses more slowly than epiglottitis, causes subglottic swelling and a barking cough, and is often accompanied by signs of viral upper respiratory infection. It can rarely progress to bacterial tracheitis, an emergent airway infection. Unlike croup, which rarely requires intubation, bacterial tracheitis usually requires intubation, frequent suctioning, and antibiotics. When severe, croup requires treatment with racemic epinephrine, steroids, and observation.

2. Epiglottitis—Epiglottitis classically progresses rapidly with a toxic-appearing, drooling child sitting in the upright position with the neck hyperextended. Abrupt, complete airway obstruction can occur with minimal stimulation of the patient. When suspicion is high for epiglottitis, supplemental oxygen should be supplied and the patient transported with minimal disturbance to the operating room, where the epiglottis can be directly visualized. More than half of the patients with epiglottitis will require intubation, which is best done in the operating room by the most experienced intubator before airway obstruction occurs. If intubation fails, tracheostomy must be performed on an emergency basis, preferably by a pediatric otorhinolaryngologist. Treatment includes antibiotics and intravenous fluids after the airway is secured (see Chapter 50).

▶ Management of Foreign Bodies in the Airway

Management of foreign bodies in the airway is dictated by the location of the object and the patient's age and condition. Most airway obstructions due to foreign bodies occur between the ages of 1 and 5 years. More than 3000 deaths annually are due to this disorder.

Assessment begins with observation for tachypnea, air movement, stridor, retraction, agitation or lethargy, and cyanosis. Auscultation and chest x-ray may be helpful. Examination of the oropharynx may reveal the foreign body. If the foreign body is visible, the airway may be cleared with a manual sweep. Blind sweep is not recommended. If the patient is coughing, do not interfere; the normal reflexes often clear the airway. Oxygen should be administered to all patients with foreign body aspiration.

If there is total obstruction, attempt the Heimlich maneuver in patients older than 1 year; in younger children, back blows and chest thrusts are recommended. If these methods are unsuccessful, position the airway to optimize patency. Attempt to remove the object under direct observation with a laryngoscope. If this is unsuccessful, a surgical airway may be necessary to relieve subglottic obstructions. Removal in the operating room with rigid bronchoscope may be the only option.

Management of the partially obstructed airway must be individualized. Bronchial obstructions often do not require intubation, and compromise may be subacute. If there is air movement and the object cannot be visualized on direct observation, the safest method for removal is under general anesthesia with the rigid bronchoscope. Take care not to cause complete obstruction while inserting the laryngoscope or bronchoscope.

▶ Management of Airway in Trauma Patients

A. Patients with Unstable Cervical Spines or Facial Injuries

When airway control must precede definitive stabilization of the spine, oral intubation with RSI and in-line maintenance of the C-spine has been proved safe and effective. It is the method of choice in the trauma patient with suspected spinal injury. However, most large series report no bad neurologic outcomes with any technique that is carefully done. Other options for airway control include blind techniques such as nasal or digital intubation, use of lighted accessories, and transtracheal methods. The decision must be individualized based on the patient's level of consciousness and injuries, the urgency of the need for airway control, and the intubator's skill with various techniques.

Patients with severe facial and upper neck trauma present significant challenges to the emergency physician. If RSI techniques are attempted, the emergency physician should be prepared to switch immediately to a surgical airway or a bridge device to allow ventilation in the event that bag–valve–mask ventilation proves difficult or ineffective. If the airway is predicted from the beginning to be difficult, an awake intubation using topical anesthetics and intravenous sedation may be the best approach.

B. Patients with Head Trauma

Intubation of patients with severe head trauma (GCS ≤ 8) is indicated to treat hypoventilation and hypoxia and to protect and control the airway in patients who are unstable or combative and agitated enough to require paralysis for necessary studies and procedures. Additionally, it is the only way to hyperventilate the patient to a lower P_{CO_2} as part of the treatment for severely elevated intracranial pressure and imminent herniation. Approach to the airway must take into account other potential traumatic injuries to the midface, C-spine, soft tissues of the neck, and respiratory tract. Oral intubation with the RSI protocol is generally recommended. If the RSI protocol is used, lidocaine, 1.5 mg/kg intravenously, may attenuate the rise in intracranial pressure. Although succinylcholine is reported to raise intracranial pressure, it remains the recommended agent for neuromuscular blockade in the setting of head trauma because it allows for rapid control of the airway and initiation of treatment. Other sedative options available to attenuate the rise in intracranial pressure associated with laryngoscopy include fentanyl and etomidate. Vecuronium, an NDNMB, is administered at 0.01 mg/kg as a small priming dose to eliminate muscle fasciculations associated with succinylcholine use.

Cummins RO et al: Guidelines 2000 for cardiopulmonary resuscitation and emergency cardiovascular care. American Heart Association Currents 2000;(Fall):1 (update of advanced cardiac life support guidelines).

Levy RJ et al: Managing the airway in the critically ill patient—Pediatric issues. Crit Care Clin 2000;16:489 [PMID: 10941587] (review of the management of the difficult airway in the pediatric patient).

Newth C et al: The use of cuffed versus uncuffed endotracheal tubes in pediatric intensive care. J Pediatr 2004;144:333–337 [PMID: 15001938] (prospective, observational study of ET types used in a pediatric intensive care unit).

Sullivan KJ, Kissoon N: Securing the child's airway in the emergency department. Pediatr Emerg Care 2002;18(2):108–124 [PMID: 11973505] (review of emergent pediatric airway management).

Verghese ST, Hannallah RS: Pediatric otolaryngologic emergencies. Anesthesiol Clin North Am 2001;19(2):237–256 [PMID: 11469063] (review of management of foreign bodies in the airway).

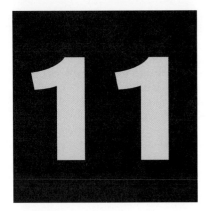

Shock

William F. Young, Jr., MD

Shock is a state of severe systemic reduction in tissue perfusion characterized by decreased cellular oxygen delivery and utilization as well as decreased removal of waste byproducts of metabolism. Hypotension, although common in shock, is not synonymous to shock. One can have hypotension and normal perfusion, or shock without hypotension in a patient who is usually very hypertensive. Shock is the final preterminal event in many diseases. Progressive tissue hypoxia results in loss of cellular membrane integrity, a reversion to a catabolic state of anaerobic metabolism, and a loss of energy-dependent ion pumps and chemical and electrical gradients. Mitochondrial energy production begins to fail. Multiple organ dysfunction follows localized cellular death, and organism death follows. Despite recent advances in treatment, mortality remains high: > 50% in cardiogenic shock and > 35% in septic shock.

PATHOPHYSIOLOGY OF SHOCK

Blood pressure is determined by the formula BP = systemic vascular resistance (SVR) × cardiac output (CO), where CO = heart rate (HR) × stroke volume (SV). SV = end diastolic volume (EDV) minus end systolic volume (ESV). EDV is the filled ventricular volume prior to systolic contraction averaging about 100 cc in many adults. ESV is residual blood left in the ventricle after emptying during systole averaging about 40 cc. Therefore, the determinants of blood pressure are vascular resistance, HR, preload volume, and contractility (see Figure 11–1). SVR is the vascular "tone" and is a large determinant of diastolic blood pressure. EDV is largely determined by preload volume that augments SV via Frank–Starling curves where increases in diastolic filling volumes increase CO. ESV is determined largely by cardiac contractility and it decreases as the heart ejects a greater percentage of its diastolic volume. For example, one can increase SV by increasing preload (EDV) with volume or decreasing ESV with increased contractility. The ejection fraction ((EDV – ESV)/EDV) thus increases.

The initial derangement precipitating a state of shock might be (1) vasodilation (causing a decreased SVR) from sepsis, anaphylaxis, drugs, or cervical cord lesion, (2) extremes of HR, (3) loss of preload volume (causing decreased EDV) from blood or volume loss, or (4) loss of contractility (increasing the ESV) from heart failure. Compensatory mechanisms come into play and provide many of the clinical clues to early shock.

The initial compensatory mechanisms depend on the initial insult. (1) Vasodilation with loss of SVR generally causes a compensatory tachycardia and thirst. Despite systemic tissue hypoxemia, the skin remains perfused and is warm initially. (2) Blood or fluid loss (decreasing EDV) causes a reflex increase in SVR, which increases diastolic BP, narrowing the

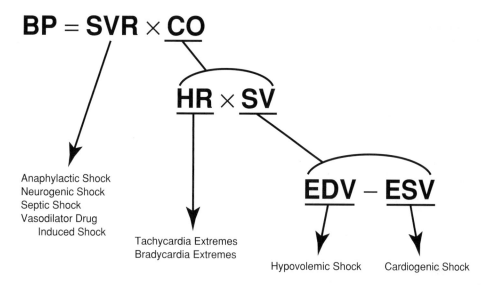

BP = blood pressure, SVR = systemic vascular resistance, HR = heart rate, SV = stroke volume, EDV = end diastolic volume (i.e. preload), ESV = end systolic volume (i.e. contractility)

▲ **Figure 11-1.** Determinants of blood pressure.

pulse pressure, increases sympathetic cholinergic sweating and makes the patient pale, thirsty, and cool. As volume loss increases, tachycardia and hypotension ensue. (3) Loss of contractility also is compensated by increases in SVR to maintain blood pressure with similar symptoms.

Once compensatory mechanisms fail, irreversible shock occurs with irreversible cell death, microcirculation plugging, and free radical generation. There is loss of autonomic regulation due to local nitric oxide vasodilator generation, and even with complete correction of blood volume (for example, in hypovolemic shock), tissue function, and organ function are not restored, causing eventual death.

CAUSES OF SHOCK

The major classical classification of shock includes (1) hypovolemic, (2) cardiogenic, (3) distributive, and (4) obstructive shock. The first three involve a primary derangement in EDV, ESV, and SVR, respectively, while obstructive shock is usually a problem with SV due to mechanical obstruction to preload. Causes of "obstructive shock" are usually classified as hypovolemic or cardiogenic. Common causes of each type are listed in Table 11–1.

CLINICAL PRESENTATION

There is no one clinical or biological test to determine shock. If compensatory mechanisms are functioning early in shock, one may not see hypotension but instead an anxious patient still maintaining a blood pressure. In these early stages (called preshock) symptoms can be subtle, but provide an opportunity for early intervention. Waiting for full-blown shock leads to a loss of precious time, and an aggressive proactive approach should be pursued.

During the early or preshock state, pale, cool, moist skin reflects compensatory elevated SVR in hypovolemic and cardiogenic shock. The pulse pressure narrows (with a slight decrease in systolic blood pressure and rise in diastolic blood pressure) and patient anxiety increases. Blood is shunted preferentially from "nonessential" skin and gastrointestinal (GI) tract to heart and brain. After a 20–30% volume loss in hypovolemic shock, tachycardia increases, urine volumes decrease with decreased renal blood flow, and the patient becomes more agitated. In cardiogenic shock, left-sided heart failure manifests as pulmonary edema and right-sided heart failure manifests as peripheral edema with elevated jugular venous distention (JVD).

In distributive shock, the primary problem is loss of vascular tone with erythematous warm skin despite hypotension. Tachycardic response is variable and early on, the heart may be hyperdynamic. This is the "warm patient in shock."

In full-blown shock, patients become agitated and finally decrease their mental status. Hypotension occurs and may be profound. The patient has tachypnea until respiratory failure occurs and has a metabolic acidosis due to elevated lactic acid from anaerobic metabolism. At the cellular level, tissue oxygen extraction is maximal and is reflected in decreased mixed venous O_2 saturation. Multiple organ failure follows. Irreversible shock follows if treatment is not aggressive.

Table 11–1. Causes of Shock.

A. Hypovolemic shock
  1. Blood loss
    a. Traumatic hemorrhage
      1. Exsangination (e.g. Scalp)
      2. Hemothorax
      3. Hemoperitoneum
      4. Fracture (femur & pelvis)
    b. Nontraumatic hemorrhage
      1 GI bleed
      2. AAA rupture
      3. Ectopic pregnancy rupture
  2. Volume loss
    a. Burns
    b. Skin integrity loss (TEN)
    c. Vomiting
    d. Diarrhea
    e. Hyperosmolar states (DKA)
    f. Third spacing (e.g., Ascites)
    g. Decreased intake
B. Cardiogenic shock
  1. Dysrhythmia
    a. Bradycardias and blocks
    b. Tachycardias
  2. Cardiomyopathy
    a. Infarction
    b. RV infarction
    c. Dilated cardiomyopathy
  3. Mechanical
    a. Valvular
      1. Aortic insufficiency from dissection
      2. Papillary muscle rupture from ischemia
    b. Ventricular aneurysm rupture
    c. Free wall ventricle rupture
C. Distributive shock
  1. Anaphylactic shock
  2. Septic shock
  3. Neurogenic shock
  4. Drug induced vasodilation
  5. Adrenal insufficiency
D. Obstructive shock
  1. Tension pneumothorax
  2. Pericardial disease
    a. Pericardial tamponade
    b. Constrictive pericarditis
  3. Massive pulmonary embolism
  4. Auto PEEP from mechanical ventilation

INITIAL EVALUATION OF SHOCK

In the initial evaluation of a patient in preshock, one must ask: Is the patient in shock or headed that way? It is ill advised to wait for severe hypotension in the patient who is still compensating for their shock before aggressively intervening. The clinician's first priority is to maintain vital functions while exploring the potential causes of shock. One

should also consider early decontamination if the patient has been exposed to a toxin.

ABCs open the airway and maintain adequate ventilation/oxygenation with high flow oxygen. Airway adjuncts such as the nasopharyngeal airway may help, but one must anticipate worsening of the airway with time. If the patient cannot protect the airway, has a GCS score < 9 in trauma, has extremes of respiratory rate or is hypoxic despite supplemental oxygen, endotracheal intubation is indicated. Relieve any tension pneumothorax based on clinical grounds (below). Establish multiple short-length, large-bore peripheral IV access and place on a cardiac monitor in a critical care area of the ED. Central venous access and arterial catheter placement should be considered, but should not delay resuscitation. Intravenous access in shock can be challenging and intraosseous access may be timely. Remove clothes and keep the patient warm. Next, try to determine if there is a readily recognizable and potentially reversible cause of the patient's condition?

▶ Is There a Reversible Condition?

Is there traumatic blood loss? Stop visible hemorrhage, look for cavitary bleeding in the chest (CXR, ultrasound (U/S)), abdomen (FAST exam), or pelvis from pelvic fracture or disruption or long-bone fracture. If pelvic or long-bone fractures are present, immobilize these injuries by wrapping the pelvis with a sheet in the case of a pelvic fracture or for femur fracture, immobilization of the extremity in an external traction device.

Is there nontraumatic blood loss? Check for a pulsatile abdominal mass (abdominal aortic aneurysm, AAA) or perform bedside U/S of the abdomen; check for GI bleed (hematemesis or melena).

Is there a dysrhythmia? Monitor and obtain an ECG. Cardiovert an unstable tachydysrhythmia and begin external cardiac pacing for unstable bradydysrhythmias.

Is there a tension pneumothorax? Check for decreased unilateral breath sounds, tracheal deviation away from pneumothorax, and a hyperresonant hemithorax. Perform needle decompression followed by chest tube thoracostomy.

Is there cardiac tamponade? Check for JVD, muffled heart sounds, low ECG voltage, and electrical alternans and perform bedside U/S if available. Perform pericardiocentesis if U/S demonstrates a pericardial effusion in the patient in shock.

Is there evidence of massive pulmonary embolism? In the patient at risk for pulmonary embolism (PE), is there hypoxemia with signs of acute right ventricular overload (bedside echocardiography)? Consider thrombolytics or surgical intervention.

Is there overt anaphylaxis? Look for angioedema, laryngeal edema with stridor, wheezing, and hives.

Is the spinal cord injured? Check for a motor/sensory level of paralysis/anesthesia. Trauma patients should be logrolled maintaining cervical spine precautions to examine the back for injury and check for gross rectal bleeding or loss of rectal tone.

Is the problem with SVR? If the skin is warm, despite hypotension, think sepsis, neurogenic, anaphylactic shock, or medication overdose (β-blocker or calcium channel blocker overdose).

OBTAIN HISTORY CLUES TO THE CAUSE OF SHOCK

There may be historical clues to the patient's condition. Check for potential unsuspected trauma, unsuspected or known pregnancy, new medications, allergies, overdose, or depression. Look for potential drug interactions such as those of sildenafil and nitroglycerin. Obtain a travel history (SARS) and tampon-use history (toxic shock syndrome); chest pain and dyspnea may imply acute coronary syndrome or PE. Fever or hypothermia might signify sepsis.

GIVE A FLUID CHALLENGE

Unless the patient is in severe pulmonary edema from cardiogenic shock, a fluid challenge of 20 cc/kg of isotonic crystalloid is a reasonable next step after the ABCs have been evaluated and overt causes addressed as above.

OBTAIN APPROPRIATE LABS

Important early labs include complete blood count, coagulation studies, electrolytes, BUN, creatinine, arterial blood gas, and serum lactate. Note that the *venous* blood gas and *pulse oximetry* may be inaccurate in shock. In septic shock, obtain pan cultures. Obtain urinalysis in all patients and perform urine pregnancy testing in all women of child-bearing age. Type and crossmatch the patients for packed RBCs. In cardiogenic shock, obtain cardiac enzymes.

OBTAIN APPROPRIATE IMAGING

A chest radiograph and ECG are valuable initial examinations with further testing dictated by clinical suspicion. Bedside U/S can have a key role with evaluation of pericardial fluid and hemoperitoneum but complex imaging studies should wait until the patient is resuscitated.

Hopefully, by this time you have some idea as to the nature of the type of shock and further therapy and evaluation can be tailored to the potential cause.

SPECIFIC SHOCK CONDITIONS

▶ Hypovolemic Shock

The treatment objectives in hypovolemic shock are to stop the bleeding or fluid loss and to replace the blood or fluid.

In traumatic hemorrhage, direct pressure is usually effective in stopping external hemorrhage. Shock from hemothorax or hemoperitoneum requires urgent operative intervention. Massive blood loss from a pelvic fracture might improve with manual stabilization in a sling (or sheet tied around the pelvis) or embolization via angiography. Femur fractures should be splinted with an external traction device. Rapid EMS transport is essential with therapy done enroute.

A crystalloid infusion of normal saline or lactated Ringer's solution of 20 cc/kg should be given with general resuscitation measures described above. There has been no demonstrated advantage of albumin or other colloids over crystalloids. Hypertonic (7.5%) saline infusion (with or without dextran) has shown promise but is still largely of unproven benefit. Crystalloids continue to have the advantage of cost and availability.

Blood should be given early in hemorrhagic shock patients not readily responding to crystalloid infusion of 40 cc/kg. Choice is based on the time frame: For immediate need in an unstable patient, use un-crossmatched O-negative packed RBCs. If time allows, use type-specific red blood cells or typed and crossed packed RBCs. It is worthwhile knowing at your institution the time frames for when these various blood products are available. Although the ideal ratio of packed RBCs: FFP: Platelets remains unclear, a massive transfusion protocol should involve all blood components. One protocol recommends the use of RBC : FFP: platelet ratio of 1:1:1 with one unit of cryoprecipitate given for every two units of RBC's. While more than one synthetic blood substitute has been studied in recent years, because of questions related to efficacy and safety, none have been approved for use nor available in the treatment of hemorrhagic shock.

The concept of "permissive hypotension" requires rapid surgical intervention and remains unproven, although overly aggressive fluid resuscitation might dislodge clots, interfere with the clotting cascade, and exacerbate bleeding. The goal of resuscitation should be to maintain a reasonable perfusion while aggressively stopping the source of bleeding.

Nontraumatic hemorrhagic shock from ectopic pregnancy or AAA rupture requires operative intervention. Patients with GI bleeding should have a nasogastric tube placed to reduce gastric size and monitor bleeding along with a proton pump inhibitor, H2 blockade (for gastric bleeding) and/or octreotide infusion (for variceal bleeding). Endoscopy will likely be necessary for any patient exhibiting signs of shock and upper GI bleeding. Shock from fluid loss or third spacing should respond to crystalloid infusion.

Monitor for signs of successful resuscitation (Table 11–2), but realize that many patients suffering hemorrhagic shock require operative intervention.

Geeraedts LMG, Kaasjager HAH, van Vugt AB et al: Exsanguination in trauma: a review of diagnostics and treatment options. Injury 2009;40:11–20 [PMID 19135193].

Table 11-2. Signs of a Successful Initial Resuscitation.

1. Improved blood pressure
2. Improving level of consciousness
3. Improving peripheral perfusion
4. Decreasing tachycardia
5. Decreasing lactate
6. Normalizing pH

Chen YJ, Scerbo M, Kramer G: A review of blood substitutes: examining the history, clinical trial results, and ethics of hemoglobin-based oxygen carriers. Clinics 2009;64:803–813 [PMID 19690667].

Spahn DR, Cerny V, Coats TJ, et al: Management of bleeding following major trauma: a European guideline. Crit Care 2007; 11:R17 [PMID 17298665].

▶ Cardiogenic Shock

Cardiogenic shock from tachydysrhythmias should be treated with cardioversion. Bradydysrhythmias require immediate transcutaneous pacing, although atropine may be tried first for sinus bradycardia or second-degree type I (Wenckebach) block. Myocardial infarction (MI) (particularly anterior STEMI) remains the most common cause of cardiogenic shock, complicating 7–10% of all acute MIs mortality remains high (>50%) for these patients and the incidence is increasing. Most patients have extensive and multivessel disease. Although many patients develop pump failure from loss of myocardium, there is some contribution by a systemic inflammatory response syndrome (SIRS) and abnormally decreased ventricular compliance.

Treatment of cardiogenic shock includes general supportive measures of oxygen, aspirin, heparin, and "gentle" fluid challenges (250 cc) if there is no overt pulmonary edema. A search for a surgically correctable mechanical cause such as septal rupture or valvular incompetence should be done with early echocardiography. Glycoprotein IIb/IIIa inhibitors have shown a risk/benefit in favor of treatment. Avoid nitrates, β-blockers and calcium-channel blockers. Clopidogrel can be delayed since some patients will require emergent CABG. Pulmonary artery catheter insertion is necessary to guide therapy and further fluid/pressor therapy.

Early mechanical ventilation has been shown to decrease mortality and should be considered to decrease the work of breathing and reverse acidosis. This can be done invasively with endotracheal intubation or noninvasively via continuous positive airway pressure.

Vasopressors are often needed. Dopamine, titrated to hemodynamic response (hopefully with pulmonary artery catheter data guidance), can be started at 5 μg/kg/min, increasing to 15 μg/kg/min, where α vasoconstrictor effects predominate. Norepinephrine is preferred by some because of its potency and improved efficacy in a recent study. Dobutamine, which causes mild vasodilation and increased contractility, can also be added (often in concert with dopamine).

For patients with STEMI, revascularization by PCI or emergent CABG is preferred to fibrinolysis if the former is available and can be done within 90 minutes of presentation. If revascularization is not available in a timely manner, fibrinolysis with augmentation of blood pressure with vasopressors and / or intra-aortic balloon pump (IABP) should be done with prompt transfer to PCI/CABG capable facilities. IABP insertion augments diastolic blood pressure, improving coronary artery perfusion and better delivery of fibrinolytics to the coronary arteries. Although at high risk for early death, cardiogenic shock is treatable and has a reasonable prognosis for recovery.

Right ventricular infarction, often occurring in the setting of an inferior MI involving the right coronary artery, can be complicated by hypotension. Infarction of the right ventricle causes the ventricle to stiffen, requiring a greater preload to stretch the noncompliant muscle. Decreased right ventricle function decreases CO to the left ventricle via the lungs causing hypotension, especially if given a vasodilator like nitroglycerin. Inferior MIs do not usually cause pump failure, and hypotension in this setting should be examined with right-sided ECG leads and a fluid challenge. Right ventricular infarction is confirmed when 1 mm of ST elevation is noted in lead V4R or when the ST-segment elevation in lead III exceeds the ST elevation in lead II.

Van dr Werf F, Bax J, Betriu A et al: Management of acute myocardial infarction in patients presenting with persistent ST-segment elevation. Eur Heart J 2008;29:2909–2945 [PMID 19004841].

Backer DD, Biston P, Devriendt J et al: Comparison of Dopamine and Norepinephrine in the treatment of shock. NEJM 2010;362:779–789 [PMID 20200382].

Antman EM et al: ACC/AHA guidelines for the management of patients with ST-elevation myocardial infarction—executive summary: a report of the American College of Cardiology/ American Heart Association Task Force on Practice Guidelines (Writing Committee to Revise the 1999 Guidelines for the Management of Patients With Acute Myocardial Infarction). Circulation 2004;110:588 [PMID: 15358047].

Reynolds HR, Hochman JS: Cardiogenic shock: current concepts and improving outcomes. Circulation 2008;117:686–697 [PMID 18250279].

Den Uil CA, Lagrand WK, Valk SD et al: Management of cardiogenic shock: focus on tissue perfusion. Curr Prob Cardiol 2009;34:330–349 [PMID 19591748].

▶ Anaphylactic Shock

One of the most frightening causes of shock is the patient in anaphylaxis where the airway is obstructing, ventilation is compromised with bronchospasm, and the blood pressure is low. Treatment should be aggressive and proactive. The airway is at risk in anaphylaxis due to angioedema, tongue, or laryngeal edema. Patients with anaphylaxis are likely to be among the most challenging with regard to airway management. These patients can rapidly deteriorate and become "can't intubate, can't ventilate" airway disasters (see Chapter 10). In rapidly advancing airway obstruction, early intubation is advised. In these patients, because of difficulties with standard intubation techniques, a surgical airway may be needed. Patients with bronchospasm should receive aggressive treatment with β-agonist aerosol or epinephrine (see below). Systemic vasodilation causes hypotension, and aggressive fluid resuscitation is needed using crystalloids.

Treatment includes removal of any known antigen, early administration of epinephrine, β-agonist aerosol, H1 and H2 histamine receptor blockade, and steroids. For mild to moderate symptoms, epinephrine can be given 0.3–0.5 preferably IM lateral thigh (pediatrics use 0.01 mg/kg/dose). For life-threatening symptoms, use 0.5–1 cc of 1:10,000 solution (50–100 μg) IV slowly. For a safer and titratable infusion, mix 1 mg epinephrine in 250 D_5W for a 4 μg/mL drip and start at 1–10 μg/min titrating to response. Albuterol by nebulizer may also be used as a bronchodilator. Diphenhydramine 50 mg IV or IM (pediatric 1–2 mg/kg) and ranitidine 50 mg IV (or famotidine 20 mg) provide histamine blockade. A stress dose of steroids completes the primary treatment. In patients on β-blockers, glucagon 1–2 mg IV can be used to bypass β receptors. Mild cases, after a 6-hour observation, can be discharged with a prescription for a self-injector of epinephrine for future life-threatening symptoms. Patients need to be encouraged to use this potential lifesaving self-treatment. Moderate to severe cases require admission.

Simons EFR, Camargo CA: Anaphylaxis: rapid recognition and treatment. http://www.uptodate.com. Updated 1/2010 (last accessed on 4/1/2010).

Sampson HA et al: Symposium on the definition and management of anaphylaxis: Summary report. J Allergy Clin Immunol 2005;115:584 [PMID: 15753908].

▶ Septic Shock

Septic shock is sepsis induced hypotension despite volume resuscitation and lies at the extreme end of a continuum from sepsis (infection plus SIRS), severe sepsis (sepsis plus organ dysfunction and hypoperfusion) and finally septic shock. It is a clinical syndrome complicating infections and is caused by an exaggerated release of inflammatory mediators causing widespread organ dysfunction. The hallmark is the SIRS which is defined as two or more of the following: (1) temperature > 38°C or < 36°C, (2) HR > 90 bpm, (3) respiratory rate > 20 breaths per minute, or $Paco_2$ < 32 (4) WBC > 12,000 cell/mm³ or < 4000 cell/mm³ or > 10% bands). In septic shock, SIRS is associated with decreased SVR with an early hyperdynamic compensation followed by impaired contractility from myocardial depressants and

hypoxemia. Elevated serum lactate levels (> 4) provide early evidence of tissue hypoperfusion.

Gram-negative rods are the classic cause of septic shock but increasingly gram-positives, viral, and fungal infections contribute. Patients with trauma, wounds, diabetes, extremes of age, and those whose immune systems are depressed by chemotherapy, cancer, or renal disease are at greatest risk. The cause might also be a toxemia from staphylococcal or streptococcal infection. Menstruating females and patients with wounds are at risk for toxic shock syndrome caused by TSST 1 (toxic shock syndrome toxin 1) from tampons or from wounds. These patients have SIRS, hypotension, and an erythematous rash. Frequent occult sites of infection include the biliary tree, urinary tract, retroperitoneum, and perirectal areas. A lumbar puncture will reveal meningitis.

Treatment begins with the general principles outlined above. Patients are resuscitated, given goal-directed therapy, targeted antimicrobials, and, if present, drainage of any abscess. Early endotracheal intubation should be done to decrease the work of breathing and ensure oxygen delivery. Etomidate inhibits glucocorticoid synthesis, but has neutral hemodynamic effects and can be used (once) for induction. Ketamine should also be considered as a sedative agent during induction because of its favorable hemodynamic profile in the critically ill patient. Goal-directed therapy requires central venous and arterial monitoring, sedation with or without paralysis, optimization of central venous pressures (CVP) to 8–12 mm Hg first with fluids using a "give bolus, check patient response" method, optimization of mean arterial pressure (MAP) with fluid and vasopressors, and optimization of mixed venous oxygen content to > 70% by adding initiation of vasopressor therapy or transfusion to a hematocrit > 30. Dopamine is commonly used as the initial vasopressor but norepinephrine, with its α activity, might be a better choice. Vasopressin shows some promise, but data are limited. Keys to therapy are aggressive volume resuscitation and early antibiotic use with supportive care.

Antibiotics should be given as early as possible after recognizing sepsis; appropriate cultures should be obtained prior to antibiotic administration, covering the most likely pathogens based on the most likely site and immune competence of the patient. A third or fourth generation cephalosporin or plus vancomycin is a reasonable choice for an immunocompetent patient. Anaerobic coverage is helpful in intra-abdominal infections and adding a macrolide for pneumonia is reasonable. Immune incompetent patients require overlapping coverage for gram-positive and gram-negative aerobes and anaerobes and possibly viral or fungal causes.

Removal of any abscess or foreign body is important and might necessitate amputation, foreign body removal or incision, and drainage. High-dose steroids have been shown to be harmful in septic shock and most patients in septic shock should not receive stress dose steroids due to side effects and lack of proven efficacy. Aggressive glucose control insulin therapy with its risk for recurrent hypoglycemia is also not recommended.

Recombinant human-activated protein C (drotrecogin alfa or RHAPC) although very costly is indicated as an adjunctive treatment for septic shock in those with severe sepsis and high risk of death (APACHE II scores > 25 or multiorgan failure), because its use is associated with a significant risk of bleeding RHAPC should not be used in patients with an elevated baseline risk of bleeding, those with a history of recent surgery or intracranial hemorrhage. Unfortunately, giving antiendotoxin antibodies or nitric oxide synthase inhibitors has not been shown to be effective.

Brunkhorst FM, Engel C, Bloos F et al: Intensive insulin therapy and pentastarch resuscitation in severe sepsis. New England Journal of Medicine 2008;358:125–139 [PMID 18184958].

Jones AE, Puskarich MA: Sepsis-induced tissue hypoperfusion. Crit Care Clin 2009;25:769–779 [PMID 19892252].

Dellinger RP, Levy MM, Carlet JM et al: Surviving sepsis campaign: International guidelines for management of severe sepsis and septic shock. Crit Care Med 2008;36:296–327 [PMID 18158437].

Morrell MR, Micek ST, Kollef MH: The management of severe sepsis and septic shock. Infect Dis Clin N Am 2009;23:485–501 [PMID 19665079].

Schmidt GA, Mandel J: Management of severe sepsis and septic shock in adults. http://www.uptodate.com (last accessed on 4/1/20100).

Sprung CL, Goodman S: Steroid therapy of septic shock. Crit Care Clin 2009;25:825–834 [PMID 19892255].

▶ Neurogenic Shock

Loss of vascular tone due to paralysis from a cervical cord spinal lesion can cause hypotension and shock. In trauma, however, any patient, even with paralysis, should be assumed to have an alternate source of hemorrhage before assigning the hypotension to neurogenic shock. Loss of feedback loops of autonomic ganglia cause less reflex tachycardia even in the face of hypotension. Neurogenic shock should not be confused with spinal shock, which is due to transient spinal cord dysfunction after injury manifest as loss of spinal reflexes such as the bulbocavernosus. Spinal shock clouds the prognosis from cord injury until spinal reflexes return.

Clinically, patients with neurogenic shock present with warm skin, hypotension (often marked if the patient is tilted in reverse Trendelenburg), and a variable tachycardia response (in a patient with a cervical spine level of injury). Treatment revolves around an aggressive evaluation of other potential causes of shock and includes a fluid challenge of 20 cc/kg × 2. A reasonable endpoint is an MAP > 90 mm Hg.

If volume replacement is unsuccessful, vasopressors with α activity should be given. The key point is to not assume that the cause is only neurogenic shock until all other sources of traumatic shock have been excluded.

▶ Drug-induced Vasodilation

β-Blockers and calcium channel blocker overdose or overuse can precipitate hypotension and shock. Hypotension and warm skin without any compensatory tachycardia is the hallmark of presentation. Glucagon 5–10 mg, IV, followed by an infusion of 2–5 mg/h will improve β-blocker toxicity and calcium channel blocker toxicity. Calcium gluconate 10% will improve calcium channel toxicity at a dose of 10–20 cc. Either cause of shock may require atropine or pacing. Of course, general decontamination with charcoal is helpful as well as fluid resuscitation.

▶ Obstructive Shock

Tension pneumothorax, pericardial tamponade, and massive PE are often termed *obstructive shock*, although all three impair ventricular filling and CO.

Tension pneumothorax is a clinical not radiographic diagnosis characterized by unilateral decreased breath sounds, unilateral chest hyperresonance, and tracheal deviation in the setting of respiratory distress and shock. Treatment is immediate needle decompression followed by chest tube thoracostomy placement.

Pericardial tamponade likewise should be considered early in the evaluation of undifferentiated shock. Patients with blunt or penetrating chest trauma can rapidly decompensate with minimal bleeding into the pericardium, while those with uremia and cancer usually develop an effusion over time. Symptoms include hypotension, elevated right side pressures (JVD) pulsus paradoxus (a fall in systolic blood pressure in inspiration), and Kussmaul's sign (increased jugular venous pressure on inspiration). Bedside U/S is extremely sensitive in detecting pericardial fluid and can be instrumental in guiding pericardiocentesis, although in the patient in extremis, blind pericardiocentesis might be lifesaving.

Massive PE presents as chest pain, syncope, tachypnea, and hypotension with signs of acute right ventricular overload with JVD and ECG changes. Fluid administration might worsen right ventricular failure and should be given only cautiously. Blood pressure should be augmented with an appropriate vasopressor such as norepinephrine 0.5–1 μg/min titrated to response. Immediate surgical embolectomy is sometimes effective but not usually feasible. Shock complicating PE is an indication for thrombolytics if no other contraindication exists.

The Multiply Injured Patient

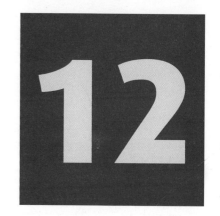

Julia Martin, MD, FACEP

Immediate Management of Life-Threatening
Problems
  Preparation
  Initial Assessment
  Hemorrhagic Shock
Emergency Treatment of Specific Disorders
  Injuries to the Neck Region
  Tension Pneumothorax
  Flail Chest

Pulmonary Contusion
Cardiac Tamponade
Myocardial Contusion
Traumatic Aortic Rupture
Abdominal Trauma
Head Trauma
Genitourinary Trauma
Extremity Trauma
Spinal Trauma

IMMEDIATE MANAGEMENT OF LIFE-THREATENING PROBLEMS

(See Figure 12–1.) The primary goal in providing care to the trauma patient is effective resuscitation while minimizing the time from injury to definitive care.

PREPARATION

Trauma care begins at the scene of the incident. It is important for hospitals to have good working relationships with local fire departments and emergency medical services (EMSs) to ensure that proper care is provided early. Preparation efforts should be coordinated between the emergency departments and the local EMS systems including prehospital protocols related to the treatment and transport of trauma patients. Transport protocols should incorporate decision-making guidelines including information regarding transporting patients to the most appropriate facility and the proper use of air medical transport. Prehospital providers should be trained to detect specific injuries and know the mechanism of forces that could predict the possibility of severe injury (Table 12–1). Prehospital personnel should provide early notification to the emergency department for all major trauma patients to allow emergency department preparedness.

Injury-scoring systems, such as the Glasgow Coma Scale (GCS), Trauma Score, and Revised Trauma Score, may be used to help quantify the degree of injury (Figure 12–2).

Maintain a high index of suspicion with pediatric, geriatric, and obstetric patients. Their physiologic responses to major trauma differ from those of other patients, and their injuries are often missed or delayed in diagnosis. Early transfer to definitive care improves outcomes in these patient groups.

Emergency department response should include a stepwise notification system to alert local surgeons or trauma teams and ancillary services such as X-ray, computed tomography (CT) scan, laboratory, blood bank, and operating room personnel. Initial stabilization and resuscitation is done most effectively if a well-organized team approach is used. The key to an organized system is the designation of a person in charge to oversee the total care of the patient. The team leader should assign specific tasks to emergency department team members. It is important for everyone to understand their roles, know where equipment is located, adhere to universal precautions, and keep noise and extraneous conversation to a minimum. Constant reassessment of the patient and maintenance of a high index of suspicion for possible injuries are important in the evaluation and resuscitation of trauma patients.

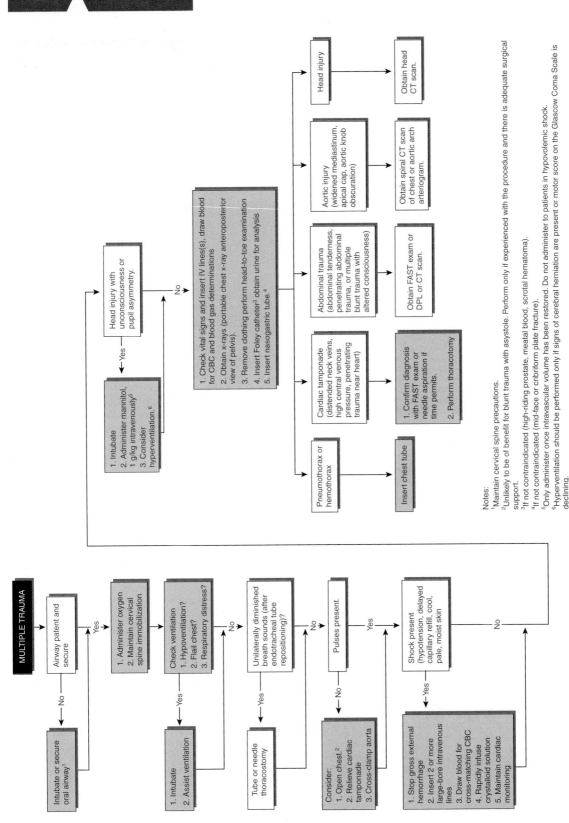

▲ **Figure 12–1.** Assessment of the patient with multiple injuries. DPL, diagnostic peritoneal lavage; FAST, focused assessment with sonography for trauma.

Table 12–1. Definitions of Major Trauma.

Mechanism of Injury	Clinical Information
Falls > 20 ft	Systolic blood pressure < 90 mm Hg
Rollover motor vehicle collision Crash speed >40 mph	Respiratory rate <10/min or >29/min
Auto-pedestrian or auto-bicycle collision	Glasgow Coma Scale score <10
Ejection of patient	Penetrating trauma other than distal extremity
Occupant fatality same vehicle Major auto deformity (greater than 20 inches intrusion) Blast Injury	Combination of 2nd- or 3rd-degree burns over > 15% of the body and multiple trauma Trauma score < 13 Revised trauma score < 11 Pelvic fractures paralysis

INITIAL ASSESSMENT

The initial assessment consists of a rapid primary survey, initiation of resuscitative measures, followed by a secondary survey. The primary survey includes evaluation of the airway, breathing, and circulation and a brief neurologic examination. During the initial assessment, assess the patient for injuries or conditions that would indicate the patient's care needs require a higher level of care at a trauma center. Early initiation of transfer to the most appropriate trauma facility reduces morbidly and mortality in critically ill or injuries patients. Delay in transfer of theses patients for local diagnostic work-up delays their arrival to definitive care facility and potentially increases morbidity and mortality. Problems identified in the primary assessment should be corrected immediately. Several tasks should occur simultaneously such as assessing the patient; initiating resuscitation; placing the patient on the cardiac monitor, pulse oximetry, and supplemental oxygen; and initiating intravenous lines. Rapid stabilization of airway, breathing, circulation, and neurologic status is paramount for patient survival.

1. Primary Survey

▷ Assessment of ABCs

A. Airway

Airway management and maintenance of adequate oxygenation are extremely important in the multiply injured patient (See also Chapter 10). Shock leads to an oxygen deficit, which increases the body's demands and necessitates the need for supplementary oxygen. Cervical spine immobilization is considered part of airway management in trauma patients. To open the airway, a modified jaw thrust should be used with cervical spine control. An oropharyngeal or nasopharyngeal airway is useful to help maintain an airway. The nasopharyngeal tube may be used in semiconscious patients with an intact gag reflex. The oropharyngeal airway should be used only in unconscious patients without a gag reflex; otherwise, it may induce vomiting.

Obtain a definitive airway in any patient who is not breathing, has inadequate ventilation or oxygenation, has

A Glasgow Coma Scale

Eye opening	Spontaneous	4
	To verbal command	3
	To pain	2
	None	1
Verbal responsiveness	Oriented	5
	Confused	4
	Inappropriate words	3
	Incomprehensible sounds	2
	None	1
Motor response	Obeys	6
	Localizes	5
	Withdraws (pain)	4
	Flexion (pain)	3
	Extension (pain)	2
	None	1
	Total: _____	

B Revised Trauma Score

Respiratory rate (breaths/min)	10–29	4
	> 29	3
	6–9	2
	1–5	1
	0	
Systolic blood pressure (mm Hg)	> 89	4
	76–89	3
	50–75	2
	1–49	1
	No pulse	0
Glasgow conversion scale	13–15	4
	9–12	3
	6–8	2
	4–5	1
	< 4	0
	Total: _____	

▲ **Figure 12–2.** Trauma scores used to quantify degree of injury. **(A)** Determine total on Glasgow Coma Scale. **(B)** Convert Glasgow Coma Scale total to Revised Trauma Score points and determine Revised Trauma Score total.

an unprotected airway without a gag reflex, or has a decreased level of consciousness with a GCS score less than 8. Emergency department providers should be knowledgeable about and skilled with a variety of surgical and nonsurgical methods of securing an airway. Patients with inadequate ventilation and oxygenation require bag-mask-ventilation until intubation is accomplished. Tracheal intubation may be accomplished by two methods: nasotracheal or orotracheal. Both methods require good cervical spine immobilization including manual stabilization of the neck. With adequate training and experience, rapid-sequence induction (RSI) intubation offers many advantages in the multiply injured trauma patient. RSI involves the use of paralytics to rapidly achieve muscle relaxation and sedatives to render the patient unconscious and unaware of laryngoscopy and intubation. Use of paralytics helps protect against a rise in intracranial pressure associated with laryngoscopy, and with good manual cervical spine stabilization there is less risk of additional cervical spine injury. The use of paralytics and sedation requires a good working knowledge of the medications' indications, their side effects, and their contraindications, in order to minimize complications associated with the procedure. Being well trained in backup airway maneuvers, such as the laryngeal mask airway, lighted stylet, fiberoptic intubation, and surgical airway options, is imperative prior to initiating RSI in a patient. RSI is relatively contraindicated in patients who cannot be ventilated with a bag-valve-mask if intubation proves difficult or impossible. If orotracheal or nasotracheal intubation is unsuccessful, a surgical airway such as a cricothyrotomy should be performed.

B. Breathing

Assess adequacy of ventilation by inspecting the chest wall for adequate expansion; looking for paradoxical rise of the chest, flail segments, and sucking wounds; and noting labored respirations or auxiliary muscle use. Auscultate the lungs for the presence of symmetrical breath sounds.

If breath sounds are unilaterally diminished and the patient is intubated, consider withdrawing the endotracheal tube 2–3 cm in case the tip is residing in a mainstem bronchus, and then recheck the breath sounds. Persistently, diminished breath sounds imply pneumothorax or hemothorax. If the patient is hypotensive, in shock, or laboring to breathe, perform a tube thoracostomy immediately. Should a delay exist before this can occur, decompress the chest with a 14-gauge angiocatheter or other catheter-clad needle inserted in the second intercostal space at the midclavicular line. A stable patient with diminished breath sounds may await a chest X-ray for confirmation prior to decompression with a needle or thoracostomy tube.

Treat a sucking chest wound by sealing the wound with an occlusive dressing (eg, petrolatum-impregnated dressing) at three points and then performing a tube thoracostomy (not through the chest wall defect). Adequacy

of ventilation can be confirmed with arterial blood gas measurements.

C. Circulation

Rapidly assess blood pressure and pulse. A narrowed pulse pressure suggests hypovolemic shock. Hypotension is suggestive of severe intravascular depletion. Rapidly evaluate the abdomen because it is frequently a source of significant hemorrhage in the multiply injured patient. Severe pelvic fracture or pelvic ring disruptions can be associated with massive intrapelvic hemorrhage. Give the patient crystalloid initially and then blood, if needed, to improve perfusion.

1. Traumatic arrest—If spontaneous cardiac activity is not detected by palpation of the carotid artery, begin cardiopulmonary resuscitation immediately. If the patient has penetrating chest trauma and arrives by EMS with Cardiopulmonary Resuscitation (CPR) in progress, assess the patient for signs of life. If there are no signs of life and no cardiac electrical activity present, no further resuscitative effort should be made. If there are signs of life and the patient has been pulseless for less than 15 minutes, consider emergency thoracotomy. Only experienced physicians trained in emergency thoracotomy should perform this procedure. If the patient has been pulseless longer than the abovementioned time limits or arrives with CPR in progress from blunt trauma, regardless of the cardiac rhythm, thoracotomy is not indicated and has not been shown to improve survival. Initiate closed chest compressions with volume resuscitation with crystalloids and cardiac drugs per advanced cardiac life support guidelines (Chapter 9).

2. External hemorrhage—Stop obvious external hemorrhage using direct pressure with sterile dressings. Scalp wounds, even small ones, can produce significant blood loss if not controlled. Sometimes direct pressure and dressings are not sufficient. For uncontrolled scalp wound hemorrhage, the wound should be closed with sutures, staples, or, if available, Raney scalp clips, preferably using sterile technique. If a nonsterile technique is used, the wound should be reopened and inspected carefully, cleansed, and then definitively closed using sterile technique when the patient stabilizes. Bleeding vessels should not be clamped indiscriminately. Rarely will compression be insufficient to control an exsanguinating arterial hemorrhage from an extremity. A blood pressure cuff inflated proximal to the wound can serve as an effective tourniquet temporarily until surgical control of the bleeding can be achieved. Recent studies indicate tourniquet use in uncontrolled extremity injuries, particularly if placed before shock is clinically evident, can be life saving with little limb complications.

3. Shock—(See also Chapter 11) Shock is defined as inadequate tissue perfusion and is further classified as mild, moderate, or severe, based primarily on clinical criteria. Cool, pale skin; diaphoresis; delayed capillary refill (>2s); tachycardia; and mental status changes are reliable indicators of shock. Hypotension and oliguria are presumed to be due to shock until proved otherwise. Do not assume that perfusion is adequate on the basis of a supine pulse and blood pressure alone, because these signs may not change until late in shock. This is particularly true in young healthy adults—who are the most common victims of multiple trauma. Patients taking β-blockers (or other medications that blunt the normal response to adrenergic stimulation) may not exhibit tachycardia despite profound shock.

Shock in the traumatized patient is due to hypovolemia from hemorrhage in the majority of the cases. Cardiac tamponade and tension pneumothorax are conditions that can cause shock, which must be excluded rapidly in the assessment of hypotensive trauma patients. Spinal cord or brain injury may contribute or (rarely) may cause shock without concurrent volume loss. In a trauma patient, shock should be treated as hypovolemic shock with volume infusions until other causes of shock are found.

Brief Neurologic Examination

A quick neurologic examination may be accomplished by using the GCS (see Figure 12–2). The GCS allows for quick assessment of the patient's level of responsiveness to determine if he or she is awake and alert; responds to verbal stimuli with eye opening or following of commands; responds to painful stimuli (eg, sternal rub, muscle, or tendon squeeze) by appropriate movement, localization, or posturing; or is unresponsive.

Assess the patient's pupils for symmetry, size, and reactivity. An asymmetrically enlarged pupil in an unresponsive patient may imply transtentorial herniation, which should be treated with endotracheal intubation along with the other interventions to reduce intracranial pressure such as short-term hyperventilation and administration of mannitol (Chapter 22).

2. Initial Resuscitation

Evaluation and treatment must proceed rapidly and simultaneously. During the primary survey, correct any identified problems immediately. Place the patient on a cardiac monitor, including pulse oximetry with supplemental oxygen administered. Initiate intravenous lines and order initial laboratory studies. Place a Foley catheter after examination of the perineal area and rectal examination. Do not insert a urethral catheter if there is obvious injury to the external genitalia, obvious urethral bleeding, scrotal hematoma, a malpositioned or high-riding prostate on rectal examination, or difficulty in passing the catheter. Monitoring of urine output is important in evaluating the patient's response to resuscitative efforts. Urinary output below 0.5 cc/kg/h indicates significant hypovolemia.

Intravenous Access

Insert multiple large-bore (≥16 gauge) catheters in a patient with profound shock. Initiate at least two intravenous lines. Consider a large-bore central line to administer large amounts of fluids rapidly or to monitor central venous pressure in patients with poor peripheral venous access in profound shock, in the elderly, and in patients with significant comorbid disease. If peripheral IV is not easily obtainable, proximal humerus intraosseous line should be started. Studies have shown that intraosseous lines are fast to place and can be used for volume resuscitation or medication administration when peripheral IV is difficult.

Laboratory Tests

Consider blood specimens for hematocrit or complete blood count (CBC), electrolyte measurements, renal function tests, and coagulation (prothrombin and partial thromboplastin times). Obtain a urine sample for gross blood. Obtain a pregnancy test from female patients of child-bearing age. If abdominal trauma is present, consider laboratory studies for liver enzymes and lipase. If severe shock is evident or suspected, type and crossmatch for four units of packed red blood cells, and obtain an arterial blood gas and serum lactate. Base deficit and or lactate can be useful in determining the presence and severity of shock. Serial measurement of these can be useful in monitoring the response to therapy. Trauma patients have high rates of alcohol and drug use, and a blood alcohol level or urine drug screen may be useful in evaluating patients with altered mental status.

Fluid Resuscitation

If clinical evidence of shock is present, initiate intravenous infusion of crystalloid solution. Give up to 2 L of crystalloid solution to support intravascular volume before giving blood. Give crossmatched or type-specific blood, if available, to a patient in persistent shock unresponsive to crystalloids. If typed and crossmatched blood is not available, then give type O blood. Reserve type O-negative blood for females younger than 50 years; all others should receive type O-positive.

Initial Radiographic Studies

During the acute phase of evaluation and resuscitation, the most valuable X-rays are those of the chest and pelvis. These X-rays assist in the evaluation of potential injuries associated with a large amount of blood loss. Although spine X-rays are important, the spine can be protected from further injury by adhering strictly to spinal immobilization precautions during the initial evaluation and resuscitation.

Large hemorrhages can also be found in the abdominal cavity. The abdomen can be rapidly evaluated in the unstable trauma patient by using bedside emergency ultrasound and performing a FAST (focused assessment with sonography for trauma—see Chapter 6) exam to look for free fluid. In stable trauma patients, a contrasted CT scan of the abdomen and pelvis provides useful information regarding the extent of specific organ injuries. Because ultrasound and CT scan are poor in evaluating bowel injuries, maintain a high index of suspicion so that this type of injury is not overlooked, especially in pediatric patients.

Ongoing Evaluation and Resuscitation

Frequently reassess a multiply injured trauma patient for evidence of new or ongoing signs of shock. In the multiply injured patient, hemorrhage is the most common cause of shock. Even so, it is important to conscientiously assess the patient for other underlying causes of shock. Early surgical consult is important for any trauma patient with signs of shock. Splint fractures, administer antibiotics and tetanus toxoid when needed, and keep patients warm. Pay close attention to the prevention of further injury. Avoiding infection, hypothermia, coagulopathy, and ongoing blood loss is important for minimizing possible mortality and morbidity.

Kortbeek JB et al: Advanced trauma life support, the evidence for change, 8th ed. J Trauma 2008;64(4):1638–1650 [PMID: 18545134].

Paxton JH, Knuth TE, Klausner HA: Proximal humerus intraosseous infusion: A preferred emergency venous access. J Trauma 2009;67(3):606–611 [PMID: 19741408] (Great article on use of intraosseous infusions when peripheral IV is not obtainable.).

Kragh JF et al: Survival with emergency tourniquet use to stop bleeding in major limb trauma. Annal Surg 2009;249(1):1–7 [PMID:19106667] (Great article regarding use of tourniquets).

HEMORRHAGIC SHOCK

ESSENTIALS OF DIAGNOSIS

▶ Evidence of external blood loss
▶ Injuries with associated internal blood loss
▶ Tachycardia
▶ Decreased level of consciousness
▶ Decreased urine output
▶ Delayed capillary refill
▶ Hypotension (late sign)

General Considerations

Defined as inadequate tissue perfusion due to decreased cardiac output secondary to blood loss. Hemorrhagic shock accounts for the overwhelming majority of trauma patients in shock. Clinical signs are due to compensatory mechanisms. For example, excess sympathetic nervous system stimulation causes tachycardia and peripheral vasoconstriction, whereas decreased peripheral and renal blood flow result in decreased urine output, pallor, delayed capillary refill, and weak peripheral pulses.

Clinical Findings

A. Obvious Sources of Blood Loss

Identify and control external hemorrhage during the primary survey. Logroll trauma patients to examine their backs. A single hematocrit may provide a baseline but is not helpful in detecting acute occult hemorrhage. Serial hematocrits over several hours are useful in determining continued blood loss, because a single initial value may be deceivingly normal.

B. Hidden Sources of Internal Blood Loss

Major sources of occult blood loss are as follows:

1. Thorax—Each hemithorax may contain 1–2 L of blood, primarily as a result of a pulmonary laceration or laceration of intercostal vessels or internal mammary artery due to either penetrating or blunt trauma. Suspect hemothorax in cases of shock associated with decreased or absent breath sounds or when dullness to percussion is present on the affected side. A supine chest X-ray may only show haziness over the hemithorax.

2. Abdomen—Assume intra-abdominal hemorrhage in patients in shock with a normal chest X-ray and no external sources of bleeding. Abdominal distention is a late and unreliable sign. Kehr's sign is referred pain to left shoulder due to diaphragmatic irritation associated with hemoperitoneum and splenic injuries. Cullen's sign (periumbilical ecchymosis) is a late finding in intra-abdominal hemorrhage. Use a FAST exam to examine unstable patients. Stable patients should undergo CT scan of the abdomen.

3. Retroperitoneum—The retroperitoneum can accumulate approximately 4 L of blood before tamponade occurs, and retroperitoneal hemorrhage may not be detected by abdominal ultrasound. Grey–Turner's sign (flank ecchymosis) is a late finding on physical examination of retroperitoneal hemorrhage. CT scan of the abdomen and pelvis is necessary to confirm the diagnosis.

4. Pelvis—Pelvic fractures may result in extensive bleeding from the bone itself or from disruption of the presacral venous plexus. Identification of the definitive source of bleeding requires CT scan with IV contrast or angiography, which has the advantage of allowing embolization of vascular bleeding.

5. Soft tissues (ie, thigh, upper arm, calf)—Between 1 and 4 L of blood can accumulate in the soft tissues due to long bone fractures and may not be immediately apparent on physical examination.

▶ Treatment

A. Direct Pressure

Obvious external hemorrhage can usually be controlled with direct pressure over the bleeding site or over a proximal artery. If bleeding can not be controlled with direct pressure or pressure on proximal artery, placement of proximal tourniquet should be considered. Never blindly place a clamp into a wound.

B. Indirect Pressure

Immediate temporary stabilization of an unstable pelvis fracture can decrease the pelvic volume and help tamponade bleeding. Pelvic stabilization can be accomplished by internally rotating the lower legs and tying them together with a sheet, followed by another sheet tied around the pelvis itself. There are several commercial devices available for use as well.

C. Supportive Measures

Guidelines for volume resuscitation are set forth in Chapter 11.

1. Crystalloid solutions—Normal saline and lactated Ringers are traditionally the intravenous solutions of choice. There is no evidence to support the use of colloids in initial trauma management. Initiate blood products if the patient's hemodynamic response is not favorable after the first 2 L of crystalloids, particularly if there is significant blood loss.

2. Blood products—The amount of blood or blood products given depends on the clinical situation and the patient's response to fluid resuscitation. Traditionally, it has been recommended that the hematocrit should be kept at around 30% (35–40% in elderly patients and those with pre-existing cardiopulmonary disease). Newer studies advocate the use of Massive transfusion protocols for patients who require multiple units of PRBCs. It has been noted that 65% of patients requiring massive transfusion develop coagulopathy with mortality rates in this group exceeding 50%. Massive transfusion protocols significantly reduce mortality and morbidity in traumatized platelets. While the optimal amounts and ratios of RBCs, platelets and fresh frozen plasma are still being studied, current data support the use of a 1:1:1 ratio with one unit of cryoprecipitate given for every two units of RBCs.

3. Warming of blood—Hypothermia is a common side effect of transfusion of stored blood. New combination pressure infusers and fluid warmers are ideally designed to avoid hypothermia during aggressive fluid resuscitation of trauma patients.

▶ Disposition

Admit patients for surgery or observation as indicated.

Shaz BH, Dente CJ, Harris RS, MacLeod JB, Hillyer CD: Transfusion management of trauma patients. Anesth Analg 2009;108(6):1760–1768 (Review) [PMID: 19448199] (Nice review of current data regarding massive transfusions).

▼ EMERGENCY TREATMENT OF SPECIFIC DISORDERS

INJURIES TO THE NECK REGION

See also Chapter 23.

ESSENTIALS OF DIAGNOSIS

- ▶ Immobilize to prevent further injury
- ▶ Examine neck for both blunt and penetrating trauma
- ▶ Evaluate neck for expanding hematoma, crepitus, subcutaneous air, external hemorrhage, trachea deviation from the midline, and cervical spine tenderness or deformity

1. Cervical Spine

▶ Clinical Findings

See Chapter 23 and Spinal Trauma section at the end of this chapter.

▶ Treatment

Maintain in-line axial immobilization with a cervical collar if a cervical spine injury is suspected (Chapter 23).

▶ Disposition

Admit all patients with injury to neck structures, other than minor blunt or superficial penetrating injuries.

2. Upper Airway

▶ Clinical Findings

Injury to the upper airway is characterized by hoarseness or aphonia, apnea or respiratory distress, stridor, subcutaneous emphysema, or bubbling of blood during inspiration and expiration in open neck wounds.

▶ Treatment and Disposition

Early definitive airway management using RSI or crico-thyrotomy may be lifesaving if indicated. If the airway is exposed, intubate directly through the wound. If subcutaneous emphysema is present, assume a tracheobronchial injury is present and attempt to pass the endotracheal tube distal to the site of injury if possible.

All patients with injuries to the upper airway require admission.

3. Esophagus

▶ Clinical Findings

Esophageal injury is uncommon, even in penetrating trauma. Difficulty swallowing and neck pain are common, but overt clinical signs may be minimal initially. Chest X-ray may reveal pneumomediastinum, but definitive diagnosis requires esophagoscopy or contrasted swallowing studies.

▶ Treatment and Disposition

Insert a nasogastric tube and administer broad-spectrum antibiotics (ie, penicillin). Obtain surgical consultation.

4. Vascular Injury

▶ Clinical Findings

Blunt trauma to the head and neck are risk factors for carotid and vertebral artery injuries. Early recognition and treatment can reduce the risk of stroke in patients with these injuries. Traumatic injuries at risk for arterial injury include: C1-3 fractures, C-spine fracture with subluxation, fractures involving the foramun transversarium. CTA (CT angiography) san of the neck is useful in the diagnosis of arterial injuries associated with blunt trauma to the head and neck.

Penetrating trauma to the neck may also result in vascular injuries. The neck is divided into three anatomic zones (see Figure 23–2). Zone I is below the cricoid cartilage, zone II is between the cricoid and the angle of the mandible, and zone III is above the angle of the mandible. Clinical findings of a vascular injury are variable and may be subtle or absent initially. Traditionally, surgical exploration was advocated for all zone II injuries deep to the platysma and for others with clinical indications (expanding hematoma, active bleeding, diminished carotid pulsation, hemoptysis, crepitus, dysphonia, hematemesis, dysphagia, or Horner syndrome). Some researchers advocate selective management with angiography, Gastrografin swallow, and esophagoscopy. Because of difficulties in accessing the major vascular structures in zone III and especially zone I, arteriography (Table 12–2) and the other studies mentioned above continue to be utilized for evaluation of injuries in these zones.

Table 12–2. Indications for Arteriography Following Trauma.

Penetrating neck injuries: zones I and III and selected zone II
Suspected thoracic aortic rupture after indeterminate CT scan of the chest or transesophageal echocardiography
Pelvic fractures with massive hemorrhage
Penetrating extremity trauma associated with an abnormal pulse or Doppler pressure index such as the ankle-brachial index or wrist-brachial index
Knee dislocation

▶ Treatment and Disposition

Treat hemorrhagic shock as indicated (Chapter 11). Prompt surgical consultation with or without arteriography is essential.

Tisherman SA et al: Clinical practice guideline: Penetrating zone II neck trauma. J Trauma 2008;64(5):1392–1405 [PMID: 18469667] (Excellent review of the ligature and applying it to a clinical guideline in the management of penetrating neck trauma.).

TENSION PNEUMOTHORAX

See also Chapter 24.

ESSENTIALS OF DIAGNOSIS

- ▶ Respiratory distress
- ▶ Asymmetrical lung sounds
- ▶ May or may not have external signs of trauma to chest wall
- ▶ Tracheal shift is late sign
- ▶ Distended neck veins may not be present in patients with hypovolemic shock

▶ General Considerations

Tension pneumothorax interferes with venous return to the heart and thus decreases cardiac output and perfusion. Oxygenation is also impaired. A simple pneumothorax can be converted to a tension pneumothorax during positive pressure ventilation.

▶ Clinical Findings

Tension pneumothorax is manifested by respiratory distress, distended neck veins, contralateral tracheal shift, asymmetry of breath sounds, and percussion tympany.

Chest X-ray confirms the diagnosis; however, tension pneumothorax is a clinical diagnosis and treatment should not be delayed while waiting for radiographs. Profound shock and cardiac arrest may be refractory to usual treatment unless the tension is relieved. Therefore, if a tension pneumothorax is clinically suspected, and an appropriate mechanism of injury is identified, emergency tube thoracostomy should be performed.

► Treatment

Tension pneumothorax may be treated initially by inserting a large-bore (ie, 14 gauge) needle into the second intercostal space, in the midclavicular line on the affected side. A rush of air confirms the diagnosis. If the tension pneumothorax is due to an open pneumothorax creating a one-way valve (ie, sucking chest wound), then application of an occlusive dressing sealed on three sides can prevent the development of further tension. Definitive treatment is tube thoracostomy in the fifth intercostal space, in the midaxillary line, as soon as possible (Chapters 7 and 24).

► Disposition

Hospitalization is required for all patients with tension pneumothorax.

FLAIL CHEST

See also Chapter 24.

ESSENTIALS OF DIAGNOSIS

► Paradoxical chest wall motion
► Respiratory distress
► If signs of hypoxia or ventilatory failure are present, intubation is required

► Clinical Findings

Flail chest is diagnosed clinically with careful inspection and palpation revealing paradoxical motion of the flail segment (inward movement with inspiration and outward movement with expiration).

► Treatment

The goal is the maintenance of adequate ventilation and careful fluid resuscitation, because the underlying injuries are sensitive to both inadequate resuscitation of shock and fluid overload. In some patients, flail chest can be managed without mechanical ventilation; however, intubation and mechanical ventilation may be necessary at the first sign of ventilatory failure or hypoxia. All patients with flail chest should receive supplemental oxygen.

► Disposition

All patients with flail chest require hospitalization in an intensive care unit and may eventually require intubation as pulmonary contusions worsen and the increased work of breathing and pain contribute to poor respiratory function.

PULMONARY CONTUSION

See also Chapter 24.

ESSENTIALS OF DIAGNOSIS

► Respiratory distress
► Worsening hypoxia with time
► Radiographic findings often delayed in comparison to a rapid decline in respiratory function based on clinical examination
► Diffuse pulmonary opacities on chest X-ray

► General Considerations

Pulmonary contusion is one of the most common potentially lethal injuries to the chest, with respiratory failure developing over time. The severity of injury generally peaks between 48 and 72 hours.

► Clinical Findings

The diagnosis of pulmonary contusion is based on chest X-ray findings of diffuse opacities following traumatic chest trauma. A high index of suspicion is required, because radiographic findings may be delayed more than 24 hours. CT scan of the chest can confirm the diagnosis earlier than does the chest X-ray.

► Treatment

Careful monitoring of oxygenation and ventilation (including oxygen saturation and arterial blood gases) is required. Administer supplemental oxygen as indicated. Any patient with significant hypoxia (PaO_2 < 65 or oxygen saturation < 90%) despite high-flow supplemental oxygen should be intubated and mechanically ventilated. Associated medical conditions (ie, chronic obstructive pulmonary disease, renal failure) increase the likelihood that a patient will require early intubation and ventilatory assistance.

Disposition

Hospitalize all patients for observation and monitoring.

CARDIAC TAMPONADE

See also Chapters 24 and 34.

ESSENTIALS OF DIAGNOSIS

► Hypotension

► Jugularvenous distensionmay or may not be present

► Muffled heart sounds

► Electrical alternans on electrocardiogram

► Positive FAST exam for pericardial fluid

General Considerations

Cardiac tamponade most commonly results from penetrating injuries and interferes with diastolic filling, thus leading to inadequate cardiac output and end-organ perfusion.

Clinical Findings

The classic presentation consists of the Beck triad, although this is not always present. The triad includes hypotension, jugular venous distention, and muffled heart tones. However, jugular venous distention is common in supine patients without tamponade and may not be seen in hypovolemic patients with tamponade. In addition, muffled heart sounds are difficult to hear during a noisy resuscitation. Although not commonly seen, electrical alternans on electrocardiogram (ECG) (positive and negative QRS axis alternating with each beat) is pathognomonic for the condition. A FAST exam can rapidly confirm the diagnosis (Chapter 6).

A. Penetrating Injury

Suspect cardiac tamponade in any patient with penetrating trauma to one of the hemithoraces, because it has been estimated to occur in approximately 2% of patients with anterior penetrating chest injury. However, injury to the heart can occur even with remote wounds (ie, abdomen, back, and flank), and especially following gunshot injuries.

B. Blunt Trauma

Blunt anterior chest trauma occasionally causes tamponade, with blood originating from injuries to the heart itself, the great vessels, or pericardial vessels. Associated myocardial contusion is common, and the clinical findings of tamponade may be delayed.

Treatment

If cardiac tamponade is suspected before the patient is in extremis, a FAST ultrasound with pericardial views is useful in confirming the diagnosis. Pericardiocentesis (Chapter 34) may be beneficial as temporary treatment; however, all patients with a positive pericardiocentesis after trauma require open thoracotomy to further evaluate the heart and great vessels.

If shock is rapidly progressive despite treatment or if cardiac arrest occurs due to tamponade, immediate emergency thoracotomy is required in order to decompress the pericardium (Chapter 34).

Disposition

Hospitalization is required for all patients with traumatic pericardial effusions.

MYOCARDIAL CONTUSION

See also Chapter 32.

ESSENTIALS OF DIAGNOSIS

► High-velocity blunt chest trauma

► New conduction abnormalities on electrocardiogram

► Hypotension

► Wall motion abnormalities on echocardiogram

Clinical Findings

Suspect myocardial contusion (better known as blunt cardiac injury) in any patient who sustains high-velocity blunt chest trauma. The classic mechanism is an unrestrained driver in a head-on motor vehicle collision, in which a bent steering wheel or deformed steering column results. Clinically important sequelae include hypotension and wall motion abnormalities on two-dimensional echocardiography, although significant conduction abnormalities may be the most potentially lethal manifestations and usually occur in the first 12 hours following injury. Unlike myocardial infarction, the contused area usually heals completely; however, a significant number of patients may have a clinically significant decrease in cardiac output. The diagnosis is initially evaluated via ECG; unexplained sinus tachycardia is the most common finding. Other ECG abnormalities associated with the condition include arrhythmias (both atrial and ventricular), ST and T wave changes, and heart blocks. Echocardiogram and elevated levels of cardiac enzymes have also been used to evaluate myocardial contusion, although they are not usually recommended as screening tools because they are unreliable and do not predict complications.

Treatment

Treat arrhythmias as indicated (Chapter 34). Obtain serial ECGs to assess for changes (including premature ventricular contractions, atrial fibrillation, bundle branch block, and ST-segment abnormalities).

Disposition

There is evidence that hemodynamically stable patients younger than 55 years, with normal ECGs and no significant medical history, can be discharged to home. However, all other patients with significant blunt chest trauma should be considered for admission with continuous cardiac monitoring and observation for 12–24 hours.

TRAUMATIC AORTIC RUPTURE

See also Chapters 24 and 40.

ESSENTIALS OF DIAGNOSIS

▶ Mechanism of injury at risk for aortic rupture

▶ X-ray findings consistent with aortic rupture

▶ Positive definitive diagnostic study such as CT scan, aortography, or transesophageal echocardiogram

Clinical Findings

The diagnosis of traumatic aortic rupture requires a high index of suspicion, based on mechanism of injury (eg, deceleration injuries, pedestrian struck by a vehicle, falls > 30 ft) and radiographic findings. Making the diagnosis can be difficult because specific signs and symptoms are frequently absent and the physical examination is neither sensitive nor specific.

A. Symptoms and Signs

Pseudocoarctation, with blood pressure higher in the upper extremities than in the lower extremities, diminished femoral pulses; or a new harsh systolic murmur suggests the possibility of aortic injury. However, up to 50% of patients are without external evidence of chest trauma.

B. X-ray Findings

The following findings on chest X-ray indicate aortic injury:

- Widened mediastinum (>8 cm on supine X-ray).
- Tracheal or nasogastric tube deviation to the right.
- Widening of the right paratracheal stripe (>5 mm).
- Depression of the left main-stem bronchus.

- Indistinct aortic knob.
- Left apical capping.

C. Other Imaging Studies

Helical CT scanning of the chest with intravenous contrast is highly sensitive for aortic injury. However, many sources still list aortography as the gold standard for diagnosis. Transesophageal echocardiogram (TEE) has also been reported to have very high sensitivity and specificity for thoracic aortic injury. Although not widely practiced for evaluation of traumatic aortic injury, TEE can be performed in the unstable patient either in the emergency department or in the operating room.

Treatment and Disposition

Patients with significant blunt chest trauma and possible aortic rupture should be hospitalized for surgical consultation, diagnostic studies, and immediate surgery if indicated. Unstable patients require immediate thoracotomy. Otherwise, support blood pressure with intravenous crystalloids and blood, and maintain hematocrit at greater than 30%. Maintain systolic blood pressure at 100–120 mm Hg, and use β-blockade (ie, esmolol) and after load reduction (ie, nitroprusside) to control hypertension.

El-Chami MF, Nicholson W, Helmy T: Blunt cardiac trauma. J Emerg Med 2008;35(2):127–133 [PMID: 17976783].

ABDOMINAL TRAUMA

See also Chapter 25.

ESSENTIALS OF DIAGNOSIS

▶ Mechanism of injury

▶ Abdominal tenderness, distension, rigidity, or bruising

▶ FAST exam, DPL, or CT scan is diagnostic

▶ Laboratory studies: cbc, lactate

General Considerations

Significant amounts of blood may be present in the abdominal cavity without any dramatic change in appearance or abdominal dimensions. Injuries may be blunt (related to compression or crushing injury or deceleration) or penetrating. In blunt injuries, the spleen is the most commonly injured organ, and in penetrating injuries, the liver and small bowel are the most commonly injured organs.

▶ Clinical Findings

History, including the mechanism of injury, and physical examination suggestive of abdominal injury should undergo further diagnostic studies. Laboratory studies include complete blood count, electrolytes, lactate, serum alcohol, urine drug screen, and urine pregnancy test as indicated. Radiographic studies may include FAST exam and/or CT scan of the abdomen with intravenous, contrast.

A. Stable Patients

Hemodynamically stable patients may be sent to the radiology suite for CT scanning of the abdomen. A negative CT scan does not completely rule out bowel injuries. Patients suspicious for bowel injury should be admitted with serial abdominal examinations.

B. Unstable Patients

Hemodynamically unstable patients should remain in the emergency department and undergo FAST examination. If the FAST exam is positive and the patient subsequently stabilizes, then CT scanning of the abdomen with intravenous contrast can be performed for further diagnosis and assessment of the extent of injury. Otherwise, the unstable patient with a positive FAST exam requires laparotomy. If the initial FAST exam is negative, but a high index of suspicion for intra-abdominal injury remains, serial FAST exams may be performed.

▶ Treatment and Disposition

Treatment is determined by the results of the above-noted studies and may include operative or nonoperative treatment of specific organ injuries depending on the injury severity and the patient's stability. Serial abdominal examinations or serial FAST exams are indicated for patients undergoing nonoperative treatment of intra-abdominal organ injury.

Deunk J et al: Predictors for the seletion of patients for abdominal CT after blunt trauma: A proposal for a diagnostic algorithm. Ann Surg 2010;25(3):512–520 [PMID: 20083993].

HEAD TRAUMA

See also Chapter 22.

▶ Clinical Findings

A. Symptoms and Signs

Suspect head injury in any trauma patient with cranial lacerations or hematomas, and in any patient with an altered mental status with or without focal neurologic findings.

Examine the scalp and cranium for evidence of lacerations, hematomas, or other structural deformities (ie, depressions). Examine the nose and ears for any clear fluid, which must be assumed to be cerebrospinal fluid. Physical examination findings suggestive of a basilar skull fracture include hemotympanum, cerebrospinal fluid leakage from the nose or ears, a postauricular hematoma (Battle's sign), bilateral periorbital ecchymosis (raccoon eyes), or seventh cranial nerve palsy.

B. Neurologic Examination

Perform a rapid and directed neurologic examination on all patients. The GCS is used to quantify neurologic findings and allows a uniformed, standardized description of head injury severity. It assesses eye opening and verbal and motor responses. This standardized format allows for rapid identification of changes in neurologic status on subsequent evaluation. In addition, the following factors should be evaluated:

- Level of consciousness—a simplified approach uses the AVPU mnemonic (awake, responds to verbal or painful stimuli, and unresponsive).
- Pupillary response, extraocular movements, and the presence or absence of decorticate or decerebrate posturing.
- General motor function and motor response to painful stimuli.
- Deep tendon reflexes, including assessment of Babinski reflex.

Serial neurologic examinations are used to identify changes in neurologic status.

C. Imaging Studies

CT scan of the head without contrast should be performed on all patients suspected of having a closed head injury following trauma, especially if there is a history of more than a momentary loss of consciousness, amnesia, persistent vomiting, or severe headache.

▶ Treatment

An initial goal is to achieve euvolemic fluid status, because fluid overload or dehydration can be detrimental. In addition, the goal is to maintain a Pco_2 of 35–40 mm Hg, with hyperventilation indicated only for impending uncal herniation. Even when hyperventilation is indicated, the Pco_2 needs to be maintained above 25 mm Hg. Mannitol may be given as an osmotic diuretic for signs of increasing intracranial pressure. Decompressive craniotomy or burr holes may be indicated for extremely rapid neurologic deterioration.

Chesnut RM. Care of central nervous system injuries. Surg Clin North Am 2007;87(1):119–156 [PMID: 17127126].

Ropper AH, Gorson KC. Clinical practice. Concussion. N Engl J Med 2007;356(2):166–172 (Review) [PMID: 17215534].

GENITOURINARY TRAUMA

See also Chapter 26.

ESSENTIALS OF DIAGNOSIS

▶ Evidence of pelvic injury or fracture
▶ Blood at urinary meatus, scrotal or perineal hematoma, high-riding prostate, or vaginal lacerations

▶ Clinical Findings

Injuries such as pelvic fractures are often associated with genitourinary injuries. Initial physical examination findings suggestive of genitourinary injury include blood at the urinary meatus, scrotal or perineal hematoma, or a high riding, ballotable prostate on rectal examination in males. Patients with blood at the urethral meatus should undergo a retrograde urethrogram prior to insertion of an indwelling urinary catheter to identify injuries anterior to the urogenital diaphragm. If a catheter is placed and gross hematuria is identified, then obtain a cystogram to identify injuries posterior to the urogenital diaphragm. Renal or ureteral injuries in hemodynamically stable patients are evaluated by CT scan of the abdomen with intravenous contrast. CT cystogram can be obtained at the same time and is useful if bladder injury is suspected.

▶ Treatment

Treat shock as indicated. Consult urology for any urological injury.

▶ Disposition

Hospitalize patients as required. Obtain urologic consultation. Hematuria without identifiable genitourinary or renal structural abnormalities may be followed by a urologist on an outpatient basis.

Ramchandani P, Buckler PM. Imaging of genitourinary trauma. AJR Am J Roentgenol 2009:192(6):1514–1523 (Review) [PMID: 19457813].

EXTREMITY TRAUMA

See also Chapter 28.

ESSENTIALS OF DIAGNOSIS

▶ Deformities
▶ Swelling, soft tissue ecchymosis
▶ Abnormal neurovascular examination
▶ Early splinting decreases further damage

▶ General Considerations

The goal in the initial assessment and management of extremity injuries is to rapidly identify injuries that pose a threat to life or limb. Early definitive management can prevent or limit complications from extremity injuries that can lead to long-term loss of function.

▶ Clinical Findings

During the secondary survey, examine all bones and joints and obtain X-rays at 90° angles to one another of areas of suspected injury.

Crush injuries are characterized by massive swelling and soft tissue ecchymosis and are suggested by the mechanism of injury. They place the patient at risk for developing a compartment syndrome, with immediate or delayed neurovascular compromise.

▶ Treatment

Pain control is of utmost importance. Splinting of fractures (Chapter 28) prevents excessive fracture site motion, which helps control blood loss, reduce pain, and prevent further soft tissue or neurovascular damage. Cover open fractures with sterile saline-moistened dressings. Administer intravenous antibiotics (ie, cefazolin, 1 g ± penicillin and aminoglycoside depending on the type and severity of contamination) and tetanus prophylaxis if indicated. Obtain orthopedic consultation.

If compartment syndrome is suspected, compartment pressures should be measured (>35 mm Hg exceeds the tissue perfusion pressure and suggests impending neurovascular compromise). Fasciotomy may be required. Evaluate patients for rhabdomyolysis via measurement of creatinine kinase and urine myoglobin. Treatment of associated myoglobinuria consists of aggressive fluid resuscitation and osmotic diuresis to maintain high renal tubular volume and urine flow. Alkalinization of the urine with sodium bicarbonate reduces the precipitation of myoglobin in the renal tubules.

Disposition

Hospitalize patients for observation or surgery as indicated.

Morshed S et al: Delayed internal fixation of femoral shaft fracture reduces mortality among patients with multisystem trauma. J Bone Joint Surg AM 2009;91(1):3–13 [PMID: 19122073].

O'Tolle RV et al: Resuscitation before stabilization of femoral fractures limits acute respiratory distress syndrome in patients with multiple traumatic injuries despite low use of damage control orthopedics. J Trauma 2009;67(5):1013–1021 [PMID: 19901662].

SPINAL TRAUMA

See also Chapter 27.

ESSENTIALS OF DIAGNOSIS

- ▶ Immobilize to prevent further damage
- ▶ Direct spinal tenderness on physical examination
- ▶ Swelling or deformity over spine
- ▶ Neurologic deficits in extremities
- ▶ Sensory loss
- ▶ Decreased rectal sphincter tone or perineal sensation

General Considerations

Cervical spine immobilization is accomplished with a semi-rigid cervical collar and maintaining logroll precautions and is required until vertebral or spinal cord injuries are excluded. Patients should be log rolled off EMS spine boards as soon as possible but maintained with spinal precautions.

Patients left on long spine boards even for short periods of time are at risk to develop significant skin breakdown and other complications related to the use of ridged spine boards.

Clinical Findings

Evaluation consists of logrolling the patient to examine the entire spine, including a rectal examination to evaluate rectal sphincter tone and perineal sensation. Evaluate any painful areas radiographically, and perform a detailed motor and sensory examination on all extremities. Neurologic deficits may or may not be present initially; therefore, a high index of suspicion must be maintained while in-line spinal immobilization is continued.

Treatment and Disposition

Immobilization and hospitalization are required for patients with evidence of spinal trauma, with the exception of alert and oriented patients with a thoracolumbar strain or those with a cervical strain, who may be discharged to home in a cervical collar with outpatient follow-up in 1–2 weeks for reevaluation for possible ligamentous injury. Orthopedic or neurologic consultation is indicated for fractures or neurologic deficits. Despite the use of high-dose methylprednisolone in spinal cord injury as "a standard of care," there are significant concerns regarding methodologically for the primary studies. Multiple complications have been reported with the use of high dose steroids. Both the neurosurgical guidelines and the Consortium for Spinal Cord Medicine clinical practice guideline consider the use of high-dose methylprednisoloone to be a treatment option and not a standard.

Tsutsumi S, Ueta T, shibaK, Yamamoto S, Takagishi K. Effects of the Second National Acute Spinal Cord Injury Study of high-dose methylprednisolone therapy on acute cervical spinal cord injury-results in spinal injuries center. Spine 2006;31(26):2992–2996 [PMID: 17172994].

Wuermser LA et al: Spinal cord injury medicine. 2. Acute care management of traumatic and nontraumatic injury. Arch Phys Med Rehabil 2007;33(3 suppl 1):S55–S61 [PMID:17321850].

Respiratory Distress

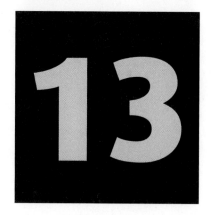

13

C. Keith Stone, MD

Immediate Management of Life-Threatening Problems	Further Diagnostic Evaluation
Cardiac Arrest	Emergency Treatment of Specific disorders
Severe Upper Airway Obstruction	Chest Wall Defects
Altered Mental Status with Shallow Breathing	Pulmonary Collapse
Tension Pneumothorax	Loss of Functional Lung Parenchyma
Massive Aspiration	Airway Disease
Severe Pulmonary Edema	Pulmonary Vascular Disease
Severe Asthma, Chronic Obstructive Pulmonary Disease	Miscellaneous Conditions

IMMEDIATE MANAGEMENT OF LIFE-THREATENING PROBLEMS

See Figure 13–1.

▶ Assess Severity and Give Immediate Necessary Care

Patients in severe respiratory distress should receive simultaneous evaluation and therapy (see Figure 13–1). Providing and maintaining an adequate airway is the first consideration. Quickly assess the severity of distress by noting the patient's general appearance. Patients struggling to breathe demonstrate a greater use of chest and accessory muscles than the normal quiet use of the diaphragm. Any patient with severe respiratory distress should receive immediate oxygen supplementation during assessment and treatment. Rapidly perform a focused examination of the oropharynx, neck, lungs, heart, chest, and extremities. A plain film chest X-ray (CXR) with PA and lateral views, if possible, provides valuable information and should be obtained as soon as possible.

▶ Assess Adequacy of Oxygenation

A. Pulse Oximetry

Bedside pulse oximeters measure the percent saturation of oxygen in capillary blood. Pulse oximetry is particularly useful during procedural sedation and during attempts at endotracheal intubation because of the real-time availability of the information. However, this information is incomplete because pulse oximeters do not measure the PCO_2 or detect the presence of hypoventilation leading to respiratory acidosis.

B. Arterial Blood Gases

Arterial blood gases provide, in essence, the same information about arterial oxygen saturation as does pulse oximetry, but are necessary to provide valuable information about the effectiveness of ventilation. The blood gas provides measurement of pH, PO_2, and PCO_2. Arterial blood gases should be obtained in patients who are in severe respiratory distress, especially if pulse oximetry identifies that they require high concentrations of oxygen.

CARDIAC ARREST

▶ Clinical Findings

In unresponsive patients, check for airway patency and properly position the head and jaw to open the airway (Chapter 9). Evaluate respiratory effort and assist ventilations if inadequate. Ventricular fibrillation results in rapid loss of consciousness usually within 5–10 seconds. Such patients

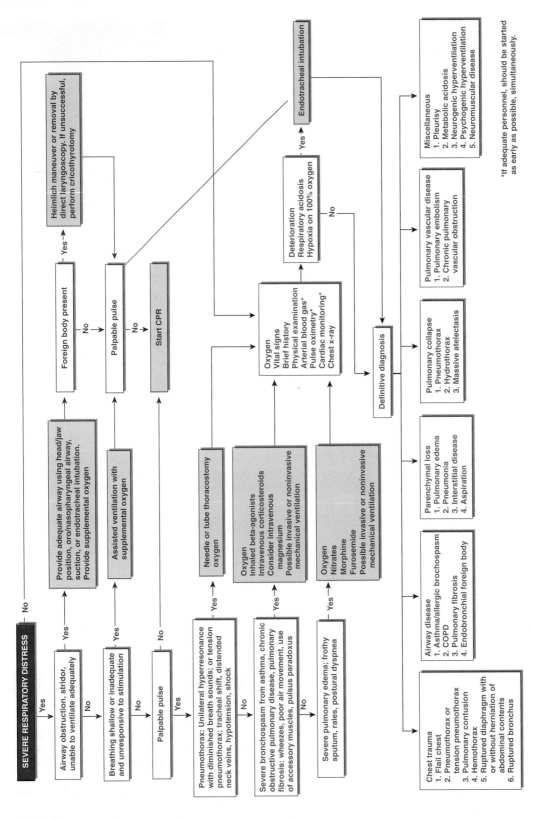

▲ Figure 13–1. Management of severe respiratory distress.

usually become apneic but may have perfunctory respiratory effort while unconscious. Such agonal breathing will be shallow and ineffective. It is important to recognize the situation as a primary cardiac event. The treatment is immediate defibrillation.

Basic and advanced life support is covered in Chapter 9.

SEVERE UPPER AIRWAY OBSTRUCTION

See also Chapter 10.

▶ Clinical Findings

Unless the patient has progressed to apnea unwitnessed, high-grade upper airway obstruction is usually obvious from pronounced stridorous respirations. Retractions of the supraclavicular and suprasternal areas of the chest indicate that there is significant obstruction. Patients with complete airway obstruction will not be able to breathe or speak. Patients may have a visible swelling or mass in the neck. The tongue may be swollen, as may other structures in the mouth. Laryngoscopy may reveal a foreign body, tumor, or other obstruction in the larynx or trachea.

▶ Treatment

(See also Chapter 9). Upper airway obstruction is most often due to soft tissue swelling secondary to infection or angioedema. Therapy should be directed to reduce the edema either by cooling or by vasoconstriction and treating the underlying infection or allergy. Epinephrine, either topically, by inhalation, or parentally, is the most effective medication for angioedema but caution should be exercised because of the associated cardiovascular effects. Direct laryngoscopy coupled with the use of forceps is the best method of removing obstructing foreign bodies. Obstructing liquids and particulate matter can be removed with a rigid suction device with a blunt tip (Yankauer). Foreign bodies such as meat may be removed by the Heimlich maneuver. A physician skilled in difficult airway management should care for these patients and may use adjuncts such as fiberoptic intubating bronchoscopy for diagnosis or securing the airway. If less invasive methods fail, immediate cricothyrotomy or tracheostomy is required (Chapter 7).

▶ Disposition

Patients with easy, uncomplicated removal of an obstructing foreign body may be sent home following a period of observation with instructions to eat more slowly, chew more thoroughly, and swallow more carefully. Patients who have lost consciousness but otherwise appear well should be examined and observed in the emergency department and hospitalized only if symptoms develop or persist. Some patients will have aspirated some material into the lungs, and hospitalization is appropriate if significant aspiration is suspected.

ALTERED MENTAL STATUS WITH SHALLOW BREATHING

▶ Clinical Findings

Altered mental status in a patient with obvious respiratory distress may be due to carbon dioxide retention or profound tissue hypoxia. However, the patient may have unlabored shallow respirations. Absence of a gag reflex (unprotected airway) or severe hypercapnia or hypoxemia on arterial blood gas studies (ie, respiratory failure) together with clinical assessment of underlying causes of altered mental status support the necessity for endotracheal intubation in the emergency department.

▶ Treatment

Ventilatory support should be given until endotracheal intubation can be accomplished. Provide high-flow (10–15 L/min) supplemental oxygen by nonrebreather mask or bag-valve-mask ventilation, as indicated.

As soon as oxygenation and carbon dioxide exchange have been partially corrected by assisted ventilation, the patient should be intubated. An endotracheal tube provides a definitive airway by preventing aspiration and facilitating effective respiratory support. If there is doubt about the need for intubation, err on the side of intubation. Evaluation and treatment of other causes of altered mental status should follow airway management (Chapters 17–20 and 37).

▶ Disposition

Hospitalize these patients for further diagnosis and treatment.

TENSION PNEUMOTHORAX

▶ Clinical Findings

Tension pneumothorax may develop as a result of trauma or may occur during positive pressure ventilation. Spontaneous pneumothorax (SP) rarely produces a tension pneumothorax. Specific physical signs of tension pneumothorax include shift of the trachea to the contralateral side, and distended neck veins. Often these signs are difficult to appreciate, especially during a tense and sometimes chaotic trauma resuscitation. Clinical suspicion is the key to the diagnosis.

▶ Treatment

Provide supplemental oxygen 100% by mask. Tube thoracostomy (Chapter 7) is the definitive treatment. Needle decompression should be rarely, if ever, be required. Tube thoracostomy can be justified by clinical examination without a CXR and is usually preferable to needle decompression. If a delay in performing tube thoracostomy is unavoidable and the patient is in severe distress, a large-bore (14–16-guage) needle may be placed through the second intercostal space in the midclavicular line. A rush of air verifies successful decompression of the hemithorax. Follow needle decompression with tube thoracostomy when the situation permits.

▶ Disposition

Hospitalize these patients for further treatment.

MASSIVE ASPIRATION

▶ Clinical Findings

If the patient with severe respiratory distress has vomitus with particulate matter in the oropharynx, significant aspiration is likely. Aspiration may be observed sometimes during airway procedures. Vomitus, tube feedings, or particulate food particles may be observed in the oropharynx or suctioned from the airway. Following such an episode, the patient with aspiration will typically become hypoxic with tachypnea and respiratory distress. Fever and tachycardia frequently occur. Hypotension may develop. An infiltrate, sometimes extensive, usually appears on CXR especially in the dependent areas of the lungs. Aspiration pneumonia is a common cause of respiratory morbidity and mortality in elderly and debilitated patients.

▶ Treatment

The airway should be suctioned to clear the aspirated material. Administer oxygen to correct hypoxia. Chemical pneumonitis resulting from aspiration does not require antibiotics but there is usually such difficulty in distinguishing aspiration pneumonitis from bacterial pneumonia that most clinicians begin treatment with broad-spectrum antibiotics. Corticosteroids have no proven value in the treatment of aspiration pneumonia and, in fact, may be deleterious.

▶ Disposition

Hospitalize these patients for definitive treatment.

SEVERE PULMONARY EDEMA

See also Chapters 33 & 35.

▶ Clinical Findings

Patients with acute pulmonary edema present with severe dyspnea and labored breathing. This may be the presenting manifestation of cardiac disease, may represent decompensation of previously managed congestive heart failure (CHF), or be noncardiac in origin. Most patients

have rales at the base of both lungs but in some cases, all one can appreciate is wheezing, prolonged expiration, and diminished breath sounds. Most of these patients are elderly or have known cardiac disease such as cardiomyopathy, coronary artery, or valvular heart disease. Jugular venous distension and lower extremity edema are unreliable predictors of the presence and severity of pulmonary congestion. The CXR will usually demonstrate interstitial (Figure 13–2) and sometimes alveolar edema. The work of breathing is greatly increased when the lungs are congested and edematous. Varying degrees of hypoxia are usually present. Brain natriuretic peptide (BNP) testing is helpful, especially in differentiating CHF from COPD. A level of greater than 100 pg/dL is consistent with acute decompensated heart failure. The level of BNP correlates with the severity of CHF.

▶ Treatment

Patients should be treated with 100% oxygen by a nonrebreather mask. Furosemide should be given with the initial dose of 40 mg. Doses of 80–160 mg should be used if the patient already takes diuretics or has renal insufficiency. Severe hypertension is usually present and is responsible for much of the reduced cardiac output and high left atrial pressure. Reducing it rapidly is a priority. Nitroglycerin by intravenous infusion is the best choice of a vasodilator in this setting starting at 5–10 μg/min. A higher dose may be used if the blood pressure is very high. Sublingual nitroglycerin should be used prior to establishing the infusion.

Angiotensin-converting enzyme inhibitors are important in the long-term management of heart failure but their role in the acutely decompensated patient is yet unclear. β blockers are useful in the long-term management of CHF but are best avoided in the acutely decompensated patient. Bilevel positive airway pressure (BiPAP) with an expiratory level of 5 cm H_2O and an inspiratory level of 15 cm H_2O is most commonly used to provide noninvasive ventilatory support and my obviate the need for endotracheal intubation.

▶ Disposition

Many of these patients are severely ill on presentation but improve dramatically with treatment. Most will still need to be hospitalized. The presence of chest pain, hypotension, or arrhythmia increases the risk of complications. Some patients with mild exacerbations of CHF that are referable to an easily reversible cause, such as medication noncompliance, may be discharged if they respond well to treatment.

SEVERE ASTHMA, CHRONIC OBSTRUCTIVE PULMONARY DISEASE

See also Chapter 33.

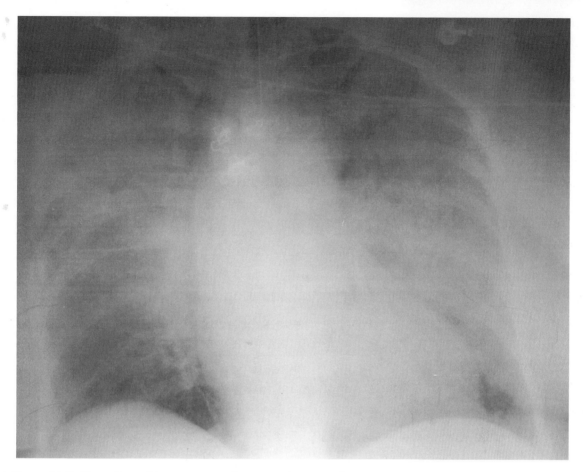

▲ **Figure 13-2.** The radiographic appearance of severe pulmonary edema.

▶ Clinical Findings

Patients with asthma or chronic obstructive pulmonary disease may present with severe dyspnea and respiratory distress. However, dyspnea in this group of patients is less likely to be postural and cough is more common and troublesome. Patients with asthma or chronic obstructive pulmonary disease usually have wheezing on auscultation of the chest. Also common are tachypnea, tachycardia, cyanosis, chest hyperexpansion, and globally diminished breath sounds. Severe episodes are characterized by inability to speak in full sentences, oxygen saturations < 92%, use of accessory muscles, pulsus paradoxus, confusion, and a quiet chest on auscultation. CXR shows only hyperexpanded lung fields unless another pathologic process such as bacterial pneumonia is present. These patients frequently have viral or (rarely) bacterial tracheobronchitis, or exposure to an allergen has exacerbated their chronic underlying disease. Peak expiratory flow rate is the most practical objective test of airway obstruction and the response to treatment available.

▶ Treatment

A. Oxygen

Give oxygen, 1–3 L/min, to raise arterial saturation to at least 95% or Po_2 to between 60 and 80 mm Hg without causing respiratory depression and a marked increase in arterial Pco_2. Pulse oximetry is preferred, but arterial blood gas analysis may be indicated to help direct therapy. Noninvasive ventilation may be attempted to avoid tracheal intubation and mechanical ventilation. However, intubation may be necessary if a patient is in acute respiratory failure.

B. β-Adrenergic Sympathomimetic Bronchodilators

In adults, β-adrenergic sympathomimetic bronchodilators should be given in aerosol form if possible; otherwise, they may be given parenterally. A typical regimen is albuterol, 0.2–0.3 mL in 3 mL normal saline, delivered by nebulizer every 20–30 minutes. β-agonists may be nebulized in combination with ipratropium bromide (0.5 mg, up to three doses). For patients who are able to use them properly, metered-dose inhalers are as efficacious as nebulized therapy.

In general, parenteral therapy offers little benefit over nebulization, except in the most extreme cases. If used, parenteral therapy includes epinephrine, 0.2–0.3 mL (1:1000 dilution) every 20–30 minutes subcutaneously, or terbutaline, 0.25 mg subcutaneously every 2–4 hours. Parenteral therapy may have value in younger patients with severe exacerbation. However, parenteral administration of sympathomimetics can produce marked tachycardia and may induce myocardial ischemia, especially in elderly patients or those with preexisting coronary artery disease. Therefore, they should be used cautiously in this group and be withheld if chest pain or extreme tachycardia develops.

C. Corticosteroids

Corticosteroids should be given early to patients who do not respond adequately to nebulized or parenteral β-adrenergic agents. The recommended regimen is methylprednisolone, 125 mg intravenously initially, or prednisone, 60 mg orally. If the patient is to be discharged from the emergency department, a short course of oral steroids may be considered.

D. Magnesium Sulfate

Magnesium sulfate has a bronchodialiting effect that may be of benefit in asthma. Its use should be reserved for life-threatening bronchospasm, which is refractory to all other interventions. Adult dosing of magnesium sulfate is 1–2 g intravenously over 15–30 minutes; pediatric dosage is 40 mg/kg intravenously. Effects are short-lived after the infusion is discontinued. Blood pressure should be monitored and the infusion stopped if hypotension occurs. Intravenous calcium should be immediately available to counteract cardiac dysrhythmias related to magnesium. Deep tendon reflexes will be lost once serum magnesium concentration reaches 7–10 mEq/L (normal concentration is 1.5–2.0 mEq/L); the infusion should be stopped if reflexes are lost. At higher concentrations, respiratory depression and cardiac arrest may occur. However, the dose used for asthma is relatively low (approximately one-fourth the dose used in preeclampsia).

▶ Disposition

Hospitalize patients with significant bronchospasm that does not respond promptly to treatment, or those with moderate bronchospasm that fails to improve after several hours of treatment.

Further management of patients with these disorders is discussed in Chapter 33.

Barnard A: Management of an acute asthma attack. Aust Fam Physician 2005;34:531–534 [PMID: 15999162].

Hammer J: Acquired upper airway obstruction. Paediatr Respir Rev 2004;5:25–33 [PMID: 15222951].

Holley AD, Boots RJ: Review article: management of acute severe and near-fatal asthma. Emerg Med Australas 2009;21:258–268 [PMID:19682010].

Jessup M, Abraham WT, Casey DE et al: 2009 focused update: ACC/AHA guidelines for the diagnosis and management of heart failure in adults. Circulation 2009;119:1977–2016 [PMID: 19324967].

Keel M, Meier C: Chest injuries-what is new? Curr Opin Crit Care 2007;13:674–679 [PMID: 17975389].

Maher TM, Wells AU: Acute breathlessness. Br J Hosp Med 2007;68:M40–M43 [PMID: 17419463].

Masip J: Non-invasive ventilation. Heart Fail Rev 2007;12:119–124 [PMID: 17492379].

Paintal HS, Kuschner WG: Aspiration syndromes: 10 clinical pearls every physician should know. Int J Clin Pract 2007;61:846–852 [PMID: 17493092].

Leigh-Smith S, Harris T. Tension pneumothorax—time for a re-think? Emerg Med J 2005;22:8–16 [PMID: 15611534].

▼ FURTHER DIAGNOSTIC EVALUATION

A. Diagnostic Information

After supplemental oxygen has been started and life-threatening problems have been corrected, proceed as follows:

1. Obtain brief history directed toward cardiopulmonary disease and comorbidities, including potential triggers or causes, previous similar episodes, previous need for mechanical ventilation, and duration of this attack of dyspnea.

2. Obtain complete list of prescribed and unprescribed medications (current and recent past), including most recent dosage history and history of steroid use.

3. Conduct physical examination of the heart, lungs, abdomen, extremities, and other areas as indicated.

4. Obtain complete blood count, urinalysis, serum creatinine or blood urea nitrogen, serum electrolytes, and glucose, depending on the patient's history and examination findings.

5. Monitor pulse oximetry and peak expiratory flow rate and conduct dyspnea scale assessment. Arterial blood gas may be performed on the basis of pulse oximetry or concomitant clinical findings.

6. Order CXR and electrocardiogram, if indicated.

7. Order additional indicated tests such as D-dimer or other imaging studies (ie, chest computed tomography [CT] scan, ventilation–perfusion scan).

B. Interpretation of Diagnostic Data

Information gathered from the history, physical exam, and ancillary testing, usually will allow the emergency physician to identify the cause of dyspnea (further discussed below and in Table 13–1).

Table 13–1. Esseyntials of Diagnosis of Diseases Causing Dyspnea and Respiratory Distress.[a]

Disorder	Specific Condition	Onset History	Symptoms Other Than Dyspnea	Sans	Chest X-ray	Comment
Chest wall defect	Flail chest	Trauma	Pain with respiration	Paradoxical motion of chest wall	Rib fractures	Coexistent pneumothorax common
	Muscular weakness	Gradual onset	Weakness of other muscles	Weakness of nonrespiratory muscles	Normal	Diminished inspiratory force
Pulmonary	Pneumothorax.	Sudden onset; occasionally trauma	Cough and chest pain common	Tympany and decreased breath sounds; decreased blood pressure and tracheal shift if tension	Lung collapse; mediastinal shift if tension	
	Hydrothorax	Gradual onset		Dullness and decreased breath sounds	Pleural effusion (decubitus views)	
	Atelectasis	Variable onset		Variable	Signs of atelectasis	
Loss of functional lung parenchyma	Pulmonary edema	Usually abrupt onset (hours to days)	Cough common; dyspnea on exertion, paroxysmal nocturnal dyspnea, orthopnea	Bibasilar rales (occasional wheezing); jugular venous distention with or without peripheral edema	Bilateral, alveolar infiltrates, often symmetric	Most common cause is cardiogenic, in which case the patient will have associated signs of heartfailure
	Pneumonia	Usually abrupt onset (hours to days)	Cough, pleurisy common	Rales with or without dullness over affected areas; fever	Patchy alveolar infiltrates, usually asymmetric	Leukocytes and often bacteria sputum
	Diffuse interstitial disease	Previous dyspnea common	Cough	Often dry rales	Interstitial disease (or negative)	Patient often a ware of diagnosis
	Aspiration	Abrupt onset; history of vomiting	Cough	Vomitus in oropharynx, or on endotracheal suction	Normal or infiltrate	Usually associated with coma or obtundation, underlying disease
Airway disease	Upper airway obstruction	Often sudden onset	Hoarseness or aphonia	Inspiratory stridor	Normal	Soft tissue X-rays of neck may be helpful
	Asthma	Usually previous attacks	Wheezing	Wheezing; hyperinflation and decreased breath sounds in status asthmaticus	Hyperinflation	Patient usually aware of diagnosis
	Chronic obstructive lung disease and cystic fibrosis	Previous dyspnea common; onset variable	Cough, wheezing	Wheezing; hyperinflation and decreased breath sounds	Hyperinflation; occasional pneumonitis	Clubbing with cystic fibrosis; patient usually aware of diagnosis
Pulmonary vascular disease	Acute pulmonary embolism	Abrupt onset	Cough, pleurisy, hemoptysis	Tachycardia; occasionally signs of acute cor pulmonale	Usually normal; occasionally infiltrates, atelectasis, elevated hemidiaphragm. "Hampton's hump"	Ventilation-perfusion lung scan, CT angiogram, pulmonary arteriogram for diagnoses, D-dimer

(continued)

Table 13–1. Esseyntials of Diagnosis of Diseases Causing Dyspnea and Respiratory Distress.[a] (*Continued*)

Disorder	Specific Condition	Onset History	Symptoms Other Than Dyspnea	Sans	Chest X-ray	Comment
	Repeated small pulmonary emboli	Gradual onset	Rarely, pleurisy or chest pain	Occasionally signs of cor pulmonale	Rarely helpful	May require formal pulmonary function tests for diagnosis
Miscellaneous	Pleurisy	Often abrupt	Pleuritic pain	Rub (about 80%)	Normal	Rule out pulmonary embolism
	Metabolic acidosis	Gradual onset	Often not dyspneic	Hyperventilation	Normal	Low arterial blood pH and bicarbonate
	Neurogenic		Usually not dyspenic	Sign of cardiac or neurologic disease	Normal	Stroke, heart failure are usual causes
	Psychogenic	Previous attacks common; abrupt onset with stress	Circumoral and acral tingling	Tetany	Normal	Relief obtained with rebreathing system (e.g., paper bag). Low P_{CO_2}

[a] The most helpful tests or findings are shaded.

▶ Disposition

(See also Miscellaneous Conditions, below.) If the clinical workup suggests a significant acute abnormality, but an exact diagnosis cannot be made that would permit specific therapy to be started, hospitalize the patient even if the clinical status would not otherwise warrant hospitalization. Sometimes more than one abnormality is present in the same patient (eg, acute exacerbation of chronic bronchitis and pneumonia).

▼ EMERGENCY TREATMENT OF SPECIFIC DISORDERS

CHEST WALL DEFECTS

1. Flail Chest

▶ Clinical Findings

Flail chest is an uncommon condition from blunt force trauma that is usually apparent on physical examination as a painful paradoxical motion of the rib cage or sternum (inward with inhalation and outward with exhalation). Crepitation or subcutaneous emphysema may be noted on examination together with decreased breath sounds on the affected side. A full trauma evaluation should be undertaken to identify any associated injuries.

▶ Treatment

Provide supplemental oxygen. Use a bag-mask to support ventilation of patients with obvious hypoventilation.

Continuously monitor pulse oximetry. Intubation for respiratory support need not be performed immediately if the patient demonstrates adequate ventilation and oxygenation. However, endotracheal intubation and positive-pressure ventilation are likely to be required for hypoxia or hypoventilation due to pain should trigger intervention. Provide analgesia (morphine, 1–4 mg intravenously, or fentanyl, 25–50 μg intravenously), and watch carefully for signs of respiratory depression.

▶ Disposition

All patients with flail chest injuries require hospitalization and consideration for ICU admission for aggressive pulmonary toilet and pain control.

2. Neuromuscular Diseases

▶ Clinical Findings

Patients with dyspnea or respiratory distress associated with progressive neuromuscular disease usually have hypoventilation (decreased pulse oximetry readings or arterial blood gases showing hypoxemia and hypercapnia) and objective weakness of other muscle groups, though the latter is not always present. Among many possible causes are Guillain–Barré syndrome, myasthenia gravis, hypokalemic periodic paralysis, botulism, and tick paralysis.

▶ Treatment and Disposition

Evaluate respiratory status using pulse oximetry, arterial blood gas analysis, and pulmonary function tests (eg, vital

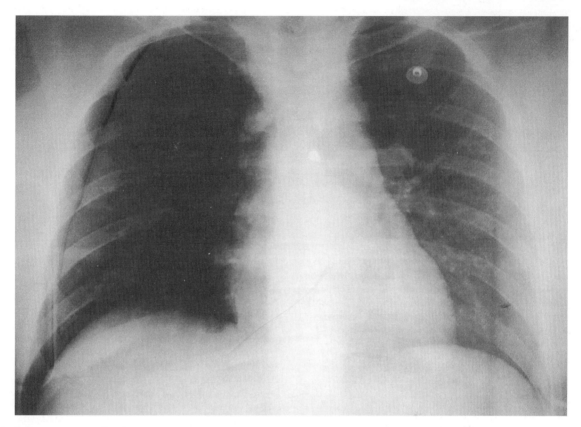

▲ **Figure 13–3.** Small right-sided pneumothorax.

capacity and maximal inspiratory force). Intubation may be postponed if initial blood gas levels are satisfactory. Specific therapy should focus on the neuromuscular disease (Chapter 37). Immediate hospitalization is usually indicated.

PULMONARY COLLAPSE

Moderate degrees of pulmonary collapse that do not cause severe respiratory distress or obvious physical findings can be apparent on CXR. Treatment depends on the specific cause as discussed below.

1. Pneumothorax

▶ Clinical Findings

Clinically, pneumothorax is classified as spontaneous or traumatic. SP is divided into primary SP (no underlying lung disease) or secondary SP (clinically apparent underlying lung disease). The patient often has chest pain and respiratory distress, with decreased breath sounds and tympany elicited by chest percussion of the affected side. The degree of dyspnea or respiratory distress depends on the amount of collapse

and on the degree of pressure (ie, tension pneumothorax). CXR shows lung collapse and air in the pleural space (Figure 13–3). Small amounts of fluid may also be present in the pleural space. Tension pneumothorax presents in a similar manner, and late findings include shift of the mediastinum away from the involved side, distended neck veins, hypotension, and shock.

▶ Treatment and Diposition

Immediate thoracostomy is indicated for bilateral pneumothoraces. Unilateral tension pneumothorax, should be treated with immediate needle decompression or throacostomy based on the clinical evaluation, do not wait for CXR confirmation.

A. Primary Spontaneous Pneumothorax

Patients that present with a first time SP that is small defined as < 20% or apical < 3 cm and minor symptoms should not be treated and can be discharged home with close outpatient follow up. For larger first time SP > 20%, or > 3 cm apical or with major symptoms, simple manual aspiration or catheter aspiration connected to a Heimlich valve is the preferred treatment. If a follow-up CXR demonstrates persistent lung reexpansion, the patient may be discharged with close follow-up and instructions to return if symptoms reappear. If aspiration fails, patients are best treated by thoracostomy tube in the emergency department before hospitalization. Patients with a first recurrence of primary SP should be treated as detailed below for secondary SP.

B. Secondary Spontaneous Pneumothorax

An air evacuation procedure should be done and the patient should be admitted for observation and recurrence prevention treatment. Immediate insertion of a chest tube is preferred over the use of catheter aspiration to evacuate the pleural space.

C. Traumatic Pneumothorax

Most patients with a pneumothorax secondary to chest trauma should be treated with chest tube insertion. Large bore tubes (28–36 Fr.) should be used if there is an associated hemothorax. If the patient will require positive pressure ventilation, a chest tube is mandatory. All patients with traumatic pneumothorax should be hospitalized.

2. Hydrothorax and Hemothorax (Pleural Fluid or Blood)
▶ Clinical Findings

Fluid in the pleural space results in pulmonary collapse. Small amounts of air may be present as well. The patient shows moderate dyspnea or respiratory distress and has dullness with chest percussion of the affected side. CXR is diagnostic (Figure 13–4).

▶ Treatment

A. Hydrothorax

If dyspnea of acute onset is thought to be secondary to hydrothorax, immediate drainage in the emergency department is indicated. A needle or small-gauge catheter should be used if the fluid is watery. Viscous effusions may require tube thoracostomy. No more than 1–2 L should be removed at any one time because of the risk of expansion injury to the lung. The fluid should be sent for analysis (pH, specific gravity, cell count, glucose, protein, lactate dehydrogenase, and amylase), culture (for *Mycobacterium tuberculosis* and other bacteria), and cytologic studies.

B. Hemothorax

In hemothorax due to penetrating trauma, autotransfusion may be indicated. Otherwise, thoracentesis or tube thoracostomy (or both) should be done, followed by investigation into the source of bleeding (eg, aortic angiography, exploration) as indicated (Chapter 24).

▶ Disposition

Hospitalization is required for all patients except those with chronic recurrent pleural effusions of known cause and without significant hypoxia or respiratory impairment.

3. Massive Atelectasis
▶ Clinical Findings

Atelectasis is alveolar collapse that is not due to pneumothorax or hydrothorax. Decrease in chest motion on the affected side, dullness to percussion, and decreased to absent breath sounds are noted. Dyspnea, tachycardia, and cyanosis may be present. The disorder is evident radiologically as an increase in density of the collapsed lung, with reduced volume of the involved hemithorax (narrowed rib interspaces, elevated hemidiaphragm, and mediastinal shift to the side of involvement).

▶ Treatment

In general, patients with atelectasis exhibit some degree of respiratory distress, which can be quite variable. In the rare patient with respiratory failure, respiratory support (administration of oxygen and usually also assisted ventilation) should be initiated in the emergency department. Administration of oxygen is indicated for patients with hypoxia on pulse oximetry while the underlying cause is determined.

▶ Disposition

Hospitalization is required unless the process is known to be chronic and nonprogressive.

LOSS OF FUNCTIONAL LUNG PARENCHYMA

A number of conditions can produce acute or chronic dyspnea through loss of functional pulmonary parenchyma.

The hallmarks of diseases causing loss of functional lung parenchyma are inspiratory rales (crackles) on physical examination, dullness to percussion, auscultatory pitch changes (eg, egophony and bronchial breath sounds), and one or more infiltrates on CXR. These disorders may be divided into those associated with (1) pulmonary edema, (2) pneumonia (including aspiration pneumonia), and (3) interstitial disease. Pulmonary contusion following blunt chest trauma is covered in Chapter 24.

In patients with dyspnea, several processes may be occurring simultaneously. For example, aspiration pneumonia may be a combination of chemical pulmonary edema and bacterial pneumonia, with varying degrees of airway obstruction; viral pneumonias are often inter-stitial in their early phases; and cardiogenic pulmonary edema starts as interstitial edema before progressing to the alveolar filling stage. Additionally, it may be difficult to differentiate these conditions initially in the emergency department (eg, pneumonia from pulmonary edema).

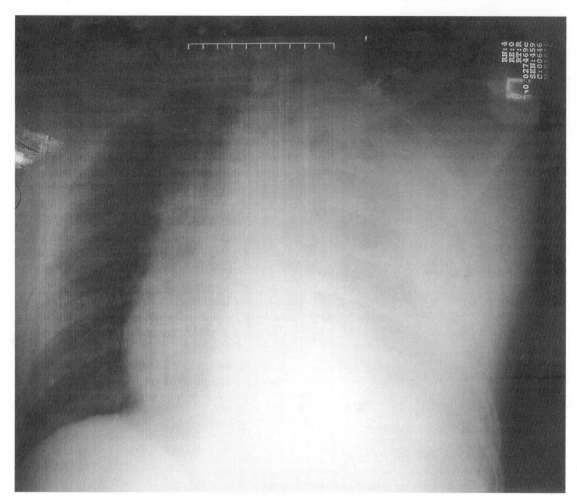

▲ **Figure 13–4.** Large left-sided hemothorax.

1. Pulmonary Edema

▶ Clinical Findings

The clinical presentation of less severe pulmonary edema is similar to that associated with the more severe form discussed above. Patients generally are less dyspneic and have a history of symptoms and signs such as paroxysmal nocturnal dyspnea, gradually increasing peripheral edema, and intermittent chest pain if the pulmonary edema is cardiogenic. Noncardiogenic edema usually begins more abruptly and is more severe than the cardiogenic form. CXR shows cephalization (Figure 13–5).

▶ Treatment

Give oxygen as needed. Additional treatment depends on whether the diagnosis is cardiogenic or noncardiogenic

pulmonary edema (Chapters 33 and 35). A trial of BiPap may obviate the need for endotracheal intubation. However, intubation may be required if hypoxemia cannot be corrected.

▶ Disposition

Many patients with dyspnea from acute pulmonary edema require hospitalization. Some patients with chronic or recurrent pulmonary edema (usually cardiogenic) can potentially be managed on an outpatient basis.

2. Pneumonia

See also Chapter 42.

▶ Clinical Findings

Patients with pneumonia generally give a history of fever and cough; dyspnea is a secondary or late symptom. Production

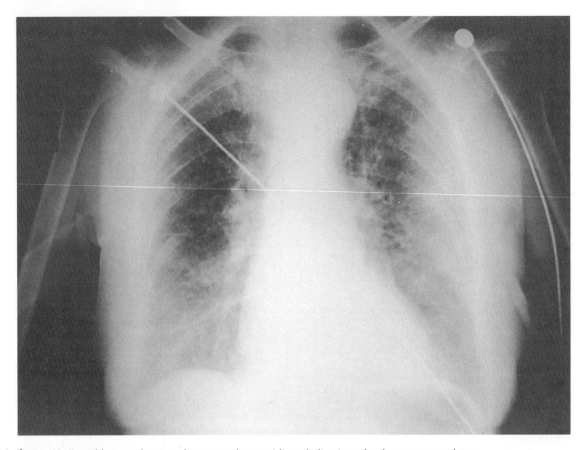

▲ **Figure 13–5.** Mild-to-moderate pulmonary edema with cephalization of pulmonary vasculature.

of purulent sputum and pleuritic chest pain are common. Physical examination usually shows a febrile patient with localized rales and dullness on percussion, often associated with signs of consolidation (egophony, bronchial breath, and vocal sounds). In children, fever and cough are the only constant symptoms.

CXR (Figure 13–6) shows one or more infiltrates, except in patients with early pneumonia or concomitant dehydration, in whom observation and rehydration over 4–6 hours generally will make the infiltrates visible on X-ray. Immunosuppressed patients may also have pneumonia without infiltrates.

Patients with AIDS may develop pneumonia due to *Pneumocystis carinii*. Despite cough, fever, dyspnea, and hypoxemia (or an elevated alveolar-arterial PO_2 gradient calculated from arterial blood gas data), the clinical findings may be few and X-ray findings extremely subtle or normal. However, typical X-ray findings, if present, are a diffuse heterogeneous alveolar or interstitial infiltrate.

▶ **Treatment**

Begin antibiotics promptly based on the clinical situation; community acquired, or health care associated pneumonia.

See Chapter 42 for a more extensive discussion of evaluation and treatment of pneumonia.

▶ **Disposition**

Hospitalization is warranted for all seriously ill patients, for very young or very old patients, for patients with significant concurrent illnesses, for unreliable patients, and for patients with pneumonia of unknown cause. Patients with *Pneumocystis* pneumonia should be admitted.

Adolescents and young adults with mild viral, mycoplasmal, or pneumococcal pneumonia usually can be managed on an outpatient basis (Chapter 42).

3. Diffuse Interstitial Pulmonary Disease

See also Chapter 33.

▶ **Clinical Findings**

Most patients with interstitial pulmonary disease have a history of chronic dyspnea, are aware of their diagnosis, and come to the emergency department because of recent worsening of

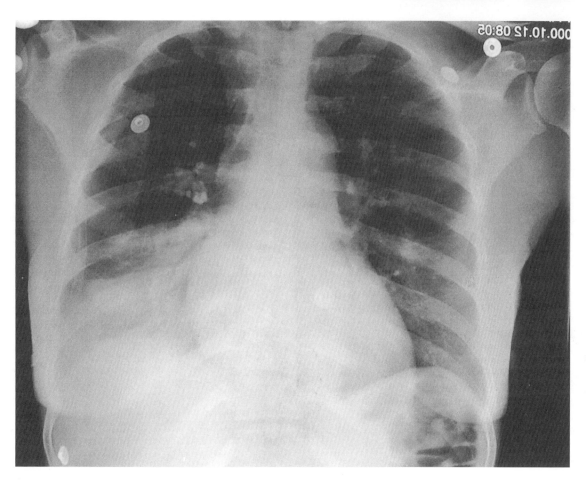

▲ **Figure 13–6.** Radiographic appearance of a right lower lobe pneumonia.

symptoms. If the patient has not sought medical attention previously, interstitial pulmonary disease may be suspected if the physical examination shows diffuse "dry" rales, the CXR shows interstitial infiltrates, and arterial PCO_2 and PO_2 are low.

▶ Treatment

Supportive care is the only treatment recommended in the emergency department.

▶ Disposition

Hospitalization should be considered for all newly diagnosed patients and for patients with known interstitial disease with significant recent increase in dyspnea or hypoxemia.

4. Aspiration

▶ Clinical Findings

Aspiration may present clinically as pneumonia without obvious prior aspiration or as respiratory distress *with*

obvious aspiration (vomitus in mouth and on clothing and elsewhere). This latter presentation is more common in patients with altered mental status.

▶ Treatment

Supportive care should be given immediately in all cases. If obvious aspiration has occurred, clearing the airway is the most important emergency measure. This is best accomplished with a large-bore, hard-tipped suction device. Endotracheal intubation for better airway control and pulmonary toilet should be considered, as should emergency bronchoscopy.

▶ Disposition

Hospitalize all patients. The patient's initial status is not a reliable guide to the need for hospitalization, because pulmonary function may worsen progressively for 24–72 hours after aspiration.

AIRWAY DISEASE

Obstruction to airflow (airway obstruction) is a principal manifestation of all types of airway disease.

1. Upper Airway Obstruction

Lesions of the oropharynx, larynx, or trachea may occlude the airway sufficiently to cause dyspnea.

▶ Clinical Findings

Upper airway obstruction usually causes pronounced stridor (obstruction of inspiratory airflow equal to or greater than expiratory airflow), which may be accentuated by forced ventilatory efforts. The stridor may be accompanied by intercostal, suprasternal, or supraclavicular retractions or other signs of increased respiratory effort. The diagnosis can be made with lateral soft-tissue X-rays of the neck. In some cases, fiberoptic laryngoscopy is helpful.

Causes of upper airway obstruction include foreign bodies, tonsillar hypertrophy, croup, epiglottitis, anaphylaxis with laryngeal edema, retropharyngeal abscess, and tumors. If epiglottitis is suspected, obtain a lateral neck X-ray before attempting to visualize the upper airway directly (Chapter 32). Young children may aspirate small objects (eg, beads, coins, or peanuts) that lodge in the trachea or main-stem bronchus. Wheezing may be mistaken for bronchospastic disease. An expiratory CXR is diagnostic, showing unilateral hyperexpansion on the affected side due to the ball-valve effect of the obstructing object (which may not be visible).

▶ Treatment

A foreign body should be removed if present. Anaphylaxis with laryngeal edema requires immediate subcutaneous or intramuscular injection of epinephrine, 0.5–1.0 mg (0.5–1.0 mL of 1:1000 solution). Alternatively, give 0.1–0.2 mg (1–2 mL of 1:10,000 solution) intravenously. Repeat in 3–10 minutes as needed (Chapter 11). Additionally, administration of diphenhydramine, 25–50 mg intramuscularly or intravenously, or selective histamine blockers such as famotidine, 20 mg intravenously, will block further histamine release. Discharged patients should receive diphenhydramine, 25 mg orally every 6 hours for 24–48 hours, to prevent recurrence.

Surgical cricothyrotomy may be emergently required if obstruction progresses. Occasionally patients with hereditary angioedema (due to C1q esterase inhibitor deficiency) will present with signs and symptoms similar to those of allergic anaphylaxis. These patients are affected little by epinephrine and require C1q esterase inhibitor replacement (or fresh-frozen plasma if C1q esterase inhibitor is unavailable).

Children with epiglottitis (Chapter 50) should not receive direct or indirect laryngoscopy in the emergency department, because laryngeal spasm may precipitate complete obstruction. They should be carefully intubated in the operating room with surgeons present who can perform an emergency tracheostomy if needed. Adults with epiglottitis are less prone to sudden airway obstruction but should be admitted and monitored closely. Both children and adults should receive intravenous antibiotics.

▶ Disposition

Patients with dyspnea from documented or suspected upper airway obstruction require hospitalization unless the problem is chronic, mild, and nonprogressive or is due to a foreign body that can be removed in the emergency department. Successfully treated upper airway obstruction due to anaphylaxis may recur when epinephrine wears off. Therefore, a 4–6-hour period of observation (or hospitalization) is advisable.

2. Asthma, Chronic Obstructive Pulmonary Disease

(See also Chapter 33). In these disorders, expiratory airflow tends to be reduced proportionally more than the inspiratory flow. Patients with dyspnea caused by these types of airway disease usually have a history of respiratory symptoms and are aware of their diagnosis.

▶ Clinical Findings

Cough is commonly a feature, although sputum production is variable. Most of these patients have wheezing on auscultation, which is accentuated during forced expiration. Other findings are similar to those discussed earlier in this chapter.

▶ Treatment

The therapy discussed under treatment of severe forms of these disorders is also of value in less severe presentations.

▶ Disposition

Hospitalization is indicated for patients with severe or rapidly worsening dyspnea that does not respond to a few hours of treatment in the emergency department. Patients with asthma who are discharged home should receive corticosteroid therapy: oral for those with moderate symptoms, and oral or inhaled for those with minor symptoms.

PULMONARY VASCULAR DISEASE

Dyspnea from pulmonary vascular disease may be one of the most difficult diagnostic problems confronting the emergency physician. The manifestations of pulmonary vascular disease are extremely varied in character and severity, and there is a significant risk of labeling patients with these illnesses as hysterical personalities or malingerers.

Acute Pulmonary Embolism

See also Chapter 33.

▶ Clinical Findings

Patients with acute pulmonary embolism and infarction usually have dyspnea, tachypnea, pleuritic chest pain, tachycardia, hypoxemia, and hypocapnia. Low-grade fever, cough, hemoptysis, and wheezing may also be present. Pulmonary infiltrates, occasionally with effusion, may be seen on X-ray.

Patients with embolization without infarction have similar manifestations but often without pulmonary infiltrates, fever, and hemoptysis. In massive pulmonary embolization, crushing anterior chest pain, dyspnea, severe hypoxemia, syncope, shock, and cardiac arrest are common. Patients with right-sided endocarditis and other causes of septic pulmonary embolization usually have high fever and rigors associated with symptoms of embolization; the CXR often shows multiple, scattered infiltrates that frequently cavitate after several days of illness.

▶ Diagnosis

Progressive, noninvasive evaluation strategies that consider specific risk factors and physical findings (Wells Criteria) have replaced invasive methods of diagnosis. Serum D-dimer, venous lower extremity Doppler ultrasound, spiral CT, CT angiography, and ventilation–perfusion scanning have significantly decreased the need for conventional pulmonary angiography in suspected pulmonary embolism.

▶ Treatment

Give oxygen. Give morphine as necessary for pain. Treat shock if present. Heparin should be started (unless contraindicated) if embolization is strongly suspected. For adults, give a bolus of 80 units/kg followed by an infusion of 18 units/kg/h adjusting the rate to maintain the prothrombin time at 1.5–2 times control values. Selected patients may be appropriate for low-molecular-weight heparin therapy (enoxaparin sodium, 1 mg/kg subcutaneously every 12 hours or fondaparinux 5 mg SQ for < 50 kg patient, 10 mg SQ for > 100 kg patient, and 7.5 mg SQ for all others). Thrombolytic therapy should generally be reserved for patients with moderate to severe right ventricular dysfunction. See Chapter 33 for further discussion on management.

▶ Disposition

Patients with suspected or documented pulmonary embolization almost always require hospitalization.

MISCELLANEOUS CONDITIONS

1. Pleurisy

▶ Clinical Findings

Pleurisy and pleuritic pain from any cause may produce a sensation of dyspnea. Even conditions such as rib fractures that produce pleuritic pain in the absence of significant underlying pulmonary parenchymal abnormalities may cause splinting and atelectasis sufficient to produce hypoxemia. When pleural fluid forms, the pain and friction rub may lessen or disappear. Pleurisy is often part of a viral syndrome (which may occasionally be accompanied by pericarditis). Fever, myalgias, headache, nasal congestion, or flu-like symptoms may be present. A CXR is required to exclude underlying lung disease, pleural effusion, or pneumothorax.

▶ Treatment

Other than measures for relief of pain, therapy must be directed toward the underlying lesions.

▶ Disposition

Hospitalization is required if the patient is severely hypoxemic (arterial $PO_2 \leq 60$ mm Hg as a new finding), if parenteral analgesia is required for pain relief, or if the underlying disease requires hospital treatment.

2. Metabolic Acidosis

▶ Clinical Findings

Metabolic acidosis (eg, diabetic ketoacidosis, salicylate overdose) can produce secondary hyperventilation that may be taken for dyspnea or respiratory distress. Arterial blood gas analyses usually show a normal or high PO_2, marked hypocapnia (PCO_2 of 10–20 mm Hg), and metabolic acidosis (low serum bicarbonate concentration).

▶ Treatment and Disposition

Treatment depends on the underlying condition. Patients almost always require hospitalization for management of the underlying cause of metabolic acidosis (Chapter 44).

3. Neurologic Hyperventilation

Primary central nervous system disease can produce a variety of abnormal breathing patterns, including central hyperventilation and Cheyne–Stokes respiration, any of which could be mistaken for respiratory distress. Cheyne–Stokes respiration may also occur when the circulation is slowed, as in heart failure.

▶ **Clinical Findings**

The diagnosis is based on finding obvious neurologic or cardiac disease consistent with the respiratory pattern. The arterial PO_2 is usually normal; PCO_2 may be low or high.

▶ **Treatment**

No treatment of the respiratory condition is required.

▶ **Disposition**

Disposition depends on the underlying disease.

4. Psychogenic Hyperventilation and Pulmonary Neurosis

▶ **Clinical Findings**

Patients with psychogenic hyperventilation usually present with a history of acute dyspnea and anxiety, often precipitated by personal or environmental factors. Hyperventilation to the point of tetany is diagnostic. Lightheadedness (due to cerebral vasoconstriction) and circumoral or limb paresthesias are often present. Another helpful feature is that the dyspnea often improves with exercise. Patients can be calmed enough to speak, whereas in organic dyspnea, patients may not be capable of speech. There are usually no abnormalities on the screening database other than a low arterial PCO_2, normal or high arterial PO_2, and elevated pH. Most of these patients can be diagnosed in the emergency department as having neuroses, but the possibility of pulmonary vascular disease must be considered.

▶ **Treatment**

There is no specific treatment. Reassurance is usually helpful. Patients with symptomatic hypocapnia (circumoral tingling, carpopedal spasm, tetany) or marked respiratory alkalosis (pH > 7.55) should breathe into an airtight bag for several minutes to relieve hypocapnia.

▶ **Disposition**

The patient should be referred to a pulmonary clinic or internist for complete evaluation and reassurance.

Baumann MH, Noppen M: Pneumothorax. Respirology 2004;9:157–164 [PMID: 15182264].

Hammer J: Acquired upper airway obstruction. Paediatr Respir Rev 2004;5:25–33 [PMID: 15222951].

Karmy-Jones R, Jurkovich GJ: Blunt chest trauma. Curr Probl Surg 2004;41:211–380 [PMID: 15097979].

Kelly AM: Treatment of primary spontaneous pneumothorax. Curr Opin Pulm Med 2009;15:376–379 [PMID: 19373088].

Maher TM, Wells AU: Acute breathlessness. Br J Hosp Med 2007;68:M40–M43 [PMID: 17419463].

Noppen M, De Keukeleire T: Pneumothorax. Respiration 2008;76:121–127 [PMID:18708734].

Pettiford BL, Luketich JD, Landreneau RJ: The management of flail chest. Thorac Surg Clin 2007;17:25–33 [PMID:17650694].

Rahimtoola A, Bergin JD: Acute pulmonary embolism: an update on diagnosis and treatment. Curr Probl Cardiol 2005;30:61–114 [PMID: 15650680].

Chest Pain

14

Martin R. Huecker, MD

Daniel J. O'Brien, MD, FACEP, FAAEM

▼ IMMEDIATE MANAGEMENT OF LIFE-THREATENING PROBLEMS

See Figure 14–1.

INITIAL MANAGEMENT

▶ Airway, Breathing, Circulation

A. Begin Supplemental Oxygen

Give oxygen by nasal cannula or face mask, pending further evaluation.

B. Begin Continuous Cardiac Monitoring

Begin cardiac monitoring with pulse oximetry and treat life-threatening arrhythmias (Chapters 9 and 34).

▶ Look for Markedly Abnormal Hemodynamics

A. Clinical Findings

Look for signs of shock. Altered sensorium, pale clammy skin, oliguria, and respiratory distress may result from arterial hypotension and poor peripheral perfusion.

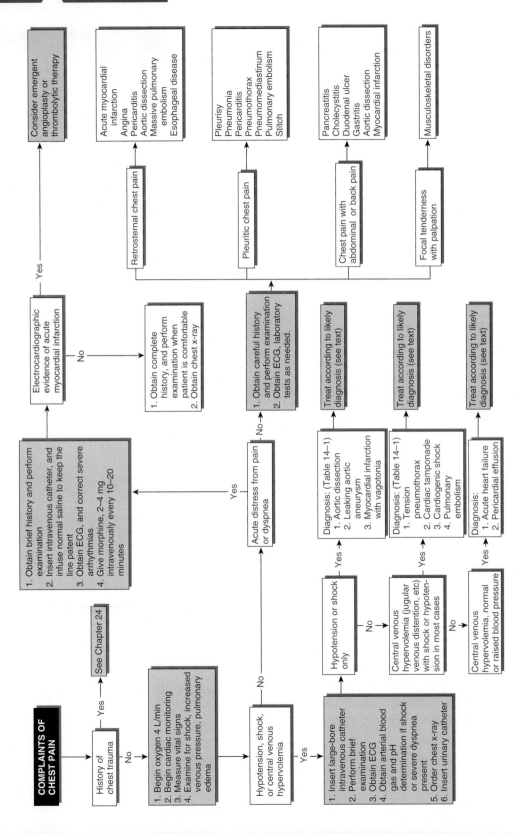

▲ **Figure 14–1.** Management of complaints of chest pain.

MANAGEMENT OF THE PATIENT WITH CHEST PAIN AND ABNORMAL HEMODYNAMICS

▶ Treatment and Disposition

A. Immediate Measures

Insert two large-bore (≥16-gauge) intravenous catheters. Intraosseous (IO) access is acceptable and compatible with all resuscitation infusions including thrombolytics. Obtain blood for a complete blood count (CBC), markers of cardiac injury, and basic metabolic panel (electrolytes, glucose, renal function). Begin administration of intravenous fluids based on estimate of intravascular fluid volume.

1. Hypovolemic shock—Infuse 250–500 mL of intravenous crystalloid solutions (normal saline or lactated Ringer's). Monitor the response (blood pressure, urine output, sensorium).

2. Central venous hypervolemia (with or without shock or hypotension)—Pending more precise diagnosis, infuse normal saline to keep the intravenous catheter patent or place a saline lock IV.

Briefly examine the pulmonary and cardiovascular systems, and palpate the abdomen for presence of a pulsatile mass. Obtain a 12-lead electrocardiogram (ECG). Obtain arterial blood for blood gas and pH determinations. Avoid unnecessary arterial punctures if the patient is a candidate for thrombolytic therapy for acute myocardial infarction. Obtain a portable chest radiograph. Insert a urinary catheter.

B. Hypotension or Shock Present

1. Central venous hypovolemia—Hypovolemia is manifested by collapsed neck veins, clear lung fields on physical examination or chest X-ray, and absence of peripheral edema. Table 14–1 lists the differentiating features of the three most important conditions causing chest pain with hypotension with central venous hypovolemia.

If the diagnosis is uncertain, treatment should be oriented primarily toward aortic dissection (Chapter 40). Type and crossmatch for 6–10 units of packed red blood cells. Expand intravascular volume with administration of intravenous crystalloid solution. Consider inserting a central venous catheter. For severe hypovolemia with shock, up to 3 L of crystalloid solution may be given rapidly (over 30–60 minutes) to restore normal hemodynamics until crossmatched blood is available. If there is no response to crystalloid solution, type-specific or universal donor blood (O negative, low antibody titer, or erythrocyte antigens) may be used pending the availability of crossmatched blood. Maintain blood pressure with continued infusion of blood and crystalloid solution. Obtain emergency vascular or thoracic surgical consultation.

Pulse deficits, an abdominal mass, or occult hematuria indicate aortic aneurysm or dissection. Obtain a portable chest X-ray and if the patient is stable consider computed tomography (CT) scan of the chest or abdomen and pelvis if indicated. Bedside ultrasound, if available, can be of great assistance in the diagnosis and management of these patients.

Management of thoracic aortic dissection consists of β-blockade (esmolol) to maintain heart rate less than 60–80 beats/min and vasodilators (nitroprusside) to maintain a systolic blood pressure less than 120 mm Hg, establishing the β-blockade first. Dissections involving the ascending aorta are managed surgically, while those not involving the ascending aorta are generally managed medically. For medical management, hospitalize the patient in an intensive care setting immediately for further evaluation and treatment.

2. Central venous hypervolemia—Superficial veins (especially neck veins) are distended; pulmonary and peripheral edema may be present. See Table 14–2 for guidelines to differential diagnosis.

A. TENSION PNEUMOTHORAX—(See Chapter 24) Consider tension pneumothorax immediately because this condition

---

Table 14–1. Differentiating Features of Conditions Causing Chest Pain with Hypovolemia.

Diagnosis	History	Examination	ECG	X-Rays
		Findings		
Myocardial infarction with vagotonia	Crushing chest pain; nausea	Bradycardia; stable hypotension	Acute infarction pattern and bradycardia	Nonspecific
Aortic dissection	Tearing chest pain; back pain; often history of hypertension	Tachycardia; pulse deficits; progressive hypotension	Nonspecific or may show ischemia or infarction pattern, left ventricular hypertrophy	Widened mediastinum; pleural fluid. CT scan is more sensitive than X-ray
Leaking upper abdominal aortic aneurysm	Chest and epigastric pain	Tachycardia; pulsatile epigastric mass	Nonspecific	CT scan or ultrasound is more sensitive than X-rays

Table 14–2. Distinguishing Features of Conditions Causing Chest Pain, Hypotension, or Shock in Association with Distended Neck Veins.

Diagnosis	Helpful Distinguishing Features
Tension pneumothorax	Hyperresonant hemithorax with decreased breath sounds; chest X-rays diagnostic, trachea deviates away from affected side
Cardiac tamponade	Faint heart sounds; ECG with diffuse low voltage or electrical alternans. Pulmonary edema rare. Echocardiography diagnostic
Cardiogenic shock (arrhythmogenic)	ECG or cardiac monitor shows severe bradycardia or tachycardia (ventricular rate <50 beats/min, usually <40 beats/min, usually >180 beats/min). Signs of myocardial ischemia may also be present
Cardiogenic shock (myocardial)	Pulmonary edema almost always present. ECG almost always shows pattern diagnostic of infarction
Pulmonary embolism (massive)	Physical examination, ECG, and chest X-ray show signs of right heart strain. Chest X-ray may show infiltrates, effusion, or truncation of pulmonary vasculature. Confirm diagnosis by ventilation-perfusion scanning, spiral CT scan of chest or pulmonary arteriography

may be quickly and reliably differentiated from the others and is easy to treat. Look for marked respiratory distress, tracheal deviation away from the affected side, and a hyperresonant hemithorax with markedly decreased or absent breath sounds on the affected side. Chest X-ray confirms the diagnosis, but treatment should not be delayed to obtain a chest X-ray. Treatment consists of the insertion of a thoracostomy tube if one is readily available (Chapter 7). Otherwise, a 14-gauge needle inserted in the second intercostal space at the midclavicular line or in the fourth intercostal space at the anterior axillary line relieves tension in the chest until a thoracostomy tube can be inserted. Hospitalize the patient for further care.

B. CARDIAC TAMPONADE—(See Chapter 24) Cardiac tamponade should also be diagnosed early because treatment is reasonably effective but differs markedly from that for cardiogenic shock, heart failure, or pulmonary embolism. Look for hypotension, jugular venous distension, and muffled heart sounds (Beck triad). Electrocardiographic manifestations may include low voltage on all leads, electrical alternans, or diffuse ST-segment elevation typical of pericarditis. A narrow pulse pressure and pulsus paradoxus may also be present. Pulmonary edema is rare. Because acute tamponade does not cause cardiomegaly, chest X-ray is not helpful. Definitive diagnosis by noninvasive

methods is best done by bedside emergency ultrasound or formal echocardiography. Attempt volume expansion with intravenous administration of 500–1000 mL of crystalloid solution over 20–30 minutes if the diagnosis is confirmed (this therapy is disastrous for cardiogenic shock). If the initial trial succeeds in elevating the blood pressure, volume expansion may be repeated once in a patient whose systolic blood pressure subsequently drops to less than 90 mm Hg.

Obtain emergency cardiothoracic consultation for therapeutic pericardiocentesis, which should be performed in the operating room or under echocardiographic or fluoroscopic guidance. If rapid, progressive hypotension develops and the patient fails to respond to volume expansion perform immediate pericardiocentesis (under ultrasound guidance if available) (Chapter 6). Hospitalize the patient at once in an intensive care unit.

C. CARDIOGENIC SHOCK (ARRHYTHMOGENIC)—See Chapter 35 for further details on the diagnosis and treatment of cardiac arrhythmias.

Severe bradydysrhythmia (heart rate usually <40 beats/min)—Give atropine, 0.5 mg intravenously; if necessary, repeat every 5–10 minutes up to a total dose of 0.04 mg/kg. An external transcutaneous pacemaker (Chapter 7) may be applied to increase the heart rate until a percutaneous transvenous pacemaker can be inserted, if indicated. Epinephrine infusion can be used for patients that do not respond to atropine. Begin an infusion at 2–10 μg/min and titrate to patient response. Assess intravascular volume and support as needed. Dopamine can be used to support blood pressure and increase myocardial contractility. Infuse at a rate of 10–20 μg/kg/min by continuous intravenous infusion. It may be administered with epinephrine or administered alone. Titrate the dose to patient response. Consider IV glucagon, 3 mg initially, followed by infusion at 3 mg/hour for patients with hypotension and bradycardia from either B-blocker or calcium channel blocker overdose.

Severe tachydysrhythmia (heart rate usually >150 beats/min)—Immediate cardioversion is the treatment of choice for tachydysrhythmia-induced shock. Deliver 50–100 J of synchronized direct current counter shock initially, and increase the shock by 50–100 J increments if there is no response. (If the patient is STABLE ie, no alteration in mental status, no chest pain, no shock or hypotension see Chapter 34).

D. CARDIOGENIC SHOCK (MYOCARDIAL INFARCTION)—(See also Chapter 34) In patients with no evidence of pulmonary edema, ensure adequate intravascular volume; give intravenous crystalloid solution, 250–500 mL over 30 minutes. If blood pressure improves, maintain the infusion at a rate of 100–200 mL/h. Avoid unnecessary arterial punctures in patients who may be candidates for thrombolytic therapy.

Give dobutamine 5–20 mcg/kg/min IV continuous infusion, dopamine 5–20 mcg/kg/min IV continuous infusion; increase by 1–4 mcg/kg/min q10–q30 minutes to optimal response, or a combination of both if no change in blood pressure occurs or if severe shock or pulmonary edema is present initially. Dobutamine is the drug of choice for treatment of cardiogenic shock due to pump failure. *Caution:* Observe for signs of dysrhythmia.

Give morphine, 2–4 mg intravenously every 5–20 minutes, until pain and dyspnea are controlled. If hypotension is a concern, then fentanyl may be used for pain. Carefully monitor the patient's respiratory status.

Nitroglycerin should generally be avoided in patients in cardiogenic shock or blood pressure less than 90 mm Hg systolic.

Consider aspirin 325 mg orally if aortic dissection is unlikely. In patients with aspirin allergy or expected deferred catheterization clopidogrel may be used.

Obtain cardiology consultation immediately if an acute infarction pattern is evident on the 12-lead ECG. Emergency reperfusion therapy with thrombolytic agents or percutaneous coronary intervention has been shown to be of benefit in decreasing the mortality rate and the size of the infarct. If thrombolytic therapy is to be used (Chapter 35), it should be initiated in the emergency department by the emergency physician, avoiding the delay necessitated by obtaining cardiologic consultation or transporting the patient to the coronary care unit. Hospitalize the patient immediately in a coronary care or intensive care unit.

E. MASSIVE PULMONARY EMBOLISM—(See Chapter 33) Because massive pulmonary embolism is a difficult diagnosis to confirm rapidly, every attempt should be made to exclude other causes of chest pain with shock. Consider an emergency echocardiogram if available. Findings consistent with massive pulmonary embolism include right ventricular hypokinesis and dilation. Right ventricular dysfunction from pulmonary embolism predicts increased mortality and the need for thrombolytic therapy.

Administer 250–500 mL of normal saline over 20–30 minutes in an effort to elevate systolic blood pressure. The dose may be repeated if the trial is successful and if heart failure does not develop. In the rare patient with hypotension without central venous hypervolemia, a fluid challenge should also be given, but a larger dose (500–1000 mL of normal saline instead of 300–500 mL) may be administered.

Give dopamine (see above). If clinical signs strongly suggest pulmonary embolism and thoracic dissection has been ruled out (computerized tomography may be useful in definitively establishing either of these diagnoses), begin heparin (unfractionated or a low-molecular-weight heparin) (see Pulmonary Embolism, below, and Chapters 33 and 34). Obtain pulmonary consultation, and consider thrombolytic therapy.

C. Hypotension or Shock not Present

Central Venous Hypervolemia—Superficial veins (especially neck veins) are distended. Pulmonary and peripheral edema is common. Blood pressure is normal or (more commonly) elevated.

Acute exacerbation of congestive heart failure is the most common cause. It occasionally results from acute myocardial infarction (acute cardiogenic pulmonary edema), and less commonly from acute myocarditis or pericardial effusion.

A. NITROGLYCERIN—Nitroglycerin may be quickly administered either sublingually (0.4 mg) or transdermally (nitroglycerin ointment 1.25–2.5 cm) (½–1 inch). An intravenous nitroglycerin infusion may be started in the emergency department. Monitor the blood pressure closely, and if hypotension develops, place the patient in the Trendelenburg position and decrease the infusion rate. Avoid nitrates in patients taking any selective phosphodiesterase 5 inhibitor (sildenafil [Viagra], tadalafil [Cialis], or vardenafil [Levitra]).

B. FUROSEMIDE—Give furosemide, 0.5–1.0 mg/kg, by bolus intravenous injection. The initial effect of rapid preload reduction is of immediate benefit; diuresis occurs later.

C. MORPHINE—Give morphine, 2–4 mg intravenous, and repeat every 5–10 minutes until pain and dyspnea are relieved.

D. ASPIRIN—Give aspirin, 160–325 mg chewed, if not contraindicated. If the patient has an allergy to aspirin, use clopidogrel, 75 mg orally.

E. ANGIOTENSIN-CONVERTING ENZYME (ACE) INHIBITORS—Captopril and enalapril are associated with reduced admission rates to the intensive care unit and decreased endotracheal intubation rates. Acutely, reduction in preload and afterload has been reported. For oral or sublingual captopril, a one-time dose of 12.5 or 25 mg is given; enalapril is given as a 1.25 mg intravenous infusion over 5 minutes. Avoid using ACE inhibitors in patients who are hypotensive, pregnant, hyperkalemic, or have renal insuffiency.

F. POSITIVE PRESSURE VENTILATION—If the patient continues to deteriorate, consider early noninvasive positive pressure ventilation (BiPAP or CPAP); this approach may even prevent the need for endotracheal intubation.

G. INOTROPIC AGENTS—Short-term inotropic therapy can improve hemodynamic parameters. These agents may be beneficial for patients who are unable to receive conventional therapy. Milrinone or dobutamine are reasonable choices.

H. NESIRITIDE—Has been shown by meta-analysis to actually increase mortality but can be considered in patients who cannot tolerate nitroglyerin. It is costly and has no additive benefit to nitroglycerin.

I. HOSPITALIZATION—Hospitalize the patient immediately in an intensive care setting.

MANAGEMENT OF THE PATIENT WITH SEVERE CHEST PAIN AND NORMAL HEMODYNAMICS

▶ Clinical Findings

The patient is in acute distress because of chest pain but is neither hypotensive nor in shock.

▶ Differential Diagnosis by Location and Quality of Pain

Evaluation of patients who complain of chest pain but are not in severe distress should proceed in a systematic fashion. The single most useful means of evaluation is the carefully elicited history supplemented by examination of the heart, lungs, abdomen, and peripheral vessels in conjunction with electrocardiography and chest X-ray. Consider most of the diagnostic possibilities at least briefly in every patient who presents with chest pain (Table 14–3).

A. Retrosternal Discomfort

Retrosternal discomfort, especially if it is a tightness, pressure, or "squeezing" pain, should suggest serious underlying disease, for example, myocardial infarction, unstable angina due to atherosclerosis or valvular heart disease, pericarditis, dissection of the aorta, or pulmonary embolism. When the abovementioned diagnoses are excluded, esophageal disease (eg, spasm, esophagitis) is the most common cause of retrosternal distress (see below). Because esophageal disease is relatively benign and rarely requires hospitalization, the more serious causes of retrosternal discomfort must be excluded with a high degree of certainty before concluding that the pain is of esophageal origin.

B. Pleuritic Pain

Pain that is markedly worse on inspiration should suggest pleurisy associated with pneumonia, pulmonary embolism, or isolated pleuritis. The pain of pneumothorax, pneumomediastinum, ruptured esophagus, and pericarditis frequently has a pleuritic component. The fleeting pain of a "stitch in the side" is often pleuritic in nature as well. Chest pain due to myocardial infarction may have a pleuritic component.

One of the most serious causes of pleuritic chest pain, pulmonary embolism, is also one of the most difficult to diagnose given the widely varied presentations of the disease with nonspecific history and physical examination findings. Because of the increased mortality associated with misdiagnosis, consider pulmonary embolism in all patients presenting with pleuritic chest pain (Chapters 33 and 35).

C. Back or Abdominal Pain with Chest Pain

Abdominal pain that is inferior to the xiphoid process and associated with chest pain should suggest intra-abdominal disease, dissecting aortic aneurysm, or possibly myocardial ischemia. In stable patients, CT scan of the chest and abdomen with intravenous contrast can reliably exclude the diagnosis of dissecting or ruptured aortic aneurysm. Even after aortic catastrophes are excluded, patients with chest pain often require hospitalization or admission to an observation unit to rule out myocardial ischemia.

D. Musculoskeletal Discomfort

Musculoskeletal disease with chest pain (Tietze's syndrome, rib fracture) is usually associated with marked tenderness localized over the affected site. Patients with chest pain referred from intrathoracic structures may also have some associated tenderness of superficial structures. Most patients with chest pain from musculoskeletal disorders can receive treatment in the emergency department and be discharged for outpatient follow-up care.

E. Chest Pain Unit

An emerging method of evaluation of chest pain in the Emergency Department is the Chest Pain Unit. Various structures can be utilized, but most are protocol-driven observation units intending to screen low risk patients for cardiac origin of chest pain. Often located in the ED proper, the Chest Pain Unit is a virtual observation unit holding patients in preparation for some form of noninvasive stress testing.

The protocols usually include serial electrocardiograms, serial markers of cardiac injury, telemetry, and risk stratification. Certain exclusion criteria typically apply: existing coronary artery disease, diabetes mellitus, stimulant induced chest pain, and sometimes female patients. These populations are thought to have higher likelihood of silent ischemia, reduced exercise tolerance, or increased risk of adverse events when undergoing stress testing.

The Chest Pain Unit will likely grow in sophistication and see more widespread use in the future of emergency medicine. In centers with large indigent populations who may have difficulty obtaining outpatient follow up, emergency physicians will increasingly incorporate this observational method. As an alternative to hospital admission, this diagnostic modality offers a cost-effective means of observing and testing low-risk patients.

Table 14-3. Diagnostic clues to cause of chest pain.[a]

Cause	History						Signs	Other Abnormalities	Other Comments
	Previous Attacks of Similar Pain	Pain			Duration	Common Associated Findings			
		Location	Character	Onset					
Angina	Usually	Restrosternal, radiating to arms, neck, back, or epigastrium	Squeezing, dull ache	Often with stress or exercise	2–10 min up to 20–30 min	Occasionally dyspnea; dizziness and syncope rare	Often none. S_4 occasionally	ECG often normal between attacks	Relieved by nitroglycerin
Acute myocardial Infarction	In some cases	Restrosternal, radiating to arms, neck, back, or epigastrium	Squeezing, dull ache, increase with time	No precipitating factor necessary	>30 min	Nausea and vomiting, diaphoresis, dyspnea	Heart failure, restlessness, shock; cardiac examination often normal	ECG may be diagnostic or normal	Elevated CK, CK-MB isoenzymes and Troponin I or T. Normal isoenzymes levels on one determination do not exclude diagnosis
Mitral valve prolapse	Usually	Variable	Variable	Variable	Variable; usually hours	Dyspnea, dizziness common; syncope in some	Midsystolic click or murmur in most cases	ECG may shown inverted T waves on leads II, III, and aVF. Echocardiogram is diagnostic	Arrhythmia or sudden death may occur. Usually seen in young women, high-arched palate or chest or spine deformities may be present
Aortic stenosis	May have occurred	Like angina	Like angina	Like angina	Like angina	Syncope, dyspnea	Systolic ejection murmur transmitted to carotid arteries; delayed carotid pulse	ECG usually shows left ventricular hypertrophy. Echocardiography and angiocardiography are diagnostic	More common in older men
Aortic regurgitation	May have occurred	Like angina	Like angina	Like angina	May be prolonged	Dyspnea	Diastolic murmur transmitted to carotid arteries. Water-hammer and Quincke's pulse. Wide arterial pulse pressure	ECG may be normal or may show left ventricular hypertrophy. Echocardiographyand angiocardiography are diagnostic	History of rheumatic heart disease, connective tissue disease, or syphilis
Pericarditis	May have occurred	Retrosternal	Variable; often pleuritic and relieved by sitting	Variable	Hours to days	Variable	Pericardial friction rub in many	ECG may be diagnostic, nonspecific, or normal. Echocardiography often shows fluid	Recent history of upper respiratory Infection

(continued)

Table 14–3. Diagnostic clues to cause of chest pain.[a] (*Continued*)

Cause	History — Previous Attacks of Similar Pain	History — Pain — Location	History — Pain — Character	History — Pain — Onset	History — Pain — Duration	Common Associated Findings	Signs	Other Abnormalities	Other Comments
Aortic dissection	No	Retrosternal and back	Tearing, maximal at onset	Sudden	Variable	Myocardial infarction, stroke, limb ischemia, syncope	Stroke, absent pulses, hematuria, shock	Chest X-ray may show widened mediastinum or be normal. ECG may show acute myocardial infarction. Pulsatile abdominal mass	Angiography or CT scan is definitive. Hypertension or connective tissue disease may be present
Pleurisy	In some cases	Variable; usually lateral thorax	Pleuritic	Usually sudden	Variable	Subjective dyspnea	Often none. Occasionally friction rub, low-grade fever	Occasionally pleural effusion	
Pneumothorax	May have occurred	Variable	Variable often pleuritic	Usually sudden	Variable	Dyspnea and cough; shock if tension pneumothorax is present	Tachycardia, lung collapse with or without mediastinal shift	Chest X-ray is diagnostic but needs careful examination	Negative lung scan, spiral chest CT scan, or pulmonary angiogram
Pneumomediastinum	No	Retrosternal	Variable; often pleuritic	Usually sudden	Variable	Dyspnea	Mediastinal crunch	Chest X-ray is diagnostic. Pneumothorax common	Consider esophageal perforation as cause
Pulmonary hypertension	Usually	Retrosternal	like angina	like angina	Variable	Dyspnea, fatigue, exercise syncope	Loud P_2, right ventricular lift	ECG show right heart strain. Chest X-rays shows signs of pulmonary hypertension	
Pulmonary embolism	May have occurred	Variable; usually lateral thorax	Usually strong pleuritic component	Usually sudden	Minutes to hours	Dyspnea, cough, and tachypnea; hemoptysis sometimes	Friction rub or splinting in some	Hypoxemia and hypocapnia. Chest X-ray usually abnormal, but findings are not specific	Abnormal ventilation-perfusion radionucleotide lung scan, spiral CT chest, or pulmonary angiogram
Pneumonia	Rare	Over affected lobe	Pleuritic	Variable	Variable	Fever and chills, cough, dyspnea, sputum production	Fever, rales with or without consolidation, friction rub	Infiltrates on chest X-ray; purulent sputum	

(*continued*)

Table 14-3. Diagnostic clues to cause of chest pain.[a] (*Continued*)

		History							
		Pain							
Cause	Previous Attacks of Similar Pain	Location	Character	Onset	Duration	Common Associated Findings	Signs	Other Abnormalities	Other Comments
Esophagitis Esophageal spasm Hiatal hernia	Usually	Retrosternal or epigastrium	Changes with eating	Usually gradual	Variable	Gastrointestinal symptoms	None	Positive barium swallow or endoscopy	Relieved by antacids, H2 blockers, or proton pump inhibitors
Perforated esophagus	No	Retrosternal	Severe	Usually sudden	Variable	Variable	Subcutaneous emphysema, mediastinal crunch	Chest X-ray usually shows pneumomediastinum, pneumothorax, or pleural effusion. Esophagogram or esophagoscopy is diagnostic	History of severe retching or vomiting or esophageal trauma or instrumentation.
Perforated duodenal ulcer	No, or milder pain of ulcer	Retrosternal to epigastrium	Severe	Variable	Variable	Variable	Epigastric pain. May have prominent findings of peritoneal irritation	Free air in peritoneum; elevated amylase	Rare as cause of chest pain
Pancreatitis	May have occurred	Retrosternal to epigastrium	Variable	Variable	Hours to days	Vomiting, anorexia	Epigastric or upper quadrant tenderness	Markedly elevated serum lipase or amylase	Rare as cause of chest pain
Cholecystitis	Usually	Right upper quadrant; occasionally epigastrium or retrosternal	Variable	Usually sudden	Hours to days	Vomiting, anorexia, fever	Epigastric or right upper quadrant tenderness	Abnormal liver function tests. Sonography usually diagnostic	Rare as cause of chest pain
Musculoskeletal disorder (eg, Tietze's syndrome, stitch), rib fracture	Variable	Costochondral junction; retrosternal and lateral	Pleuritic ache, "sticking" sensation	Gradual to sudden	Variable; fleeting for stitch	Splinting	Tender (or, rarely, swollen), costosternal junction, especially first and second ribs. Point tenderness over affected ribs	None.	Relieved by lidocaine-corticosteroid injection.

[a]The shaded areas are the most helpful diagnostically.

MANAGEMENT OF SPECIFIC DISORDERS CAUSING CHEST PAIN

CARDIOVASCULAR DISORDERS

ACUTE CORONARY SYNDROME

See Chapter 35.

MYOCARDIAL INFARCTION

See Chapter 35.

MITRAL VALVE PROLAPSE

ESSENTIALS OF DIAGNOSIS

▶ Has late systolic click

▶ Palpitations are the most frequent complaint

▶ Clinical Findings

Consider mitral valve prolapse in any patient with a mitral regurgitation murmur or clicks (without other known heart disease or other cause of chest pain) who presents with recurring atypical chest pains. The ECG may show nonspecific T-wave abnormalities. Echocardiography is required for definitive diagnosis.

▶ Treatment

No specific emergency therapy is required. Although life-threatening arrhythmias may occur, they are rare. β-blocker therapy (eg, metoprolol, 50 mg orally twice daily) may be offered to patients who are uncomfortably symptomatic.

▶ Disposition

Refer patients to a cardiologist or primary care physician for definitive evaluation and management.

AORTIC STENOSIS AND REGURGITATION

ESSENTIALS OF DIAGNOSIS

▶ Classic triad: angina, syncope, and heart failure

▶ Crescendo–decrescendo systolic murmur is classic finding in aortic stenosis, loudest at second right intercostal space

▶ Aortic regurgitation is a high-pitched, blowing decrescendo diastolic murmur

▶ Clinical Findings

A. Aortic Stenosis and Regurgitation

Aortic stenosis may have a latent period of 10–20 years. Symptoms may develop gradually and eventually culminate in the classic triad of chest pain, heart failure, and syncope. Aortic regurgitation chest pain occurs less often than in patients with aortic stenosis. However, nocturnal angina, often accompanied by diaphoresis, may occur when the heart rate slows and arterial diastolic pressure falls to extremely low levels.

Chest pain in patients with severe aortic stenosis or regurgitation is clinically similar to that of angina and is probably the result of a similar mechanism, that is, relative myocardial ischemia secondary to diminished coronary blood flow.

Anginal pain in a patient with aortic valve disease may indicate that hemodynamically significant abnormalities of the valve are present, with a higher risk of impending sudden death. Murmurs of aortic stenosis or regurgitation are present on physical examination, often with adjunctive findings indicating severe valvular disease (eg, thrill over the carotid artery, wide pulse pressure; see Table 14–3).

▶ Treatment

Provide symptomatic treatment pending further evaluation for definitive treatment. Begin oxygen, 4 L/min, by nasal cannula, and obtain an ECG. Insert an intravenous catheter (18–20 gauge) and begin an infusion of normal saline to keep the catheter open or insert a saline lock IV. Give nitroglycerin, 0.3–0.4 mg sublingually, for pain. Patients with aortic stenosis may be hemodynamically very sensitive to nitrates. If nitroglycerin is not effective, give morphine, 2–4 mg intravenously as tolerated. Monitor the patient closely and discontinue medication if any signs of decompensation develop.

▶ Disposition

Hospitalization is warranted because of the imminent risk of decompensation or sudden death. Patients should be evaluated for cardiac catheterization or valve replacement with or without coronary bypass.

PERICARDITIS

See Chapter 35.

AORTIC DISSECTION

See Chapter 40.

PULMONARY DISORDERS

PLEURISY AND PLEURODYNIA

See also Chapter 33.

ESSENTIALS OF DIAGNOSIS

▶ Coxsackievirus b is the most common cause
▶ Sudden lancinating chest pain
▶ Associated with fever, malaise, and headaches

Clinical Findings

Patients with idiopathic pleurisy or pleurodynia are generally young, and the onset of illness is acute, with severe pleuritic chest pain. Apart from low-grade fever in some patients and possible friction rub, other findings on physical examination are usually normal. Chest X-ray may show a small pleural effusion, with or without a small pulmonary infiltrate. Viruses (especially enteroviruses) are the usual causative agents.

An accurate diagnosis of pleurisy is important because its symptoms are similar to those of pulmonary embolism. Pleurisy is often a diagnosis of exclusion.

Treatment

Pleurisy and pleurodynia are benign, self-limited diseases, and only symptomatic measures are necessary. Although aspirin is sufficient for most patients, indomethacin, 25–50 mg orally three times daily, is reported to be more effective.

Disposition

Hospitalization is rarely indicated (only for relief of severe pain). Refer patients to an outpatient clinic for tuberculin testing and repeat chest X-ray.

SPONTANEOUS PNEUMOTHORAX

See Chapter 33.

TRAUMATIC PNEUMOTHORAX

See Chapter 25.

PNEUMOMEDIASTINUM

See also Chapter 33

ESSENTIALS OF DIAGNOSIS

▶ "Crunch" of subcutaneous air is felt on examination
▶ Chest X-ray is diagnostic
▶ Retrosternal pain

Clinical Findings

Pneumomediastinum is frequently associated with pneumothorax. It is characterized by severe boring pain located retrosternally or in adjacent areas; the pain sometimes radiates to the back. Chills, fever, and shock may be present, especially if there is concurrent mediastinitis. A mediastinal "crunch" on auscultation or air in the mediastinum on chest X-ray is diagnostic.

Treatment

Give oxygen by nasal cannula or mask. Insert an intravenous catheter and keep it open with normal saline. Give morphine for pain.

Treat pneumothorax with tube thoracostomy as indicated. Evaluate the patient thoroughly to rule out serious underlying disease, ruptured bronchus, or a ruptured esophagus. Rupture of the esophagus is invariably associated with mediastinitis.

Disposition

Hospitalize patients for observation and examination to rule out serious precipitating factors such as rupture of the trachea, bronchus, or esophagus. Refer patients with chronic or recurrent pneumomediastinum for outpatient care.

PULMONARY HYPERTENSION

See also Chapter 33

ESSENTIALS OF DIAGNOSIS

▶ Dyspnea, exertional syncope, and exertional chest pain
▶ Evidence of right ventricular failure almost always present
▶ Prominent P_2 (pulmonic) heart sound
▶ Doppler echocardiography can help make diagnosis

Clinical Findings

Severe or sudden onset of significant pulmonary hypertension may cause an oppressive retrosternal sensation or frank angina associated with dyspnea on exertion. A history of easy fatigability, weakness, syncope on exertion, and hemoptysis may be elicited. A loud P_2 and right ventricular lift on physical examination suggest pulmonary hypertension. The ECG may reveal strain in the right side of the heart or cor pulmonale (right axis deviation; depressed ST segment and inverted T waves in leads II, III, aVF, and V1–5; and tall, peaked P waves in leads II, III, and aVF). On chest X-ray a large right ventricle or large pulmonary vessels are diagnostic.

▶ Treatment

No specific treatment is available for pulmonary hypertension. Administer oxygen for hypoxia and treat other abnormalities (bronchopulmonary infection, recurrent pulmonary emboli, heart failure) that may be exacerbating the pulmonary hypertension.

▶ Disposition

Hospitalization is indicated for patients with severe pain, hypoxia, or severe heart failure. Refer patients to a cardiologist for complete evaluation to rule out repairable lesions and to evaluate patients for treatment with anticoagulants or other investigational treatments.

PULMONARY EMBOLISM

See Chapter 33.

PNEUMONIA

See Chapter 42.

GASTROINTESTINAL DISORDERS

ESOPHAGEAL DISORDERS

▶ Clinical Findings

Esophageal disorders such as esophagitis, spasm, motility disorders, and gastroesophageal reflux frequently cause retrosternal chest pain that can be difficult to differentiate from pain due to cardiac causes. When cardiac disease is excluded, esophageal disorder is the most common cause of chest pain. Characteristic features of chest pain of esophageal origin include pain that is burning in nature, often radiates along the sternum, is made worse by lying down and relieved by sitting, may be induced by swallowing, and often persists for hours after a shorter episode of more intense pain. Rest, sublingual nitroglycerin, "GI cocktails," and calcium channel blockers can relieve pain of both cardiac and esophageal origin and should not be used as diagnostic aids. Because cardiac disease is more life threatening, cardiac causes of chest pain must be excluded with a high degree of certainty before attributing the symptoms to an esophageal disorder.

Diagnostic tests include barium swallow, endoscopy, manometry, and pH monitoring. Definitive emergency diagnosis of the esophageal disorder is seldom warranted.

▶ Treatment

General symptomatic treatment can be offered to patients who are in discomfort because the specific esophageal disorder is not usually known at the time of the emergency visit. A trial of viscous lidocaine, 15 mL mixed with 15 mL of an antacid given orally, can be tried for acute relief. Clinicians are cautioned to avoid attributing chest pain symptoms to an esophageal cause based entirely on improvement in chest discomfort after a "GI cocktail." Other measures include eating frequent small meals, using antacids, avoiding food before sleep, and using bed blocks (10–15 cm [4–6 in] high) under the head of the bed. If gastroesophageal reflux is suspected, H_2-receptor blocker or proton pump inhibitor therapy may be tried.

▶ Disposition

If an esophageal disorder is diagnosed as the cause of chest pain and cardiac disease or other life-threatening conditions can be excluded with confidence, refer the patient for outpatient care within 1–2 weeks.

PERFORATED ESOPHAGUS

See also Chapter 24

 ESSENTIALS OF DIAGNOSIS

▶ Severe chest pain
▶ Pain increased with swallowing or breathing
▶ Chest X-ray may reveal air within the mediastinum, pleural cavity, pericardium, or subcutaneous tissue

▶ Clinical Findings

Esophageal perforation is marked by agonizing retrosternal chest pain associated with pneumomediastinum, pneumothorax, pneumonia, or purulent pleural effusion. A recent history of severe retching, vomiting (Boerhaave's syndrome), or endoscopy is often present. The diagnosis is confirmed by an esophagogram using water-soluble contrast medium or esophagoscopy.

▶ Treatment

See Chapter 24.

▶ Disposition

Hospitalize the patient in a critical care unit for resuscitation, physiologic monitoring, limiting the extent of mediastinal contamination (NPO and nasogastric tube decompression), broad-spectrum antibiotics, and usually surgical treatment.

PERFORATED STOMACH OR DUODENUM

See also Chapter 15

ESSENTIALS OF DIAGNOSIS

▶ Often a history of peptic ulcer disease
▶ Vomiting is common
▶ Acute distress
▶ Acute abdominal X-ray may reveal free air in the abdomen

▶ Clinical Findings

Perforation distal to the esophagus is characterized by sudden onset of severe pain that is usually epigastric but may be retrosternal and may radiate to the back. A history of chronic epigastric pain or ulcer disease often is present. Epigastric tenderness and diminished or absent bowel sounds may be found. If peritonitis has supervened, rebound tenderness and a rigid abdomen are present. Air under the diaphragm may be seen on an X-ray. Serum amylase or lipase levels may be elevated as a result of posterior perforation into the pancreas. Leukocytosis with a shift to the left often is present.

▶ Treatment

Insert a large-bore intravenous catheter, and give crystaloid solutions intravenously to support blood pressure. Give morphine for pain.

Insert a nasogastric tube and begin continuous suction. Obtain urgent surgical consultation and begin prophylactic intravenous antibiotics (see Table 15–1).

▶ Disposition

Hospitalize the patient at once for emergency surgery.

PANCREATITIS

See Chapter 15.

CHOLECYSTITIS

See Chapter 15.

MUSCULOSKELETAL DISORDERS

COSTOCHONDRAL SEPARATION, RIB FRACTURES, AND INTERCOSTAL MUSCLE STRAIN

See also Chapter 24.

ESSENTIALS OF DIAGNOSIS

▶ Pain associated with movement
▶ X-rays may reveal a fractured rib
▶ Often a history of trauma

▶ Clinical Findings

In this group of musculoskeletal disorders, pain is usually worse with movement and breathing. A history of minor trauma, strenuous exercise, or severe coughing often is present. Pain is localized and elicited by palpation. Chest X-ray may be normal or may show rib fractures if they are present.

▶ Treatment

Oral analgesics and nonsteroidal anti-inflammatory drugs (NSAIDs) are effective for analgesia. Local heat alone may provide relief. Narcotic analgesics may be required if respiratory effort is affected because of pain. Splinting is generally not recommended for rib fractures, because it may impair respiratory function and promote atelectasis or pneumonia. For patients with rib fractures, ensure that a pneumothorax is not present on X-ray.

▶ Disposition

Refer the patient for outpatient follow-up if pain is severe or persistent.

DISK DISEASE: CERVICAL AND THORACIC

ESSENTIALS OF DIAGNOSIS

▶ Pain radiates from neck or back to arms
▶ Paresthesia in fingers
▶ Weakness in arm with decreased reflexes

▶ Clinical Findings

Disk disease may cause paroxysmal pain radiating from the back of the neck into the arms and fingers. The pain is aggravated by coughing, sneezing, and straining. Neck movement is restricted by cervical muscle spasm. The patient may have paresthesias and pain in the fingers, weakness of hand and forearm muscles, and decreased biceps and triceps reflexes. Narrowing of the vertebral interspace may be seen on a plain film, and magnetic resonance imaging confirms the diagnosis.

Treatment

Treatment is symptomatic. Superficial heat may relax muscles and be of value. A soft cervical collar is recommended only for acute soft-tissue neck injuries and should not exceed 3–4 days of continuous use.

Disposition

Hospitalization is rarely required, even for patients with severe disk disease. Outpatient follow-up by a spinal surgeon is recommended. Mild cases can be treated on an outpatient basis.

TIETZE'S SYNDROME: COSTOCHONDRITIS

ESSENTIALS OF DIAGNOSIS

▶ Remember that cardiac pain also can be reproducible by palpation
▶ Pain is localized to a specific point

Clinical Findings

Tietze's syndrome affects the costochondral or chondrosternal junctions with localized tenderness.

Treatment

Pain usually is relieved by NSAIDs or other oral analgesics.

Disposition

Refer the patient for outpatient follow-up if pain is severe or persistent.

MUSCLE SPASM: "STITCH"

ESSENTIALS OF DIAGNOSIS

▶ History of trauma or exercise

Clinical Findings

The patient complains of aching pain, usually in localized areas but sometimes more generalized. Pain often increases with movement and palpation. A history of minor trauma or strenuous exercise may be present. Chest radiograph is normal.

Treatment

Massage, heat, and other local treatments are effective. Aspirin or other NSAIDs are useful.

Disposition

Refer the patient for outpatient follow-up as needed. A search for more serious illnesses (eg, myositis, arthritis, Pancoast tumor) may be necessary in recurrent or persistent cases that have no obvious cause.

MISCELLANEOUS DISORDERS

INTRATHORACIC NEOPLASM

ESSENTIALS OF DIAGNOSIS

▶ History of fever, night sweats, and weight loss
▶ Cough or hemoptysis
▶ Chest X-ray may reveal a mass

Clinical Findings

Intrathoracic neoplasm is suggested by a mass seen on chest X-ray with no other explanation for the chest pain.

Treatment

Give analgesics and other supportive measures as required.

Disposition

Depending on their general condition, patients with intrathoracic neoplasms should be either hospitalized or referred for timely evaluation by a pulmonologist.

VARICELLA ZOSTER

See also Chapter 48.

ESSENTIALS OF DIAGNOSIS

▶ Vesicles in a dermatomal pattern
▶ Does not cross midline
▶ Pain may precede vesicles

Clinical Findings

In the pre-eruptive stage of zoster, pain felt on the skin surface in dermatomal distribution may occur several days before the characteristic skin lesions (clusters of clear, fluid-filled vesicles in a dermatomal distribution) appear. Pain is typically unilateral and does not cross the midline. Hypoesthesia in dermatomal distribution may also be present.

The appearance of the skin lesions confirms the diagnosis. Rarely, patients may present with pain as the only manifestation of the disease; in such patients, a rise in antibody titer is diagnostic.

▶ Treatment

Give analgesics as necessary; narcotics may be required for relief. Acyclovir, 800 mg orally five times daily for 7–10 days, or famciclovir, 500 mg orally three times a day for 7 days, if given within 72 hours of onset, may alleviate symptoms, shorten the duration of illness, and reduce the incidence of postherpetic neuralgia, a special concern in elderly patients. Local nerve block with long-acting anesthetics (eg, bupivacaine [Marcaine, Sensorcaine]) is effective and obviates the need for narcotics and their associated side effects. It may also decrease the incidence and severity of postherpetic neuralgia. Prednisone, 60 mg orally daily (tapered over 2 weeks), may also decrease the incidence and severity of postherpetic neuralgia in elderly patients.

▶ Disposition

Patients with severe cases (extensive localized disease, dissemination, immunosuppression) may require hospitalization for pain control and possible treatment with intravenous acyclovir. Other patients may be referred for outpatient evaluation and continued treatment (analgesia).

ACC/AHA 2006 guidelines for the management of patients with valvular heart disease: a report of the American College of Cardiology/American Heart Association Task Force on Practice Guidelines (writing committee to revise the 1998 Guidelines for the Management of Patients With Valvular Heart Disease): developed in collaboration with the Society of Cardiovascular Anesthesiologists: endorsed by the Society for Cardiovascular Angiography and Interventions and the Society of Thoracic Surgeons. American College of Cardiology/American Heart Association Task Force on Practice Guidelines; Society of Cardiovascular Anesthesiologists; Society for Cardiovascular Angiography and Interventions; Society of Thoracic Surgeons, Bonow RO, Carabello BA, Kanu C et al: Circulation. 2006;114(5): e84–e231 [PMID: 16880336].

Amsterdam EA, Kirk JD, Diercks DB et al: Exercise testing in chest pain units: rationale, implementation, and results.Cardiol Clin 2005;23(4):503–516 (vii. Review) [PMID: 16278120].

Avora RR, Venkatesh P, Molnar J: Short- and long- term mortality with nesiritide. Am Heart J 2007;152:1084 [PMID: 17161057].

Aziz S, Ramsdale DR: Acute dissection of the thoracic aorta. Hosp Med 2004;65(3):136–142 [PMID: 15052903].

Brady WJ et al: Electrocardiographic diagnosis of acute myocardial infarction. Emerg Med Clin North Am 2001;19(2):295 [PMID: 11373980].

Bushnell J, Brown J: Evidence-based emergency medicine/rational clinical examination abstract. Clinical assessment for acute thoracic aortic dissection. Ann Emerg Med 2005;46(1):90–92 [PMID: 15988435].

Campillo-Soto A et al: Spontaneous pneumomediastinum: descriptive study of our experience with 36 cases. Arch Bronconeumol 2005;41(9):528–531 [PMID: 16194517].

Chinnaiyan KM, Raff GL, Goldstein JA: Cardiac CT in the emergency department. Cardiol Clin 2009;27(4):587–596 (Review) [PMID: 19766915].

Collins SP, Hinckley WR, Storrow AB: Critical review and recommendations for nesiritide use in the emergency department. J Emerg Med 2005;29(3):317–329 [PMID: 16183453].

Diercks DB, Kirk JD, Amsterdam EA: Chest pain units: management of special populations. Cardiol Clin 2005;23(4):549–557 (viii. Review) [PMID: 16278124].

Diercks DB, Kirk JD, Lindsell CJ et al: Door-to-ECG time in patients with chest pain presenting to the ED. Am J Emerg Med 2006;24:1 [PMID: 16338501].

Duvernoy CS, Bates ER: Management of cardiogenic shock attributable to acute myocardial infarction in the reperfusion era. J Intensive Care Med 2005;20(4):188–198 [PMID: 16061902].

Eichinger S, Weltermann A, Minar E et al: Symptomatic pulmonary embolism and the risk of recurrent venous thromboembolism. Arch Intern Med 2004;164:92 [PMID: 14718328].

Ekelund U, Forberg JL: New methods for improved evaluation of patients with suspected acute coronary syndrome in the emergency department. Emerg Med J 2007;24(12):811–814 (Review). [PMID: 18029508].

Fedullo PF, Tapson VF: Clinical practice. The evaluation of suspected pulmonary embolism. N Engl J Med 2003;349(13): 1247–1256 [PMID: 14507950].

Fesmire FM, Decker WW, Diercks DB et al: Clinical policy: critical issues in the evaluation and management of non-ST-segment elevation acute coronary syndromes. Ann Emerg Med 2006;48:270 [PMID: 16934648].

Goodacre S, Locker T, Morris F et al: How useful are clinical features in the diagnosis of acute, undifferentiated chest pain? Acad Emerg Med 2002;9:203 [PMID: 11874776].

Gutterman DD: Silent myocardial ischemia. Circ J 2009;73(5): 785–797 (Review) [PMID: 19703877].

Halpern EJ: Triple-rule-out CT angiography for evaluation of acute chest pain and possible acute coronary syndrome. Radiology 2009;252(2):332–345 (Review).

Hillen TJ, Wessell DE: Multidetector CT scan in the evaluation of chest pain of nontraumatic musculoskeletal origin. Radiol Clin North Am 2010;48(1):185–191 [PMID: 19995636].

Hollander JE, Gibson CM, Pollack CV Jr: Hospitals with and without percutaneous coronary intervention capability: considerations for treating acute coronary syndromes. Am J Emerg Med 2009;27(5):595–606 (Review) [PMID: 19497467].

Howlett JG: Acutely decompensated congestive heart failure: new therapies for an old problem. Expert Rev Cardiovasc Ther 2005;3(5):925–936 [PMID: 16181036].

Iakobishvili Z et al: Does current treatment of cardiogenic shock complicating the acute coronary syndromes comply with guidelines? Am Heart J 2005;149(1):98–103 [PMID: 15660040].

Karcz A, Korn R, Burke MC et al: Malpractice claims against emergency physicians in Massachusetts: 1975–1993. Am J Emerg Med 1996;14:341 [PMID: 8768150].

Kontos MC: Evaluation of the emergency department chest pain patient. Cardiol Rev 2001;9(5):266 [PMID: 11520450].

Kucher N, Goldhaber SZ: Management of massive pulmonary embolism. Circulation 2005;112(2):e28–e32 [PMID: 16009801].

Lange RA, Hillis LD: Clinical practice. Acute pericarditis. N Engl J Med 2004;351(21):2195–2202 [PMID: 15548780].

Limkakeng AT, Halpern E, Takakuwa KM: Sixty-four slice multidetector computed tomography: The future of ED cardiac care. Am J Emerg Med 2007;25:450 [PMID:17499666].

Mohammed AA, Januzzi JL Jr: Clinical applications of highly sensitive troponin assays. Cardiol Rev 2010;18(1):12–19 [PMID: 20010334].

Morrow DA, Cannon CPNACB Writing Group M et al: National Academy of Clinical Biochemistry laboratory medicine practice guidelines: Clinical characteristics and utilization of biochemical markers in acute coronary syndromes. Circulation 2007;115:e356 [PMID: 17384001].

Ng SM et al: Ninety-minute accelerated critical pathway for chest pain evaluation. Am J Cardiol 2001;88:611 [PMID: 11564382].

Phillips K, Luk A, Soor GS, Abraham JR, Leong S, Butany J: Cocaine cardiotoxicity: a review of the pathophysiology, pathology, and treatment options. Am J Cardiovasc Drugs 2009;9(3):177–196 (Review) [PMID: 19463023].

Pope JH, Aufderheide TP, Ruthazer R et al: Missed diagnoses of acute cardiac ischemia in the emergency department. N Engl J Med 2000;342:1163 [PMID:10770981].

Rahimtoola A, Bergin JD: Acute pulmonary embolism: an update on diagnosis and management. Curr Probl Cardiol 2005;30(2):61–114 [PMID: 15650680].

Rubin LJ: Primary pulmonary hypertension, review of the treatments. N Engl J Med 1997;336:111 [PMID: 8988890].

Rubins JB: The current approach to the diagnosis of pulmonary embolism: lessons from PIOPED II. Postgrad Med 2008;120(1):1–7 (Review) [PMID: 18467802].

Rubinshtein R, Halon DA, Gaspar T et al: Usefulness of 64-slice cardiac computed tomographic angiography for diagnosing acute coronary syndromes and predicting clinical outcome in emergency department patients with chest pain of uncertain origin. Circulation 2007;115:1762 [PMID: 17372178].

Shiga T, Wajima Z, Apfel CC et al: Diagnostic accuracy of transesophageal echocardiography, helical computed tomography, and magnetic resonance imaging for suspected thoracic aortic dissection: systematic review and meta-analysis. Arch Intern Med 2006;166:1350 [PMID: 16831999].

Spodick DH: Acute cardiac tamponade. N Engl J Med 2003;349(7):684–690 [PMID: 12917306].

Stankus SJ, Dlugopolski M, Packer D: Management of herpes zoster (shingles) and postherpetic neuralgia. Am Fam Physician 2000;61:2437 [PMID: 10794584].

Stein PD, Fowler SE, Goodman LR et al: Multidetector computed tomography for acute pulmonary embolism. N Engl J Med 2006;354:2317 [PMID:16738268].

Stern S, Bayes de Luna A: Coronary artery spasm: a 2009 update. Circulation 2009;119(18):2531–2534 (Review) [PMID: 19433770].

Thygesen K, Alpert JS, White HD et al: Universal definition of myocardial infarction. Circulation 2007;116:2634 [PMID: 17951284].

Troughton RW, Asher CR, Klein AL: Pericarditis. Lancet 2004;363:717 [PMID: 15001332].

Launbjerg J, Fruergaard P, Hesse B et al: Long-term risk of death, cardiac events and recurrent chest pain in patients with acute chest pain of different origin. Cardiology 1996;87:60 [PMID: 8631047].

Vial CM, Whyte RI: Boerhaave's syndrome: diagnosis and treatment. Surg Clin North Am 2005;85(3):515–524, ix [PMID: 15927648] (Review).

Wang CS et al: Does this dyspneic patient in the emergency department have congestive heart failure? JAMA 2005;294(15): 1944–1956 [PMID: 16234501].

Wells PS, Anderson DR, Rodger M et al: Excluding pulmonary embolism at the bedside without diagnostic imaging: management of patients with suspected pulmonary embolism presenting to the emergency department by using a simple clinical model and d-dimer. Ann Intern Med 2001;135:98 [PMID: 11453709].

Woo KM, Schneider JI: High-risk chief complaints I: chest pain-the big three. Emerg Med Clin North Am 2009;27(4):685–712 x (Review) [PMID: 19932401].

Zalenski RJ, Shamsa F, Pede KJ: Evaluation and risk stratification of patients with chest pain in the emergency department. Predictors of life-threatening events. Emerg Med Clin North Am 1998;16:495 [PMID: 9739772].

Abdominal Pain

15

Justin Coomes, MD

Melissa Platt, MD[1]

Immediate Management of Life-Threatening Problems
Further Evaluation of the Patient with Abdominal Pain
   History
   Physical Examination
   Laboratory Examination
   Radiologic Examination
Additional Measures for the Management of
Acute Abdomen
Management of Specific Disorders Causing Abdominal Pain
   Intestinal Disorders
   Hepatobiliary Disorders

Vascular Disorders
Urinary Disorders
Acute Pancreatitis
Gynecologic Disorders
Primary Peritonitis
Retroperitoneal Hemorrhage
Conditions Causing Acute Abdominal Pain
that are not Amenable to Surgery

IMMEDIATE MANAGEMENT OF LIFE-THREATENING PROBLEMS

See Figure 15–1.

▶ Perform a Brief Examination

First, determine if the patient is stable or not. Distinguishing stability or instability is best performed pragmatically through multiple, simultaneous steps.

1. Look at the patient and identify if the patient is ill appearing.

2. Evaluate responsiveness, focusing on eye opening, and verbal and motor responses.

3. Assess airway, breathing, and circulation.

4. Record and review a complete set of vital signs.

5. Gauge perfusion to the brain and extremities.

6. Continue the physical examination with inspection of the abdomen, looking for signs of an acute abdomen: rebound tenderness, board-like rigidity or guarding, or an obvious pulsatile mass.

7. If appropriate, perform a rectal examination earlier than later, inspecting for blood.

8. In the acute patient, emergency bedside ultrasound is helpful in identifying aortic aneurysm/dissection, intraperitoneal fluid, and/or IVC collapse (volume status).

9. If instability is confirmed, measures to stabilize the patient must be taken immediately.

Caution—A number of patients presenting to the ED with abdominal pain will have a source of that pain outside the abdomen, anatomically, as when epigastric or upper abdominal pain is caused by an acute myocardial infarction, pulmonary embolus, or pneumonia. Occasionally, abdominal pain is due to a metabolic derangement, as is the case with diabetic ketoacidosis. In brief, the differential diagnosis should extend beyond intra-abdominal pathology.

▶ Identify Candidates for Urgent Surgery

Some patients with abdominal pain will require surgical evaluation. Those requiring early surgical evaluation or

[1]This chapter is a revision of the chapter by Melissa Platt, MD, Samir Doshi, MD, & Eric Telfer, MD, from the 6th edition.

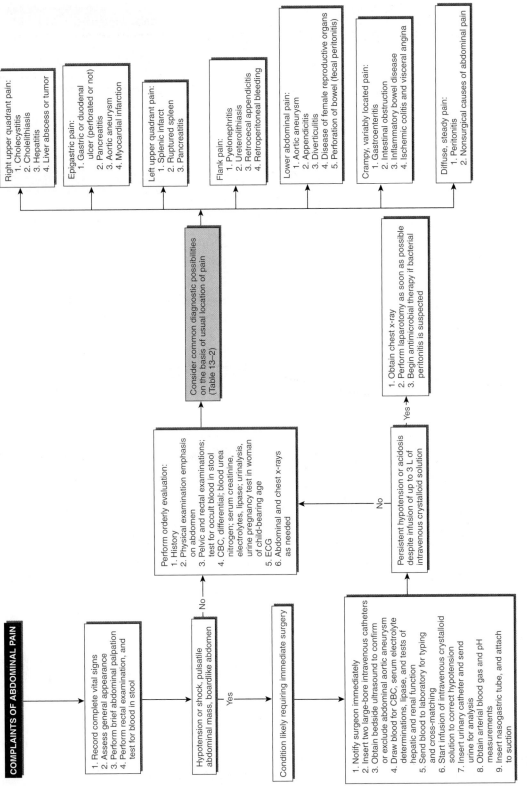

▲ **Figure 15-1.** Algorithmic approach to complaints of abdominal pain.

intervention include patients with an acute abdomen, a pulsatile abdominal mass, or shock with abdominal pain. If hypotension or hemodynamic instability is present with abdominal pain, especially with gastrointestinal bleeding or a rigid abdomen, there is a strong possibility of underlying life-threatening pathology, and surgical consultation should be immediately sought. One of the most critical decisions an ED physician can make is whether a surgeon should be involved or not. Therefore, it is of paramount importance to consider this question early and frequently throughout the evaluation.

▶ Treat Shock

Treat hypotension or frank shock (Chapter 11).

1. Give oxygen at a rate of 2–10 L/min by nasal cannula or mask. Keep oxygen saturation above 95%.

2. Insert two large-bore (≥16-gauge) intravenous catheters in an upper extremity.

3. Obtain blood for a complete blood count (CBC) with differential, serum electrolyte measurements, lipase measurement, renal function tests, liver function tests, serum pregnancy test, serum lactate, and a rapid bedside glucose test. Also, send a tube of blood for typing and crossmatching.

4. Consider emergency bedside ultrasound to evaluate for free intraperitoneal fluid and aortic aneurysm.

5. Immediately begin rapid infusion of crystalloid solution. Titrate rate of infusion to the blood pressure; initially, give a 1-L bolus over 10–20 minutes (adult dose). Remember to exercise caution in patients with congestive heart failure.

6. Insert a urinary catheter to monitor urine output, a sensitive indicator of visceral blood flow. Send a urine sample for analysis.

7. Obtain a blood gas to assess the patient's acid–base status and overall physiologic condition.

8. Insert a nasogastric tube if the patient shows evidence of intestinal obstruction. Also consider NG placement if peritonitis, severe ileus, or gastrointestinal bleeding are suspected.

9. Obtain a 12-lead ECG and begin continuous cardiac monitoring.

10. If bacterial peritonitis or perforated viscous is suspected, begin broad-spectrum antibiotics after appropriate cultures have been obtained (Table 15–1).

Note: Persistent shock despite fluid resuscitation in the patient with acute abdominal pain requires urgent laparotomy. Some patients will not be such that they can be stabilized prior to surgical intervention and must be taken for emergency intervention despite instability. Early surgical consultation is imperative.

Table 15–1. Antimicrobials for the Acute Abdomen.[a]

Minor to Moderate Disease	
Drug	**Dose**
Ampicillin-sulbactam	3.0 g IV every 6 hours
Metronidazole PLUS Cefazolin OR Ciprofloxacin OR Levofloxacin OR	500 mg IV every 6 hours 1.5 g IV every 8 hours 400 mg IV every 12 hours 750 mg IV daily
Moxifloxacin	400 mg IV daily
Ertapenem	1 g IV daily
Ticarcillin-clavulanate	3.1 g every 6 hours
Severe Disease	
Drug	**Dose**
Imipenem	500 mg IV every 8 hours
Meropenem	1 g IV every 8 hours
Piperacillin-Tazobactam	4.5 g IV every 8 hours
Ampicillin AND Metronidazole	2 g IV every 6 hours 500 mg IV every 8 hours
Aztreonam AND Metronidazole	2 g IV every 6 hours 500 mg IV every 8 hours

[a]Drug doses from 2009 EMRA Antibiotic Guide, edited by Brian J. Levine, MD.

▼ FURTHER EVALUATION OF THE PATIENT WITH ABDOMINAL PAIN

After the patient has been stabilized, reassess as described below unless immediate surgery is required (Table 15–2).

The importance of a good, thorough history cannot be overemphasized. The initial assessment and plan will be based on the physician's initial "stability" assessment and the meticulous history obtained thereafter. That history is crucial in helping the physician decide what laboratory and radiographic studies to acquire, what the differential diagnosis is, whether the patient needs surgical evaluation, whether the patient requires admission, etc.

HISTORY

The approach offered here is intended for nontraumatic abdominal pain. A history of abdominal trauma requires a different diagnostic approach, which has been discussed in Chapter 25. Pelvic pain in the female has been discussed in more detail in Chapter 38.

▶ Mode of Onset of Abdominal Pain

See Figure 15–2 and Table 15–2.

Table 15–2. Differential Diagnosis of the Common Causes of Acute Abdominal Pain.

Disease	Location of Pain and Prior Attacks	Mode of Onset and Type of Pain	Associated Gastrointestinal Symptoms	Physical Examination	Helpful Tests and Examinations
Acute appendicitis	Periumbilical or localized generally to right lower abdominal quadrant	Insidious to acute and persistent	Anorexia common; nausea and vomiting in some	Low-grade fever, epigastric tenderness initially; later, right lower quadrant	Slight leukocytosis; CT scan of the abdomen or ultrasound of the appendix may be helpful if diagnosis is uncertain
Intestinal obstruction	Diffuse	Sudden onset; Crampy	Vomiting common	Abdominal distention; high-pitched rushes	Dilated, fluid-filled loops of bowel on abdominal X-ray; CT scan with contrast
Perforated duodenal ulcer	Epigastric; history of ulcer in many	Abrupt onset; steady; worse when supine	Anorexia; nausea and vomiting	Epigastric tenderness; involuntary guarding	Upright abdominal X-ray shows air under diaphragm; CT scan
Diverticulitis	Left lower quadrant; history of previous attacks	Gradual onset; steady or crampy	Mild diarrhea common	Fever common; mass and tenderness in left lower quadrant	CT scan shows inflammation
Inflammatory bowel disease	Diffuse; primarily in lower abdomen; prior attacks common	Gradual onset; often crampy	Diarrhea common, often with blood and mucus	Fever; diffuse abdominal tenderness	Blood and leukocytes in stool; CT scan; abnormal results on proctosigmoidoscopy or barium enema
Acute cholecystitis	Epigastric or right upper quadrant; may be referred to right shoulder	Insidious to acute	Anorexia; nausea and vomiting	Right upper quadrant tenderness; may have fever	Right upper quadrant sonography shows gallstones, gall bladder wall thickening or pericholecystic fluid; radionucleotide scan shows nonvisualization of the gallbladder
Biliary colic	Intermittent right upper quadrant; prior attacks common	Often abrupt onset; dull to sharp	Anorexia; nausea and vomiting common	Right upper quadrant tenderness	Sonography shows gallstones
Ischemic colitis	Epigastric; diffuse; prior attacks common	Often abrupt; crampy	Diarrhea, commonly bloody	Diffuse abdominal tenderness; vascular disease elsewhere	Barium enema shows "thumbprinting" of mucosa; CT scan; visceral angiography shows vascular obstruction
Ruptured abdominal aortic aneurysm	Epigastrium and back	Abrupt; sharp and severe	Variable; may be none	Hypotension or shock; abdominal aneurysm; pulsatile mass	Sonography, CT scan, or angiography shows aneurysm
Rupture of spleen	Left upper quadrant or diffuse; may be referred to left shoulder; history of trauma common	Abrupt; severe	Usually none	Hypotension or shock; peritonitis; left upper quadrant tenderness; fractured left ribs in some	CT scan or liver–spleen scan shows rupture; U/S shows free fluid
Renal colic	Costovertebral or along course of ureter	Sudden; severe and sharp	Frequently nausea and vomiting	Flank tenderness	Hematuria; noncontrast CT scan of the abdomen or excretory urogram (obstruction, hydronephrosis)

(continued)

Table 15–2. Differential Diagnosis of the Common Causes of Acute Abdominal Pain. (*Continued*)

Disease	Location of Pain and Prior Attacks	Mode of Onset and Type of Pain	Associated Gastrointestinal Symptoms	Physical Examination	Helpful Tests and Examinations
Acute pancreatitis	Epigastric penetrating to back	Acute; persistent, dull, severe	Anorexia; nausea and vomiting common	Epigastric tenderness	Elevated serum lipase; CT scan shows pancreatic inflammation
Acute salpingitis	Bilateral adnexal; later, may be generalized	Gradually becomes worse	Nausea and vomiting may be present	Cervical motion elicits tenderness; mass if tubo-ovarian abscess is present	Ultrasound can rule out tubo-ovarian abscess
Ectopic pregnancy	Unilateral early; may have shoulder pain after rupture	Sudden or intermittently vague to sharp	Frequently none	Adnexal mass; tenderness	Pelvic ultrasound reveals adnexal mass or blood; positive pregnancy test

A. Abrupt Onset

The abrupt onset of severe abdominal pain should suggest a vascular accident or a rupture of a hollow viscus, especially if its severity is maximal at onset. On the other hand, pain that begins abruptly, but is only moderately severe at the time of onset, and worsens rapidly with time suggests nephrolithiasis, acute pancreatitis, mesenteric thrombosis, or small-bowel strangulation. If the pain is of lower abdominal or pelvic origin, ruptured ectopic pregnancy or ovarian follicle cyst should also be considered in females (Chapter 38).

B. Gradual Onset

Gradual onset of slowly worsening pain is the characteristic of peritoneal inflammation or infection. Patients with appendicitis or diverticulitis often report a gradual onset of pain that escalates.

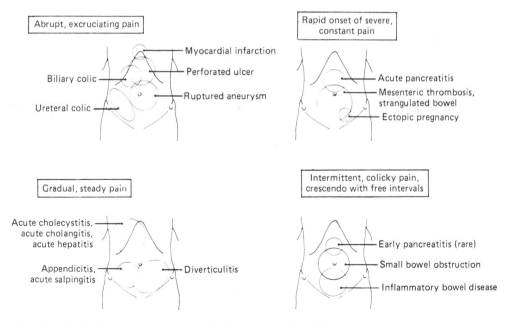

▲ **Figure 15–2.** Correlation between nature of abdominal pain and underlying condition. (Reproduced, with permission, from Way LW (editor): *Current Surgical Diagnosis & Treatment,* 9th ed. Lange, 1991.)

▶ Character of Pain

See Figure 15–2.

A. Severe Pain

Severe abdominal pain may be caused by many conditions, including renal colic, biliary colic, and various vascular conditions such as myocardial infarction, mesenteric ischemia, and rupture of an abdominal aortic aneurysm. Other conditions that cause severe pain include acute pancreatitis, perforation of a hollow viscus, and peritonitis.

B. Dull Pain

Dull, vague, poorly localized pain is typically gradual in onset. When these two findings are coupled, they suggest an inflammatory process or a low-grade infection, appendicitis, or diverticulitis, for example.

C. Intermittent Pain with Cramps

Intermittent, crampy abdominal pain is common in gastroenteritis. Crampy pain that occurs in regular cycles, rising and falling in a crescendo fashion, is more characteristic of a mechanical small-bowel obstruction, especially if pain-free intervals are present.

D. Absence of Pain

Occasionally, a patient will complain of a sense of abdominal fullness with a notion that a bowel movement will provide relief. A bowel movement, whether spontaneous or induced, usually fails to relieve discomfort, however. This is known as the "gas stoppage" sign and is characteristic of retrocecal appendicitis. It may also be present when any inflammatory lesion is walled off from the free peritoneal cavity.

▶ Location of Pain

The parietal peritoneum is innervated by somatic nerve fibers, producing pain that is generally well localized. In contrast, pain arising from visceral fibers alone tends to be poorly localized. Common examples of conditions associated with visceral pain sensation are hollow viscus distention and visceral ischemia.

A. Localized Abdominal Pain

(See Table 15–2.) In general, when abdominal pain becomes localized, it does so over or near the involved viscus, the right lower quadrant pain of appendicitis or the right upper quadrant pain of cholecystitis, for example. On the other hand, anatomic variants (eg, retrocecal appendix) must be kept in mind, and one must maintain a wide differential, considering all the possible etiologies of the pain.

B. Radiation of Pain or Shift in Localization

Radiation of pain or shift in localization of pain has particular diagnostic significance.

1. Shoulder pain—Ipsilateral diaphragmatic irritation by air, blood, or infection in the peritoneal cavity can cause shoulder pain. A classic example is cholecystitis, which may be associated with right shoulder pain.

2. Diffuse periumbilical and epigastric pain—Diffuse periumbilical and epigastric pain that gradually localizes to the right lower quadrant is a classic sign of appendicitis. With early appendicitis, only the visceral peritoneum surrounding the appendix is inflamed, and the localization is therefore poor. As the inflammation spreads to the parietal peritoneum, the pain localizes to the right lower quadrant. The retrocecal appendix, which is found in 15% of cases, is an important exception, with pain remaining poorly localized secondary to lack of parietal peritoneum involvement.

3. Pain radiating from the flank—Pain radiating from the flank to the groin or genitalia usually signifies ureteral colic, as seen in urolithiasis. The physician must also consider testicular pathology such as testicular torsion in any male patient with abdominal pain, whether that pain radiates to the groin or not.

▶ Anorexia, Nausea, and Vomiting

Anorexia, nausea, and vomiting are common with abdominal pain, especially abdominal pain having its source in the upper abdomen; nonetheless, severe intra-abdominal processes can occur without any of these symptoms. For example, one may retain a normal appetite with appendicitis if the appendix is isolated from the peritoneum, as may be the case with a retrocecal appendix or an appendix that is isolated by omentum.

Nausea and vomiting are infrequently the initial or dominant symptoms with surgical acute abdomen, making these symptoms preceding abdominal pain more indicative of less acute conditions such as food poisoning, gastroenteritis, acute gastritis, and acute pancreatitis. However, these symptoms may have developed after initial onset of pain in abdominal emergencies by the time the patient has sought medical attention.

▶ Fever and Rigors

Fever is common with many causes of abdominal pain, usually suggesting infection. Fever with continual rigors is most common in infections of the biliary and urinary system (eg, cholangitis and pyelonephritis). Fever with chills, jaundice, and hypotension suggests suppurative cholangitis, a surgical emergency. High fever with peritoneal signs in a female patient with no apparent general systemic illness otherwise is suggestive of acute salpingitis with pelvic peritonitis. Interestingly, appendicitis with high fever and rigors

Table 15–3. Routine for Physical Examination of Acute Abdomen.

Inspection
Auscultation
Palpation
    Examination of hernial rings and male genitalia
    Cough tenderness
    Rectus muscle spasm
    One-finger palpation
    Costovertebral angle tenderness
    Deep palpation
Percussion
Special signs (iliopsoas and obturator signs, etc)
Pelvic and rectal examinations

is uncommon unless peritonitis, most likely from viscus perforation, has developed. Recall that absence of fever is common in the elderly and immunosuppressed patients.

▶ Diarrhea, Constipation, and Obstipation

Constipation and obstipation may suggest intestinal obstruction or ileus but are usually not the primary symptoms in acute surgical intra-abdominal disease. Diarrhea, though common with gastroenteritis, is a nonspecific symptom that can be associated with colitis, diverticulitis, appendicitis, and salpingitis.

PHYSICAL EXAMINATION

The basic steps of the physical examination of the acute abdomen are outlined in Table 15–3. Remember that physical findings may be subtle in elderly or immuno-compromised patients.

▶ Inspection

The abdominal examination starts with visual inspection of abdomen and external genitalia. Significant findings include masses, distention, pregnancy, previous surgical scars, ecchymosis, a board-like abdomen, and stigmata of severe hepatic disease.

▶ Auscultation

While a silent abdomen, ie, complete absence of audible peristalsis, is thought to signify diffuse peritonitis, peristalsis may persist in the face of established peritonitis. Also, note that because peristalsis is related to meal intake, it may be necessary to listen for as long as 2–3 minutes to establish the absence of peristalsis, especially in those who have not eaten in quite a while. In general, it must be understood that auscultation may be less contributory to diagnosis, especially with findings of absent or normal bowel sounds. Even so, high-pitched bowel sounds can be suggestive of bowel obstruction.

▶ Palpation

A. Examine Hernial Rings and Genitalia

Examine the inguinal and femoral canals and the genitalia, primarily looking for incarcerated hernias that may be causing intestinal obstruction. This must be done by asking the patient to cough but should be done gently so as to cause as little discomfort as possible. It is optimal if this portion of the examination can take place with the patient standing as well.

B. Elicit Cough Tenderness

In most acute inflammatory conditions arising within the abdomen, coughing elicits pain in the involved area. Directing the patient to point one finger to the area of pain provides objective localization of the lesion. With this information, the examiner can proceed to examine the abdomen and deliberately examine last the area now known to be most tender.

C. Feel for Spasm of Rectus Abdominis Muscle (Guarding)

The next step is to establish the presence or absence of true muscle spasm by gently depressing the rectus abdominis muscle without causing pain. Have the patient flex their knees at 90° to aid in relaxation of the abdominal muscles. The patient is then asked to take a long, slow breath. If the spasm is voluntary, the muscle will immediately relax underneath the gentle pressure of the palpating hand. If there is true spasm, the muscle will remain taut and rigid through the respiratory cycle. This maneuver alone may be sufficient to establish the presence of peritonitis.

Except for rare neurologic disorders, renal colic, or rectus muscle injury, only peritoneal inflammation produces abdominal muscle rigidity. In renal colic, the spasm is confined to the entire rectus muscle on the involved side. This distinction is important because marked rigidity of the entire length of one rectus muscle with relaxation of the opposite rectus cannot occur in peritonitis as the peritoneal cavity is not compartmentalized. In generalized peritonitis, both muscles are usually involved to the same degree.

D. Perform One-Finger Palpation

Abdominal tenderness must be assessed with one finger, because it is impossible to localize peritoneal inflammation accurately if palpation or tenderness is done with the entire hand. Careful one-finger palpation, beginning as far away as possible from the area of tenderness elicited by coughing and gradually working toward it, will usually enable the examiner to delineate the area of abdominal tenderness precisely. In early acute appendicitis, this area is often no larger than 2–3 cm in diameter. Diffuse abdominal tenderness without involuntary rigidity of musculature suggests gastroenteritis or some other inflammatory process of the intestines without peritonitis. It is helpful if the examiner divides the abdomen into four quadrants during this section of the examination and tries to localize the area of pain.

Do not test for peritoneal inflammation by looking for classic rebound tenderness (deep palpation of the abdomen with abrupt release). This maneuver yields little additional information, often causes considerable discomfort, and may limit further examination.

E. Look for Costovertebral Angle Tenderness

Gentle percussion of the costovertebral angles should follow palpation. This should elicit pain in individuals with pyelonephritis, retroperitoneal abscesses, and retrocecal appendicitis. Excessively vigorous percussion is not helpful in localizing tenderness and may limit further examination.

F. Perform Deep Palpation

Having established the presence or absence of muscular rigidity and localized the area of tenderness, the examiner now palpates more deeply for the presence of abdominal masses. Often, it is difficult to perform a reliable physical examination of the abdomen in an anxious patient. Some patients are so anxious that they begin to guard with voluntary contraction of the abdominal musculature before the examiner performs even light palpation. This barrier to palpation can occasionally be overcome by palpating with a stethoscope during auscultation of bowel sounds or by asking the patient to flex the legs at the hips and knees.

Among the more common lesions identifiable by careful palpation in patients with acute abdominal pain are the distended, tender gallbladder found in acute cholecystitis, the right lower quadrant tender mass of appendicitis with early abscess formation, the left lower quadrant mass of sigmoid diverticulitis, and the midline pulsatile mass of abdominal aortic aneurysm.

▶ Percussion

Percussion aids in determining size and density of underlying matter. It can be used in estimation of liver, spleen, or bladder size and in differentiating etiologies of abdominal distention, specifically organomegaly, ascites, and obstruction.

▶ Special Signs

Several maneuvers in physical examination may help localize an acute abdominal lesion.

A. Iliopsoas Sign

The patient flexes the thigh against the resistance of the examiner's hand. A painful response indicates an inflammatory process involving the psoas muscle.

B. Obturator Sign

The patient's thigh is flexed to a right angle and gently rotated, first internally and then externally. If pain is elicited, an inflammatory lesion involving the obturator muscle (pelvic appendicitis, diverticulitis, pelvic inflammatory disease) is present.

C. Murphy's Sign (Inspiratory Arrest)

As the patient takes a slow, deep breath, the examiner elicits an abrupt cessation in inspiration by deep palpation of the right upper quadrant. This finding is suggestive of cholecystitis.

▶ Pelvic and Rectal Examination

The importance of pelvic and rectal examination cannot be overstressed. The pelvic examination in women provides essential information not revealed by other maneuvers. Evaluation of lower abdominal pain in women is discussed further in Chapter 38.

Examination of stool for gross or occult blood must be considered in patients with abdominal pain. Occult blood may result from intestinal tumors, inflammatory bowel disease, ischemic bowel disease, and lesions of the upper gastrointestinal tract. More specifically in men, rectal examination plus simultaneous lower abdominal palpation often reveals masses or localized pain not disclosed by abdominal examination alone.

▶ Bedside Abdominal Ultrasound

Bedside ultrasound is increasingly used as an adjunct to the physical exam in the emergency department. It is now a required component of training for all emergency medicine residencies. Uses include:

1. Focused Abdominal Sonography for Trauma (FAST exam).
2. Identification of free peritoneal fluid including blood, pus, or ascites.
3. Measurement of the cross-sectional abdominal aortic diameter to identify dissection or aneurysm.
4. Transvaginal and/or transabdominal ultrasound for identification of an intrauterine pregnancy, ectopic pregnancy, and other anatomic gynecological pathologies.
5. Identification of gall stones, a dilated common bile duct, or pericholecystic fluid.
6. Evaluation for hydronephrosis.
7. Testing of IVC collapse to evaluate intravascular volume status.

Such testing will be increasingly widespread as the skills required become commonplace among emergency physicians.

LABORATORY EXAMINATION

CBC with differential, lipase measurements, and urinalysis are indicated in most cases. Electrolyte determinations and tests of renal function are especially important if vomiting, diarrhea, hypotension, or shock are present. Liver function testing can be helpful in patients with suspected liver or gallbladder disease.

▶ Blood Count

The hematocrit reflects changes both in plasma volume and red cell volume. It is diagnostically most useful if markedly elevated (indicating dehydration) or depressed (indicating anemia). Furthermore, the hematocrit can be followed to assess for, or estimate the degree of, blood loss. The hematocrit should be corrected toward normal values in preparation for surgery in hemodynamically unstable patients.

The white cell count may be helpful if it is significantly elevated. However, it is neither sensitive nor specific. Normal or even low counts can occur in established peritonitis or sepsis (although usually with a marked shift to the left), and elevated counts may occur in gastroenteritis. A shift to the left on a blood smear may be a clue to an inflammatory reaction in the presence of a normal or only moderately elevated white count. Recall that in elderly and immunosuppressed patients the count may be low or normal.

▶ Serum Amylase and Lipase

Patients with abdominal pain and elevated lipase usually have acute pancreatitis. Although serum amylase is often still obtained, lipase is both more sensitive and specific than serum amylase and has greater diagnostic value. Serum amylase may also be elevated in other conditions such as obstruction, mesenteric ischemia, perforated viscus, renal failure, ectopic pregnancy. If pancreatitis is suspected, ordering lipase alone may be sufficient. Unfortunately, the degree to which either marker is elevated cannot predict the severity of the condition or any associated complications of pancreatitis.

Smith RC, Southwell-Keely J, Chesher D: Should serum pancreatic lipase replace serum amylase as a biomarker of acute pancreatitis? ANZ J Surg 2005;75(6):399–404 [PMID: 15943725].

▶ Hepatic Function Tests

Hepatic function testing is indicated for patients who have right upper quadrant pain or tenderness, jaundice, light-colored stools, or tea-colored urine and for patients in whom hepatitis is a possibility.

▶ Urine

Urinalysis (including microscopic examination of the sediment) is critical in ruling out urinary tract infection, urolithiasis, and uncontrolled diabetes. Low urine specific gravity associated with severe vomiting may be the earliest clue to renal disease. While hematuria strongly suggests urolithiasis, urolithiasis with complete obstruction of the ureter is occasionally associated with normal results on urinalysis.

Positive findings on urinalysis require cautious evaluation. Lower abdominal inflammatory conditions such as appendicitis or pelvic inflammatory disease can cause pyuria, and there are countless etiologies for hematuria.

▶ Serum Electrolytes and Tests of Renal Function

Serum electrolyte determinations and tests of renal function are required to document the nature and extent of fluid losses if vomiting or diarrhea has been significant or if the illness has lasted for more than 48 hours with diminished oral intake. An elevated blood urea nitrogen may also be noted with gastrointestinal bleeding.

▶ Pregnancy Test

A pregnancy test should be obtained in all women of childbearing age unless pregnancy is physically impossible (eg, complete hysterectomy and bilateral oophorectomy). Women with a history of pelvic infection, current intrauterine device use, prior ectopic pregnancy, and failed tubal ligation are at increased risk for ectopic pregnancy.

▶ Electrocardiogram

A 12-lead ECG should be obtained in patients with epigastric or upper abdominal pain in whom no clear cause of the pain is identified and cardiac ischemia is a possibility. This is especially true in the elderly or other populations that may have atypical presentations.

▶ Peritoneal Fluid

In peritoneal dialysis or chronic liver disease patients, examination of the peritoneal fluid is often warranted if abdominal pain, tenderness, and fever are present.

RADIOLOGIC EXAMINATION

Radiologic examination may provide important evidence for diagnosis of acute abdominal disease. Close cooperation between the radiologist and the emergency physician is essential.

▶ Suggested Studies

Abdominal radiographs can be helpful in the evaluation of patients with suspected bowel obstruction, volvulus, or hollow viscus perforation and in children or mentally handicapped adults with possible foreign body ingestion. Renal stones > 3 mm in size may also be seen.

▶ Interpretation

When the films are reviewed, the following questions should be asked: (1) Are the outlines of the liver, spleen, kidneys, and psoas muscles clearly defined? (2) Are the peritoneal fat lines identifiable? (3) Is the gas pattern in the stomach, small bowel, and colon within normal limits? (4) Is there evidence of air outside the bowel or beneath the diaphragm? (5) Is there air in the biliary ducts and ductules? (6) Are there abnormal opaque shadows such as gallstones, ureteral stones, fecaliths or calcification in lymph nodes, pancreas, aorta, or other soft tissue masses?

On the basis of these observations, the following important pieces of evidence may be obtained.

A. Gas Patterns

Dilated loops of small bowel with air–fluid levels and no gas in the colon are indicative of small-bowel obstruction (Figure 15–3).

B. Cecum and Sigmoid

Marked dilatation and rotation of the cecum or sigmoid are typical of volvulus.

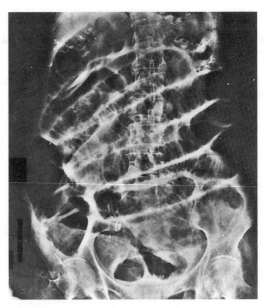

▲ **Figure 15–4.** Upright abdominal X-ray showing dilated loops of small bowel with air–fluid levels and no gas in the colon. Patient had small-bowel obstruction. (Reproduced, with permission, from Way LW (editor): *Current Surgical Diagnosis & Treatment*, 9th ed. Lange, 1991.)

C. Dilatations

Marked dilatation of the entire colon suggests colonic obstruction. Massive dilatation of the colon in acute colitis indicates toxic megacolon. Distention of both the small and the large bowel is characteristic of ileus, peritonitis, and pseudo-obstruction of the bowel (Figure 15–4). The differentiation between distended small and large bowel may at times be difficult. In advanced cases, the clinical signs may be more reliable than X-rays in the differentiation between intestinal obstruction and peritonitis.

D. Air in Abnormal Locations

Except following laparotomy, laparoscopy, or recent percutaneous gastrotomy tube placement, free air under the diaphragm usually indicates a perforated viscus, most commonly seen in perforated duodenal or gastric ulcer (Figure 15–5). Massive amounts of air beneath the diaphragm suggests colonic perforation. An encapsulated air shadow outside the contours of small or large bowel may indicate localized perforation of the intestine. Air in the biliary tract is diagnostic of a free communication between some portion of the gastrointestinal tract and the biliary tree; if evidence of intestinal obstruction is also present, this pattern is the characteristic of gallstone ileus. Rarely, free air

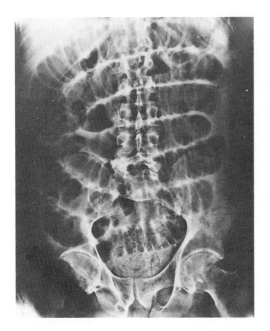

▲ **Figure 15–3.** Abdominal X-ray showing dilated loops of small and large bowel without air–fluid levels, typical of diffuse peritonitis. (Reproduced, with permission, from Way LW, ed. *Current Surgical Diagnosis and Treatment*, 11th ed. New York, NY: McGraw-Hill; 2003.)

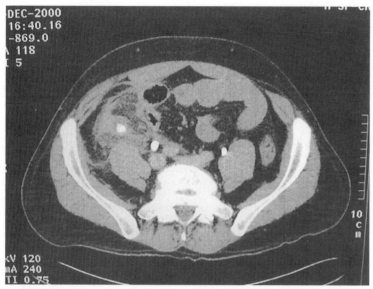

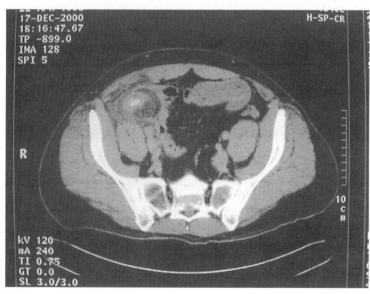

▲ **Figure 15–5.** CT scan of the abdomen with oral and intravenous contrast in a patient with right lower quadrant pain. The study demonstrates a calcified appendolith (**A** and **B**) with associated stranding in the right lower quadrant. A dilated, fluid-filled appendix is noted (**C**).

in the peritoneum, presumably from the genital tract, may be seen in asymptomatic or minimally symptomatic women with no signs of apparent underlying disease.

E. Calcifications and Opacities

X-rays of the abdomen may establish the presence of gallstones, ureteral stones, pancreatic calcification, retroperitoneal calcification, and vascular calcification. Such findings must be carefully correlated with the history and physical examination to establish their significance.

▶ Special Studies

(See Table 15–4.) Special X-ray contrast studies, ultrasonography, or computed tomography (CT) scans may be helpful.

A. Barium Enema

In cases of intussusception, barium or air contrast enema is diagnostic and often therapeutic. Otherwise, avoid barium enema if possible in the presence of undifferentiated acute

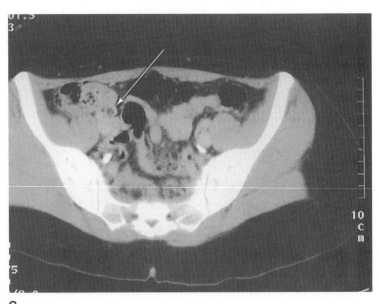

▲ **Figure 15–5.** *(Continued)*   **C**

abdominal disease and peritonitis. In rare cases, a contrast enema is necessary to establish a diagnosis of sigmoid volvulus or colonic obstruction.

B. Ultrasonography

Ultrasonography is a useful, noninvasive technique for evaluating the gallbladder, biliary ducts, pancreas, appendix, kidneys, abdominal aorta, and portions of the male and female reproductive tract. It is probably the best single diagnostic test for evaluating patients with right upper quadrant pain (see Table 15–4).

C. Computed Tomography

CT scan has emerged as a frequently used modality for diagnosis of gastrointestinal, genitourinary, and vascular pathology. Studies can be performed with or without contrast. Options for contrast enhancement include oral, rectal, intravenous, and any combination thereof. A noncontrast renal stone protocol CT scan may be performed if a physician suspects renal stones.

CT scan of the abdomen is frequently obtained to gain information about not only the solid organs and retroperitoneal structures but also the hollow organs of the abdomen. There is currently much debate over the need to IV and/or oral contrast in abdominal CT scanning (see section on appendicitis).

D. Angiography

Angiography use has become less frequent in evaluation for abdominal aortic aneurysm and solid viscus injury with

advent of CT scan. Nonetheless, mesenteric angiography remains useful in localization of massive lower gastrointestinal bleed.

▼ ADDITIONAL MEASURES FOR THE MANAGEMENT OF ACUTE ABDOMEN

▶ Repeated Examination

Repeat abdominal examinations are essential for proper evaluation of abdominal pain in the emergency setting. While this is true for all patients with abdominal pain, it can form the cornerstone of the decision-making process when the diagnosis is uncertain. Frequent inquiries about progression or change in symptoms combined with repeated examinations of the abdomen and, occasionally, repeat laboratory tests can prevent unnecessary operations without risking dangerous delays.

▶ Intravenous Fluids and Withholding Oral Intake

Intravenous fluids are indicated to replace volume deficiency, mainly secondary to gastrointestinal or vascular losses or poor intake, in most patients with abdominal pain. Also, it is recommended to withhold oral intake, at least initially.

▶ Relief of Pain

Parenteral analgesics should be administered expeditiously to relieve severe pain. Evaluation of acute abdominal

Table 15–4. Definitive Diagnosis of Conditions Causing Acute Abdominal Pain.

Usual Location of Pain	Condition	Most Sensitive and Specific Signs and Diagnostic Tests
Right upper quadrant	Cholecystitis	Right upper quadrant sonogram; radionuclide scan
	Biliary colic	Right upper quadrant sonogram
	Cholangitis	Right upper quadrant sonogram
	Hepatitis	Liver function tests, especially transaminases
	Liver abscess or tumor	Right upper quadrant sonogram; CT scan; radionuclide liver scan
	Right lower lobe pneumonia	Chest X-ray
Epigastrium or midline	Peritonitis	Smear and culture of peritoneal fluid; laparoscopy or laparotomy
	Pancreatitis	Serum lipase; CT scan
	Duodenal perforation	Upright or left decubitus flat plate of abdomen; CT scan with water-soluble oral contrast media
	Abdominal aortic aneurysm	Sonogram; CT scan
	Myocardial infarction	ECG; CK/troponin isoenzymes
Left upper quadrant	Rupture of spleen	Ultrasound; CT scan of abdomen
Flank	Pyelonephritis	Urinalysis and Gram's stain of urine; urine culture
	Renal colic	Urinalysis; noncontrast CT scan of abdomen; excretory urogram
Lower abdomen	Appendicitis	CT scan; sonogram; laparoscopy or laparotomy
	Diverticulitis	CT scan with oral and intravenous contrast
	Ectopic pregnancy	Pelvic sonogram; laparoscopy or laparotomy; positive urine pregnancy test
	Salpingitis	Pelvic sonogram
	Ruptured ovarian follicle cyst	Pelvic sonogram
Diffuse or variable	Gastroenteritis	Stool smear and culture
	Intestinal obstruction	History and examination; supine and upright abdominal X-ray
	Volvulus and intestinal strangulation	Supine and upright abdominal X-ray
	Intestinal perforation	Supine and upright abdominal X-ray; CT scan with intravenous and water-soluble oral contrast
	Ischemic colitis	CT scan; visceral angiography; barium enema
	Idiopathic inflammatory bowel disease	CT scan with intravenous and water-soluble oral contrast
	Retroperitoneal hemorrhage	CT scan
	Mesenteric thrombosis	Visceral angiography; laparotomy; CT with intravenous and water-soluble oral contrast

disease can be performed more accurately after severe pain is relieved and the patient can cooperate. In addition, studies have demonstrated no adverse effects on the ability to diagnose acute surgical conditions when patients with an acute abdomen receive narcotics. In fact, diffuse tenderness may become more localized and masses may become more obvious to palpation.

▶ Emesis Control and Nasogastric suctioning

In addition to adequate control of pain, patients will frequently require control of emesis. Initially, this may be in the form of parenteral antiemetics, but in refractory cases or in patients with high suspicion for obstruction, nasogastric suction is necessary.

Antimicrobials

Antimicrobial agents should be withheld until the diagnosis is at least tentatively established, except in the presence of obvious signs of systemic infection (high fever, rigors, hypotension). In obscure cases, antibiotic therapy may mask progression of disease and lead to serious complications with increased illness (eg, appendicitis).

Surgical Consultation

Early surgical consultation is helpful for both the patient and the surgeon. Because the surgeon, like the emergency physician, must rely on repeated examinations for diagnosis, the earlier the observation begins, the faster a definitive diagnosis can be made. Furthermore, delays in consultation may allow worsening of the condition, with possible disastrous sequelae.

Thomas SH et al: Effects of morphine analgesia in diagnostic accuracy in emergency department patients with abdominal pain: a prospective, randomized trial. J Am Coll Surg 2003;196:18 [PMID: 12517545].

▼ MANAGEMENT OF SPECIFIC DISORDERS CAUSING ABDOMINAL PAIN

INTESTINAL DISORDERS

1. Appendicitis

Clinical Findings

Classically, the initial symptom is poorly localized abdominal pain around the epigastrium or umbilicus. Later, the pain shifts from the periumbilical or epigastric region to the right lower quadrant over McBurney's point. Anorexia, nausea, vomiting, and a low-grade fever are typical features as well, but do not have to be present. Abdominal tenderness and guarding in the right lower quadrant are characteristic on physical examination. Variations from the classical picture are common, especially in retrocecal appendicitis, where the pain commonly remains poorly localized. Laboratory testing may show a moderately elevated white cell count. Individual clinical and laboratory descriptors are weak discriminators of appendicitis if used independently.

Abdominal CT has become a widely accepted tool in the evaluation of patients with possible appendicitis (see Figure 15–5C). The sensitivity and specificity of the abdominal CT scan with oral and IV contrast in the evaluation of appendicitis are 93 and 93%, respectively. Rectal contrast seems to show the highest sensitivity at 97%. Scans performed without any contrast have a sensitivity of 92.7%, with a specificity of 96.1%. Ultrasonography of the appendix may be helpful either as an initial test pre-CT or if the

diagnosis is uncertain. Sensitivity and specificity are 83 and 93%, respectively. In skilled hands, a positive ultrasound may be used to avoid unnecessary CT scanning, but a negative one is insufficient to rule out the disease.

Treatment and Disposition

The patient should be hospitalized and prepared for surgery. Administer appropriate analgesia and intravenous crystalloid solution to replace any volume deficits. For intact appendices, only perioperative antibiotics are required. However, a ruptured appendix will require IV antimicrobial therapy continuing well into the hospital stay.

Anderson BA, Salem L, Flum DR: A systemic review of whether oral contrast is necessary for the computed tomography diagnosis of appendicitis in adults. Am J Surg 2005;190(3):474–478 [PMID: 16105539].
Doria AS, Moineddin R, Kellenberger CJ et al: US or CT for diagnosis of appendicitis in children and adults? A meta-analysis. Radiology 2006;241(1):83–94 [PMID: 16928974].
Hlibczuk V, Dattaro JA, Jin Z et al: Diagnostic accuracy of non-contrast computed tomography for appendicitis in adults: a systematic review. Ann Emerg Med 2010;55(1):51–59 [PMID: 19733421].

2. Intestinal Obstruction

Clinical Findings

The patient usually complains of intermittent, poorly localized, crampy pain that tends to be associated with altered bowel function. Change in character to constant and severe pain may be a sign of perforation or bowel ischemia. Vomiting is frequently bilious and will be feculent with distal and long-standing obstruction. On examination, the abdomen is typically distended and tender with auscultation of high-pitched bowel sounds. Bowel sounds may be absent in ileus or distal obstruction. Dilated loops of bowel with air–fluid levels on flat and upright abdominal X-rays support the diagnosis (see Figure 15–3). Occasionally, X-ray findings are absent, and the diagnosis is based on clinical suspicion or abdominal CT scan with oral contrast.

Treatment and Disposition

Nasogastric suction and intravenous hydration should be initiated with electrolyte monitoring. Early surgical consultation is important. The patient should be hospitalized for further evaluation and possible surgery. Some cases will resolve without surgery.

3. Perforated Peptic Ulcer

Clinical Findings

Perforation of a peptic ulcer usually causes sudden severe upper abdominal pain. The pain of perforation may subside

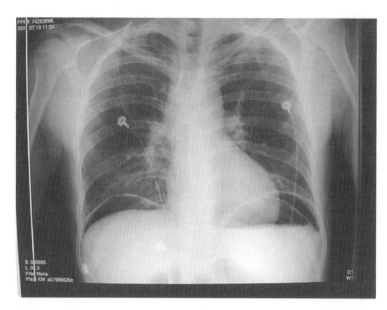

▲ **Figure 15–6.** Upright anteroposterior chest X-ray demonstrating pneumoperitoneum from a perforated peptic ulcer.

when peritoneal secretions dilute the leaking gastric contents. However, it will later return, progressively worsening. Referred shoulder pain may occur secondary to diaphragmatic irritation. The patient is usually in severe distress with shallow breathing and knees drawn up to the chest in an effort to minimize pain. Upper abdominal tenderness is accompanied by board-like rigidity of the abdomen. Evaluation of any perforation should include a three-view acute abdominal series including an upright chest, as well upright and lateral decubitus abdominal films. This may show free air under the diaphragm (Figure 15–6). When abdominal radiographs are non-diagnostic and perforation is suspected, abdominal CT scan with oral and intravenous contrast can be diagnostic (see Chapter 16).

▶ Treatment and Disposition

Insert a nasogastric tube for drainage of gastric acid. Administer crystalloid solution intravenously to correct volume depletion. Initiate broad-spectrum intravenous antibiotics (Table 15–1). Hospitalize for immediate surgery.

4. Perforation of the Bowel
▶ Clinical Findings

Perforation of the bowel is accompanied by sudden or explosive onset of severe, agonizing mid- or lower-abdominal pain. Shock may be present and can be profound. Nausea and vomiting are common. The abdomen is rigid and tender. Fever may be high and is often accompanied by leukocytosis. A history of diverticulitis can often be elicited. As above, a three-view abdominal series should be ordered and will show similar findings.

▶ Treatment and Disposition

Treat shock with intravenous crystalloids. Obtain blood and urine cultures. Begin antimicrobials (see Table 15–1). Hospitalize for immediate surgery.

Langell JT, Mulvihill SJ: Gastrointestinal perforation and the acute abdomen. Med Clin North Am 2008;92:599–625 [PMID:18387378].

5. Diverticulitis
▶ Clinical Findings

Patients typically report lower abdominal pain that is gradual in onset. The pain tends to localize to the left lower quadrant with associated tenderness, but may be midabdominal or in the right lower quadrant. Fever is typically of low grade, and may be accompanied by a mild leukocytosis. Other findings may include abdominal tenderness, a palpable abdominal mass, alterations in bowel function (either constipation or frequent defecation), and heme-positive stools. Plain films are usually normal or nonspecific; the diagnostic procedure of choice is abdominal CT scan.

▶ Treatment and Disposition

Most patients should be hospitalized for administration of intravenous fluids, IV antimicrobial treatment (see Table 15–1), and further observation. A subset of reliable patients in which peritoneal signs, intractable vomiting, and signs of systemic infection are absent may be candidates for outpatient treatment with oral antibiotics provided good follow-up is possible. Both gram negative aerobic and anaerobic bacteria should be covered.

6. Intestinal Strangulation
▶ Clinical Findings

Intestinal strangulation occurs most frequently in volvulus or femoral hernia and occasionally in inguinal hernia. Onset of pain is usually rapid. Pain increases in severity and may be intermittent and colicky. The patient may complain of an urge to defecate. The abdomen is distended, rigid, and diffusely tender. Exquisite tenderness is present in the region of strangulation. Shock appears early. Other findings usually include nausea and vomiting, high fever, and leukocytosis. In the case of volvulus, findings on abdominal X-ray may be diagnostic. Additional imaging options include CT scan and barium enema.

▶ Treatment and Disposition

The patient should be hospitalized and prepared for surgery immediately.

7. Gastroenteritis

See also Chapter 36.

▶ Clinical Findings

The patient complains of mild to severe cramping and pain that may have come on gradually or abruptly. There may be nausea and vomiting, retching, and diarrhea, in any combination. These symptoms usually precede the onset of pain, in contrast to conditions requiring surgery, in which pain is usually the first symptom. Abdominal examination reveals generalized discomfort. Also in contrast to situations requiring surgery, involuntary guarding, localized tenderness, and peritoneal signs are absent. Fever is generally not present or mild, although patients with shigellosis typically have high fever and rigors. The patient may be dehydrated. Stool should be tested for blood, examined microscopically for leukocytes, and sent for culture if the patient has prolonged or severe diarrhea associated with fever.

▶ Treatment and Disposition

Severely ill or dehydrated patients should be hospitalized. Mild to moderately ill patients can be sent home with instructions for rehydration. If symptoms persist or worsen, patients should receive follow-up evaluation.

8. Inflammatory Bowel Disease
▶ Clinical Findings

The patient typically complains of abdominal cramps and intermittent bloody diarrhea. A history of previous episodes may be given, and a long history of colitis may be present. Weight loss, fever, and anemia may be present. Cramps may develop gradually or suddenly. Abdominal examination will vary with etiology and severity of disease. Infectious causes (eg, *Shigella* sp., *Clostridium difficile*, *Campylobacter* sp., *Entamoeba histolytica*) should be systematically ruled out.

▶ Treatment and Disposition
A. For the Seriously Ill Patient or for Uncertain Diagnosis

Treat hypotension or shock with administration of intravenous crystalloids. Give nothing by mouth. Nasogastric suction may be helpful if the patient is vomiting, in addition to antiemetics. Abdominal radiographs or CT scan may provide important information about possible complications such as perforation, bowel obstruction, toxic megacolon, or intraperitoneal abscess. Hospitalize the patient for definitive diagnosis and treatment. Indications for hospitalization are uncertain diagnosis, shock, fever, toxic megacolon, anemia, or gross blood in the stool. Surgical consultation should be obtained for significant hemorrhage, perforation, abscesses, or toxic megacolon.

B. For the Ambulatory Patient with Certain Diagnosis

For patients under the care of a gastroenterologist, discuss the options with the patient's physician regarding outpatient treatment with oral antibiotics, steroids, and other antiinflammatory medications such as sulfasalazine. Patients with mild to moderate disease may be restarted on maintenance therapy or have their currently therapy modified.

Baumgart DC, Sandborn WJ: Inflammatory bowel disease: clinical aspects and established and evolving therapies. Lancet 2007;369:1641–1657 [PMID: 17499606].

HEPATOBILIARY DISORDERS

1. Biliary Colic
▶ Clinical Findings

Biliary colic is due to intermittent obstruction of the biliary tree, usually at the cystic duct, by stones. The pain occurs in discrete episodes (frequently after ingestion of food), which usually begin abruptly and subside gradually over a few hours. During an attack, persistent abdominal pain extends all the way across the upper abdomen but tends to be more severe on the right. Pain may be referred to the scapula. A careful history often reveals prior attacks of similar pain. Abdominal examination shows right upper quadrant tenderness and, occasionally, a palpable gallbladder. A right upper quadrant sonogram will show gallstones (see Figure 15–7) or

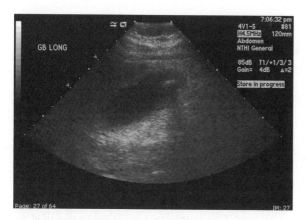

▲ **Figure 15–7.** Right upper quadrant ultrasound showing a gallbladder containing a gallstone. This study demonstrates a gallstone with distinctive posterior shadowing.

a dilated gallbladder or cystic duct. Dilation of the common bile duct is commonly seen with choledocholithiasis.

Treatment and Disposition

In the absence of acute cholecystitis, ascending cholangitis, choledocholithiasis, or pancreatitis, no specific immediate treatment is required. However, pain should always be brought under control. Patients must also be able to tolerate oral hydration and nutrition. Refer for possible elective cholecystectomy and provide appropriate analgesics and antiemetics.

2. Acute Cholecystitis
Clinical Findings

Acute cholecystitis presents very similarly to biliary colic, but the patient's symptoms become persistent and more severe. The discomfort may be moderate to severe and prostrating with associated anorexia, nausea, and vomiting. Low-grade fever and leukocytosis are usually present. In some cases, the gallbladder is palpable.

Ultrasonography of the abdomen demonstrating gallstones, dilatation of the intra or extrahepatic bile ducts or thickening of the gallbladder wall, and pericholecystic fluid (if present) confirms the diagnosis of acute cholecystitis. Ultrasonography is the preferred diagnostic technique because it is sensitive, specific, rapid, inexpensive, and without adverse effects. A sonographic Murphy's sign, specific tenderness of the gallbladder noted during the ultrasound examination, has a sensitivity of 88% and a specificity of 80% for acute cholecystitis. A recent prospective analysis of bedside ultrasound showed similar sensitivity and specificity to that of an ultrasound done in radiology. Nonvisualization

of the biliary tract on nuclear imaging (HIDA) is also diagnostic.

Treatment and Disposition

Give nothing by mouth. Insert a nasogastric tube and attach it to continuous suction if the patient is vomiting. Anti-emetics typically have little effect in these patients. Give intravenous crystalloids and parenteral analgesics. Administer empiric antibiotics if the patient has systemic signs of infection such as fever. Hospitalize and obtain surgical consultation.

Caddy GR: Gallstone disease: symptoms, diagnosis and endoscopic management of common bile duct stones. Best Pract Res Clin Gastroenterol 2006;20(6):1085–1101 [PMID: 17127190].

Elwood DR: Cholecystitis. Surg Clin North Am 2008;88(6): 1241–1252 [PMID: 18992593].

Summers SM, Scruggs W et al: A prospective evaluation of emergency department bedside ultrasonography for the detection of acute cholecystitis. Ann Emerg Med 2010;56:123–125 [PMID: 20138397].

3. Acute Suppurative Cholangitis
Clinical Findings

Acute suppurative cholangitis, a complication of cholecystitis, is a surgical emergency commonly accompanied by bacteremia and septic shock. Symptoms include abdominal pain, jaundice, fever, mental confusion, and shock. The classic Charcot triad of fever, jaundice, and right upper quadrant pain is seen in 50–70% of patients. The addition of shock and mental confusion (Raynaud's Pentad) is rare with an incidence of only 3.5–7.7%. Right upper quadrant sonography is the diagnostic procedure of choice and may show dilated, obstructed intrahepatic biliary ducts.

Treatment and Disposition

Severity has recently been divided into three grades. Grade I responds to initial medical treatment. Grade II does not respond, but does not show signs of organ dysfunction. Grade III is associated with dysfunction in at least one organ system (ie requiring a vasopressor for blood pressure support).

Treat shock with intravenous crystalloids. Administer broad-spectrum antimicrobials intravenously. Insert a Foley catheter to monitor urine output. Emergent surgical consultation should also be obtained.

Lee JG: Diagnosis and management of acute cholangitis. Nat Rev Gastroenterol Hepatol 2009;6:533–541 [PMID: 19652653].

Wada K, Takada T, Kawarada Y et al: Diagnostic criteria and severity assessment of acute cholangitis: Tokyo guidelines. J Hepatobiliary Pancreat Surg 2007;14:52–58 [PMID: 17252297].

4. Hepatic Abscess

▶ Clinical Findings

When liver abscess results from other intra-abdominal infections (a pyogenic abscess), increasing toxicity with high fever, chills, nausea, vomiting, jaundice, and a deteriorating clinical picture are seen. Right upper quadrant pain may be present. Patients typically present acutely, however, a chronic onset with hepatomegaly may be seen.

With primary (amebic) liver abscesses (caused by *E. histolytica*), onset is insidious and it may be several weeks before the disease becomes fulminant. High fever and leukocytosis often accompany the abscess. The liver becomes enlarged and is often tender. Many patients with amebic liver abscesses do not have intestinal amebiasis; hence, stool examination for parasites is not helpful. Right upper quadrant sonography, CT scan, or liver scan is diagnostic. CT-guided aspiration also can assist in diagnosis.

▶ Treatment and Disposition

Hospitalize the patient immediately for evaluation and treatment by percutaneous drainage or surgical exploration. Obtain blood for culture and amebic serology and initiate antimicrobial therapy.

Krige JE, Beckingham IJ: ABC of diseases of the liver, pancreas, and biliary system, liver abscesses and hydatid disease. Br Med J 2001;322:537–540 [PMID: 11230072].

5. Hepatitis

▶ Clinical Findings

The majority of cases of hepatitis are asymptomatic. When symptomatic, it is often manifested with anorexia, abdominal pain, malaise, nausea and vomiting, and dark urine. Fever, jaundice, and hepatomegaly are also usually present. Liver function tests show elevated bilirubin and hepatic enzymes (AST [SGOT], ALT [SGPT], and alkaline phosphatase). The white cell count is low or normal. Coagulation studies should also be checked as hepatitis can lead to coagulopathy. If acetaminophen toxicity is a possibility, serum levels should be ordered.

The most common causes are viral infection and alcohol. The history, physical examination, and amino-transferase levels can be used to differentiate viral and alcoholic hepatitis. In alcoholic hepatitis, AST (SGOT) levels are the same or higher than ALT (SGPT) levels. With viral hepatitis, the opposite is true.

▶ Treatment and Disposition

Most cases of hepatitis are treated symptomatically, giving fluids and antiemetics, as well as correcting any electrolyte imbalances. Stable patients can be referred to a primary-care physician and receive treatment at home. The patient should be instructed to maintain hydration, strict hygiene, and to avoid potential hepatotoxins (alcohol or acetaminophen). Severely ill patients with persistent vomiting, dehydration, hypoglycemia, hepatic encephalopathy, or significant coagulopathy (prothrombin time > 15) should be hospitalized. With suspected acetaminophen-toxicity, *N*-acetylcysteine should be given (see Chapter 47).

Stravitz TR: Critical management decisions in patients with acute liver failure. Chest 2008;134:1092–1102 [PMID: 18988787].

VASCULAR DISORDERS

1. Ruptured Aortic Aneurysm

▶ Clinical Findings

Rupture of an abdominal aneurysm is accompanied by severe abdominal pain of sudden onset that often radiates into the back. In some patients, pain is confined to the flank, low back, or groin. Syncope, usually secondary to blood loss and lack of cerebral perfusion, often occurs as well. After the initial hemorrhage, pain may lessen and faintness may disappear, but these symptoms recur and progress until shock finally supervenes. While dissection is occurring, a discrete pulsatile abdominal mass or unequal lower extremity pulses may be palpated. If rupture occurs in the retroperitoneum, a poorly defined midabdominal fullness, periumbilical ecchymosis (Cullen sign), or flank ecchymosis (Grey–Turner's sign) may be noted. Bedside ultrasound can rapidly confirm the diagnosis (see Figure 15–8), but ruptured aneurysms are difficult to visualize and may still be missed. Most patients with a leaking or ruptured abdominal aortic aneurysm are too unstable to be diagnosed by CT scan. A chest X-ray should also be obtained to evaluate the thoracic aorta.

▶ Treatment and Disposition

See also Chapter 40.

Obtain intravenous access in the form of at least two large-bore peripheral catheters or a central venous catheter. Collect necessary laboratory studies, including type and crossmatch for packed red blood cells. Treat shock with intravenous crystalloids followed by whole blood as soon as available. Obtain immediate surgical consultation, as mortality is virtually 100% without surgical intervention.

Assar AN, Zarins CK: Ruptured abdominal aortic aneurysm: a surgical emergency with many clinical presentations. Postgrad Med J 2009;85:268–273 [PMID: 19520879].

Chaikof EL, Brewster DC, Dalman RL et al: The care of patients with an abdominal aortic aneurysm: The Society for Vascular Surgery practice guidelines. J Vasc Surg 2009;50(4 Suppl):S2–S49 [PMID: 19786250].

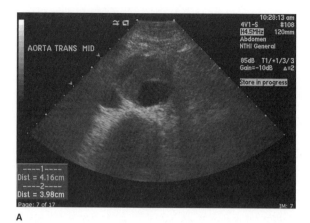 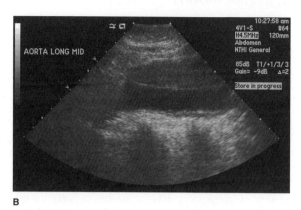

▲ **Figure 15–8.** Ultrasound of the abdominal aorta in transverse (**A**) and longitudinal (**B**) views. These studies show a thrombus in an aortic aneurysm with a diameter greater than the aorta itself.

2. Ischemic Colitis

▶ Clinical Findings

The pain is abrupt in onset, of varying degrees of severity, and may be localized or diffuse. A history of similar attacks is often present. Most patients present with sudden cramping abdominal pain and diarrhea. Exam may reveal mild to moderate tenderness to palpation over the affected area. Rectal exam shows hemoccult positive stool. Severe colitis is usually accompanied by bloody diarrhea and may present with peritoneal signs. Ischemic areas may progress to gangrene if the ischemia is sufficiently severe; if ischemia is milder, the areas may heal, often with stricture formation.

Routine laboratory tests do not show specific abnormalities. Confirmatory studies include sigmoidoscopy or colonoscopy, barium enema, and visceral angiography. CT is the most often utilized imaging modality.

▶ Treatment and Disposition

Treat shock and hemoconcentration with intravenous crystalloids. Administer appropriate antimicrobials (see Table 15–1). Hospitalize for further diagnostic testing and possible surgery.

Theodoropoulou A, Koutroubakis IE. Ischemic colitis: clinical practice in diagnosis and treatment. World J Gastroenterol 2008;14(48):7302–7308 [PMID: 19109863].

3. Mesenteric Ischemia

▶ Clinical Findings

The patient usually complains of the sudden onset of severe, diffuse abdominal pain in the mid- or lower abdomen.

The pain is poorly localized, out of proportion to examination, and severe, often not relieved by narcotics. Onset can be variable in thrombotic, versus embolic, source of ischemia. Nausea, vomiting, and diarrhea, with gross or occult blood in the stool, may be present. Initially, physical findings are frequently absent. As the condition progresses, abdominal distention and signs of systemic toxicity develop. Marked leukocytosis, hemo-concentration, azotemia, and acidosis are commonly associated with mesenteric ischemia. Whereas traditional angiography has been the historic gold standard, CT angiogram has increased in popularity since the onset of multi-row detector CT. Additional findings available by CT (such as bowel wall thickening or organ infarction) have lead to a sensitivity and specificity of 96 and 94%, respectively.

▶ Treatment and Disposition

Hospitalize and obtain immediate surgical consultation. Treat shock and hemoconcentration with intravenous crystalloids and administer antimicrobials (see Table 15–1).

Herbert GS, Steele SR, (et al): Acute and Chronic Mesenteric Ischemia. *Surg Clin North Am.* 2007; 87:115–1134, (PMID:17936478)

4. Rupture of the Spleen

See also Chapter 25.

▶ Clinical Findings

The spleen is the intra-abdominal solid organ most commonly injured in blunt trauma, with rupture usually due to trauma to the left lower rib cage. Occasionally, the spleen may rupture after trivial or overlooked injury, usually when pathologic enlargement has occurred (eg, infectious mononucleosis, AIDS, leukemia). Blood leaking into the peritoneal cavity causes abdominal pain and tenderness that may radiate to the left side of the neck or left shoulder (Kehr's sign). However, patients occasionally present without abdominal symptoms.

Tachycardia, hypotension, and falling hematocrit are present, and shock may develop. Palpation of the left upper quadrant or left 9th and 10th ribs may reveal tenderness. Splenomegaly is also a common feature. Emergent bedside ultrasound, specifically the FAST examination (Chapters 6 and 25), can rapidly identify intraperitoneal fluid, which in the setting of blunt trauma must be assumed to represent blood. CT scan of the abdomen is useful for diagnosis and grading of splenic injury severity in stable patients. CT may demonstrate active extravasation if ongoing bleeding is occurring.

▶ Treatment and Disposition

Obtain large-bore intravenous access, collect necessary laboratory studies, and treat shock with intravenous crystalloids. When available, administer packed red blood cells for further resuscitation. Hospitalize all patients with major splenic injury or rupture. Hemodynamically stable patients with less severe splenic injuries may be observed nonoperatively. Patients with hypotension and shock require emergent splenectomy.

Renzulli P, Hostettler A, Schoepfer AM et al: Systematic review of atraumatic splenic rupture. Br J Surg 2009;96(10):1114–1121 [PMID: 19787754].

URINARY DISORDERS

1. Renal Colic

See also Chapter 39.

▶ Clinical Findings

Renal colic is usually characterized by sudden, severe flank pain, often radiating laterally around to the groin, followed by hematuria. A constant, dull ache between episodes may be present. Associated nausea, vomiting, and restlessness are common. A history of passage of stones may be present. The patient is often in severe, writhing pain. Examination reveals costovertebral angle tenderness with a relatively benign abdominal examination. Urinalysis is the first step, providing useful information about the presence of blood, crystals, and/or infection. It can be followed by a urine culture if infection is suspected. Imaging is not always necessary if the patient has a history of stones and a clinical diagnosis can be made. Abdominal X-ray will frequently reveal renal calculi, as most, but not all, are radiopaque. Noncontrast helical CT scan of the abdomen (with 5 mm or less slices) has replaced the intravenous pyelogram as the standard diagnostic modality for the evaluation of renal colic (Figure 15–9). It is helpful in identifying the size and location of ureteral stones. Another benefit of noncontrast CT scan is that alternative diagnoses such as appendicitis or diverticulitis may be identified.

▶ Treatment and Disposition

Pain can often be controlled with NSAIDs or narcotics. Oral (if possible) or IV fluids are also recommended. Absolute criteria for admission include obstructing stones

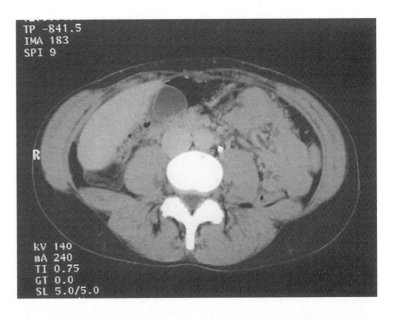

▲ **Figure 15–9.** Noncontrast CT scan of the abdomen in a patient with left flank pain. Study demonstrates a dense calcification (ureterolithiasis) involving the mid portion of the left ureter, confirming the diagnosis of renal colic.

with signs of infection, renal dysfunction related to bilateral obstruction, intractable nausea/vomiting, pain requiring parenteral analgesics, extravasation of urine, and hypercalemic crisis. Other, relative indications include obstruction high in the urinary tract, leukocytosis, renal disease, and comorbidities making outpatient treatment difficult. Patients with small stones (<5 mm) can receive treatment on an ambulatory basis, with appropriate oral analgesia, hydration, and follow-up care with a primary-care physician or urologist. Larger stones (>5 mm) may require urologic intervention.

Worcester EM, Coe FL: Nephrolithiasis. Prim Care 2008;35(2): 369–391,vii [PMID: 18486720].

2. Pyelonephritis

See also Chapter 42.

▶ Clinical Findings

Patients with pyelonephritis typically have flank pain, dysuria, urinary urgency, urinary frequency, fever, and sometimes rigors. Malaise, nausea, and vomiting are commonly present as well. Tenderness is usually over the costovertebral angle or occasionally the abdomen. The pain is typically dull and gradual in onset. Urinalysis and urine culture should be obtained.

▶ Treatment and Disposition

A patient who is severely ill (vomiting, high fever, rigors), pregnant, very young, very old, immunocompromised, or who has known anatomic abnormalities of the genitourinary tract requires hospitalization for observation, intravenous hydration, and parenteral antibiotics. Out-patient therapy is appropriate for those who can be informed of the culture results, are tolerating oral intake and are reliable to return if their condition worsens. Sequential therapy using an initial parenteral dose of antibiotic followed by an oral regimen as an outpatient is often recommended.

Ramakrishnan K, Scheid D: Diagnosis and management of acute pyelonephritis in adults. Am Fam Physician 2005;72(11):2182 [PMID: 15768623].

ACUTE PANCREATITIS

▶ Clinical Findings

Acute pancreatitis is characterized by acute onset of severe, unrelenting epigastric pain radiating to the back that tends to be worst when supine. Occasionally, pain can present in the right upper quadrant. Nausea and vomiting are usually present. In severe cases, the patient may be in shock. A predisposing condition (alcoholism, gallstones, glucocorticoid administration, or diabetes mellitus) may be present. Abdominal examination reveals decreased or absent bowel sounds and tenderness usually greatest in the epigastrium. Elevated serum amylase and lipase levels, mild fever, and leukocytosis are often present. As discussed previously, lipase has better specificity and sensitivity for pancreatitis than amylase. If the diagnosis is uncertain, abdominal CT scan can often demonstrate changes pathognomonic of pancreatitis with sensitivity and specificity of 87–90 and 90–92%, respectively.

▶ Treatment and Disposition

Initial treatment involves aggressive crystalloid infusion and appropriate parenteral analgesia. Obtain additional pertinent laboratory studies including CBC, electrolytes, glucose, calcium, LDH, and hepatic and renal function tests. Give nothing by mouth.

Patients with severe pain or persistent vomiting should be hospitalized for analgesia, intravenous hydration, and correction of electrolyte abnormalities. Even if they are not acutely ill, patients with no history of pancreatitis should be hospitalized for evaluation and treatment. Patients with chronic and recurrent pancreatitis may not require hospitalization if they can take fluids by mouth and do not require parenteral analgesics; these patients should be instructed to maintain a clear liquid diet and have close follow-up in 24–48 hours.

Frossard JL, Steer ML, Pastor CM: Acute pancreatitis. Lancet 2008;371(9618):143–152 [PMID: 18191686].

GYNECOLOGIC DISORDERS

See also Chapter 38.

1. Ectopic Pregnancy with Rupture

▶ Clinical Findings

An ectopic pregnancy should be considered in any woman of child-bearing age who presents with abdominal pain. The classic triad of symptoms in ectopic pregnancy (abdominal pain, amenorrhea, and vaginal bleeding or spotting) is not present consistently. Risk factors should be included in the history, including prior ectopic pregnancy, history of STDs (especially PID), smoking, IUD use, progestin-only birth control pills, and implanted progestin contraception. Prior to rupture the pain may be vague or intermittent and possibly difficult to localize. Once the ectopic has ruptured, the patient will experience sudden, continuous, and severe unilateral abdominal or pelvic pain that may be referred to the shoulder. There may be occasional nausea and vomiting, but usually no fever. Postural hypotension or shock may be found on initial examination. Pelvic examination often reveals a unilateral doughy mass and tenderness on movement of the cervix. Pelvic sonography has a sensitivity of 84.4% and a specifity of 98.9%. It may reveal free fluid and/or an adnexal mass. A quantitative serum hCG is positive in almost all cases. In the emergency department, it can be used to correlate with ultrasound results. Further, serial hCG levels can be used to followed suspected ectopic as an outpatient if diagnosis is uncertain.

▶ Treatment and Disposition

Treat shock or hypotension with intravenous crystalloids and blood if necessary. Hospitalize the patient for emergent surgical intervention (Chapter 38).

Nama V, Manyonda I: Tubal ectopic pregnancy: diagnosis and management. Arch Gynecol Obstet 2009;279:443–453 [PMID: 19039599].

2. Acute Salpingitis (Pelvic Inflammatory Disease)

See also Chapter 42.

▶ Clinical Findings

There are a wide variety of presentations for salpingitis. Patients typically report a gradual onset of pelvic and lower abdominal pain frequently with associated vaginal discharge and/or bleeding. Headache, nausea and vomiting, and lassitude with high fever and tachycardia may also be present. Exquisite tenderness to bimanual examination is typical, particularly with cervical motion. Adnexal fullness or mass (tubo-ovarian abscess) may be present. However, these signs are neither highly sensitive nor specific. A pelvic sonogram showing a tubo-ovarian abscess is diagnostic. A serum pregnancy test should be performed in all patients.

▶ Treatment and Disposition

The CDC recommends empiric treatment in sexually active young women experiencing pelvic or lower abdominal pain if a cause cannot be found or if one of the following are present on pelvic exam:

- Cervical motion tenderness OR
- Uterine tenderness OR
- Adnexal tenderness

Hospitalization of patients with pelvic inflammatory disease is recommended for the following situations: diagnosis is uncertain (eg, cannot exclude appendicitis); abscess is suspected; patient has severe symptoms such as nausea, vomiting, or high fever; patient is pregnant; patient has failed outpatient treatment; patient is unable to follow up; or patient is immunocompromised (eg, HIV with low CD4

count). Surgery may be necessary if abdominal symptoms persist or if the patient's condition deteriorates.

See Chapter 42 for treatment regimens.

CDC Sexually Transmitted Disease Treatment Guidelines, 2006. http://www.cdc.gov/std/treatment/2006/pid.htm. Bethesda, MD (last accessed on 2/12/2010).

Haggerty CL, Ness RB: Diagnosis and treatment of pelvic inflammatory disease. Women's Health (Lond Engl) 2008;4(4): 383–397 [PMID: 19072503].

3. Ruptured Ovarian Follicle Cyst

▶ Clinical Findings

Patients with ruptured ovarian follicle cyst experience sudden, severe pelvic, or lower abdominal pain. Gastrointestinal symptoms are usually absent, and the patient is afebrile without leukocytosis. Tenderness may be elicited over the affected ovary. There should be no masses on pelvic examination, and the serum pregnancy test should be negative.

▶ Treatment and Disposition

Provide adequate analgesia and keep the patient under observation in the hospital until the diagnosis is confirmed. If the diagnosis can be confirmed by ultrasound and there are no other complicating factors, the patient may be discharged with close follow-up. Operation is not usually necessary.

Bottomley C, Bourne T: Diagnosis and management of ovarian cyst accidents. Best Pract Res Clin Obstet Gynaecol 2009;23(5): 711–724 [PMID: 19299205].

4. Ovarian Torsion

▶ Clinical Findings

Torsion of the ovary is characterized by sudden unilateral lower abdominal or pelvic pain of moderate or severe intensity that is often made worse by a change in position. The pain may radiate into the groin, back, or flank. Nausea and vomiting may be present. A history of ovarian abnormalities such as cysts or masses may be present. No imaging modality has been found to have excellent sensitivity or specificity. Currently, ultrasound with Doppler is the most-commonly utilized. However, negative imaging cannot rule out torsion, especially in cases with strong clinical suspicion. Surgical consultation is recommended in such cases.

▶ Treatment and Disposition

The patient should be hospitalized for observation and possible surgery.

Oltmann SC, Fischer A, Barber R et al: Cannot exclude torsion—a 15 year review. J Pediatr Surg 2009;44(6):1212–1217 [PMID: 19524743].

5. Endometriosis

▶ Clinical Findings

Patients with endometriosis usually have a history of dysmenorrhea and previous cyclic attacks of cramps and pains in the lower abdomen and possibly in the flank. Pain is worse with menses. Onset of symptoms may be gradual or sudden if there is associated bleeding. Dyschezia and dyspareunia are often present. Aching pelvic discomfort and general tenderness on pelvic examination suggest endometriosis.

▶ Treatment and Disposition

If symptoms are mild, give the patient analgesics and refer her to the obstetrics and gynecology department for follow-up. If pain is severe, the patient should be hospitalized for evaluation and possible surgery.

Mounsey AL, Wilgus A, Slawson DC: Diagnosis and management of endometriosis. Am Fam Physician 2006;74(4):594–600 [PMID: 16939179].

PRIMARY PERITONITIS

▶ Clinical Findings

Primary peritonitis occurs almost exclusively in patients with preexisting large-volume ascites, especially those with cirrhosis or nephrotic syndrome. The symptoms and signs vary, but fever, abdominal pain, and tenderness are common. The most helpful tests are blood culture and abdominal paracentesis for Gram-stained smear, CBC, and fluid culture. A polymorphonuclear (PMN) cell count of more than 250/mm^3 is highly suspicious for spontaneous bacterial peritonitis and is an indication for initiation of empiric antibiotics. Most cases of primary bacterial peritonitis demonstrate positive blood cultures, peritoneal fluid leukocyte counts over 1000/mm^3 (with a predominance of PMNs), and bacteria on Gram-stained smears of culture. Peritoneal fluid smears and cultures may be negative when the disease process is present.

▶ Treatment and Disposition

All patients with suspected or confirmed acute peritonitis should be hospitalized for diagnostic evaluation and treatment. Treat shock, if present, with intravenous crystalloids. Culture blood and peritoneal fluid first, then begin broad-spectrum parenteral antimicrobials.

Koulaouzidis A, Bhat S, Saeed AA: Spontaneous Bacterial Peritonitis. World J Gastroenterol 2010;15(9):1042–1049 [PMID: 20143473].

RETROPERITONEAL HEMORRHAGE

▶ Clinical Findings

Retroperitoneal hemorrhage is a rare condition that may occur with major trauma or secondary to minor trauma in individuals with defective clotting factors resulting from medication or disease. It may also occur after invasive femoral procedures, such as coronary artery catheterization. Back pain and abdominal pain may be present, and the psoas sign is often positive. Abdominal CT scan localizes the bleeding in most cases.

▶ Treatment and Disposition

Treat shock with intravenous crystalloids and cross-matched whole blood as soon as available. Correct coagulation defects with administration of platelets or clotting factors as needed. Hospitalize patients with active hemorrhage, clotting abnormalities, or severe pain.

▼ CONDITIONS CAUSING ACUTE ABDOMINAL PAIN THAT ARE NOT AMENABLE TO SURGERY

A variety of conditions not amenable to surgery may cause abdominal pain. Aside from common conditions such as pyelonephritis, salpingitis, myocardial infarction, lobar pneumonia, and diabetic ketoacidosis, a number of these conditions are capable of mimicking abdominal disorders requiring surgery. Most of these conditions simulate acute diffuse peritonitis. Helpful differential diagnostic tests are listed in Table 15–4.

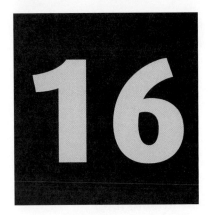

Gastrointestinal Bleeding

Timothy G. Price, MD, FACEP, FAAEM[1]
Zachary E. Armstrong, MD

For the majority of patients presenting with gastrointestinal (GI) bleeding, hematemesis, hematochezia, or melena will be the chief complaint. Occasionally, patients may present with only dizziness, weakness, or syncope. If no obvious cause of shock is present, gastric lavage and a rectal examination should be performed promptly as part of the initial assessment. The severity of blood loss must be assessed quickly so that lifesaving therapeutic interventions can be instituted. Factors that increase the morbidity and mortality are hemodynamic instability, ongoing symptoms, inability to clear bleeding with lavage, age over 60, and other comorbidities.

IMMEDIATE MANAGEMENT OF LIFE-THREATENING BLEEDING

See Figure 16–1.

ASSESS THE RATE AND VOLUME OF BLEEDING

Any patient presenting to the emergency department with ongoing hematemesis or hematochezia is at significant risk of exsanguination, and prompt volume resuscitation must begin at once. Proceed with initial stabilization procedures as described below.

CONDUCT INITIAL ASSESSMENT

Place the patient in a monitored bed and obtain a full set of vital signs including oxygen saturation. If the initial systolic blood pressure is greater than 100, and the pulse is less than 100 beats/min in the supine position, consider obtaining orthostatic blood pressure and pulse rate measurements.

[1]This chapter is a revision of the chapter by Alicia Haywood, MD, Tammy Ray, MD, & Timothy G. Price, MD FACEP FAAEM from the 6th edition.

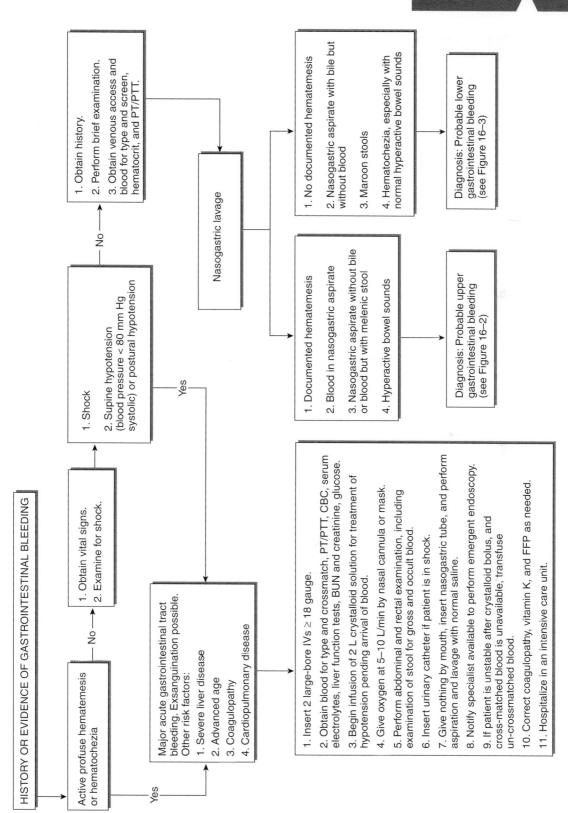

▲ **Figure 16–1.** Immediate management of life-threatening bleeding. BUN, blood urea nitrogen; FFP, fresh frozen plasma; PT, prothrombin time; PTT, partial thromboplastin time.

HISTORY OR EVIDENCE OF GASTROINTESTINAL BLEEDING

Active profuse hematemesis or hematochezia

— No →

1. Obtain vital signs.
2. Examine for shock.

Yes ↓

Major acute gastrointestinal tract bleeding. Exsanguination possible. Other risk factors:
1. Severe liver disease
2. Advanced age
3. Coagulopathy
4. Cardiopulmonary disease

1. Shock
2. Supine hypotension (blood pressure < 80 mm Hg systolic) or postural hypotension

— No →

1. Obtain history.
2. Perform brief examination.
3. Obtain venous access and blood for type and screen, hematocrit, and PT/PTT.

Yes ↓

1. Insert 2 large-bore IVs ≥ 18 gauge.
2. Obtain blood for type and crossmatch, PT/PTT, CBC, serum electrolytes, liver function tests, BUN and creatinine, glucose.
3. Begin infusion of 2 L crystalloid solution for treatment of hypotension pending arrival of blood.
4. Give oxygen at 5–10 L/min by nasal cannula or mask.
5. Perform abdominal and rectal examination, including examination of stool for gross and occult blood.
6. Insert urinary catheter if patient is in shock.
7. Give nothing by mouth, insert nasogastric tube, and perform aspiration and lavage with normal saline.
8. Notify specialist available to perform emergent endoscopy.
9. If patient is unstable after crystalloid bolus, and cross-matched blood is unavailable, transfuse un-crossmatched blood.
10. Correct coagulopathy, vitamin K, and FFP as needed.
11. Hospitalize in an intensive care unit.

Nasogastric lavage

1. Documented hematemesis
2. Blood in nasogastric aspirate
3. Nasogastric aspirate without bile or blood but with melenic stool
4. Hyperactive bowel sounds

Diagnosis: Probable upper gastrointestinal bleeding (see Figure 16–2)

1. No documented hematemesis
2. Nasogastric aspirate with bile but without blood
3. Maroon stools
4. Hematochezia, especially with normal hyperactive bowel sounds

Diagnosis: Probable lower gastrointestinal bleeding (see Figure 16–3)

▶ Recognize Risk Factors for Severe Gastrointestinal Bleeding

Signs, symptoms, or history that may indicate ongoing hemorrhage are as follows:

- Profuse hematemesis or hematochezia
- Hypotension, tachycardia, or signs of shock
- Postural hypotension, tachycardia, or lightheadedness
- Possible aortoenteric fistula (history of abdominal aortic aneurysm repair or palpable pulsating abdominal mass)
- Known or suspected esophageal varices
- Previous history of GI bleeding
- History of diverticulosis

▶ Initial Stabilization Procedures

As with any emergency, always address your patient's ABCs first.

A. Assess Need for Airway Management

Consider endotracheal intubation for patients with ongoing massive hematemesis or if signs and symptoms of shock are present, If immediate airway control is not needed, provide supplemental oxygen as needed to maintain oxygen saturation at greater than 93%.

B. Obtain Venous Access

Insert two large-bore intravenous catheters (18 gauge or larger) into peripheral veins. If peripheral access cannot be obtained, consider placement of a central venous line.

C. Begin Fluid Resuscitation

Rapidly bolus either warmed lactated Ringer's or normal saline to restore intravascular volume.

D. Assess the Need for Immediate Blood Transfusion

For persistent hypotension despite the infusion of 2 L of crystalloid, consider immediate transfusion of cross-matched blood if available. If not, then transfuse O-negative blood until cross-matched blood is available. There should be a lower threshold to transfuse for elderly patients or those with known cardiac dysfunction. Continue transfusion to maintain systolic blood pressure at greater than 90 mm Hg.

E. Perform Laboratory Studies

Send blood for complete blood count. Type and cross-match blood for two to six units, depending on the extent of bleeding and the patient's status. Measure prothrombin and partial thromboplastin time to assess for any coagulopathy. Measure serum electrolytes and renal and liver functions.

Blood urea nitrogen is elevated in many patients with upper GI bleeding. Venous blood gas and lactate may be helpful in assessing tissue perfusion status. Whenever possible, draw the patient's blood for analysis prior to transfusion for accurate coagulation studies.

F. Perform Electrocardiogram

Obtain an electrocardiogram (ECG) for any patient older than 50 years; for any patient with a history of ischemic heart disease or significant anemia; and for any patient with chest pain, shortness of breath, or severe hypotension. If the initial ECG demonstrates ongoing ischemia in the face of ongoing GI bleeding, then consider immediate transfusion of packed red blood cells. If a patient's initial hematocrit is less than 30% and he or she has a history of ischemic heart disease, consider early transfusion. Maintain a low threshold of suspicion for myocardial infarction (MI), as patients suffering MIs subsequent to massive bleeding may not experience chest pain.

G. Physical Examination

Perform a complete physical examination, including general appearance and mental status; cardiac examination; pulmonary examination; abdominal examination (including noting surgical scars, distention, auscultation for bruits that may indicate an aneurysm, palpating organ size); and skin changes such as pallor, moisture, telangiectasia, ecchymoses, and petechiae. Rectal examination for hemorrhoids or fissures and stool examination for occult blood are essential.

H. Insert Nasogastric or Orogastric Tube

If hematemesis has not been documented, prepare the nasal passageway and posterior pharynx with topical anesthetic, place a nasogastric tube, and lavage with room temperature normal saline (cold fluids may impede normal coagulation) until aspirate is clear. Persistent bleeding during lavage indicates potential life-threatening upper GI bleeding, and immediate consultation with a gastroenterologist or surgeon should be obtained. Lavage prior to endoscopy may improve visualization during endoscopic procedure, especially in the fundus.

If persistent bleeding is noted and the endoscopist gives instructions to do so, place a nasogastric tube for gastric lavage with increments of 200–300 mL of either saline or tap water. The patient should be in the left lateral decubitus position with the bed in the reverse Trendelenburg position. Lavage until the return is clear. Administration of erythromycin IV will stimulate gastric motility and will also help to clear the stomach of blood prior to endoscopy to improve visualization during the procedure.

I. Perform Bladder Catheterization

If a patient is in shock or has a history of cardiac or renal dysfunction, insert a Foley catheter into the bladder to monitor urinary output. Order a urine analysis to assess for hematuria, which may indicate an abdominal aneurysm.

J. Withhold All Fluids and Antacids

Patients waiting for endoscopy should receive nothing by mouth. Antacids may impair adequate visualization during endoscopy.

K. Correct Coagulopathy

Patients taking Coumadin or those who show signs of hepatic failure (eg, jaundice) may require vitamin K and fresh frozen plasma to correct coagulopathy before bleeding can be controlled.

L. Seek Early Consultation

After initial stabilization of the patient, contact the on-call general surgeon or gastroenterologist for either immediate endoscopy and therapy or further instructions. If emergent endoscopic services are unavailable at the treating facility, the emergency physician should find an accepting physician at a facility capable of providing these services and arrange rapid transport.

▶ Disposition

On the basis of certain clinical criteria such as age, co-morbid disease, presenting vital signs, laboratory data, and availability of next-day follow-up, a subgroup of patients with GI hemorrhage can be discharged home. This decision should be made with the gastroenterologist. Intensive care unit admission should be reserved for patients with continued bleeding, abnormal vital signs, significant co-morbid disease, or need for transfusion therapy and for those at increased risk for rebleeding (ie, esophageal varices).

DETERMINE SITE OF BLEEDING

Once the patient is stabilized, attempt to determine the bleeding site if it is not already obvious. In 90% of patients presenting with GI hemorrhage, the bleeding has an upper GI source (ie, proximal to the ligament of Treitz). In about 80–85% of patients with GI hemorrhage, the bleeding will cease prior to the patient's arrival in the emergency department.

▶ Diagnostic Characteristics of Upper Gastrointestinal Bleeding

(See Figure 16–2) The incidence of upper GI bleeds is 50–150/100,000 with a predominance in males and the elderly.

A. Hematemesis

Hematemesis (excluding hemoptysis or swallowed blood from epistaxis) is observed during upper gastrointestinal bleeding. Nasogastric lavage usually reveals aspirate which is grossly bloody or guaiac positive.

The aspirate will be negative in approximately 10% of patients with a duodenal source of GI hemorrhage. A duodenal source cannot be excluded unless gastric lavage contents reveal bile. Even if bile is returned, the bleeding may have resolved spontaneously prior to arrival. If a patient reports unwitnessed hematemesis and gastric lavage is inconclusive, consultation with a gastroenterologist for early endoscopy is warranted.

B. Melena and Hematochezia

Melena is usually due to bleeding from an upper GI source. Hematochezia from an upper source usually indicates severe hemorrhage and corresponds with significant increases in mortality, need for transfusion, complications, and need for surgery.

▶ Diagnostic Characteristics of Lower Gastrointestinal Bleeding

The incidence of lower GI bleeds is 20/100,000 and are again more frequent in males and the elderly.

A. Hematochezia

Hematochezia is usually due to bleeding distal to the Ligament of Treitz. An upper GI source is found for suspected lower GI bleeding in up to 15% of patients presenting with hematochezia. In these instances, consider aortoenteric fistula (in patients with abdominal aortic aneurysm repair) or duodenal ulcer.

B. Melena

Melena is rarely associated with lower GI bleeding except when motility in the intestinal tract is decreased. Bismuth salicylate and iron supplementation may also result in black stools or pseudo-melena.

C. Bright Red Blood

When seen as streaks on stool or on toilet paper after wiping, bright red blood usually indicates a hemorrhoidal or anal fissure source of bleeding. If the patient complains of painful bowel movements anal fissures are most likely.

D. Absence of Bleeding

Spontaneous cessation of bleeding occurs in about 80–85% of cases without intervention, although cessation can be intermittent, and bleeding can restart at any time.

▼ FURTHER EVALUATION OF GASTROINTESTINAL BLEEDING

The unstable patient should be rapidly resuscitated and stabilized prior to completing a detailed history and physical examination. Once the patient's hemodynamic status has

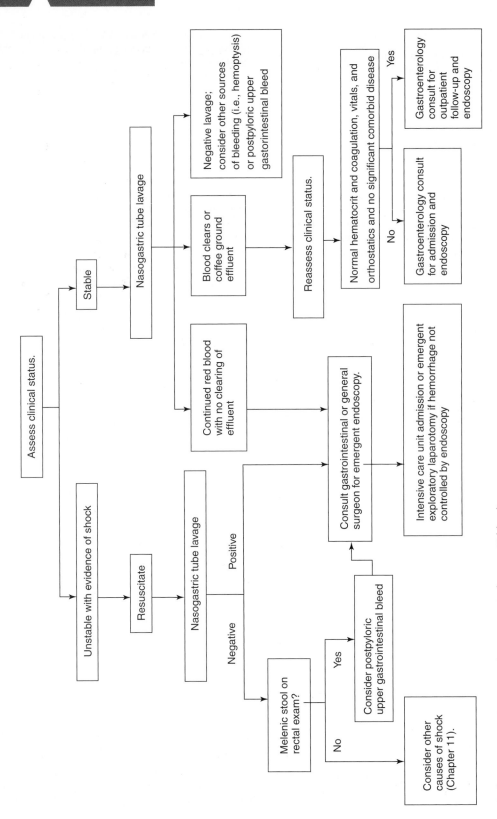

▲ **Figure 16-2.** Hematemesis or suspected upper GI bleeding.

stabilized, a more thorough examination should be done. For the patient not in extremis and those otherwise stable, this examination can be performed during the initial assessment.

▶ History

Inquire about history of GI bleeding, esophageal varices, alcohol or non-steroidal anti-inflammatory drug (NSAID) use, oral anticoagulation, recent weight loss, change in caliber of stools, abdominal aneurysm repair, liver disease, or abdominal surgery. Recent vigorous retching or vomiting prior to onset of hematemesis suggests the presence of Mallory–Weiss tears. Inquire about history of hemorrhoids, anal fissures, or rectal trauma (eg, rectal intercourse, placement of foreign objects in rectum).

In immunocompromised patients, bleeding may be related to Kaposi sarcoma, lymphoma, or cytomegalovirus ulcerations. Visceral Kaposi sarcoma is usually associated with cutaneous lesions.

▶ Physical Examination

A. Vital Signs

Reassess vital signs every 15 minutes or more frequently as needed.

B. Cardiopulmonary Examination

Evaluate the patient for any evidence of cardiac dysfunction (ie, murmurs, rubs, gallops, arrhythmias). Listen to the lungs for abnormal sounds that may be suggestive of heart failure or an infectious process.

C. Abdominal Examination

Tenderness to palpation in the epigastrium is common with gastritis or peptic ulcer disease. Any patient who has had multiple episodes of vomiting may also have diffuse tenderness of the abdomen. Any elderly patient whose complaints of abdominal pain are out of proportion to the examination should be suspected of having mesenteric ischemia. Significant tenderness or peritoneal signs may indicate perforation and warrant immediate surgical consultation. Auscultation of hyperactive bowel sounds may be observed in an upper GI bleed as the presence of blood will stimulate peristalsis.

Examine the patient for signs of chronic liver disease (hepatosplenomegaly, ascites, spider angiomas, enlarged abdominal vessels, jaundice, hepatojugular reflux, asterixis, palmar erythema). Although the presence of liver disease constitutes a higher likelihood of esophageal varices, one should make no assumptions regarding the etiology of the bleeding. GI bleeding will be from another identifiable source in 50% of patients with known esophageal varices. Inspect the patient for surgical scars that indicate previous abdominal surgery or possible vascular repair.

D. Integument Examination

The presence of telangiectasias of the skin (particularly the digits) and lips may indicate Osler–Weber–Rendu disease (hereditary hemorrhagic telangiectasia), which causes GI bleeding secondary to vascular malformations.

E. Rectal Examination

Obtain a stool sample for hemoccult testing, and check for evidence of hemorrhoids or anal fissures.

▶ Special Examinations

A. Upper Gastrointestinal Bleeding

1. Endoscopy—Endoscopy is the most accurate diagnostic tool for upper GI bleeding; it locates the source of bleeding in 75–95% of patients. If the patient is actively bleeding, endoscopy should be performed as soon as possible. If the patient is stable and has no active bleeding, endoscopy should generally be performed within 24 hours. Endoscopic hemostasis techniques offer therapeutic benefit to the patient and result in improved outcomes.

2. Upper gastrointestinal series—An upper GI series plays no role in the evaluation of upper GI bleeding. Contrast material may obscure the endoscopist's view preventing adequate evaluation.

3. Angiography—Angiography is used in only about 1% of patients with upper GI bleeding. It may be useful if endoscopy cannot identify a bleeding source even when active bleeding is suspected.

B. Lower Gastrointestinal Bleeding

1. Colonoscopy—Colonoscopy is considered by many endoscopists to be the modality of choice for diagnosis as well as for therapeutic intervention. A definitive diagnosis is made in approximately 75% of cases. Epinephrine injection can be performed if active bleeding sites are identified.

2. Anoscopy/proctosigmoidoscopy—Examination of the rectum and distal sigmoid colon should be undertaken as soon as the patient has been stabilized. If there is evidence of hemorrhoidal bleeding and no blood is noted above the rectum, the bleeding source is in the rectum. The presence of blood above the rectum reliably indicates bleeding from a more proximal site.

3. Barium enema—Barium enema is not used as a diagnostic study for lower GI bleeding. The barium would interfere not only with endoscopic visualization but also with visceral angiography, should that be necessary.

4. Mesenteric angiography—If the bleeding rate is estimated to be greater than 0.5–1 mL/min, angiography allows for selective embolization or vasopressin infusion. Complications associated with angiography include contrast-induced renal failure, arterial dissection, and bowel infarction. This test should be ordered only after consultation with a general surgeon or gastroenterologist.

5. Technetium red cell scintigraphy—Technetium bleeding scans may be indicated if the bleeding rate is greater than 0.1 mL/min. A portion of the patient's red blood cells are labeled with technetium-99m and reinfused, followed by scanning. The scan can be repeated periodically to help localize the bleeding site within the GI tract. This testing modality can be used prior to angiography to increase the yield and decrease the risk associated with the procedure. These examinations are usually performed after consultation with an endoscopist.

▶ Monitoring for Rebleeding

A. Gastric Lavage

After placement of a nasogastric tube, continue reassessment for rebleeding by using intermittent low continuous suction. Bright red blood or clots in the aspirate are an indication for gentle gastric lavage. Overly vigorous lavage can cause gastric erosions. Continued bleeding or rebleeding is an indication for emergent endoscopy.

B. Stool

Record frequency, color, and approximate amount of stool passed by the patient. Continued passage of bright red, maroon, or melenic stools may indicate need for further studies or transfusion.

C. Hemoglobin and Hematocrit

Frequent checking of hemoglobin and hematocrit (every 4 hours) is essential in patients with active bleeding after they are hemodynamically stabilized. Often the initial hematocrit is normal. After fluid resuscitation and equilibration of intravascular volume, the hemoglobin and hematocrit should be rechecked.

Almela P et al: Outpatient management of upper digestive hemorrhage not associated with portal hypertension: a large prospective cohort. Am J Gastroenterol 2001;96:2341 [PMID: 11513172].

Fallah MA et al: Acute gastrointestinal bleeding. Med Clin North Am 2000;84:1183 [PMID: 11026924].

Jensen DM et al: Urgent colonoscopy for the diagnosis and treatment of severe diverticular hemorrhage. N Engl J Med 2000;342:78 [PMID: 10631275].

Lee SD et al: A randomized controlled trial of gastric lavage prior to endoscopy for acute upper gastrointestinal bleeding. J Clin Gastroenterol 2004;38:861–865 [PMID: 15492601].

Lefkovitz Z: Radiology in the diagnosis and therapy of gastrointestinal bleeding. Gastroenterol Clin 2000;29:489 [PMID: 10836191].

O'Neil BB et al: Cinematic nuclear scintigraphy reliably directs surgical intervention for patients with gastrointestinal bleeding. Arch Surg 2000;135:1076 [PMID: 10982513].

Podila PV et al: Managing patients with acute, nonvariceal gastrointestinal hemorrhage: development of a clinical care pathway. Am J Gastroenterol 2001;96:208 [PMID: 11197254].

Shetzline MA et al: Provocative angiography in obscure gastrointestinal bleeding. South Med J 2000;93:1205 [PMID: 11142458].

Cappell, MS: A study of the syndrome of simultaneous acute upper gastrointestinal bleeding and myocardial infarction in 36 patients. Am J Gastroenterol 1995;90:1444–1449 [PMID: 7661167].

▼ EMERGENCY TREATMENT OF SPECIFIC DISORDERS CAUSING UPPER GASTROINTESTINAL BLEEDING ·

ESSENTIALS OF DIAGNOSIS

▶ May present with hematemesis or melena; massive upper GI bleeding may have hematochezia.

▶ Peptic ulcer disease accounts for 50% of upper GI bleeding; consider initiating proton-pump inhibitor therapy.

▶ Endoscopy is frequently diagnostic and often therapeutic.

Table 16–1 lists the most likely sites of upper GI bleeding. Figure 16–2 is an algorithm for identification of the bleeding site. Esophagogastroduodenoscopy (EGD) is the procedure of choice for the patient with acute hemorrhage or the stable

Table 16–1. Top Causes of Upper Gastrointestinal Tract Hemorrhage in Patients Undergoing Diagnostic Endoscopy at the San Francisco General Hospital Over 3 Years.

Source of Hemorrhage	Severity of Hemorrhage (%)
Mild-Moderate (n = 246 patients)	
Duodenal ulcer	31
Gastric ulcer	15
Esophagitis	12
Severe (n = 140 patients)	
Esophageal varices	31
Mallory-Weiss tear	19
Duodenal ulcer	15
Gastric ulcer	14

patient without active bleeding. Specific conditions and their management are discussed below.

PEPTIC ULCER DISEASE

Peptic ulcer disease accounts for approximately half of all episodes of upper GI bleeding (see Table 16–1).

▶ Clinical Findings

Patients with peptic ulcer disease usually present with epigastric to left upper quadrant pain. This pain is frequently described as burning. Depending on the location of the ulcer, this pain can be made worse or even better with food. Many patients have had dyspeptic symptoms for years. Up to 40% of patients may not relate pain prior to onset of bleeding.

The severity of bleeding determines the clinical presentation:

- Acute: Sudden onset with massive hemorrhage with symptoms and signs suggestive of shock upon presentation.
- Chronic: Increased fatigue, weakness, occult blood in stool, and anemia due to slow bleeding may be the only symptoms among elderly patients with ulcer disease.

▶ Treatment

Provide emergent management as discussed above, in the Immediate Management of Life-Threatening Bleeding section. All patients with known peptic ulcer disease should be given a proton-pump inhibitor such as omeprazole or rabeprazole. If the patient has suspected peptic ulcer disease, consider initiating treatment with a proton-pump inhibitor in the emergency department.

Somatostatin is an endogenous peptide that reduces splanchnic blood flow and GI motility, inhibits acid secretion, and may have gastric cytoprotective effects. Octreotide is a synthetic analogue of somatostatin that, when used in the presence of upper GI hemorrhage, may reduce the risk of continued bleeding from actively bleeding peptic ulcer disease. With a very short half-life, it is typically given as a bolus of 50–100 μg followed by an infusion of 25–50 μg/h.

Patients should be instructed not to smoke, consume alcohol, or use NSAIDS, aspirin, or caffeine on a regular basis. Recurrent or persistent hemorrhage requires evaluation for surgical intervention.

▶ Disposition

Patients with active bleeding, tachycardia, hypotension, anemia, age greater than 65 years, or significant co-morbid disease should be admitted for evaluation and observation. If none of these risk factors are present, and close follow-up with a gastroenterologist can be arranged within 24–48 hours, the patient may be discharged home. All patients should

be given a proton pump inhibitor as an outpatient, if not already prescribed by their primary care physician.

GASTRITIS

Gastritis is a more frequently recognized entity with the advent of upper endoscopy as the preferred diagnostic modality in the evaluation of upper GI bleeding. Gastritis is commonly associated with alcohol ingestion as well as aspirin, caffeine, and NSAID use. Esophagitis and duodenitis may also coexist as findings on endoscopy. The presence of esophagitis on endoscopy indicates dysfunction of the gastroesophageal sphincter with reflux of gastric secretions.

▶ Clinical Findings

Although gastritis is asymptomatic in many cases, patients may experience anorexia, nausea, dyspepsia, pain, and immediate postprandial emesis. The diagnosis is made by endoscopy and cannot be reliably made by an upper GI series. Gastritis rarely results in massive bleeding by itself, but it can occur in the presence of portal hypertension and coagulopathies.

▶ Treatment

Provide therapy as directed above. Continue nasogastric lavage until brisk bleeding has resolved.

For non-bleeding, clinically suspected gastritis, a trial of an antacid with viscous lidocaine ("GI cocktail") may provide quick relief. Consider prescribing a proton-pump inhibitor or recommending any of the many over-the-counter histamine H2 antagonists (eg, ranitidine, famotidine).

Instruct patients to avoid aspirin, NSAIDS, caffeine, and alcohol until re-evaluated by their primary care physician.

▶ Disposition

Patients with active bleeding should be hospitalized and receive treatment as outlined above. For patients who meet previously mentioned criteria for discharge, ensure timely follow-up with either their doctor or a gastroenterologist.

MALLORY–WEISS SYNDROME

Tears in the esophageal mucosa and submucosa that usually occur after forceful retching and vomiting are responsible for approximately 10% of acute upper GI bleeding. Hematemesis is present in 85% of patients on presentation. Bleeding usually resolves spontaneously, but 3% of deaths from upper GI bleeding have been attributed to Mallory–Weiss tears.

▶ Clinical Findings

In addition to retching and vomiting, this disorder has been reported following chest compressions, coughing, sneezing, or even straining with bowel movement. Many cases have no discernible predisposing factor. Alcohol abuse is a significant risk factor. EGD is the diagnostic gold standard.

▶ Treatment

Provide emergency management as outlined earlier. Nasogastric lavage until clear. For persistent bleeding, consult with an endoscopist for emergent EGD with possible therapeutic epinephrine injection, coagulation, or embolization of the vessel. A proton-pump inhibitor or sucralfate may be used to reduce acid or bile that may impair healing of the mucosal tear. Also consider treating precipitating factors such as antiemetics for nausea and vomiting. Prognosis is good and most patients stop bleeding spontaneously with healing of the mucosal tear in 48–72 hours.

▶ Disposition

For bleeding that does not resolve spontaneously, hospitalize the patient for observation and treatment.

ESOPHAGEAL VARICES

Patients with underlying liver disease and portal hypertension are at increased risk for esophageal or gastric variceal bleeding. Approximately 40% of these patients will experience a variceal bleed with mortality rates of 30–50%. Alcohol-induced and viral cirrhosis are the most common cause of esophageal varices in the United States, but parasitic infestations of the liver are a frequent cause of cirrhosis in underdeveloped countries.

▶ Clinical Findings

Upper GI bleeding secondary to varices cannot be clinically diagnosed on the basis of signs and symptoms alone. As mentioned earlier, in approximately 50% of patients with known varices who present with GI bleeding, the bleeding is from a source other than the varices. Endoscopic verification is mandatory for accurate diagnosis and treatment.

▶ Treatment

A. Emergency Measures

Provide emergent resuscitative efforts as outlined above.

B. Airway Management

If the patient has altered mental status or profuse hematemesis, protective endotracheal intubation is recommended.

C. Monitor Cardiovascular Status

If the patient is unstable and has significant co-morbid disease, consider invasive monitoring of central venous pressure and arterial blood pressure.

D. Medical Therapy

In general, a nasogastric tube is inserted to monitor the amount of GI hemorrhage and to facilitate endoscopy by evacuation of gastric contents including blood. The immediate use of octreotide has been proven effective in controlling bleeding. Octreotide decreases splanchnic and hepatic blood flow as well as transhepatic and variceal pressures. Vasopressin has fallen out of favor because of its systemic effects and risk of ischemia.

E. Endoscopic Therapy

Sclerotherapy involves the injection of various sclerosing agents to promote thrombus formation. Band ligation uses endoscopically placed rubber bands, which block blood flow and promote thrombus formation. Both therapies work well in over 90% of patients, but band ligation is associated with fewer complications.

F. Balloon Tamponade

In rare circumstances it may be necessary to insert a Sengstaken–Blakemore tube to tamponade uncontrolled hemorrhage prior to endoscopic confirmation. Patients must be intubated prior to insertion of the tube.

▶ Disposition

Essentially all patients with variceal bleeding are admitted to an intensive care area for further observation and treatment.

HEMOBILIA

Hemobilia can occur secondary to trauma, hepatic tumors, gallstones, and parasites. It can cause bleeding into the biliary tract, resulting in upper GI bleeding.

▶ Clinical Findings

Hemobilia presents as GI bleeding. During EGD, bleeding is noted from the ampulla of Vater. Bleeding is typically mild. Angiography can further delineate the bleeding site.

▶ Treatment and Disposition

Patients should be hospitalized for observation and treatment. Embolization via interventional radiographic technique is the therapy of choice.

AORTIC ANEURYSM (AORTOENTERIC FISTULA)

▶ Clinical Findings

Upper GI bleeding in the presence of an abdominal aortic aneurysm (or graft) should be assumed to be secondary to an aortoenteric fistula until proven otherwise.

Bleeding may be moderate at first, but profuse hemorrhage will eventually occur unless proper treatment is given. If the patient has a GI bleed and a history of an abdominal aortic aneurysm or graft repair, or if the history and physical examination are suggestive of such, obtain immediate surgical consultation after performing initial resuscitation. If the patient is hemodynamically unstable, emergent surgery is indicated. Consider bedside ultrasonography followed by computed tomography scan for confirmation in the stable patient.

Treatment

Stabilize as previously outlined and obtain immediate surgical consultation.

Disposition

All patients with the diagnosis mentioned above should be admitted to an intensive care setting with evaluation by a surgeon.

Almela P et al: Outpatient management of upper digestive hemorrhage not associated with portal hypertension: a large prospective cohort. Am J Gastroenterol 2001;96:2341 [PMID: 11513172].

Sharara AI et al: Medical progress: gastroesophageal variceal hemorrhage. N Engl J Med 2001;345:669 [PMID: 11547722].

Fallah MA et al: Acute gastrointestinal bleeding. Med Clin North Am 2000;84:1183 [PMID: 11026924].

Podila PV et al: Managing patients with acute, nonvariceal gastrointestinal hemorrhage: development of a clinical care pathway. Am J Gastroenterol 2001;96:208 [PMID: 11197254].

EMERGENCY TREATMENT OF SPECIFIC DISORDERS CAUSING LOWER GASTROINTESTINAL BLEEDING

 ESSENTIALS OF DIAGNOSIS

▶ Patients present with hematochezia; 10% may be from an upper GI source.

▶ 80–85% of lower GI bleeding resolves spontaneously.

▶ Sigmoidoscopy or colonoscopy can diagnose most sources of lower GI bleeding.

General Considerations

Lower GI bleeding is most commonly a result of diverticular disease, followed by angiodysplasia, colonic ulcers, and other miscellaneous causes. The most common cause depends on the patient's age. In the adolescent or young adult, Meckel's diverticulum, inflammatory bowel disease, and polyps are the most likely causes. In adults up to 60 years, diverticula, inflammatory bowel disease, and neoplasms are the more common causes. In patients older than 60 years, angiodysplasia, diverticula, and neoplasms predominate.

In 80–85% of patients with lower GI bleeding, the bleeding resolves spontaneously, often making it difficult to locate the source of bleeding. Massive bleeding can occur from any site in the lower GI tract, although diverticular bleeding originates in the colon.

DIVERTICULOSIS

Clinical Findings

Although typically asymptomatic, patients with diverticulosis may present with cramping, lower abdominal pain, and left lower quadrant tenderness to palpation. Tenesmus, constipation, or diarrhea may be associated with diverticulosis. Massive bleeding may occur acutely without any signs or symptoms of diverticulitis.

Treatment and Disposition

(See Figure 16–3) Perform emergency stabilization as outlined above. Colonoscopy is becoming the modality of choice for initial evaluation in many cases after bowel prep. If massive hemorrhage is present, surgery may be necessary. Selective angiography with embolization is also an option for bleeding control. Most patients should be admitted for further observation and treatment.

ANGIODYSPLASIA

Clinical Findings

Angiodysplasia is characterized by painless bleeding that may be mild or massive. Signs may range from occult blood in stools to melena to hematochezia. Most patients are older than 60 years and have a history of cardiac or renal disease.

Approximately 90% of bleeding caused by angiodysplasia spontaneously ceases. For bleeding rates 0.1 mL/min or greater, technetium red cell scan is fairly reliable, although the diagnostic modality of choice may vary between consultants. Colonoscopy may reveal spider angioma-like lesions.

Treatment and Disposition

Stabilize the patient as previously discussed. Electrocoagulation has shown good results for treatment of bleeding lesions visualized during colonoscopy. If bleeding is localized via radionucleotide scanning, then embolization through angiography can be curative in many cases. Angiography can also provide accurate localization of the bleeding when surgical intervention is necessary.

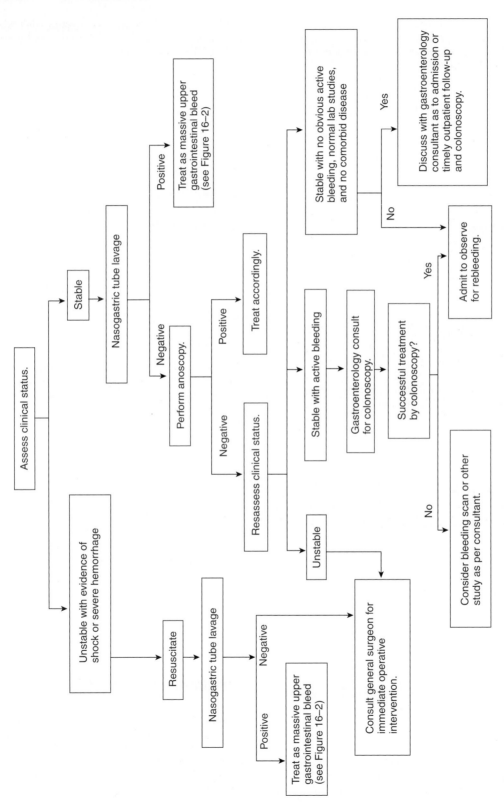

▲ **Figure 16-3.** Hematochezia or suspected lower GI bleeding.

Hospitalize patients for further work-up and observation as directed by the consultant.

HEMORRHOIDS

▶ Clinical Findings

Bleeding is usually the first symptom of internal hemorrhoids. Hemorrhoids are the most common cause of hematochezia in adults. There may be a history of straining on defecation, and the patient will present with frank hematochezia often mixed with well-formed, normal-appearing stools. Occasionally, recurrent bleeding can result in marked anemia. Exsanguinating hemorrhage is rare unless portal hypertension is present. The diagnosis should be confirmed by proctoscopy in the emergency department. Careful anoscopy must be done to fully visualize hemorrhoids. If a flexible fiberoptic sigmoidoscope is used, retroflexion of the insertion tube is necessary to ensure good visualization of the anorectal junction.

▶ Treatment

A. Medical Measures

Most early cases can be managed with high-roughage diet, local measures (sitz baths, suppositories for hemorrhoids), and stool softeners (psyllium, dioctyl sodium sulfosuccinate).

B. Surgical Measures

Surgery is required occasionally to arrest hemorrhage not controlled by medical measures.

▶ Disposition

Hospitalize patients for surgery to arrest persistent brisk bleeding. It is prudent to hospitalize patients with portal hypertension as well. Otherwise, refer patients for outpatient follow-up.

COLONIC POLYPS

▶ Clinical Findings

Painless rectal bleeding and discovery of a polyp on sigmoidoscopy, colonoscopy, or barium enema confirm the diagnosis of colonic polyposis.

▶ Treatment

For significant bleeding, see Immediate Management of Life-Threatening Bleeding section. If bleeding persists, the polyps should be removed immediately.

▶ Disposition

Hospitalization is necessary if bleeding persists. If bleeding has stopped, patients can be referred for elective polypectomy.

COLITIS

▶ Clinical Findings

The chief findings are abdominal cramps, diarrheal stools containing blood and mucopurulent material, fever, weight loss, and anemia. On sigmoidoscopy, the rectal mucosa is eroded and friable. Infectious causes of colitis (particularly *Shigella, Campylobacter, Entamoeba histolytica, Clostridium difficile,* and *Salmonella*) must be ruled out.

Occasionally, particularly in elderly patients, ischemic colitis can occur with brisk hematochezia. Differentiation from idiopathic or infectious colitis is often possible on sigmoidoscopy. Ischemic colitis rarely, if ever, involves the rectum, whereas other forms of colitis almost always involve the rectum.

▶ Treatment

See Emergency Management of Life-Threatening Bleeding section. Medical measures can usually control most symptoms in mild to moderate cases. Surgery is reserved for severe problems.

▶ Disposition

Severe cases are medical emergencies requiring immediate hospitalization. Mild cases can be referred for outpatient evaluation and treatment after stool samples have been collected for evaluation for enteric pathogens.

CROHN'S DISEASE

▶ Clinical Findings

Frank blood is seen in about one-third of patients with Crohn's disease, but massive bleeding is unusual. Patients have abdominal pain, anorexia, diarrhea, weight loss, and fatigue. There may be fever and sepsis.

Fistula formation, fissures, and hemorrhoids are common. However, Crohn's disease may not involve the rectum or sigmoid. A normal proctosigmoidoscopic examination does not exclude the disease.

▶ Treatment

Severe exacerbations of Crohn's disease should be managed medically with bowel rest, nasogastric suction, and IV fluids. Surgery is rarely indicated, when massive bleeding is not controlled by medical measures. Amebic disease must be excluded before corticosteroids are used.

▶ Disposition

Patients with severe bleeding or systemic symptoms (fever, weight loss) must be hospitalized for observation and treatment. Patients with mild disease can be referred for outpatient follow-up.

SOLITARY RECTAL ULCER

▶ Clinical Findings

Rectal ulcer is an unusual lesion associated with rectal prolapse. It may result from straining at stool. The patient passes blood and mucus per rectum. Many patients are elderly and have chronic constipation.

▶ Treatment and Disposition

Offer general measures to aid defecation (eg, hydration, stool softeners). Surgery should be avoided. Refer the patient for outpatient evaluation and follow-up.

MECKEL'S DIVERTICULUM

▶ Clinical Findings

The incidence of Meckel's diverticulum is approximately 2% of the population. About 25% of patients with Meckel's diverticulum become symptomatic and 25% of these patients have lower GI bleeding. This disorder usually occurs before age 2 years and rarely after age 10 years. Symptoms may mimic acute appendicitis. Hemorrhage is the most common complication followed by intestinal obstruction. Meckel's diverticulum may be diagnosed by technetium pertechnetate scintigraphy or angiography.

▶ Treatment and Disposition

Hospitalize patients for observation, because surgery may be required for severe bleeding, intestinal obstruction, diverticulitis, and umbilicoileal fistulas.

Fallah MA et al: Acute gastrointestinal bleeding. Med Clin North Am 2000;84:1183 [PMID: 11026924].

Jensen DM et al: Urgent colonoscopy for the diagnosis and treatment of severe diverticular hemorrhage. N Engl J Med 2000;342:78 [PMID: 10631275].

O'Neil BB et al: Cinematic nuclear scintigraphy reliably directs surgical intervention for patients with gastrointestinal bleeding. Arch Surg 2000;135:1076 [PMID: 10982513].

Cappell MS et al: Initial management of acute upper gastrointestinal bleeding: from initial evaluation up to gastrointestinal endoscopy. Med Clin North Am 2008;92:491–509 [PMID: 18387374].

Lee J et al: Acute lower GI bleeding for the acute care surgeon: current diagnosis and management. Scand J Surg 2009;98:135–142 [PMID: 19919917].

Coma

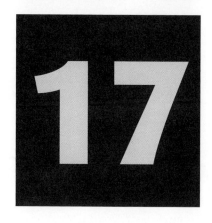

Dylan B. Medley, MD
James E. Morris, MD, MPH

▼ IMMEDIATE MANAGEMENT OF LIFE-THREATENING PROBLEMS

See Figure 17–1.

▶ General Considerations

Coma is defined as the total absence of arousal and awareness lasting at least 1 hour associated with injury or functional disruption of the ascending reticular activating system in the brainstem or bilateral cortical structures. Comatose patients demonstrate no eye opening, speech, or spontaneous movements, and motor activity elicited by painful stimuli (if present) is abnormal or reflexive rather than purposeful. Coma must be differentiated from other pathologic changes in consciousness such as brain death, vegetative state, and delirium, although it may be difficult to do so in the emergency department.

INITIAL MANAGEMENT

Initial management of the comatose patient involves the same steps needed to manage any critically ill patient presenting to the emergency department. Immediate assessment and support of airway, breathing, and circulation should be performed before efforts to diagnose or address specific causes of coma are undertaken, with the caveat that consideration may be given to postponing intubation until administration of empiric therapy for coma. Empiric therapy, often abbreviated by the acronym "D.O.N.T." consists of IV dextrose, supplemental oxygen, IV naloxone, and thiamine. Dextrose (50 mL of 50% solution in adults) reverses coma secondary to hypoglycemia and is indicated if rapid testing of blood glucose is unavailable. Oxygen therapy should be initiated to immediately correct possible hypoxemic induced coma. Naloxone (0.4–2.0 mg IV) rapidly reverses coma and respiratory depression secondary to narcotic overdose but because of short half-life, multiple doses may be required. Thiamine (100 mg IV) is commonly given along with dextrose to avoid precipitating Wernicke encephalopathy in predisposed patients. Flumazenil (0.2 mg/min IV) specifically antagonizes benzodiazepines but is not routinely given empirically as it may precipitate seizures that are then refractory to benzodiazepines. It may be indicated in iatrogenic coma secondary to excess benzodiazepine administration.

If coma persists following the administration of naloxone and dextrose, definitive management of airway and breathing should be considered. IV access with two large-bore IVs should be obtained and blood pressure (especially hypotension) managed aggressively. A complete set of vital signs, including temperature and pulse oximetry, is essential to avoid missing coma complicated by severe hypo- or hyperthermia and hypoxia. Cervical spine immobilization should be maintained if there is any suspicion of trauma. A focused

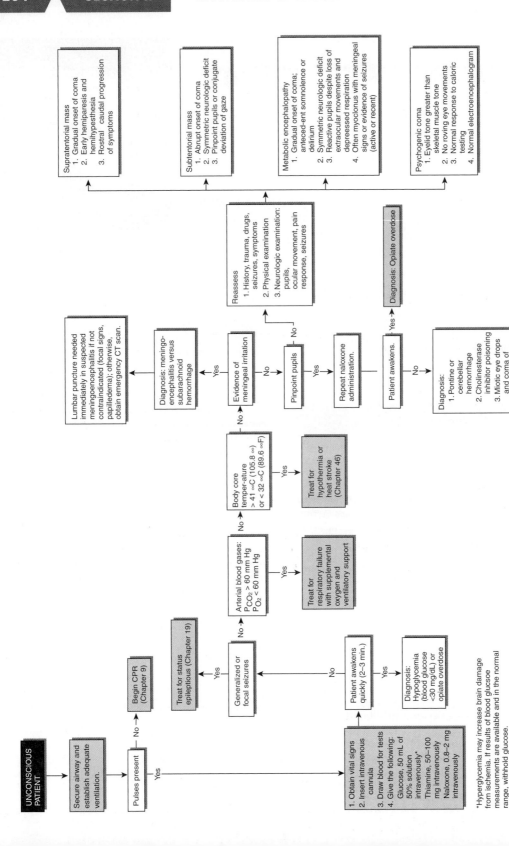

▲ **Figure 17–1.** Approach to the unconscious patient.

Table 17–1. Glasgow Coma Scale.

Component	Score	Adult	Child <5 years	Child >5 years
Motor	6	Follows commands	Normal spontaneous movements	Follows commands
	5	Localizes pain	Localizes to supraocular pain (>9 months)	
	4	Withdraws to pain	Withdraws from nailbed pressure	
	3	Flexion	Flexion to supraocular pain	
	2	Extension	Extension to supraocular pain	
	1	None	None	
Verbal	5	Oriented	Age-appropriate speech/vocalizations	Oriented
	4	Confused speech	Less than usual ability; irritable cry	Confused
	3	Inappropriate words	Cries to pain	Inappropriate words
	2	Incomprehensible	Moans to pain	Incomprehensible
	1	None	No response to pain	
Eye opening	4	Spontaneous	Spontaneous	
	3	To command	To voice	
	2	To pain	To pain	
	1	None	None	

physical examination should be performed to evaluate for potential precipitating factors (evidence of drug use, systemic trauma, etc). Obtaining additional history from friends, relatives, bystanders, and EMS personnel is essential.

NEUROLOGIC ASSESSMENT

Neurologic assessment in comatose patients is of paramount importance, and a structured evaluation should be conducted as soon as possible once immediate threats to life have been addressed. Level of consciousness, cranial nerve examination, and motor examination should be performed.

Lateralizing deficits and a rostrocaudal progression of brainstem dysfunction are seen with structural lesions, while involuntary movements are suggestive of a metabolic cause of coma. Although originally developed for traumatic brain injury, the Glasgow Coma Scale (GCS) has been shown to have predictive value in many different types of coma. Both total and component (eye, verbal, motor) scores should be documented (see Table 17–1).

Cranial nerve examination (especially pupillary response) is an essential part of the neurologic examination and may assist in determining the level of brainstem dysfunction (see Table 17–2). Normal pupillary function

Table 17–2. Brainstem Reflexes.

Reflex	Examination Technique	Normal Response	Brainstem Location
Pupils	Response to light	Direct and consensual restriction	Midbrain
Oculocephalic	Turn head from side to side	Eyes move conjugately in direction opposite to head	Pons
Vestibulo-oculocephalic	Irrigate external auditory canal with cold water	Nystagmus with fast component away from stimulus	Pons
Corneal reflex	Stimulation of cornea	Eyelid closure	Pons
Cough reflex	Stimulation of carina	Cough	Medulla
Gag reflex	Stimulation of soft palate	Symmetric elevation of soft palate	Medulla

Table 17-3. Signs of Increased Intracranial Pressure and Herniation Syndromes.

Sign	Mechanism	Type of Herniation
Coma	Compression of midbrain tegmentum	Uncal, central
Pupillary dilation	Compression of ipsilateral third nerve	Uncal
Miosis	Compression of the midbrain	Central
Lateral gaze palsy	Stretching of CN VI	Central
Hemiparesis	Compression of contralateral cerebral peduncle	Uncal
Decerebrate posturing	Compression of the midbrain	Central, uncal
Hypertension, bradycardia	Compression of the medulla	Central, uncal, cerebellar
Abnormal breathing	Compression of the pons or medulla	Central, uncal, cerebellar

and eye movements may be seen in lesions rostral to the midbrain. Pupillary abnormalities (especially unilateral) may be an early indicator of herniation, and pupillary function should be assessed frequently when increased intracranial pressure (ICP) is a concern. Symmetrically reactive pupils that are unusually large or small are commonly secondary to drug ingestions.

Motor examination should focus on the presence of movements and whether they are involuntary, reflexive, or purposeful. Purposeful movements such as localization require some degree of cortical processing, while reflexes are stereotypical responses that occur in the absence of cortical input. Structural lesions may result in posturing. Decerebrate posturing, characterized by extension of both upper and lower extremities, is seen in lesions caudal to the midbrain. Decorticate posturing, characterized by flexion of the upper extremities and extension of the lower extremities, is seen in lesions rostral to the midbrain.

INCREASED INTRACRANIAL PRESSURE AND HERNIATION

Herniation syndromes result from increased ICP and lead to brainstem compression, manifested by arterial hypertension, bradycardia, and respiratory irregularities (Cushing triad). Herniation may be classified as uncal, central, or cerebellar (see Table 17–3). Increased ICP commonly results from a space-occupying lesion such as a tumor or hematoma but may also result from cerebral edema secondary to trauma, infection, or severe metabolic derangements.

Treatment of increased ICP focuses on maintaining cerebral perfusion pressure, defined as mean arterial pressure (MAP) minus ICP. The goal is to keep CPP > 70–80 mm Hg. The Monro-Kellie principle states that the volume within the skull is fixed and contains three components: brain, blood, and CSF. Increase in the amount of these components (eg, cerebral edema, hematoma, hydrocephalus) or the addition of other components (eg, tumor) results in increased ICP. Using this principle, treatment is aimed at either reducing the volume of the components or expanding the volume available through surgical decompression.

Emergency department care of herniation consists initially of prompt recognition and maximizing resuscitation. Hypoxia and hypotension must be avoided and other adverse systemic factors such as hyperglycemia and fever treated aggressively. The patient's head should be elevated at 30° and adequate sedation and analgesia provided. Seizure prophylaxis should be considered, particularly when paralytics have been given. When available, further treatment should be guided by ICP monitoring. In the absence of ICP monitoring, hyperventilation to a $Paco_2$ of 30–35 mm Hg should be initiated, followed by mannitol (0.25–1.0 g/kg IV) or hypertonic saline (2 mL/kg of 7.5% solution IV). If the ICP remains high and craniectomy is not indicated or not available, barbiturates may be used to decrease cerebral metabolism and thus cerebral blood flow. Induced hypothermia to 32–34°C has been shown to effectively lower otherwise refractory ICP.

Jiang JY: Clinical study of mild hypothermia treatment for severe traumatic brain injury. J Neurotrauma 2009;26:399–406 [PMID: 19260782].

FURTHER EVALUATION OF THE COMATOSE PATIENT

The differential diagnosis of coma is broad and includes primary cerebral disorders (bilateral/diffuse, unilateral with mass effect, and brain-stem disorders) as well as a number of systemic derangements (see Table 17–4).

History

History should be obtained from whatever sources are available, including friends, bystanders, police, and EMS personnel. Crucial points include the following:

- Recent head trauma, even seemingly trivial
- Drug use (including alcohol), recent or past
- Past medical history, including a history of seizures, diabetes, cirrhosis, or other neurologic disease
- Medications, including narcotics and benzodiazepines use
- Precomatose activity and behavior (headache, confusion, vomiting)

Table 17–4. Etiology of Coma and Altered Consciousness.

Primary cerebral disorders
Bilateral or diffuse hemispheric disorders
    Traumatic brain injury
    Ischemic
    Hemorrhagic (subarachnoid hemorrhage, intraventricular
        hemorrhage)
    Hypoxic-ischemic encephalopathy
    Cerebral venous thrombosis
    Malignancy
    Meningitis/encephalitis
    Generalized or complex partial seizures; status epilepticus
    Hypertensive encephalopathy
    Posterior reversible encephalopathy syndrome
    Acute disseminated encephalomyelitis
    Hydrocephalus
Unilateral hemispheric disorders (with displacement of midline
    structures)
    Traumatic (contusions, subdural hematoma, epidural hematoma)
    Large hemispheric ischemic stroke
    Primary intracerebral hemorrhage
    Cerebral abscess
    Brain tumor
Brain stem disorders (pons, midbrain)
    Hemorrhage, infarction, tumor, trauma
    Central pontine myelinolysis
    Compression from cerebellar infarct, hematoma, abscess, tumor
Systemic derangements causing coma
Toxic
    Medication overdose/adverse effects
    Drugs of abuse
    Exposures (carbon monoxide, heavy metals)
Metabolic
    Systemic inflammatory response syndrome/sepsis
    Hypoxia
    Hypercapnia
    Hypothermia
    Hypoglycemia
    Hyperglycemic crises (DKA, NHHS)
    Hypo/hypernatremia
    Hypercalcemia
    Hepatic failure
    Renal failure
    Wernicke encephalopathy
Endocrine
    Panhypopituitarism
    Adrenal insufficiency
    Hypo/hyperthyroidism

- Sudden versus gradual onset of coma
- Other individuals with similar symptoms

▷ Physical Examination

The physical examination (other than the neurologic examination) should focus on ruling out other threats to life such as hypovolemia and systemic trauma. Evidence of trauma elsewhere on the body is presumptive evidence of head trauma in the comatose patient.

▷ Imaging

Non-contrast head CT is an integral part of the workup for coma that is not obviously related to hypoglycemia, overdose, or other metabolic cause, and should be strongly considered in any patient who remains comatose after dextrose and naloxone. Contrast-enhanced head CT or MRI may be indicated in certain patient populations.

▷ Laboratory Evaluation

Electrolytes, LFTs, CBC, UA, glucose, urine/serum toxicology screens, thyroid function studies, BUN/Cr, and ABG should be obtained early in the evaluation of coma. Lumbar puncture and CSF analysis should be performed if not contraindicated (eg, mass lesions or other evidence of increased ICP) in patients for whom the cause of coma is unclear or in whom an infectious cause or SAH is suspected. ECG should be obtained and cardiac monitoring instituted to eliminate cardiac arrhythmias as a contributing factor. An EEG should be obtained when possible, especially in intubated patients receiving paralytics and in those for whom nonconvulsive status epilepticus is a consideration.

Stevens RD, Bhardwaj A: Approach to the comatose patient. Crit Care Med 2006;34:31–41 [PMID: 16374153].

Wilber ST: Altered mental status in older emergency department patients. Emerg Med Clin North Am 2006; 24:299–316 [PMID: 16584959].

▼ EMERGENCY TREATMENT OF SPECIFIC DISORDERS CAUSING COMA

STRUCTURAL LESIONS

1. Intracerebral Hemorrhage

See also Chapter 37.

 ESSENTIALS OF DIAGNOSIS

▶ Headache, nausea, vomiting
▶ Hypertension
▶ Focal neurologic deficit with signs of increased ICP

▷ General Considerations

Intracerebral hemorrhage (ICH) can be classified as primary (unrelated to congenital or acquired lesions) or secondary

Table 17–5. Primary ICH Syndromes

Location	Findings
Basal ganglia	Contralateral motor deficits, gaze paresis, aphasia
Thalamus	Contralateral sensory loss
Cerebellum	Nausea, vomiting, ataxia, nystagmus, AMS, ipsilateral gaze/facial palsy
Pons	Coma, pinpoint pupils, autonomic instability, quadriplegia, altered respiratory patterns

(related to vascular malformations, tumors, or other lesions). The vast majority of primary ICH is related to hypertension and occurs in characteristic areas of the brain: cerebral lobes, basal ganglia, thalamus, pons, and cerebellum. Secondary ICH is more variable in location. Smoking, advanced age, and anticoagulant use are other risk factors for ICH. Early hematoma growth is more common than previously thought and is most likely responsible for sudden deterioration within the first 6 hours of initial presentation. Cytotoxic and vasogenic edema surrounding the hemorrhage may result in ischemia and are likely responsible for delayed deterioration.

▶ **Clinical Findings**

Presentation is related to the size and location of the hemorrhage (see Table 17–5). Patients with large areas of hemorrhage are often comatose on arrival. The majority of patients with brainstem or cerebellar hemorrhage present with a decreased level of consciousness necessitating intubation. Headache is universally present in awake patients and may accompany other signs of increased ICP. Seizures occur in 10% of all ICH but in 50% of patients with lobar hemorrhage. Most patients are hypertensive on presentation, even if previously normotensive. Non-contrast CT scan is the diagnostic study of choice with CT angiography being useful in certain patient populations.

▶ **Treatment and Disposition**

Care is primarily supportive and aimed at reducing ICP and controlling blood pressure. Aggressive blood pressure control using IV labetalol, esmolol, or nicardipine should be instituted with a target SBP < 180 mm Hg or MAP < 130 mm Hg. CPP should be maintained > 70. Patients on anticoagulants should receive reversal agents (FFP and vitamin K for warfarin, protamine for heparin) promptly. The use of prothrombin complex concentrate, factor IX complex concentrate, and rFVIIa have been shown to reverse the elevation of the INR very rapidly (often within 1–2 hours) and is faster to prepare than FFP. Corticosteroids are contraindicated. Prompt neurosurgical consultation should be

obtained for all patients with declining neurological status or evidence of hydrocephalus on CT scan. Cerebellar hemorrhages > 3 cm require surgery. Hemorrhages in typical locations may not need further diagnostic evaluation and are rarely amenable to surgery. All patients should be admitted for further care.

Broderick J et al: Guidelines for the management of spontaneous intracerebral hemorrhage in adults: 2007 update: a guideline from the American Heart Association/American Stroke Association Stroke Council, High Blood Pressure Research Council, and the Quality of Care and Outcomes in Research Interdisciplinary Working Group: The American Academy of Neurology affirms the value of this guideline as an educational tool for neurologists. Stroke 2007;38:2001–2023 [PMID: 17938297].

Hemphill JC. Treating warfarin-related intracerebral hemorrhage: is fresh frozen plasma enough? Stroke 2006;37:6–7 [PMID: 16306461].

Rincon F, Mayer SA: Clinical review: Critical care management of spontaneous intracerebral hemorrhage. Crit Care 2008;12:237 [PMID 19108704].

2. Subdural Hematoma

 ESSENTIALS OF DIAGNOSIS

▶ Headache
▶ Confusion
▶ Depressed level of consciousness
▶ Hyperdense crescent-shaped (biconcave) extra-axial collection of blood on CT scan

▶ **General Considerations**

The possibility of subdural hematoma must be considered in any comatose patient. Trauma is the most common cause, but in about 25% of cases, there is no history or evidence of trauma. Elderly patients are particularly likely to present with absent or trivial trauma. Other risk factors include history of alcoholism, seizures, and coagulopathics.

▶ **Clinical Findings**

Symptoms and signs are notoriously nonspecific, nonlocalizing, or absent and may be either stable or rapidly progressive. The frequency of bilateral hematomas makes localization of the lesion even more difficult, as does the coexistence of associated cerebral contusion. Hemiparesis, when present, is contralateral to the lesion in approximately 60% of cases, and ipsilateral pupillary dilatation occurs in approximately 75% of cases. Seizures may occur. When associated with trauma, a subdural hematoma is most frequently found contracoup to the side of injury. CT scan is the diagnostic study of choice, revealing a hyperdense extra-axial crescent-shaped collection of blood, which rarely crosses the falx or tentorium. Sub-acute lesions (2–3 weeks) may appear as isodense, and patients receiving anticoagulation may demonstrate layering of blood in acute-on-chronic subdural hematoma.

▶ Treatment and Disposition

Immediate hospitalization and emergency neurosurgical consultation are indicated. Unstable patients with rapid worsening (minutes to hours) of their neurologic deficit thought to be due to an expanding subdural hematoma should be treated for increased ICP as discussed previously. Steroids have not been shown to be beneficial.

3. Epidural Hematoma

ESSENTIALS OF DIAGNOSIS

- ▶ Headache
- ▶ History of trauma with overlying skull fracture
- ▶ Classic lucid interval: "talk and die"
- ▶ Lens-shaped (biconvex) extra-axial collection of blood on CT scan

▶ General Considerations

Epidural hematoma is a collection of blood between the dura and the inner table of the skull and occurs almost exclusively in the setting of trauma. The majority of epidural hematomas occur in the temporoparietal region secondary to laceration of the middle meningeal artery. Occipital epidural hematomas may progress rapidly and extend beneath the tentorium, resulting in apnea.

▶ Clinical Findings

Symptoms are progressive. The classic presentation of head trauma followed by a brief loss of consciousness, return to alertness ("lucid interval"), then worsening headache and vomiting with subsequent coma is seen in only 1/5 of patients. Non-contrast CT scan is the diagnostic study of choice, revealing a hyperdense lenticular (biconvex) collection of blood that does not cross suture lines, differentiating it from a subdural hematoma. Ipsilateral pupillary dilation and contralateral hemiparesis are ominous findings suggestive of impending herniation. When associated with trauma, hematoma is most frequently found on the coup side of the injury.

▶ Treatment and Disposition

Immediate neurosurgical consultation is required. In the event a neurosurgeon or CT confirmation of the diagnosis is unavailable and the patient is herniating, a burr hole performed ipsilateral to the area of trauma (or to the dilated pupil if external trauma is not apparent) may be life-saving. Care is otherwise supportive and aimed at decreasing ICP.

4. Cerebral Infarction

ESSENTIALS OF DIAGNOSIS

- ▶ Hemiparesis
- ▶ Hemisensory losses
- ▶ Aphasia (dominant hemisphere)

▶ General Considerations

The brain swelling of cerebral edema following massive hemispheric infarction can produce contralateral hemispheric compression or transtentorial herniation that will result in coma. Such cerebral swelling becomes maximal 48–72 hours after the infarct.

▶ Clinical Findings

The principal findings are hemiparesis or hemisensory loss (and aphasia if the dominant hemisphere is involved). Evolving transtentorial herniation progresses slowly over many hours or several days to stupor and coma. Non-contrast CT scan is the initial diagnostic test of choice.

▶ Treatment and Disposition

Hemicraniectomy may be life-saving in younger patients. Patients who are comatose from massive cerebral infarction have likely progressed to coma secondary to increased ICP rather than the infarction itself, and initial treatment is supportive and aimed at lowering ICP. Blood pressure management is controversial; in severe hypertension (SBP > 220 mm Hg, DBP > 120 mm Hg), IV labetalol or nicardipine are preferred with a goal of reducing the SBP by 15% in first 24 hours.

Adams Jr H et al: Guidelines for the early management of adults with ischemic stroke: a guideline from the American Heart Association/ American Stroke Association Stroke Council, Clinical Cardiology Council, Cardiovascular Radiology and Intervention Council, and the Atherosclerotic Peripheral Vascular Disease and Quality of Care Outcomes in Research Interdisciplinary Working Groups. Stroke 2007;38:1655–1711 [PMID: 17515473].

5. Basilar Artery Occlusion

ESSENTIALS OF DIAGNOSIS

- ▶ Coma, altered mental status
- ▶ Respiratory pattern irregular
- ▶ Pupillary abnormalities, absent or abnormal horizontal eye movements
- ▶ Hemiparesis, hyperreflexia, positive Babinski sign

▶ General Considerations

Basilar artery thrombosis and embolic occlusion are relatively common vascular syndromes that cause coma because of direct involvement of the penetrating arteries supplying the central core of the brain stem. Patients are usually elderly and often have a history of hypertension or transient ischemic attacks or evidence of other atherosclerotic vascular disease.

▶ Clinical Findings

Basilar artery transient ischemic attacks are characterized by (in order of frequency of occurrence) dizziness, diplopia, weakness and ataxia, slurred speech, and nausea and vomiting. Basilar artery occlusion causes coma in half of affected patients, and almost all present with some alteration of consciousness. Focal subtentorial signs are present from the onset, and the respiratory pattern is irregular. Pupillary abnormalities vary with the site of the lesion. Skew deviation of the eyes is common. Horizontal eye movements are absent or asymmetric during the doll's eye maneuver or caloric testing. Conjugate eye deviation, if present, is directed away from the side of the lesion and toward the hemiparesis. Vertical eye movements in response to the doll's eye maneuver may be intact. Symmetric or asymmetric motor signs (hemiparesis, hyperreflexia, and Babinski sign) may be present. The classic "locked in syndrome" is characterized by complete quadriplegia, lower cranial nerve palsy, and mutism with retained consciousness and vertical gaze. CT scan of the head with CT angiography is the diagnostic study of choice, with MRA useful in special populations.

▶ Treatment and Disposition

Current therapy recommendation is recanalization with intravenous or intra-arterial thrombolytics in combination with mechanical manipulation, depending on the institution. While specific guidelines are lacking, time to recanalization is of prognostic importance. In situations where recanalization may be delayed, "bridging therapy" with IV abciximab has shown to improve survival. Even with aggressive treatment, mortality ranges up to 70%. Hospitalize the patient for treatment and supportive care.

Lindsberg PJ, Mattle HP: Therapy of basilar artery occlusion: a systematic analysis comparing intra-arterial and intravenous thrombolysis. Stroke 2006;37:922–928 [PMID: 16439705].

Nagel S et al: Therapy of acute basilar artery occlusion: intraarterial thrombolysis alone vs bridging therapy. Stroke 2009;40:140–146 [PMID: 18927446].

6. Brain Tumor

ESSENTIALS OF DIAGNOSIS

- ▶ Headache
- ▶ Focal weakness
- ▶ Altered mental status
- ▶ Seizures
- ▶ Papilledema
- ▶ CT scan, MRI findings

▶ General Considerations

Coma is seldom the presenting symptom in primary or metastatic tumors of the CNS, although coma may result from seizures induced by the tumors. Acute bleeding into a tumor may also result in coma secondary to a sudden increase in ICP.

▶ Clinical Findings

The patient typically has a history of days to weeks of headache, focal weakness, and altered or depressed consciousness. Papilledema is present in 25% of cases. CT scan (noncontrast followed by contrast-enhanced if needed) is the initial diagnostic study of choice.

▶ Treatment and Disposition

Glucocorticoids (Dexamethasone 10 mg IV) are remarkably effective at reducing surrounding edema and should be initiated early in consultation with neurosurgery. Hospitalization for supportive care and further evaluation is indicated.

Roger EP, Butler J, Benzel EC: Neurosurgery in the elderly: brain tumors and subdural hematomas. Clin Geriatr Med 2006;22:623–44 [PMID: 16860250].

7. Brain Abscess

 ESSENTIALS OF DIAGNOSIS

► Fever (often low grade)
► Leukocytosis
► Contrast-enhanced CT scan or MRI findings of intracranial mass

General Considerations

Brain abscess accounts for only 2% of intracranial masses. Brain abscess should be considered in patients who are immunocompromised who develop changes in mentation. Bacterial brain abscesses most commonly are the result of contiguous spread of infection from the oropharynx, middle ear, and paranasal sinuses. Cranial trauma and hematogenous spread from distant infection are also causes.

Clinical Findings

Progression to stupor and coma may be rapid, occurring over days or, rarely, hours. Symptoms include headache (~70%), mental status changes (70%), focal neurological deficits (> 60%), and seizure (25–35%) at time of presentation. The usual signs of infection are frequently absent. The temperature is normal in half of patients, and the white blood cell count is below 10,000/mL in over one-fourth of patients. CT scan (non-contrast followed by contrast-enhanced if needed) or MRI will reveal almost all abscesses. Lumbar puncture is contra-indicated.

Treatment and Disposition

Initiate antibiotic therapy early, prior to imaging if possible when the clinical suspicion for CNS infection is high. Antibiotic choice should cover anaerobes as well as aerobes, and coverage for fungal or other organisms may be indicated depending on the patient's history. Empiric therapy with a combination of vancomycin 1.0–1.5 g IV plus metronidazole 7.5 mg/kg IV plus a third- or fourth-generation cephalosporin is indicated. Carbapenems can be used in placed of the combination of cephalosporins and metronidazole. Neurosurgical consultation should be obtained with operative intervention necessary of abscesses > 2.5cm. The use of steroids remains controversial and is generally deferred for this indication. Seizure prophylaxis should be initiated early during hospitalization.

Honda H, Warren DK. Central nervous system infections: meningitis and brain abscess. Infect Dis Clin N Am 2009;23:609–623 [PMID: 19665086].

METABOLIC ENCEPHALOPATHIES

 ESSENTIALS OF DIAGNOSIS

► Progressive somnolence
► Intoxication, toxic delirium
► Agitation, stupor, coma
► Headache
► Symmetric neurologic findings
► Reactive pupils
► Hypoventilation, abnormal respiratory pattern
► Loss of extraocular movements

Clinical Findings

Metabolic encephalopathies are characterized by a period of progressive somnolence, intoxication, toxic delirium, or agitation, after which the patient gradually sinks into a stuporous and finally comatose state. Headache is not an initial symptom of metabolic encephalopathy except in the case of meningitis or poisoning due to organophosphate compounds or carbon monoxide.

Neurologic examination fails to reveal focal hemispheric lesions (hemiparesis, hemisensory loss, aphasia) before loss of consciousness. Neurologic findings are symmetric except in some patients with hepatic encephalopathy and hypoglycemic coma, which may be accompanied by focal signs (especially hemiparesis) that may alternate sides. Asterixis may be present.

The hallmark of metabolic encephalopathy is reactive pupils (a midbrain function) in the presence of impaired function of the lower brain stem (eg, hypoventilation, loss of extraocular movements), an anatomically inconsistent set of abnormalities. Respiratory patterns in metabolic coma vary widely and may help establish the cause of coma.

Treatment and Disposition

Treatment depends entirely on the cause of coma. All patients require hospitalization for supportive care and specific therapy.

1. Hypoglycemia

See also Chapter 43.

General Considerations

Unlike other organs, the brain relies mainly on glucose to supply its energy requirements. Abrupt hypoglycemia rapidly interferes with brain metabolism and quickly produces symptoms. Insulin and oral hypoglycemic drug overdose are the most common causes of hypoglycemia.

▶ Clinical Findings

Signs of sympathetic nervous system activity (tachycardia, sweating, and anxiety) may warn patients of impending hypoglycemia, although these signs may be masked by β-blockers and may be absent in patients with diabetic autonomic neuropathy. Common neurologic abnormalities are delirium, seizures, focal signs that often alternate sides, stupor, and coma. Hypoglycemic coma may be tolerated for 60–90 minutes, but once the stage of flaccidity with hyporeflexia has been reached, glucose administration within 15 minutes is mandatory to avoid irreversible damage.

▶ Treatment and Disposition

Give glucose, 50 mL of 50% solution intravenously (adult dose). Once the diagnosis of hypoglycemia is confirmed by analysis of blood drawn before treatment, give an additional 50 mL as needed or begin an infusion of dextrose 5% in water. Subcutaneous or intramuscular glucagon should be considered in patients in which IV access cannot be obtained. Although case reports of octreotide use in hypoglycemia have been shown to be effective, the indications and dosage have not clearly been defined. Patients should be observed for 1–2 hours after glucose supplementation has been discontinued to ensure that hypoglycemia does not recur before they are discharged from the hospital. In some cases, hospitalization may be necessary, especially if hypoglycemia recurs despite treatment or in the event of long-acting insulin or oral hypoglycemic agent overdose (eg sulfonylureas).

Rowden AK, Fasano CJ: Emergency management of oral hypoglycemic drug toxicity. Emerg Med Clin N Am 2007;25:347–356 [PMID: 17482024].

2. Hypoxemia
▶ Clinical Findings

Hypoxemia produces brain damage only as a result of concomitant cerebral ischemia. Cerebral blood flow diminishes and brain ischemia occurs when the arterial Po_2 falls to 20–45 mm Hg. In cerebral anoxia due to cardiac arrest, where the duration can be timed precisely, 4–6 minutes of asystole begins to result in permanent CNS damage. Following asystole, the pupils dilate rapidly and become fixed, and tonic posturing is observed. A few seizure-like tonic–clonic movements are common.

▶ Treatment and Disposition

Treatment of hypoxemia depends on the cause. Support cardiac output and maintain arterial Po_2 above 60 mm Hg by supplemental oxygen or mechanical ventilation. Induction of mild hypothermia (~33°C) after cardiac arrest has been shown to improve survival and neurological outcome. Hospitalize all patients for diagnosis and treatment.

Arrich J, Holzer M, Herkner H, Müllner M: Hypothermia for neuroprotection in adults after cardiopulmonary resuscitation. Cochrane Database Syst Rev 2009;7:CD004128 [PMID: 19821320].

3. Drug Overdose

See also Chapter 47.

Drug overdose is one of the most common causes of coma in patients presenting to the emergency department. Many drugs may be implicated, including sedative–hypnotics, opiates, tricyclic antidepressants, and antiepileptics. Details of management can be found in Chapter 47.

▶ Ethanol Intoxication

Alcohol intoxication produces a metabolic encephalopathy similar to that produced by sedative–hypnotic drugs, although nystagmus during wakefulness and early impairment of lateral eye movements are not as common. Peripheral vasodilatation is a prominent manifestation and produces tachycardia, hypotension, and hypothermia.

In individuals who are not chronic alcoholics, stupor occurs when blood alcohol levels reach 250–300 mg/dL, and coma occurs when levels reach 300–400 mg/dL. Because alcohol has significant osmotic pressure (100 mg/dL = 22.4 mOsm), alcohol intoxication is one cause of hyperosmolality.

Management is discussed in Chapter 47. Patients should be observed until improvement has occurred with normal orientation and judgment, and satisfactory coordination. Hospitalize patients who have abnormalities that would usually require hospitalization (eg, metabolic abnormalities, Wernicke encephalopathy).

▶ Narcotic Overdose

In narcotic overdose, hypoventilation is almost always present, along with pinpoint pupillary constriction and absent extraocular movements in response to the doll's eye maneuver. Pinpoint pupils are also associated with other disorders that must be ruled out: use of miotic eye drops, pontine hemorrhage, Argyll-Robertson pupils from syphilis, and organophosphate insecticide poisoning.

Narcotic intoxication is confirmed by rapid pupillary dilation and awakening after administration of a narcotic antagonist such as naloxone, 2 mg, by rapid IV injection or intranasally. *Note*: Patients who have overdosed on certain narcotics (eg, propoxyphene) may not respond to 2 mg and may require 4 mg or more. The duration of action of naloxone varies with the dose and route of administration (20–90 minutes). Repeat doses are frequently necessary, especially following intoxication with long-acting narcotics (eg, methadone).

Treatment of drug overdose and poisoning is outlined above and discussed in more detail in Chapter 47. Hospitalization should be considered for patients who do not recover completely in the emergency department or who have taken long-acting narcotics.

Merlin MA, Saybolt M, Kapitanyan R, Alter SM, Jeges J, Liu J, Calabrese S, Rynn KO, Perritt R, Pryor PW: Intranasal naloxone delivery is an alternative to intravenous naloxone for opioid overdoses. Am J Emerg Med 2010;28:296–303 [PMID: 20223386].

▶ γ-Hydroxybutyrate

γ-Hydroxybutyrate is a CNS depressant and can induce coma. The drug has become popular at rave parties and has also been called the "date rape drug." Detection of the drug is difficult, because most of it is eliminated through the lungs. Treatment is primarily supportive and may involve endotracheal intubation. Some patients require hospitalization for prolonged supportive care.

4. Hepatic Encephalopathy
▶ Clinical Findings

Hepatic encephalopathy can occur in patients with severe acute or chronic liver disease. Jaundice need not be present. In the patient with preexisting liver disease, encephalopathy may develop rapidly following an acute insult such as gastrointestinal hemorrhage or infection. Patients with surgical portacaval shunts are especially predisposed to encephalopathy.

Mental status is altered and ranges from somnolence to delirium or coma. There is increased muscle tone; hyperreflexia is common. Prominent asterixis occurs in the somnolent patient. Seizures, either generalized or focal, occur infrequently. Ammonia levels correlate poorly with disease severity. Hyperventilation with respiratory alkalosis is nearly universal and may be demonstrated by measuring arterial blood pH. CSF is normal but may appear xanthochromic in patients with serum bilirubin levels higher than 4–6 mg/dL.

▶ Treatment and Disposition

Emergency department care is supportive. Treatment aimed at decreasing intestinal ammonia absorption (lactulose, neomycin) may be initiated but should not take the place of hospitalization for definitive treatment. Studies on induced hypothermia in acute liver failure are inconclusive to this point.

Stravitz RT, Larsen FS: Therapeutic hypothermia for acute liver failure. Crit Care Med 2009;37:S258–264 [PMID: 19535956].

5. Hyponatremia

Delirium and seizures are common presenting features of hyponatremia. Hyponatremia may cause neurologic symptoms when serum sodium levels are below 120 mEq/L, and symptoms are common with levels below 110 mEq/L. When the serum sodium level falls rapidly, symptoms occur at higher serum sodium levels.

▶ Treatment and Disposition

The diagnosis and treatment of these entities are discussed in Chapter 44. Hospitalization is mandatory in symptomatic patients.

6. Hypothermia/Hyperthermia
▶ Clinical Findings

Hypothermia and hyperthermia are associated with symmetric neurologic dysfunction that may progress to coma. All comatose patients must have rectal temperature taken with an extended-range thermometer if the standard thermometer fails to register.

A. Hypothermia

Internal body temperatures below 26°C (78.8°F) uniformly cause coma; hypothermia with core temperatures above 32°C (89.6°F) does not cause coma. Body temperatures of 26–32°C (78.8–89.6°F) are associated with varying degrees of obtundation. Pupillary reaction will be sluggish below 32°C (89.6°F) and lost below 26.5°C (80°F).

B. Hyperthermia

Internal body temperatures above 41–42°C (105.8–107.6°F) are associated with coma and may also rapidly cause permanent brain damage. Seizures are common, especially in children.

▶ Treatment and Disposition

Diagnostic and treatment measures for both hypothermia and hyperthermia are discussed in detail in Chapter 46. Hospitalization is mandatory.

7. Meningoencephalitis

See also Chapter 42

▶ Clinical Findings

The classic triad of fever, neck stiffness, and altered mental status is poorly sensitive for bacterial meningitis (40%). Any patient with altered mental status, seizure, focal neurologic deficit, or evidence of increased ICP should undergo neuroimaging prior to lumbar puncture to minimize the risk of herniation. CSF pleocytosis is common although depending on the stage of the disease, the differential may be variable. CSF glucose < 40 mg/dL is more consistent with bacterial meningitis.

▶ Treatment and Disposition

Start antibiotic therapy immediately based on clinical findings, prior to obtaining imaging. Current recommendations are for vancomycin with a third-generation cephalosporin, and dexamethasone (0.6 mg/kg) should be given with or before antibiotic administration. Hospitalization is indicated for all patients with meningitis who present in coma or in whom bacterial meningitis cannot be excluded.

Van de Beek D, de Gans J, McIntyre P, Prasad K: Corticosteroids for acute bacterial meningitis. Cochrane Database Syst Rev 2007;1: CD004405 [PMID: 17253505].

OTHER DISORDERS CAUSING COMA

1. Subarachnoid Hemorrhage

See also Chapter 37.

ESSENTIALS OF DIAGNOSIS

- ▶ Sudden onset of severe headache
- ▶ Nausea and vomiting
- ▶ Photophobia, visual changes

▶ General Considerations

Aneurysmal subarachnoid hemorrhage (SAH) accounts for 80% of all cases of nontraumatic SAH. Risk factors include cigarette smoking, hypertension, cocaine and alcohol use, first-degree relatives with a history of SAH, female sex, African–American race, and connective tissue disorders.

▶ Clinical Findings

Typical presentation of SAH involves nausea or vomiting (77%), sudden onset of severe headache (74%), meningismus (35%), photophobia, and may include decreased level of consciousness. A "thunderclap" headache may signify a sentinel leak, and the headache may resolve relatively quickly. The patient may lose consciousness at onset (53%) or may experience a seizure (20%). Retinal hemorrhages may be present on fundoscopic examination and blood pressure is usually markedly elevated. Noncontrast enhanced CT scan of the head is the initial diagnostic study of choice. Because the diagnostic sensitivity of CT scanners is only 98–100% for SAH within the first 12 hours, current recommendations are to follow a negative CT with CSF analysis. If CSF is normal (no xanthochromia, no elevated RBCs), SAH is effectively excluded. Positive or indeterminate CSF findings require CT angiography or traditional angiography to rule out the presence of an aneurysm.

▶ Treatment and Disposition

Emergency department care is supportive. After stabilization, the patient should be admitted or transferred for definitive therapy by neurosurgery for craniotomy and clipping or interventional radiology for coiling. Blood pressure should be treated aggressively to be kept within normal limits until the aneurysm has been secured. Nimodipine (60 mg), an oral calcium channel antagonist, is commonly used to prevent delayed vasospasm and can be initiated in the emergency department.

Bederson JB, Connolly ES Jr, Batjer HH, Dacey RG, Dion JE, Diringer MN, Duldner JE Jr, Harbaugh RE, Patel AB, Rosenwasser RH; American Heart Association: Guidelines for the management of aneurysmal subarachnoid hemorrhage: a statement for healthcare professionals from a special writing group of the Stroke Council, American Heart Association. Stroke 2009;40:994–1025 [PMID: 19164800].

2. Seizure

See also Chapter 19.

ESSENTIALS OF DIAGNOSIS

- ▶ Patient is unresponsive to pain
- ▶ Nonfocal neurologic examination
- ▶ Babinski sign (transient)
- ▶ Todd paralysis
- ▶ Signs of recent seizure: tongue trauma, incontinence, rapidly clearing anion gap lactic acidosis

▶ General Considerations

Coma resulting from seizure disorders is usually not a difficult diagnostic problem, because recovery of consciousness is rapid following the end of the seizure. Prolonged postictal coma (several hours) followed by several days of confusion may occur after status epilepticus, in patients with brain damage (eg, multiple cerebral infarctions, head trauma, encephalitis, mental retardation) and in patients with metabolic encephalopathy that alters consciousness and induces seizures (eg, hyponatremia, hyperglycemia). Nonconvulsive status epilepticus is more common than previously thought and should be considered in any patient with no other apparent cause of coma, especially in those with a history of seizure disorder.

▶ Clinical Findings

Patients may initially be unresponsive to deep pain and exhibit sonorous respirations. The neurologic examination is usually nonfocal, although Babinski sign may be transiently present. Uncommonly, there may be focal abnormalities (Todd paralysis) referable anatomically to the focus of seizure activity in the brain.

Other evidence of a recent seizure may be present, such as trauma to the tongue from biting, incontinence, or a rapidly clearing anion gap (lactic) acidosis. The rapid resolution of coma in a patient with a witnessed seizure or known seizure disorder should suggest the diagnosis of the postictal state as the cause of coma. Coma that is at first thought to be postictal but fails to improve should prompt an investigation for underlying processes contributing to mental status depression, including metabolic encephalopathy, underlying diffuse brain damage, encephalitis, and structural lesion. Appropriate investigations could include measurements of serum electrolytes, calcium, and magnesium; CT scan; and lumbar puncture.

▶ Treatment and Disposition

Treatment depends on the underlying cause of the seizure. Be alert for metabolic causes and treat them appropriately. See Chapter 19 for details of management. Immediate hospitalization is required for all cases of status epilepticus and prolonged postictal coma and for seizures due to metabolic causes that are not quickly correctable.

3. Psychogenic Coma

ESSENTIALS OF DIAGNOSIS

▶ Patient is unresponsive
▶ Normal physical examination
▶ Flaccid symmetric decreased muscle tone
▶ Normal and symmetric reflexes
▶ Normal Babinski
▶ Nystagmus with ice water calorics
▶ Normal electroencephalogram findings

▶ Clinical Findings

Psychogenic coma is a diagnosis of exclusion that should be made only after careful documentation. The general physical examination should elicit no abnormalities; neurologic examination generally reveals flaccid, symmetrically decreased muscle tone, normal and symmetric reflexes, and the normal downward response to Babinski plantar stimulation. The pupils are normal in size (2–3 mm) or occasionally larger and respond briskly to light. Lateral eye movements elicited with the doll's eye maneuver may or may not be present, because visual fixation can suppress this reflex.

▶ Differentiating Psychogenic Coma from Organic Coma

A. Eye Movements

The slow, conjugate roving eye movements of patients in metabolic coma cannot be imitated and, if present, are incompatible with a diagnosis of psychogenic unconsciousness.

B. Eyelid Tone

The slow, often asymmetric and incomplete eyelid closure commonly seen in organic forms of coma following passive opening of the lids cannot be mimicked. In addition, the patient with psychogenic coma usually shows some voluntary muscle tone of the eyelids during passive opening by the examiner.

C. Ice Water Caloric Response

A helpful objective test in diagnosing psychogenic unconsciousness is the caloric test: there is no response at all or tonic deviation to the side of the irrigation in organic coma, but nystagmus occurs in psychogenic coma. Because the quick (return) phase of nystagmus requires an intact cortex, its presence is incompatible with a diagnosis of true coma.

D. Electroencephalogram

The electroencephalogram in psychogenic coma is that of a normal, awake person. In coma due to other causes, it is invariably abnormal.

▶ Treatment and Disposition

Obtain psychiatric consultation. Hospitalization may be required.

Bazakis AM, Kunzler C: Altered mental status due to metabolic or endocrine disorders. Emerg Med Clin North Am 2005;23: 901–908 [PMID: 15982551].

Chen JW, Wasterlain CG: Status epilepticus: pathophysiology and management in adults. Lancet Neurol 2006;5:246–256 [PMID: 16488380].

Manno EM, Atkinson JL, Fulgham JR, Wijdicks EF: Emerging medical and surgical management strategies in the evaluation and treatment of intracerebral hemorrhage. Mayo Clin Proc 2005;80:420–433 [PMID: 15757025].

Mas A: Hepatic encephalopathy: from pathophysiology to treatment. Digestion 2006;73:86–93 [PMID: 16498256].

Mayer SA, Brun NC, Broderick J, Davis S, Diringer MN, Skolnick BE, Steiner T; Europe/AustralAsia NovoSeven ICH Trial Investigators: Safety and feasibility of recombinant factor VIIa for acute intracerebral hemorrhage. Stroke 2005;36:74–79 [PMID: 15569871].

Mayer SA, Rincon F: Treatment of intracerebral haemorrhage. Lancet Neurol 2005;4:662–672 [PMID: 16168935].

Rathlev NK, Medzon R, Lowery D, Pollack C, Bracken M, Barest G, Wolfson AB, Hoffman JR, Mower WR: Intracranial pathology in elders with blunt head trauma. Acad Emerg Med 2006;13:302–307 [PMID: 16514123].

Suarez JI, Tarr RW, Selman WR: Aneurysmal subarachnoid hemorrhage. N Engl J Med 2006;354:387–396 [PMID: 16436770].

Vincent JL, Berre J. Primer on medical management of severe brain injury. Crit Care Med 2005;33:1392–1399 [PMID: 15942361].

van de Beek D, de Gans J, Tunkel AR, Wijdicks EF: Community-acquired bacterial meningitis in adults. N Engl J Med 2006;354:44–53 [PMID: 16394301].

Wills B, Erickson T: Drug- and toxin-associated seizures. Med Clin North Am 2005;89:1297–1321 [PMID: 16227064].

CRITERIA FOR BRAIN DEATH

Brain death is defined as the irreversible loss of function of the brain, including the brain stem. Before a patient may be evaluated for the diagnosis of brain death, the patient must meet certain criteria:

- Clinical or neuroimaging evidence of catastrophic CNS event compatible with the clinical diagnosis of brain death
- Exclusion or correction of medical conditions that may confound clinical assessment:
  - Acid–base disorders
  - Severe electrolyte disorder
  - Endocrinopathies
  - Absence of drug intoxication/poisoning
  - Patient core temperature > 32°C (90°F)

Once these criteria have been met, the patient can be tested for the diagnosis of brain death. If the patient meets the following criteria, the patient is observed for at least 6 hours and clinical testing is repeated. If patient testing remains unchanged, a diagnosis of brain death can be made.

- Coma (unresponsiveness): no cerebral motor response to pain

- Absence of brain-stem reflexes (all of the below):
  - No pupillary response to light
  - No oculocephalic reflex (doll's eyes maneuver)
  - No response to cold water calorics
  - No corneal reflexes
  - No jaw reflex
  - No grimacing to painful stimulus
  - No gag reflex
  - No cough response to tracheal/bronchial stimulation
  - Apnea over 8 minutes with Pco_2 > 60 mm Hg

Confirmatory testing may be used when complicating factors are present such as severe facial trauma, preexisting pupillary abnormalities, or toxic drug levels. Confirmatory tests result in findings that are consistent with brain death and are not diagnostic. The standard confirmatory tests include cerebral angiography, transcranial Doppler ultrasonography, technetium-99m-hexamethylpropyleneamine brain scan, and somatosensory-evoked potentials. In some cases these tests may aid in the diagnosis and in others they may confuse the picture. Documentation of the diagnosis of brain death should include the cause and irreversibility of the condition, the absence of brain-stem reflexes, the absence of any motor response to pain, the formal apnea test results, and the justification for and results of any confirmatory tests. The initial and repeat examinations should be included. Currently most authorities feel that the same criteria above can be used for full-term infants more than 7 days old. Criteria for premature and newborns are still unclear.

Manno EM, Wijdicks EF: The declaration of death and the withdrawal of care in the neurologic patient. Neurol Clin 2006;24:159–169 [PMID: 16443137].

Wijdicks EF, Rabinstein AA, Manno EM, Atkinson JD: Pronouncing brain death: contemporary practice and safety of the apnea test. Neurology 2008;71:1240–1244 [PMID: 18852438].

Syncope

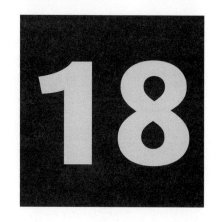

18

C. Keith Stone, MD

Margaret Strecker-McGraw, MD, FACEP

Andrew Juergens, MD

IMMEDIATE MANAGEMENT OF LIFE-THREATENING PROBLEMS CAUSING SYNCOPE

CARDIAC ARREST

See also Chapter 9.

▶ Clinical Findings

Loss of consciousness due to cardiac arrest (ventricular fibrillation or asystole) from any cause occurs in 3–5 seconds if the patient is standing or within 15 seconds if the patient is recumbent. The patient usually rapidly regains consciousness if adequate cardiac output is restored promptly; most patients who regain consciousness within 12 hours will recover without neurologic sequelae.

▶ Treatment and Disposition

Initiate cardiopulmonary resuscitation; see Chapter 9 for further details. Immediate hospitalization in an intensive care unit for evaluation and treatment is required.

CARDIAC ARRHYTHMIAS

See also Chapter 34.

▶ Clinical Findings

See Table 18–1 for common causes of cardiac and neurologic related syncope. Palpitations, fatigue, dyspnea, or chest pain may precede loss of consciousness. Atypical chest pain (mainly nonexertional, left precordial, sharp, and of variable duration) suggests mitral valve prolapse.

Rapid ($\geq$160 beats/min), slow ($\leq$50 beats/min), or irregular pulse must be carefully investigated. Tachycardia of 180–200 beats/min will produce syncope in half of healthy persons. In patients with underlying heart disease or atherosclerosis, tachycardia as fast as 135 beats/min or bradycardia as slow as 60 beats/min may result in loss of consciousness.

Chest auscultation with the patient in various positions (eg, sitting, left lateral decubitus, squatting) may disclose abnormal murmurs and clicks in the case of mitral valve prolapse. The electrocardiogram (ECG) may confirm the

Table 18–1. Common Causes of Syncope Due to Cardiopulmonary and Cerebrovascular Disease.

Cardiac arrest due to any cause
Acute myocardial infarction
Cardiac dysrhythmias
  Tachyarrhythmias
    Supraventricular
      Paroxysmal atrial tachycardia
      Atrial flutter
      Atrial fibrillation
      Accelerated junctional tachycardia
    Ventricular
      Ventricular tachycardia
      Ventricular fibrillation
  Bradyarrhythmias
    Sinus bradycardia
    Sinus arrest
    Second-degree or complete (third-degree) heart block
    Implanted pacemaker failure or malfunction
  Mitral valve prolapse (click-murmur syndrome)
  Prolonged QT interval syndromes
  Brugada syndrome
  Sick sinus syndromes (tachycardia–bradycardia syndrome)
  Drug toxicity (especially digitalis, quinidine or procainamide,
    propranolol, phenothiazines, tricyclic antidepressants, potassium)
Cardiac inflow obstruction
  Left atrial myxoma or thrombus
  Constrictive pericarditis or cardiac tamponade
  Tension pneumothorax
Cardiac outflow obstruction
  Aortic stenosis
  Pulmonary stenosis
  Hypertrophic obstructive cardiomyopathy (idiopathic hypertrophic
    subaortic stenosis)
Severe pulmonary hypertension due to any cause
  Pulmonary hypertension
  Acute pulmonary embolus
Cerebrovascular syncope
  Basilar artery insufficiency
  Subclavian steal syndrome
  Migraine
  Takayasu's disease
  Carotid sinus syncope
  Orthostatic hypotension

diagnosis of arrhythmia, heart block, sick sinus, or prolonged QT interval. However, a single ECG, obtained when the patient is asymptomatic, is frequently normal or nondiagnostic. A diagnosis can be firmly established only by demonstrating arrhythmias during symptomatic periods.

Treatment and Disposition

Patients with syncopal attacks thought to be due to structural cardiac disease or an arrhythmia should be hospitalized for further evaluation.

EVALUATION OF THE CONSCIOUS PATIENT WITH A HISTORY OF SYNCOPE

The emergency department evaluation of the patient presenting with syncope consists of a careful history, a physical examination that includes orthostatic blood pressure measurements, and a 12-lead ECG. The initial goal should be to identify life-threatening causes of syncope.

▶ Confirm that Loss of Consciousness was Caused by Syncope

Syncope is a symptom characterized by transient, self-limited loss of consciousness. It is associated with a loss of postural tone, usually resulting in falling. Syncope must be differentiated from other symptoms such as dizziness, presyncope, and vertigo, all of which do not result in loss of consciousness. Typically syncopal episodes are brief, lasting no longer than 20 seconds. Recovery from syncope is usually characterized by almost immediate restoration of appropriate behavior and orientation. Syncope should not be confused with other causes of loss of consciousness such as seizure hypoxia, hyperventilation, hypoglycemia, and intoxications.

▶ Rule Out Blood Loss

In the *awake* patient with a history of one or more episodes of loss of consciousness, rule out blood loss due to various causes such as aortic aneurysm rupture, vaginal or gastrointestinal bleeding.

A. Measure Blood Pressure and Pulse

Supine hypotension (systolic blood pressure < 90 mm Hg) or severe peripheral vasoconstriction should be considered evidence of hemorrhagic shock until proven otherwise (Chapter 11).

Orthostatic vital signs should be obtained, though they may be contraindicated in patients who have supine hypotension; those in shock; and those with severe altered mental status, spinal injuries, or pelvic and lower extremity injuries. Measure blood pressure and pulse after the patient has been lying down for 3 minutes. Record blood pressure, pulse, and symptoms again after the patient has been standing for 1 minute. A positive test for orthostatic hypotension is an increase of pulse of 30 beats/min or more, or a decrease in systolic blood pressure of 20 mm Hg or less than 90 mm Hg. The presence of symptoms such as dizziness or syncope should also be noted as a positive test. Many conditions can produce postural hypotension in the absence of hypovolemia (Table 18–2). The utility of orthostatic vital signs in children is questionable.

B. Gain Venous Access

Use an intravenous catheter (≥18 gauge), and administer a crystallized solution (eg, normal saline) as needed. If

Table 18–2. Causes of Orthostatic Hypotension.

```
Drug-induced
  Phenothiazines (chlorpromazine, etc)
  Tricyclic antidepressants (amitriptyline, etc)
  Antihypertensives
  Diuretics
  Nitrates (nitroglycerine, etc)
  Levodopa
  Monoamine oxidase inhibitors
Peripheral neuropathies (see Chapter 16)
  Diabetic
  Amyloid
Hypovolemia or hemorrhage
Addison's disease
Acute or chronic spinal cord injury
Degenerative diseases of the central nervous system
  Parkinsonism
  Shy-Drager syndrome (anhidrosis, sphincter dysfunction,
    impotence)
Posterior fossa tumors
Sequelae of surgical sympathectomy
```

blood loss is suspected and the hematocrit or hemoglobin is normal, a repeat determination after volume repletion may confirm blood loss. Serial CBCs may be helpful in detecting active bleeding, and a dextrose test may be helpful if the history or physical examination suggests hypoglycemia.

C. Look for Possible Gastrointestinal Tract Bleeding

Nasogastric intubation may be indicated in suspected gastrointestinal tract bleeding or in syncope with unexplained postural hypotension. Check stool specimens for blood (gross and microscopic).

D. Consider Other Possible Causes of Bleeding

Consider pelvic bleeding (eg, ruptured ectopic pregnancy) or trauma, especially that is not visually obvious, such as splenic, hepatic, retroperitoneal, or pelvic injury. Look for a history of anticoagulant use.

▶ Determine Presence or Absence of Related Symptoms

A. Syncope Associated with Cardiac Arrhythmias or Conduction Abnormalities

Obtain an ECG. This quick, easy, noninvasive test is indicated in all cases of syncope except for those with an otherwise clear cause. ECG abnormalities suggesting an arrhythmic cause of syncope are listed in Table 18–1.

B. Syncope Associated with Prominent Abdominal or Pelvic Pain

Patients with abdominal or pelvic pain may have hypovolemic syncope secondary to gastrointestinal hemorrhage, leaking aortic aneurysm, or ruptured ectopic pregnancy. Aortic dissection and rupture of a viscus into the peritoneal cavity may also produce syncope initially by vagal stimulation or later as a result of blood loss.

C. Syncope Associated with Chest Pain or Dyspnea

Consider myocardial infarction, pulmonary embolism (PE), tension pneumothorax, or dissecting aortic aneurysm.

D. Syncope Associated with Neurologic Symptoms (eg, Headache, Vertigo, Diplopia)

Consider possible neurologic cause such as basilar artery insufficiency, migraine, and subclavian steal syndrome. Loss of consciousness as an isolated symptom is rarely if ever caused by basilar artery ischemia.

▶ Further Evaluation of Syncope

A detailed, accurate history from the patient, family, observers, or ambulance attendants is the most important factor in making the diagnosis. A head computed tomography (CT) scan must be obtained in the emergency department if the patient has focal neurologic findings or a history suggestive of subarachnoid hemorrhage as the etiology of syncope. The most helpful features are the following.

A. Epileptic Aura

History of an epileptic aura preceding the loss of consciousness or a period of confusion (postictal state) upon regaining consciousness strongly suggests seizures as the diagnosis (see Chapter 19). This aura must be differentiated from symptoms of decreased cerebral blood flow (eg, those occurring before a syncopal episode or as a result of orthostatic hypotension or cardiac arrhythmia).

B. Position of the Patient at Time of Loss of Consciousness

Episodes beginning when the patient is lying down suggest seizure or cardiac arrhythmia, whereas orthostatic hypotension and vasovagal syncope occur when the patient is standing or sitting up.

C. Syncope Related to Active Physical Exertion

Syncope following active physical exertion is frequently noted in cardiac outflow obstruction (eg, aortic stenosis, hypertrophic obstructive cardiomyopathy, myxoma) and is elicited occasionally in patients with cardiac arrhythmias or pulmonary vascular disease.

D. Other Causes of Syncope

Micturition and coughing are associated with distinctive syncopal syndromes. Simple fainting may occur during the first trimester of pregnancy and must be differentiated from syncope due to blood loss from ectopic pregnancy. Rare causes of syncope include glossopharyngeal neuralgia, hyperventilation, psychiatric causes, and Meniere's disease (look for associated hearing loss and vertigo).

E. Disposition

Deciding whether to admit the patient with syncope is based on two different objectives: admission for diagnosis or for treatment. When the cause of syncope remains unknown, a risk assessment can be used for the admission decision. The following risk factors warrant consideration for hospitalization: (1) suspected or known heart disease, (2) ECG abnormalities suspicious for arrhythmic syncope, (3) syncope with onset during exercise, (4) family history of sudden death, (5) syncope causing severe injury, and (6) older age and associated comormidities. Reasons for admission/of patients who require treatment include the following: (1) syncope due to cardiac arrhythmia, ischemia, or structural cardiac disease; (2) cerebrovascular accident or focal neurologic deficits; and (3) severe orthostatic hypotension.

Chen LY, Benditt DG, Shen WK: Management of syncope in adults: an update. Mayo Clin Proc 2008;83:1280–1293 [PMID: 18990328].

Huff JS, Decker WW, Quinn JV, Perron AD, Napoli AM, Peeters S, Jagoda AS: Clinical policy: critical issues in the evaluation and management of adult patients presenting to the emergency department with syncope. Ann Emerg Med 2007;49:431–444 [PMID: 17371707].

Miller TH et al: Evaluation of syncope. Am Fam Physician 2005;72:1492 [PMID: 16273816].

▼ EMERGENCY EVALUATION OF SPECIFIC DISORDERS CAUSING SYNCOPE

NEURALLY MEDIATED SYNCOPE

Neurally mediated syncope is a broad category involving an inappropriate vasodilation or bradycardia in response to a stimulus that results in a loss of postural tone. Common precipitating factors are shown in Table 18–3. It is often used synonymously with vasovagal syncope, also this is but one subtype. It may have a visceral (eg, micturition and defecation) or emotional component. Carotid sinus syncope is classified as a form of neurally mediated syncope.

Table 18–3. Common Factors Precipitating of Neurally Mediated Syncope.

Emotional upset
Sight of blood
Sudden exposure to cold
Prolonged motionless standing
Medical or surgical procedures
Injury
Pain
Blood loss
Cough
Micturition
Migraine
Carotid sinus pressure
Early pregnancy

VASOVAGAL SYNCOPE

 ESSENTIALS OF DIAGNOSIS

► Usually occurs when patient is standing or sitting
► Lasts 10 seconds to a few minutes
► Associated with lightheadedness, nausea, pallor, sweating, and blurred vision
► No postictal period

▶ General Considerations

Vasovagal disorders account for most episodes of syncope. Physiologic decreases in both arterial pressure and heart rate mediated by parasympathetic tone combine to produce central nervous system hypoperfusion and subsequent syncope. Prolonged cerebral hypoxia with resultant tonic–clonic movements is more likely to occur if the patient remains upright.

▶ Clinical Findings

Vasovagal episodes begin in a standing or sitting position and only rarely in a supine position.

A. Prodrome

The prodrome lasts from 10 seconds to a few minutes and includes weakness, lightheadedness, nausea, pallor, sweating, salivation, blurred vision, and tachycardia.

B. Syncope

Brain hypoperfusion causes dimming of vision; the patient then loses consciousness and sinks to the ground. Examination reveals an unconscious individual who is pale and is sweating and who has dilated pupils and a slow, weak pulse. With loss of consciousness, bradycardia replaces tachycardia.

C. Associated Symptoms

Abnormal movements may be noted during the period of unconsciousness. These are mainly tonic or opisthotonic. These may be accentuated by prolonged periods of decreased cerebral blood flow or hypoxia, as may occur if the patient remains seated or is held up by others.

D. Postsyncopal Findings

The patient is lucid and awake seconds to less than a minute after sinking to a recumbent position; a postictal confusional state is absent unless a seizure has occurred. However, nervousness, dizziness, headache, nausea and vomiting, pallor, and perspiration may persist for hours.

E. Recurrence

Syncope may recur, especially if the patient stands up within 30 minutes after the attack. Syncope due to a specific precipitating factor (eg, cough) may be reproduced in the emergency department.

▶ Treatment

After ruling out more serious causes of syncope and addressing concomitant issues such as trauma from a fall, reassurance and a recommendation to avoid precipitating factors are usually all that is necessary. Cough suppression and sitting down to urinate are helpful in posttussive and micturitional syncope. Adequate nutrition and hydration should be encouraged.

▶ Disposition

Refer the patient to an outpatient clinic or primary care physician after a period of observation and confirmation of the diagnosis in the emergency department.

CAROTID SINUS SYNCOPE

▶ Clinical Findings

Carotid sinus syncope classically results from pressure on an abnormally sensitive carotid sinus by a tight collar, neck mass, enlarged cervical nodes, or tumor. This pressure causes vagal stimulation that slows the sinoatrial and atrioventricular nodes and inhibits sympathetic vascular tone. The resulting bradycardia and systemic hypotension then produce syncope. The syndrome may be reproduced in the emergency department by pressure on the carotid sinus for 5–10 seconds while the patient is both supine and erect: cardiac monitoring or ECG documents the induced bradyarrhythmia. Such pressure may also produce syncope resulting from cerebral ischemia if the examiner compresses the artery

contralateral to an occluded carotid. Syncope is then due to cerebral hypoperfusion secondary to cerebrovascular disease and not to carotid sinus hypersensitivity.

▶ Treatment and Disposition

The patient with syncope should be placed supine and pressure on the carotid sinus relieved (eg, loosening a tight collar). Refer the patient to an outpatient clinic or primary care physician for evaluation.

CARDIOPULMONARY SYNCOPE

▶ General Considerations

A cardiovascular origin for syncope is suggested when it occurs during recumbency, during or following physical exertion, or in a patient with known heart disease. Loss of consciousness in cardiac disease is most often due to an abrupt decrease in cardiac output, with subsequent cerebral hypoperfusion producing symptoms identical to those of fainting. Such cardiac dysfunction may result from rhythm disturbances (bradyarrhythmias or tachyarrhythmias), cardiac inflow or outflow obstruction, acute myocardial infarction, intracardiac right-to-left shunts, leaking or dissecting aortic aneurysms, or acute pulmonary embolus. Table 18–1 lists some of the more common cardiopulmonary causes of syncope.

CARDIAC INFLOW OBSTRUCTION

ESSENTIALS OF DIAGNOSIS

▶ Suspect with syncope due to change in position
▶ Look for physical examination findings—cardiac findings, engorged neck veins, weak pulse, or hypotension

▶ Clinical Findings

Patients with atrial or ventricular myxomas and atrial thrombi usually present with embolization but may also have sudden loss of cardiac output and syncope; syncope occurring with change in position is classic but uncommon. A left atrial myxoma often mimics mitral stenosis but is occasionally manifested by mitral regurgitation murmur. Mitral valve prolapse may also cause syncope.

Constrictive pericarditis or cardiac tamponade causes reduced cardiac output and may result in syncope. Any maneuver or drug that decreases heart rate or venous return will further impair cardiac output. The diagnosis is suggested by the presence of engorged neck veins, clear lung fields on chest X-ray, weak pulse, and hypotension. Tension pneumothorax reduces cardiac output by decreasing venous return and may produce syncope. There is usually a history of chest trauma or chronic pulmonary disease with bullae. Chest X-ray and physical examination confirm the diagnosis.

▶ Treatment and Disposition

Patients with syncope thought to be due to cardiac inflow obstruction require hospitalization.

CARDIAC OUTFLOW OBSTRUCTION

ESSENTIALS OF DIAGNOSIS

▶ Consider with syncope related to exertion
▶ Look for cardiac physical findings

1. Aortic Stenosis

Loss of consciousness secondary to congenital or acquired severe stenosis may occur in all age groups. Exertional syncope occurs as a result of cerebral hypoperfusion due to exercise-induced vasodilation in the presence of a fixed cardiac output. Two other pathophysiologic events are recognized: (1) acute transient left ventricular failure with normal sinus rhythm and (2) transient arrhythmia or cardiac standstill, causing an acute drop in cardiac output. Sudden death may result. Autonomic insufficiency also has been reported in these patients. Reflex peripheral vascular vasodilation (presumably due to left ventricular baroreceptor activity) has been demonstrated in the absence of cardiac arrhythmia.

▶ Clinical Findings

Syncope usually follows exercise and is often associated with dyspnea, anginal chest pain, and sweating. Physical findings that occur with hemodynamically severe aortic stenosis include the following:

• Characteristic midsystolic ejection murmur (often associated with a palpable thrill).

• Sustained and prolonged left ventricular lift.

• Paradoxically split second sound.

• Delayed upstroke and reduced amplitude (pulsus parvus et tardus) on the carotid pulse.

▶ Treatment and Disposition

Promptly hospitalize all patients with symptomatic aortic stenosis (angina, congestive heart failure, or syncope) to evaluate them for possible valve replacement. Median survival time following the initial episode of syncope due to aortic stenosis in the patient who does not receive a prosthesis is 1.5–3 years.

2. Pulmonary Stenosis

▶ Clinical Findings

Severe pulmonary stenosis may produce syncope, especially following exertion. A hemodynamic process similar to that of aortic stenosis is responsible. Physical findings include right parasternal lift, systolic ejection murmur at the upper left sternal border, a prominent S_4, and a conspicuous wave in the jugular venous pulse.

▶ Treatment and Disposition

Immediate hospitalization is required, because the pathophysiology and prognosis of this condition are similar to those of aortic stenosis.

3. Hypertrophic Cardiomyopathy

ESSENTIALS OF DIAGNOSIS

▶ Syncope with exercise, dyspnea on exertion, and chest pain
▶ Cardiac findings including systolic ejection murmur, S_4, and perhaps a thrill

▶ Clinical Findings

Symptoms include syncope with exercise, dyspnea on exertion, and chest pain. Physical findings include a prominent fourth heart sound, ventricular lift, transient arrhythmias, and systolic ejection murmur and perhaps a thrill, both of which increase with exertion and with decreased left ventricular chamber size (eg, as produced during the Valsalva maneuver). Echocardiography confirms the diagnosis.

▶ Treatment and Disposition

Hospitalize the patient for further evaluation and treatment.

PULMONARY VASCULAR DISEASE

▶ Clinical Findings

A. Pulmonary Hypertension

Syncope or near syncope may be found in patients with pulmonary hypertension. Progressive dyspnea and chest pain, palpitations with a loud P_2, tricuspid regurgitation, and right ventricular heave are often found.

B. Pulmonary Embolism

Syncope is found in a subset of patients with a pulmonary embolism. The syncope may be recurrent and is more often found in women. PE patients with syncope may have a higher incidence of angiographic obstruction, new right incomplete bundle branch block, and cardiac arrest when compared to patients without syncope.

▶ Treatment and Disposition

Provide supplemental O_2 via face mask or assisted ventilation. Treat with heparin by continuous infusion or subcutaneous low molecular heparin. Consider thromboembolic agents in patients who are hemodynamically unstable or have massive PE. Admission of unstable patients to an ICU is appropriate. See Chapter 33 for further details.

CEREBROVASCULAR SYNCOPE

Although syncope resulting from cerebrovascular disease is often diagnosed, such an association is uncommon because both cerebral hemispheres and the brain-stem reticular formation must be compromised before consciousness is lost.

BASILAR ARTERY INSUFFICIENCY

▶ Clinical Findings

Atherosclerotic occlusive disease of the extracranial vertebral artery is usually insidious with disabling or fatal consequences. Symptoms of vertebrobasilar insufficiency are often not well recognized by physicians, leading to delays in treatment. Vertebrobasilar ischemic symptoms are often positional and may be associated with stereotypical movement such as extension of the neck or rotational movement of the head in a particular direction. Basilar artery insufficiency manifests as a cluster of symptoms with the most common being vertigo and visual dysfunction. Episodic perioral numbness or paraesthesia, ataxia, dysarthria, syncope, headache, nausea, vomiting, tinnitus, and cranial nerve dysfunction can also be found.

▶ Treatment and Disposition

Accurate diagnosis is often difficult. Neurological consultation is recommended. Hospitalization is recommended and treatment with aspirin should be started although the effective dose has not yet been clarified.

SUBCLAVIAN STEAL SYNDROME

▶ Clinical Findings

Subclavian artery steal is caused by stenosis of the subclavian artery proximal to the takeoff of the vertebral artery. This causes a retrograde flow in the ipsilateral internal mammary artery and the vertebral arteries. Symptoms of subclavian artery steal may include vertigo and syncope with left arm exertion, angina, or ulcerated or gangrenous fingers.

Blood pressures measured in the upper extremities are nearly always unequal. The average difference is a 45-mm Hg decrease in systolic pressure in the arm supplied by the stenotic vessel.

▶ Treatment and Disposition

If subclavian steal is suspected, vascular consult is warranted. Elective hospitalization should be considered.

MIGRAINE

(See also Chapter 20.) Syncope occurs in a minority of patients with migraines. It usually manifests as a gradual loss of consciousness in the context of other migraine symptoms and is typically associated with familial hemiplegic migraine. Basilar artery migraine presents with syncope typically proceeded by visual blackening, vertigo, or diplopia.

ORTHOSTATIC HYPOTENSION

Orthostatic hypotension is a physical finding, not a disease. Multiple medical conditions can cause an abnormal response to positional change. Maintenance of blood pressure during position change is complex, and neurohumoral, cardiac, vascular, neurologic, and muscular responses must occur quickly. If response is abnormal, blood pressure and organ perfusion can be reduced with resultant symptoms of CNS hypoperfusion. This includes weakness, nausea, headache, lightheadedness, dizziness, blurred vision, fatigue, tremulousness, palpitation, vertigo, and impaired cognition. Orthostatic hypotension may result from multiple disorders; the more common causes are listed in Table 18–2.

▶ Clinical Findings

Syncope often occurs following rapid change in the upright position, that is, from lying to sitting or from sitting to standing. Prolonged motionless standing, especially after exercise, or standing after prolonged bed rest, may also cause syncope. Patients usually describe lightheadedness, dimming of vision, weakness, and a fainting sensation. True vertigo does not occur.

Blood pressure that is significantly lower (>20 mm Hg systolic difference) when the patient is standing than when he or she is supine is diagnostic. Orthostatic tachycardia may be present as well.

A stool sample should be evaluated for the presence of blood. CBC may reveal anemia or hemoconcentration due to blood loss or dehydration, respectively. Electrolyte determinations should be made to detect abnormalities produced by dehydration or drugs. Serum drug levels should be obtained as indicated.

▶ Disposition

Hospitalize the patient if postural hypotension is currently producing symptoms and cannot be easily corrected in the emergency department or if an acute underlying cause of hypotension is discovered. If postural hypotension is corrected and no acute pathology persists, the patient may be discharged to an outpatient clinic or their primary care physician.

▼ MISCELLANEOUS RARE CAUSES OF STATES OF SYNCOPE

HYPERVENTILATION

ESSENTIALS OF DIAGNOSIS

- ▶ Diagnosis of exclusion
- ▶ Numbness and tingling (especially circumoral)
- ▶ Muscle twitching and carpal pedal spasm

▶ General Considerations

Psychogenic hyperventilation is a frequent cause of altered consciousness (eg, faintness, lightheadedness) but rarely culminates in syncope. Acute anxiety is the usual cause. The disorder is usually benign, but serious cardiopulmonary causes of hyperventilation or subjective dyspnea must be ruled out (Chapter 13).

▶ Clinical Findings

Common symptoms include lightheadedness, shortness of breath, numbness and tingling (especially circumoral or acral), muscular twitching, and in severe cases, carpal pedal spasm. Positive Chvostek and Trousseau tests are noted during the acute stage. Respiratory alkalosis without other abnormalities (eg, metabolic acidosis) is noted on arterial blood gas analysis. Symptoms are reproduced by hyperventilating in a controlled setting (eg, emergency department).

▶ Treatment and Disposition

Reassure the patient, and alleviate underlying anxiety. If the patient is acutely hyperventilating, ask the patient to count to 3 slowly between breaths. Patients experiencing a panic attack may benefit from alprazolam, 0.25–0.5 mg orally. Rebreathing from a paper bag is no longer recommended because of the potential risk of hypoxia.

PSYCHIATRIC CAUSES

ESSENTIALS OF DIAGNOSIS

- ▶ Diagnosis can be made only after careful exclusion of other causes
- ▶ Presence of bizarre postures or movements

▶ General Considerations

Psychiatric causes of syncope include major depression, general anxiety disorder, and panic disorder. Fainting is also a known manifestation of somatization disorder. Alcohol and drug abuse can lead to syncopal episodes. Malingering may be a factor; patients may use the episodes of feigned unconsciousness to manipulate other people for secondary gain. Patients with factitious disorder also may fake unconsciousness, but they do so for psychological reasons.

▶ Clinical Findings

Features that suggest psychiatric causes of syncope are lack of any prodrome, presence of bizarre postures or movements, lack of pallor, and prolonged unconsciousness. Many patients will have a well-documented history of psychiatric responses to stress. Without such a history, a psychogenic cause can be made only after thorough evaluation has excluded other causes of syncope.

▶ Treatment and Disposition

Refer the patient to an outpatient clinic or primary care physician for follow-up.

Aronow WS: Aortic stenosis. Compr Ther 2007;33:174–183 [PMID: 18025609].

Benditt DG, Nguyen JT: Syncope: therapeutic approaches. J Am Coll Cardiol 2009; 53:1741–1751 [PMID: 19422980].

Brignole M: Diagnosis and treatment of syncope. Heart 2007;93:130–136 [PMID: 17170354].

Carabello BA, Paulus WJ: Aortic stenosis. Lancet 2009;373: 956–966 [PMID: 19232707].

Catanzaro JN, Makaryus AN, Rosman D, Jadonath R: Emotion-triggered cardiac asystole-inducing neurocardiogenic syncope. Pacing Clin Electrophysiol 2006;29:553–556 [PMID: 16689856].

Chen EH, Hollander JE: When do patients need admission to a telemetry bed? J Emerg Med 2007;33:53–60 [PMID: 17630076].

Dovgalyuk J, Holstege C, Mattu A, Brady WJ: The electrocardiogram in the patient with syncope. Am J Emerg Med 2007;25:688–701 [PMID: 17606095].

Freeman R: Clinical practice. Neurogenic orthostatic hypotension. N Engl J Med 2008;358:615–624 [PMID: 18256396].

Gopinathannair R, Mazur A, Olshansky B: Syncope in congestive heart failure. Cardiol J 2008;15:303–312 [PMID: 18698538].

Kuriachan V, Sheldon RS, Platonov M: Evidence-based treatment for vasovagal syncope. Heart Rhythm 2008;5:1609–1614 [PMID: 18984541].

Levine E, Rosero SZ, Budzikowski AS, Moss AJ, Zareba W, Daubert JP: Congenital long QT syndrome: considerations for primary care physicians. Cleve Clin J Med 2008;75:591–600 [PMID: 18756841].

Napolitano C, Priori SG: Brugada syndrome. Orphanet J Rare Dis 2006;1:35 [PMID: 16972995].

Quinn J, McDermott D, Stiell I, Kohn M, Wells G: Prospective validation of the San Francisco Syncope Rule to predict patients with serious outcomes. Ann Emerg Med 2006;47:448–454 [PMID: 16631985].

Williams L, Frenneaux M: Syncope in hypertrophic cardiomyopathy: mechanisms and consequences for treatment. Europace 2007;9:817–822 [PMID: 17522079].

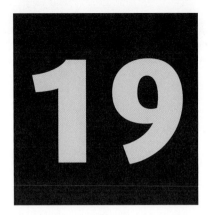

Seizures

C. Keith Stone, MD

▼ IMMEDIATE MANAGEMENT OF LIFE-THREATENING PROBLEMS

STATUS EPILEPTICUS

 ESSENTIALS OF DIAGNOSIS

▶ A prolonged seizure lasting 5–15 minutes
▶ Continuous or multiple seizures without intervening periods of consciousness

▶ Clinical Findings

A prolonged seizure lasting more than 5 minutes, or multiple seizure episodes without intervening periods of consciousness defines status epilepticus. Search carefully for seizure activity in the comatose patient. Manifestations may be subtle (eg, deviation of head or eyes; repetitive jerking of fingers, hands, or one side of the face).

A. Protect the Airway

Insert a nasopharyngeal airway. Administer 100% oxygen by nasal cannula or non-rebreathing face mask and monitor with pulse oximetry. Prepare for possible endotracheal intubation in the event that anticonvulsants fail to terminate the seizure.

B. Insert an Intravenous Catheter

Obtain blood specimens for glucose, electrolytes, magnesium, and calcium determinations; hepatic and renal function tests; and complete blood count; as well as 3–4 tubes of blood for possible toxicology screen or determination of drug levels (including anticonvulsants if patient is known or suspected to be taking them).

C. Rule-Out Hypoglycemia

Obtain a bedside glucose and give glucose, 50 mL of 50% solution IV if the patient is hypoglycemic. *Note*: If malnutrition is suspected, give thiamine, 100 mg IV, slowly prior to, or at the same time as, glucose.

D. Pharmacological Treatment Protocol

1. First-line Agent—

A. BENZODIAZEPINES—Give lorazepam, 2–4 mg (0.05–0.1 mg/kg) IV every 3–4 minutes to 8 mg total in adults and an additional dose of 0.05 mg/kg can be given in children. Diazepam, 5–10 mg (0.25 mg/kg) IV every 3–4 minutes up to 30 mg total dose in adults and 5 mg in children. These drugs have been shown to be equally effective as first-line choices. Lorazepam has a longer duration of action compared to diazepam. Because of this property, lorazepam is currently considered the drug of choice. If venous access cannot be obtained, diazepam can be given rectally, endotracheally, or intraosseously, or midazolam, 0.2 mg/kg, can be given intramuscularly.

2. Second-line Agent—

A. PHENYTOIN OR FOSPHENYTOIN—If the seizure persists after adequate doses of benzodiazepines, give phenytoin 20 mg/kg by IV infusion at a rate of 50 mg/min or slower. If the seizure persists, an additional 10 mg /kg is given. Infusion of phenytoin at more rapid rates (especially if given into centrally placed IV lines) can precipitate cardiac arrhythmias or hypotension. These unwanted hemodynamic and cardiac side effects can be avoided by the use of fosphenytoin, a prodrug of phenytoin. Fosphenytoin dosages are expressed as phenytoin equivalents (PE). Advantages of fosphenytoin are that it can be administered faster than phenytoin (150 PE/min) and be given intramuscularly if needed. The standard dose is 20 mg PE/kg IV.

3. Refractory Status Eepilepticus—There is no accepted standard definition of refractory status epilepticus (RSE). A seizure that continues after the administration of first and second-line treatment within 60 minutes of onset of status is considered RSE. An alternate definition is a seizure that is refractory to loading or protracted maintenance doses of at least three anti-epileptics. Consider one of the following pharmacologic agents for patients with RSE. Intubation will most likely be required for all except valproate and levetiracetam. Continuous EEG monitoring should be considered while using these agents.

A. PHENOBARBITAL—Administer phenobarbital at a dose of 10–20 mg/kg. Beware of both hypotension and respiratory depression. Endotracheal intubation is often necessary.

B. MIDAZOLAM—Administer midazolam in a loading dose of 0.2 mg/kg followed by an infusion of 0.1–0.4 mg/kg/h. Hypotension is rare compared to propofol.

C. PROPOFOL—Propofol, a short-acting nonbarbiturate sedative hypnotic is given at a dose of 1–2 mg/kg load followed by an infusion of 6–12 mg/kg/h. Some evidence exists to show that propofol is superior to midazolam and the shorter acting barbiturates to terminate RSE.

D. VALPROIC ACID—Successful termination of RSE has been reported with valproic acid administration. Give a loading dose of 20–25 mg/kg IV followed by an infusion of 2 mg/kg/h. The chief advantage of this agent is the excellent safety profile and the ease of administration. Intubation may be avoided when using this agent.

E. LEVETIRACETAM—RSE has shown to be effective in RSE. Give a dose of 500–2000 mg over 30–60 minutes. The drug has attractive features for RSE with almost no drug interactions, rare allergic reactions and minimal respiratory and cardiovascular effects with IV dosing.

F. PENTOBARBITAL—Pentobarbital given at a loading dose of 12 mg/kg followed by and infusion of 5 mg/kg/h titrated up to burst suppression on EEG. Hypotension and myocardial depression are prominent side effects.

E. Measure Arterial Blood Gases and PH

Arterial blood Pco_2 is a sensitive indicator of the adequacy of ventilation (hypercapnia is present in proportion to the degree of hypoventilation). Metabolic acidosis due to lactic acidosis resulting from status epilepticus is commonly present for as long as 1 hour after a seizure. This acidosis requires no treatment. Acidosis lasting longer than 1 hour should prompt a search for other causes (Chapter 44).

F. Maintain Ventilation

Patients in status epilepticus or those given anticonvulsant medications that are strong respiratory depressants may require endotracheal intubation to protect the airway and maintain adequate ventilation. Monitor arterial blood gas measurements to assess adequacy of oxygenation and ventilation.

G. Rule Out Meningitis

Perform lumbar puncture immediately to rule out meningitis if fever (body temperature > 38.5°C [>101.2°F]) or nuchal rigidity is present. However, the muscle activity of status epilepticus alone produces transient fever higher than 38.5°C (>101.2°F) in up to 79% of patients. Hyperthermia should be treated with passive cooling measures. Status epilepticus may also produce a mild transient cerebrospinal fluid pleocytosis.

H. Search for the Underlying Cause of Seizure

Common causes of seizures of acute onset are listed in Table 19–1.

▶ Prevention of Injury

Prevent injury to the patient during the seizure by padding the environment. Do not use rigid restraint (fractures may result) or insert objects into the patient's mouth during the seizure.

Table 19–1. Common Causes of Seizures of Acute Onset.

Disorder	Comment
Primary central nervous system disorders idiopathic epilepsy	Onset uncommon after age 25
Head trauma	Especially acute trauma or when associated with depressed skull fracture or subdural hematoma
Stroke	Especially hemorrhagic stroke
Central nervous system mass lesion	Primary or metastatic tumor; brain abscess; arteriovenous malformation
Metabolicor systemic disorders cerebral hypoperfusion (hypoxia)	Cardiopulmonary arrest; cardiac dysrhythmia; severe hypotension, etc (Chapters 7, 9, 34).
Meningitis, encephalitis	Acute or chronic; bacterial, viral, fungal, parasitic, etc (Chapter 40)
Hyponatremia	Serum sodium usually less than 120 mEq/L and often less than 110 mEq/L (Chapter 42)
Hypoglycemia	Serum glucose usually less than 40 mg/dL (Chapter 41)
Hyperosmolality	Serum osmolality usually greater than 300 mOsm/L (Chapter 42)
Hypertensive encephalopathy	Blood pressure usually greater than 250/150 mm Hg; seizures may occur at lower pressures (usually > 160/100 mm Hg) when hypertension occurs suddenly (eg, in children with acute renal failure) (Chapter 34)
Uremic encephalopathy	
Hepatic encephalopathy	Respiratory alkalosis nearly always present
Eclamptogenic toxemia	Develop and utilize a protocol for managing pregnancy-related seizures
Acute drug overdose	Especially with tricyclic antidepressants, theophylline (aminophylline), phencyclidine (PCP), lidocaine, phenothiazines, isoniazid (Chapter 45)
Acute drug withdrawal	Anticonvulsants, ethanol, or sedative-hypnotic drugs (with habituation to daily doses of 600-800 mg secobarbital or its equivalent)
Benign febrile convulsions of childhood	Do not occur after age 5; always consider other causes
Hyperthermia	Internal body temperature usually above 41-42°C (105.8-107.6°F); *immediate* reduction of body temperature to 39°C (102.2°F) is mandatory (Chapter 44)

American College of Emergency Physicians: Clinical policy: critical issues in the evaluation and management of adult patients presenting to the emergency department with seizures. Ann Emerg Med 2004;43:605–625 [PMID: 15111920].

Kanke S, Hamer HM, Rosenow F: Status epilepticus: a critical review. Epilepsy Behav 2009;15:10–14 [PMID: 19236943].

Marik PE et al: The management of status epilepticus. Chest 2004;126:582 [PMID: 15302747].

Millikan D, Rice B, Sillbergleit R: Emergency treatment of status epilepticus: current thinking. Emerg Med Clin North Am 2009;27:101–113 [PMID: 19218022].

Möddel G, Bunten S, Dobis C, Kovac S, Dogan M, Fischera M, Dziewas R, Schäbitz WR, Evers S, Happe S: Intravenous levetiracetam: a new treatment alternative for refractory status epilepticus. J Neurol Neurosurg Psychiatry 2009;80:689–692 [PMID: 19448097].

▼ EVALUATION OF THE CONSCIOUS PATIENT WITH SEIZURES

▶ General Considerations

Seizures can result from a primary central nervous system disorder or may be a manifestation of a serious underlying metabolic or systemic disorder. The distinction is critical, because therapy must be directed at the underlying disorder as well as at control of the seizure.

Clinically, seizures are diagnosed by episodes of loss of consciousness or depressed consciousness and a period of confusion or disorientation (postictal state) following it. The most common type of seizure is generalized tonic–clonic seizure. Firm diagnosis of subtler types of seizures like absence

Table 19–2. Emergency Evaluation of the Patient with Seizures.

Vital signs
  Pulse: Rule out dangerous cardiac dysrhythmia, including cardiac arrest
  Blood pressure: Rule out postural hypotension and shock
  Body temperature: Rule out hyperthermia (>41-42°C [105.8-107.6°F])
History
  Trauma
  Previous seizures
  Drug or alcohol use
Medications
  Physical examination
  Papilledema
  Focal neurologic signs
  Evidence of systemic disease
  Heart murmur
Laboratory and special examinations
  Serum glucose: Hypoglycemia or hyperglycemia
  Arterial blood gases: Hypoxemia, hypercapnia, acidosis
  Electrocardiogram: Cardiac arrhythmia
  Serum electrolytes: Hyponatremia or hypernatremia
  Approximate serum osmolality calculation (normal range: 270-290 mOsm/L):

$$\text{Osmolality} = 2(\text{Na}^+ \text{ mEq/L}) + \frac{\text{Glucose mg/dL}}{18}$$

  Complete blood count with differential
  Serum calcium and magnesium measurements
  Hepatic and renal function studies
  Lumbar puncture (if signs of increased intracranial pressure are absent)
  Blood and urine samples for toxicologic studies (if indicated)
  Computed tomography scan (if focal signs are present)

or complex partial may require an electroencephalogram. New onset seizures require a comprehensive ED evaluation (Table 19–2) to find the underlying cause. Patients with a known seizure disorder who present with a seizure require a much less exhaustive investigation depending on the clinical presentation.

NEW ONSET SEIZURE

▶ Laboratory Evaluation

A comprehensive laboratory evaluation in an otherwise healthy adult with a new onset seizure (who has returned to baseline) is not indicated. Determination of serum sodium and glucose is indicated. A serum pregnancy test is indicated in women of child-bearing age. If the patient has a persistent change in mental status or a focal neurologic deficit, a comprehensive lab evaluation should be considered. Lumbar puncture should be considered if CNS infection is suspected based on clinical presentation (Chapter 42).

▶ CT Scan

When feasible, a CT scan of the head should be performed on all patients with new onset seizures. Deferred outpatient neuroimaging (CT scan or MRI) can be considered if reliable follow-up can be arranged from the ED.

▶ Antiepileptic Therapy

In general, patients with a first seizure, who have returned to baseline, do not need to be started on antiepileptic therapy. Evidence exists that they do not decrease the incidence of recurrent seizure and may actually increase the incidence of a second seizure.

▶ Disposition

Patients with a new onset seizure, who have returned to baseline, have a normal CT scan and lab evaluation can be safely discharged with outpatient follow-up and instructions not to drive or operate machinery. Patients with abnormal head CT scans or persistent focal abnormalities should be hospitalized so that diagnostic studies can be performed and the patient observed.

KNOWN SEIZURE DISORDER

▶ Laboratory Evaluation

Laboratory studies other than measurement of anticonvulsant levels are rarely required in the patient with a history of seizure if they have returned to baseline. If the patient has a persistent change in mental status or a focal neurologic deficit, a comprehensive lab evaluation should be considered.

▶ CT Scan

A CT scan of the head in the patient with a known history of seizures is rarely indicated. If the patient has returned to baseline and has a nonfocal neurologic examination, there is no indication for brain imaging. All others should undergo CT scan if feasible.

▶ Antiepileptic Therapy

The measurement of anticonvulsant levels will assist in guiding therapy. Consider giving loading doses and restarting maintenance doses in patients that have sub-therapeutic levels. Avoid adjusting anticonvulsant doses in patients who are subtherapeutic since noncompliance is common. In patients with therapeutic levels refer the patient for early outpatient follow-up for consideration of adding an additional agent to their regimen.

▶ Disposition

Patients with established seizure disorders may be sent home if they have returned to baseline, if the seizures have not recurred, and if no acute abnormalities are found. They should be referred to their regular source of medical care within a few days. All others should be hospitalized.

American College of Emergency Physicians: Clinical policy: critical issues in the evaluation and management of adult patients presenting to the emergency department with seizures. Ann Emerg Med 2004;43:605–625 [PMID: 15111920].

Smith PE, Cossburn MD: Seizures: assessment and management in the emergency unit. Clin Med 2004;4:118–122 [PMID: 15139727].

EMERGENCY TREATMENT OF SPECIFIC SEIZURES TYPES

GENERALIZED SEIZURES

MYOCLONIC AND TONIC—CLONIC (GENERALIZED CONVULSIVE SEIZURES)

Generalized seizures with obvious motor components are usually not difficult to diagnose and should be treated as described above. If status epilepticus ensues, the motor component may become subtle in some cases, and may be mistaken as a postictal period. If consciousness is not regained within 20 minutes of the termination of convulsions, the diagnosis of subtle status epilepticus should be considered. It is important to recognize subtle status epilepticus as it bears a dismal prognosis, even when compared to other forms of nonconvulsive status epilepticus.

ABSENCE

Absence seizures usually present with limited or no motor activity despite impairment of consciousness. Patients can be comatose, but frequently present as lethargic or confused. These seizures may be mistaken for complex partial seizures when automatisms are present. It is more common in females than males and is divided into childhood (onset around 6 years old) and juvenile (onset around 12 years old). Therapy consists of valproate given in an IV loading dose of 25 mg/kg in 50 mL NS over 10 minutes. If the patient is on valproate, a level should be drawn and the dose adjusted accordingly. Both absence and complex partial seizures may lead to nonconvulsive status epilepticus if untreated.

COMPLEX PARTIAL SEIZURES

A detailed history may be required to make this diagnosis. Symptoms vary depending on the anatomic location of the seizure focus. Some patients will experience behavioral or sensory symptoms, as apposed to motor and postural symptoms, prior to generalization of their seizure. Patients may present with automatisms; however, they are usually more pronounced than those of absence seizures. These patients

may progress to nonconvulsive status epilepticus. Treatment is identical as for convulsive seizures.

Duncan JS, Sander JW, Sisodiya SM, Walker MC: Adult epilepsy. Lancet 2006;367:1087–100 [PMID:16581409].

Hughs JR: Absence seizures: a review of recent reports with new concepts. Epilepsy Behav 2009;14:404–412 [PMID: 19632158].

SECONDARY CAUSES OF SEIZURES

INTRACRANIAL HEMORRHAGE

(See also Chapter 37.) Intracerebral hemorrhage is the most common form of hemorrhagic stroke and results in major disability or death. Bleeding occurs primarily in the brain parenchyma and seizure is common. Prolonged seizure activity leads to increased intracranial pressure, cerebral metabolic demands, release of excitatory neurotransmitters and cerebral acidosis. Morbidity in this population is directly related to the duration of seizure activity. Recommended therapy for these patients includes lorazepam for cessation of seizure activity followed by a loading dose of phenytoin or fosphenytoin. If seizure activity continues, additional benzodiazepines may be needed. If barbiturates are required for seizure control, invasive airway management should be considered.

MASS LESIONS

In addition to simple mass effect, many neurophysiologic changes occur in response to the presence of a neoplastic process in the brain. This results in seizures that are potentially less responsive to standard therapy. Seizure may present as the first symptom of a brain tumor. The risk is the most in tumors that are central in location and have slow growth. Clinical trials have shown poor control with standard antiepileptic drugs (AEDs) and current recommendations include therapy for symptomatic patients only. Benzodiazepines and phenytoin or fosphenytoin are appropriate for patients who are seizing. No clear benefit has been shown with AEDs for seizure prophylaxis in this patient population.

FEVER

(See also Chapter 50.) Febrile seizures are the most common type of seizures in the pediatric population affecting between 2 and 14% of children worldwide. Most occur in children between the ages of 6 months and 5 years with a peak incidence around 18 months. These generalized seizures usually last less than 15 minutes and are considered fairly benign and are known as simple febrile seizures. Greater attention should be paid to children with complex febrile seizures which is defined as focal seizure, seizure activity greater than 15 minutes or with multiple seizures in close succession. Other causes of seizure with fever must also be investigated, such as herpes encephalitis and bacterial meningitis. Antipyretics do not prevent seizures, but should still be employed for febrile children. The use of AEDs for chronic control of febrile seizures is currently a topic of debate and most studies show no benefit. Benzodiazepines should be used for patients with an active seizure.

ALCOHOL WITHDRAWAL

Alcohol withdrawal seizures, in and of themselves, are not epilepsy and should be treated symptomatically with benzodiazepines alone. The alcoholic patient may have other reasons for seizure, however, including head injury, poor nutrition, metabolic disturbances and toxic exposures. Attention to these and other possible causes must be made in order to miss other life-threatening conditions in this high-risk population.

Patients with alcohol withdrawal typically have seizures 6–48 hours following cessation of alcohol intake. No AEDs have been shown to be effective preventing this syndrome. Phenytoin is clearly ineffective; phenobarbital and lorazepam, while useful in theory, have not demonstrated efficacy in controlled studies. Benzodiazopines should be used to abort active seizures. Chronic anticonvulsant administration is not necessary for alcohol withdrawal seizures alone. Hospitalization for alcohol withdrawal seizures is usually not needed if the patient can be reliably observed (eg, at a detoxification center or by family or friends) and the seizures treated with benzodiazepines.

ECLAMPSIA

(See also Chapter 38.) Eclampsia is a new onset type seizure in the clinical setting of a women with preeclampsia and no known seizure history. Eclampsia presents with generalized tonic–clonic seizures most commonly; however, simple and complex partial seizure may also be found. Status epilepticus is rare. Significant risk to the mother and fetus mandates delivery as soon as possible. Treatment of eclamptic seizures includes magnesium sulfate 4–6 gm IV loading dose over 15 to 20 minutes followed by a continuous infusion of 2 g/h. Magnesium sulfate has been shown to be superior to benzodiazepines and phenytoin and should be the first-line drug for eclamptic seizures.

Eclampsia may also present in the intrapartum and postpartum periods (usually occurring in the first 48 hours). Late postpartum eclampsia may occur between 48 hours and 4 weeks postpartum. CT scanning is considered appropriate as intracranial hemorrhage is a rare complication of eclampsia.

DRUG OVERDOSE

(See also Chapter 47.) Many different drugs can cause seizures. Overdose of isoniazid theophylline, organophosphates and cocaine commonly cause seizures. Treat symptomatic patients with supportive measures and benzodiazepines initially. A detailed history to discover the exact toxin may lead to more specific therapy, including administration of an antidote.

Fetveit A: Assessment of febrile seizures in children. Eur J Pediatr 2008;167:17–27 [PMID: 17768636].

Hughes JR: Alcohol withdrawal seizures. Epliepsy Behav 2009;15:92–97 [PMID: 19249388].

Karumanchi SA, Lindheimer MD: Advances in the understanding of eclampsia. Curr Hypertens Rep 2008;10:305–312 [PMID: 18625161].

Reid AY, Galic MA, Teskey GC, Pittman QJ: Febrile seizures: current views and investigations. Can J Neurol Sci 2009;36:679–686 [PMID: 19960745].

Sperling MR, Ko J: Seizures and brain tumors. Semin Oncol 2006;33:333–341 [PMID: 16769422].

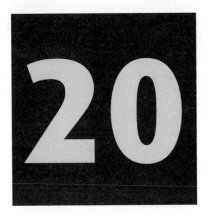

Headache

C. Keith Stone, MD

IMMEDIATE EVALUATION AND MANAGEMENT OF HEADACHE CAUSED BY LIFE-THREATENING CONDITIONS

See Figure 20–1.

Has Head Trauma Occurred?

If recent head trauma has occurred, evaluation of this problem takes precedence (Chapter 22).

Have Seizures Occurred?

Patients may have headache following one or more grand mal seizures. However, because the seizures may themselves be due to serious underlying disease (eg, subdural hematoma), evaluation of this problem takes precedence (Chapter 19).

Are There Focal Neurologic Abnormalities?

The presence of new focal neurologic abnormalities with headache, especially if papilledema is present as well, is strongly suggestive of a mass lesion (tumor, hematoma, abscess). Computed tomography (CT) scan or magnetic resonance imaging (MRI) should be done as soon as possible to make the diagnosis. Further evaluation is discussed in Chapter 37.

Is Headache New or of Acute Onset?

The single most important item of information to obtain from a patient with headache is whether the headache is new or acute in onset. A new headache is one occurring in a patient without a history of headaches, or a novel pattern or quality of pain in a patient with a history of headaches. A headache that is acute in onset is far more likely to have underlying pathology that may be life-threatening requiring prompt investigation.

Is The Complaint Consistent with Meningitis or Meningeal Irritation?

If the headache is acute or subacute in onset, subarachnoid hemorrhage or meningitis must be suspected. The usual manifestations are signs of meningeal irritation (stiff neck; positive Kernig and Brudzinski signs) and fever. These findings may be minimal or even absent in very young or very old patients. Seizures, confusion, or coma may be present as well.

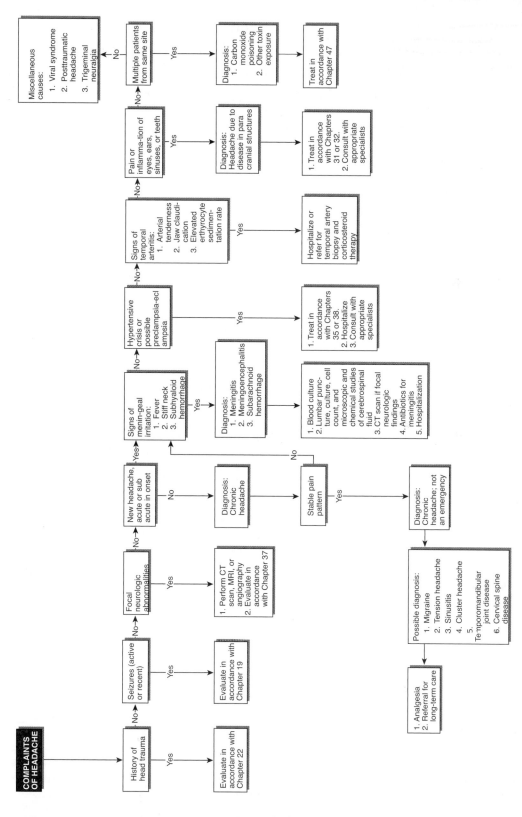

▲ **Figure 20–1.** Management of complaints of headache.

Subarachnoid hemorrhage should be strongly suspected in a patient with abrupt onset of headache that is unique to the patient's experience, especially if meningeal irritation or focal neurologic findings are present. An emergency CT scan is the initial test of choice. However, as many as 2% of patients with subarachnoid hemorrhage can have a normal CT scan within the first 12 hours after the hemorrhage begins. If the diagnosis is unclear, lumbar puncture should be performed.

Meningitis should be strongly suspected in a patient who presents with headache accompanied by fever, especially if signs of meningeal irritation are present. Antibiotic therapy should be started as soon as possible (based on microorganisms most common for each age group) before the CT scan or lumbar punctures are performed (Chapter 42). However, if there are signs of focal neurologic findings in a patient with fever, a brain abscess should be suspected and the lumbar puncture (but not antibiotics) should be delayed until a CT scan is performed.

▶ Is Headache Due to Hypertensive Encephalopathy or Preeclampsia-Eclampsia?

Moderate elevations of blood pressure alone seldom cause headache; however, severe hypertension as seen in hypertensive crises and eclampsia can be associated with headache. If hypertension is present and the patient is pregnant or has signs of cerebral dysfunction (confusion, obtundation, or coma) or other end-organ damage (retinitis; nephritis with proteinuria), a life-threatening emergency exists.

Note: In pregnancy, a slight increase in blood pressure may be more significant than in the nonpregnant patient. See Chapter 34 (see Hypertensive Crisis) or Chapter 38 (see Eclampsia).

▶ Is This Temporal Arteritis?

Temporal arteritis is a rare but treatable disease with serious sequelae that must be considered in every elderly patient with new headache. The principal manifestations are headache with temporal artery tenderness (not found in every case) and a markedly elevated erythrocyte sedimentation rate. Sudden irreversible monocular blindness may occur. If this condition is suspected, immediate treatment with steroids is indicated and hospitalization should be considered to confirm the diagnosis by means of temporal artery biopsy.

▶ Is Headache Due to Disease in Paracranial Structures?

New or acute headaches are often caused by disease in the eyes, ears, sinuses, or teeth. Look carefully for iritis or acute glaucoma (Chapter 31) or for sinusitis, otitis media, or dental caries or abscess (Chapter 32). Treatment should be focused on the primary condition.

▶ Are There Multiple Patients from the Same Vicinity?

Multiple patients from the same vicinity with complaint of headache suggest carbon monoxide poisoning or other toxin exposure. Patients should be questioned specifically about heating sources (eg, gas heat or oven), burning materials (eg, charcoal) in poorly ventilated areas, use of household cleaners, or other chemical exposure. Specific treatment of carbon monoxide poisoning and other toxin exposure is discussed in Chapter 47.

▶ Disposition

Even after careful initial history and physical examination, the diagnosis may not be apparent in the patient with new headache. Patients with recent onset of new headache should be hospitalized if there is any suspicion of a life-threatening process. Increasing severity of subacute headache over days or weeks, even without focal signs, suggests serious intracranial disease, and the patient should undergo appropriate diagnostic procedures. Subacute headaches without progressive symptoms and chronic headaches may be referred and evaluated on a nonemergency basis.

Bederson JB, Connolly ES, Batjer HH et al: Guidelines for the management of aneurysmal subarachnoid hemorrhage: a statement for healthcare professionals from a special writing group of the Stroke Council, American Heart Association. Stroke 2009;40:994–1025 [PMID: 19164800].

Lipton RB, Bigal ME, Steiner TJ, Silberstein SD, Olesen J: Classification of primary headaches. Neurology 2004;63: 427–435 [PMID: 15304572].

Somad D, Meurer W: Central nervous system infections. Emerg Med Clin Am 2009;27:89–100 [PMID: 13218021].

▼ APPROACH TO THE DIAGNOSIS OF HEADACHE

▶ Pain-Sensitive Structures and Their Projections

Headache is caused by traction, displacement, inflammation, or distention of pain-sensitive structures in the head or neck. Disorders of the scalp, teeth, eyes, and ears and of the mucous membranes of the nose, sinuses, and oropharynx can produce pain. Pain-sensitive structures about the calvarium include the scalp and its blood vessels, the neck muscles, and the upper cervical nerves. The skull, brain, and most of the dura are not pain sensitive. In general, discrete intracranial lesions above the cerebellar tentorium produce pain in trigeminal distribution (anterior to ears), whereas lesions in the posterior fossa project pain to the second and third cervical dermatomes (posterior to ears).

▶ History

A. Time of Onset

Chronic headache (duration of months or more) is usually not due to a serious disorder, but headache of acute onset or of a changing pain pattern demands prompt evaluation in the emergency department. If the patient has a chronic headache disorder, determine whether the present headache differs from or is identical to the patient's chronic problem. Headaches in the early morning or those causing waking may indicate an increase in intracranial pressure and prompt an evaluation for intracranial tumor.

B. Family History of Headaches

Primary headache disorders such as migraine and tension headaches commonly have a family history of headaches.

C. Location of Pain

1. Migraine or the cluster variant—Hemicranial or retroocular pain.

2. Tension headache—Commonly diffuse, occipital, or bandlike pain.

3. Mass lesion headache—Often focal ("right here").

4. Trigeminal neuralgia—Stabbing pain localized to the second or third division of the trigeminal nerve.

D. Quality of Pain

1. Migraine or the cluster variant—Commonly described as throbbing and often preceded by prodromal symptoms or auras, for example, scintillating scotomas or other visual changes.

2. Tension headache and mass lesion headache—Usually steady pain.

3. Trigeminal neuralgia—A shooting or stabbing character.

E. Timing

1. Mass lesion headache—Commonly maximal on awakening.

2. Cluster variant of migraine—Frequently awaken patients from sleep and often recur at the same time of day or night.

3. Tension headache—May develop at regular intervals, especially with recurrent stressful situations.

F. Factors Influencing Severity

1. Migraine or the cluster variant—Frequently relieved by pressure on the ipsilateral temporal or carotid artery; by darkness, sleep, or vomiting; or during pregnancy.

2. Mass lesion headache—Often exacerbated by events such as coughing and sneezing that transiently raise intracranial pressure.

G. Precipitating Factors

1. Tension headache—Tension, emotional stress, and fatigue.

2. Migraine—Hunger, nitrite-containing foods (hot dogs, salami, sausage), chocolate, aged cheeses, bright lights, menses, alcohol, caffeine, monosodium gluta-mate, aspartame, and insomnia.

3. Cluster variant of migraine—Alcohol.

4. Trigeminal neuralgia and the jaw claudication of temporal arteritis—Chewing and eating.

H. Associated Symptoms

Nausea or vomiting is common with migraine and post-traumatic headache syndromes and may be seen late in the course of mass lesions. Photophobia is prominent with migraine headache but occurs also with meningitis, especially viral (aseptic) meningitis. Myalgias of pericranial muscles (eg, posterior neck muscles) often accompany tension headaches and viral syndromes. Rhinorrhea and lacrimation during headache typify the cluster variant of migraine and are ipsilateral to the pain.

I. Previous Diagnostic Tests

Has the headache that the patient is presenting with previously been evaluated, and what tests (CT scan, MRI, lumbar puncture, pertinent laboratory data) have been performed?

J. Response to Medication

Find out what medications have worked in the past for this patient and if the patient commonly takes medications for prevention of headache. Clinical response of decreased pain to a medication should no be used as a lone indicator of a benign etiology of the headache.

▶ Physical Examination

A. Vital Signs

1. Fever—The presence of fever supports a diagnosis of meningitis, encephalitis, or headache associated with viral infection. A low-grade fever may also occur in temporal arteritis.

2. Blood pressure—Hypertension per se rarely causes headache, but chronic hypertension is the major risk factor for stroke, especially intracerebral hemorrhage. Intracerebral hemorrhage may be associated with acute headache. Blood pressure may be markedly elevated during hypertensive encephalopathy or as a result of preeclampsia–eclampsia, subarachnoid hemorrhage, or brain-stem stroke.

B. Skin

Neurofibromas or café au lait spots of Recklinghausen disease may be associated with benign or malignant intracranial tumors.

Cutaneous angiomas sometimes accompany arteriovenous malformations of the central nervous system; rupture results in subarachnoid hemorrhage and acute headache.

C. Scalp and Head

1. Temporal arteries—Note nodularity or tenderness compatible with temporal arteritis.

2. Sinuses—Note tenderness, erythema of overlying skin, or nasal discharge.

3. Temporomandibular joints—Look for tenderness or limitation of motion.

4. Orbits—A bruit heard when the stethoscope is placed on the eyeball over closed eyelids may suggest intracranial arteriovenous malformation.

D. Neck and Back

1. Muscle spasm—Cervical muscle spasm may be a sign of tension or may occur with migraine.

2. Meningeal signs—Can the patient touch chin to sternum? If not, is the limitation of motion mainly in the anteroposterior direction, suggesting meningeal irritation, or in all directions, as is common with cervical spine disorders? Is there any discomfort, neck flexion, or contralateral knee flexion during straight leg raising (Kernig sign)? Most important, is there even slight flexion of the knee (Brudzinski sign) during passive neck flexion?

Meningeal signs may be absent or difficult to demonstrate in the early stages of subacute meningitis and may be very minimal in very young or older patients. Several hours may elapse before evidence of meningeal irritation develops after subarachnoid hemorrhage, and these signs disappear if the patient lapses into deep coma.

E. Neurologic Examination

Unilateral cranial nerve, cerebellar, motor, or reflex abnormalities suggest a diagnosis of intracranial mass lesion.

F. Miscellaneous Physical Findings

Papilledema, the hallmark of increased intracranial pressure, should always be sought. Acute confusion or altered consciousness is common after subarachnoid hemorrhage and with purulent meningitis.

G. Indications for Imaging in the ED

The following are indications to order no contrast CT scans in patients presenting to the ED with an acute headache:

1. Abnormal neurologic exam to include altered mental status, cognitive impairment, or a focal deficit.

2. Patients experience a new severe headache of sudden onset.

3. HIV positive patients with a presentation of a new headache.

Edlow JA, Panagos PD, Godwin SA, Thomas TL, Decker WW: American College of Emergency Physicians: clinical policy: critical issues in the evaluation and management of adult patients presenting to the emergency department with acute headache. Ann Emerg Med 2008;52:407–436 [PMID: 18809105].

Go S: Nontraumatic headaches in the Emergency Department: a systematic approach to diagnosis and controversies in two "big ticket" entities. Mo Med 2009;106:156–161 [PMID 19397118].

Lamar AJ: Not all morning headaches are due to brain tumours. Pract Neurol 2009;9:80–84 [PMID: 19289557].

Peters KS: Secondary headache and head pain emergencies. Prim Care 2004;31:381–393 [PMID: 15172513].

▼ MANAGEMENT OF SPECIFIC DISORDERS CAUSING ACUTE HEADACHE

SUBARACHNOID HEMORRHAGE

ESSENTIALS OF DIAGNOSIS

▶ Sudden onset of severe headache
▶ Nuchal rigidity is seen in most patients but can take hours to develop

Acute onset of severe headache with maximum intensity in just a few minutes, that is unlike any headache that the patient has experienced previously, is suspicious for subarachnoid hemorrhage. Subarachnoid hemorrhage usually results from rupture of an aneurysm or arterial venous malformation. The diagnostic test of choice is a noncontrast CT scan. However, 2% of patients with subarachnoid hemorrhage can have a normal CT scan within the first 12 hours after the hemorrhage begins. As a result, a lumbar puncture should be performed if the CT is normal and the diagnosis is still suspected. A detailed discussion of subarachnoid hemorrhage is found in Chapter 37.

Bederson JB, Connolly ES, Batjer HH et al: Guidelines for the management of aneurysmal subarachnoid hemorrhage: a statement for healthcare professionals from a special writing group of the Stroke Council, American Heart Association. Stroke 2009;40:994–1025 [PMID: 19164800].

Edlow JA, Panagos PD, Godwin SA, Thomas TL, Decker WW: American College of Emergency Physicians:clinical policy: critical issues in the evaluation and management of adult patients presenting to the emergency department with acute headache. Ann Emerg Med 2008;52:407–436 [PMID: 18809105].

CEREBROVASCULAR ACCIDENT (STROKE)

See also Chapter 37.

ESSENTIALS OF DIAGNOSIS

- ▶ Sudden-onset focal neurologic deficit
- ▶ Symptoms related to vasculature involved

▶ Clinical Findings

Thrombotic or embolic strokes may be associated with mild to moderate nonthrobbing headaches and are present in 14% of strokes. The headache may precede or accompany the stroke.

▶ Treatment and Disposition

Treat stroke as described in Chapter 37. Hospitalize the patient for evaluation and treatment.

Yew K: Acute stroke diagniosis. Am Fam Physician 2009;80:33–40 [PMID: 19621844].

MENINGITIS AND MENINGOENCEPHALITIS

See also Chapter 42.

ESSENTIALS OF DIAGNOSIS

- ▶ Headache, fever
- ▶ Nuchal rigidity

▶ Clinical Findings

Headache, confusion, and nuchal rigidity developing over hours to days are classic features of meningitis. However, in rapidly progressive pyogenic meningitis, fever and altered consciousness are the most prominent presenting signs. In patients with subacute meningitis, headache is an early symptom that may precede nuchal rigidity and other meningeal signs. The headache of meningitis is continuous and throbbing and, although generalized, usually most prominent over the occiput. The pain is increased by head shaking, jugular vein compression, or any other maneuver that increases intracranial pressure. Pain is not relieved by changes in posture. Neck stiffness and other signs of meningeal irritation must be sought with care, because they may not be obvious early.

If meningitis or meningoencephalitis is suspected, perform a lumbar puncture (Chapter 7) and obtain blood for culture. A neuroimaging study should be obtained prior to lumbar puncture if any of the following is present: (1) papilledema, (2) altered mental status, and (3) focal or lateralizing neurologic findings.

▶ Treatment

A. Antimicrobials

Begin antibiotics immediately and do not delay awaiting blood draws or performance of a lumbar puncture. The choice of drug depends on the clinical circumstances and the age of the patient (see Chapter 42).

B. Supportive Care

General supportive care should be initiated in the emergency department. Protect the patient's airway and provide padded bed rails or restraints for agitated or delirious patients. If seizures have occurred, start anticonvulsant therapy. Concomitant corticosteroid treatment in bacterial meningitis has been shown in children to decrease the incidence of residual hearing impairment when caused by *Haemophilus influenzae* type B but not *Streptococcus Pneumoniae* or *Neisseria meningitidis*. Consider steroid therapy in children older than 1 month with suspected meningitis. There is also evidence to support steroid use in adults with meningitis.

▶ Disposition

Immediate hospitalization is warranted except perhaps in the case of a patient with aseptic (viral) meningitis who appears well, can be observed at home by a third party, and has close follow-up within 24 hours for reexamination.

Edlow JA, Panagos PD, Godwin SA, Thomas TL, Decker WW: American College of Emergency Physicians: clinical policy: critical issues in the evaluation and management of adult patients presenting to the emergency department with acute headache. Ann Emerg Med 2008;52:407–436 [PMID: 18809105].

Somand D, Meurer W: Central nervous system infections. Emerg Med Clin North Am 2009;27:89–100 [PMID: 19218021].

POSTURAL (POSTLUMBAR PUNCTURE) HEADACHE

ESSENTIALS OF DIAGNOSIS

► Follows lumbar puncture
► Headache exacerbated by the upright position
► Headache relieved by laying down

► Clinical Findings

Postural headache may follow lumbar puncture, especially if a large gauge, medium bevel, cutting spinal needle is used. Studies have shown that the larger the needle diameter, the higher the incidence of postdural puncture headache. This type of headache is worse in the upright position and nearly absent in recumbency. The onset of headache is usually within the first 24–48 hours and rarely occurs later. The site of the headache may be bifrontal, occipital, or in the neck and upper shoulders.

► Treatment and Disposition

Recumbency for 18–24 hours is often recommended but there is no evidence that it is beneficial. Adequate hydration and analgesics are usually sufficient management. For more persistent cases, IV caffeine can be tried. Referral to an anesthesiologist for an epidural blood patch may be of benefit.

Williams J, Lye DC, Umapathi T: Diagnostic lumbar puncture: minizing complications. Intern Med J 2008:38:587–591 [PMID: 18422562].

MANAGEMENT OF SPECIFIC DISORDERS CAUSING SUBACUTE HEADACHE

POSTTRAUMATIC HEADACHE

ESSENTIALS OF DIAGNOSIS

► History of head trauma
► May have associated dizziness, vertigo, insomnia

► Clinical Findings

Headache caused by head injury may begin immediately or within weeks after trauma. Chronic posttraumatic headache is defined as a headache that continues for more than 3 months after the trauma occurs. The symptoms are not necessarily proportionate to the severity of the traumatic event. Associated dizziness, vertigo, insomnia, depression, and personality change may occur. This constellation of symptoms is referred to as posttraumatic syndrome. Posttraumatic headache usually presents no special diagnostic or distinguishing features, although it may be suggestive of tension headache or migraine. Pain usually remits after days to weeks but occasionally persists for years.

► Treatment and Disposition

The character of the headache dictates the treatment of posttraumatic headache. The pharmacologic treatments for migraine and tension headache are appropriate for posttraumatic headache and should be chosen by the constellation of the patient's symptoms. Hospitalization is not indicated for posttraumatic headache, although referral for prophylactic therapy is indicated if symptoms persist.

Packard RC: Current concepts in chronic post-traumatic headache. Curr Pain Headache Rep 2005;9:59–64 [PMID: 15625027].

TRIGEMINAL NEURALGIA

ESSENTIALS OF DIAGNOSIS

► Excruciating, stabbing, facial pain
► Pain in the distribution of the trigeminal nerve

► Clinical Findings

Trigeminal neuralgia is distinguished by repetitive, brief unilateral facial pain confined to the distribution of the trigeminal nerve. Lightning-like stabs of excruciating pain characteristically recur over seconds to minutes and spontaneously abate. Occurrence during sleep is rare. Sensory stimulation (eg, touch, cold, wind, talking, chewing) of trigger zones about the cheek, nose, or mouth precipitates paroxysms of pain.

Trigeminal neuralgia usually develops after the fourth decade and is more common in women than men. Pain-free intervals may last minutes to weeks, but permanent spontaneous remission is rare. Pain is confined mainly to areas supplied by the second or third divisions of the trigeminal nerve (maxillary and mandibular areas of the face). Involvement of the first division of the trigeminal nerve (the forehead) or bilateral disease occurs in less than 5% of cases.

► Treatment

Phenytoin, 250 mg IV over 5–10 minutes, may abort an acute attack. Remission of symptoms with carbamazepine occurs in so many patients that it has been used as a diagnostic test. Begin with 100 mg orally twice daily, and increase by 100 mg every other day until the patient is pain free or side effects develop.

Baclofen (Lioresal, others) is also beneficial and has synergistic effects when used with carbamazepine or phenytoin. Lamotrigine (Lamictal) has also been shown to be useful in the treatment of trigeminal neuralgia, with a starting dose of 25 mg daily with an increase of 25 mg each week until a maintenance dose is reached.

Narcotic therapy has been shown to be of little use because of the brief duration of the pain. Surgical referral may be indicated for patients who do not respond to conventional pharmaceutical intervention.

▶ Disposition

Neurologic referral for evaluation and treatment is appropriate. Hospitalization is not usually indicated.

Cheshire WP: Trigeminal neuralgia: diagnosis and treatment. Curr Neurol Neurosci Rep 2005;5:79–85 [PMID: 15743543] (A review of diagnostic and treatment for trigeminal neuralgia.).

Liu JK, Apfelbaum RI: Treatment of trigeminal neuralgia. Neurosurg Clin N Am 2004;15:319–334 [PMID: 15246340] (A review of treatment of trigemnal neuralgia with focus on surgical intervention.).

INTRACRANIAL MASS

ESSENTIALS OF DIAGNOSIS

- ▶ Mild to moderate headache increasing in frequency or duration
- ▶ Becomes associated with a focal neurologic deficit

▶ Clinical Findings

Headache due to primary or metastatic intracranial tumor is usually mild to moderate in severity and described as deep, aching, and initially intermittent. Pain is maximal on awakening and during episodes of increased intracranial pressure (eg, coughing, sneezing, or straining at stool). Headaches increase in frequency and duration over weeks to months and become associated with focal neurologic signs. One-third to one-half of patients with brain tumor present with this classic history. A CT scan obtained with IV contrast will usually confirm the diagnosis. MRI, which is more sensitive, may be used as well.

▶ Treatment and Disposition

If an intracranial mass lesion is found to be the cause of headache, urgent neurologic or neurosurgical consultation is indicated. Hospitalization may be required for initiation of treatment. The distinction between primary and metastatic tumor is essential.

Chandana SR, Movva S, Arora M, Singh T: Primary brain tumors in adults. Am Fam Physician 2008;77:1423–1430 [PMID: 18533376].

IDIOPATHIC INTRACRANIAL HYPERTENSION (PSEUDOTUMOR CEREBRI)

ESSENTIALS OF DIAGNOSIS

- ▶ Papilledema
- ▶ Increased intracranial pressure
- ▶ Nonspecific brain imaging study

▶ Clinical Findings

Idiopathic intracranial hypertension is a syndrome characterized by papilledema, increased intracranial pressure (with normal CSF), and a nonspecific brain imaging study demonstrating normal or small-sized ventricles. Women, specifically obese women, are affected much more commonly than men; the peak incidence occurs in the third decade. Diffuse headache is almost invariably a presenting symptom. Complaints of diplopia and blurred vision or transient visual obscuration occur in more than 60% of cases. Moderate to severe papilledema is seen in over 40% of affected persons. The diagnosis is made when the patient has symptoms of increased intracranial pressures, no localizing symptoms, a nonspecific or normal imaging study and CSF pressures are elevated over 250 mm of H_2O with otherwise normal CSF findings.

The course in idiopathic cases is generally self-limited over several months, but visual loss may occur. Differentiation from space-occupying intracerebral mass lesions is critical and can be achieved by CT scan.

▶ Treatment and Disposition

Hospitalization is necessary for evaluation and treatment in patients with newly diagnosed idiopathic intracranial hypertension in the emergency department. Appropriate treatments include repetitive lumbar punctures, carbonic anhydrate inhibitors (acetazolamide), thiazide diuretics, and corticosteroids for visual complaints. Surgical maneuvers, including lumbar-peritoneal shunting or optic nerve sheath decompression, may be required. Patients who present to the emergency department with a known diagnosis of pseudotumor cerebri should receive treatment in consultation with the patient's neurologist, neurosurgeon, or ophthalmologist.

Binder DK, Horton JC, Lawton MT, McDermott MW: Idiopathic intracranial hypertension. Neurosurgery 2004;54:538–552 [PMID: 15028127].

TEMPORAL ARTERITIS (GIANT CELL ARTERITIS)

 ESSENTIALS OF DIAGNOSIS

▶ Older than 50 years
▶ Unilateral headache
▶ Usually tender over the temporal artery
▶ Elevated erythrocyte sedimentation rate
▶ Unilateral vision loss if treatment is delayed

▶ Clinical Findings

Temporal arteritis, although uncommon in the general population, is the most common form of systemic vasculitis. The disease preferentially involves large- to medium-sized arteries. It affects women twice as often as men and is rarely seen before the age of 50 years. Nonspecific signs and symptoms are typical: malaise, myalgia, weight loss, arthralgia, and fever. The headache is classically of rapid onset, unremitting, and located over the temporal arteries. It is often unilateral. Associated scalp tenderness may be a prominent complaint, especially when patients lie with their head on a pillow or brush their hair. Pain during chewing (jaw claudication) is strongly suggestive of temporal arteritis. Permanent unilateral blindness, usually sudden in onset, occurs in about half of patients if treatment is delayed; half of patients so affected go on to develop bilateral blindness.

The temporal arteries may be normal on examination, although focal tenderness, thickening, nodularity, or decreased pulsation may be found. The diagnosis should be suspected if the erythrocyte sedimentation rate is more than 50 mm/h.

The diagnosis can be established by demonstration of vasculitis in biopsy specimens of an affected artery. The biopsy specimens must be carefully examined (multiple sections) because involvement is segmental.

▶ Treatment

Temporal arteritis responds dramatically to corticosteroid treatment. Begin prednisone, 40–60 mg/d orally, as soon as the diagnosis is suspected. Biopsy should be obtained within 2–3 days after beginning corticosteroids. Patients presenting with visual loss warrant immediate ophthalmology consult and should receive IV steroids in the emergency department.

▶ Disposition

For patients with severe symptoms or visual loss, hospital admission is urgently indicated for evaluation and treatment with IV steroids. Patients with minimal symptoms may be discharged with oral prednisone but should make arrangements for close follow-up and biopsy within 3 days.

Chew SS, Kerr NM, Danesh-Meyer HV: Giant cell arteritis. J Clin Neurosci 2009;16:1263–1268 [PMID: 19586772].

MANAGEMENT OF SPECIFIC DISORDERS CAUSING CHRONIC HEADACHE

TENSION HEADACHE

 ESSENTIALS OF DIAGNOSIS

▶ Gradual onset
▶ Bilateral pressure or tightening about the head
▶ No nausea or vomiting

▶ Clinical Findings

Tension headache is the most prevalent form of headache. It has significant societal impact with lost workdays and reduced effectiveness when at work. Women are affected slightly more commonly than men. The age at onset is usually at age 25–30. Headaches are often associated with emotional stress and have no prodrome. The pain typically comes on gradually, is bilateral, occipital, or frontal in location, and is described as a tight band or pressure about the head. The pain is constant and nonthrobbing and persists for hours or for the entire day. Nausea and photophobia are frequent accompanying symptoms but are milder than that with migraine. Vomiting is not a feature of tension-type headache. Neurologic examinations are normal.

▶ Treatment

The treatment approach for tension headaches in the emergency department is pharmacotherapy. Nonsteroidal antiinflammatory drugs remain the therapy of choice in abortive treatment of tension headache. Combination medications that contain caffeine, analgesics, and sedatives have been found to be effective. Muscle relaxants (cyclobenzaprine, methocarbamol) may be appropriate when muscle tension appears to play a strong role. Referral for prophylactic treatment with antidepressants (amitriptyline) and incorporation of a "wellness" component is appropriate for patients expressing depression or anxiety as precipitants to their headaches.

Disposition

If simple measures are not successful, neurologic referral may be necessary. Hospitalization is not indicated.

Bendtsen L, Jensen R: Tension-type headache. Neurol Clin 2009;27:525–535 [PMID: 19289230].

Krusz JC: Tension-type headaches: what they are and how to treat them. Prim Care 2004;31:293–311 [PMID: 15172508].

MIGRAINE

ESSENTIALS OF DIAGNOSIS

▶ Throbbing-type pain
▶ Associated nausea, vomiting, and photophobia are common
▶ May have associated neurologic symptoms

General Considerations

Migraine headache is a primary brain disorder in which neural events result in vasodilation of blood vessels that causes pain and further nerve activation. Most cases occur in women, there is an inherited predisposition, and onset may be as early as the first decade. Recurrent vomiting during childhood may be the earliest manifestation of migraine. A family history of migraine is commonly present.

Clinical Findings

Migraine headaches are classified as being with aura (formerly called classic migraine) or without aura (formerly called common migraine).

In migraine without aura headache, pain is throbbing or pulsing, unilateral, and of moderate or severe intensity. Associated symptoms include nausea and vomiting, photophobia, or phonophobia. Continuing pain may cause cervical muscle contraction, leading to an erroneous diagnosis of tension headaches.

Migraine with aura is preceded by transient neurologic symptoms (the aura). The most common auras are visual disturbances: hemianopic field defects, scotomas, and scintillations that enlarge and spread peripherally. Other aura may include sensory symptoms or dysphasic speech disturbance. As the aura fades, vasodilatation occurs producing the headache that has identical characteristics as migraine without aura.

Attacks may be precipitated by certain foods such as tyramine-containing cheeses, wine, meats with nitrite preservatives, chocolate containing phenylethylamine, and monosodium glutamate (a flavor enhancer). Fasting, emotion, menses, drugs (especially oral contraceptive agents and vasodilators such as nitroglycerin), and bright lights may also trigger attacks.

Treatment

A. Analgesics and Analgesic Combinations

These drugs remain appropriate first-line therapy for acute migraine attacks. Commonly patient will have tried at least one or several analgesics prior to presentation to the emergency department. Appropriate analgesics include aspirin, nonsteroidal anti-inflammatory drugs, and combination medications that contain caffeine, analgesics, and sedatives. Opiates should be avoided because they can exacerbate gastrointestinal symptoms and have a high abuse potential.

B. Dopamine Antagonists (Antiemetics)

Several dopamine antagonists have been shown to be effective in aborting acute migraine headaches. Prochlorperazine and metoclopramide are most widely used. Prochlorperazine dosing is 10 mg IV. Side effects include hypotension and akathisia. Metoclopramide is also effective in doses of 10 mg IV.

C. Triptans

The triptans have an advantage of being selective pharmacologic agents for the treatment of migraine headaches. These compounds are serotonin 5-HT receptor agonists. All of these drugs have been shown to be effective in aborting acute migraine headaches. However, they have significant side effects including coronary artery constriction leading to myocardial infarction. These drugs cannot be used in patients with a history of ischemic heart disease, uncontrolled hypertension, or cerebrovascular disease. The following triptans can be used in the treatment of migraines in the emergency department:

- Sumatriptan—4–6 mg subcutaneously, which may be repeated after 1 hour; or 25–100 mg orally, which may be repeated after 2 hours.

- Naratriptan—1–2.5 mg orally, which may be repeated after 4 hours.

- Almotriptan—6.25–12.5 mg orally, which may be repeated after 2 hours.

- Rizatriptan—5–10 mg orally, which may be repeated after 2 hours.

- Zolmitriptan—1.25–2.5 mg orally, which may be repeated after 2 hours.

D. Ergot Derivatives

Ergot preparations have been used widely in the past for the acute treatment of migraine headaches. These drugs have complex pharmacology, and there is little evidence to support their use. With the effectiveness of dopamine antagonists and triptans, ergot preparations should be abandoned for abortive therapy in the emergency department.

E. Prophylactic Drugs

Prophylactic therapy may be useful in preventing migraine headaches, but it should not be initiated in the emergency department. Patients should be referred to a neurologist for evaluation for preventive treatment.

▶ Disposition

Referral to a neurologist or primary care physician is indicated. Hospitalization (other than a brief stay in the emergency department for parenteral medication) is rarely needed.

Sprenger T, Goadsby PJ: Migrainepatogenesis and state of pharmacological treatment options. BMC Med 2009;7:71. [PMID19917094].

Lawrence EC: Diagnosis and management of migraine headache. South Med J 2004;97:1069–1077 [PMID: 15586597].

CLUSTER HEADACHE

ESSENTIALS OF DIAGNOSIS

▶ Clusters of daily attacks separated by week to months of pain-free intervals

▶ Attacks consist of severe unilateral headache

▶ Associated cranial autonomic symptoms include lacrimation, miosis, conjunctivalinjection, nasalcongestion, and rhinorrhea

▶ Clinical Findings

Cluster headache is a syndrome of distinct attacks of severe, unilateral headache with ipsilateral cranial autonomic symptoms. The autonomic symptoms may include ptosis, lacrimation, miosis, conjunctival injection, nasal congestion, and rhinorrhea. It is more common in men than in women and begins later in life than migraine headaches.

Pain occurs in distribution of the trigeminal nerve and most commonly in the ocular, frontal, and temporal areas. Each attack builds in intensity over 10–15 minutes and may last up to 3 hours. Attacks recur one to three times daily, often at nearly the same time for periods of 2–12 weeks that may be separated by headache-free interval remission periods that average 6 months to 2 years. A subset of patients experience chronic cluster headaches without remission. These patients have attacks for more than 1 year without remission or with remissions lasting less than 14 days. Episodes may be precipitated by alcohol or vasodilator-type drugs. Nitroglycerin challenge can be diagnostic, producing a typical headache in 30–60 minutes.

▶ Treatment

Standard treatment for acute attacks is oxygen (7 L/min for 15 min) delivered by face mask; this treatment has a reported 70% response rate. Sumatriptan subcutaneously or intranasally, although contraindicated in patients with known cardiovascular disease, has proved effective: more than 90% of patients experience complete or near complete relief. Less effective agents such as dihydro-ergotamine and ergotamine are also commonly used. Lidocaine, 20–60 mg given intranasally, provides some relief within 10 minutes in most patients, but complete relief is rare.

Due to the severity, reoccurrence, and chronicity of attacks, transitional therapy should follow treatment for the acute headache. Transitional treatment should be initiated at the first sign of an attack and continued for 2 weeks past the last attack. Agents for transitional therapy include corticosteroids (prednisone 60–80 mg/d tapered over 2 weeks), naratriptan 2.5 mg twice daily, and ergotamine 2 mg at bedtime or twice daily. Surgical interventions on the cranial parasympathetic system or on the trigeminal nerve have been recommended for intractable chronic cluster headaches that have become resistant to medical management.

▶ Disposition

Neurologic referral is indicated.

Beck E, Sieber WJ, Trejo R: Management of cluster headache. Am Fam Physician 2005;71:717–724 [PMID: 15742909].

Rozen TD: Cluster headache: diagnosis and treatment. Curr Pain Headache Rep 2005;9:135–140 [PMID: 15745625].

Arthritis & Back Pain

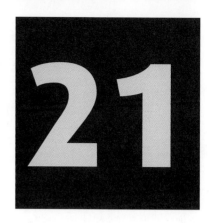

Ryan P. Woods, MD
Jason Seamon, DO, MHS, FACEP, FAAEM[1]

EVALUATION OF THE PATIENT WITH ACUTE ARTHRITIS

See Figure 21–1.

Is the Patient Systemically Ill?

Whenever a patient with acute joint pain also presents with fever, rigors, systemic symptoms, or signs of involvement of additional organ systems, careful evaluation is necessary to rule out potentially life-threatening processes such as infection or diffuse vasculitis. Hospitalization and consultation for evaluation of rheumatic or infectious disease are usually required for patients with arthritis and systemic symptoms. Obtain blood cultures, and perform the evaluation outlined below.

Is This Disseminated Gonococcal infection?

In young adults, hematogenous gonococcal infection is one of the most common causes of acute arthritis. Arthritis may be the sole manifestation of disseminated gonococcal infection. Skin lesions are few and are found on the extremities, frequently around a joint, and are pustular or hemorrhagic, rarely bullous. Gram-stained smears of material contained in the pustules may reveal gram-negative diplococci within polymorphonuclear neutrophils. Tenosynovitis classically involves tendons of the hand or foot. The primary (mucosal) site of gonococcal infection is often asymptomatic. If disseminated gonococcal infection is suspected, culture of blood and secretions from the pharynx, rectum, and urethra or cervix should be obtained.

Is There Arthritis on Joint Examination?

Ascertain by careful examination whether acute joint pain is due to an intra-articular process. Is there redness, diffuse warmth, effusion, or painful limitation of active and passive

---

[1] This chapter is a revision of the chapter by Terry C. Hermance and L. Richard Boggs, from the 6th edition.

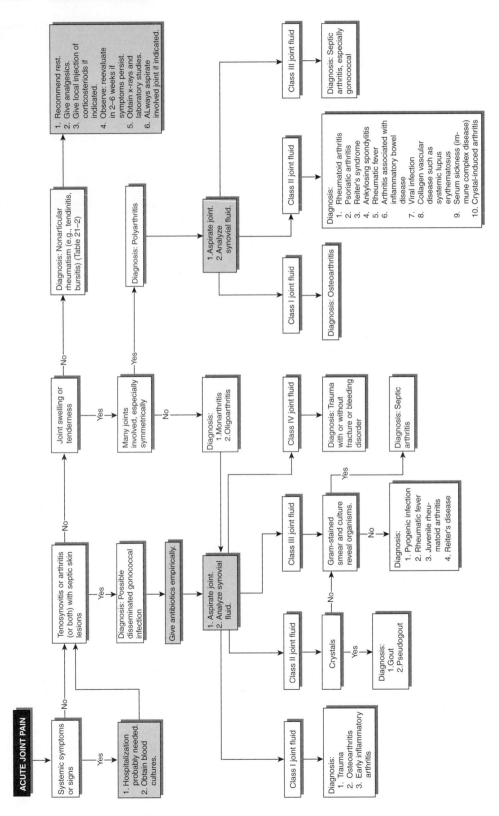

▲ Figure 21-1. Assessment of patients with acute joint pain.

motion? If the joint is not involved, consider cellulitis, tenosynovitis, bursitis, or other periarticular lesions.

Is the Process Oligoarticular or polyarticular?

Involvement of 1–3 joints in an asymmetric pattern is generally considered a characteristic of oligoarthritis, although this asymmetric involvement may occur early in some polyarticular conditions such as juvenile rheumatoid arthritis. Common causes of oligoarthritis include infection, crystal deposition (eg, gout), and trauma. The polyarthritis syndromes involve many joints, usually in a symmetric fashion.

Perform Arthrocentesis

If one of the affected joints is acrally located (eg, wrist, elbow, knee, ankle), arthrocentesis should be attempted in the emergency department, using local anesthesia and sterile technique (Chapter 6). A specialist and/or ultrasound guidance should be considered for arthrocentesis of the shoulders and hips. The joint fluid should be analyzed and the results should be used to classify the arthritis according to the scheme in Table 19–1.

Classification of Arthritis

See Table 21–1.

A. Noninflammatory (Class I)

Acute arthritis in the presence of normal joint fluid usually indicates trauma, or osteoarthritis. Rarely, early joint

aspiration in inflammatory arthritis produces a similar result.

B. Inflammatory (Class II)

Inflammatory arthritis may be present in acute gout, pseudogout, Reiter syndrome, rheumatoid arthritis, and rheumatic fever. Gram stain and culture of synovial fluid should be done to rule out early infectious arthritis.

C. Septic (Class III)

Purulent joint fluid (class III) is seen almost exclusively in bacterial and fungal infections. Gram stain of joint fluid may help to identify the causative organism before cultures become positive.

D. Hemorrhagic (Class IV)

Hemorrhagic joint fluid is seen in trauma with or without fracture; the presence of fat globules suggests fracture. A tear in the anterior cruciate ligament is the most common cause of hemarthrosis in the knee when no fracture is present. Other frequent causes of hemarthrosis include peripheral meniscus tears and patellar dislocations (with medial retinaculum tears). Hemorrhagic effusion is more likely to be associated with acute pain than is the noninflammatory effusion that can occur with minor joint trauma, because blood within the joint space generally causes an inflammatory reaction. Hemorrhagic fluid is also seen in hemophilia and in synovial neoplasms.

Table 21–1. Classification of Abnormal Synovial Fluid.

Type of Joint Fluid	Viscosity	Clarity	Color	Leukocyte Count (per μL)	Gram Stain and Culture	Other Findings
Normal	High	Clear	Light yellow	<200	Negative	...
Noninflammatory (class I)	High	Clear	Light yellow	<4000	Negative	...
Inflammatory (class II)	Low	Cloudy	Dark yellow	>2000–<50,000	Negative	Crystals are diagnostic of gout or pseudogout (differentiate with polarizing microscopy); usually seen with class II joint fluid
Septic (class III)	Low	Cloudy	Dark yellow	Usually > 50,000	Usually positive[a]	Bacteria on culture or Gram-stained smear. Usually seen with class III joint fluid but may be seen with class II; rarely, class I
Hemorrhagic (class IV)	Variable	Cloudy	Pink-red	Usually > 2000[b]	Negative	Fat globules strongly suggest intraarticular fracture and are usually seen with class IV joint fluid

[a]Most common exception is gonococcal infection (only about 25% of cases have positive culture or Gram stain).
[b]Many red cells also found.

EMERGENCY TREATMENT OF SPECIFIC CONDITIONS CAUSING ACUTE ARTHRITIS—MONARTHRITIS OR OLIGOARTHRITIS

MONARTHRITIS OR OLIGOARTHRITIS

TRAUMATIC ARTHRITIS

ESSENTIALS OF DIAGNOSIS

► Effusions often develop immediately after trauma
► Fever or other systemic signs or symptoms are not present

▶ Clinical Findings

Severe joint pain associated with trauma is usually related temporally to an obvious injury. Mild pain may occur some time after the injury. Fever and other systemic signs usually are not present. The presence of noninflammatory or hemorrhagic synovial fluid confirms the diagnosis. Because patients with septic arthritis may also give a history of recent trauma, Gram stain and culture of fluid routinely should be performed.

The presence of many small fat globules in hemorrhagic joint fluid strongly suggests intra-articular fracture; X-rays should be carefully scrutinized to locate occult fractures. Well-localized tenderness over a bone is an important sign of fracture (Chapter 28). Scaphoid fractures are particularly difficult to locate and require careful correlation with clinical findings (eg, localized tenderness in the anatomic snuffbox). X-rays that show only joint effusion or periarticular soft tissue swelling are consistent with occult fractures or other joint injuries such as spontaneously reduced dislocations, ligamentous injuries, meniscus tears, avulsion fractures, and osteochondral fractures. Joint effusions that accumulate immediately following trauma are uniformly hemorrhagic and usually do not require arthrocentesis for diagnostic purposes.

▶ Treatment and Disposition

Splinting, protection from weight bearing, and follow-up care are essential. Analgesia may be needed. See Chapter 28 for more specific details and guidelines for treatment and disposition.

ACUTE GOUTY ARTHRITIS

ESSENTIALS OF DIAGNOSIS

► Presence of negative birefringent urate crystals in joint fluid and a negative Gram stain and culture
► Uric acid level is not helpful for diagnosis in an acute attack

▶ Clinical Findings

Patients with acute gouty arthritis have monarthritis or oligoarthritis with class II or class III joint fluid, urate crystals in the synovial fluid, and a negative synovial culture.

A. Symptoms and Signs

There is sudden onset of warmth, hyperemia, induration, and extreme pain in a joint, most commonly the metatarsophalangeal joint of the great toe. The next most commonly involved joint is the knee. Although most patients present with only one painful joint, several joints may be involved.

B. Laboratory Findings

Elevated serum uric acid concentration is supporting evidence of gouty arthritis, although during an acute attack the serum urate level may be normal. Therefore, a uric acid level should not be ordered. Definitive diagnosis requires use of a polarizing microscope to demonstrate characteristic negative birefringence of urate crystals in the synovial fluid.

▶ Treatment
A. Nonsteroidal Anti-inflammatory Drugs

Indomethacin or other nonsteroidal anti-inflammatory drugs (NSAIDs) may be indicated if a diagnosis of gout is well established. Aspirin is contraindicated, because small doses may cause hyperuricemia.

1. Indomethacin—Give 50 mg orally every 8 hours for 2 days. Then reduce the dosage to 25 mg 3–4 times daily for 3 days. Peptic ulcer disease is a contraindication to indomethacin.

2. Other drugs—Alternatives to indomethacin include ibuprofen 600 mg orally every 6 hours, naproxen 500 mg orally every 12 hours, may be used. Other NSAIDs, such as ketorolac in appropriate doses, can also be effective in acute gout.

B. Colchicine

Oral or intravenous colchicine, if administered within 24 hours of acute arthritis, can provide dramatic relief. Colchicine should not be used in patients with renal or hepatic dysfunction. Response to colchicine also strongly supports a diagnosis of gout.

1. Oral treatment—Give colchicine, 0.6 mg every hour until pain has resolved, a maximum dose of 4–6 mg is reached, or side effects of nausea and diarrhea cannot be tolerated.

2. Intravenous treatment—Gastrointestinal toxicity can be reduced by giving colchicine, 1–2 mg intravenously in 50 mL of normal saline over 20 minutes; repeat this dose every 6 hours until the patient is asymptomatic or to a total dose of 4 mg. After a full course of colchicine, no further doses should be administered for 1 week.

C. Corticosteroids

Corticosteroids are useful in patients who cannot take NSAIDs or colchicine. Prednisone, 40 mg daily for 1–3 days followed by a slow taper over 1–2 weeks, is recommended. Alternatively, a single dose of adrenocorticotropic hormone or corticotrophin, 40 units intramuscularly, boosts the patient's endogenous steroid production and can provide relief from a gouty flare-up.

3. Disposition

Hospitalization is rarely necessary. The patient should receive follow-up evaluation in a few days.

ACUTE PSEUDOGOUT

ESSENTIALS OF DIAGNOSIS

▶ Calcium pyrophosphate crystals in the joint

▶ Clinical Findings

Patients with acute pseudogout have acute oligoarthritis with class II joint fluid and calcium pyrophosphate crystals in the synovial fluid. Pseudogout simulates gout in middle-aged or elderly patients. It differs from gout in that the knee is the most commonly involved joint.

Serum uric acid levels are usually normal. Chondrocalcinosis may be present, although not necessarily in the acutely involved joint. The presence of chondrocalcinosis, however, regardless of location, is not diagnostic. Definitive diagnosis depends on the presence of calcium dihydrate (pyrophosphate) crystals in synovial fluid.

▶ Treatment

Aspiration of the joint is often adequate for relief of symptoms. NSAIDs may be helpful (see Acute Gouty Arthritis, above). Unlike patients with gouty arthritis, patients with acute pseudogout do not respond as well to colchicine.

▶ Disposition

Hospitalization is rarely necessary. Refer the patient to a primary care physician.

SEPTIC ARTHRITIS

ESSENTIALS OF DIAGNOSIS

▶ Joint is painful, erythematous, and tender
▶ Systemic symptoms: fever and chills are common
▶ Definitive diagnosis by aspiration of the joint. Fluid may demonstrate the infecting organism by Gram stain or culture

▶ General Considerations

Septic arthritis is one of the more common causes of oligoarthritis, but often only one joint is affected. The most frequent pathogen in septic oligoarthritis is the gonococcus, which, although difficult to demonstrate in joint fluid, often produces typical pustular skin lesions or tenosynovitis. The most common pathogen in monarticular septic arthritis is *Staphylococcus aureus*. Another common pathogen is *Streptococcus* spp. In intravenous drug users and immunocompromised hosts, gram-negative and anaerobic organisms may be seen.

▶ Clinical Findings

Patients with septic arthritis show evidence of infection in the joint (bacteria on Gram-stained smear or culture, or rapid response to antimicrobial therapy). Class III joint fluid is usually present.

A. Symptoms and Signs

Patients with septic arthritis usually present with a severe monarticular process characterized by marked pain, erythema, and tenderness. The onset of septic arthritis is usually less precipitous than that of gout. A few patients with staphylococcal or gonococcal arthritis may present with two or more involved joints. Acute migratory oligoarthritis followed in 1–2 days by acute arthritis localized to one or two joints is especially suggestive of gonococcal arthritis. If multiple joints are involved in septic arthritis, the distribution is usually asymmetric. Systemic symptoms and signs of infection (eg, fever, chills, leukocytosis) are common.

B. Laboratory Findings

A definitive diagnosis is established by demonstrating the infecting organism in synovial tissue or joint fluid. Joint fluid shows high leukocyte counts, usually over 50,000/mL. The higher the white blood cell count in joint fluid, the greater the likelihood of bacterial or fungal arthritis. The glucose content of synovial fluid is usually reduced. If no antimicrobial therapy has been given, smears and cultures of joint fluid usually reveal organisms.

In gonococcal arthritis, however, Gram-stained smears and even cultures of joint fluid are frequently negative, although in most cases, cultures of exudate from the cervix, urethra, pharynx, or rectum demonstrate gonococci. In gonococcal arthritis, the diagnosis may also be confirmed by prompt response to antimicrobial therapy (Chapter 42).

▶ Treatment

A. Joint Aspiration

Aspiration of the joint is essential. Obtain cultures of blood and joint fluid. If gonococcal arthritis is suspected, cervical, urethral, and possibly pharyngeal and rectal cultures should be obtained. If sepsis is considered likely, as much fluid as possible should be removed from the joint.

B. Antibiotics

Begin an antibiotic deemed appropriate based on clinical findings and Gram-stained smears. Narrow the antibiotic coverage once results of Gram stain, culture, and sensitivities are reported. The treatment of gonococcal arthritis is discussed in more detail in Chapter 42.

▶ Disposition

Hospitalize all patients with suspected or documented septic arthritis and start them on intravenous antibiotics. Consult an orthopedic surgeon for possible incision and drainage of the infected joint. Patients with mild gonococcal arthritis often can be discharged early and given antibiotics to be taken orally, provided that they are reliable patients and that careful follow-up can be ensured.

Mathews CJ, Weston VC, Jones A et al: Bacterial septic arthritis in adults. Lancet 2010;375:846–855 [PMID: 20206778].

OLIGOARTHRITIS OR POLYARTHRITIS

OSTEOARTHRITIS (DEGENERATIVE JOINT DISEASE)

ESSENTIALS OF DIAGNOSIS

▶ Usually polyarticular involvement. Most commonly involves hips, knees, spine, and distal and proximal interphalangeal joints

▶ Systemic signs and symptoms (fever and chills) should be absent

▶ Radiographs usually demonstrate cartilage changes with osteophytes

▶ Clinical Findings

Osteoarthritis is a chronic, progressive disease that is characterized by focal areas of loss of articular cartilage in synovial joints, associated with varying degrees of osteophyte formation, subchondral bone change, and synovitis. Osteoarthritis commonly affects load-bearing areas of bone. The clinical features of pain, increased age, stiffness, decreased movement, muscle wasting, and cracking of joints (crepitus) combined with radiographic findings of joint space narrowing, osteophytes, irregular joint surfaces, and bony sclerosis are used in making the diagnosis. Osteoarthritis is usually polyarticular but can be monarticular. The most commonly infected joints are knee, hip, cervical and lumbar spine, and distal and proximal interphalangeal joints. This condition is strongly correlated with age, infrequently seen before the fifth decade of life and rising in prevalence with increasing age.

▶ Treatment and Disposition

In the emergency department, newly diagnosed osteoarthritis must be carefully distinguished from the septic joint. Once osteoarthritis is diagnosed, patients should be discharged with medication and exercise instructions. First-line treatment is acetaminophen, 2000 mg every 24 hours in divided doses. Acetaminophen is as effective for osteoarthritis as NSAIDs and has fewer side effects. If NSAIDs are prescribed, select ibuprofen, 600 mg every 6 hours, as initial therapy. If patients are at high risk for gastrointestinal bleeding, selective use of a COX-2 inhibitor may be considered. Tramadol and opioid analgesics may be considered if the patient fails more conservative analgesic treatment. Patient education, aerobic exercise, swimming, walking, and range of motion exercises have all shown benefits in knee and hip osteoarthritis. Patients should follow up with their primary care physician within 1 week.

DeAngelo NA, Gordon V: Treatment of patients with arthritis related pain. JAOA 2004;104:2–5 [PMID: 15602034].

Dieppe PA, Lohmander S: Pathogenesis and management of pain in osteoarthritis. Lancet 2005;365(3963):965–973 [PMID: 15766999].

RHEUMATIC FEVER AND POSTSTREPTOCOCCAL REACTIVE ARTHRITIS

ESSENTIALS OF DIAGNOSIS

► Evidence of recent streptococcus infection
► Constitutional symptoms: fever, malaise
► Often oligoarthritis with associated cardiac involvement, subcutaneous nodules, and erythema marginatum

Rheumatic fever or poststreptococcal reactive arthritis may present early as acute monarticular joint pain. Acute rheumatic fever is diagnosed using the revised Jones criteria (Table 21–2). Poststreptococcal reactive arthritis will have only some of the Jones criteria and is usually oligoarticular. Carditis is rare, and the arthritis tends to be severe and recurrent and poor responsive to aspirin and other NSAIDs. Patients should be hospitalized if rheumatic fever is suspected. Initial treatment is penicillin and salicylates.

Hahn RG, Knox LM, Forman TA: Evaluation of poststreptococcal illness. Am Fam Physician 2005;15:1949–1954 (Review) [PMID: 15926411].

Table 21–2. Revised Jones Criteria for Diagnosis of Rheumatic Fever.[a]

Major criteria
Pericarditis, myocarditis, or endocarditis
Chorea
Subcutaneous nodules
Erythema marginatum
Polyarthritis
Minor criteria
Fever
Arthralgias
Laboratory findings: elevated sedimentation rate, evidence of preceding streptococcal infection (increased titer of antistreptolysn O), increased C-reactive protein
History of rheumatic fever or rheumatic heart disease; increased PR interval on ECG

[a]The presence of two major or one major and two minor criteria with supporting evidence of recent infection with group A streptococcus indicates a high probability of rheumatic fever.

POLYARTHRITIS

RHEUMATOID ARTHRITIS

ESSENTIALS OF DIAGNOSIS

► Often subacute joint pain
► Usually symmetric polyarthritis
► Radiographs demonstrate juxta-articular osteoporosis and later cartilage erosions

► Clinical Findings

Rheumatoid arthritis generally presents as a symmetric, chronic polyarthritis with prominent involvement of proximal interphalangeal and metacarpophalangeal joints, often with ulnar deviation. Distal interphalangeal joints are not involved.

A. Symptoms and Signs

Rheumatoid arthritis is a common cause of subacute joint pain involving multiple joints in adults. Although symmetric involvement is classic, the disease may begin with asymmetric involvement. In a typical acute presentation, joints may only be warm, tender, or swollen.

B. Laboratory Findings

Rheumatoid factor is positive in 85% of patients; therefore, a negative test does not rule out rheumatoid arthritis. Elevated erythrocyte sedimentation rate and C-reactive protein are also common but nonspecific findings.

C. X-ray Findings

Early X-ray examination generally reveals soft tissue swelling and juxta-articular osteoporosis. Erosions are seen later.

► Treatment

Aspirin and other NSAIDs have proven effective for the initial treatment of rheumatoid arthritis. However, the simultaneous administration of other drug classes in addition to NSAIDs is now common. For example, steroids, gold, penicillamine, methotrexate, cyclosporine, and sulfasalazine are being used. Initial management in the emergency department should consist of aspirin or NSAIDs in appropriate doses with urgent rheumatologist follow-up or consultation for additional prescriptions if indicated.

► Disposition

The patient should be referred early to a rheumatologist or primary care physician. Consider admission for patients with severe systemic involvement (eg, disabling polyarthritis, fever, or weight loss) or vasculitis.

SPONDYLOARTHROPATHIES

Spondyloarthropathies are a cluster of chronic inflammatory rheumatic diseases that include psoriatic and intestinal arthritis, Reiter syndrome, and ankylosing spondylitis. They are not associated with rheumatoid factor but have a strong association with HLA-B27. Anatomic sites include the following: the entheses (sites of ligament and tendon insertion into bone), the sacroiliac joints, limb joints, and nonarticular sites (eg, gut, skin, and eye).

1. Psoriatic Arthritis and Intestinal Arthritis

ESSENTIALS OF DIAGNOSIS

► Common in patients with psoriasis or inflammatory bowel disease

► Clinical Findings

Psoriatic arthritis is an inflammatory arthritis seen in up to 40% of patients with psoriasis. Nail involvement (pitting, dystrophy, or onycholysis) is a clue to the diagnosis. The arthritis occurs before psoriasis is seen in 15% of patients. Intestinal arthritis is an inflammatory arthritis seen in patients with ulcerative colitis or Crohn's disease. In one study, this form of arthritis occurred in approximately 40% of patients. The arthritis can be in the limb joints or the sacroiliac.

► Treatment and Disposition

Initial treatment is with NSAIDs. Sulfasalazine should be added if the patient cannot take or does not respond to NSAIDs.

2. Reiter Syndrome

ESSENTIALS OF DIAGNOSIS

► Usually affects young males
► Arthritis, conjunctivitis, and urethritis
► Arthritis is polyarticular and asymmetric, developing after chlamydial urethritis or bacterial gastroenteritis

► Clinical Findings

Reiter syndrome is a reactive arthritis with the classic triad of arthritis, conjunctivitis, and urethritis ("can't see, can't pee, can't climb a tree"). It is most commonly seen in men aged 15–35 years. The arthritis affects primarily the weight-bearing joints of the lower extremities. Reactive arthritis occurs within 1 month of a genitourinary (*Chlamydia trachomatis*) or enteral (*Shigella, Salmonella, Yersinia, Campylobacter*) infection. It is asymmetric and polyarticular. Arthrocentesis reveals a class II inflammatory joint fluid.

► Treatment and Disposition

NSAIDs are the mainstay of treatment. Tetracycline improves recovery time for reactive arthritis due to *Chlamydia* but not for enteral causes. The typical reactive arthritis lasts 4–5 months, but patients can develop chronic or recurrent arthritis.

Winterfield LS, Menter A, Gordon K, Gottlieb A: Psoriasis treatment: current and emerging directed therapies. Ann Rheum Dis 2005;64:ii87–ii90 [PMID: 15708946].

3. Ankylosing Spondylitis

ESSENTIALS OF DIAGNOSIS

► Patients younger than 40 years
► Back pain of gradual onset
► Stiffness worse in morning
► X-rays show sacroiliitis

► Clinical Findings

Ankylosing spondylitis is the most common spondyloarthropathy. Its classic findings include the following: gradual onset, age less than 40 years, back pain and morning stiffness worse with inactivity and made better with exercise, at least 3 months' duration, and radiographic evidence of sacroiliitis. Often a history of uveitis can be elicited.

An asymmetrical arthritis is manifested in peripheral joints because areas of enthesitis (Achilles and plantar fascia) are commonly involved. Arthrocentesis reveals a class II inflammatory joint fluid. Some patients will have constitutional complaints of malaise, decreased appetite, and fever.

► Treatment and Disposition

NSAIDs and strengthening exercises are used for treatment. Follow-up with a rheumatologist should be arranged.

VIRAL ARTHRITIS

General Considerations

Viral arthritis is acute, symmetric, and polyarticular. The two most common viruses causing secondary arthritis are rubella and hepatitis B. Mumps, adenoviruses, enteroviruses, and Epstein–Barr viruses have also been implicated. The arthritis is caused by deposition of immune complexes that cause an inflammatory reaction.

Clinical Findings

Diagnosis is made from the history of the patient. A recent viral infection or vaccination can aid in diagnosis. The most frequently affected joints are the proximal interphalangeal joints, metacarpophalangeal joints, knee, and ankle. The symptoms are usually self-limiting after several weeks but can last years.

Treatment and Disposition

Treatment is symptomatic and includes NSAIDs. Refer patients to their primary care physician.

SYSTEMIC LUPUS ERYTHEMATOSUS

ESSENTIALS OF DIAGNOSIS

- ▶ Arthritis associated with other systemic symptoms: rash, fever
- ▶ Positive anti-double-stranded DNA or positive antinuclear antibody test

Clinical Findings

Almost all patients with systemic lupus erythematosus will have arthritis. Patients usually also have fever, rash, or other features of the disease. Diagnosis in patients who present only with arthritis requires demonstration of a positive antinuclear antibody test or anti-double-stranded DNA test along with other criteria set forth by the American Rheumatism Association.

Treatment and Disposition

The acute arthritis of systemic lupus erythematosus is treated with NSAIDs. Patients should be referred to a rheumatologist for diagnostic evaluation and appropriate care.

NONARTICULAR RHEUMATISM

In the emergency evaluation of joint pain, it is important to distinguish between true articular (arthritis) and extra-articular (tendonitis and bursitis) causes.

TENDONITIS

ESSENTIALS OF DIAGNOSIS

- ▶ Pain and tenderness more localized to the tendon
- ▶ Although rare, always consider infectious causes of inflammation

Clinical Findings

In contrast to diffuse pain, warmth, and tenderness across an arthritic joint, tendonitis generally produces more localized pain that is reproduced with stretching of the affected tendon. Tendonitis is thought to be caused by repetitive overuse resulting in damage and inflammation to the tendon and surrounding structures. If the history reveals a puncture or laceration over a tendon with erythema, pain along the tendon, fever, and severe pain on minimal passive tendon motion, an infectious process must be ruled out.

Treatment

A. Adjunctive Measures

Relative rest from exacerbating activities, effective splinting, and ice as needed are the mainstays of treatment. NSAIDs and an exercise program to maintain joint motion and build muscle strength are helpful.

B. Local Injection

Local injection of anesthetic and depot glucocorticoid preparations may be appropriate for some patients (see Bursitis, below). However, this procedure should be performed only by an individual skilled in the procedure, because complications (eg, local atrophy and rupture of the tendon) can result if corticosteroids are errantly injected into a weight-bearing tendon.

C. Antimicrobials

Suspicion of an infectious tendonitis requires orthopedic consultation for possible incision and debridement and hospital admission for appropriate intravenous antibiotics to cover presumptive staphylococcal and streptococcal species.

Disposition

Most patients with tendonitis can receive treatment on an outpatient basis, with referral to an orthopedist if necessary.

BURSITIS

ESSENTIALS OF DIAGNOSIS

▶ Inflammation localized to the bursa, not the entire joint

▶ Common sites involved are elbow and prepatellar area

▶ Consider infection as cause of inflammation, especially if systemic symptoms such as fever and chills are present

▶ Clinical Findings

A bursa is a sac normally containing a thin film of synovial fluid that cushions the interface between bone with ligaments and the overlying skin. Bursitis is inflammation of the bursa. Like tendonitis, bursitis may be due to trauma or infection (most commonly found in the olecranon and prepatellar bursa) or may be idiopathic. Clinical findings are pain, tenderness, and swelling of the involved bursa.

▶ Treatment

A. Aspiration

The olecranon and prepatellar bursa should be aspirated for diagnosis and treatment if fluctuance and infectious signs are present.

B. Antibiotics

Septic bursitis is usually due to *S. aureus* and, pending results of culture and susceptibility testing, patients have traditionally been treated with a penicillinase-resistant, β-lactamase-resistant antimicrobial (eg, nafcillin, 150 mg/kg/d intravenously in 4–6 divided doses; or cefazolin, 60 mg/kg/d intramuscularly or intravenously in three divided doses). Given the prevalence of Community Acquired MRSA, vancomycin (1 gm IV every 12 hours) should be considered as the initial parenteral antibiotic for inpatients and trimethoprim/sulfamethoxazole (two DS tablets by mouth every 12 hours) should be considered for outpatient treatment of septic bursitis.

C. Anti-inflammatory Agents

NSAIDs, combined with rest, are most effective.

D. Corticosteroid Injection

Locally injected corticosteroids are useful in treatment of aseptic bursitis. However, injections should be given only by physicians skilled in the procedure because complications can include infection.

E. Surgery

Septic bursitis rarely requires incision and debridement.

▶ Disposition

Patients with septic bursitis require intravenous antibiotics either via home parenteral therapy or in the hospital. Patients with aseptic bursitis may be discharged with primary care follow-up within 1 week.

Brent LH: Ankylosing spondylitis and undifferentiated spondyloarthropathy. Available at: www.emedicine.com/med/topic2700.htm

Easton BT: Evaluation and treatment of the patient with osteoarthritis. J Fam Pract 2001;50:791 [PMID: 11674913].

Kaplan J: Gout and pseudogout. Available at: www.emedicine.com/emerg/topic221.htm

Khan MA: Update on spondyloarthropathies. Ann Intern Med 2002;136:896 [PMID: 12069564].

Laupland KB, Davies HD: Olecranon septic bursitis managed in an ambulatory setting. The Calgary Home Parenteral Therapy Program Study Group. Clin Invest Med 2001;24:171 [PMID: 11558851].

Meader RJ: Acute rheumatic fever. Available at: www.emedicine.com/med/topic2922.htm

Sack K: Monoarthritis: differential diagnosis. Am J Med 1997;102(Suppl 1A):30S [PMID: 9217557].

Smith HR: Rheumatoid arthritis. Available at: www.emedicine.com/med/topic2024.htm

Torralba KD, Quismorio FP: Soft tissue infections. Rheum Dis Clin North Am 2009;35:45–62 (Review) [PMID: 19480996].

EVALUATION OF THE PATIENT WITH ACUTE BACK PAIN

See Figure 21–2.

▶ Perform Baseline Evaluation

An established routine for evaluating patients with acute back pain will ensure that life-threatening disease is not missed. Patients who do not fit into the categories mentioned below are likely to have acute back pain due to a nonemergent cause (eg, disk disease, facet syndrome, strains, and sprains) without underlying disease.

A. History

1. Is trauma present or did a precipitating event occur?—Often the patient reports trauma or a precipitating event causing acute back pain. In patients with chronic back problems, even minor trauma such as a cough can cause acute back pain.

2. Is visceral disease present?—The emergency physician's first goal should be to identify emergent causes of back

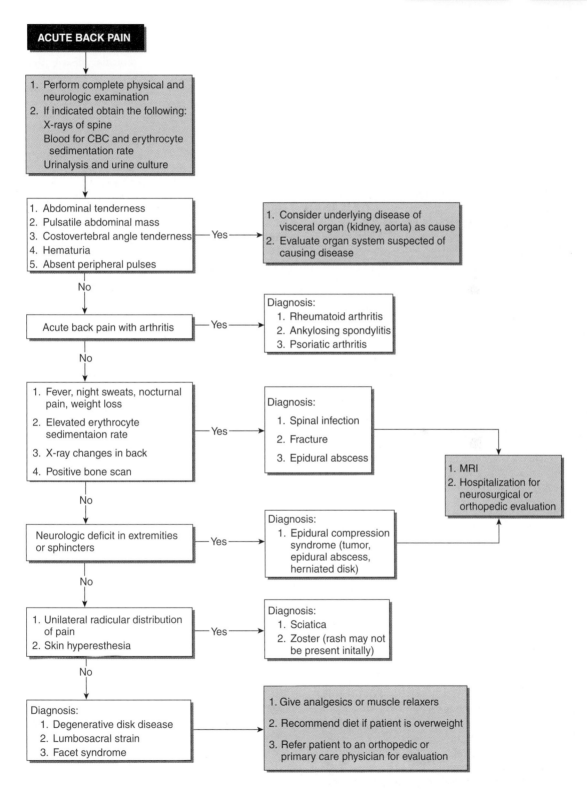

▲ **Figure 21-2.** Assessment of patients with acute back pain.

Table 21–3. Nonorthopedic (visceral) Causes of Acute Back Pain.

Diagnosis	Common Clinical Findings
Pyelonephritis	Flank pain, fever, pyuria, dysuria
Nephrolithiasis	Flank pain, hematuria
Abdominal Aortic Aneurysm	Hypotension, pulsatile mass, abnormal emergency bedside ultrasound or CT scan
Aortic Dissection	Absent pulses, hematuria, abnormal chest X-ray
Pancreatitis	Elevated serum lipase, tender abdomen, pancreatic calcifications
Ruptured Abdominal Viscus	Tender abdomen, air under diaphragm
Retroperitoneal Hemorrhage	Tachycardia, hypotension, decreased hemoglobin/hematocrit

pain and to exclude nonorthopedic causes (Table 21–3). Evaluation and treatment should then focus on the organ thought to be involved.

3. Are red flags present?—Red flags in the history will help the emergency physician recognize associated life threats. In patients younger than 18 years, consider spondylolysis, spondylolisthesis, infection, tumor, and developmental disorders. In patients older than 50 years, consider aortic abdominal aneurysm, fracture, and malignancy first. A history of trauma or chronic steroid use increases the possibility that back pain is related to a vertebral fracture. If bowel or bladder incontinence, saddle anesthesia, or bilateral neurologic deficit is reported, then an epidural compression syndrome (ie, spinal cord compression, cauda equina, or conus medullaris syndrome) is likely and must be investigated emergently. Weight loss, night pain, fever, chills, history of cancer, or intravenous drug use is concerning for malignant or infectious causes of back pain. Patients with a previous history of surgical intervention or recent instrumentation may also be at risk for significant pathology.

4. Is associated arthritis present?—When back pain is associated with arthritis (oligoarthritis or polyarthritis), both disorders are usually due to the same cause. For example, ankylosing spondylitis commonly causes peripheral and vertebral arthritis concurrently. Evaluate these patients and provide treatment as if they had acute arthritis.

5. Is a neurologic deficit present?—A new neurologic deficit in association with back pain, saddle anesthesia, or decreased rectal tone may indicate an epidural compression syndrome due to infection, tumor, or disk disease and calls for emergent management. An emergent magnetic resonance imaging (MRI) study should be obtained and consultation with a neurosurgeon should be considered

immediately. These patients may require hospitalization for diagnosis and treatment.

6. Does the pain have a radicular distribution?—Unilateral back pain in a nerve root distribution suggests preeruptive zoster or nerve root compression. Refer the patient for follow-up care after providing appropriate analgesics.

B. Examination

Examine the back for deformity, tenderness, and range of motion; test for limitation of straight-leg raising; and evaluate gait. Examine the heart, peripheral pulses, lungs, and abdomen. Perform a neurologic evaluation that includes reflexes, muscle strength, sensory examination of the legs and perineum, and assessment of rectal sphincter strength. Pay particular attention to vital signs because fever, tachycardia, or hypotension suggests a serious or possibly life-threatening cause of back pain. A rectal examination does not have to be performed in every patient with back pain, but it must be performed in all patients who have neurologic complaints or deficits. Red flags in the physical examination include decreased rectal tone, saddle anesthesia, motor weakness, and absent reflexes. These findings indicate possible epidural compression syndrome. A herniated disc is strongly suggested in the setting of diminished reflexes and positive straight-leg and crossed straight-leg raise tests.

C. X-ray and Laboratory Findings

Obtain plain X-rays of the spine for patients with trauma and spinal tenderness, for children or adolescents with atraumatic back pain, and when red flags for infection or malignancy are present. MRI may be indicated to rule out an epidural compression syndrome. Laboratory studies such as complete blood count (CBC) with differential, erythrocyte sedimentation rate, C-reactive protein and urinalysis should be performed if red flags are present. Patients with uncomplicated acute lumbosacral strains of less than 1 month's duration usually do not require imaging or laboratory testing.

D. Disposition

See below under specific conditions.

▼ **EMERGENCY TREATMENT OF SPECIFIC CONDITIONS CAUSING BACK PAIN**

TRAUMATIC BACK PAIN

Back pain associated with trauma may imply a fracture or dislocation of the thoracic or lumbar spine. The patient should remain flat on his or her back and be moved only by logroll. Perform a careful examination for other injuries. After the examination is completed, logroll the patient, maintaining in-line spinal immobilization. If a spine board is present, remove it at this time to avoid soft tissue injury. With the patient on his or her side, carefully palpate the thoracic and lumbar spine for tenderness and deformity, and perform a rectal exam. Roll the patient back to a supine position, and obtain a careful neurologic exam. Order thoracic and lumbar spine X-rays if appropriate. Other evaluation and treatment should proceed as indicated depending on the injuries present (Chapters 10 and 25). Special consideration for the gravid patient would include gentle positioning onto the left side while maintaining spinal immobilization. This technique is thought to improve venous return by limiting IVC compression.

ACUTE LUMBOSACRAL STRAIN AND CHRONIC DEGENERATIVE DISK DISEASE

ESSENTIALS OF DIAGNOSIS

▶ Often pain develops after lifting or twisting

▶ No associated constitutional symptoms (such as fever or weight loss)

▶ Normal neurologic examination

▶ X-rays may show evidence of chronic degenerative disk disease

▶ Clinical Findings

A. Symptoms and Signs

Acute lumbosacral strain and chronic degenerative disk disease differ only in their chronicity. The pain is typically a deep steady pain in the mid or low back that may be episodic. It is commonly unilateral and may radiate into the buttocks and posterior thigh. Pain is relieved by bed rest and aggravated by activity. There should be no red flags in the history or physical exam.

B. Physical Examination

The physical examination may show normal results or may disclose one or more of the following: increased lumbar lordosis, scoliosis, limited back motion, asymmetric lateral bending, local deep tenderness, or tight hamstring muscles. Red flags, including positive stretch tests, are not present.

C. Laboratory Findings

CBC, urinalysis, and erythrocyte sedimentation rate are not indicated. If obtained, they are normal.

D. X-ray Findings

X-rays are not indicated. If obtained, they may be normal or may show one or more of the following signs of degenerative disk disease: disk space narrowing, horizontal anterior

osteophytes, spondylolisthesis, posterior facet subluxation, sclerosis, or spurs.

▶ Treatment

A. Analgesics

Give drugs (NSAIDs or acetaminophen). Consider the opioids or a muscle relaxer for patients who cannot tolerate NSAIDs. If opioids are required, limit duration to less than 1 week and arrange close follow-up. If adequate pain control is not possible in the emergency department, consider hospitalization.

B. Bed Rest

Bed rest is no longer indicated. Patients should resume normal activities as tolerated by pain. Research indicates that back exercises are not beneficial in the acute setting, and patients who perform activities as tolerated recover more quickly than those who are on bed rest.

C. Muscle Relaxers

If spasm of the lumbar musculature is present, muscle relaxers for the first several days may be helpful. These agents generally cause sedation.

D. Diet

Weight loss is important if obesity is a causative factor in acute lumbosacral strain.

▶ Disposition

Hospitalization is rarely required. Refer the patient to a primary care physician or orthopedist if symptoms do not improve within 2 weeks. Patients must have instructions to return to the emergency department or their physician if any of the following red flags develop: new neurologic symptoms, bowel or bladder incontinence, worsening pain, fever, or night pain.

SCIATICA

ESSENTIALS OF DIAGNOSIS

▶ Often acute on chronic flare-ups of pain

▶ Radiation of pain in radicular fashion along the distribution of the sciatic nerve

▶ Positive straight- and crossed-leg raise tests

Sciatica usually represents an acute episode in a chronic degenerative process. Patients may have a history of chronic episodic low back pain.

Table 21–4. Neurologic Findings in Herniated Lumbosacral Disk.

Disk	Root	Motor Findings	Sensory Findings	Reflexes	Sciatic Stretch Tests
L5–S1	S1	Weak foot evertors and plantar flexors	Decreased response on lateral side of foot and leg	Achilles jerk depressed or absent	Strongly positive
L4–5	L5	Weak extensor hallucis iongus	Decreased response on mid dorsum of foot	No changes	Moderately positive
L3–4	L4	Weak knee extension	Decreased response on medial foot and anteromedial leg	Knee jerk depressed or absent	May be negative

▶ Clinical Findings

Pain usually begins abruptly, often with trivial trauma such as sneezing. The pain is often described as stabbing or shooting; is worse with coughing, Valsalva maneuver, or sitting; and is often incapacitating. Radiation in the distribution of the sciatic nerve is common. The main distinguishing feature of sciatica is radicular pain that extends below the knee. It affects 2% of patients with acute low back pain. In most cases it is caused by herniation of the nucleus pulposus, known most commonly as a herniated disc, that compresses a nerve root. Sciatica is 88% specific for a herniated disc. Other causes include intraspinal tumor or infection, foraminal stenosis, piriformis syndrome, and lumbar spinal stenosis.

The radicular pain is usually only in one leg and may be characterized by paresthesias, loss of sensation, or motor weakness (Table 21–4); 95% of herniated discs occur at the L4–L5 or L5–S1 levels. The most common pathologic findings of the L5 nerve root are foot drop, loss of dorsiflexion of the great toe, and pain in the great toe. Findings in S1 include heel pain, decreased plantar flexion of the great toe, and decreased ankle jerk.

The difference between lumbosacral strain and sciatica is the presence of abnormal neurologic findings, pain below the knee, and positive straight-leg and crossed straight-leg raise tests in the latter case. Plain X-rays and laboratory evaluation are not indicated for sciatica unless associated red flags for fracture, malignancy, infection, or epidural compression syndrome are present.

▶ Treatment and Disposition

Treatment is nearly the same as that for lumbosacral strain, including instructions for activity as limited only by pain. Opioids may need to be used more frequently in the short term. The only treatment difference is that selected patients with sciatica may need epidural steroid injections. Systemic steroids have no proven benefit.

Approximately 80% of patients with a herniated disc improve without surgery. Only 5–10% will require surgery. More than 50% will improve within 6 weeks with conservative therapy. Therefore, patients meeting the criteria for sciatica alone may be safely discharged to follow up with their primary physician in 2 weeks and return to the emergency department for the same reasons as listed under lumbosacral strain.

▶ Back Pain in Children

A child who presents with back pain should be evaluated carefully. Red flags include decreased activity secondary to pain, fever, and nocturnal pain. These are possible indicators of tumor or infection. If the child has recently been involved in strenuous sports or exercise programs, consider spondylolysis and spondylolisthesis. Bacteremia increases the risk of spinal infections. Therefore, a history of recent febrile illness is important. Spine X-rays should be taken of virtually every child who presents with back pain. Consider obtaining CBC, urinalysis, and erythrocyte sedimentation rate if any red flags are raised. Consider admission for further workup and observation.

EPIDURAL COMPRESSION SYNDROME

ESSENTIALS OF DIAGNOSIS

▶ Bowel or bladder incontinence
▶ Saddle anesthesia, decreased or absent rectal sphincter tone, lower extremity deficits

▶ Clinical Findings

Epidural compression syndrome is a true emergency. Consider this possibility in every patient who presents with back pain. Red flags in the history and physical examination are used to screen for this syndrome. The hallmark symptoms include urinary retention marked by overflow incontinence, saddle anesthesia, decreased rectal tone, and bilateral motor and sensory deficits. If any of these red flags is present, obtain a urinary postvoid residual. If the postvoid residual is less than 50–100 mL, then cauda equina syndrome can usually be ruled out (negative predictive value is 99.99%). However, if a patient has other significant red flags, pursue an epidural compression syndrome with imaging regardless of a normal postvoid residual. Causes include a large central disc herniation, tumors, trauma, epidural abscess, and hematomas.

▶ Treatment and Disposition

If an epidural compression syndrome is likely, start steroid therapy immediately before waiting for confirmatory MRI results. Dexamethasone is usually given in doses ranging between 10 and 100 mg intravenously depending on severity and rapidity of presentation and progression. The next step is to consult a neurosurgeon while ordering an emergent MRI. If unable to obtain an MRI scan, order a CT (computed tomography) scan with myelography.

FACET SYNDROME

Excessive overriding of lumbar or thoracic facets usually occurs as a consequence of disk space narrowing associated with degenerative disk disease. Facet syndrome is unusual and episodic and is characterized by the onset of acute scoliosis after asymmetric lifting. The diagnosis is usually made by exclusion. Patients should be instructed in the fundamentals of proper back care.

SPINAL INFECTIONS

See also Chapter 42.

ESSENTIALS OF DIAGNOSIS

▶ Usually occurs in patients with predisposition for infections: diabetic patients, intravenous drug users, transplant patients, cancer patients

▶ Fever and back pain are the hallmarks

▶ MRI or CT scan of the spine is essential

▶ General Considerations

Disk space infections today are most commonly seen in intravenous drug users, diabetics, transplant patients, and cancer patients. Vertebral osteomyelitis should be suspected in patients who have recently undergone spinal surgery and present with red flags for infection. Epidural abscess and vertebral osteomyelitis are the most common spinal infections. The organism most commonly implicated is *S. aureus.*

▶ Clinical Findings

Red flags for disk space infections are night pain, cough pain, night sweats, fever, and an elevated erythrocyte sedimentation rate. Be alert for the rare low-grade presentations of tuberculous and fungal diskitis. Systemic evidence of infection is usually present.

The typical X-ray changes of disk space narrowing with adjacent vertebral end-plate destruction do not appear until 10–14 days after onset of symptoms. Bone scans are usually positive early in the illness before X-ray changes appear. Epidural or paraspinous abscess may appear as an ill-defined mass on X-ray. If a spinal infection is suspected, an MRI scan (gold standard) or CT scan must be ordered. Blood and urine cultures should also be collected.

▶ Treatment and Disposition

Spinal infections require hospitalization and orthopedic consultation, needle aspiration for bacteriologic diagnosis, and appropriate antibiotics. Occasionally surgical drainage is required.

A neurologic deficit in association with signs of spinal infection often means that an epidural or paraspinous abscess is present. This is a major emergency demanding immediate MRI or CT myelography, consultation, hospitalization, and possibly emergent decompression.

ANKYLOSING SPONDYLITIS

See previous discussion for details of diagnosis, treatment, and disposition.

NEOPLASM

Metastatic tumor is the most common neoplastic process causing back pain. Bone marrow tumors such as multiple myeloma are second in frequency. Primary tumors of the spinal column or spinal cord are rare.

Fifty per cent of bone must be lost before a lesion is evident on plain X-rays. Multiple lesions are common. Bone scan is more sensitive for early diagnosis.

Red flags are weight loss; night pain in the absence of day pain; and a history of insidious and progressive pain that has not responded to conservative measures, especially in elderly patients. Laboratory findings may include an elevated erythrocyte sedimentation rate, significant anemia, proteinemia, and findings in other organ systems that suggest neoplasm.

ZOSTER

Preeruptive zoster may mimic degenerative disk disease. The pain of zoster is burning and dysesthetic, with striking unilateral radicular distribution that does not cross the midline. Skin hyperesthesia over the painful area is the earliest physical finding.

Aree D et al: Recognizing spinal cord emergencies. Am Fam Physician 2001;64:631 [PMID: 11529262].

Della-Giustina D et al: Back pain: cost-effective strategies for distinguishing between benign and life-threatening causes. Emerg Med Pract 2000;2(2):1.

Head Injuries

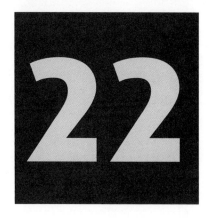

Roger L. Humphries, MD

IMMEDIATE MANAGEMENT OF LIFE-THREATENING PROBLEMS

▶ Cervical Spine Immobilization

Any patient with blunt force injury to the head should be suspected of having cervical spine injury until proven otherwise. Penetrating injuries to the torso and extremities not associated with blunt force are rarely associated with cervical spine injury. Cervical spine injury is associated with 5% of all blunt force injuries to the head; the greater the force, the greater the incidence of associated injury. Immobilization of the cervical spine during transport of a patient with potential injuries must include an appropriately sized and fitted cervical collar, head blocks, and a long, rigid spine board to which the patient is secured. Immobilize the cervical spine during evaluation by manual stabilization and logrolling the patient. Do not apply traction to the cervical spine.

▶ Airway

Hypoxia is associated with increased morbidity and mortality in trauma patients. In patients with traumatic brain injury hypoxia is an independent risk factor for mortality with a 50% higher incidence that in those without hypoxia. Hypoxia must be avoided or corrected immediately. All patients with traumatic head injury should receive 100% oxygen by high-flow nonrebreathing mask as initial therapy. Keep the airway clear by suctioning of blood and secretions as needed. Remove foreign bodies, avulsed teeth, and dental appliances. Loss of gag reflex, inability to adequately clear secretions, or Glasgow Coma Scale (GCS) score of 8 or less are all indications to secure the airway with an endotracheal tube. Use clinical judgment to determine if a patient needs to be intubated in other situations, with priority on maintaining the airway during resuscitation, evaluation, and transport. Ventilate apneic or hypoventilating patients with an Ambu bag and 100% oxygen until intubation can be accomplished. Over ventilation is also dangerous to the head injured patient as hypocarbia will lead to cerebral vasospasm and worsen outcome. Avoid using a bag to provide positive-pressure ventilation to an actively breathing patient because this induces gastric distention.

Perform intubation while maintaining manual in-line cervical immobilization without applying traction. Rapid sequence induction intubation should be strongly considered for all patients. Once sedatives and paralytics have taken effect, remove the cervical collar and maintain manual stabilization. After intubation, secure the endotracheal tube and replace the cervical collar.

Orotracheal intubation is preferred because of the technical difficulty of nasotracheal intubation as well as the complications of bleeding, elevated intracranial pressure, and possible passage of the endotracheal tube through a fractured cribiform plate into the cranium. If orotracheal intubation is not successful, intubate the patient using a retrograde Seldinger technique, fiberoptic-guided intubation, or cricothyroidotomy depending on the equipment available immediately, the clinical status of the patient and the procedures with which the physician is most skilled. In addition, consider a temporizing device, such as a laryngeal mask airway, in the patient who is difficult to intubate. After intubation, confirm endotracheal tube position by auscultation over the lung fields and epigastrium. Additional devices, such as color capnometers and aspiration devices may be used to confirm tube placement. Data show that any single test of endotracheal tube position is substantially less accurate than using two tests of position. Immediate portable chest X-ray must also be used to visualize endotracheal tube position. After successful intubation, place an orogastric tube. Avoid nasogastric tubes in patients with head trauma for the same reasons that nasotracheal intubation is to be avoided.

Any change in the patient's condition or oxygen saturation and any substantial movement of the patient, such as to or from a computed tomography (CT) gantry, necessitates revaluation of the endotracheal tube position by auscultation.

The emergency physician must be familiar with advanced airway techniques to be able to perform rapid sequence induction intubation and guarantee definitive airway access in any patient especially those with head injuries.

▶ Breathing

Once the airway is secured by intubation, assess the patient's respiratory status with an arterial blood gas. Use serial arterial blood gases and end-tidal carbon dioxide monitoring to maintain arterial Pco_2 level in the normal physiologic range. Hypercapnia is associated with increased morbidity and mortality. Hypocapnia is associated with decreased cerebral blood flow and decreased cerebral oxygen perfusion. Patients should not be hyperventilated in order to decrease Pco_2 levels, and Pco_2 should be maintained at 35 mm Hg or more. The only exception to maintaining normal ventilation and Pco_2 is as a temporizing measure in patients in extemis from impending uncal herniation. Frequently reassess the respiratory status of patients who do not require intubation. All patients with head trauma should be monitored with transcutaneous pulse oximetry during evaluation.

▶ Circulation

Hypotension is associated with increased morbidity and mortality in trauma patients. Care should be taken to maintain an adequate blood pressure, defined as a mean arterial pressure more than 90 mm Hg. Treat shock aggressively with warmed intravenous-lactated Ringer's or normal saline and blood products as needed. Avoid hypotonic fluids. Avoid glucose-containing fluids because of the risk of hyperglycemia, which is deleterious to the injured brain. Do not attribute hypotension to head injury alone. Elevated blood pressure associated with bradycardia and respiratory depression is a sign of increased intracranial pressure (Cushing's Response).

▶ Disability

Establish a GCS for any patient with a head injury. The scale measures eye opening, speech, and motor response with total scores ranging from 3 (no response in all categories) to 15 (completely normal) provides a reliable way for physicians to assess the degree of neurologic dysfunction and communicate findings to other clinicians. Repeat the GCS periodically during reassessment. In addition, measure pupillary response and symmetry and also consider doll's eye (oculocephalic) movements (unless cervical spine injury has not been excluded) and caloric stimulation (oculovestibular) tests, if needed, to gauge the patient's level of cortical and brainstem functioning. Note any asymmetry in neurologic examination or focal neurologic findings. In an unresponsive patient, motor response may be elicited by nail bed pressure. If motor responses are asymmetric, the best response is a more accurate predictor of outcome and should be used for calculating the GCS. It is particularly important to document initial neurologic examination findings prior to administering sedative or paralytic agents, if possible.

As for any patient with altered mental status, the clinician is advised to check for and treat any easily reversible causes of decreased level of consciousness including hypoglycemia (bedside fingerstick blood glucose), hypoxemia (pulse oximetry), narcotic overdose (naloxone administration), and, in malnourished or alcoholic patients, Wernicke encephalopathy (thiamine administration).

▶ Exposure

As with all trauma patients, the patient should be completely undressed and the entire body examined, including the back. Once initial examination is complete, cover the patient with warm blankets. Take care to avoid hypothermia by warming the examination room and using warm blankets and warm fluids. Rewarm the patient if he or she is already hypothermic.

▼ MANAGEMENT OF OTHER SYMPTOMS

▶ Seizures

Seizure prophylaxis in the immediate postinjury period should be considered in patients with severe traumatic brain injury including those with an initial GCS of 8 or less and in those with cerebral contusion, depressed skull fracture, intracranial hematoma, or penetrating head wound. In adults, phenytoin, fosphenytoin, or carbamazepine are the prophylactic drugs of choice. In children, phenobarbital has been used prophylactically. Treat any acute posttraumatic seizure rapidly with lorazepam, phenytoin, phosphenytoin, or phenobarbital to prevent worsening hypoxemia associated with the seizure and to limit secondary brain injury. Continuing prophylaxis for more than 7 days after the injury is of unclear benefit and therefore is not recommended.

► Combativeness

Evaluate a combative patient first for hypoxia, hypotension, hypoglycemia, and pain. Avoid physical restraints if possible, or, if needed, use them only long enough to allow for proper sedation and analgesic administration. Patients should never be allowed to struggle against restraints. Occasionally, patients who cannot be controlled with sedation and analgesia alone will require paralysis and endotracheal intubation for protection of the spine and to accomplish diagnostic studies.

► Pain Control

After initial evaluation, do not withhold sedatives and analgesics. Narcotics and benzodiazepines are safe and effective medications for sedation and analgesia and should be used in doses high enough to be effective. Care must be taken to ensure that patients who are paralyzed and intubated have sufficient analgesic and sedative medications.

► Systemic Hypertension

If blood pressures are elevated, evaluate the patient for adequate sedation and analgesia. As mentioned previously, in a severely brain-injured patient, hypertension associated with bradycardia is an ominous sign of elevated intracranial pressures. Isolated systemic hypertension that is high enough to constitute a hypertensive urgency or emergency is rare. If present, systemic hypertension should be treated with caution to avoid rapid decrease in blood pressure or decrease in blood pressure below 10% of initial values.

► Intracranial Hypertension

Elevations of intracranial pressure are heralded by bradycardia and hypertension (Cushing's Response), signs of transtentorial herniation, or progressive neurologic deterioration without other attributable causes. Mannitol (0.25–1.0 g/kg bolus) is the drug of choice for treating elevated intracranial pressure. It is vitally important to maintain serum osmolality below 320 mOsm and maintain euvolemia with intravenous fluid replacement during mannitol administration. Elevation of serum osmolality above 320 mOsm can lead to a reversal of the osmotic gradient with subsequent increase in cerebral edema. Mannitol administration should be initiated in consultation with a neurosurgeon, if possible.

Chesnut RM: Care of central nervous system injuries. Surg Clin North Am 2007;87(1):119–156 [PMID: 17127126].

▼ EMERGENCY TREATMENT OF SPECIFIC HEAD INJURIES

SOFT TISSUE INJURIES

Although often dramatic in nature, soft tissue injuries of the head cause little long-term sequel and most can be easily managed in the emergency department. However, soft tissue injuries of the head can be an indicator of possible significant intracranial injury. For example, one study found that any sign of trauma above the clavicles is an independent predictor of possible intracranial abnormality on CT scan.

1. Scalp Lacerations

ESSENTIALS OF DIAGNOSIS

► Diagnosed through inspection and palpation
► May be significant source of blood loss
► Evaluate for underlying skull fracture

► Clinical Findings

Scalp lacerations are primarily diagnosed by palpation and a visual inspection of the patient's scalp. A complete and thorough examination of the scalp must be performed to find any evidence of laceration or hematoma. Once a laceration is located, palpate the area thoroughly to determine if any signs of skull fracture are present. Because the scalp has tremendous vascularity, scalp lacerations can be a source of significant blood loss.

► Treatment

Most scalp lacerations can be easily closed with either staples or simple interrupted sutures. Clipping of the hair may facilitate easier closure. Alternatively, water-soluble lubricating jelly (eg, Surgilube) may be used to keep hair out of the laceration during closure. Shaving of the scalp may lead to increased risk of infection. The scalp is highly vascular and may be closed up to 12 hours after initial injury. Any patient with a scalp laceration and alteration of consciousness should undergo CT scanning prior to closure of the scalp laceration. The wound should be copiously irrigated with normal saline before closure. Occasionally, layered closure with absorbent sutures may be required (Chapter 30).

► Disposition

Patients with scalp lacerations and no other complications may be discharged safely to home. Follow-up should occur in 3–5 days for recheck; the staples or sutures may be removed in 7–10 days.

2. Hematoma

ESSENTIALS OF DIAGNOSIS

▶ Diagnosed by inspection and palpation
▶ Strongly consider CT scan

▶ Clinical Findings

Scalp hematoma is diagnosed by palpation and visual inspection. In isolation a hematoma has little long-term significance but may be an indicator of more serious intracranial abnormality especially in children under 2 years of age when the hematoma is located in a nonfrontal scalp location. Patients with scalp hematoma and significant mechanism of injury or alteration in level of consciousness should undergo CT scanning.

▶ Treatment

A scalp hematoma is treated primarily like a hematoma or contusion in any other part of the body. Ice, elevation, and nonsteroidal antiinflammatory drugs should be the mainstay of treatment. Aspiration of a scalp hematoma has little, if any, benefit and should rarely be attempted.

▶ Disposition

Patients with only a scalp hematoma may be safely discharged home and referred for standard follow-up.

SKULL FRACTURES

Skull fracture is strongly associated with other more serious intracranial abnormalities. Studies have shown that 40–100% of all intracranial abnormalities are associated with skull fracture. Unless open and or depressed, the skull fracture itself, however, is typically of little clinical consequence to the patient.

1. Closed Skull Fractures

ESSENTIALS OF DIAGNOSIS

▶ Use CT scan for diagnosis because CT shows fractures and other associated injuries

▶ Clinical Findings

Closed fractures of the skull are detected primarily on noncontrast CT scan. Because these fractures are often associated with more serious injury, it is prudent to evaluate the injury with CT scan rather than plain skull X-rays.

▶ Treatment

There is no specific treatment for linear skull fractures. Close observation is recommended to detect the development of an epidural hematoma after an initially negative CT scan.

▶ Disposition

Consider admission or extended observation for patients with isolated closed skull fractures and no evidence of brain injury.

2. Open Skull Fractures

ESSENTIALS OF DIAGNOSIS

▶ Use CT scan for diagnosis because CT shows fractures and other associated injuries
▶ Underlie scalp lacerations
▶ High risk of infection

▶ Clinical Findings

Open fractures underlie scalp lacerations and are often palpated during evaluation of the scalp laceration. These fractures have a serious risk of infection. Definitive diagnosis is made with noncontrast CT scan, and more serious intracranial abnormality should be ruled out. Open skull fracture is likely if pneumocephalus is noted on CT scan (Figure 22–1).

▶ Treatment

Because the indications for antibiotics are controversial in patients with open skull fractures, discuss the decision to initiate antibiotics with the neurosurgeon who will be definitively managing the problem.

▶ Disposition

Hospitalize all patients with open skull fracture.

3. Depressed Skull Fractures

ESSENTIALS OF DIAGNOSIS

▶ Often found with inspection or palpation
▶ Use CT scan for diagnosis because CT shows fractures and other associated injuries

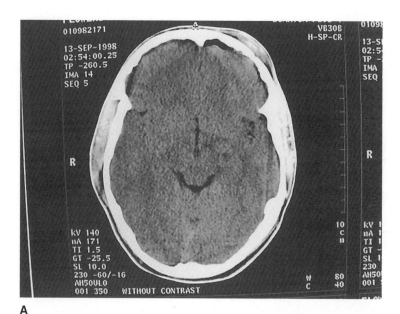

A

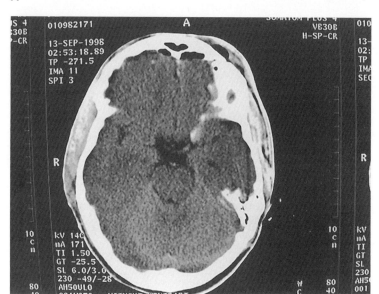

B

▲ **Figure 22–1.** Depressed right temporal and nondepressed left frontal skull fractures not well visualized on typical brain windows (**A** and **B**) but clearly seen on bone windows. Also note the associated frontal pneumocephalus.

▶ Clinical Findings

Depressed skull fractures are often palpable or visible during examination. However, swelling around the area of the injury can mask a depressed skull fracture and make it appear to be a simple hematoma. Like all skull fractures, depressed skull fractures are often associated with more serious intracranial injury, and patients need to be evaluated accordingly. Noncontrast CT scan is the test of choice to determine whether the patient has intracranial injury or depressed skull fracture (Figure 22–2).

▶ Treatment

Depressed skull fractures without intracranial injury represent a cosmetic situation. Open depressed skull fractures are at high risk of infection, similar to open nondepressed skull fractures.

▶ Disposition

Patients should be admitted to the hospital for observation and referred to the appropriate surgical subspecialist for possible elevation of the depression and debridement if the fracture is open.

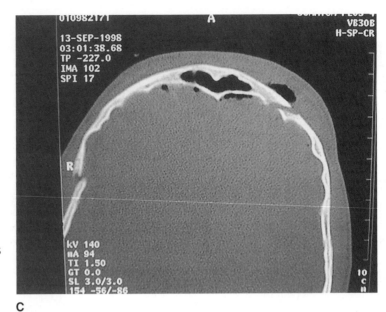

▲ **Figure 22-1.** *(Continued)*
Depressed right temporal and
nondepressed left frontal skull fractures
not well visualized on typical brain
windows but clearly seen on bone
windows (**C**). Also note the associated
frontal pneumocephalus.

C

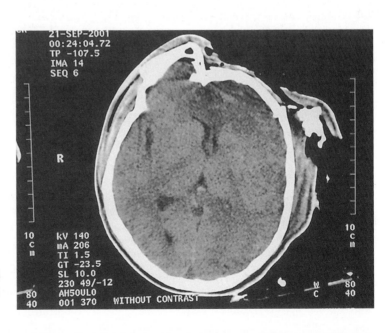

▲ **Figure 22-2.** Severely depressed frontal
skull fracture with significant impingement
on the frontal lobes.

4. Basilar Skull Fractures

ESSENTIALS OF DIAGNOSIS

▶ Use CT scan for diagnosis because CT shows fractures and other associated injuries; however, some basilar skull fractures may be missed on CT

▶ Associated with hemotympanum, Battle sign, raccoon's eyes, cerebrospinal fluid leaking from ear or nose, or hearing loss

▶ Clinical Findings

Basilar skull fractures are skull fractures at the base of the skull, typically at the petrous portion of the temporal bone. Clinical signs include hemotympanum, Battle sign (ecchymosis along the mastoid area of the skull), raccoon's eyes (periorbital ecchymosis), cerebrospinal fluid leak from the nose or ear, or hearing loss. Patients with any of these signs should undergo noncontrast CT evaluation for possible basilar skull fracture and to rule out more serious intracranial abnormality.

▶ Treatment

Antibiotics are controversial and have unproven benefit in preventing meningitis in patients with basilar skull fracture. The decision to administer antibiotics should be made in consultation with the neurosurgeon to whom the patient is referred. If desired, an intravenous antibiotic such as cefazolin is a common choice.

▶ Disposition

Patients with documented basilar skull fracture or significant signs of a basilar skull fracture should be admitted for observation. If a more serious intracranial abnormality is present, obtain neurosurgical consultation.

INTRACRANIAL INJURY

1. Epidural Hematoma

ESSENTIALS OF DIAGNOSIS

▶ Classic history of brief loss of consciousness followed by transient lucid interval

▶ Arterial bleeding source

▶ Diagnosis made by CT scan, which shows a biconvex hematoma

▶ Requires rapid neurologic evaluation for decompression

An epidural hematoma is a collection of blood and clot between the dura mater and the bones of the skull. Sources of bleeding from epidural hematoma include the meningeal arteries (often the middle meningeal artery) or occasionally the dural venous sinuses. These bleeds generally have a lenticular (biconvex) shape. Patients with epidural hematoma may have an initial, brief loss of consciousness followed by a lucid interval during which they may be neurologically intact. This interval is then followed by rapid clinical deterioration. All patients with epidural hematoma typically require rapid intervention by a neurosurgical specialist. An epidural hematoma represents a space-occupying lesion to the brain, often from a high-pressure arterial source. Therefore, rapid expansion of this hematoma can lead to herniation of brain contents. Patient outcome is directly related to the patient's level of consciousness on presentation and to the time until decompression of potential space-occupying lesions (Figure 22–3).

2. Subdural Hematoma

ESSENTIALS OF DIAGNOSIS

▶ Venous bleeding source

▶ Diagnosis made by CT scan, which shows concave hematoma following the contour of the cortex

▶ May be chronic, acute, or acute on chronic

▶ Admit for neurosurgical evaluation

A subdural hematoma also represents a space-occupying lesion. This lesion, however, lies in the space between the dura mater and the arachnoid mater and usually conforms to the contour of underlying cerebral cortex (Figure 22–4). The source of bleeding is often the bridging veins, which are more likely to tear in patients with significant brain atrophy (eg, elderly or alcoholic patients). These patients can develop large chronic subdural hematomas with minimal neurologic deficit. A subdural hematoma may or may not require surgical drainage. Acute bleeds can develop in areas of chronic subdural hematoma (often from new trauma) and cause neurologic deterioration (Figure 22–5). All patients with subdural hematoma should receive prompt neurosurgical evaluation.

3. Cerebral Contusion

ESSENTIALS OF DIAGNOSIS

▶ Diagnosis made by CT scan

▶ Associated edema may require intervention

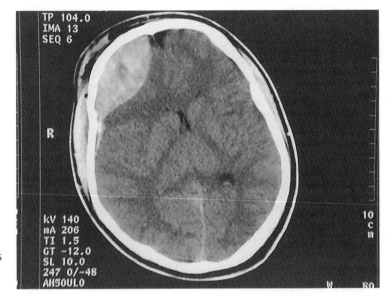

▲ **Figure 22-3.** Large acute right frontal epidural hematoma with associated mass effect on the frontal lobes and slight midline shift.

Cerebral contusion represents a non-space-occupying discrete lesion within the brain matter itself. These lesions are less likely to lead to herniation than are other types of intracranial lesions. Significant edema can occur around areas of cerebral contusion, which can lead to increased intracranial pressure and midline shift. Typically no surgical intervention is required for cerebral contusion. However, if the contusion is large enough and significant shift occurs, then intracranial pressure monitoring may be instituted by the neurosurgical specialist.

4. Traumatic Subarachnoid Hemorrhage

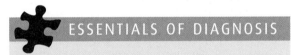

ESSENTIALS OF DIAGNOSIS

▶ Diagnosis made by CT scan
▶ Can lead to elevated intracranial pressure owing to cerebrospinal fluid obstruction

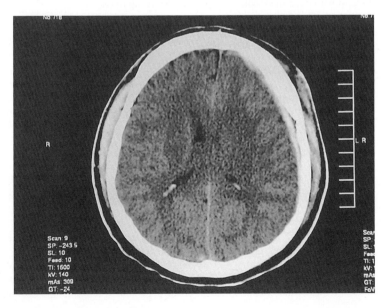

▲ **Figure 22-4.** Small left subdural hematoma with effacement of the left lateral ventricle.

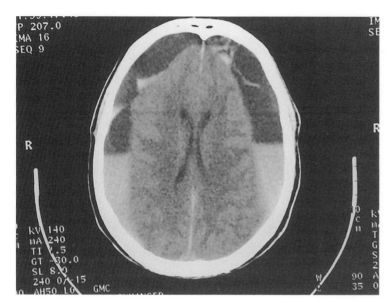

▲ **Figure 22–5.** Bilateral acute on chronic subdural hematoma with significant mass effect compressing both cerebral hemispheres. Note the acute component of the hematoma layering posteriorly (dependent position).

It was once thought that subarachnoid hemorrhage was relatively rare and had a poor outcome. However, it appears now that subarachnoid hemorrhage in a traumatic setting is much more common than previously believed. Traumatic subarachnoid hemorrhage is not a space-occupying lesion but can lead to increasing intracranial pressure, primarily by blocking the outflow of cerebrospinal fluid from the third and fourth ventricles in the brain. Patients with asymptomatic subarachnoid hemorrhage may be admitted for observation and no further intervention. Patients with altered level of consciousness or other neurologic findings may require intracranial pressure monitoring in the critical care unit setting (Figure 22–6).

5. Diffuse Axonal Injury

ESSENTIALS OF DIAGNOSIS

▶ Diagnosis made by CT scan demonstrating blurring of gray- to white-matter margin, punctate cerebral hemorrhages, or cerebral edema

▶ Associated with posttraumatic coma

Shearing forces from sudden deceleration during blunt trauma can cause severe intracranial injury. Diffuse axonal injury is a frequent cause of posttraumatic coma. This injury is typically manifested on noncontrast CT by a blurring the margin between the gray and white matter, punctate hemorrhages often in the internal capsule, and cerebral edema (Figure 22–7).

MINOR HEAD INJURIES

The vast majority of the nearly 8 million patients that present to North American emergency departments with head trauma have minor head injuries and are conscious and talking. The primary goal in evaluating patients with potential head injury is to determine if an intracranial abnormality is present and then to determine if that injury requires surgical intervention. There has long been controversy as to which patients require CT scanning. Of patients presenting to the emergency department with head injury and a GCS of 15, 6–8% have an intracranial abnormality. The vast majority of these injuries are nonsurgical, but they may have long-term cognitive implications for the patient. There are currently few widely accepted recommendations as to when a patient requires CT scanning in the setting of head trauma. In addition, the ionizing radiation of CT scanning is not benign. Brenner estimates that the lifetime risk of a fatal cancer related to a 1 year old child undergoing a single CT scan of the head is 1 in 1500 (for a 10 year old the mortality risk is 1 in 5000). Clinicians must decide for each patient if the risk of a CT scan of the head outweighs the risk that a clinically important brain injury will be missed if the study is not performed.

The emerging practice over the last 10 years has been to obtain a CT scan whenever a patient has had an alteration in the level of consciousness at any time or amnesia to the event of injury. One recent study compared the performance of six clinical decision rules utilizing criteria that may allow CT scans to be safely foregone in a small to moderate percentage of these patients. The long list of variables that were used to determine the need for a CT scan in the setting of trauma in adult patients included: GCS < 15, amnesia (anterograde or retrograde), suspected

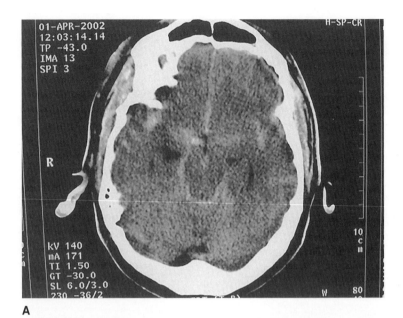

A

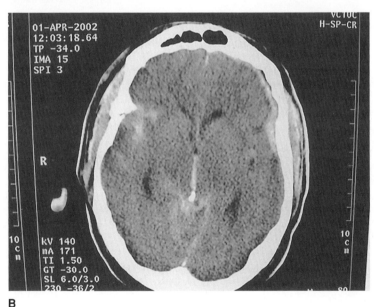

▲ **Figure 22–6.** Right temporal traumatic subarachnoid hemorrhage (**A–D**) with extension into basal cistern (**A**), third ventricle (**B**), and lateral ventricles (**C** and **D**). Also note the moderate-sized left frontotemporal subdural prominently seen in **B–D**.

B

skull fracture, vomiting, age ≥ 65 (60 in one study), coagulopathy, focal deficit, seizure, loss of consciousness, visible trauma, headache, injury mechanism, intoxication, and previous neurosurgery. All of the clinical decision rule studies had 95% confidence interval sensitivities in the range of 93–100% for finding clinically significant neurosurgical lesions. The Canadian Head CT Rule is one of the most widely studied decision rules. Its sensitivity for detecting a clinically important brain injury was 100% (95% confidence interval of 98–100%). According to this

rule which applies only to patients between 16 and 64 years of age, computed tomography of the head is required for patients with minor head injury (defined as GCS 13–15 and witnessed loss of consciousness, amnesia, or confusion) if any of the following variables are present:

- GCS <15 at 2 hours post-injury

- Suspected open or depressed skull fracture or any sign of basilar skull fracture

- Two or more episodes of vomiting

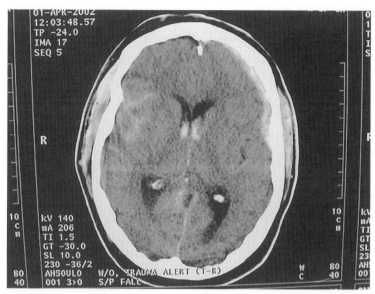

C

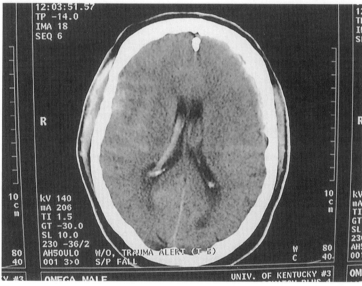

D

▲ **Figure 22-6.** (Continued)

- Amnesia before impact of 30 minutes or more
- Dangerous mechanism defined as
  - Pedestrian struck by motor vehicle
  - Occupant ejected from motor vehicle
  - Fall from an elevation of three or more feet or five stairs

This rule does not apply to patients with a history of a bleeding disorder or those taking warfarin. Importantly, the more clearly clinicians can understand the risk of a condition being present, the better he or she can limit the risk of the evaluation of each patient.

A significant question often arises regarding whether the injury is a concussion and what type of postconcussion restrictions are needed. Concussion is often wrongly thought of as transient loss of consciousness if CT findings are negative. Most current precaution guidelines, of which there are many, consider concussion to be a trauma-induced alteration in mental status that may or may not

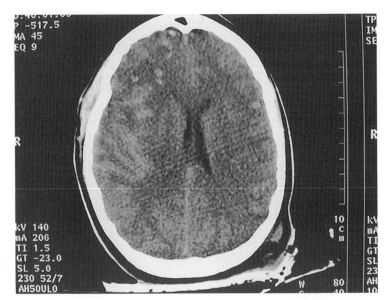

▲ **Figure 22–7.** Diffuse axonal injury with punctate hemorrhages (mainly right frontal), changes of generalized edema with poor gray–white matter discrimination in the right hemisphere, and mass effect on the right lateral ventricle.

include loss of consciousness. The primary hallmarks of concussion are confusion and amnesia. Concussion is of significant importance because long-term neuropsychiatric testing on athletes who have sustained frequent concussions has shown that multiple concussions over a lifetime can lead to cognitive impairment. As a result, guidelines have been developed that grade concussion and recommend activity level by an athlete who undergoes concussion. Although these guidelines have not been fully used with nonathlete patients, some of these guidelines can be used to guide the outcome of nonathlete patients. Current guidelines have divided concussions into three grades (Table 22–1).

The length of time the athlete or patient should refrain from strenuous activity is based on both the grade of the concussion and the history of prior concussions. Patients with a history of prior concussions have longer restrictions. Current recommendations for immediate treatment and restrictions are also available.

Postconcussion syndrome is characterized by headache, dizziness, and cognitive impairment (memory) and occurs acutely in 50% of patients experiencing a mild traumatic brain injury. These symptoms can occur singly or with other symptoms, and they generally resolve over the initial weeks to months after a concussion.

Table 22–1. Concussion Grading and Outcomes for a First Concussion (American Academy of Neurology).

	Grade		
	1	**2**	**3**
Symptoms	Transient confusion; no loss of consciousness; concussion symptoms last less than 15 minutes	Transient confusion; no loss of consciousness; concussion symptoms last more than 15 minutes	Any loss of consciousness
Immediate treatment	Removal from contest	Removal from contest without return that day	Removal from contest and transport to nearest emergency department
Projected return	Same day after free from symptom for 15 minutes	After one full asymptomatic week	After one full asymptomatic week if loss of consciousness is brief (seconds); after two full asymptomatic weeks if loss of consciousness is prolonged (1 minute).

Table 22–2. PECARN Rule for Identification of Children at Very Low Risk of Important Brain Injury.

Important Variables
Mental status:
- GCS = 14 or altered mental status (agitation, somnolence, repetitive questioning or slow response to verbal communication)

Loss of consciousness:
- ≥5 seconds

Severe mechanism of injury
- Ejection from motor vehicle
- Death of vehicle occupant
- Vehicle rollover
- Pedestrian or unhelmeted bicyclist struck by motorized vehicle,
- Falls
  - Fall of more than 3 feet if <2 years of age
  - Fall of more than 5 feet if 2 years of age or older

Physical exam findings
- Any palpable skull fracture for children <2 years of age
- Any sign of basilar skull fracture for children 2 years of age or older

The rule recommends CT scan of the head if any of the above variables are present

The risk of clinically important brain injury if none of the above variables are present is
- <0.02% for those <2 years of age
- <0.05% for those 2 years of age or older

Kuppermann N, Holmes JF, Dayan PS et al: Identification of children at very low risk of clinically-important brain injuries after head trauma a prospective cohort study. Lancet 2009; 374:1160–1170 [PMID: 19758692].

SPECIAL CONSIDERATIONS FOR PEDIATRICS

Although it is difficult to determine when adult patients need further workup after minor brain injury, the question is even more difficult to resolve for pediatric patients. Smaller children (younger than 2 years) present a greater challenge to evaluate for possible loss of consciousness, transient confusion, and amnesia. Some conservative guidelines favor obtaining a noncontrast CT scan of the head on any child under age 2 years with any sign of trauma to the head, including minor hematomas and scratches. Given the risk of ionizing radiation to a child's developing brain as well as the increased risk of a lethal neoplasm later in life (up to 1 in 1500 children with a head CT scan), it is unacceptable to indiscriminately scan all children with minor head injury. A recent validated decision rule by Kupperman et al and the Pediatric Applied Research Network (PECARN) was described to identify children at very low risk of clinically important brain injuries (see Table 22–2).

The use of this rule has the potential to reduce CT utilization in children with minor traumatic brain injury by 56% while maintaining a very high sensitivity for clinically important brain injury. Considering that the consequences

of obtaining negative head CTs in young children include increased rates of fatal cancer and possibly decrements in cognitive functioning, it is extremely important to limit the use of CT in children to only those patients likely to benefit from the performance of the test.

INDICATIONS FOR HOSPITALIZATION

In general, patients with minor head injury who have no clinical history findings that suggest neurologic injury, no neurologic abnormality on examination, and if performed, a normal CT scan can be discharged to home. Patients who have persistent amnesia, persistent alteration in level of consciousness, or any abnormality on CT scan should be admitted for observation. Patients with severe traumatic brain injuries with or without significant mass or space-occupying lesions should receive immediate neurosurgical consultation and be admitted to an ICU (including intracranial pressure monitoring for GCS < 9) or taken to the operating room on an emergency basis for decompression of space-occupying lesions.

DISCHARGE INSTRUCTIONS

Various methods have been proposed for ongoing evaluation after discharge of patients with minor head injury. These methods have ranged from having the patient's caregiver evaluate the patient every 30 minutes to once per night. None of these discharge instructions has been validated in any prospective manner. Currently, with relatively frequent use of CT scan, the possibility of return for worsening head injury is unlikely. It is not unusual, however, for patients to present with postconcussive symptoms days or weeks after a minor head injury. Discharge instructions for these patients should include being aware of any nausea or vomiting, alteration in level of consciousness, and any seizure activity.

The interval at which patients should be reevaluated is unclear. Patients with minimal clinical findings or negative CT scan and a history not suggestive of or not including loss of consciousness or amnesia are unlikely to have a significant space-occupying lesion. The exception may be the patient with an epidural hematoma during the lucid interval. Therefore, patients with minor head injury should be closely observed in the emergency department and carefully reevaluated prior to discharge.

INTOXICATED PATIENTS

Intoxicated patients frequently present to the emergency department after being found unresponsive or with a decreased level of consciousness. Alcoholic patients are at increased risk of obtaining a head injury secondary to ataxia, frequent falls, and other types of trauma. A detailed examination looking for signs of head trauma, pupillary abnormalities, or other lateralizing neurologic deficits is critical in early identification of head injuries in intoxicated patients. Frequent reexamination is also important to ensure that an intoxicated patient's level of consciousness is improving over time. Watch carefully for any deterioration in the level of consciousness or the development of new deficits, which should prompt an emergency noncontrast CT scan for further evaluation.

American Academy of Neurology: Practice parameter: the management of concussion in sports (summary statement). Neurology 1997:48:581 [PMID: 9065530].

Chang BS, Lowenstein DS: Practice parameter: antiepileptic drug prophylaxis in severe traumatic brain injury: Report of the Quality Standards Subcommittee of the American Academy of Neurology. Neurology 2003;60;10–16 [PMID: 12525711].

Coombs JB, Davis RL: A synopsis of the American Academy of Pediatrics' practice parameter on the management of minor closed head injury in children. Pediatr Rev 2000;21:413 [PMID: 11121498].

Hay del MJ et al: Indications for computed tomography in patients with minor head injury. N Engl J Med 2000;343:100 [PMID: 10891517].

Jogoda AS et al: Clinical policy: neuroimaging and decision-making in adult mild traumatic brain injury in the acute setting. Ann Emerg Med 2002;40:231 [PMID: 12140504].

Ratial B, Costa J, Sampaio C: Antibiotic prophylaxis for preventing meningitis in patients with basilar skull fracture. Cochrane Database Syst Rev 2006;25(1):CD004884 [PMID: 16437502].

Schutzman SA et al: Evaluation and management of children younger than two years old with apparently minor head trauma: proposed guidelines. Pediatrics 2001;107:983 [PMID: 11331675].

Servadel F et al: Defining acute mild head injury in adults: a proposal based on prognostic factors, diagnosis and management. J Neurotrauma 2001;18:657 [PMID: 11497092].

Simon B et al: Pediatric minor head trauma: indications for computed tomographic scanning revisited. J Trauma 2001;51:231 [PMID: 11493779].

Smally AJ: Management of minor closed head injury in children. Pediatrics 2001;107:1231 [PMID: 11388318].

Woodcock RJ, Davis PC, Hopkins KL: Imaging of head trauma in infancy and childhood. Semin Ultrasound CT MR 2001;22:162 [PMID: 11327530].

Kupperman N et al: Identification of children at very low risk of clinically important brain injuries after head trauma: a prospective cohort study. Lancet 2009;374:1160–1170 [PMID: 19758692].

Stein SC, Fabbri A, Servadei F, Glick H: A critical comparison of clinical decision instruments for computed tomography scanning in mild closed traumatic brain injury in adolescents and adults. Ann Emerg Med 2009;53:180–188 [PMID: 18339447].

Brenner DJ: Estimating cancer risks from pediatric CT: going from the qualitative to the quantitative. Pediatr Radiol 2002;32:228–231 [PMID: 11956700].

Maxillofacial & Neck Trauma

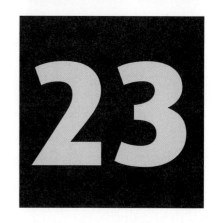

Alicia A. Shirakbari, MD

Marshall Hall, MD

▼ IMMEDIATE MANAGEMENT OF LIFE-THREATENING CONDITIONS

Emergency management of life-threatening associated conditions is described in Chapter 12.

AIRWAY

Evaluate the patient's entire airway with direct visualization while maintaining immobilization of the cervical spine (C-spine) with a cervical collar. The patient should remain fully immobilized until spinal column injury is ruled out.

Diligent continuous monitoring of the airway should be performed for any patient with significant maxillofacial or neck trauma, as airway compromise can be abrupt. Keep a low threshold for intubation of any patient with impending airway obstruction. Soft tissue swelling and edema may result in delayed airway compromise. Warning signs include hoarseness, subcutaneous emphysema of the neck, laryngeal pain, visible edema, or the presence of an expanding hematoma.

Perform a jaw thrust to allow for ventilation while aggressively clearing and suctioning the obscuring material. The chin lift maneuver is contraindicated in any patient with potential cervical spinal trauma. Rapid-sequence intubation (RSI) with in-line C-spine stabilization is the preferred method of securing an airway in any patient without contraindications. Avoid using paralytics if the patient's facial trauma might preclude successful bag-valve-mask ventilation. Intubation with sedatives alone is an alternative. Fiberoptic and videolaryngoscopic intubations are difficult in maxillofacial trauma patients secondary to poor visualization resulting from blood, secretions, and vomitus in the airway. LMA should only be considered as a bridging device when immediate ventilation is needed and only used until a definitive airway can be established. Surgical airways and direct laryngoscopy are still the best options for definitive airway management. Nasogastric (NG) or orogastric tube placement if facial trauma is present, should be performed after intubation for gastric decompression.

▶ Laryngeal Airway Injury

Hoarseness, dysphonia, edema, persistent pain below the hyoid bone or crepitance over the thyroid cartilage implies a laryngeal injury. Presence of these signs necessitates a definitive airway. Endotracheal intubation is not contraindicated but may be difficult in this situation secondary to disruption and displacement of normal anatomic structures. If direct laryngoscopy is impossible, a cricothyroidotomy with prompt revision to a tracheostomy is the preferred alternative.

▶ Tracheal Airway Injury

Tension pneumothorax or persistent air leak from chest tube may indicate a tracheal or bronchial injury. A chest X-ray may demonstrate signs of an occult upper airway injury by demonstration of mediastinal air. Bronchoscopy may be necessary for definitive diagnosis. Endotracheal intubation is not contraindicated in injury to the trachea below the cricothyroid membrane and should be attempted. Preparations for a surgical airway should be ongoing simultaneously. Tracheotomy below the trauma is the preferred alternative and should be performed immediately after the initial attempt at endotracheal intubation fails. Endotracheal or tracheostomy tubes may also be placed during diagnostic bronchoscopy if necessary.

▶ Intubation Through a Traumatic Opening

Dashboard trauma to the neck in motor vehicle accidents and "clothes-line" injuries from motorcycle or skiing injuries can sever the soft tissue of the neck and the tracheal cartilage leaving a defect sufficient for intubation. Often this site is the laryngotracheal junction adjacent to the cricoid cartilage. Intubation of this defect is the preferred method of securing an airway in these patients, as endotracheal intubation will often result in the tube exiting the neck through the defect. A small-lumen (6.0 or smaller) ET tube can be inserted directly into the wound. If impossible, convert to tracheotomy.

BREATHING

▶ Treat Tension Pneumothorax and Pneumothorax

See Chapter 24.

▶ Maintain Oxygenation and Ventilation

After securing an airway, monitor gas exchange with periodic arterial blood gases. Patients with concomitant lung injury may require higher FIO_2 and positive endexpiratory pressure (PEEP) to maintain oxygenation. Cervical cord transection resulting in paralysis of the diaphragm or intercostal muscles precludes a strong cough making it difficult to tolerate secretions. Aggressive suctioning may be necessary.

CIRCULATION

▶ Control Hemorrhage

Neck trauma with vascular injury may present with moderate to large hematomas, a pulsatile stable hematoma, pulse deficits, or a bruit. Look for any mediastinal changes on chest X-ray. Expanding hematomas can cause rapid airway compromise and necessitate intubation. Never remove impaled foreign bodies, as they may be preventing massive hemorrhage.

A. Pressure

Direct firm pressure is the mainstay of stopping bleeding on the face and neck. Circumferential neck dressings are contraindicated as they may act as a noose if edema or hematomas worsen and will inevitably increase intracranial pressure (ICP).

B. Pressure and Clamping

If direct pressure alone fails, clamping with hemostats or suturing with a "figure of eight" stitch can control arterial bleeds. Direct visualization of the artery must be achieved before this is attempted to avoid vagus or phrenic nerve injury. Never blindly clamp large amounts of tissue.

C. Foley Catheter Balloon Tamponade (FCBT)

If bleeding cannot be controlled with direct pressure then consider balloon tamponade. A foley catheter is inserted into the wound in the direction of active bleeding. Inflate the balloon with saline until bleeding stops or resistance develops. Gently pull back on the foley providing traction and compression. The need for FCBT does not imply a definitive vascular injury. If no vascular injury is detected in angiography then balloon catheter can be removed after 48–72 hours in the operating room.

▶ Treat Shock

Hypotension (SBP < 90 mm Hg) and shock (cool, pale skin, abnormal mentation) may be due to blood loss (hypovolemic shock) or poor sympathetic tone below a spinal cord lesion (neurogenic/spinal shock). The etiology of shock in the vast majority of trauma patients is hypovolemia.

A. Hypovolemic Shock

See Chapter11 for a more detailed discussion of shock. If hypovolemic shock is present, place two large-bore (16-gauge) intravenous catheters. If this fails, immediately place a triple-lumen central line with the largest internal diameter available. Obtain blood for a complete blood count, coagulation profile, electrolytes, renal function tests, and a type and crossmatch. Immediately infuse 2 L of isotonic crystalloid. If the systolic blood pressure remains below 90 mm Hg, infuse two units of un-crossmatched packed red blood cells (crossmatched if available). Continue administering blood products and crystalloid to improve hemodynamic stability while simultaneously arranging transfer of care to a trauma center.

B. Neurogenic Shock

Hypotension and bradycardia are hallmark signs of neurogenic shock due to spinal cord injury. Sympathetic interruption results in unopposed vagal tone. This must be differentiated from "spinal" shock which is a temporary loss of spinal reflex activity below the level of cord injury. Keeping the patient supine is often adequate to maintain adequate blood pressure, as little sympathetic tone is required. However, in the patient with persistent hypotension, infuse crystalloids to maintain a mean arterial pressure above 70 torr. Vasopressors should be used when hypotension inadequately responds to volume resuscitation. Phenylephrine is the therapy of choice. Atropine can be used for severe bradycardia.

DISABILITY

▶ Suspect Spinal Cord Injury

Patients with blunt head trauma or multiple injuries from blunt or penetrating trauma should be assumed to have vertebral column injuries until proven otherwise. Complete immobilization in a cervical collar and on a spine board should be maintained until radiographically and/or clinically cleared. If neurological deficits are present, although controversial, some clinicians will consider starting methylprednisolone within 8 hours of injury. A 30 mg/kg bolus followed by 5.4 mg/kg/h infusion over next 23 hours.

▼ FURTHER DIAGNOSIS AND EVALUATION

NECK TRAUMA

▶ Type of Trauma

A. Penetrating Neck Trauma

Penetrating neck trauma management will vary depending on the anatomical zone. Please see Figure 23–1.

1. Knife wounds—Stab wounds to the neck can injure a variety of vital structures and require extensive diagnostic tests and/or surgical exploration depending on the location of the injury and associated symptoms. Leave any impaled objects in place as they may be providing local tamponade. If not present, determine the character of the weapon, its length, and the direction of entry to help assess the depth

and extent of injury. Avoid nasogastric or orogastric tube placement as this may rupture contained pharyngeal hematomas.

2. Bullet wounds—High velocity missiles follow direct trajectory pathways. These bullet wounds can generate blast effect and secondary injury from bullet and bone fragmentation. Low velocity missiles are unpredictable and the path of trajectory does not appear to coincide with entrance or exit wounds. All structures in the neck must be evaluated including the airway, esophagus, vessels, and nerves. Surgical exploration is often necessary as well, depending on location.

B. Blunt Neck Trauma

Blunt trauma is most often associated with tracheal, laryngeal, or C-spine trauma due to the ability of each to fracture. Softer structures such as vessels and the esophagus are rarely injured. If injury occurs, it may manifest as hematomas and hematemesis, due to shearing of vessels. Occasionally, blunt carotid or vertebral injury can result in symptoms typically associated with cerebrovascular accidents and have a high associated mortality. Pneumomediastinum can indicate esophageal or airway injury. See Figure 23–2.

▶ Location of the Injury

The location of a neck injury is critical to its treatment. Any injury penetrating the platysma should be described as in zone I, II, or III (Figure 23–3) and explored by a surgeon, not in the ED. The inferior border of zone I is the suprasternal notch and clavicles and the superior border is the inferior portion of the cricoid cartilage. Zone II extends from the inferior border of cricoid cartilage to the angle of the mandible. Classically, all zone II neck injuries penetrating the platysma warranted surgical exploration. With the combination of conventional angiography, CT angiography, CT scan, 2D Doppler, and esophagoscopy, exploration is now more selective. Zone III extends from the angle of the mandible to the base of the skull. Zone I and III injuries are not surgically explored. They present the problem of proximal and distal control of bleeding, respectively.

▶ Airway Injury

Injuries perforating the airway may manifest with air leak, subcutaneous pneumomediastinum or pneumothorax with persistent air leak despite chest tube placement. Other injuries including laryngeal fracture or tracheal contusion can present with stridor, hoarseness, painful phonation, hemoptysis, or hemothorax. Always monitor the patient's airway. Bronchoscopy should be performed in any suspected airway injury. A high level of suspicion followed by bronchoscopy will identify the occult injury. Evaluate the C-spine with plain radiographs or CT scan when injury is suspected.

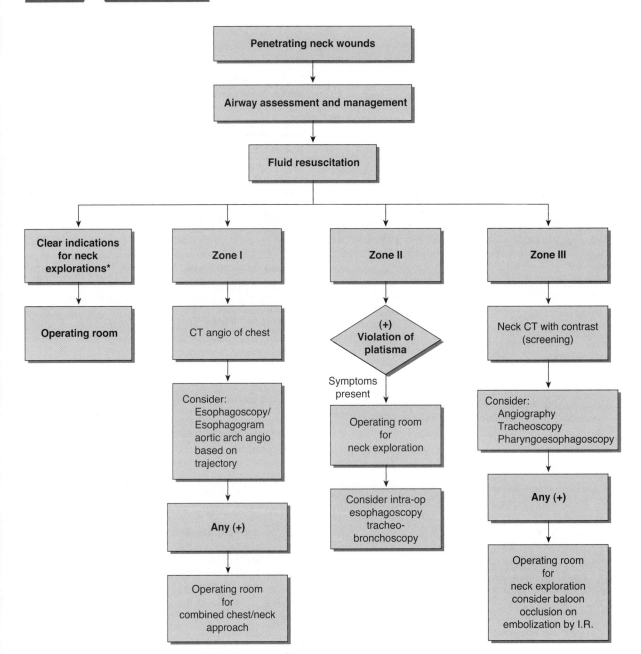

▲ Figure 23-1. Flow diagram of penetrating neck trauma.

▶ Esophageal Injury

Esophageal injury manifests as hematemesis, dysphagia, odynophagia, soft tissue crepitus, saliva leak from wound, blood in nasogastric tube, prevertebral air on lateral C-spine, or pneumomediastinum on chest X-ray. Esophagogram with water-soluble contrast may reveal the injury but esophagoscopy is often necessary if symptoms persist despite a negative study.

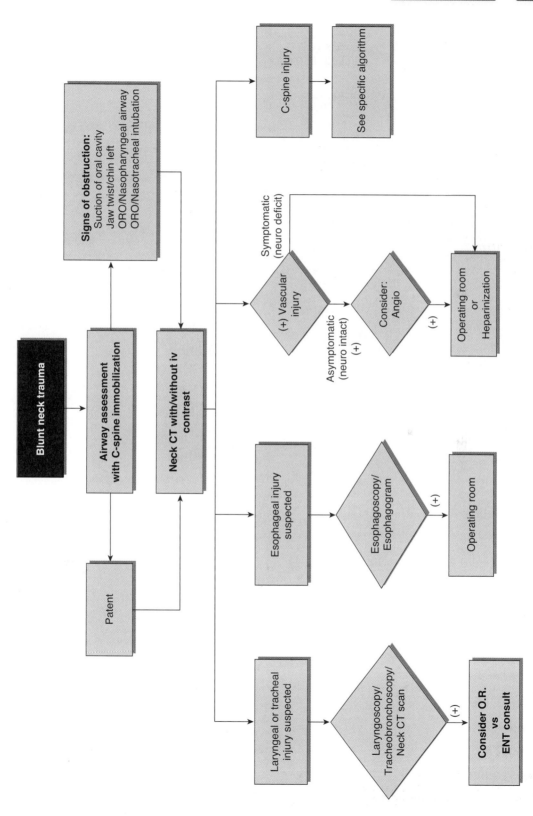

▲ **Figure 23–2.** Flow diagram of blunt neck trauma.

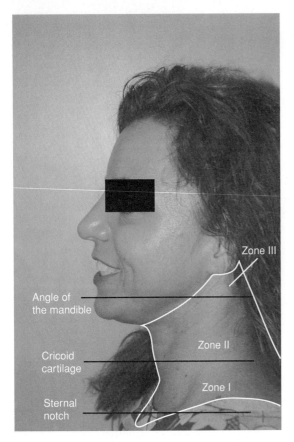

▲ **Figure 23–3.** Zones of the neck for describing traumatic injury.

Vascular Injury

While external bleeding is obvious, vascular injuries may be more insidious. An expanding hematoma may compress the trachea causing dyspnea. Palpate for a pulse deficit, bruit or thrill. Doppler ultrasound may be used as a screening test in low risk patients. Penetrating vascular injuries must be classified into zone I, II, or III. Zones I and III usually require angiography. The use of CT angiography is becoming more prevalent secondary to availability and being able to provide clinician with visualization of adjacent anatomic structures. However, conventional angiography remains the gold standard for identification of vascular injury. A trauma or cardiothoracic vascular surgeon should be involved immediately in suspected vascular injury as decompensation may occur rapidly.

Nerve Injury

Test all nerves in the neck at risk for injury.

A. Vagus, Recurrent Laryngeal

Voice abnormalities, vocal cord asymmetry, hoarseness.

B. Spinal Accessory

Sternocleidomastoid and trapezius weakness, inability to shrug shoulder of affected side and rotate chin against resistance to the opposite side.

C. Hypoglossal

Deviation of the protruded tongue to the side of the injury.

D. Phrenic

Use of respiratory accessory muscles, asymmetry of the diaphragm on chest X-ray.

Disposition

All penetrating neck trauma deep to the platysma should have immediate surgical consultation and admission to the hospital. Blunt neck trauma with no symptoms of airway, esophageal, vascular, or nervous injury can be discharged safely. Always evaluate the C-spine and chest adequately in any neck injury.

MAXILLOFACIAL TRAUMA

Type of Injury

Blunt trauma is the most common form of injury to the face followed by soft tissue lacerations and high velocity missile injuries. CNS involvement is common in missile injuries to the face and should take priority after the patient's airway, breathing and circulation are assessed.

Airway Injury

Mandibular fractures and traumatic facial injuries are often associated with difficult airways. If simple removal of debris and jaw-thrust maneuver fail, secure an airway with endotracheal intubation, cricothyroidotomy, or tracheostomy, in that order of preference. Avoid NG tubes if maxillary trauma exists.

Vascular Injury

Direct pressure is typically sufficient to stop any facial bleeding but pharyngeal packing may be necessary in some cases. Secure an airway before packing the mouth and pharynx. Avoid clamping facial arteries, as they are adjacent to important and difficult-to-visualize nerves.

Nerve Injury

Test all nerves of the face at risk for injury. Early diagnosis of nerve injury is crucial, as edema and pain may obscure examination as time passes.

A. Facial Nerve

1. Temporal branch—Frontalis muscle: inability to wrinkle the forehead.

2. Zygomatic branch—Orbicularis oculi: inability to shut eyes tightly.

3. Buccal branch—All smiling muscles: inability to smile widely, wrinkle nose, or elevate the upper lip.

4. Marginal mandibular branch—Lower lip depressors: inability to pucker or hold cheeks full of air.

B. Trigeminal Nerve

Sensory deficit to any part of the entire face or upper neck.

C. Auditory Nerve

Sensorineural hearing loss.

D. Lingual

Sensory loss to the anterior 2/3 of the tongue.

E. Hypoglossal

Deviation of the protruded tongue to the injured side.

Parotid Gland Injury

Evaluation of the parotid gland is essential if there is any chance of injury. Laceration of Stensen's duct results in a difficult-to-repair salivary fistula if left untreated. Probe the duct with a lacrimal probe entering through the buccal opening. If the probe exits through the laceration, surgical repair is necessary. See Figure 23–4 as it demonstrates the area of high probability for Stensen's duct as well as facial nerve injury. Consultation with a maxillofacial surgeon for any suspected parotid injury is recommended.

Mouth Injuries

The presence of malocclusion suggests a mandible fracture. Inspect and palpate the hard palate, in order to identify any bony irregularity or instability which may be present in maxillary fractures. Check for crepitus upon moving the teeth and for loose or missing teeth, which can be an airway hazard if aspirated. Closely inspect the soft tissues including the lips, tongue, gingiva, buccal mucosa, floor of the mouth, and posterior pharynx for injury.

Eye Injury

An irregular pupil or hyphema on gross examination may indicate a ruptured globe. Fundoscopic exam will reveal a difficult-to-visualize optic nerve and posterior pole. Slit lamp exam may demonstrate a shallow anterior chamber. If a ruptured globe is suspected, apply a rigid shield, administer prophylactic antibiotics, and consult an ophthalmologist. Diplopia, enophthalmos, or subcutaneous emphysema may indicate an orbital blowout fracture. Bilateral periorbital ecchymoses ("raccoon eyes") are a sign of a basilar skull or ethmoid fracture. Diagnose all of these fractures definitively with a facial CT scan. Evert the

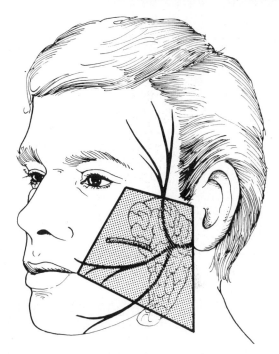

▲ **Figure 23–4.** Area of the face where facial lacerations may injure the parotid gland, Stensen's duct, or facial nerve branches.

lids, removing any foreign bodies, and stain the eye with fluorescein to reveal corneal abrasions. All ocular trauma patients should receive a slit lamp exam if possible.

Nasal Injury

Look into the nares and remove any blood clots or debris that may obscure a clear view. Assess for possible septal hematoma as this requires emergent drainage if present. Palpate the nasal bone for crepitus. Epistaxis is common with nasal injuries and may obscure full examination. Control any active epistaxis with nasal packing. Watch for aspiration of blood from the posterior nasopharynx if the bleeding is significant. Search for CSF rhinorrhea, which would necessitate a CT of the brain and neurosurgical consultation. There is no reliable way to distinguish CSF from thin nasal mucous in the ED.

Ear Injury

Blunt ear trauma often creates occult injury. Inspect the tympanic membrane (TM) for rupture and the canal for lacerations. Hemotympanum, blood in the external canal, CSF otorrhea, posterior auricular hematoma (Battle's sign), facial nerve palsies, and sensorineural hearing loss can indicate a temporal bone fracture. Inspect the external ear. Subperichondrial hematomas are usually obvious and must be drained to prevent "cauliflower ear." Close any auricle lacerations making sure to determine if cartilage is involved. If the cartilage is in need of repair, do not put a suture directly through the auricular cartilage. Sutures should be gently placed in the perichondrium in order to approximate underlying cartilage. Once repair is done, apply Vaseline gauze or saline soaked cotton balls that conform to the ear's anatomy. Place gauze behind ear for posterior support. Cover packed anterior ear with bulky fluffed gauze. Wrap the head in a firm, conforming dressing to prevent further hematoma formation and to secure dressing in place.

▶ Disposition

(See each specific condition in this chapter for details.) Open fractures and virtually any significant injury to the eye, ear, or salivary gland should be hospitalized and treated by the appropriate specialty. Uncomplicated fractures, simple lacerations, and contusions can be safely discharged with appropriate follow-up.

EMERGENT MANAGEMENT OF SPECIFIC INJURIES

 ESSENTIALS OF DIAGNOSIS

▶ Note any obvious jaw swelling or asymmetry
▶ Have the patient bite down and ask, "Do your teeth feel normal and line up correctly? Do you have any pain in your jaw or ears?"

FACIAL FRACTURES

MANDIBLE FRACTURES

▶ General Considerations

The mandible is a U-shaped bone with left and right components fused together at the symphysis in the anterior midline. It is fractured more frequently than any other bone on the face except the nasal bone. The mandible is divided into five anatomic regions which are used to describe the location of any fractures or other abnormalities. These regions include the body, angle, ramus, parasympheseal, coronoid, and condyle. The mandibular condyle forms the mandibular portion of the temporomandibular joint. As always, when managing a known or suspected mandible fracture, evaluation of the airway is paramount. Trauma to the face can cause airway obstruction through soft tissue swelling or anatomic distortion from severely displaced fractures or concomitant craniofacial injury. Because of the force required to fracture the mandible, other injuries must be ruled out, specifically C-spine injuries, other facial fractures, and traumatic brain injury.

▶ Clinical Findings

Mandible fractures almost always present with pain in at least one area of the jaw. In addition to pain as a presenting symptom, malocclusion (the subjective sensation by the patient that the maxillary teeth and mandibular teeth do not align correctly when the mouth is closed) is a very common complaint. This is especially true in displaced fractures of the mandible. Other symptoms include trismus, mucosal lacerations, and dysphagia.

When concern exists for a mandible fracture, the physical exam must include close inspection of the mouth and auditory canals. Mandible fractures can disrupt the gingival and dislodge teeth intraorally creating a grossly open fracture that requires more aggressive treatment. In cases of posterior dislocation of the temporomandibular joint, the anterior wall of the auditory canal can be disrupted, creating an open dislocation.

▶ Imaging

Panorex and computed tomography of the face are the two principal methods of imaging the mandible when concern for fracture exists. Panorex exposes the patient to less radiation but is less sensitive in detecting mandible fractures. Panorex does not adequately image other facial bones. CT of the face increases radiation exposure to the patient but is a more sensitive exam. CT of the face also has the added benefit of enabling visualization of other facial bones in addition to the mandible. If there is a low pretest probability of mandible fracture and no need to image the other bones of the face, a Panorex may be used to limit radiation exposure. However, if cases of high pretest probability based on clinical exam and mechanism, or if other bones of the face need to be imaged, a CT scan should be utilized for radiologic diagnosis. When the patient is in a cervical collar then a CT scan should be used in order to maintain C-spine precautions prior to clearance.

▶ Treatment

A. Tetanus Prophylaxis

In open mandible fractures, administer tetanus toxoid to patients without immunization in the last 5 years.

B. Antimicrobial Prophylaxis

As in oral infections, the chosen antibiotic should cover both oral aerobes and anaerobes. Penicillin 2–4 million units IV, clindamycin 600–900 mg IV, or erythromycin 500–1000 mg IV is preferred, in that order.

C. Relocate the Jaw

If a TMJ dislocation is present, place the thumbs on the inferior molars and relocate with firm downward and backward pressure (Figure 23–5).

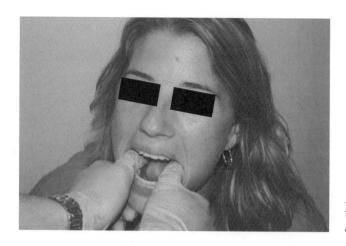

▲ **Figure 23–5.** Relocation of the temporomandibular joint. Use firm downward and backward pressure with the thumbs.

D. Immobilize the Jaw

Patients in considerable pain may find relief if a Barton bandage is used. A Barton bandage is created by wrapping an elastic bandage around the top of the head and below the mandible. This immobilizes the mandible and serves a similar purpose as a splint.

▶ Disposition

Open fractures, complex fractures associated with dislocation, grossly displaced fractures, or any injury with potential for airway compromise should be seen by a maxillofacial surgeon as these injuries commonly require surgical fixation. Ideally, all patients with mandibular fractures should be treated definitively in the ED, but it is widely accepted to discharge uncomplicated fractures without concomitant injury. Provide appropriate antibiotics and analgesics and arrange follow-up within the next few days. The patient should keep the jaw fully immobilized.

MAXILLARY (LE FORT) FRACTURES

ESSENTIALS OF DIAGNOSIS

- ▶ Note any midface mobility, swelling, ecchymosis, or asymmetric deformity.
- ▶ Consider other injuries, as Le Fort fractures result from high-energy injury.

General Considerations

The Le Fort classification system of maxillary injuries was designed to describe common patterns of maxillary fractures resulting from blunt trauma. It is not all-inclusive,

and combinations of different patterns may often be seen in the same patient. Its utility lies in the ease of description to consultants and help in recognizing the need for diagnostic tests. Le Fort fractures exist only after high-energy injury; therefore, intracranial and C-spine injury should be expected in any case. Always consider the airway first.

▶ Clinical Findings

When a Le Fort fracture is present, facial trauma is obvious in most cases because of significant swelling, ecchymosis, and possible deformity. Grasping the hard palate and rocking the maxilla may reveal midface instability, but this is present only in bilateral maxillary fractures. The patient may sense malocclusion and will certainly have localized maxillary tenderness. Diplopia from orbital involvement, facial emphysema from extension into the sinuses, and cerebrospinal fluid rhinorrhea from extension into the calvarium may also be present.

▶ Imaging

Facial CT scan is the test of choice to identify maxillary fractures and determine their classification. Le Fort fractures are divided into three major types (Figure 23–6). Plain radiographs play no role in diagnosis because of their lack of sensitivity.

A. Le Fort I Fracture

(See Figure 23–6A.) Le Fort I fractures include the maxilla parallel to the alveolar process and hard palate extending posteriorly behind the maxillary molars and across the lateral wall of the maxillary sinus. Essentially, this fracture separates the maxillary teeth from the face.

Airway complications are rare in Le Fort I injuries. Malocclusion and local tenderness, swelling, and ecchymosis occur. With stress, the hard palate and upper teeth move. After identifying the fracture with a facial CT scan and ruling out concomitant injury, no specific ED management is

Anterior views

Lateral views

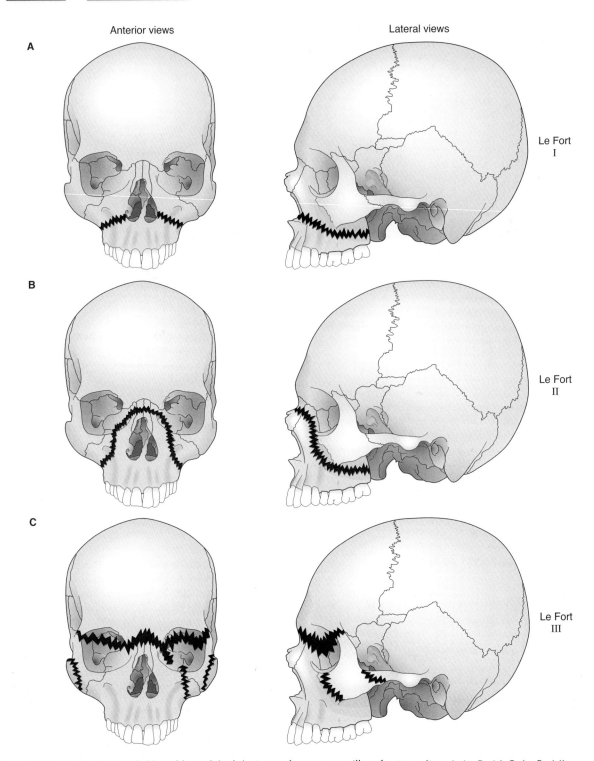

▲ **Figure 23–6.** Anterior (left) and lateral (right) views of Le Fort maxillary fracture sites. **A:** Le Fort I. **B:** Le Fort II. **C:** Le Fort III.

necessary. Consultation with a maxillofacial trauma surgeon should occur within the ED. The patient can then be safely discharged with appropriate analgesia.

B. Le Fort II Fracture

(See Figure 23–6B). Le Fort II fractures include the fracture lines of a Le Fort I fracture but now involve the bony nasal skeleton becoming a pyramidal fracture.

Once again, airway complications are rare. Malocclusion again exists along with ecchymosis of the nasal dorsum and lower eyelids. The infraorbital nerve canal is involved and injury to this nerve causes a sensory deficit below the involved lower eyelid. Stress moves the hard palate, teeth, and nose, but not the eyes. CT scan of the face is the imaging modality used to identify the fracture, and maxillofacial consultation in the ED should be used to determine the disposition of the patient. In the absence of concomitant injury, a patient may be discharged with analgesics unless surgical repair is eminent.

C. Le Fort III Fracture

(See Figure 23–6C). Le Fort III fractures define craniofacial disjunction. The fracture extends through the frontozygomatic suture lines, across the orbit and through the base of the nose and ethmoid region. The zygoma may become completely separated in some patients.

Airway complications are common with Le Fort III fractures resulting from massive edema and hematomas that can dissect into the palate, pharyngeal walls, or tonsilar pillars. Address the airway first. Nasotracheal intubation and NG tubes are contraindicated. If possible, the patient's visual acuity should be tested due to the high incidence of blindness with Le Fort III fractures. Head CT as well as C-spine imaging should accompany facial CT in all patients with this injury. A maxillofacial surgeon should determine final disposition.

ZYGOMATICOMAXILLARY COMPLEX FRACTURE

 ESSENTIALS OF DIAGNOSIS

► Lower eyelid swelling and ecchymosis
► Flattened "cheekbone"
► Diplopia with upward gaze
► Trismus

▶ General Considerations

Zygomaticomaxillary (ZMC) fractures are the second most common facial fracture. They consist of three fracture lines including the infraorbital rim, the zygomatic–frontal

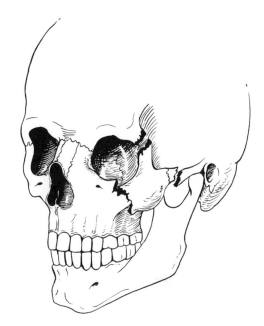

▲ **Figure 23–7.** Diagram of a zygomaticomaxillary complex fracture. Note disruption of both the lateral orbital rim and the orbital floor, as well as the zygomatic arch.

suture, and the zygomatic–temporal junction at the arch (Figure 23–7). The three fracture lines give the fracture its more common name, a tripod fracture. However, this is a quadripod structure as there is a relationship to the base of the skull as well. The ZMC fracture results from a medially directed blunt force on the cheekbone. The orbital floor is disrupted and entrapment of the inferior oblique can result, but it is not a blowout fracture and does not have the same complications. Tripod fractures do not require the high energy that Le Fort or frontal sinus fractures require so concomitant injury is less common but should not be overlooked.

▶ Clinical Findings

Most common symptoms include pain, swelling, and ecchymosis of the cheek, which may obscure the classic finding of a flattened "cheekbone." Palpable periorbital stepoffs are often present. Look for trismus and subcutaneous emphysema. Epistaxis may be present. Involvement of the infraorbital nerve as it exits its foramen may result in paresthesias of the lower eyelid, adjacent cheek, nose, and upper lip. Diplopia may result from extraocular muscle contusion, entrapment or from an orbital hematoma or "sagging" of the eyeball into the disrupted orbital floor. Upward gaze diplopia is most common. Investigate for a retrobulbar hematoma or a ruptured globe, which require immediate ophthalmologic intervention. Extraocular muscle entrapment or herniation

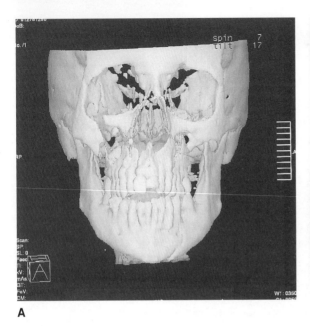
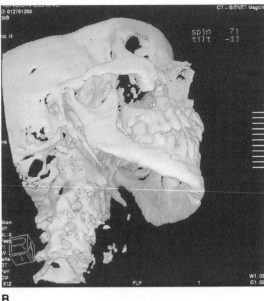

A   **B**

▲ **Figure 23–8.** Three-dimensionally reconstructed facial CT scan. **A:** Left parasymphyseal mandibular fracture. **B:** Right zygomaticomaxillary complex fracture with inferior and lateral displacement of the ZMC.

of orbital contents into the fracture is less common than in blowout fractures. Fracture extension into the paranasal sinuses is exhibited by subcutaneous emphysema.

Imaging

Plain films are not necessary. All tripod fractures should be evaluated with a facial CT scan. Three-dimensional reconstruction reveals any displacement of the fracture and guides surgical repair (Figure 23–8). Always image the C-spine if any tenderness is present.

Treatment

When ZMC fractures are diagnosed an ophthomalogic consultation should be obtained. Provide adequate analgesics and antibiotic prophylaxis if there is extension into the sinuses (penicillin, amoxicillin, fluoroquinolones, doxycycline, or clindamycin). If epistaxis is present, control the bleeding with packing or cautery.

Disposition

A maxillofacial surgeon should evaluate all ZMC fractures in the ED. Serious consideration should be given to consulting an ophthalmologist in-house as well, despite an absence of immediate ocular findings. Isolated ZMC fractures can be treated conservatively with close follow-up, adequate analgesics, and soft diet unless immediate surgical repair is planned.

ORBITAL FLOOR ("BLOWOUT") FRACTURE

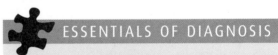

ESSENTIALS OF DIAGNOSIS

► Presence of enophthalmos
► Diplopia with upward gaze
► Decreased eye movement

General Considerations

If viewed in sagittal cross-section the orbit takes on the appearance of a cone with the base anterior and the apex posterior. The orbital walls are formed by relatively thin-walled and weak bones while the rim is formed by much thicker and stronger bone. When an external force is applied to the globe, intraorbital pressure increases to the point that one or more of the thin-walled bones of the orbit "blowout" or fracture. Interestingly, the release of pressure after an orbital blowout oftentimes prevents significant ocular trauma (Figure 23–9). The most common bone fractured is the maxillary bone which comprises the floor of the orbit. The orbital contents can be significantly displaced inferiorly after orbital blowout fracture.

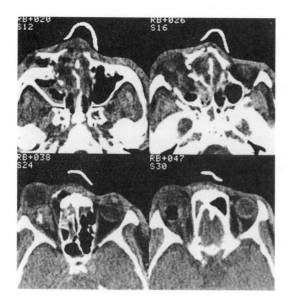

▲ **Figure 23–9.** Orbital blowout fracture (impure type) on CT scan. Sequential horizontal cuts through the mid skull show blowout fracture of the right orbit, with rupture of the orbital contents into the maxillary sinus (upper left frame). Edema of the orbital contents is causing protrusion of the right eyeball (lower left frame).

▶ Clinical Findings

Essentially all patients with an orbital blowout fracture will present with pain, and the vast majority will present with periorbital ecchymosis. A majority of patients will present with diplopia on upward gaze due to entrapment of the inferior rectus muscle. A significant proportion of patients with orbital blowout fracture will also have ipsilateral anesthesia in the V2 distribution secondary to infraorbital nerve entrapment. The most concerning clinical finding is enophthalmos as this indicates significant inferior displacement of the orbital contents through the floor. Ocular trauma frequently occurs, and a thorough examination including slit-lamp and dilated exam should be completed to investigate for lens dislocation, corneal abrasion, globe rupture, commotio retinae, or retinal detachment. If the periorbital emphysema is severe, measure the intraocular pressure and emergently consult an ophthalmologist for possible cantholysis.

▶ Imaging

CT scan of the face is the study of choice for diagnosis and management of orbital blowout fractures. CT is highly sensitive and specific in terms of diagnosis and also provides the consulting surgeon valuable information if surgical intervention is deemed necessary. Historically, radiographs of the orbits were used, but their sensitivity is unacceptably low to rely on them for diagnostic purposes.

▶ Treatment

Initial treatment in the emergency department includes appropriate tetanus prophylaxis and pain control as well as avoiding any valsalva maneuvers. Prophylactic anti-emetics may be appropriate. Give instructions to the patient to not blow their nose. Long-term treatment may be managed either nonoperatively or operatively depending on the presence of enophthalmos and extraocular muscle entrapment. If surgical management is planned, it is typically delayed 7–10 days after the initial trauma.

▶ Disposition

Emergent surgical intervention is rarely indicated. All orbital blowout fractures with significant entrapment or enophthalmos should be seen by a maxillofacial surgeon as well as an ophthalmologist for detailed ocular exam. If there is no entrapment or enophthalmos then discharge with close outpatient follow up is appropriate.

NASAL FRACTURES

ESSENTIALS OF DIAGNOSIS

► Control any epistaxis
► Identify displacement
► Discover and drain any septal hematomas

▶ General Considerations

The nasal bone is the most frequently fractured bone of the face, accounting for approximately 40% of all facial fractures. The nose is composed by cartilage distally, the frontal bones superiorly, the maxillary bone laterally, and the nasal bone anteriorly. Nasal bone fractures most commonly occur with a blow to the face in the anterior–posterior direction but can also occur with a lateral blow. An adequate cosmetic result is the chief long-term concern for nasal bone fractures.

▶ Clinical Findings

The patient will typically complain of pain in the nose, and most will have at least some epistaxis after the trauma. Patients may also complain of deformity of the nose. Referring to a photograph of the patient's face prior to the injury will assist the physician in determining the significance of any deformity. Nasal bone fractures frequently occur in conjunction with other facial fractures. If the patient has tenderness or significant ecchymosis of other areas of the face then investigations into other fractures must also take place.

Imaging

No imaging is necessary for simple nasal fractures as it is typically a clinical diagnosis. If a concomitant injury to the face is suspected then maxillofacial CT should be utilized.

Treatment

First, assess the patient's ability to breath and maintain an airway. After the airway has been addressed, next turn attention to the control of any epistaxis. Ideally, displaced fractures should be reduced immediately, however reduction prior to early fixation (3–5 days) is a reasonable alternative. An ED physician can reduce nasal fractures, but significantly displaced fractures should also be evaluated by a maxillofacial surgeon. Septal hematomas must be drained to avoid septal necrosis and disfigurement. Give the patient both oral analgesics and nasal decongestants prior to discharge.

A. Fracture Reduction

First provide analgesia. Narcotics combined with topical cocaine should be sufficient. Place cylindrical cotton or gauze soaked in cocaine solution in the patient's nose for 15 minutes. Laterally displaced fractures are reduced with simple lateral thumb pressure. Impacted fractures require both anterior and lateral manipulation with Kelly clamps or Asch septal forceps on the nasal septum (Figure 23–10). Failure to reduce requires immediate ENT consultation. Lacerations over the fracture site can be irrigated well and

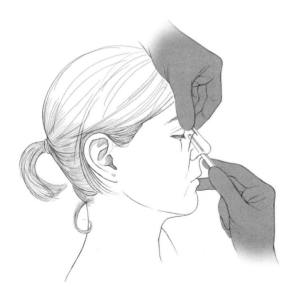

▲ **Figure 23-10.** Reduction of nasal fracture by anterior traction with forceps. (Redrawn and reproduced, with permission, from Wang MK, Macomber WB: Maxillofacial injuries. In Eichert C (editor). *Emergency Room Care*, 4th ed. Little Brown, 1981.)

primarily closed. Complex lacerations involving intranasal structures, septum, or causing significant deformity should be repaired in the ED by a consultant. As the nose harbors *Staphylococcus*, provide antimicrobial prophylaxis (amoxicillin/clavulanate, sulfa, cephalexin, or erythromycin). Secure fracture reductions simply with tape over the nasal bridge.

B. Drain Hematomas

Septal hematomas should be drained prior to discharge from the emergency department because of the high incidence of septal necrosis which causes a saddle deformity. Incise the anterior nasal mucosa with a No. 11 blade at the inferior portion of the hematoma allowing it to drain. Packing the incision following drainage is recommended so that the incision will not close. Provide prophylaxis with the same antibiotics as above.

Disposition

All nasal bone fractures can be discharged safely with analgesics if no concomitant injury is present. Follow-up with an otolaryngologist is mandatory and should be done within 1 week.

FRONTAL SINUS FRACTURES

ESSENTIALS OF DIAGNOSIS

► High-energy mechanism, consider intracranial and C-spine injury
► Rare in children, unlikely in early teens

General Considerations

A tremendous amount of energy is required to cause frontal sinus fractures. Most frontal sinus fractures are encountered in the setting of motor vehicle accidents. Because of this, frontal sinus fractures are usually associated with another craniofacial injury or traumatic injury elsewhere. Anytime a frontal sinus fracture is encountered a thorough evaluation is warranted to search for a possible secondary injury. The frontal sinus has an anterior wall (called the anterior table) just deep to the soft tissues of the face and a posterior wall (called the posterior table) that sits adjacent to the brain. Fractures of the frontal sinus can be of the anterior table alone or a combined anterior and posterior table fracture.

Clinical Findings

Contusion, swelling, and ecchymosis will be present as well as possible lacerations of the forehead and crepitus over the sinus. CSF rhinorrhea is possible if a posterior table fracture exists as a dural tear may have occurred. A dural tear may present as postnasal drip as opposed to typical CSF rhinorrhea. Anesthesia of the forehead in the setting of a frontal sinus fracture indicates damage to the supraorbital nerve. Other facial fractures, depressed skull fractures, and orbital fractures will often be present as well.

▶ Imaging

An axial and coronal CT scan of the face and head as well as C-spine imaging should be ordered on every patient. Historically, plain radiographs were utilized. However, plain radiographs have been replaced by CT as the diagnostic modality of choice because of its superior sensitivity and its ability to assist in operative planning for consulting surgeons.

▶ Treatment

Elevate the patient's head to decrease venous pressure and ICP. Antibiotics are now controversial and should be discussed with the consultant. Urgently consult a maxillofacial surgeon and neurosurgeon (with posterior table involvement) for an ED evaluation. An ophthalmologist should also be consulted if significant involvement of the orbit exists. Surgical correction is indicated for CSF rhinorrhea, open fractures, and significantly displaced fractures, posterior wall fractures. As in any trauma evaluation, maintain C-spine precautions at all times. If there are open fractures, cover the lacerations with gauze to prevent contamination.

▶ Disposition

Patients with isolated nondisplaced frontal sinus fractures may be discharged after being evaluated by a specialist and after an adequate observation period has occurred. Displaced fractures are typically admitted for surgical fixation and close observation.

TEMPORAL BONE FRACTURES

ESSENTIALS OF DIAGNOSIS

▶ Can include hearing loss, facial nerve injury, or intracranial injury

▶ External clinical signs can be absent

▶ General Considerations

Most basilar skull fractures include fractures of the temporal bone. Because the temporal bone houses the cochlea, vestibule, facial nerve canal, jugular vein, and internal carotid artery, fractures can have serious sequelae. High-energy mechanisms are usually required and are usually associated with severe brain injury which limits clinical

symptoms and signs expected from such injury. Clinical appearance, if present, includes partial or complete facial nerve palsies, conductive, sensorineural or mixed hearing loss, vertigo, dizziness, otorrhagia, CSF otorrhea, TM perforation, hemotympanum, and canal lacerations. Due to irregularity of fracture patterns, clinical features, treatment, and disposition depend on the evaluation of function more than type of fracture. Each type may be associated with intracranial bleeding, brain injury, and subsequent meningitis. Because of this, neurosurgical consultation as well as maxillofacial surgical consultation is a must.

▶ Clinical Findings

A. Longitudinal Fractures

Longitudinal fractures account for 80% of all fractures of the temporal bone. They are so named because the fracture line parallels the bone's long axis. Mastoid ecchymosis ("Battle's" sign), periorbital ecchymosis ("raccoon eyes"), hemotympanum, and bleeding into ear canal from skin and TM laceration are often seen. The TM is often torn and a step-off may be seen in the external auditory canal. CSF otorrhea is common. The ossicles may be dislocated creating conductive hearing loss. The cochlea is spared; therefore, sensorineural hearing loss is absent. Facial nerve paralysis may be present but is usually delayed. This implies a better prognosis than that for immediate paralysis, which requires surgical exploration of the nerve canal and the nerve trunk.

B. Transverse Fractures

Although less common, transverse fractures cause more severe injury to the contents of the temporal bone. The fracture usually begins in the internal auditory canal and traverses the cochlea and facial nerve canal perpendicular to the long axis of the temporal bone. Often complete sensorineural hearing loss occurs along with severe vertigo and intense nystagmus or immediate facial nerve paralysis. Over 50% of patients will have facial nerve injury. Mastoid ecchymosis ("Battle's" sign), periorbital ecchymosis ("raccoon eyes"), and hemotympanum are often seen.

▶ Imaging

CT scan of the face and head is the imaging study of choice to identify all three types of the temporal bone fractures as well as any intracranial pathology. Once again, always consider C-spine imaging.

▶ Treatment and Disposition

Patients with temporal bone fractures frequently have multiple other injuries. This can lead to delay in diagnosis and treatment. Maintain C-spine precautions until associated injury can be excluded. Once a temporal bone fracture is diagnosed then it is important to assess status of external canal by checking for blood and CSF and to evaluate facial nerve. Do not lavage external auditory canal or insert packing due to risk of introducing infection to inner ear, brain, and meninges. Immediate maxillofacial or ENT surgical consultation is required. Neurosurgery consultation should be obtained for any associated intracranial injury. All patients with temporal bone fractures should be admitted to the hospital.

DENTAL TRAUMA

TOOTH AVULSION

Tooth avulsion is complete displacement of tooth out of socket. This can result from any oral trauma and necessitates immediate action. Reimplantation success rates decrease by 1% every minute the tooth is out of the socket. The goal is to restore the tooth to its correct anatomical location in a quick and secure manner.

Rinse the tooth gently with saline. Administer local anesthesia or a regional intraoral nerve block. Replace the tooth in the socket and immediately consult a dentist or oral surgeon. If this is impossible, place the tooth in a transportation media such as Viaspan, Hank's solution, cold milk, saliva (in the patient's mouth) or saline in that preferential order. Tooth avulsion with concomitant mandible fracture is an open fracture. Consider a chest X-ray to rule out aspiration of tooth fragments.

TOOTH SUBLUXATION

Tooth subluxation is loosening of the tooth secondary to trauma. It should be treated with gentle manipulation of the tooth into its proper position. Consult a dentist or oral surgeon during the ED visit for possible splinting. Children tend to subluxate rather than fracture their primary teeth.

TOOTH FRACTURE

Rule out any fragment aspiration with a chest X-ray. Tooth fractures are best classified and treated using the Ellis classification. Ellis I fractures involve the enamel only. They require only smoothing of the rough edges and dental follow-up. Ellis II fractures involve the enamel and yellow dentin may be visible. These teeth are sensitive to air exposure and tender to touch. The exposed area should be covered with Calcium Hydroxide paste, glass ionomer or a strip of adhesive barrier (eg, Stomahesive). Dermabond is acceptable if no other material is available. A 24-hour dental follow-up is adequate. Ellis III fractures involve the enamel, dentin, and pulp and require immediate dental consultation. Cover the exposed area with Calcium Hydroxide paste or glass ionomer. Patients should be put on antibiotics that cover oral flora such as Clindamycin. Local anesthesia or nerve blocks should be considered. Avoid topical anesthetics. Panorex may be necessary to rule out alveolar ridge fractures.

EXTERNAL EAR TRAUMA

AURICULAR HEMATOMA

▶ Clinical Findings

Blunt trauma to the ear often results in bleeding between the perichondrium and auricular cartilage. This injury is common in wrestlers and boxers. If left untreated, cauliflower ear deformity will result from proliferative scarring in the hematoma site.

▶ Treatment

Administer local anesthesia or perform an auricular block. Treatment consists of needle aspiration or incision and drainage of any subperichondrial blood. Make a 1 cm incision along the natural skin folds and then evacuate the hematoma with gentle manual expression through the opening. Cover the wound with antibiotic ointment. Suture dental pledget bolsters to either side of the auricle or apply Vaseline gauze or saline soaked cotton balls that conform to the ear's anatomy. Place gauze behind ear for posterior support. Cover packed anterior ear with bulky fluffed gauze. Wrap the head in a firm, conforming dressing to prevent further hematoma formation and to secure dressing in place.

▶ Disposition

Hospitalization is not required. Antibiotics for skin flora should be prescribed. A maxillofacial surgeon should see the patient within 24 hours to be examined for reoccurrence.

LACERATIONS OF THE AURICLE

▶ Treatment

Meticulous repair of auricle lacerations is required to prevent deformity. Regional nerve blocks are preferred as local infiltration can distort anatomical landmarks. Medical literature now supports the use of epinephrine when anesthetizing the ear. Closure of the perichondrium is achieved with 6.0 synthetic absorbable suture. Sutures should not go through the cartilage but only through the perichondrium to approximate cartilage. The overlying skin should be closed with 6.0 nylon or skin tape. Cover with antibiotic ointment and a petroleum gauze dressing under light pressure. Reserve antibiotic prophylaxis for the immunocompromised, bite injuries, or contaminated wounds.

▶ Disposition

Simple lacerations can be closed in the ED and referred to a facial surgeon in 1–2 days. Complex lacerations with extensive cartilage injury or tissue loss should be closed by a maxillofacial surgeon either in the ED or in the operating room.

MIDDLE AND INNER EAR DISORDERS FOLLOWING HEAD TRAUMA

CEREBROSPINAL FLUID OTORRHEA

▶ Clinical Findings

Cerebrospinal fluid otorrhea and rhinorrhea often results from minimal head injuries. A CSF leak is indicative of a communication between the subarachnoid space and the nasal cavity or paranasal space. Eighty per cent of post-traumatic leaks occur in first 48 hours post-trauma. Patients complain of a salty or sweet taste. Clear drainage is exacerbated by valsalva maneuver. Halo sign may be present on tissue paper or bed linens. The risk of meningitis is high. A CT scan with axial and coronal views will help diagnose the injury and any concomitant intracranial bleeding or brain injury.

▶ Treatment and Disposition

Testing of fluid for the β-2 transferrin is highly sensitive and specific for CSF. Hospitalization and urgent neurosurgical consultation are indicated for all patients with CSF leakage. The use of prophylactic antibiotics is controversial.

FACIAL NERVE PARALYSIS

▶ Clinical Findings

Basilar skull fractures, direct facial injury, penetrating trauma to middle ear, barotrauma (altitude paralysis or scuba diving), and lightening injuries are all causes of traumatic facial nerve paralysis. Paralysis may be partial or complete depending on the location of the injury. Varying patterns of motor and sensory loss can occur. Examine the face for lost or decreased movement, decreased tear production, or altered sensation on the affected side of the face. CT and MRI are useful diagnostic studies. Consult a maxillofacial surgeon if any signs are present.

▶ Treatment and Disposition

Patients with facial nerve paralysis should be hospitalized and evaluated immediately by a maxillofacial surgeon.

CONDUCTIVE HEARING LOSS

▶ Clinical Findings

The ear is the most frequently damaged sense organ secondary to trauma. TM perforation, hemotympanum and ossicular chain disruptions can cause traumatic conductive hearing loss. Patients with disarticulation of ossicular chain complain of acute hearing loss. A step-off at 12 o'clock at the medial end of the ear canal is evidence of a temporal bone fracture and suggestive of ossicular dislocation. Bone conduction will be greater than air conduction in such injuries. Audiometric testing can determine whether sensorineural hearing loss is present.

▶ Treatment and Disposition

Hospitalization is not necessary. An otolaryngologist should see patients within a few days for evaluation. The majority of patients with all forms of traumatic conductive hearing loss can be managed conservatively.

SENSORINEURAL HEARING LOSS

▶ Clinical Findings

Trauma can cause both temporary (inner ear concussion) or permanent hearing loss. Acoustic trauma from gunshots, fireworks, explosions, barotraumas, traumatic TM rupture, and temporal bone fractures can all cause sensorineural hearing loss. Temporal bone fractures that traverse the cochlea may result in total permanent loss of hearing and severe vertigo for the first few days following injury.

▶ Treatment and Disposition

Control vertigo with diazepam at liberal doses. All patients should be hospitalized for urgent ENT evaluation.

VERTIGO

▶ Clinical Findings

Post-traumatic vertigo refers to dizziness after a head or neck injury. Benign positional vertigo (BPV) is common after a head injury. Patient may also develop post-traumatic Meniere's, labyrinthine "concussion," or cervical vertigo secondary to neck injury or temporal bone fracture. Occasionally, the vertigo is severe and persistent creating difficulty with walking. Nystagmus may be present as well.

▶ Treatment and Disposition

Treatment is individualized to the diagnosis. Treatment includes a combination of medications, lifestyle changes, and physical therapy. Occasionally surgery is needed. Severe vertigo can be treated with diazepam, 2–5 mg orally 2–4 times a day or meclizine at 25 mg 3–4 times a day. Hospitalization is not necessary. Refer the patient to an otolaryngologist for routine follow-up and possible additional testing.

CARE OF FACIAL LACERATIONS

See also Chapter 30.

Closure of Lacerations

Most patients are particularly concerned about scarring of the face after sustaining an open injury. Thus, primary closure, which usually results in the least noticeable scar is the preferred method of treatment for most facial lacerations. Facial laceration repair requires attention to detail and precise wound edge approximation with fine suture material to restore anatomic structure lines. Do not hesitate to request assistance from the appropriate consultant (otolaryngologist, ophthalmologist, plastic surgeon, oral and maxillofacial surgeon) if extensive tissue damage is present or the damage is adjacent to structures requiring complex closure.

Injuries to the lips specifically are common and require precise repair. Clean all debris and clotted blood with a moist sponge. The vermillion border is more easily seen when wet. Place the first suture through the vermillion border to align the two edges. It is important to also align the wet–dry mucosal surfaces in addition to the vermillion border. Repair the rest of the wound once these approximations have been made.

Replacement of Avulsed Tissue

Debridement of skin edges should be done with caution. Because of excellent blood supply to the face, tissue that appears ischemic will often revascularize. Small avulsed pieces of ear, nose, or facial soft tissue may be cleaned and replaced with a reasonable chance for survival. Larger pieces, such as subtotal avulsion of the ear or scalp, should be replaced by a surgeon using microvascular techniques. Attempts to retrieve any avulsed tissue from the scene of injury should be made.

Delay in Closing Lacerations

In general, lacerations of the eyelids, lateral orbit, nasal dorsum, and mandible should not be closed until X-rays have been taken. The lacerations may need to remain for reduction and fixation of the fracture fragments through this opening.

Because of the abundant blood supply to the area, it is acceptable to close facial lacerations that have been open for as long as 24 hours as long as the wounds are cleaned thoroughly. When delayed closure is necessary, the wound should be packed open with saline-soaked gauze until the repair can be completed. Antibiotics (cephalexin, dicloxacillin, erythromycin) should be considered in these cases.

Repair Technique

Once more extensive injuries have been excluded (ie, facial nerve or parotid duct transections), local anesthetic is infused into the wound edges or a regional block is employed. Regional blocks may be preferred, as they will not distort the wound edges. A mental nerve block is best for the lower lip and skin below the lip, an infraorbital nerve block for upper lip, lateral nose, lower eyelid and medial cheek and a supraorbital/supratrochlear nerve block for forehead lacerations. Once the wound is anesthetized, irrigation, selective debridement, and wound exploration should ensue. The extent of injury, number of layers involved, and experience with repair of facial wounds will dictate the choice of suture. Sutures of 6.0 synthetic nonabsorbable monofilament are a good choice for skin closure (nylon, polypropylene, polybutester) due to their high tensile strength and minimal inflammatory response. Synthetic absorbable suture may be used to close subcutaneous structures or mucosal lacerations. These sutures have good tensile strength and minimal inflammatory response in comparison to natural products.

An important aspect of plastic closure of such lacerations is the placement of sutures. Sutures on the face should be placed 3 mm apart and 1–2 mm from skin edge in order to achieve better cosmetic results. The angle of entry of the needle into skin should be at 90°.

Irregular lacerations, lacerations at risk for infection or lacerations in areas of significant swelling should be closed in an interrupted fashion. For linear lacerations, a running suture is acceptable. Small linear lacerations under very little tension may be closed with cyanoacrylate tissue adhesive as an alternative to sutures. Avoid mucous membranes and the eyes during the application. Do not use skin adhesives where hair is present.

Wounds should be kept clean and dry for 48 hours after suture placement. Q-tips with mild soap and water can be used to clean wounds after that time period. Peroxide and betadine should not be applied after wound repair. Patients should be informed that the overuse of topical antibiotic ointments can lessen tension of skin edges and may prevent appropriate closure. Facial skin sutures should be removed no later than 5 days after placement. An ophthalmologic suture scissor or a No. 11 blade is best for removing these fine sutures. After suture removal, the surface should be prepared with benzoin adhesive and skin tape applied (ie, Steri-Strips). This will eliminate any tension on the closure and minimize widening and hypertrophy of the scar. The patient should be told to protect the scar from sunlight for first 6 months and complete scar maturation will take 12 months. A scar revision can be performed at that time.

Brady SM: The diagnosis and management of orbital blowout fractures: update 2001. Am J Emerg Med 2001;19:147 [PMID: 11239261].

Cassada DC et al: Acute injuries of the trachea and major bronchi: importance of early diagnosis. Ann Thorac Surg 2000;69(5):1563–1567 [PMID: 10881842].

Clinical guideline on management of acute dental trauma. Available at: http://www.guidelines.gov/summary/summary.aspx?ss=15&doc_id=12105&nbr=6230. Accessed 2010

Crosby ET: Airway management in adults after cervical spine trauma. Anesthesiology 2006;104(6):1293–1318 (Review) [PMID: 16732102].

Grant JR et al: Outcomes for conservative management of traumatic conductive hearing loss. Otol Neurotol 2008;29(3): 344–349 [PMID: 18317393].

Krausz AA et al: Maxillofacial trauma patient: coping with the difficult airway. World J Emerg Surg 2009;4:21 (Published online on May 27, 2009). doi: 10.1186/1749-7922-4-21

Kucik CJ. Management of acute nasal fractures. Am Fam Physician 2004;70(7):1315–1320 [PMID: 15508543].

Kumar A, Patel S: Focus on: shock and pressors. Am Col Emerg Physicians. Available at: http://www.acep.org/webportal/membercenter/periodicals/an/2006/oct/shockpressors.htm. Accessed 2010.

Manoach S et al: Manual in-line stabilization for acute airway management of suspected cervical spine injury: historical review and current questions. Ann Emerg Med 2007;50(3): 236–245 [PMID: 17337093].

Mudry A et al: Auricular hematoma and cauliflower deformation of the ear; from art to medicine. Otol Neurotol 2009;30(1): 116–120 [PMID: 18800018].

Pinto A et al: Gunshot injuries in the neck area: ballistics elements and forensic issues. Semin Ultrasound CT MR 2009;30(3): 215–220 [PMID: 19537054].

Piya S et al: Temporal bone fractures. Emerg Rad 2009;16(4): 255–265 [PMID: 18982367].

Schneidereit NP et al: Utility of screening for blunt vascular neck injuries with computed tomographic angiography. J Trauma 2006;60(1):209–215 (discussion 215–216) [PMID: 16456458].

Stacey DH et al: Management of mandible fractures. Plast Reconstr Surg 2006;117(3):48e–60e (Review) [PMID: 16525255].

Thoma M, Navsaria PH, Edu S, Nicol AJ.: Analysis of 203 patients with penetrating neck injuries. World J Surg 2008;32(12): 2716–2723 [PMID: 18931870].

Tiwari P et al: The management of frontal sinus fractures. J Oral Maxillofac Surg 2005:63(9):1354–1360 [PMID: 16122601].

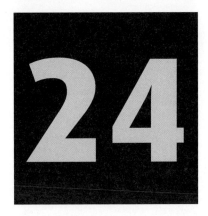

Chest Trauma

Jonathan Jones, MD
Seth Stearley, MD[1]

Up to half of all trauma patients sustain some degree of thoracic injury. Twenty to twenty-five percent of all trauma deaths are directly attributable to chest trauma. Thoracic trauma is a contributing factor in another 25% of trauma deaths.

IMMEDIATE MANAGEMENT OF LIFE-THREATENING PROBLEMS

ESTABLISH ABCS

The ABCs should be addressed as previously outlined in Chapters 9 and 10. There are specific considerations in evaluating the ABCs in the patient with blunt or penetrating chest trauma. The airway can be obstructed at any level from the pharynx to the trachea. Abnormalities in breathing can be caused by one or more of the following mechanisms: (1) impairments in the chest wall or musculature, eg, secondary to pain or because the chest wall motion is not coordinated; (2) impairments in gas exchange, secondary to atelectasis, contusion, or disruption of the respiratory tract; and (3) CNS impairments secondary to drugs or head trauma. Hypoxia is the most important feature of chest injury. Early interventions should attempt to insure that an adequate amount of oxygen is delivered to the portions of the lung capable of normal ventilation and perfusion. Abnormalities in circulation can be caused by blood loss, increased intrapleural pressure, blood in the pericardial sac, vascular disruption, or myocardial dysfunction. Since shock will most often be caused by blood loss, the first step should be to ensure adequate fluid resuscitation.

PAIN CONTROL

Pain may impair chest wall expansion and impede oxygenation. Pain should be relieved with small frequent doses of narcotic medications, eg, 2–8 mg of morphine or 50–100 μg

[1] This chapter is a revision of Chapter 22 in the 6th edition by Seth Stearley, MD, and L. Richard Boggs, MD.

of fentanyl every 30 minutes as needed. The pain level should be constantly reassessed to ensure adequate analgesia.

▼ IMMEDIATELY LIFE-THREATENING THORACIC INJURIES IDENTIFIED ON THE PRIMARY SURVEY

Several entities need to be considered in the patient with chest trauma. They can cause severe hypoxia and/or shock. The diagnoses are made clinically and need to be addressed without waiting for any diagnostic testing. Any patient presenting with any one of these entities should be treated as outlined and admitted to the hospital for further care.

TENSION PNEUMOTHORAX

Tension pneumothorax develops when a one-way valve air leak occurs from either the lung or chest wall. Air enters the pleural space but cannot escape, leading to increased intrapleural pressure, collapse of the lung, and shift of the mediastinal contents to the opposite side. Tension pneumothorax can result from blunt chest injury with resultant parenchymal lung injury, but can also be secondary to positive-pressure ventilation. Occasionally a small penetrating wound can cause a valve-like effect that allows air to enter the pleural space on inspiration but not exit on expiration. The collapse of the lung leads to right to left pulmonary shunting and resultant hypoxia. In addition, increased intrathoracic pressure and pressure on the vena cava can reduce venous return to the heart and lead to decreased cardiac output and shock.

▶ Diagnosis

Pneumothorax is characterized by respiratory distress, tachypnea, and hypoxia. There will be hyperresonance to percussion and decreased or absent breath sounds on the affected side. With tension pneumothorax, the trachea will be deviated away from the affected side. Neck veins may be distended, but this may be absent if the patient is hypovolemic. The diagnosis of tension pneumothorax is made clinically. Patients with a tension pneumothorax need immediate treatment and should not wait for X-ray. Figure 24–1 shows the chest X-ray (CXR) of a patient whose physical examination findings should have lead the physician to perform a needle decompression instead of an X-ray (not the mistake of the authors). For stable patients, in whom a pneumothorax is suspected, diagnosis is confirmed with CXR (Figure 24–2). Besides ultrasonography is quickly becoming an alternative to X-ray for rapid identification of pneumothorax. Reported sensitivity for detection of pneumothorax of 86–98% for ultrasound versus 28–75% for supine CXR makes it a potentially attractive alternative.

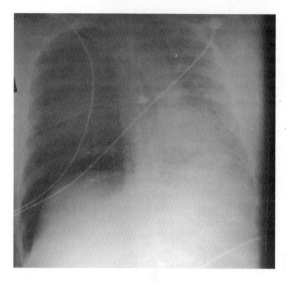

▲ **Figure 24–1.** An ill-advised CXR demonstrating tension pneumothorax. Clinical signs alone should be sufficient to diagnose this condition and avoid the life-threatening delay involved in obtaining an X-ray.

▶ Treatment

The treatment for a tension pneumothorax is immediate tube thoracostomy (Chapter 6). If a chest tube is not immediately available, needle thoracostomy with a large-bore (16-gauge or less) needle in the second intercostal space in the midclavicular line will convert the tension pneumothorax into a simple pneumothorax until a tube can be

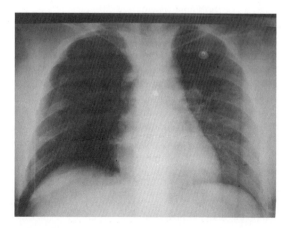

▲ **Figure 24–2.** The CXR demonstrates a large right pneumothorax with widening and deepening of the right costophrenic angle, also known as the deep sulcus sign. Occasionally this sign is the only radiographic indication of a pneumothorax in a supine patient.

placed. In this instance, the needle should be left in until a definitive chest tube can be placed. Opening the wound further with a gloved finger or a clamp can relieve a tension pneumothorax associated with a penetrating injury. For patients with a simple pneumothoraces secondary to trauma, traditional teaching has been to drain through a tube thoracostomy and admit the patient for observation. However, it has been shown that those with small pneumothoraces detected on CT scan appear at low risk for complications and may not require drainage. In addition, serial observations or simple aspiration have been shown to be safe in patients presenting later or with small simple pneumothoraces.

Di Bartolomeo S, Sanson G, Nardi G, Scian F, Michelutto V, Lattuada L: A population-based study on pneumothorax in severely traumatized patients. J Trauma 2001;51(4):677–682 [PMID: 11586158].

Miller A: Management of pneumothorax. Practitioner. 2002; 246(1631):108, 111–112 [PMID: 11852618] (Review).

Wilkerson R G, Stone M: Sensitivity of bedside ultrasound and supine anteroposterior chest radiographs for the identification of pneumothorax after blunt trauma. Acad Emerg Med 2010;17(1):11–17 [PMID: 20078434].

OPEN PNEUMOTHORAX (SUCKING CHEST WOUND)

Large penetrating wounds of the thorax result in an immediate pneumothorax. There is equilibration between intrathoracic and atmospheric pressure and so negative intrathoracic pressure cannot be generated. Effective ventilation is thus impaired since air goes through the chest wall rather than into the lung resulting in severe hypoxia. The diagnosis is obvious and therapy should be instituted immediately.

▶ Treatment

Management of an open pneumothorax should begin with assessment of the patients ABC's. All patients with a pneumothorax should be placed on 100% oxygen via nonrebreather. An occlusive dressing should be placed over the wound immediately followed by the placement of a chest tube. The occlusive dressing should be large enough to cover the wounds edges. The dressing should be taped on three side allowing air to escape from the pleural cavity but not reenter. Definitive treatment involves chest tube placement and wound closure.

MASSIVE HEMOTHORAX

Injury to the chest wall, great vessels, or lung can result in intrapleural bleeding or hemothorax. By definition, a massive hemothorax is defined by the rapid accumulation of greater than 1000–1500 ml of blood or one-third or more of the patient's blood volume in the chest cavity.

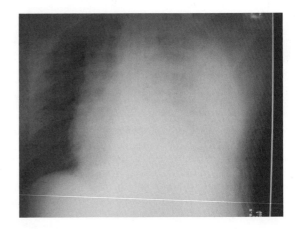

▲ **Figure 24–3.** Blunt trauma patient with left hemothorax.

Most commonly, a massive hemothorax is secondary to penetrating injury disrupting pulmonary or systemic blood vessels. In hemothorax associated with great vessel injury, 50% die immediately, 25% live 5–10 minutes, and 25% live 30 minutes or longer. Respiratory insufficiency is dependent on how much blood is lost. In massive injury, the affected lung is collapsed producing a right to left shunt. The loss of blood also leads to circulatory compromise.

▶ Diagnosis

Respiratory distress, tachypnea, and variable degree of hypoxia will be present. There will be dullness to percussion and decreased breath sounds on the affected side. Depending on the degree of blood loss, hypotension and flat neck veins may be present. Pulse pressure will be narrow. Small hemothoraces may be difficult to detect on supine patients. Diagnosis is confirmed by CXR (Figure 24–3). Small hemothoraces (<350 mL) are usually visible only as a small effusion on an upright CXR. Moderate effusions (350–1500 mL) will be seen as diffuse increase in opacity on the affected side. Large (>1500 mL) effusions will have a ground glass appearance on the supine film.

▶ Treatment

For the patients presenting with signs of massive hemothorax, tube thoracostomy should be performed immediately without waiting for diagnostic tests. For those with smaller hemothoraces, diagnosis can be confirmed before instituting therapy. Tube thoracostomy using one or two large-bore chest tubes allows for accurate assessment of current and ongoing blood loss. Autotransfusion should be considered for the patients with large bleeds (>1 L). Initial blood loss of more than 1.0–1.5 L or ongoing continuing loss of >200 mL/h for 2–4 hours requires surgery.

Mancini M. Hemothorax. Emedicine website. http://emedicine.medscape.com/article/425518-overview. Updated October 23, 2008. Accessed March 26, 2010.

Miller LA: Chest wall, lung, and pleural space trauma. Radiol Clin North Am 2006;44(2):213–224, viii [PMID: 16500204] (Review).

CARDIAC TAMPONADE

Cardiac tamponade occurs when arterial, ventricular, or atrial injury causes blood to leak into the pericardium. True tamponade is rare and most often associated with penetrating injuries. The pericardium is acutely not very distensible and tamponade can occur even with a small amount (200 mL) of blood. The increased intrapericardial pressure compresses the heart and decreases cardiac output. In addition, venous return and cardiac filling are decreased. Increased pressure may also lead to a decrease in myocardial perfusion. These factors together lead to a decrease in cardiac output. Hypotension and shock then can result.

▶ Diagnosis

Signs and symptoms of tamponade are nonspecific. Tachycardia and narrow pulse pressure are usually present. Beck's triad of hypotension, muffled heart tones, and distended neck veins is present in a minority of patients with tamponade from blunt trauma. Jugular venous distension may be absent because of coexisting hypovolemia. There are no specific findings on CXR that will confirm the diagnosis. Since tamponade can occur with a small effusion, heart size may not be significantly increased. Bedside focused assessment with sonography for trauma (FAST) examinations (Chapters 6 and 25) are performed in many emergency departments to quickly identify pericardial effusions in blunt and penetrating trauma patients. FAST examinations allow rapid detection of pericardial fluid, with high sensitivity and specificity. An emergency pericardiocentesis or thoracotomy can be lifesaving in an unstable patient with a pericardial effusion. In a stable patient, the diagnosis of pericardial effusion can be confirmed with transthoracic or transesophageal echocardiogram and define the hemodynamic impact. When ultrasound or echocardiography is not available, for the stable patient, CT scan is sensitive for detection of pericardial fluid. Cardiac dynamics are not assessable however.

▶ Treatment

Pericardiocentesis has been advocated in the past as both a diagnostic and therapeutic modality. However there are serious limitations. Pericardiocentesis has been reported to have up to 80% false negatives and 35% false positives. In acute injury, a large part of the pericardial blood may be clotted and therefore not aspirated through even a large-bore needle. Pericardiocentesis may injure the heart or other organs and may cause delays in getting definitive care.

With these caveats, in a stable patient, ultrasound-guided pericardiocentesis has been shown to be safe and reliable. In patients who are unstable or in severe shock with signs and symptoms consistent with cardiac tamponade, immediate thoracotomy allows relief of the tamponade and control of myocardial injury.

Exadaktylos AK, Sclabas G, Schmid SW, Schaller B, Zimmermann H: Do we really need routine computed tomographic scanning in the primary evaluation of blunt chest trauma in patients with "normal" chest radiograph? J Trauma 2001;51(6):1173–1176 [PMID: 11740271].

Tsang TS, Oh JK, Seward JB, Tajik AJ: Diagnostic value of echocardiography in cardiac tamponade. Herz 2000;25(8):734–740 [PMID: 11200121].

FLAIL CHEST

Flail chest occurs when a segment of the chest does not have bony contiguity with the rest of the thoracic cage. When negative intrathoracic pressure is generated on inspiration, the flail segment moves inward, thus reducing tidal volume. Usually a significant blunt force is required, eg, motor vehicle collision (MVC) or a fall from a height. The major problem is respiratory failure due to the underlying pulmonary injury.

▶ Diagnosis

The two major symptoms of flail chest are pain and respiratory distress. Tachypnea with shallow respirations secondary to pain will be seen. Paradoxical chest wall movement may not be seen in a conscious patient due to splinting of the chest wall. Crepitus is often present. Even with marked flail chest, the patient may be able to compensate initially for the reduced tidal volume by hyperventilating. When fatigue or underlying pulmonary injury develops, frank respiratory failure may supervene.

▶ Treatment

Supplemental oxygen is the first-line treatment. Pain control with intravenous morphine or fentanyl should be instituted early. Patient controlled administration (PCA) of an opiod infusion is often effective for cooperative patients. Epidural infusion of a local anaesthetic agent provides near complete analgesia allowing the patient to resume normal inspiration and cough without the risk of respiratory depression. The addition of a nonsteroidal may provide adequate relief, but should be withheld until other injuries have been excluded. Consider early intubation and mechanical ventilation in any patient with ongoing hypoxia or significant increased work of breathing. Approximately 50% of patients will need immediate intubation. Indications for early intubation include marked hypoxia, hypercapnea, or inadequate breathing. External chest wall supports (taping, sandbags) reduce pain with movement of the flail segment, but they also reduce vital capacity and may worsen respiratory function and are therefore not indicated. Surgical fixation should only be considered in cases where thoracotomy is being performed for other injuries.

Pettiford BL, Luketich JD, Landreneau RJ: The management of flail chest. Thorac Surg Clin 2007;17(1):25–33 [PMID: 17650694].

POTENTIALLY LIFE-THREATENING INJURIES IDENTIFIED ON SECONDARY SURVEY

A careful and thorough secondary survey will identify multiple non-life-threatening chest injuries. Their prompt recognition and treatment may lead to an overall reduction in morbidity and mortality.

PULMONARY CONTUSION

Pulmonary contusions are injuries of the lung parenchyma with hemorrhage and edema without associated laceration. They are the most frequent intrathoracic injuries in nonpenetrating chest trauma. They occur in approximately 30–75% of patients with significant blunt chest trauma. Pulmonary contusions typically occur at the site of impact and are often associated with other thoracic injuries such as rib fractures and flail chest, although they may occur alone. Pneumonia is the most common complication of pulmonary contusion, but their presence is a risk factor for the development of acute respiratory distress syndrome and long-term disability as well. Associated medical conditions, such as chronic obstructive pulmonary disease, increase the likelihood of complications from pulmonary contusion and should lower the threshold for early intubation.

▶ Diagnosis

Pulmonary contusion is often silent during the initial trauma evaluation. Significant traumatic mechanism as well as the presence of other associated thoracic and extrathoracic injuries should raise one's suspicion for the presence of pulmonary contusion. The most important sign of pulmonary contusion is hypoxia. The degree of hypoxemia directly correlates with the size of the contusion. Large contusions will lead to significant respiratory distress. Other clinical findings suggestive of pulmonary contusion include dyspnea, hemoptysis, tachycardia, and other evidence of chest injury such as palpable rib fractures, chest wall bruising, decreased breath sounds, or crackles on pulmonary auscultation.

Radiographic findings by CXR may range from patchy interstitial infiltrates to complete lobar opacification. CXR will initially miss a substantial number of pulmonary contusions, but as a result of ongoing hemorrhage and edema, radiographic evidence of contusion is usually apparent within 6 hours of injury. Since the size of the contusion may help predict the clinical course for the patient, thoracic CT may provide additional useful information. Animal studies suggest that CT will identify contusions in 100% of those with experimentally induced pulmonary injury; therefore, CXR should be followed by CT in the patients where suspicion for undetected injury is high and identification of the injury will alter their management.

▶ Treatment

Early recognition and treatment of pulmonary contusion is essential to preventing long-term complications. The mainstay of treatment is supportive care and consists of the careful use of intravenous fluids so as to keep the patient euvolemic, supplemental oxygen, chest physiotherapy, and if severe, the use of mechanical ventilation with positive end-expiratory pressure.

▶ Disposition

Most patients with radiographic evidence of pulmonary contusion or clinical findings suggestive of pulmonary contusion should be admitted for monitoring and respiratory support. Exceptions to this would include young adults with minor contusions and no underlying pulmonary disease.

Klein Y, Cohn SM, Proctor KG: Lung contusion: pathophysiology and management. Curr Opin Anaesthesiol 2002:15(1):65–68 [PMID: 17019186].

Miller LA: Chest wall, lung, and pleural space trauma. Radiol Clin North Am 2006;44(2):213–224, viii [PMID: 16500204] (Review).

Miller PR et al: ARDS after pulmonary contusion: accurate measurement of contusion volume identifies high-risk patients. J Trauma. 2001 Aug;51(2):223–228 [PMID: 11493778].

MYOCARDIAL CONTUSION

It is estimated that 15–20% of patients sustaining significant thoracic trauma have some degree of cardiac involvement. Myocardial contusions are distinct areas of hemorrhage that are typically subendocardial but may extend transmurally. The right ventricle is most commonly involved due to its proximity to the sternum. Contusions of the myocardium typically produce wall motion abnormalities that may lead to conduction defects, dysrhythmias, or a decrease in cardiac output leading to cardiogenic shock.

▶ Diagnosis

The clinical presentation of myocardial contusion is nonspecific. Patients are often asymptomatic but may complain of chest pain, have subtle ECG changes, or present with hypotension secondary to cardiac dysmotility. Specific standardized criteria for the diagnosis of myocardial contusion do not exist. Studies of blunt trauma patients looking for evidence of cardiac contusion have classically used one or more of the following criteria:

1. **ECG**—A normal ECG does not exclude the possibility of myocardial contusion, but it is the best screening tool. An ECG should be obtained in all patients with significant thoracic trauma, particularly if there are concomitant injuries such as flail chest, rib fractures, or pulmonary contusion. An ECG should also be obtained in trauma patients complaining of chest pain, with unexplained hypotension, and those with a history of coronary artery disease. The most common finding by ECG in myocardial contusion is sinus tachycardia (ST) followed by nonspecific ST and T wave changes. Right bundle branch block is also commonly seen. A range of dysrhythmias and conduction disturbances may be evident however, including ST elevation, atrial fibrillation, atrial flutter, premature ventricular contractions, ventricular tachycardia, ventricular fibrillation, first-degree heart block, and right bundle branch block. While a normal ECG cannot 100% exclude the presence of a myocardial contusion, the literature suggests that very few patients with normal ECGs develop complications.

2. **Biochemical markers**—There is much debate in recent literature regarding the value of obtaining cardiac enzymes in the evaluation of the patient with potential myocardial contusion. Creatine kinase MB (CK-MB) is nonspecific for cardiac injury in the setting of trauma and is often elevated in cases of skeletal muscle, diaphragm, liver, or bowel injury. Both Troponin T and Troponin I have been shown to be very specific for cardiac injury in trauma but have poor sensitivity. Cardiac enzymes have not been shown to predict the development of complications or need for hospital admission.

3. **Echocardiography**—Transthoracic and transesophageal echocardiography should not be used as screening tools for myocardial contusion. They are best used in the evaluation of patients with unexplained hypotension or persistent ECG abnormalities to exclude other potential cardiac injuries such as pericardial tamponade and ventricular rupture. While both studies will identify wall motion abnormalities that are consistent with myocardial contusion, they have not been shown to predict or prevent clinical complications.

▶ **Treatment**

There is no particular treatment for myocardial contusion other than to treat the potential complications as they arise. Patients should be monitored at all times. Dysrhythmias should be treated as discussed in previous chapters. There is no role for the administration of prophylactic antidysrhythmics. Patients who subsequently develop myocardial infarction should be treated as such, but thrombolytics should not be used in the trauma patient.

▶ **Disposition**

Asymptomatic stable patients with normal ECGs and no evidence of other thoracic injury may be safely discharged from the emergency department. Elderly patients and those with a history of coronary artery disease, significant blunt thoracic trauma, ECG changes, or hypotension should be admitted for monitoring.

El-Chami MF, Nicholson W, Helmy T: Blunt cardiac trauma. J Emerg Med 2008;35(2):127–133 [PMID: 16568196].

DIAPHRAGMATIC HERNIA

Diaphragmatic hernias have been reported in 1–5% of patients sustaining blunt chest or abdominal trauma. They result either by direct violation of the diaphragm or significant intra-abdominal or intrathoracic pressure applied to the diaphragm resulting in its rupture. The right side is affected up to three times less than the left because it is relatively well protected by the liver. Up to 50% of these injuries are missed on the initial trauma evaluation, and their delayed presentation may not be clinically significant until herniation of abdominal contents through the diaphragm results in obstruction, incarceration, strangulation, perforation, or even death. Once a tear in the diaphragm occurs, it will not heal spontaneously, allowing for the herniation of abdominal contents into the chest cavity. Delayed presentations of blunt diaphragmatic rupture have been reported up to 50 years after the primary traumatic event.

▶ **Diagnosis**

Patients with diaphragmatic hernias may be asymptomatic, particularly in the acute phase, or may present with symptoms of bowel obstruction. Delayed presentation is common with nonspecific respiratory or bowel complaints since early diagnosis is difficult to establish and often missed.

1. **CXR**—The CXR is a valuable screening tool in detecting blunt diaphragmatic rupture. The initial X-ray is interpreted as normal in up to 50% of acute cases but will be abnormal in almost 100% of those with delayed presentations. Findings on an upright CXR suggestive of diaphragmatic rupture include elevation or irregularity of the diaphragmatic border, unilateral pleural thickening, obvious herniation of abdominal contents into the chest cavity, and the presence of a nasogastric tube in the chest cavity (Figure 24–4).

2. **CT**—CT scans are often used preoperatively in the hemodynamically stable patients but have had less than satisfactory results in reporting isolated diaphragmatic injuries. Right-sided lesions are often missed because the contour of the right diaphragm is difficult to discern from the contour of the liver.

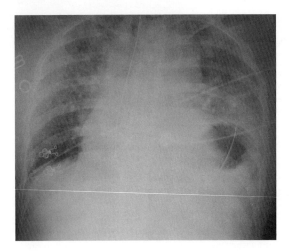

▲ **Figure 24–4.** Adult female with blunt thoracoabdominal trauma from an MVC. CXR demonstrates the nasogastric tube in the chest indicative of a ruptured left hemidiaphragm.

▶ **Treatment**

Surgical reduction of the hernia and repair of the diaphragm is mandatory in all patients with diaphragmatic rupture. Care should be taken to avoid abdominal injury when placing a chest tube in patients with concomitant hemothorax or pneumothorax.

Nursal TZ et al: Traumatic diaphragmatic hernias: a report of 26 cases. Hernia 2001;5(1):25–29 [PMID: 11387719].

Singh S et al: Diaphragmatic rupture presenting 50 years after the traumatic event. J Trauma 2000;49(1):156–159 [PMID: 10912874].

ESOPHAGEAL DISRUPTION

Esophageal disruption or perforation is an infrequent injury sustained secondary to blunt trauma. The mechanism of injury is unclear, but most occur during high-speed motor vehicle collisions and are typically associated with other serious thoracic injuries. While their occurrence is rare, the reported mortality is more than 20% because of its resultant complications of mediastinitis, which include pericarditis, pneumonitis, empyema, and even aortic erosion.

▶ **Diagnosis**

Esophageal injuries are difficult to diagnose. The symptoms and signs are often nonspecific and masked by other serious injuries. It should always be suspected in the patient with evidence of serious neck, thoracic, back, or abdominal injury. Patients may complain of throat pain, dysphagia, odynophagia, hoarseness, choking, chest pain, hematemesis, dyspnea, or continued neck pain despite appropriate treatment and immobilization. Neck redness, swelling, unexplained tachycardia, subcutaneous emphysema of the neck or chest, and bloody nasogastric tube contents may be found on physical examination.

Radiologic signs on CXR suggestive of esophageal injury include pneumomediastinum, widened mediastinum, and left pleural effusion. Gastrograffin followed by barium swallow and esophagoscopy are probably the best diagnostic tools available for the detection of esophageal perforation; however, detailed exploratory surgery may be necessary for definitive diagnosis.

▶ **Treatment**

Treatment of esophageal perforations depends on the location and the extent of the injury. Nonoperative management with drainage, antibiotics, and nutritional support may be appropriate for select injuries, but most require aggressive surgical management to prevent extensive spread of infection to the mediastinal and pleural cavities.

Monzon JR, Ryan B: Thoracic esophageal perforation secondary to blunt trauma. J Trauma 2000;49(6):1129–1131 [PMID: 11843720].

AORTIC DISRUPTION

Traumatic aortic rupture is a common cause of death in blunt trauma. Injury is typically caused by rapid deceleration and shearing forces sustained in motor vehicle accidents, falls, and crush injuries and most commonly involves the descending segment of the aorta just past the origin of the left subclavian artery. More than 80% of patients die at the scene. Another 10–20% of patients with aortic disruption will die within the first hour. Rapid diagnosis and treatment is essential for limiting the mortality associated with these injuries.

▶ **Diagnosis**

Aortic injury should be considered in all patients involved in rapid deceleration accidents such as motor vehicle collisions at speeds greater than 30 miles/h or falls from greater than 10 feet. Clinical signs and symptoms suggestive of aortic injury include chest pain, back pain, dyspnea, hoarseness, intrascapular murmur, and extremity pain caused by ischemia. Patients may be hypertensive, hypotensive, or may present with pseudocoarctation where the upper extremities are hypertensive and the lower extremities have minimal blood pressure and pulse deficits. Thirty percent of patients with traumatic aortic injury have no external signs of trauma to the chest. Other patient factors that can raise a clinician's index of suspicion for TAI include age >50,

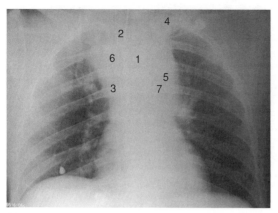

A

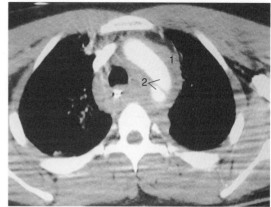

B

▲ **Figure 24–5.** **A:** CXR of hypotensive adult male injured in a high-speed MVC. Findings: (1) widened mediastinum, (2) deviation of the trachea to the right, (3) widening of the right paratracheal stripe, (4) left apical cap, (5) blurring of the aortic knob, (6) deviation of the nasogastric tube to the right, and (7) obliteration of the aortopulmonary window. **B:** Computed tomography scan of the chest demonstrates (1) periaortic hematoma and (2) a true and false aortic lumen; widening of the right paratracheal stripe is also noted. **C:** (1) Periaortic hematoma is present with (2) a small left hemothorax.

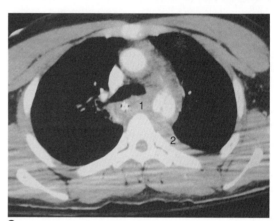

C

unrestrained driver, ejected passenger or pedestrians struck by a motor vehicle.

1. **CXR**—CXR is a screening tool for blunt aortic injury and is commonly used to determine the need for further studies. Mediastinal widening more than 8 cm is the most commonly cited abnormality on CXR that leads to further workup. Other findings suggestive of aortic injury include indistinct aortic knob, left mainstem bronchus depression, tracheal deviation to the right, nasogastric tube deviation, widening of the right paratracheal stripe (>5 mm), apical capping, and obliteration of the space between the pulmonary artery and the aorta (Figure 24–5). Despite its use as a screening tool, CXRs are normal in 2–5% of patients with aortic injury.

2. **Angiography**—Angiography has historically been the gold standard for diagnosis of aortic injury but is rarely employed in clinical practice today. Angiography is expensive, time consuming, invasive, and requires a large dye load. Because the clinical indicators for blunt aortic injury are often nonspecific, a large number of negative aortograms have been performed in the past. Over the last decade, CT of the chest has been used in the evaluation of aortic injury with angiography saved for those patients with indeterminant findings by CT.

3. **Chest CT**—CT is less expensive than angiography and can be performed much more quickly. With the newer-generation scanners and the use of intravenous contrast and consistent protocols, the sensitivity and specificity for aortic injury approaches 100%, particularly when criteria for positive scans include periaortic hematoma along with direct signs of aortic injury.

▶ **Treatment**

Treatment of blunt aortic injury includes pharmacologic management of blood pressure in combination with prompt surgical or endovascular repair.

Dyer DS et al: Thoracic aortic injury: How predictive is mechanism and is chest computed tomography a reliable screening tool? A prospective study of 1561 patients. J Trauma 2000;48(4): 673–682 [PMID: 10780601].

Nagy K et al: Guidelines for the diagnosis and management of blunt aortic injury: An EAST Practice Management Guidelines Work Group. J Trauma 2000;48(6):1128–1143 [PMID: 10866262].

O'Conor CE: Diagnosing Traumatic rupture of the thoracic aorta in the emergency department. Emerg Med J2004;21:414–419 [PMID: 15208221].

TRACHEOBRONCHIAL INJURY

Injury to the trachea or bronchus as a result of blunt trauma is relatively uncommon but can be quite severe. Approximately 80% of patients with tracheobronchial injuries die before reaching a hospital. Tracheobronchial injuries are usually the result of motor vehicle accidents and crush injuries. Right-sided bronchial injuries occur more commonly and are typically more severe, while almost 80% occur within 2 cm of the carina. The diagnosis of tracheobronchial injury is missed in at least 25% of patients during the initial trauma evaluation.

▶ Diagnosis

Failure to recognize tracheobronchial injury during the initial trauma evaluation is common. Patients may be comfortable on room air or may present in acute respiratory distress. The most common clinical symptoms and signs suggestive of injury to the trachea or bronchus are dyspnea and subcutaneous emphysema of the neck or upper thoracic region, but may also include hoarseness, hemoptysis, hypoxia, and persistent pneumothorax despite appropriate tube thoracostomy. CXR findings indicative of tracheobronchial injury include subcutaneous emphysema, pneumomediastinum, pneumothorax, and peribronchial air.

▶ Treatment

All patients in respiratory distress with suspected tracheobronchial injury should be endotracheally intubated, preferably over a bronchoscope if time allows. Blind intubation is discouraged as it may result in the complete disruption of small tracheal lacerations. Stable patients with suspected trauma to the trachea or bronchi should undergo immediate bronchoscopy for definitive evaluation and localization of the injury followed by operative repair.

Cassada DC et al: Acute injuries of the trachea and major bronchi: importance of early diagnosis. Ann Thorac Surg 2000;69(5):1563–1567 [PMID: 10881842].

Kiser AC et al: Blunt tracheobronchial injuries: treatment and outcomes. Ann Thorac Surg 2001;71(6):2059–2065 [PMID: 11426809].

▼ OTHER INJURIES

RIB FRACTURES

Rib fractures are the most common injury sustained in blunt thoracic trauma. They are usually sustained in motor vehicle accidents. Fractures of the first rib usually indicate severe trauma because of the necessary force to produce such an injury. Fractures may cause localized pain, crepitance, pain with inspiration, and dyspnea and may even cause pneumothorax or hemothorax. Mortality increases with the number of ribs involved. The pain associated with rib fractures may lead to hypoventilation, atelectasis, retained secretions, and finally pneumonia.

▶ Diagnosis

CXR is the screening tool of choice for the detection of rib fractures, although up to 50% of rib fractures cannot be detected on CXR. CT scan will often diagnose occult rib fractures. Dedicated rib views of the chest are unnecessary because they are not generally helpful in the management of patients with rib fractures.

▶ Treatment

Rapid mobilization, respiratory support, and pain management are the mainstays of treatment for the patient with multiple rib fractures. Continuous body positioning and oscillation therapy prevent hypoventilation and atelectasis by promoting redistribution of ventilation and perfusion to various lung segments. Mechanical ventilation allows for healing of the ribs and prevention of complications in the patient with respiratory failure. Incentive spirometry is excellent supportive therapy in stable patients. Pain control is paramount in facilitating adequate ventilation. Epidural anesthesia with bupivicaine controls pain without causing sedation and impairing the cough reflex.

▶ Disposition

Young, healthy patients with isolated rib fractures without evidence of other serious underlying injury may be treated with pain medications and deep breathing exercises with incentive spirometry. They do not require routine admittance or serial radiographic studies. Admission should be considered for elderly or other patients with serious underlying lung disease and isolated rib fractures. These patients have a higher complication rate due to a higher prevalence of hypoventilation, atelectasis, and pneumonia.

Easter A: Management of patients with multiple rib fractures. Am J Crit Care 2001;10(5):320–327 [PMID: 11548565].

Miller LA: Chest wall, lung, and pleural space trauma. Radiol Clin North Am 2006;44(2):213–224, viii [PMID: 16500204] (Review).

STERNAL FRACTURE

Most sternal fractures are associated with a direct blow. They are most common in postmenopausal females presumably secondary to osteopenia.

▶ Diagnosis

Pleuritic midline chest pain with focal tenderness over the sternum may be present. There may be some pain with respiration, but there should be no pulmonary compromise. Pulmonary contusions or blunt cardiac injury may accompany sternal fracture and should be considered. A rare complication of sternal fractures is a posterior sternoclavicular dislocation which can result in mediastinal displacement of the clavicular heads with accompanying superior vena caval obstruction.

▶ Treatment

In the absence of complications, therapy for sternal fractures is mainly symptomatic. Give adequate analgesia with narcotics as necessary and encourage deep breathing.

▶ Disposition

Patients with isolated sternal fractures, with no evidence of other injuries, can be safely sent home. Patients with cardiovascular complications should be admitted. Admission should also be considered for patients in whom analgesia cannot be obtained with standard doses of narcotics or those who have limited social support.

Miller LA: Chest wall, lung, and pleural space trauma. Radiol Clin North Am 2006;44(2):213–224, viii [PMID: 16500204] (Review).

Sadaba JR, Oswal D, Munsch CM: Management of isolated sternal fractures: determining the risk of blunt cardiac injury. Ann R Coll Surg Engl 2000;82(3):162–166 [PMID: 10858676] (Review).

SYSTEMIC AIR EMBOLISM

Lung trauma in which there is laceration of air passages, lung parenchyma, or blood vessels may result in a direct communication between these structures. Air can enter the pulmonary venous system as a result of a gradient caused by low pulmonary venous pressure (hypovolemia) or increased airway pressure (positive-pressure ventilation, tension pneumothorax). Pulmonary venous air embolizes systemically including coronary and cerebral circulation. Air embolization occurs most commonly after penetrating trauma.

▶ Diagnosis

There are several findings that are suggestive of air embolism. Hemoptysis, circulatory, and CNS dysfunction immediately after initiation of positive-pressure ventilation are suggestive. Focal neurologic abnormalities in the absence of head injury are common. Circulatory arrest after the initiation of mechanical ventilation suggests air embolism. Fundoscopic examination may reveal air in the retinal vessels. Air in arterial blood gases (not due to froth) is diagnostic. Transesophageal echocardiography has been suggested as a diagnostic tool.

▶ Treatment

Oxygenation is the first-line treatment. Selective lung ventilation has been advocated as a means of isolating the affected lung and stopping or minimizing the flow of gas into the circulation. Alternatively, high-frequency ventilation has been shown to be effective by allowing decreased ventilatory volumes and pressures. For moribund patients, thoracotomy and clamping of the hilum of the affected lung has been advocated. Cerebral air embolism has been treated with hyperbaric oxygen therapy, but other priorities may preclude or delay its use.

Abu-Zidan FM, Goudie A, Monaghan M: Traumatic air embolism. J Trauma 2002;52:187 [PMID: 11791075].

TRAUMATIC ASPHYXIA

Severe crush injury of the thorax or abdomen can cause retrograde flow of blood from the right heart into the great veins of the head and neck.

▶ Diagnosis

There is purplish-bluish color of the face and neck. Subconjuntival and retinal hemorrhages are common. Intracerebral bleeds are uncommon, but loss of consciousness or neurologic abnormalities can be caused by cerebral hypoxia. The clinical significance of traumatic asphyxia is the possibility of intrathoracic injuries associated with the severe crushing force.

▶ Treatment and Disposition

There is no specific therapy except oxygenation. Other injuries should be treated appropriately. Patients should be hospitalized for observation.

COMMOTIO CORDIS

Commotio cordis is the condition of sudden cardiac death or near sudden cardiac death after blunt, low-impact chest wall trauma in the absence of structural cardiac abnormality. Ventricular fibrillation is the most commonly induced arrhythmia in commotio cordis. Young male athletes aged 5–18 years are particularly at risk for this catastrophe. It has been described after blows to the chest from baseballs, softballs, hockey pucks, and other objects. Death is usually instantaneous, and successful resuscitation is uncommon.

Madias C, Maron BJ, Weinstock J et al: Commotio cordis–sudden cardiac death with chest wall impact. J Cardiovasc Electrophysiol 2007;18(1):115–122 [PMID: 17229310] (Review).

PENETRATING TRAUMA

Penetrating trauma to the chest is usually inflicted by stabbing or gunshot but can include other foreign bodies and impalement injuries as well. Stab wounds commonly injure the ascending aorta while gunshot wounds more typically injure the descending thoracic aorta, although laceration of the pericardium and any of the thoracic great vessels may occur.

Diagnosis

Information regarding the type of weapon, length or caliber of weapon, distance from the weapon, and amount of hemorrhage at the scene can be very helpful when evaluating the patient with penetrating thoracic trauma. Most patients are hemodynamically unstable and a rapid but thorough examination is essential. The ABCs should be addressed first.

During the secondary survey, the patient should be evaluated for signs of vascular injury including unequal blood pressures of the extremities, new vascular bruits, and the classic signs of pericardial tamponade: distended neck veins, muffled heart sounds, and hypotension. A CXR should be obtained immediately to identify pneumothorax, hemothorax, or foreign body. Placing radioopaque markers at the sites of wound entry and exit can be helpful in the interpretation of the CXR. Bedside emergency FAST examinations for the evaluation of pericardial tamponade can be extremely helpful in identifying the need for thoracotomy in the penetrating trauma patient with signs of shock. The same life-threatening and potentially life-threatening injuries described in blunt trauma can occur with penetrating trauma to the chest as well and should be managed as discussed in those sections.

Treatment

Significant shock should be addressed immediately with intravenous fluid boluses and blood transfusion, although there is some data to suggest that aggressive fluid resuscitation may increase the amount of uncontrolled hemorrhage and subsequent mortality. Patients with pericardial tamponade require emergent pericardial window or thoracotomy. Tube thoracostomy should be performed in all patients with evidence of pneumothorax or hemothorax. Autotransfusion is indicated in patients with large hemothoraces. Patients with initial chest tube blood loss exceeding 1500 mL, significant ongoing hemorrhage of >200 mL/h for 2–4 hours, or persistent hypotension should be taken directly to the operating room. Impaled objects should never be removed in the emergency department as they may actually provide tamponade to surrounding vascular structures. Those patients should be stabilized with removal of the object performed in the operating room. Angiography is the gold standard for the evaluation of hemodynamically stable patients at high risk for great vessel injury based on the trajectory of the wound, although CT angiography has increasingly demonstrated reliability.

Asymptomatic patients sustaining low-risk peripheral wounds with normal physical examinations and negative initial CXRs may be safely discharged to home after a 3-hour observation and repeat negative CXR. Those who develop delayed pneumothorax during this observation period require tube thoracostomy and admission.

Role of Emergency Department Thoracotomy

The role of emergency department thoracotomy is controversial. Indications for thoracotomy are (1) penetrating thoracic wound with agonal state or recent loss of vital signs, deterioration or cardiac arrest after care has been initiated, or uncontrolled hemorrhage from the thoracic inlet or out of a chest tube; (2) need for open cardiac massage or occlusion of the descending thoracic aorta to provide increased blood flow to the heart and brain prior to a laparotomy; and (3) suspected subclavian vessel injury with intrapleural exsanguination. Contraindications to thoracotomy include penetrating trauma with no signs of life in the field or blunt trauma with no signs of life on arrival in the emergency department. Thoracotomy is not indicated unless a qualified surgical backup is present.

Emergency department thoracotomy is best used in patients sustaining penetrating thoracic injuries whom have witnessed a cardiopulmonary arrest in the emergency department or lose signs of life during a short transport to the emergency department. Survival rates for cardiac injuries and stab wounds are typically better than noncardiac injuries and gunshot wounds. Thoracotomy for penetrating injuries yields an overall survival rate of approximately 11%.

Aihara R, Millham FH, Blansfield J, Hirsch EF: Emergency room thoracotomy for penetrating chest injury: effect of an institutional protocol. J Trauma 2001;50(6):1027–1030 [PMID: 11426116].

Meredith JW, Hoth JJ: Thoracic trauma: when and how to intervene. Surg Clin North Am. 2007;87(1):95–118, vii [PMID: 17127125] (Review).

Abdominal Trauma

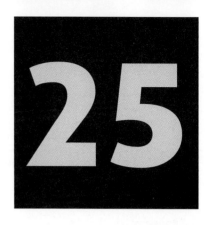

Sonya C. Melville, MD
Daniel E. Melville, MD[1]

▼ IMMEDIATE MANAGEMENT OF LIFE-THREATENING INJURIES

Abdominal injuries are potentially life-threatening and should be approached with caution. Following trauma, the abdomen may be a sanctuary for a broad spectrum of injuries that, if not discovered and corrected expeditiously, may lead to deleterious consequences. Traditionally these injuries are classified as either blunt trauma or penetrating injuries. The majority of blunt abdominal trauma is secondary to motor vehicle collisions, whereas the majority of penetrating injuries is predominantly secondary to gunshot or stab wounds. Patients with abdominal trauma require rapid assessment, stabilization, and early surgical consultation when indicated to maximize the chances of a successful outcome.

▶ Assessment

Initial management of all trauma patients is the same, and abdominal trauma is no exception. Following ATLS protocols, begin the assessment with a rapid primary survey, including evaluation of the airway, breathing, circulation, disability, and exposure.

A. Airway

Assess the airway while maintaining cervical spine immobilization until potential injury is ruled out. Jaw thrust without head extension can be used to open the airway of a trauma patient. Administer high-flow oxygen, and intubate the patient if indicated.

B. Breathing

First assess breathing by auscultating for breath sounds. Diminished or absent breath sounds should raise clinical suspicion for a possible pneumothorax. Next, inspect for asymmetry of chest wall movement, open wounds, or flail segments. Then palpate the chest wall carefully. Palpable crepitus may indicate a pneumothorax or rib fractures. Rapidly perform needle decompression or tube thoracostomy when indicated (See Chapter 24). Pulse oximetry and capnography may be useful.

C. Circulation

Assess circulation. If gross external hemorrhage is present, control with direct pressure. Assess pulses, capillary refill, and blood pressure. Obtain intravenous access, preferably with at least two large-bore (≥16-gauge) peripheral catheters. If peripheral intravenous access is inadequate or unattainable, place a central venous catheter or interosseous line. Begin fluid resuscitation. The FAST examination is important at this stage of the evaluation, especially in hemodynamically

[1]This chapter is a revision of the chapter by Roger Humphries, MD from the 6th edition.

unstable patients, where a positive FAST exam would be an immediate indication for emergency laparotomy.

D. Disability

To assess disability, complete a brief and focused neurologic examination to document the patient's current mental status. The examination should include an assessment of pupillary size and reactivity, a determination of the patient's Glasgow Coma Scale score, and notation of any focal neurologic deficits such as unilateral weakness or poor muscle tone. Ideally, assessment of disability should be performed before administering pain medications, sedatives, or paralytics.

E. Exposure

In order to complete a thorough secondary survey, the patient must be fully exposed. Completely undress the patient while taking precautions to prevent or recognize and correct associated hypothermia. Begin a more thorough secondary survey, including logrolling the patient and examining all skin folds, the back, and axillae for any signs of trauma (eg, contusions, hematomas, abrasions, or penetrating wounds). Attempt to identify all wounds and document their location. To help identify the trajectory of bullets, place a radiopaque marker (eg, paper clip) at the wound site prior to obtaining X-rays. Do not remove impaled foreign bodies because they may be providing hemostasis from a vascular injury. Most foreign body removal should be performed with surgical consultation in a more controlled setting. Describe each wound, and avoid using terms such as entrance or exit wound on initial presentation, because it is often difficult to correctly make this assessment visually. These determinations are best left to a forensic pathologist.

Any penetrating injury below the level of the nipple line warrants evaluation for intra-abdominal injury. For patients involved in motor vehicle collisions, carefully examine the chest and abdomen looking for ecchymosis or erythema in the area of the clavicles or across the abdomen. The classic "seat-belt sign" or linear bruising across the lower abdomen is a marker for intra-abdominal injury, present in approximately 25% of patients with this finding. Examine the abdomen for any tenderness, distention, rigidity, or guarding. It is often difficult to assess bowel sounds at this stage of the examination. Evaluate the pelvis for antero-posterior or lateral instability with gentle pressure; this does not require much force and should not be repeatedly performed. Examine the genitalia and look for blood at the urethral meatus, especially in males. Perform digital rectal examination in any patient with abdominal trauma to look for gross blood, assess sphincter tone, identify a high-riding prostate, and to note any other evidence of trauma. There is no role for occult blood testing acutely in a trauma. If blood at the urethral meatus or a high-riding prostate is present, placement of a urinary catheter is contraindicated and a retrograde urethrogram is required to evaluate for potential urethral injury.

▶ Treatment

A. Fluid Resuscitation

Hemodynamic support is an early goal in the treatment of trauma patient. The use of crystalloids is currently recommended in trauma resuscitation but the concept of acute fluid resuscitation is evolving and may represent an area of some controversy. Animal and human studies have demonstrated deleterious effects of aggressive fluid resuscitation, particularly if penetrating trauma is present. Rapid infusion of large amounts of crystalloids may disrupt the formation of the soft clot and dilute the clotting factors, leading to increased bleeding. The results are less clear in the setting of blunt trauma. The amount of fluid given should be tailored to each individual patient. Also, blood pressure alone is not the best indicator of the level of shock. Attempts to make the patient normotensive are not recommended. A more reasonable goal may be to obtain systolic blood pressure of 80–90 mm Hg or a mean arterial pressure of 70 mm Hg. Crystalloids remain first-line fluids, followed by infusions of packed red blood cells. Other blood products, such as fresh frozen plasma and platelets, may be indicated in potentially uncontrollable hemorrhage (eg, deep truncal injury.) Recombinant Factor VIIa is used as an adjunct to other blood products in the setting of massive hemorrhage. The CRASH-2 trial, which tested an infusion of tranexamic acid, demonstrated a 9% reduction in death for traumatized patients with suspected hemorrhage whom were given the drug within 8 hours of injury. While certainly not standard of care at this time, this treatment may become widely adopted in next few years as another option to employ in treatment of significant hemorrhage in the setting of trauma.

B. Indications for Emergency Laparotomy

Most patients with penetrating abdominal injuries will also require laparotomy given the high incidence of intra-abdominal injury once the fascia has been violated. Hemodynamically unstable patients sustaining blunt or penetrating trauma with a positive screening test (such as focused assessment with sonography for trauma [FAST] examination or diagnostic peritoneal lavage [DPL]) require laparotomy to control hemorrhage and evaluate for intra-abdominal injuries. Although there is no debate that patients with peritonitis or hemodynamic instability should undergo urgent laparotomy after penetrating trauma to the abdomen, it is also clear that certain stable patients without peritonitis may be managed without operation. Routine laparotomy is NOT indicated in hemodynamically stable patients with knife stab wounds if there is no evidence of peritonitis or diffuse abdominal tenderness. Routine laparotomy is also NOT routinely indicated in stable patients with gunshot wounds if wounds are tangential and without peritoneal signs. Initially stable blunt trauma patients with identified abdominal injuries should be carefully observed so that if they become hemodynamically unstable they can rapidly receive operative intervention. Laparoscopy for certain penetrating injuries has helped in eliminating nontherapeutic laparotomies. Patients with obvious diaphragmatic injury noted on chest X-ray require emergency laparotomy. Patients considered to be at very low risk for having intra-abdominal injury (particularly intra-abdominal injury requiring acute intervention) have no hypotension, no GCS < 14, no costal margin tenderness, no abdominal tenderness, no hematuria ≥25 RBC/hpf, no hematocrit < 30, and no femur fracture.

C. Surgical Consultation

It is imperative to seek early surgical consultation in the management of patients with abdominal trauma, especially if the patient is hemodynamically unstable. Many stable patients with blunt abdominal injuries can initially be treated with nonoperative management. Not all blunt and penetrating abdominal injuries require immediate operative intervention but the majority will require observation and repeat examinations at a minimum.

van den Elsen MJ, Leenen LP, Kesecioglu J: Hemodynamic support of the trauma patient. Curr Opin Anaesthesiol. 2010; 23(2):269-75. [PMID: 20061942].

Pepe PE, Dutton RP, Fowler RL: Preoperative resuscitation of the trauma patient. Curr Opin Anaesthesiol 2008;21(2): 216–221 [PMID: 184434].

Holcomb JB: Use of recombinant activated factor VII to treat the acquired coagulopathy of trauma. J Trauma 2005;58(6): 1298–1303 [PMID: 15995488].

Woodruff SI, Dougherty AL, Dye JL, Mohrle CR, Galarneau MR: Use of recombinant factor VIIA for control of combat-related haemorrhage. Emerg Med J 2010;27(2): 121–124 [PMID: 20156864].

Como JJ, Bokhari F, Chiu WC, Duane TM, Holevar MR, Tanoh MA, Ivatury RR, Scalea TM: Practice management guidelines for selective nonoperative management of penetrating abdominal trauma. J Trauma 2010;68(3):721–733 [PMID: 20220426].

Ahmed N, Whelan J, Brownlee J, Chari V, Chung R: The contribution of laparoscopy in evaluation of penetrating abdominal wounds. J Am Coll Surg 2005;201(2):213–216 [PMID: 16038818].

Holmes JF, Wisner DH, McGahan JP, Mower WR, Kuppermann N: Clinical prediction rules for identifying adults at very low risk for intra-abdominal injuries after blunt trauma. Ann Emerg Med 2009;54(4):575–584 [PMID: 19457583].

Shakur H, Roberts I, Bautista R et al: Effects of tranexamic acid on death, vascular occlusive events, and blood transfusion in trauma patients with significant haemorrhage (CRASH-2): a randomised, placebo-controlled trial. Lancet 2010;376:23–32 [PMID: 20554319].

▶ Diagnostic Testing

A. Laboratory Evaluation

Initial laboratory evaluation in the traumatically injured patient should include hemoglobin, hematocrit, and platelet count to establish a baseline. A blood-type and screen should be ordered in case transfusion of packed red cells is needed. A lactate level may be obtained and, if elevated, is an excellent indicator of shock. Similarly, base deficit is another indicator of shock. The role of amylase or lipase in abdominal trauma is uncertain. Elevation of liver enzymes may indicate hepatic injury. Glucose and white blood cell count are often elevated in acute trauma and are nonspecific findings. Examination of the urine may reveal gross hematuria, which typically suggests significant injury to the urogenital tract (Chapter 26).

B. Other Diagnostic Modalities

1. Plain radiography—Almost all major trauma patients require plain X-rays of the chest, pelvis, and cervical spine. Although rarely used today because of the ubiquity of computed tomography (CT) scanning, a one-shot intravenous pyelogram may be useful in patients with flank wounds or gross hematuria who are unable to undergo further diagnostic testing prior to operative intervention. Plain radiography of the abdomen is generally not helpful other than in penetrating trauma as a means of evaluating the trajectory of a retained intra-abdominal missile.

2. Diagnostic peritoneal lavage—Although DPL has largely been replaced by ultrasonography, clear indications still remain for its use. A positive DPL in hemodynamically unstable patients with potential multisystem trauma allows for expeditious interventions. A negative test in stab wounds supports observation and early discharge. The main concern regarding DPL is that it is overly sensitive for intra-abdominal blood, which has lead to a high rate of negative or nontherapeutic laparotomies. Recent literature, however, has advocated the use of DPL in conjunction with CT scanning or laparoscopy, particularly in low-velocity penetrating trauma (ie, stab wounds), to decrease the number of nontherapeutic laparotomies. If DPL is considered, it should be performed only after consultation with the trauma surgeon, who should perform this diagnostic study in most cases. Current guidelines emphasize the complimentary role of DPL, FAST, and CT scanning for trauma patients.

3. CT scanning—In the hemodynamically stable trauma patient, CT scanning is an excellent diagnostic modality that is easy to perform. If significant intra-abdominal injury is suspected and the hospital is not equipped to manage such patients, it is unwise to delay transfer in order to obtain a CT scan, assuming a reasonably expeditious transfer is possible. No diagnostic modality out performs CT in the evaluation of intraperitoneal as well as retroperitoneal injuries.

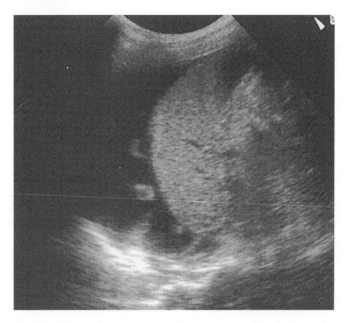

▲ **Figure 25–1.** Positive FAST examination demonstrating a large amount of fluid surrounding the spleen.

Contraindications to CT scanning in trauma patients include hemodynamic instability or clear indication for exploratory laparotomy.

4. Ultrasonography—Ultrasonography has emerged as the primary initial diagnostic examination of the abdomen in multisystem injured blunt trauma patients. Emergency ultrasonography has been studied extensively and is rapid and accurate in the identification of intraperitoneal free fluid. It is also safe in special patient populations (eg, pediatrics, obstetrics). Focused Assessment with Sonography for Trauma (FAST) has a high specificity to detect hemoperitoneum. It's main goal is to reduce time to exploratory laparotomy in blunt or penetrating abdominal trauma. FAST examination (see Chapter 6) is a bedside test that has demonstrated good accuracy with relatively minimal operator experience (at least 30 examinations). The standard FAST examination consists of an initial subxiphoid view of the pericardium, followed by examination of the right upper quadrant looking for free fluid in the Morison pouch (hepatorenal space). The Morison pouch is one of the most dependent parts of the abdomen in the supine trauma patient and often shows the first signs of intraperitoneal fluid collection (blood). Subsequently the splenorenal interface in the left upper quadrant (Figure 25–1) is evaluated, followed by the pelvis. Unlike CT, a FAST examination is rapid, can be performed at bedside in the emergency department, and is easily repeatable. In the setting of abdominal trauma, if a patient is hypotensive with a positive FAST exam, they should go directly to exploratory laparotomy. If the patient is hemodynamically stable, further testing, such as CT scan, may be indicated.

5. Laparoscopy—The use of laparoscopy, with or without CT scanning or DPL, is being studied. It is less invasive than traditional laparotomy and may shorten hospital stays and decrease patient costs, while reducing the number of nontherapeutic laparotomies. As a relatively new modality to evaluate trauma patients, laparoscopy will likely be used more frequently to determine if peritoneal penetration has occurred or if diaphragmatic injury is present in the setting of penetrating trauma. The role of laparoscopy in blunt trauma is also evolving.

Cha JY, Kashuk JL, Sarin EL, Cothren CC, Johnson JL, Biffl WL, Moore EE: Diagnostic peritoneal lavage remains a valuable adjunct to modern imaging techniques. J Trauma 2009;67(2):330–334 [PMID: 19667886].

Tsui CL, Fung HT, Chung KL, Kam CW: Focused abdominal sonography for trauma in the emergency department for blunt abdominal trauma. Int J Emerg Med 2008;1(3):183–187 [PMID: 19384513].

Inaba K, Demetriades D: The nonoperative management of penetrating abdominal trauma. Adv Surg 2007;41:51–62 [PMID: 17972556].

Ahmed N, Whelan J, Brownlee J, Chari V, Chung R: The contribution of laparoscopy in evaluation of penetrating abdominal wounds. J Am Coll Surg 2005;201(2):213–216 [PMID: 16038818].

Types of Injury

A. Blunt Abdominal Injury

Blunt injury occurs most frequently with motor vehicle collisions. Injuries occur secondary to shearing, tearing, or direct impact forces. The presence of a "seat-belt sign" is indicative of intra-abdominal injury in at least 25% of cases. It is important to ascertain if only a lap belt was used, especially in children. Lap-only restraints in children predispose them to intra-abdominal injuries such as intestinal perforations and mesenteric tears. Evaluation of the lumbar spine is also recommended as these injuries may be associated with transverse lumbar spine fractures (Chance fractures). After blunt abdominal trauma, if there is a large or moderate amount of free fluid present without evidence of solid organ injury, suspect a hollow organ injury. These patients often require laparotomy.

B. Penetrating Injuries

Any wound inferior to a line drawn transversely between the nipples should be treated as having the potential for intra-abdominal trajectory. As noted earlier, intravenous fluids should be used judiciously in the prehospital setting. Before arrival at the emergency department, patients should be given enough fluids to maintain a systolic blood pressure of 90 mm Hg, rather than a multiliter resuscitation. If penetrating injuries are present, initiate antibiotic therapy and administer a tetanus booster early in treatment.

1. Gunshot wounds—Traditional teaching mandated that all gunshot wounds with an intra-abdominal trajectory required exploratory laparotomy. Some authors have described a less aggressive approach to a carefully selected subset of patients with penetrating trauma to the abdomen including some low-velocity gunshot wounds. Nonoperative management of gunshot wounds that penetrate the peritoneum is controversial. Patients presenting with hypotension despite crystalloid resuscitation will need immediate exploratory laparotomy, blood transfusion, antibiotics to cover abdominal flora, and a tetanus booster. For hemodynamically stable patients, once intraperitoneal invasion has been ruled out, conservative management of wounds that are superficial and tangential to the abdomen may be used. Seek early surgical consultation in all cases of abdominal gunshot wounds.

2. Stab wounds—Patients with stab wounds require resuscitation as well as tetanus booster and antibiotics if intraperitoneal violation is suspected. A surgeon should conduct a wound exploration for all but the most superficial wounds, and adequate staff and lighting are required. DPL, CT scanning, and laparoscopy may be used. If peritoneal violation has been ruled out, patients may be safely discharged with local wound care instructions. If the peritoneum has been violated, traditional teaching has mandated exploratory laparotomy. Similar to the management of low-velocity gunshot wounds as mentioned above, some surgeons have begun to observe a carefully selected subset of patients with no obvious signs of intraperitoneal injury on physical examination or identified by imaging modalities such as CT scanning.

EMERGENCY TREATMENT OF SPECIFIC INJURIES

SPLENIC INJURIES

ESSENTIALS OF DIAGNOSIS

- ► Common in blunt trauma
- ► Left upper quadrant pain and tenderness, often with radiation to left shoulder
- ► May cause significant hemodynamic instability
- ► CT scan is noninvasive and sensitive in stable patients; use FAST examination or laparotomy for unstable patients
- ► Delayed rupture may occur

Splenic injuries commonly occur secondary to blunt force trauma. Patients may present with small splenic hematomas, lacerations, devascularization, or complete rupture (Figure 25–2). These injuries are further divided into grading classifications based on the severity of the injury. Most classification schemes grade the injuries based on the size and location of the laceration or hematoma and the presence of active bleeding. For example, injuries that extend into the vascular pedicle or hilum are designated higher grade and are more likely to require splenectomy.

Trauma surgeons have turned away from mandatory operative treatment of all splenic injuries toward more frequent nonoperative management. In the absence of life-threatening hemorrhage, the goal is to preserve the spleen. Hemodynamically stable patients with low-grade lesions may be observed. Nonoperative treatment is the most common method of management for patients with splenic injuries and is the most common method of splenic salvage. Patients are less suitable candidates for conservative therapy and at greater risk for nonoperative failure if they have high-grade injuries or if CT scan demonstrates free pelvic fluid. If hypotension unresponsive to 2 L of intravenous crystalloid infusion is present, blood transfusion should be given and the patient is prepared for surgery. Angiography with selective arterial embolization is used in some centers to control splenic bleeding and avoid laparotomy. All splenic injuries require consultation with a trauma surgeon and admission regardless of the severity.

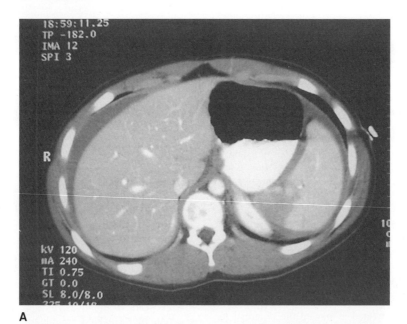

A

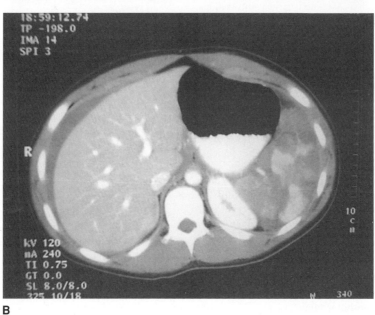

B

▲ **Figure 25–2.** Adult male blunt trauma patient with splenic injury. Multiple large lacerations of the spleen are noted with associated perisplenic hematoma. Perihepatic free fluid is also noted. **A** and **B:** Images obtained shortly after the initial bolus of intravenous contrast. Note the compression of the left kidney by the perisplenic hematoma.

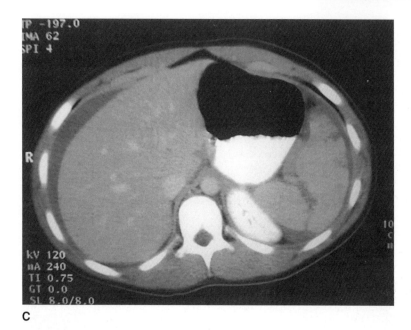

C

▲ **Figure 25–2.** *(Contined)* **C:** Image obtained after the initial bolus of intravenous (contrast) had cleared the spleen. A large laceration on the posterior surface of the spleen is more clearly visualized extending anteriorly to the hilum.

DIAPHRAGMATIC INJURIES

(For more details, see also Chapter 24).

ESSENTIALS OF DIAGNOSIS

- ► May be secondary to blunt or penetrating forces
- ► Rupture occurs predominantly on left side
- ► Often difficult to visualize on initial chest X-ray (nasogastric tube may enhance diagnosis)
- ► CT scan or laparoscopy more sensitive
- ► Delays in diagnosis lead to increased morbidity and mortality

The diaphragm may be injured by penetrating or blunt trauma. Diaphragmatic injuries are frequently difficult to detect initially. Blunt diaphragmatic rupture is a rare condition and correct diagnosis remains difficult and is occasionally made late. The presence of abdominal contents in the thorax may not be obvious on initial chest X-ray. Insertion of a nasogastric tube may facilitate the diagnosis (Figure 25–3). However, diaphragmatic ruptures may be missed even on initial CT scan. If abdominal viscera are seen in the thoracic cavity, then the diagnosis is made easy. In hemodynamically stable patients with penetrating left thoracoabdominal trauma, the incidence of injury to the diaphragm is very high and thoracoscopy or laparoscopy is recommended for diagnosis and repair of a missed diaphragmatic injury. Occult diaphragm injury after penetrating thoracoabdominal injury can be difficult to diagnose and can remain occult for months to years. Delayed diagnosis is associated with risk of hernia formation, strangulation, and high morbidity and mortality.

LIVER INJURIES

ESSENTIALS OF DIAGNOSIS

- ► Most common in blunt trauma
- ► Right upper quadrant pain and tenderness, often with radiation to right shoulder
- ► May cause significant hemodynamic instability
- ► CT scan is noninvasive and sensitive in stable patients; use FAST examination or laparotomy for unstable patients

Because of its size and location, the liver is commonly injured in blunt and penetrating abdominal trauma. Nonoperative management has become standard for > 80% of blunt liver injuries. Liver injuries can include lacerations, hematomas, or rupture (Figure 25–4). Small lacerations or

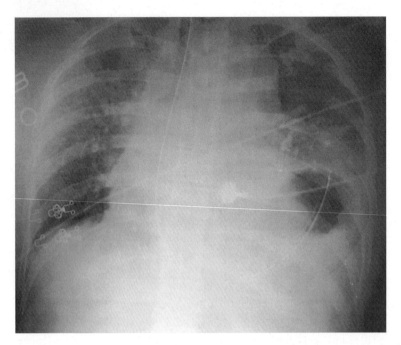

▲ **Figure 25–3.** Adult female blunt trauma patient with blurring of the left hemidiaphragm and an abnormal nasogastric tube and stomach bubble location, representing a left diaphragmatic injury.

hematomas located in the periphery of the liver (Grade I or II) are likely to be managed nonoperatively. However, nonoperative management of high grade liver injuries is associated with significant morbidity and typically is correlated with grade of the liver injury. Unstable patients with liver injuries require laparotomy to attempt hemorrhage control. Because of the significant blood supply from the hepatic artery and portal vein, large defects are technically difficult to manage and may result in exsanguination and death. In cases where operation is required, current operative management emphasizes packing, damage control, and early utilization of interventional radiology for angiography and embolization.

PANCREATIC INJURIES

ESSENTIALS OF DIAGNOSIS

► Uncommon, usually seen after blunt trauma
► Patients may present with epigastric or back pain
► Serum pancreatic enzyme levels are not sensitive or specific for injury
► CT scan is noninvasive and sensitive

Although relatively uncommon, traumatic pancreatic injury is associated with significant morbidity and mortality. It is most commonly seen with penetrating trauma. Blunt trauma to the pancreas accounts for only 26% of cases. Pancreatic injuries are rare and often difficult to diagnose. The pancreas may be lacerated or contused. Amylase levels are not specific and often not helpful, particularly early in the evaluation of the patient. CT scan or radiologist-performed ultrasound may be helpful. All patients with traumatic pancreatic injuries should be admitted.

RENAL INJURIES

(See also Chapter 26)

ESSENTIALS OF DIAGNOSIS

► Hematuria should raise suspicion for injury
► CT scan is noninvasive and sensitive in stable patients

The kidney may sustain lacerations, contusions, shattering, or devascularization injuries. In the setting of trauma, if there is no blood at the urethral meatus and no high-riding prostate, a urinary catheter is inserted to determine whether gross hematuria is present. Presence of gross hematuria is

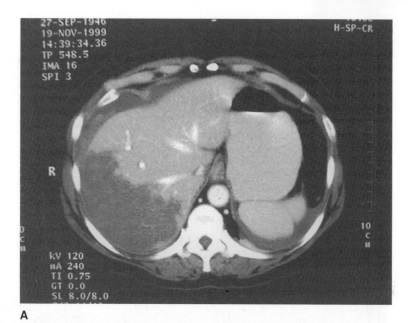

A

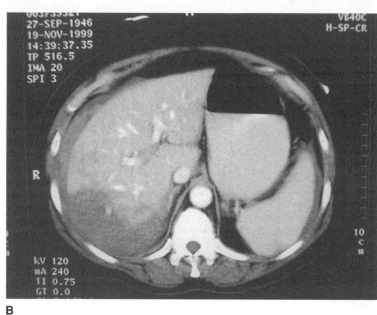

B

▲ **Figure 25–4.** Adult male blunt trauma patient with a large posterior hepatic contusion with associated perihepatic and perisplenic hemorrhage.

typically indicative of urologic injury. Microscopic analysis is not needed in adults unless the patient has been hypotensive. In children, the presence of at least five red blood cells per high-power field on microscopic examination indicates possible urinary tract injury. These findings warrant urologic consultation in the emergency department (see Figure 26–5). In patients with renal injuries chosen for nonoperative management, typical causes of failure in conservative treatment include high fever, drop in hematocrit, severe flank pain, and hemodynamic instability.

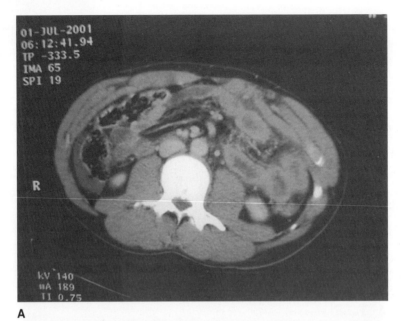

▲ **Figure 25-5.** Adult male blunt trauma patient with left-sided intra-abdominal free fluid, small bowel wall thickening, and stranding in the mesenteric fat planes. Patient underwent exploratory laparotomy and was found to have a mesenteric tear with perforated and devascularized jejunum.

BLADDER INJURIES

(See also Chapter 26)

ESSENTIALS OF DIAGNOSIS

- ▶ Most commonly seen with pelvic fractures
- ▶ Hematuria should raise suspicion for injury
- ▶ Retrograde cystogram may identify injury (as well as associated urethral injury)
- ▶ CT scan may also be used with cystogram

Bladder injuries may be either intraperitoneal or extra-peritoneal. The diagnosis is suspected in a patient with abdominal pain and gross hematuria and is confirmed with a retrograde cystogram. CT scan can also be diagnostic for traumatic intra-peritoneal bladder rupture if the "sentinel clot sign" abutting on the bladder dome can be detected and localized. Patients with intraperitoneal bladder rupture require emergent urologic consultation and immediate surgery (see Figures 26–6 and 26–7).

GASTROINTESTINAL TRACT INJURIES

ESSENTIALS OF DIAGNOSIS

- ▶ May occur with blunt and penetrating injuries
- ▶ Peritoneal signs may be delayed
- ▶ May be missed on initial plain X-rays, ultrasound, and CT scan
- ▶ May have delayed presentation (eg, duodenal hematomas)
- ▶ Strongly consider the diagnosis in patients with free fluid on CT scan but no specific solid organ injury identified

Both penetrating and blunt trauma can cause gastro-intestinal tract (GIT) injuries. Injuries to the GIT may be clinically subtle and are more common with penetrating than blunt trauma. GIT injuries occur in 30% of stab wounds and in 80% of gunshot wounds to the abdomen. In blunt trauma, an abdominal wall bruise or "seat-belt sign" should raise the level of suspicion since this finding is associated with a GIT injury in up to 25% of cases. GIT injuries may be missed on FAST examination or standard CT scan but surgically important bowel and/or mesenteric injury are accurately revealed by multidetector CT scanning (Figure 25–5). The finding of a moderate or large amount of free fluid in the abdomen on CT scan without a specific solid organ injury is highly suspicious of a hollow viscus injury. Such injury may be present even if the patient can tolerate a trial of fluids by mouth in the emergency department. The emergency physician should be cautious if this diagnosis is suspected. Give thorough instructions to the patients who are to be discharged, including planned, early follow-up care. Patients have been able to walk out of the emergency department only to return later with fever and a rigid abdomen. Rare cases of traumatic appendicitis have been reported in the literature. If injuries involving impact, or "spearing," with bicycle handlebars are present, consider evaluating the patient for a duodenal hematoma, which can often be managed conservatively with only observation in the hospital.

FLANK INJURIES

ESSENTIALS OF DIAGNOSIS

- ▶ May be associated with renal injuries
- ▶ Retroperitoneal hematoma may be false positive on DPL or ultrasound
- ▶ CT scan is noninvasive and sensitive in stable patients

Flank injuries are more difficult to manage than other types of injuries because differentiating intraperitoneal from retroperitoneal involvement can be difficult. An abdominal CT scan or one-shot intravenous pyelogram may be beneficial to diagnose ureteral or retroperitoneal injury. Hemodynamically stable patients with penetrating flank wounds with no peritonitis may need CT scan, serial physical exams, and possibly laparoscopy.

Chen ZB, Zhang Y, Liang ZY, Zhang SY, Yu WQ, Gao Y, Zheng SS: Incidence of unexplained intra-abdominal free fluid in patients with blunt abdominal trauma. Hepatobiliary Pancreat Dis Int 2009;8(6):597–601 [PMID: 20007076].

Como JJ, Bokhari F, Chiu WC, Duane TM, Holevar MR, Tanoh MA, Ivatury RR, Scalea TM: Practice management guidelines for selective nonoperative management of penetrating abdominal trauma. J Trauma 2010;68(3):721–733 [PMID: 20220426].

Ahmed N, Whelan J, Brownlee J, Chari V, Chung R: The contribution of laparoscopy in evaluation of penetrating abdominal wounds. J Am Coll Surg 2005;201(2):213–216 [PMID: 16038818].

Harbrecht BG: Is anything new in adult blunt splenic trauma? Am J Surg 2005;190(2):273–278 [PMID: 16023445].

Haan JM, Bochicchio GV, Kramer N, Scalea TM: Nonoperative management of blunt splenic injury: a 5-year experience. J Trauma 2005;58(3):492–498 [PMID: 15761342].

Bala M, Edden Y, Mintz Y, Kisselgoff D, Gercenstein I, Rivkind AI, Farugy M, Almogy G: Blunt splenic trauma: predictors for successful non-operative management. Isr Med Assoc J 2007;9(12):857–861 [PMID: 18210925].

Matsevych OY: Blunt diaphragmatic rupture: four year's experience. Hernia 2008;12(1):73–78 [PMID: 17891332].

Hanna WC, Ferri LE: Acute traumatic diaphragmatic injury. Thorac Surg Clin 2009;19(4):485–489 [PMID: 20112631].

Friese RS, Coln CE, Gentilello LM: Laparoscopy is sufficient to exclude occult diaphragm injury after penetrating abdominal trauma. J Trauma 2005;58(4):789–792 [PMID: 15824657].

Powell BS, Magnotti LJ, Schroeppel TJ, Finnell CW, Savage SA, Fischer PE, Fabian TC, Croce MA: Diagnostic laparoscopy for the evaluation of occult diaphragmatic injury following penetrating thoracoabdominal trauma. Injury 2008;39(5):530–534 [PMID: 18336818].

Stracieri LD, Scarpelini S: Hepatic injury. Acta Cir Bras 2006;21(Suppl 1): 85–88 [PMID: 17013521].

Polanco P, Leon S, Pineda J, Puyana JC, Ochoa JB, Alarcon L, Harbrecht BG, Geller D, Peitzman AB: Hepatic resection in the management of complex injury to the liver. J Trauma 2008;65(6):1264–1269 [PMID: 19077611].

Kozar RA, Moore FA, Cothren CC, Moore EE, Sena M, Bulger EM, Miller CC, Eastridge B, Acheson E, Brundage SI, Tataria M, McCarthy M, Holcomb JB: Risk factors for hepatic morbidity following nonoperative management: multicenter study. Arch Surg 2006;141(5):451–458 [PMID: 16702516].

Ahmed N, Vernick JJ: Pancreatic injury. South Med J 2009;102(12):1253–1256.

Shirazi M, Sefidbakht S, Jahanabadi Z, Asadolahpour A, Afrasiabi MA: Is early reimaging CT scan necessary in patients with grades III and IV renal trauma under conservative treatment? J Trauma 2010;68(1):9–12 [PMID: 20016434].

Shin SS, Jeong YY, Chung TW, Yoon W, Kang HK, Kang TW, Shin HY: The sentinel clot sign: a useful CT finding for the evaluation of intraperitoneal bladder rupture following blunt trauma. Korean J Radiol 2007;8(6):492–497 [PMID: 18071279].

Atri M, Hanson JM, Grinblat L, Brofman N, Chughtai T, Tomlinson G: Surgically important bowel and/or mesenteric injury in blunt trauma: accuracy of multidetector CT for evaluation. Radiology 2008;249(2):524–533 [PMID: 18796660].

Nazir S, Scarsbrook AF, Moore NR: Case of the month: flank swelling following abdominal trauma: an easily overlooked injury. Br J Radiol 2009;82(973):79–81 [PMID: 19095818].

Dissanaike S, Griswold JA, Frezza EE: Treatment of isolated penetrating flank trauma. Am Surg 2005;71(6):493–496 [PMID: 16044928].

Genitourinary Trauma

26

Brian Adkins, MD[1]

Immediate Management of Life-Threatening Injuries
Emergency Treatment of Specific Injuries
   Renal Injuries
   Ureteral Injuries

Bladder Injuries
Urethral Injuries
External Genital Injuries

IMMEDIATE MANAGEMENT OF LIFE-THREATENING INJURIES

Genitourinary injuries occur in 10–20% of major trauma patients. Most of these injuries, with the exception of renal hilar disruption or shattered kidney, are not immediately life-threatening. Because they are often accompanied by potentially life-threatening injuries to other organ systems, however, it is easy for the emergency physician to overlook and therefore miss signs or symptoms of urologic injury. Failure to diagnose and treat these injuries properly can result in significant long-term morbidity. Therefore, while evaluating the trauma patient, the physician needs to be aware of clues to genitourinary injury. These clues include (1) lumbar vertebral or lower rib fractures, (2) pelvic fractures, (3) flank pain or hematoma, (4) abnormal prostate (high riding, non-palpable, or free floating) on rectal examination, (5) blood at the urethral meatus, and (6) gross hematuria.

▶ Immediate Treatment

For all patients with blunt or penetrating trauma, evaluate airway, breathing, circulation, and disability during the primary survey as per advanced trauma life support protocol

(Chapter 12). During the secondary survey, evaluate for a boggy or high-riding prostate on rectal exam, perineal or scrotal hematoma, and any evidence of blood at the urethral meatus. If any of these signs is present, perform a retrograde urethrogram (RUG) before inserting a Foley catheter. If the signs are absent, insert a Foley catheter if indicated (ie, in unstable patients or those unable to urinate). Urethral studies should never delay diagnostic studies of, or treatment for, potentially life-threatening injuries. Figures 26–1 to 26–3 provide algorithms for managing blunt, penetrating, and pediatric urologic injury.

▶ Special Examinations and Procedures

Because of the need to determine if Foley catheter placement is safe, evaluation of the genitourinary system is generally performed in a retrograde fashion: rule out urethral injury before bladder (usually by physical exam), then bladder (by placing a Foley catheter) before ureteral or renal injury.

A. Catheterization

A Foley catheter may be placed once physical examination supports the integrity of the urethra. As mentioned previously, if any signs of urethral injury are present, perform a RUG first. If the urethrogram is negative or not indicated, a 14–16 F catheter should be placed using copious amounts of lubricating jelly and sterile technique. A folded 4 × 4 in^2

---

[1]This chapter is a revision of the chapter by Geoffrey A. Wiss, MD, Claudia Whitaker, MD, & Robert K. Dunne, MD, FACEP from the 5th edition.

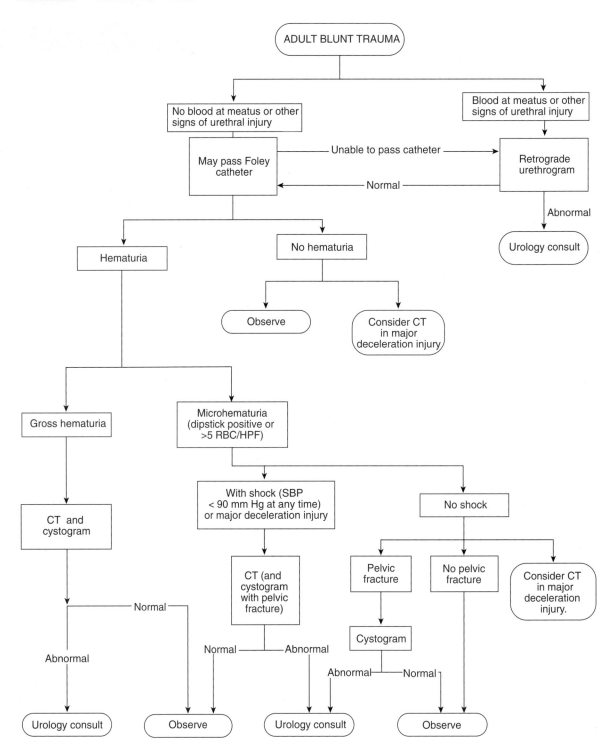

▲ **Figure 26–1.** Algorithm for staging blunt trauma in the adult. (Modified and reproduced, with permission, from Tanagho EA, McAninch JW: *Smith's General Urology*, 13th edn. Appleton & Lange, 1992.)

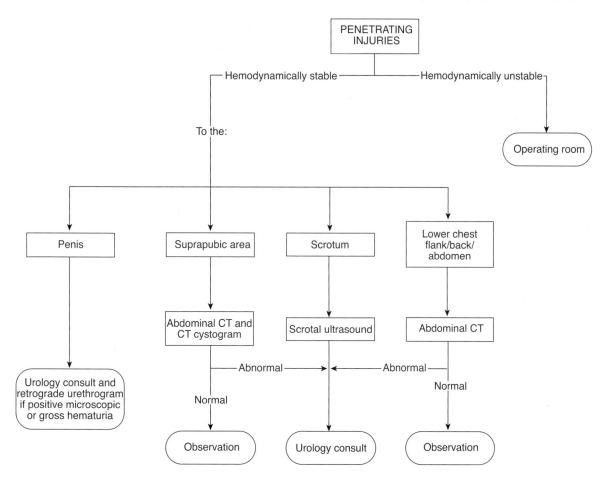

▲ **Figure 26–2.** Algorithm for staging penetrating trauma in the adult. (Modified and reproduced, with permission, from Tanagho EA, McAninch JW: *Smith's General Urology,* 13th edn. Appleton & Lange, 1992.)

gauze pad may be used to retract the foreskin in uncircumcised patients to prevent repeated unintended reduction of the foreskin over the glans with subsequent field and catheter contamination during placement. Any difficulty during placement warrants retrograde urethrography if urethral injury is a possibility. Gross or microscopic hematuria indicates possible urologic trauma, although the degree of microscopic hematuria does not correlate with the degree or location of injury.

In 1989, a 10-year prospective study established guidelines for evaluation and treatment of blunt renal trauma and the consensus opinion remains the same. Patients with gross hematuria require an imaging study. Patients with microscopic hematuria and a history of shock (systolic blood pressure < 90 mm Hg) or sudden deceleration injury should also have an imaging study performed. Those without shock or deceleration injury may be discharged home with outpatient

urology follow-up to ensure that microscopic hematuria has cleared. Patients with penetrating injuries and more than 5 red blood cells per high-power field should undergo an imaging study, although the absence of hematuria does not eliminate the need for a study. With regard to penetrating trauma, the location of the wound is more important than the presence of hematuria for predicting injury, because significant injuries (9% of patients in one study) can be present even in the absence of hematuria. In pediatric patients, the kidney is the most commonly injured intra-abdominal organ. Children are more susceptible to renal injuries than adults as their kidneys are proportionally larger and are surrounded by less perirenal fat. The ribcage is also less rigid and does not provide the extent of protection as present in adults. As a result, even microscopic hematuria from trauma requires further workup (usually by computed tomography [CT] scan) in pediatric patients. There is some controversy

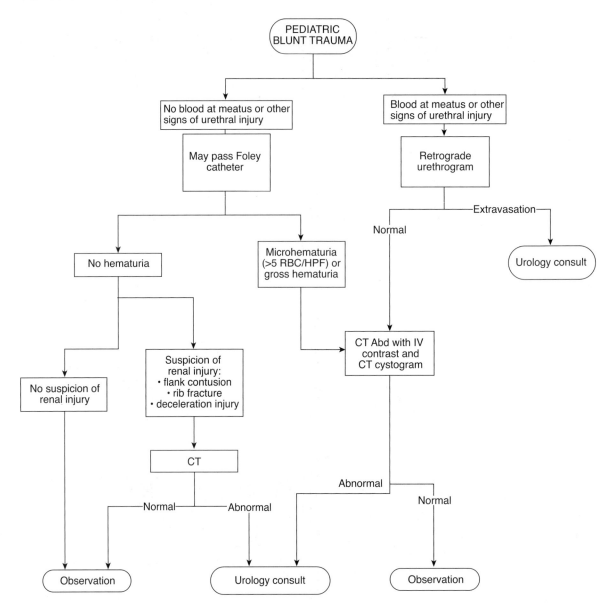

▲ **Figure 26–3.** Algorithm for the evaluation of blunt trauma in children. (Modified and reproduced, with permission, from Tanagho EA, McAninch JW: *Smith's General Urology*, 13th edn. Appleton & Lange, 1992.)

over the quantity of microscopic hematuria that necessitates further evaluation in children. A review of the current literature yielded varying cutoffs mostly ranging from 5 to 50 RBC/hpf. The authors of one retrospective review even suggested that children should be evaluated in the same manner as adults, which could potentially limit CT radiation. While this topic will likely be subject to future investigation, the current opinion is that pediatric microscopic hematuria in blunt or penetrating trauma should be considered clinically significant and prompt further evaluation.

B. Suprapubic Catheter Placement

Suprapubic catheter placement is indicated in trauma situations when Foley catheter placement is contraindicated. This usually occurs in patients with a known or suspected urethral injury who are awaiting a confirmatory study or surgical intervention. Several commercial kits are available. Most of these kits utilize placement over a guidewire. If kits are unavailable, a single-lumen central venous catheter may be used.

C. CT Scan

Helical CT scan with intravenous contrast is the study of choice for evaluating ureteral or renal trauma. Retroperitoneal structures such as the kidneys, ureters, and bladder are very well visualized by abdominal CT scanning. In the evaluation of renal trauma, CT scanning provides detailed information regarding the extent of hemorrhage, extravasation, and devascularization. The CT scan may also be used for retrograde cystography. Simply clamping the Foley catheter during an intravenous contrast pelvic CT scan is not adequate to eliminate bladder injury, because of inadequate bladder pressures and dilute dye. The technique for this study involves contrast administration into the bladder via the foley catheter.

D. Retrograde Urethrography

The RUG is the study of choice to evaluate urethral trauma. If urethral injury is suspected (eg, blood at the meatus, boggy or high-riding prostate, scrotal or perineal hematoma), urethrography should be performed prior to Foley catheter placement. The study is performed by instilling contrast medium into the urethra, usually under fluoroscopy. After a preinjection abdominal X-ray is obtained, a Cooke adapter on a 60-cc syringe is gently inserted into the urethra and approximately 20 cc of water-soluble contrast is injected over 60 seconds. If fluoroscopy is not available, an X-ray is taken during the last 10 seconds of injection. Extravasation with bladder filling denotes partial urethral tear, and extravasation with no bladder filling denotes complete urethral tear.

E. Retrograde Cystography

Similar to the IVP, the retrograde cystogram using plain radiography has essentially been replaced by the CT cystogram. In this technique, up to 400 cc of full-strength water-soluble contrast is instilled under gravity through a urethral catheter to the point of bladder contraction after a preliminary KUB. X-rays are taken with the bladder full and after complete voiding to attempt to visualize extravasation.

F. Ultrasound

Although used frequently in trauma situations to detect peritoneal blood, ultrasound does not have the sensitivity (possibly as low as 22%) to reliably detect specific renal injuries, and therefore is not recommended in the definitive workup of renal trauma.

G. Intravenous Urography

Mainly mentioned only for historical purposes, the intravenous pyelogram (IVP), which was once the standard of imaging for genitourinary trauma, has been replaced by the helical CT scan due to CT's superior sensitivity and ability to evaluate for nonurological injuries.

Brandes S, Borrelli J: Pelvic fracture and associated urologic injuries. World J Surg 2001;25(12):1578–1587 (Review) [PMID: 11775195].

Dreitlein DA, Suner S, Basler J: Genitourinary trauma. Emerg Med Clin North Am 2001;19:569 [PMID: 11554276].

Goff CD, Collin GR: Management of renal trauma at a rural, level I trauma center. Am Surg 1998;64:226 [PMID: 9520811].

Miller KS, McAninch JW: Radiographic assessment of renal trauma: Our 15-year experience. J Urol 1995;154:352 [PMID: 7609096].

Nagy KK et al: Routine preoperative "one-shot" intravenous pyelography is not indicated in all patients with penetrating abdominal trauma. J Am Coll Surg 1997;185:530 [PMID: 9404875].

Perez-Brayfield MR et al: Blunt traumatic hematuria in children. Is a simplified algorithm justified? J Urol 2002;167:2543–2547 [PMID: 11992085].

McAninch Jack W: Chapter 17: Injuries to the genitourinary tract. *Smith's General Urology*, 17th ed.2008.

Fraser J, Aguayo P, Ostlie DJ et al: Review of the evidence on the management of blunt renal trauma in pediatric patients. Pediatr Surg Int 2009;25:125–132 [PMID: 19130062].

Bjurlin MA, Fantus RJ, Mellett MM et al: Genitourinary injuries in pelvic fracture morbidity and mortality using the national trauma data bank.2009;67(5):1033–1039 [PMID:19901665].

▼ **EMERGENCY TREATMENT OF SPECIFIC INJURIES**

RENAL INJURIES

 ESSENTIALS OF DIAGNOSIS

► Often accompanied by other abdominal injuries in blunt trauma.

► Nausea, vomiting, flank ecchymosis, and lower rib or lumbar fractures suggest injury.

► No reliable markers for diagnosis, including hematuria.

► CT scan is study of choice.

▶ General Considerations

Renal injuries are the most common urologic injuries. The kidneys are not fixed in place but hang from their vascular attachments and perirenal fat and move with the diaphragm. Secured at only the vascular pedicle, the kidneys are susceptible to deceleration injury, with blunt injury five times more common than penetrating injury. Kidneys with preexisting abnormalities such as tumors, congenital lesions, or hydronephrosis may be damaged by seemingly inconsequential mechanisms.

The diagnosis of renal trauma is complicated by the frequent presence of other peritoneal injuries, as well as the absence of any accurate markers for renal injury. Hematuria may be absent with significant renal injury (especially complete ureteropelvic avulsion), and the degree of hematuria does not correlate with the degree of injury when present. Renal injuries are graded on a scale of 1 to 5 (Figure 26–4). Following a general trend for the nonoperative management of many solid organ intra-abdominal injuries, 95% of renal injuries are managed without surgical exploration. However, only a special subset of patients with high-grade renal injuries are candidates for observation without surgical repair or nephrectomy.

▶ Clinical Findings

A. Symptoms and Signs

Pain may be localized to one flank or over the abdomen, but visceral injury or pelvic fracture may obscure symptoms of renal injury. Nausea and vomiting, flank ecchymosis, lower rib fractures, or lumbar vertebral (especially transverse process) fractures may be noted. Urologic injury should be suspected in any penetrating wound to the flank or whose trajectory potentially crosses the paravertebral gutter. Extensive blood loss and shock may result from retroperitoneal bleeding. A palpable mass may indicate retroperitoneal hematoma or urinoma. If the retroperitoneum has been torn, hemoperitoneum will cause diffuse abdominal tenderness and ileus.

B. Laboratory Findings

Hematuria may or may not be present.

C. Imaging

The study of choice is a helical CT scan of the abdomen and pelvis with intravenous contrast and immediate as well as delayed images (Figure 26–5). Under no circumstances should imaging delay necessary operative intervention. Surgical exploration should replace radiographic imaging in unstable patients who require immediate surgery. In the event that CT is unavailable, IVP can be useful for diagnosing major renal injuries, although it will miss some smaller contusions and renal lacerations.

▶ Treatment

Renal contusions (85% of blunt trauma renal injuries) and minor renal lacerations (12% of such injuries) can be managed

expectantly and rarely require operative intervention. Outpatient urology follow-up is necessary to ensure that hematuria has cleared. Major lacerations (3% of blunt trauma renal injuries) may require operative intervention, although the trend is to manage these injuries conservatively when possible. Hemodynamically stable patients with active hemorrhage demonstrated on CT scanning may benefit from angiography with selective embolization. Renal pedicle injuries (arterial thrombosis or avulsion), representing 1–2% of blunt injuries, must be treated rapidly if irreversible kidney damage is to be avoided. Most surgeons believe 4 hours of warm ischemia time is the threshold of salvageability, after which the kidney has poor chance of even partial function.

Penetrating renal trauma usually requires surgical intervention. Absolute indications for surgical exploration include uncontrollable renal hemorrhage and shattered kidney or avulsion of the main renal vessels.

Harris AC et al: CT findings in blunt renal trauma. Radiographics 2001;21:S201–S212 [PMID: 11598258].

Alsikafi NF, Rosenstein DI. Staging, evaluation, and nonoperative management of renal injuries. Urol Clin North AM 2006;33: 13–19 [PMID: 16488276].

Santucci RA, Langenburg SE, Zachareas MJ et al: Traumatic hematuria in children can be evaluated as in adults. J Urol 2004;171:822–825 [PMID: 14713834].

Broghammer JA, Fisher MB, Santucci D et al: Conservative management of renal trauma: a review. Urology 2007;70:623–629 [PMID: 17991526].

Edwards NM, Claridge JA, Forsythe RM et al: The morbidity of trauma nephrectomy. Am Surg 2009; 75:1112–1118 [PMID: 19927517].

URETERAL INJURIES

ESSENTIALS OF DIAGNOSIS

▶ Usually from penetrating trauma.

▶ Patients with missed injuries may present with fever, abdominal pain, andmass.

▶ CT scan orretrograde pyelography are studies of choice.

▶ General Considerations

The least frequently injured portion of the genitourinary system is the ureter. The majority of these injuries (80-90%) result from penetrating wounds, although blunt ureteral trauma can accompany many non-urologic injuries as well. Injury to the ureter should be suspected in blunt

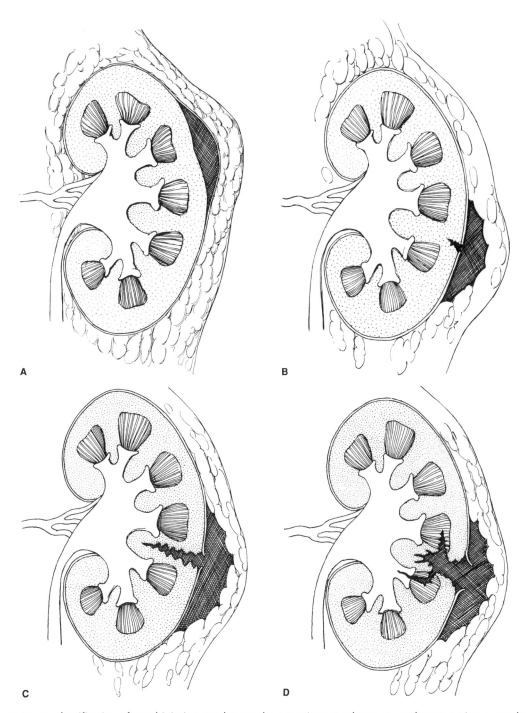

▲ **Figure 26–4.** Classification of renal injuries. Grades I and II are minor. Grades III, IV, and V are major. **A:** Grade I—Microscopic or gross hematuria; normal findings on radiographic studies; contusion or contained subcapsular hematoma without parenchymal laceration. **B:** Grade II—Nonexpanding, confined perirenal hematoma or cortical laceration less than 1 cm deep without urinary extravasation. **C:** Grade III—Parenchymal laceration extending more than 1 cm into the cortex without urinary extravasation. **D:** Grade IV—Parenchymal laceration extending through the corticomedullary junction and into the collecting system. A laceration at a segmental vessel may also be present.

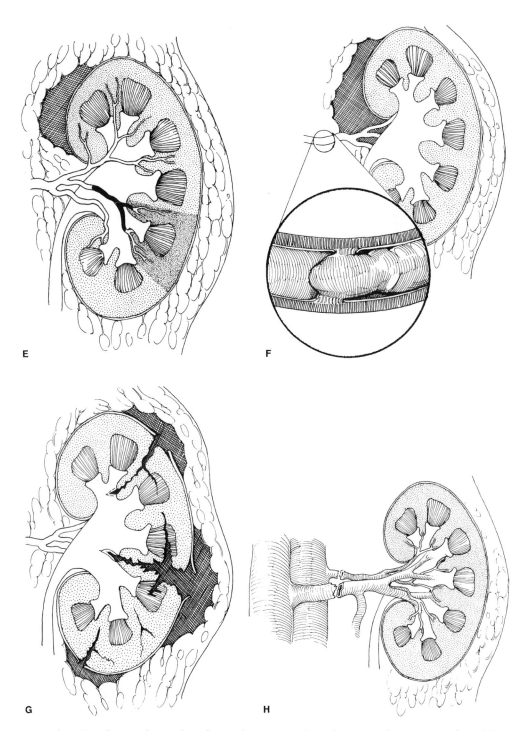

▲ **Figure 26–4.** *(Continued)* **E:** Grade IV—Thrombosis of a segmental renal artery without a parenchymal laceration. Note the corresponding parenchymal ischemia. **F:** Grade V—Thrombosis of the main renal artery. The inset shows the intimal tear and distal thrombosis. **G:** Grade V—Multiple major lacerations, resulting in a "shattered" kidney. **H:** Grade V—Avulsion of the main renal artery and/or vein. (Reproduced, with permission, from Tanagho EA, McAninch JW: *Smith's General Urology*, 16th edn. New York: McGraw-Hill, 2004.)

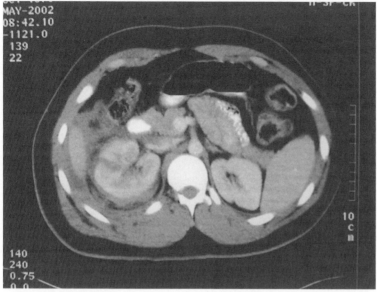

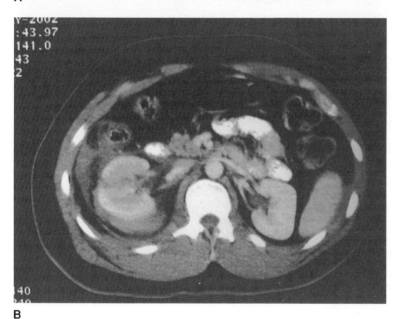

▲ **Figure 26–5.** Adult blunt trauma patient with high-grade right renal laceration and perinephric hematoma. (Note the normal appearing left kidney.)

deceleration trauma due to the kidney being torn from the ureter. This type of injury is more likely in children due to their hyperextensible vertebral column Most injuries occur in the proximal one-third of the ureter. Ureteral injuries are often diagnosed either intraoperatively or when complications arise later, because such injuries are infrequent, are difficult to diagnose, and frequently occur in the presence of other injuries.

▶ Clinical Findings

A. Symptoms and Signs

Physical examination findings are nonspecific and are usually related to associated intra-abdominal injuries, although colicky flank pain or mass may be present. Hematuria may be present but is often absent if complete ureteral transection has occurred. Use of intravenous indigo carmine dye during surgical exploration may help in the diagnosis of ureteral injury. Patients with a delay in diagnosis may present with abdominal pain, urinary urgency and frequency, fever, pyuria, and a palpable mass containing urine (urinoma) or blood.

B. Imaging

Both IVP and CT scan may miss ureteral injuries. If performed soon after injury and associated administration of resuscitative fluids, the extravasation of contrast from the ureter may show up only as a hazy, ground-glass appearance. If injuries are near the ureteropelvic junction, extension of fluid around the kidney may incorrectly lead to diagnosis of renal rather than ureteral injury. Because retrograde pyelography uses a more concentrated dye and fluoroscopy, this modality may identify injuries missed by other methods. Ultrasound is not reliable in the diagnosis of ureteral injury.

▶ Treatment

Ureteral injuries may be managed with stenting, placement of nephrostomy tube, or surgery. Delayed repair, although associated with increased incidence of infections, does not lead to increased rate of renal function loss.

Brandes S, Coburn M, Armenakas N et al: Diagnosis and management of ureteric injury: an evidence-based analysis. BJU Int 2004;94:277–289 [PMID: 15291852].

Tezval H, Tezval M, von Klot C et al: Urinary tract injuries in patients with multiple trauma. World J Urol 2007;25:177–184 [PMID: 17351781].

Pereir BM, Ogilvie MP, Gomez-Rodriguez JC et al: A review of ureteral injuries after external trauma. Scand J Trauma Resuscit Emerg Med 2010, 18:6 [PMID: 20128905].

BLADDER INJURIES

ESSENTIALS OF DIAGNOSIS

- ▶ Usually due to blunt trauma pelvic fractures.
- ▶ Gross hematuria and abdominal pain often present.
- ▶ Retrograde cystogram is the diagnostic study of choice.

▶ General Considerations

Bladder rupture most commonly occurs in association with blunt trauma and pelvic fractures, especially when the bladder is full. The rupture may occur into the intraperitoneal (Figure 26–6) or extraperitoneal space (Figure 26–7). The majority of ruptures (85%) occur into the extraperitoneal space and are often associated with pelvic fractures

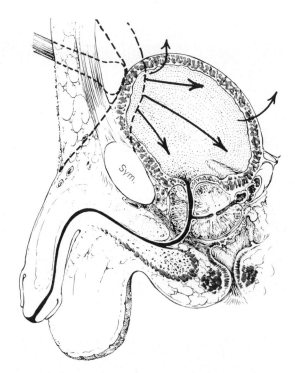

▲ **Figure 26–6.** Mechanism of vesical injury. A direct blow over the full bladder causes increased intravesical pressure and intraperitoneal rupture. (Reproduced, with permission, from Tanagho EA, McAninch JW: *Smith's General Urology*, 16th edn. McGraw-Hill, 2004.)

(60–90%). Intraperitoneal ruptures are often caused by motor vehicle collisions during which a patient has a full bladder and are more likely to occur in patients with recent alcohol intake (predisposes to full bladders), women (thinner bladder musculature), and children (bladder not protected by pelvis). Intraperitoneal bladder rupture generally occurs at the dome, the weakest area of the bladder. A combination of both intraperitoneal and extraperitoneal rupture occurs in 5–12% of patients with bladder rupture. Because blunt trauma patients who suffer bladder rupture often have multisystem injuries, the mortality has been reported at 22–44%.

▶ Clinical Findings

A. Symptoms and Signs

Gross hematuria is the most frequent finding (98%), along with lower abdominal pain and inability to void.

B. Imaging

Diagnosis of bladder injury is made by retrograde cystogram (either by conventional radiography or usually computed tomography) after urethral injury is excluded by RUG or

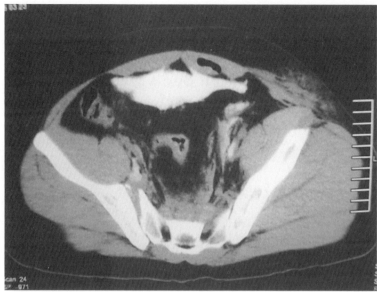

A

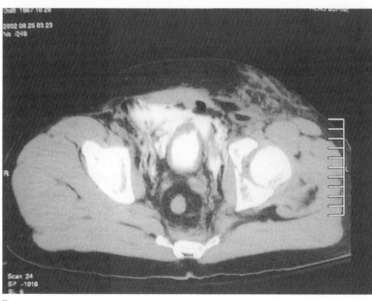

B

▲ **Figure 26–7.** Adult blunt trauma patient with extraperitoneal bladder rupture. Note the contrast extravasation in the pelvis and along the left anterior abdominal wall. As evidence of significant pelvic trauma, note **(A)** the right sacroiliac joint disruption and **(B)** the left acetabular fracture.

physical exam. The bladder should be completely distended with 300–400 cc of water-soluble contrast material instilled through a Foley catheter. Radiographs are taken after complete distention is obtained and then repeated after the bladder has been drained completely. Intraperitoneal rupture will show contrast material extending into the abdomen, outlining loops of bowel wall with extension into the paracolic gutters. Extraperitoneal rupture will show a coarse, streaked pattern of extravasation adjacent to the bladder. A postvoid view should always be obtained and is helpful in diagnosing subtle injuries that may have been obscured on initial films. However, postvoid imaging is usually not necessary with CT cystogram imaging.

▶ Treatment

Intraperitoneal ruptures and all penetrating injuries to the bladder require surgical intervention. Extraperitoneal injuries can usually be managed nonsurgically with Foley catheter drainage, followed by repeat cystogram in 10–14 days. Simple contusions or incomplete lacerations can also be managed conservatively, with Foley catheter drainage and early urologic follow-up.

Morey AF, Iverson AJ, Swan A: Bladder rupture after blunt trauma: guidelines for diagnostic imaging. J Trauma 2001;51:683 [PMID: 11586159].

Ramchandani P, Buckler PM: Imaging of genitourinary trauma. Am J Roentgenol 2009;192:1514–1523 [PMID: 19457813].

Bent C, Iyngkaran T, Power N et al: Urologic injuries following trauma. Clin Radiol 2008;63:1361–1371.

URETHRAL INJURIES

ESSENTIALS OF DIAGNOSIS

▶ Significant Injury because of frequent complications.

▶ Blood at the urethral meatus and inability to void often seen.

▶ High-riding prostate on digital rectal exam.

▶ Retrograde urethrogram is the best study.

▶ General Considerations

Urethral injuries are uncommon but are potentially the most debilitating because of the high rate of complications, such as incontinence, stricture formation, impotence, and chronic urinary tract infections. They occur most often in men secondary to blunt trauma and account for 10% of the genitourinary injuries. Urethral injuries in women are extremely rare and are usually associated with pelvic fractures. Blood at the urethral meatus is the most reliable and accurate sign of a urethral injury with a reported sensitivity of up to 93% .The amount of urethral bleeding is a poor indicator the severity of the urethral injury.

If a urethral injury is suspected, placement of a foley catheter is contraindicated until a RUG has excluded the diagnosis. If a Foley catheter has already been placed in a patient with a possible urethral injury, it should not be removed, and a urethrogram should be performed around the catheter using a pediatric feeding tube and occluding the distal urethral meatus with gentle pressure on the glans.

A special injury of note is the traumatic removal of a Foley catheter. This can occur while moving a patient or occasionally by the patient stepping on the catheter during ambulation. Significant injury can occur by this mechanism, and a urethrogram should be performed prior to reinsertion of any catheters.

1. Posterior Urethra

▶ General Considerations

The posterior urethra, consisting of the prostatic and membranous portions, is injured most commonly during blunt trauma associated with bony pelvic injuries. The urethra is usually sheared proximal to the urogenital diaphragm. The prostate then becomes displaced superiorly by the developing hematoma (Figure 26–8). Concomitant bladder injuries are associated with 35% of posterior urethral injuries.

▶ Clinical Findings

A. Symptoms and Signs

Patients will complain of abdominal or perineal pain and an inability to void. Blood at the meatus is the most frequent sign of urethral injury. The posteriorly displaced prostate will be nonpalpable or feel high riding or boggy on rectal examination.

B. Imaging

In the setting of a posterior urethral injury, the retrograde urethrogram will demonstrate extravasation of contrast material superior to the urogenital diaphragm (Figure 26–9). Once a suprapubic catheter is placed, a cystogram can be performed to assess for bladder neck injury.

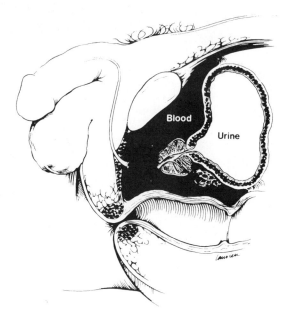

▲ **Figure 26–8.** Injury to the posterior (membranous) urethra. The prostate has been avulsed from the membranous urethra secondary to fracture of the pelvis. Extravasation occurs above the triangular ligament and is periprostatic and perivesical. (Reproduced, with permission, from Tanagho EA, McAninch JW: *Smith's General Urology*, 16th edn. McGraw-Hill, 2004.)

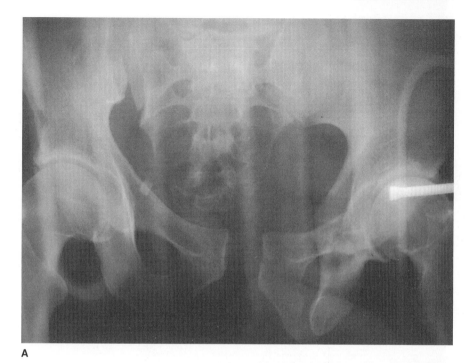

A

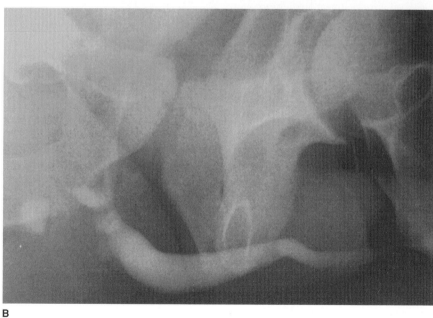

B

▲ **Figure 26–9.** Adult male blunt trauma patient with prostatomembranous urethral injury. **A:** Pubic symphysis diastasis is noted. **B:** Free extravasation and failure of contrast to fill the bladder indicate a posterior urethral disruption.

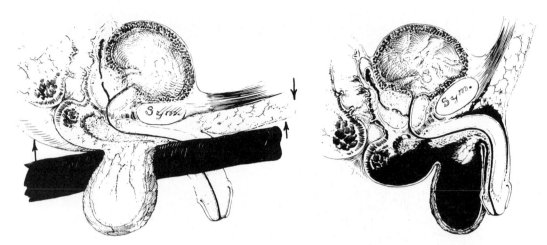

▲ **Figure 26–10.** Injury to the bulbous urethra. Left: Mechanism: Usually a perineal blow or fall astride an object; crushing of the urethra against inferior edge of pubic symphysis. Right: Extravasation of blood and urine enclosed within Colles' fascia. (Reproduced, with permission, from Tanagho EA, McAninch JW: *Smith's General Urology*, 13th edn. Appleton & Lange, 1992.)

▶ Treatment

Initial management includes suprapubic cystostomy to provide urinary drainage. Definitive treatment options vary, and urologic consultation is essential.

2. Anterior Urethra

▶ General Considerations

The anterior urethra, consisting of the bulbous and penile portions, is located below the urogenital diaphragm. Trauma to the anterior urethra is typically due to straddle injuries, penetrating injuries, a direct blow to the perineum, instrumentation, or improper Foley catheter placement (Figure 26–10).

▶ Clinical Findings

A. Symptoms and Signs

If Buck's fascia remains intact, extravasation of blood and urine will be confined to the penile shaft and perineum. With rupture of Buck's fascia, extravasation will extend along the abdominal wall, confined only by Colles' fascia, with resultant perineal "butterfly" hematoma.

B. Imaging

With anterior urethral injuries, contrast extravasation will be seen on urethrogram inferior to the urogenital diaphragm (Figure 26–11).

▶ Treatment

Long-term catheter drainage or direct reanastomosis are the most common treatment options.

Brandes S, Borrelli J: Pelvic fractures and associated urologic injuries. World J Surg 2001;25:1578–1587 [PMID: 11775195].

EXTERNAL GENITAL INJURIES

 ESSENTIALS OF DIAGNOSIS

▶ Blunt trauma to the erect penis may cause rupture with pain and deforming hematoma; evaluate for surgical repair.

▶ Blunt scrotal injuries require Doppler ultrasound studies.

▶ Genital burn injures require early Foley catheter placement to prevent edematous urethral Obstruction.

▶ Consider pelvic floor penetration and sexual assault with all vaginal lacerations.

1. Penile Rupture

Penile fractures occur from blunt trauma to the erect penis causing rupture of the corpus cavernosum. The patient typically reports a loud "cracking" sound, immediate pain, and loss of erection. Injuries to the urethra and the corpus spongiosum can also occur during penile fracture.

▶ Clinical Findings

A. Symptoms and Signs

A large hematoma will be visible on the shaft of the penis, and the axis of the shaft may be deviated.

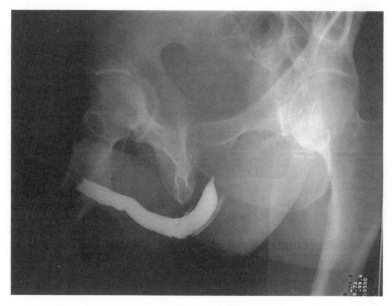

▲ **Figure 26–11.** Adult male patient with straddle injury to perineum and blood at the urethral meatus. This positive retrograde urethrogram reveals extravasation in the bulbous portion of the urethra indicative of urethral injury.

B. Imaging

Retrograde urethrogram may show extravasation if urethral injury is present.

▶ Treatment

Immediate urologic consultation is indicated for surgical repair.

2. Constriction Injuries

Constriction injuries can occur from objects placed circumferentially around the penile shaft. Occasionally these injuries are from obstructive rings placed during sexual play in adults. They require immediate removal to prevent urethral injury or neurovascular compromise. In circumcised male infants, hair is a common culprit.

3. Testicular Injuries

Blunt trauma to the scrotum may result in testicular rupture by forcefully compressing the testis against the symphysis pubis or medial thigh.

▶ Clinical Findings

A. Symptoms and Signs

Patients present with severe pain, nausea, vomiting, and extensive swelling due to hematoma formation, all of which make testicular examination difficult.

B. Imaging

The diagnostic study of choice is ultrasound examination with Doppler flow studies.

▶ Treatment

Simple hematomas can be managed conservatively with NSAIDs, scrotal elevation and sitz baths. Larger hematomas may require surgical drainage. Testicular rupture and penetrating injuries should be explored and repaired surgically. Tetanus prophylaxis and antibiotics are also recommended for penetrating injuries.

4. Skin Injuries

A degloving injury usually requires extensive surgical debridement and repair, and may require skin grafting. Scrotal lacerations can usually be closed primarily due to the elastic nature of the scrotal skin. With zipper injuries, the trapped skin can be released by cutting the sliding portion of the zipper. Scrotal lacerations can be repaired in a layered fashion once testicular injury has been ruled out. Burn injuries deserve special consideration because of the massive edema that may develop, resulting in urethral obstruction. A urethral or suprapubic catheter should be placed early during the initial resuscitative phase.

5. Female Genital Injuries

If vaginal bleeding is present, perform a speculum examination to evaluate for vaginal lacerations in addition to any injuries noted to the external genitalia. Blunt trauma to the external genitalia is rare and usually presents as vulvar hematomas. Simple lacerations can be repaired using absorbable sutures. If unable to obtain hemostasis, operative repair is indicated. In all vaginal lacerations, it is important to rule out penetration of the pelvic floor, which may indicate significant organ and vascular damage. The possibility of sexual assault must always be considered, and follow-up with a gynecologist is recommended.

Lynch TH, Martinez-Pineiro L, Plas E et al: EAU guidelines on urological trauma. European Urology 47 Eur Urol 2005;47: 1–15 [PMID: 15582243].

Martinez-Pineiro L, Djakovic N, Plas N et al: EAU guidelines on urethral trauma. Eur Urol 2010, DOI: 10.1016/j.eururo.2010.01.013 [PMID: 15582243].

Hendry WF: Testicular, epididymal and vasal injuries. BJU Int 2000;86(3):344–348 (Review) [PMID: 10930944] (Review; no abstract available).

Kadish HA, Schunk JE, Britton H: Pediatric male rectal and genital trauma: accidental and nonaccidental injuries. Pediatr Emerg Care 1998;14:95 [PMID: 9583387].

Mydlo JH, Harris CF, Brown JG: Blunt, penetrating and ischemic injuries to the penis. J Urol 2002;168(4 Pt 1):1433–1435 [PMID: 12352411].

van der Horst C, Martinez Portillo FJ, Seif C, Groth W, Junemann KP: Male genital injury: diagnostics and treatment. BJU Int 2004;93(7):927–930 (Review) [PMID: 15142139].

Vertebral Column & Spinal Cord Trauma

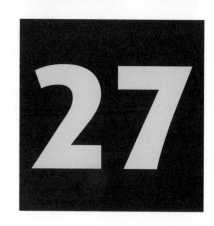

27

S. Derrick Fowler, MD

Jason Seamon, DO, MHS, FACEP, FAAEM

IMMEDIATE MANAGEMENT OF THE PATIENT WITH SUSPECTED SPINAL INJURY

▶ Suspect Spinal Cord Injury

Patients with blunt trauma, particularly those with head injury, severe mechanism, or neurologic complaints should be assumed to have spine injuries until proven otherwise. Such injuries are major causes of morbidity and mortality in the trauma patient, so thorough assessment beginning in the prehospital setting is essential. The potential instability of such injuries necessitates that the utmost care be taken not to render additional harm to these patients.

▶ Immobilization

Immobilization of the spine is essential to prevent further injury to the spinal cord. From the field, or when transferred, the patient should be on a long spine board, in a rigid cervical collar (Philadelphia) with lateral rolls and tape across the forehead. Upon arrival, logroll the patient off this board and onto the examination bed, maintaining in-line stabilization (see below). Careful immobilization should be maintained throughout resuscitation procedures, physical examination, and diagnostic evaluation.

A. Supine Position

The optimal position for examination and in-line immobilization is supine. Once in the emergency department, the patient's rigid collar should be changed to a semirigid collar (Miami-J). Remember to limit the amount of time the patient is kept on any hard surface to minimize discomfort and avoid pressure injury.

B. Lateral Position

If the patient cannot lie supine for any reason (eg, vomiting), the lateral position with careful in-line cervical stabilization is acceptable.

C. Technique for Moving the Patient

If the patient must be moved, in-line spinal stabilization should be maintained and the head and trunk rolled as one unit (logroll). Proper technique requires three individuals. The first individual stands at the head of the bed and is responsible for maintaining cervical spine immobilization and controlling the turn. The two remaining individuals stand to one side of the patient and are in charge of maintaining thoracic and lumbar spine immobilization.

▶ Establish Airway and Maintain Ventilation

As with all patients in the emergency department, initial assessment should focus on airway and breathing. However, when vertebral or spinal injury is suspected, neck alignment and immobility must be maintained during all attempts to establish adequate ventilation.

In the patient with apnea or overt respiratory failure, a definitive airway should be established immediately. Whenever possible, rapid sequence intubation is the preferred as the least traumatic and most efficient method of achieving intubation (see Chapter 10). Designate an assistant to maintain cervical spine immobilization during intubation, and minimize neck extension induced by direct laryngoscopy. Airway adjuncts such as a fiberoptic bronchoscope or videolaryngoscope, in the hands of an experienced user may further minimize neck movement. Nasotracheal intubation is an option only in the spontaneously breathing patient.

Spontaneously breathing patients with cervical spinal cord injuries can have loss of diaphragmatic and/or intercostal muscle innervation, which may cause them to tire easily, causing ineffective ventilation and progressively worsening hypoxemia and hypercapnia. In such cases, continuous pulse oximetry, close clinical observation, and serial capnography are useful adjuncts to monitor changes in ventilatory status.

▶ Establish Satisfactory Circulation

A. Shock or Hypotension

Although hypotension may be caused directly by spinal injury, hypovolemia remains more common in the setting of blunt or penetrating trauma. Therefore, shock must be presumed hypovolemic (ie, hemorrhagic) until proven otherwise (see Chapter 11). If open wounds are present, significant external hemorrhage may have occurred at the scene of the injury. Hypovolemia may also occur as a result of hemorrhage into internal compartments such as the chest or pelvis. Initial treatment of hypotension should be aimed at volume replacement using crystalloid and/or blood products.

Neurogenic shock causes hypotension as a result of loss of sympathetic tone below the level of a spinal cord injury. This can occur when there is injury at or above T6. Although this diagnosis can only be made once hypovolemia has been ruled out through appropriate examination, imaging, and laboratory studies, appropriate treatment should not be withheld during the workup. The therapeutic goal for neurogenic shock is maintenance of adequate perfusion, which is commonly refractory to volume replacement. Following fluid resuscitation of at least 2 L warmed crystalloid, start a vasopressor such as dopamine to keep the mean arterial pressure above 85–90 mm Hg. Place a Foley catheter and carefully monitor urine output, which should be equal to or greater than 30 mL/h.

B. Head Injuries

Head injuries are associated with approximately 25% of all patients with spinal cord injury. Patients with altered mental status, seizures, or cranial nerve or other focal neurologic deficits require emergency imaging of the brain after the initial assessment and stabilization of the ABCs. A noncontrast CT scan of the head is the study of choice to identify intracranial injuries. If the patient has only a history of loss of consciousness and is alert and oriented in the emergency department, head CT scan can be delayed and accomplished in conjunction with other CT scans that may be required to evaluate the patient with possible spinal injury.

▶ Minimize Neurologic Injury

A. Consider Steroids in Acute Nonpenetrating Spinal Injury

There has been heavy debate over the clinical significance of the use of corticosteroids in the treatment of spinal injury based on the NASCIS II AND NASCIS III studies. The 8th edition of the Advanced Trauma Life Support Guidelines no longer recommends methylprednisolone administration, stating "at present, there is insufficient evidence to support the routine use of steroids in spinal cord injury." In addition, the Canadian Association of Emergency Physicians no longer supports the use of steroids in the acute care of spinal cord injuries. It is important to note that, despite these conclusions, high-dose methylprednisolone remains a treatment option in acute blunt spinal cord injuries and remains widely utilized. If chosen as a treatment, give methylprednisolone, 30 mg/kg as an intravenous bolus over 15 minutes; after a 45-minute delay, begin a maintenance infusion of 5.4 mg/kg/h for 24 hours in patients receiving treatment within the first 3 hours after injury. Patients receiving treatment 3–8 hours after injury should be maintained on steroid therapy for 48 hours. Initiation of steroid treatment more than 8 hours after injury is not indicated. It is important to remember that there is risk associated with steroid therapy in both increased incidence of infection and avascular necrosis. Because of the often-limited information regarding time of injury in the initial emergency department evaluation, therapy may be instituted until injury time has been confirmed. Obtain specialty consultation as soon as possible.

Note: Steroids play no role in the treatment of penetrating spinal cord injuries.

B. Give Antibiotics for Penetrating Injuries

Patients with penetrating spinal cord injury (eg, gunshot wound) should receive prophylactic antimicrobials. Nafcillin, 200 mg/kg/d intravenously in 4–6 divided doses, is widely recommended.

▶ Treat Complications

A. Urinary Incontinence or Retention

Patients may not note bladder dysfunction after spinal trauma because of loss of sensation below the lesion. Insert an indwelling catheter whenever spinal trauma is suspected to prevent urinary retention and to aid in monitoring urine output.

B. Ileus

Paralytic ileus and gastric atony are common after spinal trauma. Give the patient nothing by mouth until spinal injury is excluded. If spinal cord injury is confirmed, a nasogastric tube connected to intermittent low-pressure suction should be placed to prevent vomiting in the acute post-injury period.

C. Aspiration

Diligent suctioning of secretions and antiemetics are essential in management of spinal trauma. Aspiration pneumonitis is a serious complication in patients with decreased respiratory function and inability to adequately protect their airway.

D. Exposure

Denervated skin is prone to the development of pressure necrosis. Remove the spine board promptly during the evaluation while continuing to maintain logroll precautions. Completely undressing the patient will not only allow for a complete examination but it will also ensure that no foreign objects such as car keys, a belt, or wallet are pushing into the skin thereby increasing the likelihood of pressure ulcer formation.

Patients with spinal cord injury are particularly susceptible to exposure and, while exposure is essential, the patient should be covered with warm blankets in the emergency department to prevent hypothermia.

▶ Take Additional Measures as Needed

A patient with spinal cord injury requires the same resuscitative measures customarily employed in major trauma. Evaluate and treat all life-threatening conditions (eg, tension pneumothorax, cardiac tamponade, hemorrhagic shock) that take precedence over definitive treatment of vertebral and spinal cord trauma (Chapter 11). In other words, follow the ABCs of trauma evaluation. Always maintain in-line spinal immobilization during resuscitation and treatment.

American College of Surgeons Committee on Trauma: Advanced Trauma Life Support for Doctors Student Course Manual. 8th ed. 2008.

Canadian Association of Emergency Physicians: Steroids in acute spinal cord injury: position statement. Can J Emerg Med 2003;5(1):7–9.

Gerling MC et al: Effects of cervical spine immobilization technique and laryngoscope blade selection on an unstable cervical spine in a cadaver model for intubation. Ann Emerg Med 2000;36:293 [PMID: 11020675].

Goldberg W et al: Distribution and patterns of blunt traumatic cervical spine injury. Ann Emerg Med 2001;38:17 [PMID: 11423806].

Vale F et al: Combined medical and surgical treatment after acute spinal cord injury: result of a prospective pilot study to assess the merits of aggressive medical resuscitation and blood pressure management. J Neurosurg 1997;87:239–246.

▼ FURTHER EVALUATION OF THE PATIENT WITH SPINAL INJURY

▶ History

Mechanism is an essential part of the history to be obtained by the patient, EMS, or any person who witnessed the event. For instance, a restrained individual in a motor vehicle collision would be more prone to a flexion/extension injury, whereas an individual who fell and landed on his or her feet would be susceptible to compression force and subsequent vertebral damage.

Complaints of back or neck pain should arouse a suspicion of spine injury and is more sensitive than pain with palpation of the spine. However, the absence of spinal pain does not eliminate the possibility of spinal injury, especially if the patient is under the influence of alcohol or other mind-altering drugs. Consider spinal injury in any patient with blunt head injury, a neurologic deficit anatomically consistent with injury at a particular spinal level, or a penetrating injury to the neck, chest, or abdomen.

▶ General Physical Examination

A brief general physical examination should precede specific assessment of neurologic function. Obtain complete vital signs, including core temperature.

Carefully examine the head, chest, heart, abdomen, and extremities for other abnormalities. Remember that patients with spinal cord injuries may show few, if any, signs or symptoms of coexisting major injury because of anesthesia below the level of the lesion. Pain, guarding, rebound tenderness, and other signs may be absent despite the presence of fractured ribs, hemothorax, hemoperitoneum, peritonitis, and other major injuries. Examination of the genitals, rectum, and perineum may reveal priapism, decreased or absent rectal sphincter tone, or diminished perineal sensation, which are all suggestive of spinal cord injury. Diligent, repeated examinations, laboratory tests, and appropriate radiologic imaging are necessary to detect unsuspected injury.

Gently but thoroughly examine the neck and spine for deformity, edema, ecchymosis, muscle spasm, or tenderness indicating possible vertebral fracture. A palpable defect in the posterior neck ligaments may be the only clue to major spinal injury.

▶ Neurologic Examination

Neurologic examination assesses the following functions: mentation, motor function, sensation, and brainstem and spinal reflexes.

A. Mentation

The spectrum of mentation includes all levels of consciousness ranging from alert to comatose. The patient's ability for mentation is best assessed by their Glasgow Coma Score (Chapter 12). This systematic evaluation is easily reproduced to monitor changes, is widely used, and easily conveyed to the neurosurgical or orthopedic consultant.

B. Motor Function

(See Table 27–1.) The American Spinal Injury Association recommends the following scale for gradation of motor strength:

- 0—No contraction or movement
- 1—Minimal movement
- 2—Active movement, but not against gravity
- 3—Active movement against gravity
- 4—Active movement against light resistance
- 5—Active movement against full resistance

1. Normal movement means that the patient moves all extremities spontaneously, purposefully (ie, in response to specific commands), and with full strength and range of motion. This would be a 5/5 on the above scale.

2. Paralysis denotes no movement of the extremity or muscle group, either spontaneously or in response to painful stimuli. Complete paralysis would be a grade of 0/5 on the above scale. (Stimuli should be applied both directly to the extremity and to the trunk, because failure to move may be secondary to hypoesthesia of the extremity.) Failure to move

Table 27–1. Motor Function Chart.[a]

Action to Be Tested	Muscle	Cord Segment	Nerves	Plexus
Shoulder Girdle and Upper Extremity				
Flexion of neck Extension of neck Rotation of neck Lateral bending of neck	Deep neck muscles (sternocleidomastoid and trapezius also participate)	C1–4	Cervical	Cervical
Elevation of upper thorax	Scaleni	C3–5	Phrenic	
Inspiration	Diaphragm			
Adduction of arm from behind to front	Pectoralis major and minor	C5–8, T1	Pectoral (thoracic; from medial and lateral cords of plexus)	Brachial
Forward thrust of shoulder	Seratus anterios	C5–7	Long thoracic	
Elevation of scapula Medial adduction and elevation of scapula	Levator scapulae Rhomboids	C3–5 C4, 5	Dorsal scapular	
Abduction of arm Lateral rotation of arm	Supraspinatus Infraspinatus	C4–6 C4–6	Suprascapular	
Medial rotation of arm	Latissimus dorsi, teres major, and subscapularis	C5–8	Subscapular (from posterior cord of plexus)	
Adduction of arm from front to back	Latissimus dorsi, teres major, and subscapularis	C5–8	Subscapular (from posterior cord of plexus)	
Abduction of arm	Deltoid	C5, 6	Axillary (from posterior cord of plexus)	
Lateral rotaion of arm	Teres minor	C4, 5		
Flexion of forearm Supination of forearm Adduction of arm Flexion of forearm Flexion of forearm	Biceps brachii Coracobrachialis Brachialis	C5, 6 C5–7 C5, 6	Musculocutaneous (from lateral cord of plexus)	

(continued)

Table 27–1. Motor Function Chart.[a] (*Continued*)

Action to Be Tested	Muscle	Cord Segment	Nerves	Plexus
Shoulder Girdle and Upper Extremity (cont.)				
Ulnar flexion of hand	Flexor carpi ulnaris	C7, 8; T1	Ulnar (from medial cord of plexus)	
Flexion of all fingers but thumb	Flexor digitorum profundus (ulnar portion)	C7, 8; T1		
Adduction of metacarpal of thumb		C8, T1		
Abduction of little finger	Adductor pollicis	C8, T1		
Opposition of little finger	Abductor digitiquinti	C7, 8; T1		
Flexion of little finger	Opponens digiti quinti	C7, 8; T1		
Flexion of proximal phalanx,	Flexor digitiquinti	C8, T1		
	Interossei			
Pronatlon of forearm	Pronator teres	C6, 7	Median (C6,7 from lateral cord of plexus; C8, T1 from medial cord of plexus)	
Radial flexion of hand	Flexor carpi radialis	C6, 7		
Flexion of hand	Palmaris longus	C7, 8; T1		
Flexion of middle phalanx of index, middle, ring, or little finger	Flexor digitorum superficialis	C7, 8; T1		
Flexion of hand	Flexor pollicis longus	C7, 8; T1		
Flexion of terminal phalanx of thumb	Flexor digitorum profundus (radial portion)	C7, 8; T1		
Flexion of terminal phalanx of index or middle finger				
Flexion of hand				
Abduction of metacarpal of thumb	Abductor pollicis brevis	C7, 8; T1	Median (C7,8 from lateral cord of plexus; C8,T1 from medial cord of plexus)	Brachial
Flexion of proximal phalanx of thumb	Flexor pollicis brevis	C7, 8; T1		
Opposition of metacarpal of thumb	Opponens pollicis	C8, T1		
Flexion of proximal phalanx and extension of the two distal phalanges of index, middle, ring, or little finger	Lumbricales (the 2 lateral)	C8, T1	Ulnar	
	Lumbricales (the second medial)	C8, T1		
	Triceps brachii and anconeus			
Extension of forearm	Brachloradialls	C6–8	Radial (from posterior cord of plexus)	
Flexion of forearm	Extensor carpi radialis	C5, 6		
Radial extension of hand	Extensor digitorum	C6–8	Radial (from posterior cord of plexus)	
Extension of phalanges of index, middle, ring, or little finger	Extensor digitiquinti proprius	C7–8		
	Extensor carpi ulnaris	C6–8		
Extension of hand		C6–8		
Extension of phalanges of little finger	Supinator			
Extension of hand	Abductor pollicis longus	C5–7		
Ulnar extension of hand	Extensor pollicis brevis	C7, 8; T1		
Supination of forearm	Extensor pollicis brevis	C7, 8		
Abduction of metacarpal of thumb	Extensor indicis proprius	C6, 8		
Radial extension of hand		C6–8		
Extension of thumb				
Radial extension of hand				
Extension of index fingure				
Extension of hand				
Trunk and Thorax				
Elevation of ribs	Thoracic, abdominal, and back	T1–L3	Thoracic and posterior lumbosacral branches	Brachial
Depression of ribs				
Contraction of abdomen				
Anteroflexion of trunk				
Lateral flexion of trunk				

(continued)

Table 27–1. Motor Function Chart.[a] (*Continued*)

Action to Be Tested	Muscle	Cord Segment	Nerves	Plexus
Hip Girdle and Lower Extremity				
Flexion of hip	Iliopsoas	L1–3	Femoral	Lumbar
Flexion of hip (and eversion of thigh)	Sartorius	L2, 3		
Extension of leg	Quadriceps femoris	L2–4		
Adduction of thigh	Pectineus	L2, 3	Obturator	Sacral
	Adductor longus	L2, 3		
	Adductor brevis	L2–4		
	Adductor magnus	L3, 4		
	Gracilis	L2–4		
Adductor of thigh	Obturator externus	L3, 4		
Lateral rotation of thigh	Gluteus medius and mininus	L4, 5; S1	Superior gluteal	
Abduction of thigh	Tensor fasciae latae	L4, 5		
Medial rotation of thigh	Piriformis	S1, 2		
Flexion of thigh	Gluteus maximus	L4, 5:S1, 2	Inferior gluteal	
Lateral rotation of thigh	Obturator intemus	L5, S1	Muscular branches form	
Abduction of thigh	Gemeli	L4, 5; S1	sacral plexus	
Lateral rotation of thigh	Quadratus femoris	L4, 5; S1		
Flexion of leg (assist in extension of thigh)	Biceps femoris	L4, 5; S1, 2	Sciatic (trunk)	Sacral
	Semitendinosus	L4, 5; S1		
	Semimembranosus	L4, 5; S1		
Dorsal flexion of foot	Tibialis anterior	L4, 5	Deep peroneal	
Supination of foot		L4, 5; S1		
Extension of toes 2–5	Extensor digitorum lingus			
Dorsal flexion of foot				
Extension of great toe and the three medial toes	Extensor digitorum brevis	L4, 5; S1		
Plantar flexion of foot in pronation	Peroneus longus and brevis	L5, S1	Superficial peroneal	
Plantar flexion of foot in supination	Gastrocnemius	L5, S1, 2	Tibial	
Plantar flexion of foot in supination	Tibialis posterior and	L5, S1		
Flexion of terminal phalanx of toes II–V	triceps surae	S1, 2		
Plantar flexion of foot in supination	Flexor digitorum longus	L5, S1, 2		
Flexion of terminal phalanx of great toe	Flexor hallucis longus	L5, S1		
Flexion of middle phalanx of toes II–V	Flexor digitorum brevis	L5, S1, 2		
Flexion of proximal phalanx of great toe	Flexor hallucis brevis	S1, 2		
Spreading and closing of toes	Small muscles of foot			
Flexion of proximal phalanx of toes				
Voluntary control of pelvic floor	Perineal and sphincters	S2–4	Pudendal	

[a]Modified from McKinley JC. Reproduced, with permission, from de Groot J: *Correlative Neuroanatomy*, 21st ed. Appleton & Lange, 1991.

at all, either spontaneously or in response to an unpleasant stimulus, may indicate paralysis due to a structural lesion (eg, fracture) or metabolic causes (eg, drug overdose). Often, failure to respond is simply due to an inadequately painful stimulus.

3. Gradation between these extremes (grade 0–5) should be described precisely, for example, "Patient extends right arm and leg, flexes left arm, and extends left leg in response to supraorbital pressure."

Avoid broad descriptive terms such as "paraparesis" or "decerebrate posturing."

C. Sensation

(See Figures 27–1 and 27–2 and Table 27–2.) Test as many sensory functions as possible in a patient with suspected spinal cord injury (in contrast to the more simple examination required for head trauma). Loss of some or all sensory functions below the lesion permits its precise anatomic

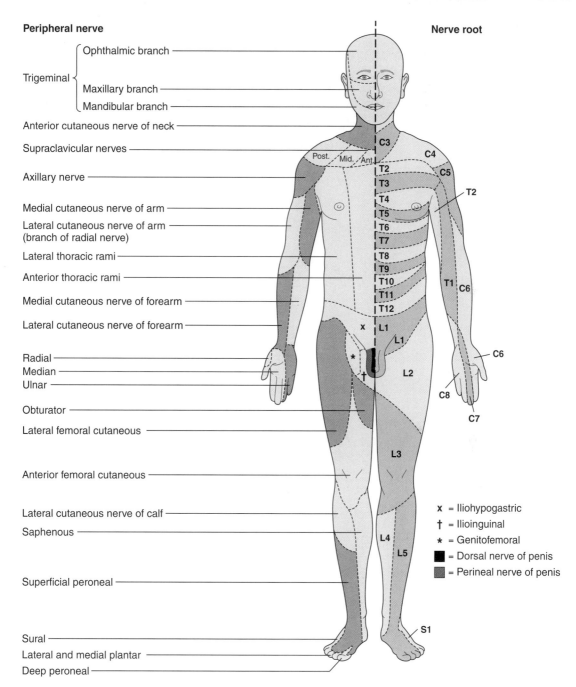

▲ **Figure 27–1.** Cutaneous Innervation (Anterior). (Reproduced, with permission, from Greenberg DA, Aminoff MJ, Simon RP: *Clinical Neurology*, 5th edn. New York: McGraw-Hill, 2002.)

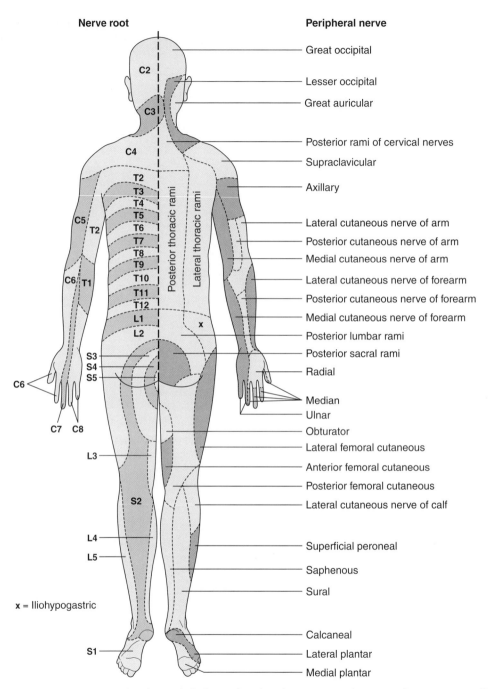

▲ **Figure 27-2.** Cutaneous Innervation (Posterior). (Reproduced, with permission, from Greenberg DA, Aminoff MJ, Simon RP: *Clinical Neurology*, 5th ed. New York: McGraw-Hill, 2002.)

Table 27–2. Commonly Used Landmarks for Testing Dermatomal Sensation.

Location	Dermatome
Second rib	C4–T2
Nipple	T4
Lower rib border	T7-8
Umbilicus	T10
Inguinal ligament	L1

localization. Perianal sensation should be tested; its presence eliminates the possibility of complete spinal cord transection and implies an improved prognosis.

1. Position, vibration, and light touch—The dorsal columns can be tested by determining response to vibration, light touch, and changes in position.

2. Pain and temperature—The ventral columns are tested by evaluating sensitivity to pain (pinprick) and temperature.

3. Impaired mentation—When mentation is impaired, a pinprick or deep painful stimulation may be the only reliable sensory test.

D. Brain-Stem Reflexes

Brain-stem reflexes are usually intact except in the case of high cervical spinal cord injury, when nystagmus (midbrain, pons), facial hypalgesia (spinal nucleus of the trigeminal nerve), and hypoventilation (phrenic nerve, intercostals) may be present.

Note: The presence of brain-stem signs should not be attributed to spinal cord injury until an intracranial lesion has been excluded.

E. Spinal Reflexes

Tendon jerks and plantar responses are usually absent below the level of an acute complete spinal cord transection (Table 27–3); asymmetry is also common. Spasticity or increased tone in muscle groups may occur with partial spinal cord injuries. Anal sphincter tone (reflex and voluntary) becomes flaccid following complete spinal cord transection. Priapism occurring soon after injury suggests immediate complete spinal cord lesion. Onset at a later time may indicate that the lesion has progressed from an incomplete to a complete stage. Sweating and skin vasomotor tone are absent below the level of a spinal cord lesion.

The bulbocavernosus reflex is dependent on an intact S1 and S2 spinal reflex. If the bulbocavernosus reflex is preserved in the presence of complete perineal sensory loss and flaccid paralysis of the lower extremities, it indicates that the period of spinal shock has passed and that the neurologic deficit is due

to a lesion above the S1 segment. Absence of the bulbocavernosus reflex may indicate either the presence of spinal shock or a spinal cord lesion including the S1 and S2 segments. Spinal shock usually resolves within 24 hours and is accompanied by return of the bulbocavernosus reflex if the S1 and S2 segments are not directly involved in the spinal cord lesion.

▶ Spinal Cord Syndromes

A. Complete Spinal Cord Lesion

The absence of sacral sparing (perianal sensation, rectal sphincter tone) indicates a complete spinal cord lesion, with recovery unlikely if the condition persists longer than 24 hours. Sacral sparing suggests an improved prognosis.

B. Partial Spinal Cord Lesions

1. Brown-Séquard syndrome—This syndrome is usually caused by penetrating injuries resulting in hemisection of the spinal cord. The findings include loss of distal ipsilateral position and vibration sense, distal ipsilateral motor loss and vasomotor paralysis, and distal loss of pain and temperature sense below T12 on the contralateral side (including the genitals and perineum).

2. Central cord syndrome—This syndrome is usually due to cervical hyperextension, involving the central gray matter and the central parts of the lateral spinothalamic tracts. Quadriplegia may result, with minimal sacral sparing. The upper extremities are more involved than the lower extremities.

3. Anterior cord syndrome—This syndrome results from cervical hyperflexion injuries. Position and vibration (posterior column functions) are preserved, but motor function, temperature, and pain sensation are lost bilaterally below the lesion.

▶ Reexamination

Neurologic examination is helpful only if it is repeated often enough to establish a diagnosis, suggest further diagnostic steps, or clearly establish a trend in neurologic function. If successive examinations indicate improvement, further specialized testing may not be necessary. Failure to improve—verified by repeated examinations—indicates that additional studies are necessary, as does progressive deterioration from a baseline established by examination done on arrival in the emergency department. It is particularly important to note progressive neurologic dysfunction if injury involves the cervical spinal cord, because respiratory failure may result.

▶ Laboratory Examination

Perform a baseline laboratory evaluation, including complete blood count (CBC), coagulation profile, basic metabolic profile, blood type, crossmatch, and urinalysis. Arterial blood gas measurements are necessary if ventilation is impaired or potentially threatened.

Table 27–3. Summary of Reflexes.[a]

Reflexes	Afferent Nerve	Center	Efferent Nerve
Superficial reflexes			
Corneal	Cranial V	Pons	Cranial VII
Nasal (sneeze)	Cranial V	Brain stem and upper cord	Cranials, V, VII, IX, X, and spinal nerves of expiration
Pharyngeal and uvular	Cranial IX	Medulla	Cranial X
Upper abdominal	T7, 8, 9, 10	T7, 8, 9, 10	T7, 8, 9, 10
Lower abdominal	T10, 11, 12,	T10, 11, 12	T10, 11, 12
Cremasteric	Femoral	L1	Genitofemoral
Plantar	Tibial	S1, 2	Tibial
Anal	Pudendal	S4, 5	Pudendal
Deep reflexes			
Jaw	Cranial V	Pons	Cranial V
Biceps	Musculocutaneous	C5, 6	Musculocutaneous
Triceps	Radial	C6, 7, 8	Radial
Periosteoradial	Radial	C6, 7, 8	Radial
Wrist (flexion)	Median	C6, 7, 8	Median
Wrist (extension)	Radial	C7, 8	Radial
Patellar	Femoral	L2, 3, 4	Femoral
Archilles	Tibial	S1, 2	Tibial
Visceral reflexes			
Light	Cranial II	Midbrain	Cranial III
Accommodation	Cranial II	Occipital cortex	Cranial III
Ciliospinal	A sensory nerve	T1, 2	Cervical sympathetics
Oculocardiac	Cranial V	Medulla	Cranial X
Carotid sinus	Cranial IX	Medulla	Cranial X
Bulbocavemosus	Pudendal	S2, 3, 4	Pelvic autonomic
Bladder and rectal	Pudendal	S2, 3, 4	Pudendal and autonomies

[a]Reproduced, with permission, from deGroot J: *Correlative Neuroanatomy*, 21st ed. Appleton & Lange, 1991.

▶ Imaging

Suspicion of spinal injury in a patient necessitates radiographic imaging, the modality of which must be chosen based on the patient's history and physical examination. In today's emergency setting, CT has become increasingly popular due to rapid and widespread availability, as well as and increased sensitivity for many injuries. In addition, the development of decision rules to help direct this endeavor have been established and validated over large patient populations.

Careful and correct interpretation of radiographs is critically important in the treatment of spinal cord injury. Many spine abnormalities (eg, minor facet fractures and nondisplaced fractures) may be more easily recognized by a radiologist. In a large study of blunt trauma patients, C-spine injuries were identified in 2.4% of patients. Three-view C-spine radiographs identified a C-spine injury in 1.5% of the patients. Radiographs were interpreted as normal in 0.9% of patients later found to have a C-spine injury.

Note: Normal radiographs do not exclude the presence of spinal cord injury. Spinal cord injury without radiographic abnormality is an uncommon but well-described condition, especially in children with flexible spinal columns and relatively larger head-to-body size ratios. In the NEXUS study—a large, observational, multicenter study—these injuries occurred in 0.07% of all blunt trauma patients and in 6% of all the patients with spinal injuries. Central cord syndrome (central hemorrhage) and spontaneously reduced dislocations can be associated with normal X-rays, as can ligamentous tears resulting from flexion–extension injuries. A thorough physical examination and a careful repeated neurologic evaluation are therefore essential in all cases.

A. Chest, Skull, and Pelvis

Portable chest and pelvis radiographs are standard in the initial evaluation of the patient with blunt spinal injury. Associated head injuries are common, and spinal injury patients often require CT scan of the head to evaluate intracranial injuries.

B. Cervical Spine

Both the National Emergency X-Radiography Utilization Study (NEXUS) criteria and Canadian C-spine Rules (CCR) have been shown reliable in terms of negative predictive value in the detection of cervical spine injury. The NEXUS criteria suggest that cervical spine imaging is unnecessary when all of the five following criteria are met:

1. No neurologic abnormalities are present
2. The patient has normal mental status
3. There is no evidence of intoxication
4. There is no posterior midline cervical spinal tenderness
5. There is no distracting painful injury

At a minimum, anteroposterior and lateral views of the C-spine extending from C1 to T1 and an odontoid (open mouth) view are required if cervical cord injury is suspected. The lateral C-spine view alone is only 79% sensitive in detecting C-spine injuries. If the segments from C6 to T1 are not visible, a "swimmer's" view should be obtained by having the patient supine, with one upper extremity abducted and extended (arm raised above head) and the opposite upper extremity adducted and extended (arm kept at side of body). The shoulder of the adducted and extended extremity is then depressed by having a person stand at the foot of the bed and pull gently on the patient's hand. The X-ray is shot upward through the axilla of the abducted, extended extremity. Oblique views increase the sensitivity of the C-spine series and are recommended by some in the evaluation of suspected cervical spinal injury. Standard oblique views require neck rotation; this can be avoided by performing a trauma oblique view, which is a modification of the oblique view. The trauma oblique view is obtained by aiming the X-ray beam at a 60° angle to the plane of the table with the patient supine (and immobilized).

Other diagnostic modalities must be used if all of the cervical vertebrae cannot be seen adequately with these techniques or if clinical suspicion for injury remains in the setting of normal radiographs. Flexion–extension views of the cervical spine are not routinely recommended in the acute evaluation of cervical instability. Any patient with a new neurologic symptom requires imaging with CT and/or MRI.

Magnetic resonance imaging (MRI), with superior ability to visualize soft tissues plays a significant role in the evaluation of the ligamentous structures of the cervical spine, as well as the spinal cord itself. Patients with neurologic symptoms not explained by radiograph or CT must undergo MRI to evaluate for cord compression or injury.

Patients with persistent cervical pain or tenderness despite normal imaging should be assumed to have a ligamentous injury. Even if the patient has a normal neurologic exam and no neurologic symptoms, continuous immobilization with a well-padded, rigid cervical collar is recommended for 14–28 days until follow-up studies such as flexion–extension radiographs or MRI can be performed.

Table 27–4 summarizes the mechanisms and common findings in many of the radiographically identifiable C-spine injury patterns.

C. Thoracic and Lumbar Spines

There are no established decision rules for imaging the thoracic and lumbar spines. However, criteria similar to that of the cervical spine are commonly applied. These criteria mandate that full radiographic evaluation be performed unless the patient is fully alert and has no evidence of midline bony tenderness; focal neurologic defect; intoxication; or painful, distracting injury. In addition, if a patient has a fracture in one portion of the spinal column, the entire spinal column should be imaged because the occurrence of an associated fracture at another level is relatively common.

D. Special Studies

1. CT scan—With advances in the speed, resolution, and the ability to reformat axial scans into two- and three-dimensional images, CT scanning of the spine has become very common and has replaced traditional plain films especially in evaluation of the C-spine. CT scan is the easiest and most sensitive imaging modality for evaluation of spinal column injury. MRI may be required for better visualization of the relationships between the spinal cord and the vertebral canal. For nonobese patients with a low pretest probability of thoracic or lumbar spinal fracture or dislocation, conventional radiographs are still an acceptable, clinically appropriate and cost effective diagnostic tool to evaluate the integrity of spinal column.

Table 27–4. Cervical Spine Injuries.[a]

Type of Injury	Injury Characteristics
Flexion-type injuries	
Simple wedge compression fracture	Anterior loss of height; intact posterior column; stable fracture
Flexion teardrop fracture	Fracture of the anteroinferior aspect of the vertebral body; disruption of anterior, middle, and posterior columns; highly unstable injury
Anterior subluxation	Disruption of posterior ligamentous complexes; potentially unstable
Bilateral facet dislocation	Anterior displacement of more than half of the anteroposterior diameter of the vertebral body; highly unstable injury
Clay shoveler's fracture	Fracture or avulsion of the spinous process; commonly seen in lower cervical vertebrae; stable injury
Flexion-rotation injuries	
Unilateral facet dislocation	Anterior displacement of less than half of the anteroposterior diameter of the vertebral body; neurologic deficits can occur; rotation may be noted by malaligned spinous processes on anteroposterior film or off-set overlap of facets ("bow-tie sign") on lateral view; usually stable
Rotary atlantoaxial dislocation	Type of unilateral facet dislocation; odontoid shows asymmetry of the lateral masses; unstable injury
Extension-type injuries	
Hangman fracture	Fracture through pedicles of C2 secondary to hyperextension; spinolaminar disruption; unstable fracture
Extension teardrop fracture	Displaced anteroinferior bony fragment avulsion secondary to traction on anterior longitudinal ligament highly unstable fracture
Fracture of the posterior arch of C1	Odontoid view demonstrates no displacement of the lateral masses; stable injury
Axial compression injuries	
Jefferson fracture	Lateral mass displacement of C1; significant prevertebral soft tissue edema; possibly unstable injury
Burst fracture of the vertebral body	Disruption of the anterior and middle columns; mandates CT scan or MRI to evaluate retropulsion; if loss of height > 25%, neurologic deficit, or retropulsion occurs, then consider it to bean unstable fracture
Complex mechanism injuries	
Atlantoaxial subluxation	Transverse ligament disruption; injury suspected if the predental space is >3.5 mm (5 mm in children); unstable injury
Atlanto-occipital dislocation	Complete disruption of all ligamentous relationships between atlas and occiput; death often occurs immediately; highly unstable
Odontoid process fractures	Type I: Avulsion of tip of dens; stable fracture
	Type II: Fracture at base of dens; unstable fracture
	Type III: Fracture extends into body of C2; unstable fracture

[a]Modified, with permission, from Hockberger RS, Kirshenbaum KJ: Spine. In Rosen P et al. (editors). *Emergency Medicine Concepts and Clinical Practice*, 5th ed., Vol. 3. Elsevier Science, 2002.

2. MRI—MRI is indicated in patients with suspected spinal cord injuries and in patients with documented cord injuries. MRI provides a detailed view of the spinal cord, associated edema or hemorrhage, and surrounding soft tissues. With information obtained from MRI scans, injuries can be followed or operative interventions for cord decompression and spinal stabilization can be planned.

E. Special Populations

Note that established decision rules do not apply to pediatric or pregnant patients. In addition, special consideration must be to limit radiation exposure in these subgroups, while still performing an adequate evaluation. When in doubt, it is best to obtain early subspecialty consultation in treating such patients. Signed informed consent is necessary when pregnant patients require radiographic imaging of the spinal column.

DISPOSITION OF THE PATIENT WITH VERTEBRAL COLUMN OR SPINAL CORD TRAUMA

▶ Clinical Findings

In vertebral fractures without spinal cord injury, there is generally focal pain and tenderness over the vertebral column. Radiographic imaging shows fractures that may be in the vertebral body, the transverse processes, or the spinous processes. Coexisting dislocation or instability may be present, however, the examination is normal.

The only patients who do not require hospitalization are those with mildly symptomatic or asymptomatic, linear, nondisplaced, stable fractures of the spinous or transverse processes, or similar fractures of the sacrum or coccyx. Such patients may be given analgesics and a cervical collar for immobilization (if fractures are in the cervical vertebrae). However, prior to discharge it is important to consult an orthopedist or neurosurgeon to make certain they are in agreement with this course of action and to ensure timely follow-up.

In contrast, spinal cord injury with or without vertebral fractures is associated with neurologic symptoms and neurologic deficit (eg, sensory deficit ending circumferentially at T8). Bony injury to the vertebrae demonstrable on radiography may or may not be apparent because severe flexion–extension injuries and bony instability from ligamentous tears may cause serious or even fatal spinal cord injury without bony abnormalities. Obtain emergent neurosurgical or orthopedic consultation.

Hospitalization is required for patients with neurologic deficit, an unstable or potentially unstable vertebral column (with or without fracture), fractures or subluxation of vertebral bodies, or severe pain requiring parenteral analgesics for relief.

WHIPLASH (HYPEREXTENSION) INJURIES (C-SPINE SPRAIN)

▶ Clinical Findings

Patients with whiplash have a history of abrupt hyperextension of the neck (usually from a motor vehicle accident), usually without loss of consciousness. Injury from hyperflexion often occurs as well. Symptoms such as neck pain or muscle spasm, headache, hoarseness, and dysphagia often do not appear until 12–24 hours after injury. Neck pain may radiate to the arms or chest. Physical examination may show tenderness of posterior neck muscles and limited range of motion. Specifically, there is no evidence of neurologic deficit. By definition, whiplash does not cause fractures that are evident on cervical X-rays, although severe injuries may rupture the anterior disk fibers and result in widened disk spaces. X-rays are usually normal but may show reversal of the normal cervical lordosis. As previously mentioned, patients may have ligamentous instability despite normal C-spine radiographs. For this reason, patients with persistent midline C-spine tenderness should be immobilized in a well-padded, rigid collar 24 h/d for 7–14 days until reexamined by a primary-care physician or spine surgeon.

▶ Treatment

Treatment consists of a rigid cervical collar, heat, and analgesics usually nonsteroidal anti-inflammatory medications are first line medications although narcotics are often required. Muscle relaxants may also be indicated. At the time of reexamination, if a ligamentous injury is present, flexion–extension views will detect subluxation. MRI can be useful to identify ligamentous injuries in patients with possible C-spine instability. If flexion–extension radiographs or MRI are abnormal, the patient should remain in the cervical collar and be referred to a spine surgeon to determine the significance of any subluxation.

▶ Disposition

Hospitalization is rarely required. Refer the patient to a primary-care physician or neurosurgeon for further evaluation.

Canadian Association of Emergency Physicians: Steroids in acute spinal cord injury: position statement. Can J Emerg Med 2003;5(1):7–9.

Ducker TB, Zeidman SM: Spinal cord injury. Role of steroid therapy. Spine 1994;19(20):2281–2287.

Frohna WJ: Emergency department evaluation and treatment of the neck and cervical spine injuries. Emerg Med Clin North Am 1999;17:739 [PMID: 10584102].

Hoffman JR et al: Validity of a set of clinical criteria to rule out injury to the cervical spine in patients with blunt trauma. N Engl J Med 2000;343:94 [PMID: 10891516].

Mower WR et al: Use of plain radiography to screen for cervical spine injuries. Ann Emerg Med 2001;38:1 [PMID: 11423803].

Panacek EA et al: Test performance of the individual NEXUS low-risk clinical screening criteria for cervical spine injury. Ann Emerg Med 2001;38:22 [PMID: 11423807].

Pollack CV et al: Use of flexion–extension radiographs of the cervical spine in blunt trauma. Ann Emerg Med 2001;38:8 [PMID: 11423804].

Ralston ME et al: Role of flexion–extension radiographs in blunt pediatric cervical spine injury. Acad Emerg Med 2001;8:237 [PMID: 11229945].

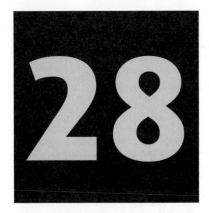

Orthopedic Emergencies

Royce Coleman, MD
Alison Reiland, MD

IMMEDIATE MANAGEMENT OF LIFE-THREATENING INJURIES

Patients with orthopedic injuries and musculoskeletal disorders constitute a large portion of patients presenting to the Emergency Department. All trauma patients should be managed initially in the same manner, with similar guiding principles of trauma care regardless of their underlying injuries. Orthopedic injuries may be dramatic, but they should not draw attention away from more critical elements of initial patient assessment and treatment. The emergency physician must assess the patient and manage injuries and based on the immediate threat to survival, evaluating each trauma patient with the primary survey, which consists of assessing the airway, breathing, circulation, disability, and exposure (ABCDEs) (Table 28–1).

Once the primary survey has been addressed, proceed to the secondary survey, which should be a thorough, but rapid physical examination from head to toe to assess for all injuries. With cervical spine precautions in place, logroll the patient, assess the posterior scalp, and examine the entire spine for tenderness or step-off deformities. Perform a digital rectal examination to evaluate for sphincter tone, gross blood, or abnormal prostate position. When evaluating the pelvis for stability, apply gentle anteroposterior and lateral compression. Visualize and go through range of motion of all joints and document all lacerations, abrasions, and contusions. Physical examination of orthopedic injuries includes inspection for deformity, color change, palpation for tenderness, range of motion, and assessment of neurovascular status. At this time, consider reduction of certain orthopedic emergencies such as a dislocated hip, knee, or any fracture or dislocation in which vascular compromise is present (Figure 28–1). Delayed reduction may lead to avascular necrosis, or other complications; therefore, if possible, reduce fractures and dislocations with neurovascular compromise before transferring the patient.

TRAUMATIC AMPUTATIONS

ESSENTIALS OF DIAGNOSIS

- ► Sharp, guillotine injuries are best candidates for reimplantation
- ► Keep amputated part clean, moisten with saline, and put on ice
- ► Do not allow part to freeze
- ► Cooling will help increase viability of amputated part up to 12–24 hours

▶ General Considerations

Patients incurring traumatic amputations should be considered for reimplantation surgery. Young healthy patients

Table 28–1. Potential Blood Loss from Closed Fractures.

Site	Amount (L)
Pelvis	1–5+
Femur	1–4
Spine	1–2
Leg	0.5–1
Arm	0.5–0.75

with sharp, guillotine injuries without crushing or avulsion damage are the best candidates for successful reimplantation. However, it is best to consider all patients as potential candidates, care for the amputated part, and make appropriate consultations or arrange for transfer.

▶ Clinical Findings

A. Symptoms and Signs

The patient presents with an amputated digit or limb.

B. X-ray Finding

Although this diagnosis is made clinically, X-rays often help delineate exactly where the injury occurred, or if underlying fractures or dislocations exist.

▶ Treatment

The amputated part should be kept clean, wrapped in a sterile dressing, moistened with sterile saline, placed in a

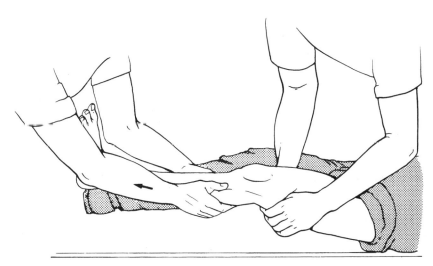

▲ **Figure 28–1.** Technique of manual traction to align an angulated fracture and correct deformity.

plastic bag, and put on ice. Do not use dry ice or allow the amputated part to freeze. Cooling the amputated part will increase the viability from 6–8 hours to approximately 12–24 hours. The injury should be treated as an open fracture, with appropriate use of antibiotics and tetanus prophylaxis.

▶ Disposition

Patients with limb amputations usually require consultation with an orthopedic, plastic, or trauma surgeon. These patients should be admitted for further surgical management, neurologic and vascular evaluation, and monitoring of blood loss. Patients with small digit amputations may be managed in the emergency department and discharged with appropriate close follow-up.

Lloyd MS, Teo TC, Pickford MA et al: Preoperative management of the amputated limb. Emerg Med J 2005;22(7):478–480 [PMID: 15983081].

COMPARTMENT SYNDROME

▶ General Considerations

A potentially devastating and subtle complication of orthopedic injuries is the development of a compartment syndrome. Although predominantly occurring in the lower extremities, a compartment syndrome can potentially occur anywhere in the body with a restricting compartment. Compartment syndromes are caused by compromised blood flow due to increased hydrostatic pressure in a closed tissue space. The lower leg has four compartments: anterior, lateral, posterior, and deep posterior. Trauma below the knee can lead to progressive swelling with eventual decreased blood flow from vascular compression as well as neurologic compromise. The immediate threat is to the viability of the tissue and nerves, but late findings can include permanent posttraumatic muscle contracture, infection, rhabdomyolysis, and renal failure.

▶ Clinical Findings

The classical findings associated with compartment syndrome are pallor, pulselessness, pain, paresthesias, and poikilothermia. Pain on passive stretching of the muscle groups and the subjective complaint of pain out of proportion to the physical findings are important findings. Decreased or absent pulses are a late and ominous sign, and the presence of a pulse does not exclude compartment syndrome. Delays in recognition of compartment syndrome are more likely to occur in sedated patients or in those with head injuries than in other patients due to altered mental status. The diagnosis can be confirmed by measuring intracompartmental pressures with a Stryker pressure monitor or

with a needle connected to an arterial line pressure monitor, although noninvasive methods such as ultrasound are being studied. Levels above 30 mm Hg are abnormal and lead to necrosis of nerve and muscle.

▶ Treatment

Initial interventions include immobilization and removal of any constricting bandages or splints, as well as being conscious of possible rhabdomyolysis and renal failure. Intracompartmental pressures greater than 30 mm Hg generally require immediate intervention with fasciotomy, preferably by a surgeon.

▶ Disposition

Patients with compartment syndrome require hospitalization for definitive surgical management.

Shadgan B, Menon M, O'Brien PJ et al: Diagnostic techniques in acute compartment syndrome of the leg. J Orthop Trauma 2008;22(8):581–587 [PMID: 18758292].

▼ GENERAL ORTHOPEDIC PRINCIPLES

FRACTURES AND DISLOCATIONS

Precise language exists to describe fractures, allowing relevant information to be communicated. The terms *closed* or *open* designate whether the skin and soft tissue overlying the fracture site are intact. The exact anatomic location should be included in the description including the name of the bone, side of the body, and standard reference points. Degrees of displacement and angulation should be described in terms of the distal structure's relationship to the more proximal part of the body. Additional modifiers include descriptions such as *comminuted* (fracture in more than two fragments), *impacted* (collapse of one fragment of bone onto another), *transverse* (fracture line at right angle to long axis of the bone), *oblique* (fracture line with angle other than right angle), and *spiral* (fracture line encircles the shaft of a long bone secondary to rotational forces). The term *valgus* refers to a deformity in which the described part is angled away from the body, whereas *varus* denotes angling toward the midline. An *avulsion fracture* occurs when a ligament or tendon pulls a fragment of bone away. *Pathologic fractures* occur in weakened areas of bone as seen with osteomalacia, cysts, carcinomas, and Paget disease. The possibility of a pathologic fracture should be considered when fractures occur with minimal trauma. *Stress fractures* occur most commonly in the lower extremity and are seen with repetitive trauma (eg, from prolonged marching or running). Stress fractures may be subtle, may be missed on initial radiographs, and may require a bone scan or other imaging modality to make the diagnosis.

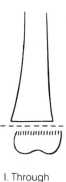 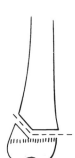 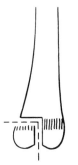 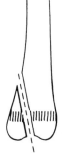 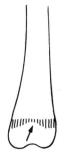

I. Through growth plate

II. Through metaphysis and growth plate

III. Through growth plate and epiphysis into joint

IV. Through metaphysis, growth plate, and epiphysis into joint

V. Crush of growth plate, may not be seen on X-ray

▲ **Figure 28-2.** Salter–Harris classification of growth plate injuries.

Dislocations are complete disruptions in the normal relationship of the articular surfaces of the bones making up a joint. They may be associated with fractures. Dislocations should be described by the relationship of the distal bone to the more proximal bone. A *subluxation* is an incomplete dislocation.

Pediatric fractures are distinguished from adult fractures due to difference in the bones of children, which are generally less dense and have increased compliance. A *Greenstick* fracture refers to an angulated fracture in which the cortex and periosteum are only disrupted on one side of the bone. *Torus* fractures (also called cortical or buckle fractures) involve a buckling of the cortex. Physeal, or growth plate injuries in children are described by the Salter–Harris classification (Figure 28–2).

Type I Injuries

The epiphysis is separated from the metaphysis without radiographic evidence of metaphyseal or epiphyseal fracture. If significant displacement is not present, type I injuries may be difficult to diagnose on initial radiographs and should be suspected if there is point tenderness over an epiphysis. Thickening of the growth plate and soft tissue swelling may be the only signs evident on X-rays. If an injury is suspected but cannot be identified on the initial films, immobilization and orthopedic follow-up are recommended.

Type II Injuries

Type II injuries are the most common physeal injuries and most often seen in older children over 10 years. The fracture line travels through the physis and is associated with an oblique fracture of the metaphysis on the opposite side from where the force was applied. The metaphyseal fragment is referred to as the Thurston–Holland sign.

Growth disturbances usually do not occur with types I and II injuries.

Type III Injuries

Type III injuries comprise a vertical fracture of the epiphysis perpendicular to the physis, extending into the growth plate. This type of injury is uncommon and most frequently occurs at the distal tibial epiphysis. To avoid the potential of growth plate arrest, the fracture must be appropriately reduced to maintain proper blood supply. Reduction is accomplished most commonly with operative fixation. If surgery is not performed, frequent rechecks and follow-up radiographs are recommended to ensure that the fracture does not become displaced after immobilization.

Type IV Injuries

Unlike types I–III, type IV injuries are the result of compressive rather than rotational or shearing forces. Vertical splitting of the epiphysis occurs, extending through the physis and metaphysis and most commonly involves the distal humerus. Type IV injuries require surgical repair, and growth plate arrest may occur even with operative fixation.

Type V Injuries

Type V injuries, which are rare, are the result of crushing forces applied to the epiphysis at the area of the physis. When seen, they occur most often at the distal tibia and the knee. Because no fracture is visible, these injuries are frequently missed on initial radiographs and are often diagnosed on follow-up visits after the shortening, and angular deformity secondary to growth plate arrest is evident. Nontraumatic causes include osteomyelitis and epiphyseal aseptic necrosis. Treatment consists of immobilization and close orthopedic follow-up.

▶ Eponyms

Even though emergency physicians are likely to be comfortable using the many eponyms that exist to describe fractures, such as Colles, Monteggia, Galeazzi, it is probably more efficient to provide orthopedic consultants with an anatomic description using the above terminology.

SPRAINS AND STRAINS

Sprains are injuries to ligaments and may be associated with a fracture. The following grading system is used to describe the severity of the injury:

- Grade I—Incomplete tear. Swelling and ecchymosis may be present. Immobilization and conservative care are indicated.

- Grade II—Significant incomplete tear. Swelling and ecchymosis are usually present as is some laxity in the joint. Immobilization and orthopedic follow-up are indicated.

- Grade III—Complete disruption. The joint is unstable. Orthopedic consultation is indicated for possible surgical repair.

When assessing joint instability, remember that joint effusions, guarding, and muscle contractions may complicate the initial clinical examination. If there is any question, a period of immobilization and follow-up examination are indicated. A strain is an injury to the muscle-musculotendinous unit. Strains are also graded according to severity. Most only require immobilization and conservative management; however, surgical repair may be necessary, and orthopedic consultation or referral should be obtained if indicated.

SPLINTING

Splints are a basic part of orthopedic care and should be applied to suspected or confirmed fractures to attempt to avoid and further damage to muscle, nerves, vessels, and skin. They are used to stabilize the injury, provide some amount of pain relief, and help prevent further injury. Some splints are designed to be temporary, such as those applied in the field by emergency medical services personnel. These splints should ideally stabilize the joint above and below the suspected injury. Attempting to correct deformities before obtaining radiographs is not recommended, unless vascular compromise is suspected.

Splints are often applied in the emergency department before the patient is discharged or admitted and are left in place until more definitive orthopedic care is instituted. All physicians should be experienced in splinting. Even if the splint is to be applied by a technician, the physician should ensure that the splint is adequately padded and the limb is stabilized in an appropriate position before the patient is discharged. In addition, the physician should reevaluate and document the limb's neurovascular status after any reduction or splinting procedure. Use of circumferential plaster (ie, casts) is strongly discouraged in the emergency department. In almost all orthopedic injuries, soft tissue swelling worsens after discharge, potentially leading to significant neurovascular compromise if a cast has been applied in the emergency department.

PROCEDURAL SEDATION

Before a fracture or dislocation is reduced, adequate analgesia and muscle relaxation must be provided. The best way to accomplish fracture or dislocation reduction is with sedation using either intravenous or intramuscular agents. Emergency departments should have specific policies in place for the administration and monitoring of patients undergoing sedation. The goal is to provide sufficient sedation for the procedure without having to administer general anesthesia.

Although controversial, most authorities recommend that before sedating a patient, ensure that the patient has fasted for 4–6 hours prior to the procedure. Necessary equipment includes at least one functioning venous catheter, continuous pulse oximetry, cardiac monitor, suction, airway intubation equipment, and a bag-valve mask. Mallampati oropharynx assessment and consideration of the patient's American Society of Anesthesiologists (ASA) categorization should be determined before beginning the procedure to ensure that the emergency physician can manage any potential airway complications resulting from sedation. In general, only ASA class I or II patients (those without serious systemic comorbid diseases) should undergo procedural sedation in the emergency department. ASA class III or IV patients should optimally receive treatment in the operating room.

Most authors recommend that patients being sedated in the emergency department receive supplemental oxygen regardless of initial oxygen saturation. The goal is to maintain an oxygen saturation above 90% at all times. It is important to remember, however, that pulse oximetry only measures oxygen saturation and does not provide any information regarding the patient's ventilation. Many clinicians now routinely utilize end-tidal CO_2 monitoring as a measure of ventilation in order to prevent hypoxemia. Many agents are available for procedural sedation. Ideally, medications should be short acting. Etomidate, 0.15mg/kg has a profound and short-lived action, which should be sufficient for most procedures. It has been reported to cause adrenal suppression, the clinical significance of which is unknown and is currently not approved for use in children. Propofol has gained widespread use in emergency medicine procedural sedation because of its rapid onset, titratable sedation effect, and quick recovery period. It also has the added advantage of antiemetic properties, which in theory would reduce the risk of aspiration during sedation. Ketamine provides distinct advantages for sedation in certain circumstances and is used commonly in children. It is effectively administered in both intravenous and intramuscular routes. It provides excellent sedation without as much risk of oversedation and hypoventilation. An alternative is the combination of agents such as midazolam and fentanyl. Be aware that a potential side effect of fentanyl is chest wall rigidity (at higher doses or with rapid boluses), which may prohibit bag-mask ventilation and may necessitate paralyzation and intubation. It is important to remember that with the use of any sedative, airway support through airway maneuvers or assisted ventilation may be needed. Adequate documentation by trained nursing staff is necessary, and sedated patients should be monitored until they can ambulate and tolerate fluids by mouth.

Cotton BA, Guillamondegui OD, Fleming SB et al: Increased risk of adrenal insufficiency following etomidate exposure in critically injured patients. Arch Surg 2008;143(1):62–67 [PMID: 18209154].

Zed PJ, Abu-Leban RB, Chan WW et al: Efficacy and patient satisfaction of propofol for procedural sedation and analgesia in the emergency department: a prospective study. CJEM 2008;10(3):196 [PMID: 18072987].

CHILD ABUSE

Unfortunately, child abuse remains a major problem in our society, with physical abuse affecting 2–5% of children in the United States. Skeletal injuries sometimes occur with abuse and may represent significant morbidity to the patient. Certain fracture patterns are commonly seen in abuse, particularly multiple fractures in varying stages of healing. Clinical suspicion of abuse should remain high whenever injured children receive treatment, particularly if fractures are found in very young patients, especially less than 3 years of age.

▶ Clinical Findings

The approach to diagnosis should be the same as for all trauma patients. Keys to potential abuse may be evident in the history, such as history inconsistent with the injuries seen or delays in seeking care (may be evidenced by callus formation at a fracture site seen on X-rays). Physical findings may include pattern injuries, old bruises, and multiple fractures in various stages of healing.

Remember that significant force is required to produce fractures in the spine, scapula, and sternum. Rib fractures are uncommon in children except in the setting of abuse, and chest radiographs should be examined carefully to identify these injuries. Spiral fractures have long been identified as red flags to alert the emergency physician of possible abuse. This is particularly true of humeral and femoral fractures in the very young; however, spiral fractures of the tibia (Toddler's fracture) may be seen with accidental injuries. Another common injury pattern in abuse is a chip fracture of the metaphysis. Pulling and twisting forces may also result in a tearing of the periosteum and cartilage at the growth plate of long bones, scapulae, and clavicles.

▶ Treatment

Treatment of specific injuries is described below. Careful documentation is encouraged.

▶ Disposition

Obtain appropriate pediatric, orthopedic, and social services consultations while the patient is still in the emergency department. If the patient's safety is in question, he or she should be admitted to the hospital or taken in to protective custody by social services until all questions have been answered and the safety of the home environment is assured. All physicians are required to report suspected child abuse.

▼ MANAGEMENT OF SPECIFIC ORTHOPEDIC INJURIES

SHOULDER GIRDLE INJURIES

STERNOCLAVICULAR JOINT DISLOCATIONS

 ESSENTIALS OF DIAGNOSIS

▶ Chest wall deformity

▶ Sternoclavicular tenderness

▶ Sternal X-rays or computed tomography (CT) aids in diagnosis

▶ May be associated with mediastinal injuries

▶ General Considerations

Dislocations of the sternoclavicular joint (SCJ) are the least commonly dislocated major joint and are associated with motor vehicle collisions or sports injuries. Anterior dislocations are most common and occur secondary to anterolateral force applied to the shoulder with a rolling movement. Posterior dislocations are associated with crushing forces applied to the chest, and 25% of posterior dislocations are associated with injuries to the superior mediastinal structures. The severity of the injury may be graded as follows:

- Grade I—Mild sprain of the sternoclavicular and costoclavicular ligaments.

- Grade II—Subluxation of the SCJ, may be anterior or posterior; associated with rupture of the sternoclavicular ligament with the costoclavicular ligament remaining intact.

- Grade III—Complete dislocation.

▶ Clinical Findings

A. Symptoms and Signs

The diagnosis can often be made clinically. Tenderness, swelling, and deformity to the SCJ will be present. Patients typically use the unaffected arm to support the affected arm across the chest. Posterior dislocations can also present with dysphagia, dyspnea, dysphonia, or upper extremity weakness.

B. X-ray Findings

Plain radiographs, including anteroposterior, oblique, and 40° cephalic tilt views aid in the diagnosis. A CT scan may be necessary and is indicated in all cases of posterior dislocations to evaluate for mediastinal injuries.

▶ Treatment

Obtain orthopedic consultation for both anterior and posterior dislocations. Anterior dislocations may be reduced in the emergency department using procedural sedation by placing a rolled towel or sheet between the scapulae and applying traction to the affected arm. A posterior dislocation may need operative repair, and early orthopedic or trauma surgery consultation is appropriate because compression of critical upper mediastinal structures such as the great vessels and trachea may occur.

▶ Disposition

Patients with anterior dislocations may be discharged in a sling and swathe. Even if the reduction is successful, the joint is often unstable and the clavicular head may dislocate again. However, because the purpose of the reduction is often more cosmetic than functional, even if reduction is unsuccessful the patient may be discharged with immobilization in a sling and orthopedic follow-up. Posterior dislocations may be reduced with traction and adduction; however, patients should be managed in consultation with a specialist and most likely will require admission.

CLAVICLE FRACTURES

ESSENTIALS OF DIAGNOSIS

- ▶ Clavicle deformity
- ▶ X-rays confirm diagnosis
- ▶ Most heal with conservative management

▶ Clinical Findings

A. Symptons and Signs

The most common mechanism causing a clavicle fracture is a direct blow to the shoulder. Often the clavicle is deformed, and some swelling, tenderness, and occasionally crepitus are present.

B. X-ray Findings

Most clavicle fractures are easily seen with a clavicle series.

▶ Treatment

Treat open fractures with antibiotics and orthopedic consultation. For closed clavicle fractures, treatment typically involves pain control, immobilization with a sling, or sling and swathe.

▶ Disposition

Most clavicle fractures heal uneventfully. Factors associated with nonunion include marked initial displacement or shortening. Patients with closed fractures may be discharged with orthopedic follow-up. Patients with open fractures require hospitalization for further management.

ACROMIOCLAVICULAR JOINT INJURIES

ESSENTIALS OF DIAGNOSIS

- ▶ Deformed and tender acromioclavicular joint (ACJ)
- ▶ May be confused with clavicle injury
- ▶ X-ray may confirm diagnosis

▶ General Considerations

Acromioclavicular joint injuries most commonly result from a direct fall onto the shoulder and account for 25% of all dislocations of the shoulder girdle. These injuries are graded according to severity:

- Type I—Sprain, minimal tear of the acromioclavicular (AC) ligament.
- Type II—small tear of AC ligament, widened joint space, coracoclavicular distance maintained.
- Type III–VI—Complete disruption of AC ligament, coracoclavicular ligament, and muscle attachments. In type III injuries, the clavicle is displaced upward, in type IV the clavicle displaces posteriorly into the trapezius, and in type V the clavicle is displaced superiorly. Type VI is rare and the clavicle displaces inferiorly.

▶ Clinical Findings

A. Symptoms and Signs

Patients should be examined in the sitting position. Often a deformity at the ACJ will be present, with swelling, tenderness, and occasionally crepitus.

B. X-ray Findings

X-rays should include anteroposterior, axillary, and 15° cephalic tilt views. Stress views are no longer recommended. Classically, separation between the acromion and the clavicle is seen in grade II and grade III injuries. Additionally, since the coraco-clavicular ligament is disrupted in a grade III injury, the distal clavicle is elevated in relation to the acromion.

▶ Treatment

Types I and II injuries are treated conservatively with a sling. Type III injuries have traditionally been treated with surgical repair; however, conservative management has been used more recently with good results.

▶ Disposition

Most patients may be discharged home. All patients should receive orthopedic referral for follow-up examination.

> Mazzocca AD, Arciero RA, Bicos J: Evaluation and treatment of acromioclavicular joint injuries. Am J Sports Med 2007;35(2):316–329 [PMID: 17251175].

SCAPULA FRACTURES

ESSENTIALS OF DIAGNOSIS

▶ Pain and tenderness over scapula

▶ May be associated with more severe intrathoracic injuries

▶ X-ray (with axillary views) confirms diagnosis

▶ General Considerations

Fractures of the scapula are uncommon, accounting for approximately 1% of all fractures. Fractures usually are secondary to direct blows or to crush injuries. Because the scapula is well protected by muscle, the presence of a fracture indicates a significant mechanism of injury and warrants evaluation for other potential injuries to the lung, chest wall, humerus, and clavicle. Acromion process and coracoid process fractures have been associated with brachial plexus injury. Scapula fractures can be classified as follows:

- Type I—Fracture of coracoid process, acromion process, or scapular spine.
- Type II—Fracture of the scapular neck.
- Type III—Intra-articular fracture involving the glenoid fossa.
- Type IV—Fracture of the body of the scapula (most common).

▶ Clinical Findings

A. Symptoms and Signs

The patient will present with pain and tenderness over the scapula. A hematoma and crepitus may also be appreciated. The patient will usually hold the affected arm close to the body.

B. X-ray Findings

Fractures may be subtle on plain radiographs. Always obtain an axillary view to help identify fractures involving the glenoid, acromion, and coracoid processes. In some instances, CT scanning may be necessary to identify subtle or intra-articular fractures. In children, the physis of the acromion may be seen on X-rays. In approximately 3% of individuals, this structure remains unfused (os acromiale) and can be mistaken for a fracture.

▶ Treatment

The majority of isolated scapula fractures are managed conservatively with a sling and swath and pain management. Intra-articular fractures such as those involving the glenoid often require surgical stabilization.

▶ Disposition

Significantly displaced fractures rarely may require surgical repair; patients with such fractures should be admitted. Patients with isolated scapular fractures may be discharged with close follow-up.

ROTATOR CUFF INJURIES

ESSENTIALS OF DIAGNOSIS

▶ Pain and decreased motion of shoulder

▶ Positive drop-arm test

▶ Plain X-ray of little value

▶ Arthrogram or magnetic resonance imaging (MRI) will confirm diagnosis

▶ General Considerations

The rotator cuff comprises four muscles: the subscapularis (internal rotation), the infraspinatus and teres minor (external rotation), and the supraspinatus (adduction). Acute tears are commonly seen with falls, either directly onto the shoulder or on an outstretched hand, but may also occur in the setting of lifting heavy objects although most tears are chronic. Rotator cuff tears occur more commonly in middle-aged to elderly males and usually involve the dominant arm.

► Clinical Findings

A. Symptoms and Signs

The patient complains of pain and decreased motion. Point tenderness over the greater tuberosity or a palpable defect may be seen. Rotator cuff tears may be evaluated by the drop arm test by passively abducting the arm to 90° and then applying pressure to the distal forearm. With significant acute tears, this will cause the patient to drop his or her arm.

B. X-ray Findings

Plain radiographs are usually of little use but should be obtained to rule out occult fractures. Superior displacement of the humeral head may be seen in complete tears but is not diagnostic.

► Treatment

Provide adequate analgesia and a sling for comfort.

► Disposition

Outpatient follow-up with scheduling of an arthrogram or MRI scan may be necessary to confirm the diagnosis. Patients may be discharged with orthopedic follow-up.

SHOULDER DISLOCATIONS

ESSENTIALS OF DIAGNOSIS

- ► Shoulder deformity, pain, and decreased movement
- ► Majority are anterior dislocations
- ► Anteroposterior, Y and axillary view X-rays confirm diagnosis
- ► Perform thorough nerve examination

► General Considerations

The shoulder is the most commonly dislocated major joint in the body. Most (approximately 95%) of these injuries are anterior dislocations and are often easily diagnosed clinically; however, in muscular individuals the clinical presentation may be less obvious. Posterior dislocations are much less common and are usually associated with violent muscle contractions as seen with seizures and electrocutions but may also occur with falls on a flexed, internally rotated arm. Posterior dislocations are often missed clinically and may also be difficult to identify on standard anteroposterior X-rays. Inferior dislocations (Luxatio erecta) have been described as a type of anterior dislocation and are rare. This occurs when the humeral head is forced below the inferior rim of the glenoid fossa.

► Clinical Findings

A. Symptoms and Signs

The patient usually holds the arm in adduction and the elbow flexed close to the body. Pain occurs with the least amount of movement. The glenoid fossa may be palpable. A complete neurologic and vascular examination of the extremity is of paramount importance. Axillary nerve function should be assessed by checking the sensation in the lateral aspect of the shoulder and testing deltoid motor function. Examine radial, ulnar, and median nerve distributions thoroughly prior to sedation and reduction. Document brachial and radial pulses. In inferior dislocations, clinically the patient will hold the arm locked overhead and abducted with the elbow flexed. This type of dislocation may also be associated with injury to the axillary artery and neuropraxis of the brachial plexus.

In posterior dislocations, the patient usually holds the affected arm against the chest in adduction and internal rotation. Abduction and external rotation are severely limited. The posterior shoulder may be prominent when viewed from above; however, this finding may be difficult to recognize, particularly in muscular individuals.

B. X-ray Findings

Obtain a shoulder series, including a scapular Y-view (Figure 28–3), which can help diagnose the direction of dislocation. Axillary views are often the most helpful if any doubt exists about the diagnosis. X-rays will also help identify associated fractures. A Hill-Sachs deformity (impaction of the posterolateral humeral head) may occur with dislocation. A fracture of the anteroinferior glenoid rim (Bankart fracture) may be seen with anterior dislocations. Bankart fractures may be subtle and identified only on CT scans.

► Treatment

Some controversy exists over the need to obtain X-rays prior to reduction of shoulder dislocations. We do not generally recommend bypassing X-rays at this time unless vascular compromise is present. In patients with chronic recurrent dislocations, the dislocations may occur without significant trauma; in this setting, consider reducing the shoulder before obtaining radiographs.

Emergency physicians should be comfortable with numerous reduction methods. The patient will often require sedation prior to the procedure and good muscle relaxation is key to successfully reductions. We prefer the external rotation–adduction technique for reduction. With the patient in an upright position, the extremity is externally rotated while gentle traction and adduction are applied at the elbow. This technique is associated with a low risk of injury and does not require a great deal of force, as do the other methods. The traction–countertraction method—in which an assistant applies countertraction with a sheet and in-line traction of the upper

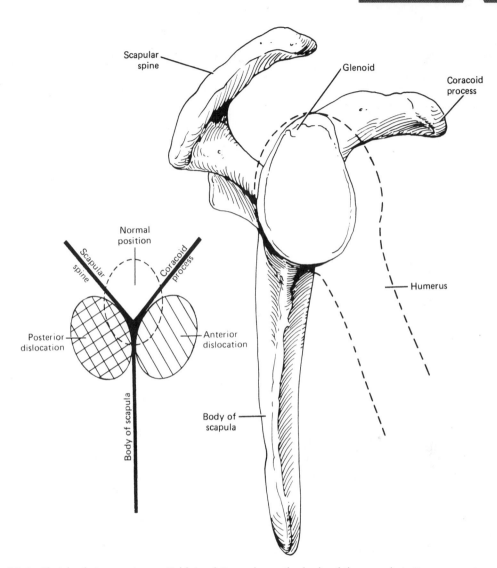

▲ **Figure 28–3.** Sketch of view on tangential lateral X-ray shows the body of the scapula in its narrowest aspect. If the patient is poorly positioned, the medial and lateral borders are not superimposed. Normally, the humeral head shadow lies directly over that of the glenoid, which may be hard to see. The position of the glenoid is indicated by the confluence of the scapular spine, the body of the scapula, and the coracoid process. A dislocated humeral head lies anterior or posterior to this point.

extremity—requires some physical strength (Figure 28–4). Do not try to pull the humerus into place. Instead place traction on the arm until the muscles fatigue and the humeral head slides in. The Stimson method achieves reduction by attaching weight to the wrist with the dislocated arm hanging over the bed to provide traction, but this method requires about 20–30 minutes. In scapular manipulation, reduction is performed by repositioning the glenoid fossa rather than the humeral head by rotating the inferior tip of the scapula medially while stabilizing the superior and medial edges. After reduction,

reevaluate neurovascular status and immobilize the shoulder with a sling and swath. Obtain postreduction X-rays.

▶ **Disposition**

Discharge patients with adequate analgesia such as non-steroidal anti-inflammatory drugs or opiates and orthopedic follow-up in 2–3 days. If any neurologic findings are present, such as a wrist drop, obtain orthopedic consultation while the patient is still in the emergency department. Most of

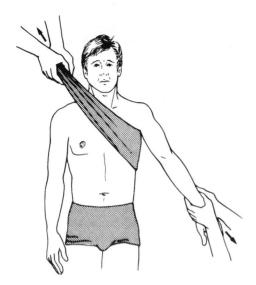

▲ **Figure 28–4.** Method of producing traction on dislocated humerus and countertraction on thorax for reduction of shoulder dislocation.

these neurologic findings are caused by a neuropraxia and usually improve over time.

Baykal B, Sener S, Turkan H: Scapular manipulation technique for reduction of traumatic anterior shoulder dislocations: experiences of an academic emergency department. Emerg Med J 2005;22(5): 336–338 [PMID: 15843700].

Kocher MS, Waters PM, Micheli LJ: Upper extremity injuries in the pediatric athlete. J Sports Med 2000;30(2):117 [PMID: 10966151].

Owens S, Itamura JM: Differential diagnosis of shoulder injuries in sports. Orthop Clin North Am 2001;32(3):393 [PMID: 11888134].

Ruotolo C, Nottage WM: Surgical and nonsurgical management of rotator cuff tears. Arthroscopy 2002;18(5):527 [PMID: 11987065].

▼ **UPPER EXTREMITY INJURIES**

HUMERUS FRACTURES

 ESSENTIALS OF DIAGNOSIS

▸ Frequent in elderly patients
▸ Pain, deformity, and decreased mobility at shoulder
▸ X-ray confirms diagnosis
▸ Conservative management

▶ General Considerations

Humerus fractures frequently occur in elderly women with a history of osteoporosis and the classic mechanism of injury involves a fall on an outstretched hand. In the Neer classification system, categories include two, three, and four part fractures.

▶ Clinical Findings

A. Symptoms and Signs

The patient usually presents with deformity at the shoulder and commonly holds the affected arm close to the body. It is important to assess vascular status because the brachial artery lies in proximity to the distal humeral shaft and associated arterial injury may be present. Assess for radial nerve injury and wrist drop, particularly with humeral shaft fractures.

B. X-ray Findings

X-rays show these injuries clearly. Proximal humerus fractures with some impaction are the most common type.

In younger patients, look for signs of a unicameral cyst or other pathologic causes of fracture.

▶ Treatment

Conservative management is generally the rule, especially in the elderly. Minimally displaced fractures constitute the majority of injuries. These patients do well with a splint, sling, and swathe (Figure 28–5), or sling and swathe alone, and adequate analgesia.

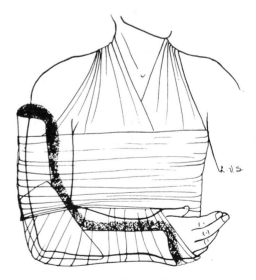

▲ **Figure 28–5.** Posterior plaster splint with sling and swathe for immobilization of elbow or forearm injuries. Abundant cast padding is first wrapped around the arm. The posterior plaster must be reinforced medially and laterally to the elbow, but neither padding nor plaster should constrict the antecubital fossa.

Disposition

Patients should have orthopedic follow-up in 3–4 days. We recommend obtaining orthopedic consultation for any young person with humeral or humeral shaft fractures while the patient is still in the emergency department. If there is displacement of a humeral shaft fracture, a hanging or gravity splint may be applied. Occasionally these patients may undergo open reduction and internal fixation (ORIF). The most common complication of proximal humerus fractures is a "frozen shoulder," or adhesive capsulitis, which can be prevented with early rehabilitation.

SUPRACONDYLAR FRACTURES

ESSENTIALS OF DIAGNOSIS

- ▶ Occurs after FOOSH
- ▶ Elbow deformity, pain, and decreased mobility
- ▶ Posterior fat pad on lateral X-ray is highly suggestive
- ▶ May have high morbidity
- ▶ Mandatory orthopedic consultation

General Considerations

Supracondylar fractures are of the distal humerus and classically occur in children, usually age 5–10, who fall on an outstretched hand with hyperextension at the elbow. If not managed properly, supracondylar fractures may predispose to serious morbidity, including complications such as Volkmann ischemic contracture.

Clinical Findings

A. Symtoms and Signs

Patients usually present complaining of elbow pain and arm swelling. A neurologic and vascular examination is important and must include notation of the function of the anterior interosseous nerve, which is a purely motor nerve serving the flexor pollicis longus, flexor digitorum profundus, and the pronator quadratus. With anterior interosseous nerve dysfunction, a patient may be unable to make an "OK sign" with the thumb and index finger and may be unable to make a fist or flex the wrist.

B. X-ray Findings

Supracondylar fractures may be subtle and at times may be suspected only by the presence of a posterior fat pad sign on a lateral elbow X-ray. Comparison views of the uninjured elbow may be of benefit if a fracture is suspected but not immediately apparent.

Treatment

All supracondylar fractures require orthopedic consultation and generally these fractures should not be reduced by emergency physicians.

Disposition

Disposition is as per orthopedic consultation. Open reduction is often required and admission is recommended for displaced fractures.

ELBOW INJURIES

ESSENTIALS OF DIAGNOSIS

- ▶ Deformity, pain, and decreased range of motion
- ▶ Assess for ulnar nerve injury
- ▶ Anteroposterior and lateral X-rays are confirmatory
- ▶ Consider fracture if posterior fat pad is present
- ▶ No X-ray needed for a simple nursemaid's elbow

General Considerations

Elbow injuries usually occur from a direct blow to the elbow, causing immobility at the elbow joint. The patient generally holds the arm in flexion, and a moderate amount of swelling is present. Both fractures and dislocations may occur. Neurovascular status and range of motion testing are important, as patients who cannot fully extend their elbow have a higher possibility of having a fracture. It is important to assess ulnar nerve function by testing sensation of palmar aspect of the fifth digit and motor function of interossei muscles of the hand because of its proximity to the elbow.

X-rays should include anteroposterior and lateral views. Always look for the presence of fat pads. A small anterior fat pad can sometimes be normal; however, the presence of a posterior fat pad is abnormal and should alert the clinician to a fracture, such as a radial head fracture in adults or a supracondylar fracture in children. *Even if a fracture is not visualized on X-ray, treat the injury as though an occult fracture is present.*

1. Olecranon Fractures

Olecranon fractures may occur by direct trauma or less commonly by contraction of the triceps while the elbow is flexed.

Clinical Findings

A. Symptoms and Signs

Pain, limited range of motion, a palpable defect or crepitus may be present. Another physical finding includes inability to extend the elbow against force.

B. X-ray Findings

Plain X-rays should be sufficient to confirm the diagnosis.

▶ Treatment

Most fractures may be treated with a long arm posterior splint with the elbow flexed at 90°, sling, and orthopedic follow-up. Displaced fractures (greater than 2-mm separation) or the presence of an ulnar nerve injury mandates acute orthopedic consultation.

▶ Disposition

Patients who do not meet criteria for surgery may be discharged home as long as orthopedic follow-up can be obtained in 1–2 days.

2. Radial Head Fractures

Radial head fractures may occur by either direct trauma or more commonly by an indirect mechanism such as a fall on an outstretched hand. Damage to the articular surface of the capitellum and collateral ligament can also occur.

▶ Clinical Findings

A. Symptoms and Signs

The patient presents with pain, particularly on supination or pronation, and with limited range of motion. Elbow extension may be limited by joint effusion.

B. X-ray Findings

It is often difficult to see a definitive fracture on plain X-rays. As mentioned previously, the presence of a fat pad (especially posterior) should raise suspicion for an occult fracture.

▶ Treatment

Simple radial head fractures are treated conservatively with analgesics and a simple sling. We recommend contacting an orthopedist for comminuted radial head fractures.

▶ Disposition

Patients may be discharged with immobilization, pain control, and orthopedic follow-up.

3. Elbow Dislocations

The elbow is the second most commonly dislocated major joint. Generally, the radius and ulna are displaced together and the dislocation is described as the relationship of the ulna to the humerus, such as posterior (which is most common), anterior, medial, or lateral. The most com-

mon mechanism is a fall, and associated fractures occur frequently.

▶ Clinical Findings

A. Symptoms and Signs

The patient often holds the elbow in 45° of flexion, and a deformity at the olecranon is usually visible. Because of the location of the brachial artery and median nerve, the patient's neurovascular status should be assessed and documented initially and reassessed frequently.

B. X-ray Findings

Examine plain radiographs for the presence of associated fractures.

▶ Treatment

If neurovascular compromise is present, perform reduction as soon as possible. Reduction can be achieved by applying traction to the wrist distally, while the humerus is stabilized (Figure 28–6). Another technique involves applying traction at the wrist while the patient lies on his or her abdomen with the affected limb hanging off the bed. After appropriate analgesia and sedation, most dislocations can be reduced in a few minutes. These injuries should be reassessed for neurovascular injury and then

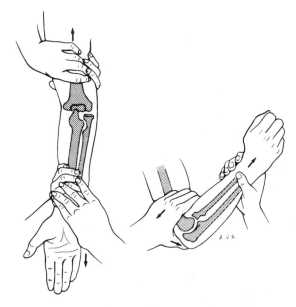

▲ **Figure 28–6.** Reduction of posterior elbow dislocation by applying manual traction on the forearm while an assistant stabilizes the humerus. If radial or lateral displacement is present, it must be corrected before reduction is completed by flexion of the elbow.

placed in a long arm splint with the elbow in flexion and sling (see Figure 28–5).

Disposition

Most patients may be discharged with adequate analgesia and orthopedic follow-up, as well as instructions to watch for signs of vascular impairment.

4. Subluxation of the Radial Head

Radial head subluxation (nursemaid's elbow) is a common injury, accounting for as many as 25% of elbow injuries in children. This injury usually occurs in the 1–3-year-old age group but may be seen up to school age and rarely in early teenagers. Subluxation occurs secondary to longitudinal traction on the arm while the elbow is extended and the arm pronated. This allows fibers of the annular ligament to slip between the radial head and the capitellum.

Clinical Findings

A. Symptoms and Signs

Generally no deformity is seen, but the child will hold the arm in passive pronation with slight flexion at the elbow. Some tenderness is present over the radial head, and the child characteristically refuses to use the arm. Although subluxation of the radial head is a common injury, obtain a thorough history to allay concerns about potential child abuse.

B. X-ray Findings

Some authors suggest that if the clinician is confident with the mechanism of injury and the physical examination, radiographs need not be obtained prior to reduction; however, others assert that X-rays should always be obtained to rule out other potential injuries. X-rays should be obtained if the child does not resume use of the arm after reduction.

Treatment

Once the diagnosis is made, reduction is usually easily performed by stabilizing the elbow with one hand and, while applying gentle pressure on the radial head, supinating the forearm and flexing the elbow. Often a click or snap will be heard. The majority of patients regain normal use of the arm within minutes. Immobilization with a sling has been suggested; however, most patients will not comply, and if the reduction is successful, the sling likely will not make much difference.

Disposition

Unsuccessful or recurrent subluxations require outpatient orthopedic consultation.

FOREARM FRACTURES

ESSENTIALS OF DIAGNOSIS

► Pain and deformity present
► X-rays are confirmatory
► Assess for concomitant dislocations

General Considerations

Forearm fractures may occur secondary to varied mechanisms but are commonly seen with direct blows or falls on an outstretched hand. The site of injury determines the physical findings. Carefully examine the patient for function of the radial, median, and ulnar nerves. Assess, document, and later reassess distal pulses and tendon function. Clinical suspicion for development of a compartment syndrome should be high and appropriate assessment performed. As noted earlier in this chapter, it is probably more useful to describe the injury anatomically; however, the forearm is an area where many common eponyms for fractures exist, for example,

- Colles' fracture—Transverse fracture of distal radius with dorsal angulation; most common wrist fracture seen in adults.
- Smith fracture—Transverse fracture of the metaphysis of the distal radius with volar displacement.
- Barton fracture—Oblique, intra-articular fracture of the distal radius, with dorsal displacement of the distal fragment along with dorsal carpus subluxation.
- Hutchinson (chauffeur's) fracture—Intra-articular fracture of the radial styloid.
- Monteggia fracture—Ulna fracture with radial head dislocation.
- Galeazzi fracture—Fracture of distal third of radius associated with dislocation of the distal radioulnar joint.

Treatment

Nondisplaced fractures are generally treated conservatively with a sugar-tong (U-shaped) splint (volar and dorsal splint from distal metacarpals going around the elbow) and orthopedic follow-up.

Disposition

Displaced fractures warrant orthopedic consultation to determine the appropriate method (open vs closed) and timetable for reduction. Displaced forearm fractures in children should be seen by the orthopedist in the emergency department.

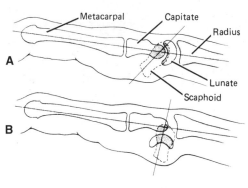
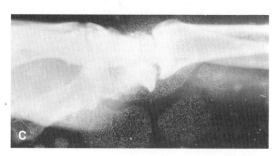

▲ **Figure 28–7. A:** Normal anatomy of the wrist. Note that the proximal end of the capitate rests in the lunate concavity. A straight line drawn through the metacarpal and capitate into the radius should bisect the lunate. The scaphoid makes an angle of 45° with the long axis of the radius. **B:** Lunate dislocation. Lunate dislocates volarly. The angle between the scaphoid and the long axis of the radius is 90° instead of the normal angle of 45°. **C:** X-ray of volar dislocation of lunate. (Reproduced, with permission, from Way LW (editor): *Current Surgical Diagnosis & Treatment*, 9th ed. Appleton & Lange, 1991.).

Appelboam A, Reuben AD, Benger JR et al: Elbow extension test to rule out elbow fracture: multicentre, prospective validation and observation study of diagnostic accuracy in adults and children. BMJ 2008;337:a2428 [PMID: 19066257].

Ring D, Jupiter JB, Zilberfarb J: Posterior dislocation of the elbow with fractures of the radial head and coronoid. J Bone Joint Surg Am 2002;84-A(4):547 [PMID: 11940613].

WRIST AND HAND INJURIES

1. Lunate or Perilunate Dislocations

ESSENTIALS OF DIAGNOSIS

▶ Occurs after FOOSH

▶ Wrist swelling, pain, and tenderness

▶ Anteroposterior and lateral X-rays of wrist are confirmatory

▶ Look for "piece-of-pie" and "spilled teacup" signs

▶ General Considerations

Lunate or perilunate dislocations usually occur from a fall on an outstretched upper extremity, causing extreme dorsiflexion.

▶ Clinical Findings

A. Symptoms and Signs

Usually the patient presents with a swollen wrist, decreased mobility, and severe pain over the dorsum of the wrist. Median nerve injuries may be seen on examination.

B. X-ray Findings

The lateral wrist view is the most important X-ray with these injuries. A line drawn through the center shaft of the radius normally bisects the lunate and capitate (Figure 28–7A). In a lunate dislocation, the radius and capitate are bisected and the lunate is displaced either dorsal or volar, giving what is sometimes referred to as a spilled teacup appearance (Figure 28–7B and C). The anteroposterior view shows a triangular-shaped lunate bone with the apex pointing toward the fingers, which is commonly referred to as the piece-of-pie sign. A perilunate dislocation occurs when the line drawn through the radius bisects the lunate only and the capitate is displaced.

▶ Treatment

This injury should be managed by providing analgesia and splinting temporarily for comfort in the emergency department. Consult an orthopedic surgeon for anatomic realignment.

▶ Disposition

Patients undergoing ORIF should be admitted until the surgeon addresses the injury. Patients with reducible injuries may be given a long arm splint and sent home after arranging a treatment plan in conjunction with a surgeon.

2. Scapholunate Dislocations

ESSENTIALS OF DIAGNOSIS

▶ Frequently missed injury

▶ Anteroposterior hand X-ray confirms diagnosis

▶ "Terry Thomas" sign (greater than 3-mm scapholunate joint space)

General Considerations

Usually occurring from a fall on an outstretched hand, a scapholunate dislocation is a commonly missed hand injury.

Clinical Findings

A. Symptoms and Signs

The patient may present with wrist swelling and decreased range of motion. Tenderness over the wrist may be present.

B. X-ray Findings

An anteroposterior view of the hand normally reveals a space between the scaphoid and lunate bone of less than 3 mm. If the distance is greater than 3 mm, then a dislocation injury is present.

Treatment

A scapholunate dislocation may temporarily be treated with analgesics and a radial gutter splint.

Disposition

Refer the patient to an orthopedic surgeon for definitive repair.

3. Carpal Bone Fractures

ESSENTIALS OF DIAGNOSIS

- ▶ Maintain high index of suspicion
- ▶ Consider scaphoid view X-rays
- ▶ Treat as fracture based on clinical findings even if X-ray findings are negative

General Considerations

Carpal bone fractures are often missed in the emergency department and require a high index of suspicion. Usually, they occur after a fall on an outstretched upper extremity. Neurovascular status should be carefully assessed. Often, even if a fracture is not seen, the injury should be treated as a fracture in order to prevent long-term sequelae such as avascular necrosis seen with scaphoid or lunate (Kienböck disease) fractures due to the tenuous blood supply of these bones. Fractures of the pisiform or the hook of the hamate can impinge on the ulnar nerve.

Clinical Findings

A. Symptoms and Signs

Carpal bone fractures usually lead to wrist and hand swelling with decreased mobility and pain. Tenderness is often seen

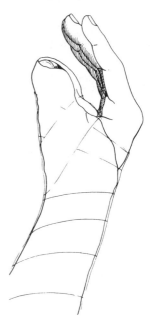

▲ **Figure 28–8.** Thumb spica splint: a slab of plaster is applied over adequate padding and secured with a loose elastic bandage.

over the injured area. If tenderness is present in the anatomic snuffbox, consider a scaphoid fracture, regardless of X-ray findings, and treat the injury appropriately.

B. X-ray Findings

Scaphoid and other carpal fractures may be seen on anteroposterior or dedicated scaphoid views. A triquetral fracture can often be seen on a lateral hand view as a small dorsal avulsion. Repeat X-rays in 1–2 weeks may often reveal a fracture that was not initially seen.

Treatment

Scaphoid fractures may be treated with a thumb spica splint (Figure 28–8); other fractures may be treated with a volar wrist splint (Figure 28–9). Due to concern for complications, including avascular necrosis, if fractures of carpal bones are suspected, they should be immobilized even if X-rays are negative.

Disposition

Patients may be discharged with analgesics and follow-up with an orthopedist in 2–3 days.

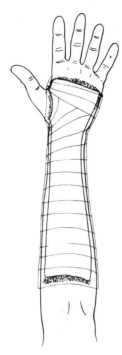

▲ **Figure 28-9.** Volar splint for immobilization of wrist injuries.

4. Metacarpal Fractures

ESSENTIALS OF DIAGNOSIS

▸ Hand swelling and pain
▸ Anteroposterior and lateral hand X-rays confirm diagnosis
▸ Assess for angulation and rotation

▶ General Considerations

The most common metacarpal fracture, known as a boxer's fracture, is through the neck of the fifth metacarpal and occurs from direct trauma such as punching an object or person. A Bennet fracture refers to an intra-articular fracture at the base of the first metacarpal. If the fracture is comminuted, then it is usually called a Rolando fracture.

▶ Clinical Findings

A. Symptoms and Signs

The patient presents with hand swelling, particularly over the dorsal surface, and tenderness over the affected bone.

Assess for rotational injury by having the patient attempt to close his or her fist. The presence of open wounds should raise the suspicion that the injury resulted from hitting teeth. These wounds should be treated as human bites, with copious irrigation and antibiotics.

B. X-ray Findings

Most metacarpal fractures should be visible on an anteroposterior or lateral view of the hand. Angulation of the fracture must be assessed in order to determine management.

▶ Treatment

If any manipulation is needed, give the patient appropriate analgesics; local lidocaine infiltration may suffice. Correct any rotational deformity by gentle traction. If angulation of the metacarpal neck requires correction, it may be accomplished with gentle traction. The easiest way to remember angulation is the 10-20-30-40 rule. These are the maximum permissable degrees of angulation that may be tolerated in the second, third, fourth, and fifth metacarpals, respectively. Fractures involving the second, third, and fourth metacarpals may be treated with a volar wrist splint (Figure 28–10). After reduction, boxer's fractures may be placed in an ulnar gutter splint (Figure 28–11) and Bennet fractures in a thumb spica splint (Figure 28–8).

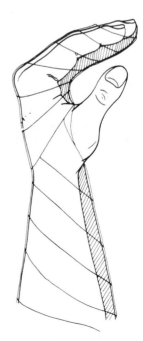

▲ **Figure 28-10.** Volar wrist and hand splint for immobilization of metacarpal shaft fractures and wrist injuries. A plaster slab is applied over adequate padding and secured with a loose elastic bandage.

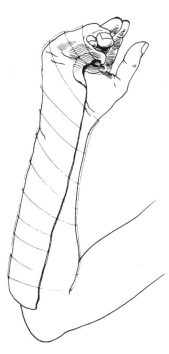

▲ **Figure 28–11.** Ulnar gutter splint for immobilization of injuries to the metacarpals of the fourth and fifth fingers. A plaster slab is applied to the ulnar border of the forearm and hand over adequate padding and is then secured with a loose elastic bandage.

 Disposition

After the injury is splinted, the patient may be sent home with adequate analgesia. We recommend arranging follow-up specifically for first metacarpal base fractures because they require operative repair.

5. Phalanx Fractures and Dislocations

ESSENTIALS OF DIAGNOSIS

▶ Finger pain, deformity, and limited mobility
▶ Finger X-rays are confirmatory

 General Considerations

Phalanx fractures and dislocations often result from a direct blow to the affected digit. They may have rotational deformities as well as angulation.

 Clinical Findings

A. Symptoms and Signs

With dislocations, an obvious deformity usually is seen. Patients with fractures may present with swelling, pain, decreased mobility, ecchymosis, and tenderness. Assess for capillary refill and sensation with two-point discrimination as well as for rotational injury.

B. X-ray Findings

Plain X-rays of the hand, including anteroposterior and lateral views, often suffice. A specific finger X-ray may also be performed.

 Treatment

Local anesthesia or digital blocks may be administered before manipulation. Reduction of dislocations and fractures can be managed with simple gentle traction. Splint these injuries with aluminum finger splints.

 Disposition

The patient may be discharged with analgesics and hand surgeon follow-up in 3–4 days.

6. Subungual Hematoma

See also Chapter 29.

ESSENTIALS OF DIAGNOSIS

▶ Painful fingernail and hematoma under nail
▶ May be associated with tuft fracture

 General Considerations

Subungual hematomas usually occur from a direct blow to the nail, such as from a hammer.

 Clinical Findings

A. Symptoms and Signs

The patient presents with a painful digit. A hematoma is easily seen under the nail.

B. X-ray Findings

Anterioposterior and lateral views of the affected digit often show a distal tuft fracture.

Treatment

Subungual hematomas are exceedingly painful injuries due to pressure, which builds under the nail plate. To decompress the hematoma, trephination is performed by using an electric cautery device. If large lacerations of the nail bed are suspected, the traditional approach has been to remove the nail, inspect the nailbed, repair any defects. After cleaning, the avulsed nail is reinserted and sutured into place as a splint to protect the nailbed and keep the proximal nail fold open.

Disposition

Antibiotics are needed if a nailbed injury is present with an open fracture; orthopedic follow-up should occur in 2–3 days. Simple hematomas may be followed up by a primary-care provider in 1 week.

7. Boutonniere Deformity

See also Chapter 29.

ESSENTIALS OF DIAGNOSIS

► Swan neck deformity of finger
► May have avulsion fracture on X-ray

General Considerations

A boutonniere deformity often occurs from forced flexion at the proximal interphalangeal joint with rupture of the central slip of the extensor tendon, causing the classic deformity.

Clinical Findings

A. Symptoms and Signs

The patient presents with swelling at the proximal interphalangeal joint. Decreased mobility and pain may also be present. While not present initially, the boutonniere deformity will develop within 2–3 weeks after an injury to the central slip extensor tendon.

B. X-ray Findings

Occasionally, an avulsion fracture of the middle phalanx may be seen on a lateral finger view.

Treatment

Splint the proximal interphalangeal joint in full extension for 4 weeks. Do not immobilize the distal joint.

Disposition

Discharge the patient with follow-up with a hand surgeon in 1 week. Give analgesics as needed.

8. Mallet Finger

See also Chapter 29.

ESSENTIALS OF DIAGNOSIS

► Flexion of distal phalanx
► May have small avulsion fracture

General Considerations

Mallet finger often occurs as a sports-related injury when the distal phalanx receives a direct blow. The injury is a disruption of the extensor tendon at the site of insertion on the distal phalanx, with subsequently unopposed flexion of the distal phalanx.

Clinical Findings

A. Symtoms and Signs

Pain is present at the distal interphalangeal joint, and the classic mallet deformity occurs, in which the distal phalanx is flexed. If not treated acutely with appropriate splinting, the swan neck deformity may develop characterized by hyperextension at the proximal interphalangeal joint and flexion at the distal interphalangeal joint.

B. X-ray Findings

Occasionally, a small avulsion fracture of the dorsal surface of the distal phalanx may be seen.

Treatment

Finger splints the distal interphalangeal joint in slight hyperextension. Commercially available splints can be used to reproduce this alignment. Continuous splinting is required for at least 4–8 weeks.

Disposition

Discharge the patient with orthopedic follow-up within 3–4 days.

9. Ulnar Collateral Ligament Rupture

ESSENTIALS OF DIAGNOSIS

► Consider in a fall while holding a ski pole
► Pain and swelling at first metacarpophalangeal joint
► X-ray may show small avulsion fracture of proximal phalanx

▶ General Considerations

Also known as gamekeeper's or skier's thumb, ulnar collateral ligament rupture of the thumb metacarpal occurs after a forceful dislocation of the proximal phalanx of the thumb radially with spontaneous relocation that results in rupture of the ulnar collateral ligament.

▶ Clinical Findings

A. Symptoms and Signs

Pain and swelling are present over the ulnar aspect of the proximal phalanx and metacarpal of the thumb. A notable finding is weak pinching ability. On examination, there is tenderness with no end point on stress testing of the metacarpophalangeal joint (Figure 28–12). Stress testing in the emergency department is usually not possible in an acute injury.

B. X-ray Findings

Occasionally an avulsion fracture of the proximal phalanx may be seen.

▶ Treatment

Apply a thumb spica splint and provide analgesics. Complete tears ultimately require surgical repair.

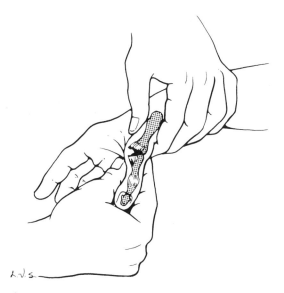

▲ **Figure 28–12.** Stress examination of the thumb metacarpophalangeal collateral ligament. The ulnar side is injured more frequently. Test both sides in extension and 30° of flexion. Compare the injured digit with the uninjured thumb. Feel for a firm end point and absence of excessive laxity.

▶ Disposition

Discharge with immobilization and orthopedic follow-up is needed for further repair.

Batrick N, Hashemi K, Freij R: Treatment of complicated subungual hematoma. Emerg Med J 2003;20(1):65 [PMID: 125333376].

Steinmann SP, Adams JE. Scaphoid fractures and nonunions: diagnosis and treatment. J Orthop Sci 2008;11(4):424–431 [PMID: 16897211].

PELVIC GIRDLE INJURIES

PELVIC FRACTURES

 ESSENTIALS OF DIAGNOSIS

- ▶ High degree of mortality
- ▶ May have large amount of bleeding
- ▶ Consider if scrotal hematoma, urethra blood, or abnormal prostate are present
- ▶ Anteroposterior films are usually confirmatory

▶ General Considerations

Pelvic fractures can be devastating injuries associated with significant mortality. The mechanism of injury in the majority of fractures is a high-velocity trauma as seen in motor vehicle collisions. Fractures may also occur with low-velocity trauma such as crush injuries and simple falls, often in elderly individuals with osteoporosis. Much of the high degree of mortality may be related to the incidence of significant associated injuries. High-energy injuries that significantly disrupt the pelvic ring commonly tear pelvic veins and arteries. Bleeding associated with these injuries can be massive with the potential for exsanguination (Table 28–1), and patients presenting with hypotension associated with pelvic fractures have a high-mortality rate.

▶ Clinical Findings

A. Symptoms and Signs

Pelvic fractures can be suggested by pain, or instability on palpation, perianal edema, pelvic edema, ecchymoses, deformities, or hematomas over the inguinal ligament or scrotum. Traditional ATLS teaching advocates that all trauma patients (especially those with pelvic fractures) receive a digital rectal examination to look for the presence of blood, to determine the position of the prostate, and for palpation of obvious fractures. Examination of the penis and testes or the vagina is necessary to evaluate for associated urologic and gynecologic

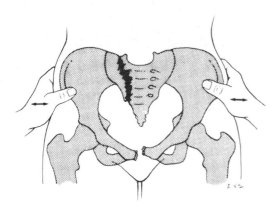

▲ **Figure 28–13.** Compression–distraction test for stability of the pelvic ring. If the iliac crests can be pressed together or pulled apart, the pelvis is unstable. With more severe instability, one hemipelvis may be displaced proximally.

injuries. If a urethral injury is suspected, do not place a urinary catheter and obtain a retrograde cystogram. If a urethral injury is present, consult with a urologist to place a suprapubic or Foley catheter (see Chapter 26). Compression to determine pelvic stability should be accomplished with gentle anteroposterior and lateral pressure (Figure 28–13).

B. X-ray Findings

X-rays should initially include an anteroposterior view. Inlet and outlet views may be helpful; however, CT scanning should be obtained to classify the extent of injury and to plan for treatment.

▶ Treatment

Fractures associated with disruption of the symphysis pubis (open book fractures) are frequently associated with massive bleeding into the pelvis. The patient should be monitored continuously with attention to the circulatory status and adequate volume replacement. Application of military antishock trousers or binders may be initiated in the prehospital setting and needs to be continued in the emergency department. A sheet wrapped around the pelvis may also be used in an attempt to stabilize the fracture and tamponade bleeding. In some cases, the orthopedist may opt to place an external fixator device. Some patients may need emergency ORIF or need to be transferred to radiology for arteriography and embolization.

▶ Disposition

Obtain orthopedic consultation in all cases. Most patients will require hospitalization. Simple nondisplaced fractures of the pubic rami may be managed conservatively on an outpatient basis. Consultation with trauma surgery, urology, and gynecology may also be necessary.

HIP INJURIES

▶ General Considerations

Hip injuries include various fractures and dislocations. As with pelvic fractures, hip injuries in young individuals are associated with high-energy trauma and may be seen with direct (falls) or indirect (knee-to-dashboard) forces. Elderly patients frequently sustain hip injuries with lower forces such as a fall from standing.

1. Hip Fractures

ESSENTIALS OF DIAGNOSIS

- ▶ Frequent in elderly patients
- ▶ Hip pain and tenderness
- ▶ Frequently limb is shortened and externally rotated
- ▶ Anteroposterior and lateral films are usually confirmatory
- ▶ Consider CT scan or MRI if X-rays are negative and diagnosis is still suspected

▶ General Considerations

Hip fractures are described anatomically as they may occur through the femoral neck, intertrochanteric, or subtrochanteric locations.

▶ Clinical Findings

A. Symptoms and Signs

The patient usually complains of groin pain. Shortening of the affected leg, with abduction and external rotation, is common but may not be obvious in cases of nondisplaced fractures. Care should be taken in the evaluation of elderly patients, because a long down time prior to obtaining help can result in dehydration, electrolyte abnormalities, or rhabdomyolysis. There is also the potential for significant blood loss and associated injuries.

B. X-ray Findings

Radiographs should include anteroposterior (with the legs in internal rotation) and lateral views. CT scanning may be necessary, particularly if acetabular involvement is suspected.

▶ Treatment

Immobilize the affected leg. If the fracture is closed and no neurologic deficits are present, in-line traction may be applied, such as a Hare splint, and is often applied in the prehospital setting.

Disposition

Monitor the patient for potential ongoing blood loss. Because of the risk of avascular necrosis of the femoral head, which occurs in 20% of these injuries, early orthopedic consultation is needed. Orthopedic consultation and admission for ORIF is warranted in the evaluation of all hip fractures.

2. Hip Dislocations

ESSENTIALS OF DIAGNOSIS

▶ Pain and deformity at hip
▶ Posterior dislocation is most common
▶ Hip or pelvic X-rays are confirmatory
▶ Patient's lower extremity is usually internally rotated and shortened

General Considerations

Hip dislocations are described by the relationship of the femoral head to the acetabulum. Dislocations may be accompanied by fractures of the acetabulum or femoral head. The vast majority (80–90%) of dislocations are posterior and typically seen by indirect forces such as knee-to-dashboard injuries in motor vehicle collisions. Anterior dislocations are less common (10–15%) and may be seen slightly more frequently in patients with hip prostheses. Central dislocation refers to the femoral head being forced through a comminuted fracture of the acetabulum. Inferior dislocations are rare and occur almost exclusively in young children. Dislocations of the hip are generally the result of significant force, and potential associated injuries should be sought.

Clinical Findings

A. Symptoms and Signs

Clinical examination in posterior dislocations generally reveals a slightly shortened extremity, adduction, and internal rotation, with the hip and knee in flexion. With anterior dislocations where the femoral head can dislocate medially toward the obturator foramen or laterally toward the pubis, and findings include abduction, external rotation, and flexion of the hip.

B. X-ray Findings

Obtain anteroposterior and lateral views to confirm the diagnosis and rule out associated fractures.

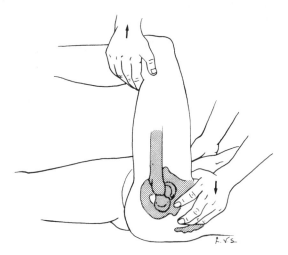

▲ **Figure 28–14.** The Allis technique for reduction of posterior hip dislocation. Both hip and knee are flexed 90°. An assistant stabilizes the pelvis while the operator pulls the femur anteriorly, rotating it slightly internally and externally to aid reduction, which is acheived mainly by firm steady traction.

Treatment

Hip dislocations require urgent reduction to decrease the risk of avascular necrosis, traumatic arthritis, joint instability, and neurologic sequel. Posterior hip dislocations are commonly reduced by the Allis technique (Figure 28–14). After adequate sedation, the patient is placed supine and an assistant stabilizes the pelvis. The hip and knee are flexed to 90° while upward traction and slight rotation are applied. Once the dislocation is reduced, the leg is extended.

An alternative method is the Stimson technique. The patient is placed prone with the leg extended over the edge of the bed. With an assistant stabilizing the pelvis, downward traction is applied with gentle rotation. The assistant then applies pressure over the greater trochanter toward the acetabulum.

Disposition

Once the dislocation is reduced by either method, the leg should be extended and placed in traction until postreduction X-rays can be obtained. Obtain orthopedic consultation for all hip dislocations.

Brooks RA, Ribbans WJ: Diagnosis and imaging studies of traumatic hip dislocations in the adult. Clin Orthop 2000;377:15 [PMID: 10943181].

Sharma OP, Oswanski MF, Rabbi J et al: Pelvic fracture risk assessment on admission. Am Surg 2008;74(8): 761–766 [PMID: 18705583].

Yang EC, Cornwall R: Initial treatment of traumatic hip dislocations in the adult. Clin Orthop 2000;377:24 [PMID: 10943182].

LOWER EXTREMITY INJURIES

FEMORAL SHAFT FRACTURES

ESSENTIALS OF DIAGNOSIS

▶ Pain and deformity of femur

▶ May lose large amount of blood in thigh

▶ Anteroposterior and lateral X-rays of femur are confirmatory

▶ Clinical Findings

Fractures of the femoral shaft occur most commonly with high-energy trauma. Fractures occurring with minimal trauma should alert the emergency physician to the possibility of a pathologic fracture.

A. Symptoms and Signs

As noted earlier, significant bleeding may occur secondary to femoral shaft fractures and up to 3L of blood can be lost in the thigh (see Table 28–1). The patient typically presents with tenderness and deformity of the thigh. Evaluate and document the neurovascular status. Although not as common as with lower leg fractures, significant soft tissue swelling can occur; therefore, frequent reexaminations should be performed to assess for the development of compartment syndrome.

B. X-ray Findings

Anteroposterior and lateral views should confirm the diagnosis. Adequate visualization of the knee and hip on these films is important because associated fractures are common.

▶ Treatment

Adequate pain control and fluid resuscitation is indicated. In-line traction, either skeletal traction or an external traction device, should be applied to the leg.

▶ Disposition

Obtain orthopedic consultation for admission and ORIF (usually with an intramedullary rod).

KNEE JOINT INJURIES

The knee is a large synovial hinge joint and is the most commonly involved joint in orthopedic injuries seen in the emergency department. The knee has a complex architecture of bone, muscle, ligament, and cartilage. The bones of the knee joint include the distal femur, proximal tibia, and patella. The fibula is not a part of the knee joint but serves as the attachment point for the lateral collateral ligament. The bones offer little stability to the joint, and the knee relies on the soft tissue components for proper function.

The medial collateral ligament originates from the medial femoral epicondyle and inserts on the medial aspect of the tibia just distal to the tibiofemoral joint. The medial collateral ligament provides stability to valgus stresses (Figure 28–15A) and helps stabilize the medial meniscus. The lateral collateral ligament originates from the lateral femoral epicondyle and inserts onto the proximal fibula, providing resistance to varus forces (Figure 28–15B). The cruciate ligaments are located within the intercondylar notch and are named anterior and posterior by their attachment to the tibia at the tibial spines. The cruciate ligaments protect against anterior and posterior displacement of the knee.

The menisci are cartilages positioned on the tibia. The menisci help dissipate forces within the knee joint and help prevent abnormal movement of the tibia and femur. The hamstring muscles (semitendinous, semimembranous, and the two heads of the biceps femoris) are the main flexors of the knee. The quadriceps muscles (vastus medialis, vastus

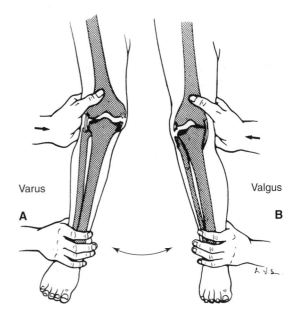

Varus

A

Valgus

B

▲ **Figure 28–15.** Varus **(A)** and valgus **(B)** stress tests for rupture of the medial and lateral collateral ligaments of the knee. More laxity than in the uninjured knee or lack of a firm end point constitutes a positive test. Pain and muscle guarding may make interpretation difficult.

lateralis, vastus intermedius, rectus femoris) combine to form the quadriceps tendon, which inserts onto the superior patella and the retinaculum of the joint capsule and functions in extension of the knee joint.

It is important to assess neurovascular status for knee injuries. The collateral circulation is tenuous, and the popliteal artery is responsible for the blood supply to the lower leg. The popliteal artery is tethered above at the hiatus of the adductor magnus and below at the soleus muscle. This tethering makes the popliteal artery susceptible to injury from traction forces as seen with dislocations as well as disruption from fractures or penetrating wounds.

The emergency department evaluation of an acute knee injury frequently involves obtaining plain X-rays, with anteroposterior, lateral, and sunrise view. Several clinical decision rules exist to aid the emergency physician in determining which patients need X-rays acutely. The Pittsburgh rules note that mechanism of injury (such as blunt trauma and falls), patient age (older than 55 years or younger than 12 years), and inability to walk at least four weight-bearing steps are predictors of fractures that require radiographic evaluation. The Ottawa rules identify five indications for radiographs of the knee: age greater than 55 years, isolated tenderness of the patella, tenderness of the head of the fibula, inability to flex the knee to 90°, and inability to transfer weight for four steps. Both sets of rules have demonstrated high sensitivity in predicting injuries and may be helpful to the emergency physician in the evaluation of the acutely injured knee.

1. Patella Fractures

ESSENTIALS OF DIAGNOSIS

▶ May be secondary to direct blow or traction injury

▶ Pain and tenderness are commonly seen

▶ May disrupt extensor mechanism

▶ Plain X-rays are usually sufficient

▶ Bipartite patella may be misinterpreted as fracture

▶ General Considerations

The patella is the largest sesamoid bone in the body and may be fractured by direct forces such as falls and by indirect forces. Significant fractures of the patella may disrupt the extensor mechanism of the knee. The most common pattern of patellar fracture is the transverse fracture, and can be caused by a direct blow or a powerful contractile force from the quadriceps.

The patella may be dislocated or subluxed by direct forces or a hyperflexion injury, and it almost always displaces

laterally. The patella is held in place by the quadriceps tendon, the patellar ligament and the medial and lateral retinacula. This injury occurs most commonly in adolescents. Often the patient gives a history of prior subluxations that resolved spontaneously.

▶ Clinical Findings

A. Symptoms and Signs

Examination of the patient reveals pain and tenderness over the patella. A joint effusion may be present. If the patella is displaced significantly, a patellar defect may be palpable.

B. X-ray Findings

Plain radiographs including anteroposterior, lateral, and sunrise views are usually sufficient to identify the fracture; however, CT scanning or MRI may be necessary to identify occult injuries. Bipartite or multipartite patellae are congenital findings that may be confused with acute fracture.

▶ Treatment

Obtain orthopedic consultation. Simple fractures may be treated with immobilization of the knee in extension.

▶ Disposition

Patients with simple fractures may be discharged with outpatient follow-up. Open and displaced fractures require surgical repair.

2. Patella Dislocations

ESSENTIALS OF DIAGNOSIS

▶ Common in adolescents

▶ Almost always displaces laterally

▶ Obvious deformity, restriction of motion

▶ Plain X-rays are usually sufficient for diagnosis

▶ Clinical Findings

A. Symptoms and Signs

Tenderness is present on physical examination, and a deformity is usually easily seen. A joint effusion may be present.

B. X-ray Findings

Plain radiographs are usually sufficient to confirm the injury.

Treatment

Management consists of closed reduction with appropriate sedation if needed for muscle relaxation, although some dislocations can be easily reduced without sedation. This is accomplished by applying medial force to the patella while the knee is being extended.

Disposition

Discharge the patient with immobilization, crutches, and orthopedic referral for follow-up. Recurrent subluxations or dislocations may require surgical repair.

3. Distal Femur Fractures

ESSENTIALS OF DIAGNOSIS

▶ Generally represent high-energy injuries
▶ Associated hip and patella injuries are common
▶ Plain X-rays are usually sufficient
▶ Obtain arteriogramif vascular injury is suspected

General Considerations

Fractures in the distal one-third of the femur are typically described by the relationship of the fracture line to the femoral condyles. Distal femur fractures generally represent high-energy injuries.

Clinical Findings

A. Symptoms and Signs

Pain, deformity, swelling, and inability to bear weight are usually present. Associated patella and hip injuries sometimes occur and acute hemarthrosis is common and can signify intra-articular extension of the fracture or ligamentous injury.

B. X-ray Findings

Diagnosis can usually be made with standard anteroposterior and lateral views. Oblique views and CT scanning may also be needed. If vascular compromise is suspected, obtain an arteriogram.

Disposition

Distal femur fractures are significant injuries that require orthopedic consultation in the emergency department. Skeletal traction and surgical repair are frequently required.

4. Tibial Plateau Fractures

ESSENTIALS OF DIAGNOSIS

▶ Usually occur to lateral aspect
▶ May be associated with peroneal nerve and popliteal artery injuries
▶ CT scan is helpful in planning treatment
▶ High suspicion for compartment syndrome

General Considerations

Tibial plateau fractures are intra-articular fractures and may result from axial loading and varus or valgus forces. The lateral portion of the tibia is most commonly involved. The fracture significantly impairs the function of the knee joint. Popliteal artery and peroneal nerve injuries may be seen, and the neurovascular status should be monitored continuously and documented. A Segond fracture is an avulsion fracture of the lateral tibial plateau and is a marker of ACL disruption.

Clinical Findings

A. Symptoms and Signs

Pain and tenderness are usually easily elicited. A hemarthrosis or effusion may be present, and the incidence of associated ligamentous injuries is significant.

B. X-ray Findings

Diagnosis is usually made on anteroposterior and lateral X-rays, but can be difficult to identify on routine radiographs. CT scanning is often used to delineate the extent of the injury. Tomograms and MRI may also be used. If vascular injury is suspected, obtain an arteriogram.

Treatment and Disposition

Immobilize the knee, keep the patient nonweight bearing, and obtain orthopedic consultation. A compartment syndrome may accompany tibial plateau fractures, and compartment pressures should be measured if indicated.

5. Tibial Tuberosity Fractures and Osgood-Schlatter Disease

ESSENTIALS OF DIAGNOSIS

▶ Usually avulsion fracture of patella tendon
▶ Obtain orthopedic consultation to determine treatment

General Considerations

The tibial tubercle is proximal at the anterior border of the shaft and is the attachment for the ligamentum patella. These fractures generally occur secondary to strong flexion or extension of the knee against resistance. Fractures usually occur prior to closure of the epiphysis and represent an avulsion fracture caused by the patella tendon. Osgood-Schlatter disease (or tibial tubercle apophysitis) represents a chronic traction injury to the tibial tuberosity and commonly occurs in adolescents engaging in sporting activities.

Clinical Findings

Tenderness and painful swelling over the tibial tubercle is present and, based on the mechanism of injury, an effusion may be seen. Diagnosis is confirmed with plain radiographs. In adolescents, Osgood-Schlatter disease must be in the differential diagnosis. Osgood-Schlatter disease is most commonly seen in males aged 10–13 years. Its radiographic findings may be difficult to differentiate from an acute fracture. A careful history and examination will help delineate an acute injury. A hemarthrosis is not associated with Osgood-Schlatter.

Treatment and Disposition

Orthopedic consultation is necessary because tibial tuberosity fractures may require open reduction. Osgood-Schlatter disease is treated conservatively with rest, ice and analgesics, and can be treated with immobilization and, in rare cases, surgery.

6. Tibial Spine Fractures

ESSENTIALS OF DIAGNOSIS

► Not common; usually seen in children
► Usually avulsion injury from cruciate ligament
► Suspect associate ligament injury

General Considerations

Fractures of the tibial spines (intercondylar eminence) are not commonly seen. These fractures usually represent an avulsion injury by one of the cruciate ligaments. They are more commonly seen in children and most often involve the anterior tibial spine.

Clinical Findings

A. Symptoms and Signs

Localized pain and a hemarthrosis may be present. If a significant ligamentous injury has occurred, instability of the knee may be seen.

B. X-ray Findings

The presentation may be subtle and may be noted only as an incidental finding on the X-ray. Plain films will usually identify the injury. In addition, as with other intra-articular fractures of the knee, a lipohemarthrosis is often demonstrated (Figure 28–16). This finding on the lateral views of the knee is produced by the layering of different density fluids (blood and marrow fat) present within the joint. CT scanning, MRI, or arthroscopy may be needed to identify associated injuries such as cruciate ligament ruptures.

Treatment

Simple fractures are usually treated with immobilization.

Disposition

If significant ligamentous injury is present, surgery may be necessary.

7. Knee Dislocations

ESSENTIALS OF DIAGNOSIS

► May be seen with high- or low-velocity injuries
► Tenderness and joint effusion are usually present
► Assess for associated popliteal artery injury

General Considerations

Dislocations involving the tibiofemoral joint (as opposed to patellar dislocations) are an orthopedic emergency and may represent a limb-threatening injury. They are commonly seen in high-energy trauma but may also be seen with low-velocity injuries such as from falls or sports injuries. The presence of a dislocation represents significant trauma to the soft tissues (ie, ligaments, menisci, and joint capsule). As noted above, the location and anatomy of the neurovascular bundle, including the popliteal artery, popliteal vein, and common peroneal nerve places it at significant risk of injury, particularly with posterior dislocations. Tenderness and joint effusion are generally present.

Clinical Findings

A. Symptoms and Signs

Visual deformity may be obvious, but some dislocations may reduce prior to evaluation. Careful attention to the neurovascular status is indicated, and the presence of a pulse does not rule out an arterial injury. Knee dislocation

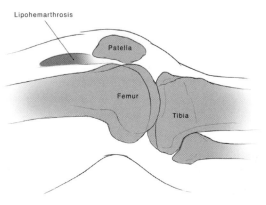

A

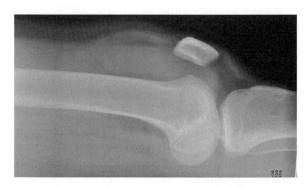

B

▲ **Figure 28–16.** A lipohemarthrosis noted on lateral radiograph of the knee in a supine patient is a specific sign of an intra-articular fracture although a fracture is not visualized. Just as oil and water separate, blood and fat from the marrow form the straight lines visualized in this radiograph.

is also associated with damage to the surrounding ligaments and menisci.

B. X-ray Findings

Plain radiographs help confirm the diagnosis. Traditionally, arteriography was recommended in all cases to identify arterial injuries, such as intimal tears, which may be clinically subtle but progress to occlusion and ischemia. Some authors recommend that serial examinations including ankle-brachial indices may be sufficient to exclude a clinically significant arterial injury. All authors agree, however, that if the arterial examination is abnormal, arteriography or Doppler studies should be obtained.

▶ Treatment

Management includes emergent reduction by in-line longitudinal traction. The neurovascular status should be monitored continuously and reassessed frequently.

▶ Disposition

Orthopedic consultation is necessary, and vascular surgical consultation may be needed. Patients for whom arteriography has not been obtained should be admitted for observation.

Gholve PA, Scher DM, Khakharia S et al: Osgood Schlatter syndrome. Curr Opin Pediatr 2007;19(1): 44–50 [PMID: 17224661].

Hollis JD, Daley BJ: 10-year review of knee dislocations: is angiography always necessary? J Trauma 2005;59(3):652–655 [PMID: 16361911].

Kleneberg EO, Crites BM, Flinn WR et al: The role of angiography in assessing popliteal artery injury in knee dislocations. J Trauma 2005;56(4):786–790 [PMID: 15187743].

8. Knee Ligament Injuries: General Considerations

 ESSENTIALS OF DIAGNOSIS

▶ Guarding and joint effusions may make diagnosis difficult in acute setting

▶ Patient may need immobilization and follow-up examination

Knee ligament injuries may range from minor sprains to complete disruptions. The more subtle injuries may be difficult to assess acutely because guarding and joint effusions may make determination of joint instability problematic. If possible, the unaffected knee should be examined before the injured knee in order to determine the patient's baseline, because some degree of laxity may be normal for an individual. After initial clinical and radiographic assessment, it is often prudent to treat the injury with a period of immobilization and crutches and to arrange for a follow-up examination. Depending on the patient's clinical situation and associated injuries, it is sometimes helpful to have the orthopedic consultant examine the patient under general anesthesia. If the patient has a grossly unstable knee with injury to multiple ligaments, consider the possibility of a spontaneously reduced knee dislocation. Serial vascular examinations including ankle-brachial indices are warranted to avoid missing an associated limb-threatening popliteal artery injury. If the vascular examination is abnormal, obtain angiography or Doppler studies for further evaluation.

9. Knee Ligament Injuries: Collateral Ligaments

The medial collateral ligament is the most commonly injured ligament in the knee and is associated with ACL injury. The mechanism of injury often involves a direct blow and sports injuries. The lateral collateral ligament is less commonly involved and occurs more often in high-energy trauma such as motor vehicle collisions.

▶ Clinical Findings

A. Symptoms and Signs

The patient usually presents with tenderness along the distribution of the ligament. Evaluate the ligament's stability by placing varus and valgus stresses (see Figure 28–15) with the knee in extension and with 30° flexion.

B. X-ray Findings

Plain radiography is of limited use but should be obtained initially to rule out associated fractures. MRI has emerged as a useful modality to evaluate these injuries but is rarely indicated in the emergency department. Orthopedic follow-up should be arranged.

▶ Treatment

Simple strains may be treated conservatively with immobilization and follow-up examination.

▶ Disposition

Patients can be discharged with immobilization and follow-up. Unstable joints will need further evaluation (eg, MRI, arthroscopy) and eventual surgical repair.

10. Knee Ligament Injuries: Cruciate Ligaments

Injuries to the cruciate ligaments usually result from direct anterior or posterior forces to the knee. Rotational forces may also injure the cruciate ligaments and are usually associated with other injuries (ie, menisci, collateral ligaments). Injuries may be associated with high- or low-energy trauma. The anterior cruciate ligament is the most commonly injured.

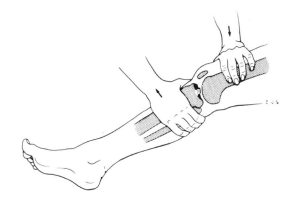

▲ **Figure 28–17.** The Lachman test for rupture of the anterior cruciate ligament. Attempt to pull the tibia forward relative to the femur while the knee is slightly flexed. Any increase in laxity compared with the uninjured knee signifies injury.

▶ Clinical Findings

A. Symptoms and Signs

Joint effusions are common, and hemarthrosis may be seen particularly with anterior cruciate ligament injuries. Stability of the anterior cruciate ligament is assessed clinically by the Lachman's test (to determine the endpoint of the tibia when pulled anteriorly with the thigh stabilized) (Figure 28–17), pivot shift ("jerk" test to detect anterolateral rotatory instability), and anterior drawer tests (to detect forward movement of the tibia relative to the femur compared to the other side). Stability of the posterior cruciate ligament is evaluated by the posterior drawer sign or the posterior sag sign (positive when the tibia sags backward with the knee flexed with muscle relaxation) (Figure 28–18).

B. X-ray Findings

Plain radiography may be unrevealing. Avulsion fractures of the tibial spines suggest a cruciate ligament tear. If the clinical examination does not reveal significant instability, outpatient follow-up examination may include MRI.

▶ Treatment

Immobilize the knee and give the patient crutches and nonweight-bearing status instructions.

▶ Disposition

Orthopedic follow-up is indicated for all significant injuries, and arthroscopy may be performed for both diagnosis and treatment.

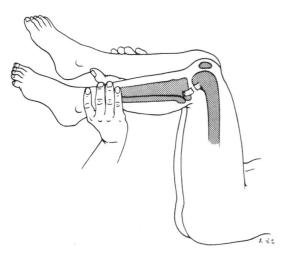

▲ **Figure 28–18.** Rupture of the posterior cruciate ligament is a likely diagnosis when the tibia of the injured knee sags posteriorly below the distal femur when the legs are held flexed 90° at the hip and knee.

11. Meniscal Tears

ESSENTIALS OF DIAGNOSIS

▶ Medial meniscus most commonly affected
▶ Patient may complain of knee locking
▶ MRI or arthroscopy may be necessary for diagnosis

▶ General Considerations

The menisci provide a gliding surface for the femoral condyles and aid in distributing stress across the joint. Meniscal tears usually occur when a rotational force is applied to the knee while the foot is planted. Because of degenerative processes, the injury producing the acute tear may not be significant. The medial meniscus is most commonly affected.

▶ Clinical Findings

A. Symptoms and Signs

The patient may complain of hearing a pop, but this finding is not specific. Joint line tenderness is usually present, and the patient may complain that the knee "locks." This locking is usually seen with a "bucket-handle" tear of the meniscus when the free central portion becomes lodged in the intercondylar notch. Clinical diagnosis is evaluated by use of the McMurray and Apley tests.

B. X-ray Findings

Plain films will not identify the tear but may be useful if associated bony injuries are suspected.

▶ Treatment

Treatment involves knee immobilization, crutches, and pain control.

▶ Disposition

Patients may be discharged from the emergency department with immobilization and orthopedic follow-up. Outpatient MRI is commonly used to make the diagnosis. Arthroscopy may be diagnostic and used to perform meniscectomy.

Roberts DM, Stallard TC: Emergency department evaluation and treatment of knee and leg injuries. Emerg Med Clin North Am 2000;18(1):67 [PMID: 10678160].

Swenson TM: Physical diagnosis of the multiple-ligament-injured knee. Clin Sports Med 2000;19(3):415 [PMID: 10918957].

12. Tendon Ruptures

ESSENTIALS OF DIAGNOSIS

▶ May disrupt extensor mechanism
▶ Quadriceps tendon is more commonly affected
▶ CT scan or MRI may be needed to confirm diagnosis

▶ General Considerations

Complete rupture of the quadriceps or patella tendon will disrupt the extensor mechanism of the knee. Injuries can occur with high-energy injuries or may be seen with low-energy trauma, particularly in the elderly, but are also classically associated with steroid use. The quadriceps tendon is more commonly ruptured compared to the patella tendon.

▶ Clinical Findings

A. Symptoms and Signs

The patient presents with a swollen and tender knee and is unable to extend the knee against resistance. A palpable defect may be appreciated.

B. X-ray Findings

Plain films may demonstrate an abnormal position of the patella. CT scanning and MRI confirm the diagnosis.

Treatment

Place the patient in a knee immobilizer until consultation is obtained.

Disposition

Management depends on the extent of the injury. Complete ruptures require surgical repair.

TIBIAL SHAFT FRACTURES

 ESSENTIALS OF DIAGNOSIS

► Most common long bone fracture
► Open fractures sometimes occur
► Plain X-rays are usually sufficient for diagnosis
► Assess for compartment syndrome

General Considerations

The tibia is the most common site of long bone fractures. The majority of these fractures will occur with associated fracture of the fibula. The tibia can be injured by a variety of forces.

Clinical Findings

A. Symtoms and Signs

Because little soft tissue is found around the tibia anteriorly, open fractures are common. Pain, swelling, and deformity are usually present. Compartment syndrome sometimes occurs with tibial injuries, and frequent reassessments should be performed.

B. X-ray Findings

Plain films are usually adequate to identify the fracture. As with all suspected long bone injuries, the joints above and below should be adequately visualized on the radiographs.

Treatment

Measure compartment pressure if a compartment syndrome is suspected clinically. Simple nondisplaced fractures may be treated with a long leg posterior splint and crutches with orthopedic follow-up.

Disposition

Open, displaced, and comminuted fractures require orthopedic consultation because they require operative management.

FIBULA FRACTURES

 ESSENTIALS OF DIAGNOSIS

► Isolated fibula fractures are uncommon
► Patient may be able to bear weight
► Assess for Maisonneuve fracture

General Considerations

Isolated fibular fractures are uncommon because they are usually seen with an associated tibia fracture. They may occur by direct blow or with rotational forces. Of particular importance is a Maisonneuve fracture, which is a fracture of the proximal fibula with an associated medial malleolus ankle fracture or ligamentous disruption of the ankle without a fracture.

Clinical Findings

A. Symptoms and Signs

The patient usually complains of pain and tenderness, and a deformity can usually be palpated. Since the fibula is a non-weight bearing bone, a patient with an isolated fibular shaft fracture may be able to walk.

B. X-ray Findings

Plain X-rays should be sufficient for the diagnosis.

Treatment

Splints or compressive dressing may be applied for comfort. A Maisonneuve fracture represents an unstable ankle injury, and requires immobilization and orthopedic consultation to determine definitive management.

Disposition

With isolated, uncomplicated fibula fractures, the patient may be discharged with instructions to advance from non-weight-bearing status to weight-bearing status as tolerated.

ANKLE JOINT INJURIES

The bones of the ankle include the distal tibia, distal fibula, and the talus. The ankle mortise is formed by the medial and lateral malleoli and the plafond (the articular surface of the distal tibia). As with the knee, the ankle relies on articular cartilage, joint capsule, and ligaments to provide joint stability. Management of ankle injuries is based on the joint's stability.

The ligaments are divided into three sets: the syndesmotic (anterior and posterior tibiofibular ligaments); the lateral collateral (calcaneofibular, anterior talofibular, and lateral tibiocalcaneal ligaments); and the medial collateral or deltoid ligaments, which are further divided into four parts (posterior tibiotalar, tibiocalcaneal, anterior tibiotalar, and tibionavicular). Ankle injuries are common and often involve a combination of bony and ligamentous injuries.

Clinical decision rules aid the emergency physician in determining whether plain radiography is needed in the evaluation of ankle or foot injuries. The Ottawa ankle rules state that ankle X-rays should be obtained if there is pain at the malleoli, inability to bear weight for four steps, and tenderness posteriorly or inferiorly at the malleoli. Ottawa foot rules recommend that X-rays be obtained if there is inability to bear weight for four steps and tenderness at the base of the fifth metatarsal or over the navicular bone. The sensitivities of the Ottawa ankle and foot rules are 98–100%.

1. Lateral Malleolar Fractures

ESSENTIALS OF DIAGNOSIS

▶ Inversion injury
▶ May include minor avulsion fractures to complete joint disruption
▶ Plain X-rays are usually sufficient for diagnosis

▶ General Considerations

Lateral malleolar fractures may range from simple avulsion fractures seen with inversion to displaced fractures with mortise disruption.

▶ Clinical Findings

A. Symptoms and Signs

The patient usually presents with point tenderness, swelling, and difficulty ambulating.

B. X-ray Findings

Plain radiographs are usually sufficient to make the diagnosis.

▶ Treatment

Simple fractures may be treated with a posterior short leg splint with stirrups (Figure 28–19), crutches with no weight bearing, and orthopedic follow-up.

▶ Disposition

Open or displaced fractures require orthopedic consultation for operative management.

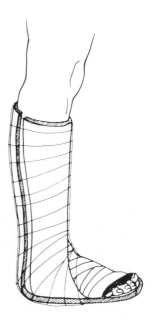

▲ **Figure 28–19.** Combined sugar-tong splint and posterior-plantar plaster slab with padding for ambulatory (nonweight-bearing) patient with foot injuries.

2. Medial Malleolar Fractures

ESSENTIALS OF DIAGNOSIS

▶ Eversion injury
▶ Often associated with deltoid ligament injury
▶ Plain X-rays are usually sufficient for diagnosis

▶ General Considerations

Medial malleolar fractures result from eversion injuries or external rotation. These fractures are frequently associated with injuries to the deltoid ligament.

▶ Clinical Findings

A. Symptoms and Signs

Pain, swelling, and difficulty in ambulating are usually present. Palpate the proximal fibula to determine whether a Maisonneuve fracture is present.

B. X-ray Findings

Plain films are usually sufficient for the diagnosis.

Treatment

Management is similar to that for lateral malleolar fractures; however, if significant injury to the deltoid ligament has occurred, the rehabilitation period will be longer.

Disposition

Patients with closed injuries may be discharged with a posterior short leg splint with stirrups (Figure 28–19), crutches with no weight bearing, and orthopedic follow-up in 2–3 days.

3. Posterior Malleolar Fractures

ESSENTIALS OF DIAGNOSIS

▶ Rare injury
▶ Usually avulsion from posterior talofibular ligament
▶ May represent significant joint instability

General Considerations

Fractures involving only the posterior malleoli are rare and usually result from an avulsion injury involving the posterior tibiofibular ligament. If isolated they may be managed conservatively as above. If these fractures are associated with other injuries or joint instability, orthopedic consultation is indicated. Bimalleolar and trimalleolar fractures should be considered unstable and mandate orthopedic consultation for surgical management.

4. Achilles Tendon Injuries

ESSENTIALS OF DIAGNOSIS

▶ May occur from direct or indirect forces
▶ Use Thompson test
▶ Orthopedic consultation is necessary

General Considerations

Rupture of the Achilles tendon is often seen in middle-aged individuals participating in sporting activities. It may be secondary to a direct blow or can occur with indirect forces as with forced dorsiflexion. The patient frequently reports hearing a pop.

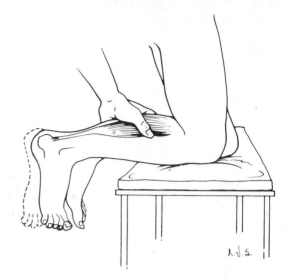

▲ **Figure 28–20.** Test for Achilles tendon continuity. Squeeze the relaxed calf while observing the amount of ankle plantarflexion thus produced. If the tendon is ruptured, less motion occurs compared with that on the uninjured side.

Clinical Findings

A. Symptoms and Signs

Localized pain and weakness in plantarflexion are present, and a deformity may be appreciated. The diagnosis is mainly clinical. To determine if the tendon has been ruptured, the emergency physician can squeeze the calf muscles with the patient prone and the knee flexed to 90° (Thompson test) or alternatively squeeze the calf muscles with the patient kneeling on a chair with both knees flexed (Figure 28–20). Absence of plantarflexion or decreased plantarflexion compared to the unaffected side suggests rupture.

B. X-ray Findings

X-rays may show thickening of the tendon. MRI will confirm the diagnosis.

Treatment

A temporary long leg or stirrup splint may be placed until consultation with orthopedics.

Disposition

Orthopedic consultation should be obtained because Achilles tendon injuries may be managed surgically or nonoperatively.

5. Peroneal Tendon Injuries

ESSENTIALS OF DIAGNOSIS

► Usually results from forced dorsiflexion
► Tenderness posterior to lateral malleolus
► CT scan or MRI may be needed to confirm diagnosis

▶ General Considerations

The peroneal tendons function in eversion, pronation, and plantarflexion. These tendons can become subluxed or dislocated by tearing of the superior retinaculum attachment on the fibula. The injury usually results from forced dorsiflexion.

▶ Clinical Findings

A. Symptoms and Signs

The patient presents with pain, swelling, and weakness on eversion. Tenderness posterior to the lateral malleolus is present.

B. X-ray Findings

A small avulsion fracture of the lateral malleolus is pathognomonic of this injury. A CT or MRI scan may be needed to confirm the diagnosis.

▶ Treatment

Treatment involves use of a posterior splint, crutches with no weight bearing, and analgesics.

▶ Disposition

Orthopedic consultation is necessary to determine appropriate management. Patients with these injuries may be discharged with appropriate follow-up, but peroneal tendon injuries often need surgical repair.

6. Ankle Dislocations

ESSENTIALS OF DIAGNOSIS

► Associated fracture often present
► Assess neurovascular status
► Dislocation may require reduction before X-rays are obtained

▶ General Considerations

An ankle dislocation represents displacement of the talus and foot from the tibia. Dislocations are described by the relationship of the talus to the tibia. They may be open or closed, and an associated fracture frequently occurs. Dislocations occur from axial loading to the foot in plantarflexion and are seen in sporting injuries and in high-energy trauma such as motor vehicle collisions.

▶ Clinical Findings

A. Symptoms and Signs

The neurovascular status should be determined quickly along with rapid reduction. The patient will have gross deformity of the ankle joint.

B. X-ray Findings

Radiographs can be used for diagnosis, but should not be delayed when skin tenting or neurovascular compromise is present.

▶ Treatment

Once the dislocation has been reduced, reassess the neurovascular status, splint the ankle, and obtain radiographs and orthopedic consultation.

▶ Disposition

These patients will frequently be admitted and should not be discharged without consultation from an orthopedist.

7. Ankle Sprains

ESSENTIALS OF DIAGNOSIS

► Anterior talofibular ligament is affected most commonly
► Swelling, ecchymosis, point tenderness
► Assess for instability of ligaments
► Ankle rules may help in determining need for X-rays
► Most are managed conservatively

▶ General Considerations

Ankle sprains most often occur secondary to significant force applied as inversion and plantarflexion. The ligament most commonly affected is the anterior talofibular ligament, accounting for approximately two-thirds of ankle sprains. The next most commonly affected ligament is the calcaneofibular ligament, and in 20% of cases both the calcaneofibular and anterior talofibular are involved. The deltoid ligament located medially is injured less often (approximately 5% of sprains). Eversion forces may initiate this injury, and sprains of the deltoid ligament typically require extended rehabilitation periods compared to the more common anterior talofibular or calcaneofibular ligament sprains. Deltoid ligament ruptures may be seen with medial malleolar fractures.

▶ Clinical Findings

A. Symptoms and Signs

The patient typically presents with a history of a fall or twisting injury. Often swelling, ecchymosis, and point tenderness are present. Grading of sprains is described earlier in this chapter. Always assess for associated injuries such as a Maisonneuve fracture or Achilles tendon rupture.

Physical examination may include the anterior drawer test. With the patient seated, the knee flexed to 90°, and the ankle in neutral position or 10° of plantarflexion, gently pull forward on the heel while pushing the lower leg posteriorly. Visualize for any deformity or feel for a clunk. This test examines the integrity of the anterior talofibular ligament. The talar tilt-test assesses the anterior talofibular and calcaneofibular ligaments. With the knee flexed to 90° and the ankle in a neutral position, invert the heel and assess for displacement of the talar head or laxity. The external rotation test is used to evaluate the distal talar syndesmotic ligaments. With the foot in neutral position and the knee flexed to 90°, rotate the foot and assess for laxity and pain laterally.

B. X-ray Findings

Use history, physical findings, and Ottawa ankle rules to determine whether radiographs are necessary. X-rays will be negative for fracture but may demonstrate soft tissue swelling. In significant ligament sprains and ruptures, the mortise may be affected.

▶ Treatment

Most ankle sprains may be treated conservatively on an outpatient basis. The RICE (rest, ice, crutches, and immobilization elevation) treatment is usually indicated. For minor injuries, immobilization with an elastic bandage and crutches may be all that is necessary. For more significant injuries, a sugar-tong or posterior plaster splint may be applied. A plaster cast should never be applied acutely because of the risk of further swelling leading to increased pain and vascular compromise. Aircasts and other commercial devices may be useful. Crutches should be used with no weight bearing initially and progressing to weight-bearing status as tolerated. Prescribe appropriate analgesics. Depending on the severity of injury, the patient may return to normal function in as

little as a few days; however, it may be several weeks until proper function is restored.

▶ Disposition

For minor injuries, treatment should be initiated as above. If symptoms resolve quickly, follow-up may not be necessary. Patients may consider follow-up with a primary-care provider for further evaluation in minor cases. Patients with significant sprains should receive treatment with immobilization and crutches as above and should be referred to an orthopedist within 1 week.

Perry JJ, Stiell IG: Impact of clinical decision rules on clinical care of traumatic injuries to the foot and ankle, knee, cervical spine, and head. Injury 2006;37(12):1157–1165 [PMID: 17078955].

Pijnenburg AC et al: Radiography in acute ankle injuries: the Ottawa ankle rules versus local diagnostic decision rules. Ann Emerg Med 2007;39:599 [PMID: 12023701].

CALCANEAL FRACTURES

ESSENTIALS OF DIAGNOSIS

- ▶ Most common tarsal bone fracture
- ▶ Axial loading, often associated with vertebral fractures
- ▶ The Boehler angle may detect subtle fractures
- ▶ Orthopedic consultation is necessary

▶ General Considerations

The calcaneus is the largest of the tarsal bones and the one most commonly fractured. The most common mechanism is axial loading from a fall. A high association exists between calcaneal fractures and other lower-extremity and vertebral fractures.

▶ Clinical Findings

A. Symptoms and Signs

The patient complains of severe pain in the heel and inability to bear weight. Ecchymosis and deformity may be present.

B. X-ray Findings

Obtain plain radiographs including anteroposterior, lateral, and axial views. Measurement of the Boehler angle on the lateral view may help to identify subtle fractures. The Boehler angle is formed by the intersection of lines drawn from the anterior and posterior elements of the superior portion of the calcaneus (Figure 28–21). The normal angle is 20–40°; an angle of less than 20° suggests a calcaneal fracture.

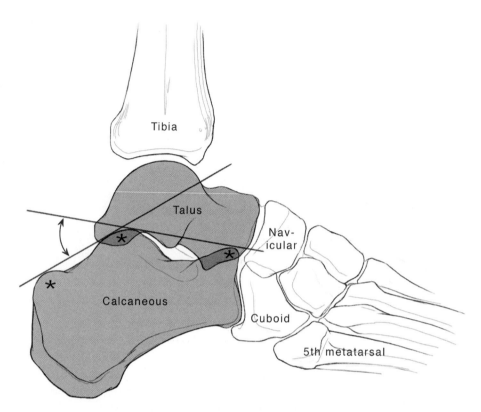

▲ **Figure 28–21.** Because calcaneal fracture lines are often subtle to visualize on foot radiographs, Boehler's Angle is used to determine if the normal anatomic relationships of the calcaneal bony prominences have been disrupted. The normal angle is 28–40° and with fracture from an axial load, the angle is reduced to less than 20°.

► Treatment

A posterior leg splint or bulky Jones splint should be applied. The patient should be given crutches and nonweight-bearing status instructions.

► Disposition

Orthopedic consultation is necessary to determine operative versus nonoperative management.

TALAR FRACTURES

ESSENTIALS OF DIAGNOSIS

- ▶ No muscle attachment on talus
- ▶ Tenuous blood supply
- ▶ CT scan or MRI may be necessary to detect subtle fractures

► General Considerations

The talus is the second largest tarsal bone and is the second most commonly injured bone after the calcaneus. The talus is the only bone in the foot with no muscle attachment; it is held in place by the malleoli and ligaments. The talus has a somewhat tenuous blood supply, and avascular necrosis is a potential with significant fractures. Other complications include infection, posttraumatic arthritis, malunion, and nonunion. Fractures may result from plantarflexion, dorsiflexion, or inversion forces. Talus fractures usually result from high-energy trauma, and associated injuries are common.

► Clinical Findings

A. Symptoms and Signs

Pain and swelling are common. Inversion and eversion are usually quite painful.

B. X-ray Findings

Plain radiographs may miss subtle fractures, and CT scanning or MRI may be necessary.

▶ Treatment

Simple fractures are treated conservatively with splinting, nonweight bearing and analgesics. Major fractures often require open reduction or prolonged nonweight-bearing immobilization.

▶ Disposition

Talar fractures require orthopedic consultation and many require ORIF.

SUBTALAR DISLOCATIONS

ESSENTIALS OF DIAGNOSIS

- ▶ Uncommon injury
- ▶ Associated with talocalcaneal and talonavicular ligament ruptures
- ▶ Plain X-rays should be sufficient for diagnosis
- ▶ Rapid reduction is indicated

▶ General Considerations

Subtalar dislocations are rare injuries and occur secondary to severe rotational forces that rupture the talocalcaneal and talonavicular ligaments, while the calcaneonavicular ligament remains intact. The dislocation is usually lateral or medial, although anterior and posterior dislocations may occur.

▶ Clinical Findings

A. Symptoms and Signs

An obvious deformity is usually visible and neurovascular status should be carefully assessed, but compromise is rare.

B. X-ray Findings

Plain radiographs including an anteroposterior view of the foot should determine the diagnosis.

▶ Treatment

The dislocation should be reduced quickly, usually via closed reduction under adequate sedation. In-line longitudinal traction should be applied to the foot and then appropriate directional force applied to correct the deformity. Direct pressure on the head of the talus can be helpful. Buttonholing of the talus through the extensor retinaculum can make reduction impossible.

▶ Disposition

After reduction, immobilization in a splint and orthopedic referral are indicated.

TARSAL INJURIES

ESSENTIALS OF DIAGNOSIS

- ▶ Isolated dislocations are rare
- ▶ Navicular fractures are most common, after calcaneal and talar fractures
- ▶ Local tenderness and swelling are common
- ▶ Plain X-rays are usually sufficient for diagnosis

▶ General Considerations

Fractures and dislocations can occur in the other tarsal bones (ie, navicular, cuboid, and the cuneiforms). Isolated dislocations are rare injuries. Fractures of the navicular are the most common in this portion of the foot. Avulsion fractures of the navicular occur when eversion stresses are exerted on the deltoid and talonavicular ligaments.

▶ Clinical Findings

Local pain and swelling are common. Plain radiographs may identify the injury; bone scans and tomography may be used to identify subtle injuries.

▶ Treatment

Immobilization with a posterior short leg splint and orthopedic referral are indicated.

TARSOMETATARSAL INJURIES (LISFRANC INJURIES)

ESSENTIALS OF DIAGNOSIS

- ▶ Uncommon injury; large amount of force is required
- ▶ Lisfranc joint
- ▶ Plain X-rays are usually sufficient for diagnosis

▶ General Considerations

The tarsometatarsal joint comprises the articulation of the first three metatarsals with the medial, middle, and lateral cuneiform bones, as well as the articulation of the fourth and fifth metatarsals with the cuboid. The tarsometatarsal joint separates the forefoot from the mid-foot and is commonly referred to as the Lisfranc joint. It functions in supination and pronation of the foot. Injuries to this joint are uncommon and generally the result of a large force applied to the foot. Dislocations can occur in part or all of this joint and are frequently associated with metatarsal and tarsal fractures.

► Clinical Findings
A. Symptoms and Signs

Pain and obvious deformity over the joint are generally present.

B. X-ray Findings

Plain films usually suffice; a lateral weight-bearing view may detect subtle injuries but is not indicated in the emergency department. Fractures at the base of the second metatarsal or the dorsal aspect of the cuboid are often associated with Lisfranc fracture dislocations.

► Treatment

These injuries are often managed with closed reduction and percutaneous wires.

► Disposition

Orthopedic consultation is necessary.

Perron AD, Brady WJ, Keats TE: Orthopedic pitfalls in the ED: lisfranc fracture-dislocation. Am J Emerg Med 2001;19:71 [PMID: 11146025].

METATARSAL FRACTURES

ESSENTIALS OF DIAGNOSIS

► Common; result from crush or twisting injuries
► Most common at base of fifth metatarsal (Jones fracture)
► Treat with posterior splint

► General Considerations

Metatarsal fractures are common, accounting for approximately one-third of foot fractures. They may occur as a result of crush injuries or twisting forces.

► Clinical Findings
A. Symptoms and Signs

A visible deformity may be present, along with tenderness and swelling.

B. X-ray Findings

A fracture involving the base of the fifth metatarsal is the most common fracture. Plain radiographs should be sufficient to make the diagnosis. Care should be taken to examine the X-rays for subtle abnormalities in the Lisfranc joint.

► Treatment

Avulsion fractures involving the tuberosity of the proximal fifth metatarsal can be splinted for comfort, or the patient may be allowed to bear weight in a hard-soled shoe. Fractures involving the metaphysis of the proximal fifth metatarsal (also known as a Jones fracture) are more prone to complication, such as nonunion, and should be immobilized in a posterior splint (see Figure 28–18).

► Disposition

Discharge the patient with orthopedic follow-up within a few days.

PHALANGEAL INJURIES

ESSENTIALS OF DIAGNOSIS

► Fractures and dislocations are common
► Pain, obvious deformity
► X-rays may be bypassed in minor injuries
► Treatment involves buddy taping

► General Considerations

Injuries to the toes are common and include both fractures and dislocations. Fractures of the phalanges are the most common fractures in the foot and frequently involve the fifth phalanx. Dislocations are rare; when seen, they most commonly occur in the metatarsophalangeal joint of the great toe.

► Clinical Findings
A. Symptoms and Signs

Pain, swelling, and deformity are usually seen.

B. X-ray Findings

X-rays usually reveal the injury. Radiographs may not be obtained for minor injuries.

Treatment

Conservative management and immobilization by taping to the adjacent toe (buddy taping) are instituted. Dislocations are usually easily reduced with adequate sedation or a digital nerve block.

Disposition

Patients with simple fractures do not require orthopedic follow-up. Complicated fractures and dislocations should be immobilized with buddy taping; patients with complicated fractures and dislocations should be referred for outpatient orthopedic follow-up.

SESAMOID FRACTURES

ESSENTIALS OF DIAGNOSIS

► Seen most commonly in flexor hallucis brevis tendon
► May be difficult to see on plain X-rays

General Considerations

Sesamoid bones commonly occur in the tendon of the flexor hallucis brevis. Fractures are not common and are usually the result of direct forces or hyperextension of the great toe.

Clinical Findings

1. Symptoms and Signs

Local pain is present.

2. X-ray Findings

Sesamoid bones are frequently unexpected findings on radiographs obtained to rule out other injuries. Sesamoid bones are not of uniform appearance, and sometimes fractures are difficult to recognize.

Treatment

Treatment is with immobilization, analgesia, and weight bearing as tolerated.

Disposition

These fractures generally do not require orthopedic evaluation; patients may be discharged to home.

COMMON PITFALLS

Missed orthopedic injuries are among the common malpractice claims in emergency medicine. Commonly missed injuries are carpal bone fractures, especially of the scaphoid. Other frequently missed injuries are posterior shoulder dislocations, hip and pelvic fractures in elderly patients, tarsometatarsal fracture dislocations, patellar tendon injuries, and compartment syndromes. Children may sustain injuries to growth plates with no radiographic evidence of injury on initial presentation. For this reason, emergency physicians should have a low threshold for immobilizing children with pain or tenderness near joints despite initially negative radiographs. Follow-up in 7–10 days should be arranged for reexamination out of the splint and possibly repeat X-rays. Patients should be advised that some nondisplaced fractures are not evident on initial radiographs and outpatient follow-up and repeat radiographs may be indicated if pain or tenderness persists.

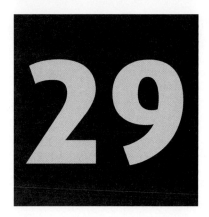

Hand Trauma

Bill Ewen, MD
Raymond G. Hart, MD, MPH[1]

▼ EMERGENCY EVALUATION AND TREATMENT

Hand injuries are one of the more common reasons for emergency department visits. Hand injuries may be isolated or part of multiple trauma. These injuries are seldom life-threatening but can result in significant disability, threatening a patient's livelihood and lifestyle. These injuries can have significant economic impact with possible loss of occupation and lost time from work. Systematic examination and initial care has a direct effect on the ultimate consequence of any hand injury. Overall, it is far better to under treat and refer than to over treat and cause avoidable iatrogenic injury or disability. The course of recovery depends on initial management.

▶ Position the Patient

A hand-injured patient may be examined while they are sitting but the environment should be calm and controlled. That does not apply to a patient with hand lacerations. It is best to examine the injured patient with a hand laceration while supine. The hand should be extended on a hand table next to the bed. The area should be clean, sterile, and have excellent lighting and all essential instruments available. It is best to have an assistant if possible for helping with lighting, positioning, and repair. There is a tendency in EM to see hand patients in hallways, chairs, and less than ideal circumstances. This must be avoided at all costs.

▶ Control Bleeding

Bleeding is controlled by direct pressure with sterile gauze packs, elevation, and, if necessary, an arterial tourniquet (eg, blood pressure cuff inflated above systolic blood pressure). *Do not use clamps unless all other measures fail.* Blind clamping of vessels can lead to further injury.

▶ Obtain History

A. Current Injuries

Ascertain the mechanism of injury by questioning the patient or others. An exact description of how the injury occurred will help determine the need for X-ray, antibiotics, urgent consultation in the ED, or in a follow-up visit. It is important to document the mechanism of injury, the time at which it occurred, and the environment in which it

[1]This chapter is a revision of the chapter by Adam Saperston, MD, MS, from the 5th edition.

occurred. Ask about the following details associated with the mechanism of injury:

- Type of injury—crush, exploding, or simple amputation.
- Lacerations—exactly what device was involved and how the lacerations were caused.
- Position of the hand at the time of the injury (ie, fingers extended or flexed).
- Presence of pain, numbness, paresthesias, weakness, discoloration, coldness, clumsiness or poor coordination, or crepitus.
- Circumstances surrounding open wounds—environment, whether inflicted in a dirty environment (ie, sewer or barnyard) or in a specific situation (ie, fight-clenched fist).

B. Relevant History

- History of prior or existing hand or upper extremity injuries or disorders. Dupuytren's fasciitis, arthritis, and benign tumors are the most common nontraumatic problems noted.
- Bleeding disorders likely to influence hemostasis (eg, hemophilia).
- Factors that might impair wound healing (eg, use of corticosteroids).
- Tetanus immunization status (Chapter 30).
- Any allergies.
- General state of health, medications, and ongoing treatments.

▶ Examine the Hand

Examination of the hand is started while the history is being taken. In the event of an open wound, proper instruments and sutures must be made ready. Sterile technique is essential at all stages of the examination and early treatment of hand injuries. A sensory examination for two-point discrimination should be done with an opened paper clip before anesthesia is used. Before beginning active examination, anesthetize the injured area of the hand, and apply and inflate a tourniquet. Be certain to remove rings from the patient's hands prior to any examination, radiographs, or procedures.

A. Anesthesia

Anesthesia must be used if a wound is to be explored or sutured. The preferred anesthetic is 1% lidocaine *without* epinephrine. It is recommended that epinephrine never be used with local anesthetics in hand injury, because it may constrict the vessels and interfere with blood flow. See Chapter 30, Wound Care for further discussion of specific techniques.

1. Digital block or wrist block—(See Figures 29–1 to 29–3.) Digital blocks are preferred for procedures done distal to the PIP joint. Half-inch (1.5-cm) needles of 25, 27, or 30 gauge should be used with small volumes of 1% lidocaine, or 0.5% bupivacaine may be used as a mix for a longer-acting anesthetic. In a digital block, use about 0.5–1.0 mL anesthetic around the digital nerve. The injection should never render the tissues tense nor be circumferential.

In blocking peripheral nerves, the physician must be familiar with the anatomy of nerve distribution and the surrounding tissues. To avoid intravascular injection, always aspirate before injecting the anesthetic agent.

2. Transthecal digital block—This block is preferred for injured digits, particularly the distal phalanx, nail bed, and volar tip. But should not be performed if there is an infection or suspicion of a flexor tenosynovitis. The digit to be blocked is extended and comfortably placed on the examination table. A 5-cc syringe with 27-gauge needle is preferred. The block should be performed with a 50:50 mixture of 1% lidocaine: 0.5% bupivacaine (see Figures 29–4). Identify the midpoint of the MCP flexion crease, insert at 90° until striking bone, then angle the tip of the needle 45° distally. Inject 2–3 cc into the flexor tendon sheath. With the tips of the opposite index and long finger palpate the infusion of medication into the sheath. In addition, the digit will gradually assume a partially flexed position. These blocks only require one needle stick. They are safe and effective. Complications are rare.

3. Local infiltration—(See Chapter 30, Figure 30–1.) Wounds can be infiltrated locally as long as the amount of anesthetic injected does not make the tissues tense.

4. Amount of solution—Systemic toxicity from over dosage may occur when large areas are anesthetized. This can be avoided by calculating the number of milligrams of drug in the volume of solution that may be required and then limiting the volume of injection so as to avoid giving a toxic dose (see Table 30–1). For example, the maximum adult dose of 1% lidocaine (10 mg/mL) without epinephrine is 300 mg (or 30 cc).

5. Inflamed areas—Anesthetic solutions should not be injected into inflamed areas unless these directly overlie an abscess that is to be drained. Such injections impair local tissue resistance to infection, may result in rapid systemic absorption because of the increased vascularity of inflamed tissues, and may be ineffective if the local tissue pH is low enough to reduce the anesthetic agent's ionic dissociation, which is essential for anesthetic activity.

B. Application of Tourniquet

An arm tourniquet should be in place when bleeding hand wounds are examined or treated. A blood pressure cuff can be used but should be inverted so that the tubes extend

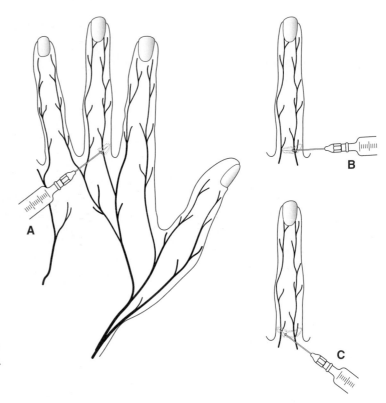

▲ **Figure 29–1.** Digital block. **A:** Use ½-in (1.5-cm) needles of 25, 27, or 30 gauge with small volume of 1% lidocaine. **B:** Use about 0.5–1.0 mL around the digital nerve. **C:** The injection should never render the tissues tense nor be circumferential.

cephalad and out of the way. First, wrap the patient's arm with cast padding, then place the cuff and inflate to 200–250 mmHg before locking (or Kelley clamps placed). This method should sufficiently occlude the brachial artery and reduce further hemorrhage. Be aware, a properly placed tourniquet will become quite painful to the patient within a few minutes and should be used only as necessary to prevent uncontrolled blood loss or allow essential evaluation of the wound.

C. Examination Sequence

By dividing the examination into four distinct steps, much useful information can be gained rapidly.

1. Observe the posture of the hand lying supine and at rest upon the examining table. Any marked variation from the normal attitude should alert the examiner to the possibility of deforming injury.

2. Observe active function of the various musculotendinous units and skeletal structures within the areas of injury. A careful examination of the flexor digitorum profundi and flexor digitorum superficialis must be performed.

3. Assess loss of sensibility by testing for sweat and for awareness of pain. Two-point discrimination is a sensitive, objective measure of sensory deficit. This may be difficult to be performed accurately, and the character and location of a wound may be more helpful than sensory nerve testing in determining nerve injury. Sensory testing must be performed before application of a tourniquet and administration of anesthetics.

4. Inspect the wound in a sterile, bloodless field with a simple 2.5-power magnifying loupes, if available. A tourniquet should be in place but should *not* be inflated until the anesthetic has become effective unless there is uncontrollable hemorrhage (see above). The examination must proceed concurrently with early treatment such as cleansing and debridement (Chapter 30) before definitive emergency treatment and suturing are done. *Note*: In handling and examining tissue, remember the importance of removal of blood clots and careful manipulation of tissues to preserve the microcirculation.

EXAMINATION OF THE HAND AND ASSESSMENT OF FUNCTION

(See Figures 29–5 and 29–6.) The hand is a highly mobile organ of extraordinary sensibility and remarkable adaptability, but it can be troubling if injured, causing permanent

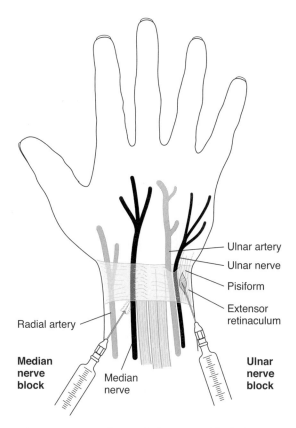

Radial artery

Ulnar artery
Ulnar nerve
Pisiform
Extensor retinaculum

Median nerve block Median nerve **Ulnar nerve block**

▲ **Figure 29–2.** Median and ulnar nerve block demonstrated on the volar surface of the left hand.

stiffness, pain, or loss of sensibility. Prevention is key and a sound knowledge of functional hand anatomy helps diagnosis and treatment of these wounds.

▶ Terminology

(See Figures 29–7.) The hand and each finger have ulnar and radial sides and palmar and dorsal surfaces. There are five digits numbered and named as follows: I (thumb), II (index), III (long or middle), IV (ring), and V (small [little]). Commonly used abbreviations for the joints of the hand are shown in the box at the beginning of the chapter. Always specify which hand is injured, and note whether it is the dominant or nondominant hand.

▶ Skin and Circulation

The skin of the palm sweats freely and is thick, tough, tethered by fascia, highly innervated, and well cushioned by fat. The dorsal skin, by contrast, is thin, very mobile, and less well supplied with sensory nerves. The arterial supply is mainly palmar. Venous and lymphatic drainage is mainly dorsal and can be impeded by dorsal injury, constriction, or taut skin.

▶ Twelve Extrinsic Flexors

See Figures 29–5.

A. Anatomy

1. Wrist flexors—There are three wrist flexors: the flexor carpi ulnaris (innervated by the ulnar nerve), the palmaris longus (median nerve), and the flexor carpi radialis (median nerve).

2. Digital flexors—There are nine digital flexors (one for each IP joint). The flexor pollicis longus (innervated by the median nerve) flexes the thumb IP joint. Flexor digitorum superficialis (sublimis) moves each PIP joint (all median nerve). Each superficialis is generally able to contract independently, because the muscles are independent for each digit.

A flexor digitorum profundus moves each DIP joint (median nerve to index and long fingers; ulnar nerve to ring and small fingers). The three ulnar profundi have a common muscle mass, and therefore one cannot contract and move one of these digit tips independently.

B. Testing of Flexors

1. Flexor carpi radialis—The flexor carpi radialis is tested by having the patient flex the wrist; it can be palpated on the radial aspect of the wrist. The flexor carpi ulnaris is also palpable when flexed. The palmaris longus is palpated by partially flexing the palm and touching the thumb and fifth digit to one another.

2. Superficialis flexors—The superficialis flexors are tested by holding three digits not being tested in full extension and directing the patient to flex the fourth one. PIP flexion indicates an intact superficialis to that finger.

3. Profundus flexors—The profundus flexors are tested by asking the patient flex the distal tip of the examined digit while immobilizing the rest of the digit at the PIP joint.

4. Flexor pollicis longus—The flexor pollicis longus is tested by having the patient actively flex the terminal phalanx of the thumb.

The flexors should be tested actively and with opposition. A partial flexor tendon laceration is best identified through opposition testing.

▶ Twelve Extrinsic Extensors

(See Figures 29–6.) All extensors are innervated by the radial nerve.

A. Anatomy

1. Central wrist extensors—The extensor carpi radialis longus and extensor carpi radialis brevis insert into the bases of the second and third metacarpals, respectively.

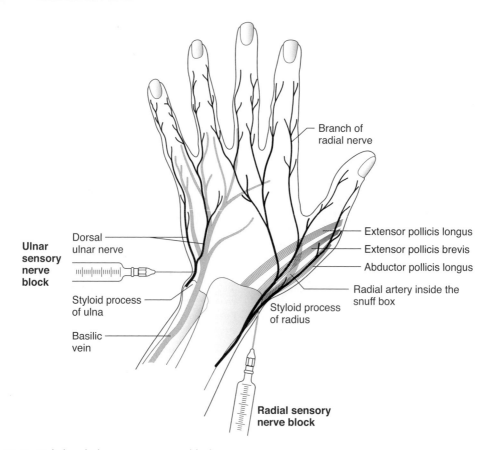

▲ **Figure 29–3.** Radial and ulnar sensory nerve block.

2. Extensor and ulnar deviator—The extensor carpi ulnaris inserts into the base of the fifth metacarpal.

3. Abductor pollicis longus—The abductor pollicis longus deviates the wrist radially and stabilizes the base of the thumb (first metacarpal). It is tested by abducting the thumb radially.

4. Two thumb extensors—The extensor pollicis brevis acts mainly at the MP joint; the extensor pollicis longus acts at the IP joint in concert with the intrinsics but, unlike the intrinsics, can extend the joint with much force and can even hyperextend it.

5. Four finger extensors—An extensor digitorum communis to each finger forms the central slip (MET) of the extensor hood.

6. Index and small fingers—The index and small fingers have independent (proprius) extensor tendons as well. These extend these fingers when the long and ring fingers are flexed.

B. Testing of Extensors

Test the extensors by asking the patient to extend the fingers at the MP joint and to extend the IP joints. The latter is achieved by action of the extensor in conjunction with the intrinsic tendons in the extensor hood. The proprius tendons of the index and small fingers always lie ulnar to the extensor digitorum communis of each.

▶ Twenty Intrinsic Muscles

A. Anatomy

Of 20 intrinsics, 15 are innervated by the ulnar nerve and five by the median nerve. In conjunction with the extensor tendon, they form the extensor hood mechanism, which is a proximally based triangular sheet of three interconnected tendons. The lateral margins ("lateral bands") are the small LETs from the intrinsic muscles. The central large tendon ("central slip") from the extrinsic extensors is called the MET, which inserts on the middle phalanx of each finger. The TET is made up of a coalescence of METs and LETs into a very thin tendon that inserts on the distal phalanx.

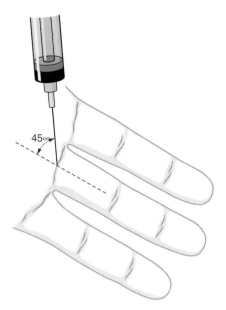

▲ **Figure 29–4.** Transthecal digital nerve block. After inserting the needle at the proximal digital crease at a 90° angle to the level of the bone, the needle is withdrawn 2–3 mm and angled 45° to the long axis of the digit as shown and the injection of anesthetic along the flexor tendon sheath is performed slowly.

In the case of the thumb, which has only two phalanges, the equivalent of the MET is the extensor pollicis brevis; the equivalent of the TET is the extensor pollicis longus. The intrinsics flex the MP and extend the IP joints and abduct and adduct the digits. Working all together, they cup the palm.

B. Testing of Intrinsics

1. Thenar and hypothenar intrinsics—The thenar and hypothenar intrinsics act to pronate the thumb and little finger and thereby cup the palm. Have the patient make the distal fat pads of the thumb and small finger meet.

2. Other intrinsics—Have the patient abduct the extended second through fifth digits; then flex these digits at the MP joints while extending the PIP and DIP joints.

▶ Examination of Nerve Injuries

The three major nerves to the hand are the radial, median, and ulnar nerves.

A. Radial Nerve

The radial nerve innervates all extensors.

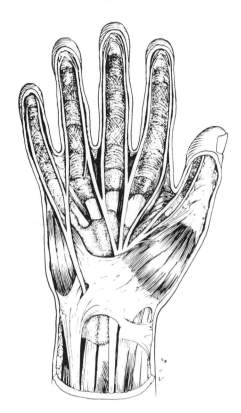

▲ **Figure 29–5.** Palmar hand with skin removed reveals flexor tendons with their sheaths and the median and ulnar nerves with their terminal sensory branches. (Modified and reproduced, with permission, from Way LW (editor): *Current Surgical Diagnosis & Treatment*, 9th ed. Appleton & Lange, 1991.)

1. Motor testing—Muscle testing is done by having the patient extend the wrist and digits (Figures 29–8C). This is best performed against opposition.

2. Sensory examination—The radial nerve gives off a sensory branch that provides sensibility for the dorsal–radial aspect of the hand (Figures 29–8A and B).

B. Median Nerve

The median nerve innervates 9 of 12 extrinsic flexors, the lumbricals to the index and long fingers, and the three muscles of the thenar eminence, which are mainly concerned with opposition.

1. Motor testing—

A. HIGH MEDIAN NERVE—Testing for high median nerve injuries is done by flexing the DIP joint of the index finger and the IP joint of the thumb (Figures 29–9).

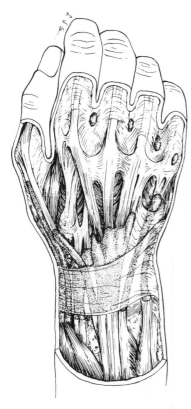

▲ **Figure 29–6.** Cutaway view of the dorsal hand demonstrates that the extensor tendons are ensheathed only at wrist level. (Modified and reproduced, with permission, from Way LW (editor): *Current Surgical Diagnosis & Treatment*, 9th ed. Appleton & Lange, 1991.)

Have the patient passively hold the fourth and fifth fingers fully flexed into the palm and follow this by full active flexion of the second and third fingers (Figures 29–9C).

Have the patient flex the thumb to touch the distal palm at the base of the fifth finger (Figures 29–9D).

B. Low median nerve—To test for low median nerve loss (eg, at the wrist), have the patient pronate the thumb, pressing the distal fat pad of the thumb against that of the ring finger. Then feel for a firm, contracted adductor pollicis brevis alongside the thumb meta-carpal.

2. Sensory examination—The median nerve provides sensibility to the radial two-thirds of the palm and the palmar surfaces of the thumb, the index, and long fingers, the radial side of the ring finger, and the dorsal surface of the middle and distal phalanges of these fingers (Figures 29–9A and B). Because of the importance of this zone of sensibility, the median nerve is called the "eye of the hand."

C. Ulnar Nerve

The ulnar nerve innervates 15 of the 20 intrinsic muscles and only three extrinsic muscles.

1. Motor testing—The intrinsics are tested by any of the following maneuvers: With the palm flat on the table, have the patient abduct and adduct the fingers, cross the fingers, or forcefully move the pointed index finger in a radial direction.

The extrinsics are tested as follows: Forcefully flex the tips of the ring and small fingers to meet the distal palm to evaluate their profundi (Figures 29–10C); then forcefully spread the fingers apart and palpate for a tensed flexor carpi ulnaris tendon at the wrist.

2. Sensory examination—The ulnar nerve innervates the radial and ulnar halves of the pads of the small finger, the ulnar half of the pads of the ring finger, and the ulnar side of the hand (Figures 29–10A and B). The additional loss of sensibility on the dorsoulnar aspect of the body of the hand signifies a high lesion well proximal to the wrist.

▶ Radiographic Examination

Severe injuries to the hand require imaging to detect fractures, dislocation, and opaque foreign material or gas. X-ray is the standard imaging modality for the majority of hand injuries; CT or MRI should be utilized in consultation with the hand/orthopedic surgeon. Special radiographs should be requested, depending on the site and direction of trauma. For example, scaphoid bone or digit-specific films should be requested as clinically indicated to improve evaluation of isolated injuries. If there is any doubt about the normalcy of the skeleton, comparable views of the opposite side should be taken for comparison. Recent literature has also demonstrated the utility of high-resolution ultrasound (HRUS) in the evaluation of common soft-tissue diseases of the hand/wrist (eg, synovitis, tendon injury) as well as detection of foreign bodies in the tissue. There is insufficient evidence for HRUS in diagnosis of fractures. This modality may be limited by the availability of an experienced upper extremity sonographer.

Allen G M et al: High-resolution ultrasound in the diagnosis of upper limb disorders: a tertiary referral centre experience. Ann Plast Surg 2008;61(3):259–264 [PMID: 18724124]

▼ EQUIPMENT AND MATERIALS FOR TREATMENT

▶ Instruments, Antiseptic solutions, and Sutures

A. Needles

Suturing should be carefully done with fine-pointed and very sharp cutting needles (eg, Ethicon P-1, P-3).

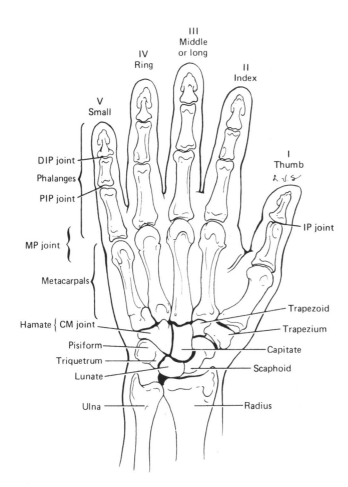

▲ **Figure 29–7.** Terminology of bones and joints of the hand.

B. Suturing Material

Fine (5-0 or 6-0) monofilament polypropylene suture material is preferred for skin closure. Only in infants and children should an absorbable suture such as 5-0 or 6-0 chromic or plain catgut be used.

C. Instruments

Fine plastic surgery forceps, retractors, clamps, and needle holders are required.

D. Skin and Wound Preparation

The skin around the wound may be sterilized as described in Chapter 30. The hand and wound may be irrigated with normal saline. Avoid prolonged soaking.

▶ Dressings, Splints, and Antibiotics

A. Inner Dressings

Petrolatum-impregnated gauze followed by a surgical gauze sponge saturated with water (tap water or sterile saline solution) is applied over the wound as the "core" dressing. The wetness draws blood from the wound and prevents dead space. None of this goes circumferentially around the digit, hand, or forearm.

A foam pad such as a Reston pad with an adherent surface on one side (or comparable substitute) is then applied over the core dressing. Soft elastic gauze (Kerlix, Kling) or cast padding to form a soft, well-padded dressing is applied over the foam pad and may go circumferentially around the part.

B. Splint

The wrist is the most important joint to splint for all major hand injuries, even if only one digit is injured. Well-padded plaster as a splint protects the hand.

For isolated pain-free dorsal injuries at the DIP or PIP joint, a tongue blade cut to the length of two phalanges and padded with gauze or foam rubber makes an excellent splint. There are ready-made aluminum splints with soft padding or other surface that are most effective. If there is a wound over the joint, such a splint should be placed on the palmar

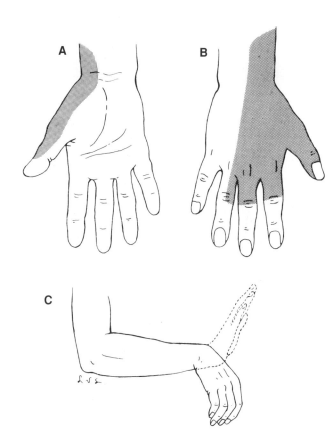

▲ **Figure 29–8. A:** Palmar and **B:** dorsal areas of autogenous radial nerve sensibility. **C:** A simple test for main trunk radial paresis.

side; if not, it is placed on the dorsum. After cutting the splint be certain that sharp edges are smoothed and padded and the patient is protected.

The most useful palmar splint consists of 10–12 layers of plaster cut to fit the involved digit or digits and extending halfway up the volar surface of the forearm. It is padded with a thin foam pad (eg, Reston) and held in place with a loosely wrapped roll of plaster of paris, bias-cut stockinet, or elastic bandage. The hand generally should be in the "position of function," that is, slight wrist extension and MP flexion, with the PIP and DIP joints in partial extension and the thumb web open (Figures 29–11). Modification must be applied to take tension off a specific wound.

C. Sling

No patient should leave the emergency department without a sling to hold the hand at the level of the heart or higher to promote venous and lymphatic drainage. Slings that hold the hand lower than the heart encourage the development of tissue edema. To avoid a tourniquet effect, the extremity should usually be outside of a sleeve.

▼ MANAGEMENT OF SPECIFIC TYPES OF HAND INJURIES

LACERATIONS

▶ Small Lacerations

Simple lacerations (superficial lacerations not extending into subcutaneous fat and not perpendicular to skin tension lines) can be closed by sterile surgical tapes (ie, Steri-Strips) or tissue adhesives. The hand and digits are so active that it is usually advisable to use suture material. Wounds that require sutures (lacerations that are parallel to skin tension lines or into subcutaneous fat) should be evaluated in a sterile, bloodless field. Splinting and elevation of the limb can help healing and reduce pain. Splinting is also important for wounds that cross joints to prevent joint stiffness or contracture from wound scarring. Follow-up with a primary care physician in 7–10 days for suture removal is appropriate. There are liquid adhesives that are effective for clean, straight laceration. Given the diminutive size of many hand/wrist lacerations encountered in the emergency

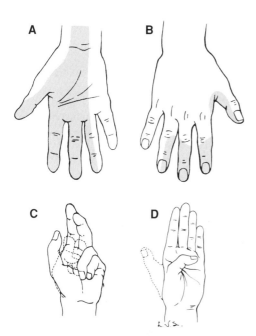

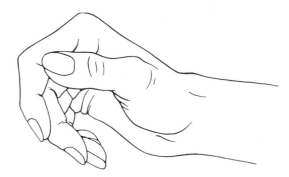

▲ **Figure 29–11.** Position of function of the hand. Note graded flexion of fingers and slight dorsiflexion of wrist.

▲ **Figure 29–9.** A and B: Autogenous median nerve sensibility is indicated by the shaded areas. The profundi of the index and long fingers (**C**) are innervated by the median nerve, as is the flexor pollicis longus (**D**).

department, it is vital to fully evaluate neurologic, tendon, and vascular functions distal to the wound. Literature suggests that significant deep structure injuries may be missed in the routine evaluation of minor hand wounds. Tendons are the most common deep structure injured in lacerations less than 3 cm, though nerve and arterial injuries are also observed.

Tuncali D et al: The rate of upper extremity deep structure injuries through small penetrating lacerations. Ann Plast Surg 2005;55(2):146–148 [PMID: 16034243].

Extensive Lacerations

Wounds should be carefully evaluated in a sterile, bloodless field. Irrigation and cleaning with tap water or sterile saline is the next step. Careful handling of tissues is essential. Approximate the wound margins with sutures. A wound should not be closed under tension. If the edges cannot be easily approximated, the wound may be left open and the patient referred to a hand surgeon for primary or delayed split-thickness grafting.

Antibiotic Therapy

Infected and grossly contaminated deep-tissue wounds (including open fractures) require extensive irrigation and may need debridement in the ER. Extensive disease should be admitted to an inpatient setting. Prompt antibiotic treatment in the ED is mandatory for infectious emergencies, along with a therapeutic course of oral antimicrobials for patients appropriate to discharge. A prophylactic course may be appropriate for less severe injuries. Although a full discussion of antibiotics for dermal lacerations is beyond the scope of this chapter, the physician should consider a

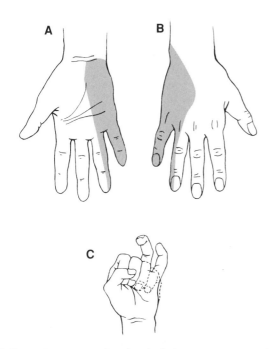

▲ **Figure 29–10.** A and B: The shaded area is innervated by the ulnar nerve. **C:** Terminal phalangeal flexion of ring and small fingers is by profundi innervated by the ulnar nerve.

short course (3–5 days) of antimicrobial coverage for typical skin pathogens. Further discussion of antibiotic therapy is included in the next sections. All penetrating injuries deserve consideration of tetanus prophylaxis.

FINGERTIP INJURIES

1. Fingertip Amputations

▶ Clinical Findings

Fingertip amputations are the most common type of amputation of the upper extremity. The location and size of the defect have to be considered. Depending on the location of the amputation, fingertip injuries can be classified into four zones. The zones have been designed to define the type of pulp damage and the existence of associated lesions of the nail bed and bone. The zone 1 lesion is a distal amputation located far from the distal phalanx tubercle. Usually the lesion is less than 1 cm in area and does not affect the nail bed or bone. Zone 2 lesions involve the nail bed and usually partial phalangeal bone disruption and exposure. In zone 3 injuries, the nail matrix is involved so that the nail growth will be followed by curved deformation. Zone 4 defines an amputation at the level of the distal phalanx, near the DIP joint. Despite the intact distal attachment of the extensor and flexor tendons at the distal phalanx, the active motion of the distal remnant is limited.

Important information to be obtained from the patient includes age, the digit injured, mechanism and time of injury, occupation, location of the wound, and hand dominance. The digit injured influences management. Most hand surgeons want to maintain the length of the thumb. The index finger is considered the next priority before other fingers. An intact pulp-to-pulp pinch mechanism is the goal.

▶ Treatment and Disposition

For zone 1 injuries with pad loss of less than 1 cm, healing by secondary intention is the simplest and often best approach. It is the treatment of choice for pediatric fingertip amputations, especially when there is no bone exposure. Initial treatment includes wound cleansing, a nonadherent sterile dressing, appropriate tetanus prophylaxis, splinting, and a bulky dressing to protect the tip. Amputations that expose the distal phalanx are usually treated as contaminated open fractures with an initial intravenous dose of a cephalosporin followed by an oral course. Patients should have appropriate follow-up care in 1–3 days for wound care check.

Fingertip amputations that have significant pad loss or bone loss (zones 2–4) usually require the expertise of a hand surgeon. Surgical options include primary closure, full- or partial-thickness skin grafts, composite grafts, flaps, and replantation. If the amputated fingertip pad has been retained, is clean, and is in good condition, it may be reattached as a full-thickness skin graft.

2. Subungual Hematoma

▶ Clinical Findings

Hematoma from blunt trauma (ie, a hammer blow) or crush injury that ruptures subungual blood vessels causes pain and dark red to black discoloration of the nail bed. An X-ray is needed to rule out a fractured phalanx.

▶ Treatment

Large subungual hematomas cause significant pain and should be evacuated via nail trephination (making a hole in the nail) with a high-temperature microcautery device or an 18-gauge needle or via complete removal of the nail. Use of heated paper clips may introduce carbon particles known as "lampblack" into the nail bed and is discouraged. Anesthesia is not usually required for trephination, and pain relief is immediate following decompression. Large subungual hematomas are often associated with significant nail bed lacerations. Many surgeons recommend removal of the nail and repair of nail bed lacerations for large subungual hematomas to promote optimal healing and normal nail growth. When the nail is removed, it should be cleaned and placed back into position, secured with sutures to function as a splint for the nail bed and to keep the proximal nail fold open.

A fracture of the distal phalanx on radiographs may technically be called an open fracture, although these injuries usually heal without complication. Osteomyelitis is not often associated with ungual tuft fractures. The risk of infection with an open fracture of the phalanx proper should be considered, and a broad-spectrum antibiotic and close follow-up are recommended.

▶ Disposition

Patients with a subungual hematoma may be discharged from the emergency department after treatment (trephination, nail removal with or without nail bed repair). All patients with subungual hematoma should be informed about the possibility of nail loss or deformity. Antibiotics are recommended for hematomas associated with tuft fractures.

3. Avulsion of Nail

▶ Clinical Findings

Avulsion of the nail results from a force elevating the tip of the nail and ripping it off its bed or from a downward crushing force sufficient to tear the base of the nail out of the eponychial sulcus, ripping open the nail bed, and carrying the nail plate on a palmar-based pedicle flap.

Treatment

Nails avulsed at the base may need to be completely removed. If such a nail is left in place, a badly lacerated nail bed that requires repair may inadvertently be overlooked. The nail also creates a dead space that promotes scarring and infection.

A. Removal of Nail

Anesthetize by digital block. Remove the avulsed nail by inserting a clamp under the distal attached portion of the nail and advancing it proximally, removing the nail by spreading the clamp. The exposed nail bed should be covered with either the original nail (as described above) or with sterile petrolatum gauze and a portion of the gauze tucked into the nail sulcus. A lacerated nail bed should be meticulously closed with 5-0 or 6-0 absorbable suture.

B. Reattachment of Distal Torn Finger Flap

If the distal portion of the finger has been torn off with the nail and has been left attached to the finger by a volar pedicle, the flap should be anatomically reduced and sutured back in position with 6-0 absorbable suture. Antibiotics should be administered.

C. Management of Fractures

Open fractures of the distal phalanx are reduced and held by soft tissue suturing. If the fracture is displaced, internal fixation with a Kirschner wire may be necessary.

Disposition

The patient should follow-up in 2–3 days for wound check and dressing change. Complicated problems should be referred to a hand surgeon and an immediate appointment made.

DISTAL EXTENSOR TENDON INJURIES[2]

1. Laceration of Extensor Tendons

Clinical Findings

Dorsal finger and hand wounds frequently result in a partially or completely lacerated extensor tendon or extensor tendon hood mechanism. The extent of injury can be determined only by adequate exposure and direct examination. Accurate assessment of a tendon can be difficult because a 90%-lacerated tendon can still retain function. A partial tendon laceration can often be discovered by testing the tendon against resistance. Strength against resistance is diminished if a partial tendon laceration exists. In addition, the patient will usually note pain with resistance. Description using the

eight zones of extensor tendon injuries will help assess and guide treatment (Figures 29–12).

Treatment

Treatment of a partial tendon laceration that is less than 50% may require no repair and be effectively treated with a protective splint. Minor extensor tendon repairs can be performed in the emergency department after careful irrigation, inspection, and debridement or later by the consultant.

If the tendon ends can be retrieved easily with minimal extension of the wound or by slight stretching of the skin, the tendon should be repaired by a simple figure of-eight suture or a crisscross suture technique with 4-0 or 5-0 suture (in infants, 6-0 nylon). This repair should ideally be performed by the hand surgeon (Figures 29–13). A padded plaster forearm splint is then applied with the digit and hand positioned so that the repair is relaxed as much as possible. No individual joint should be hyperextended, nor should all joints be simultaneously extended. The MP joint should not be immobilized in full extension, because contraction of collateral ligaments may result in fixation of the joint in extension. One or more neighboring fingers should always be immobilized with the injured digit.

Disposition

If the tendon ends are not easily retrieved, a hand surgeon should be consulted for follow-up and the patient should be seen in the next 1–2 days. In the interim, administer antibiotics for 2–3 days (see discussion of cellulitis, below).

2. Mallet Finger

ESSENTIALS OF DIAGNOSIS

- ► Suspect if bruising is present at DIP joint
- ► X-ray may be normal or show an avulsed chip at DIP joint
- ► Carefully test extension of DIP joint
- ► If left untreated, swan neck deformity may occur

Clinical Findings

Mallet finger is caused by laceration or avulsion of the extensor tendon at its insertion at the dorsum of the distal phalanx. A mallet finger commonly occurs after the distal finger is forcibly flexed, such as from a sudden blow to the tip of the extended finger. Clinically, there may be ecchymosis at the DIP joint, but tenderness and swelling may be less than anticipated. An X-ray may be normal or

[2]Flexor and proximal extensor tendon injuries are discussed with flexor tendon injuries later in this chapter.

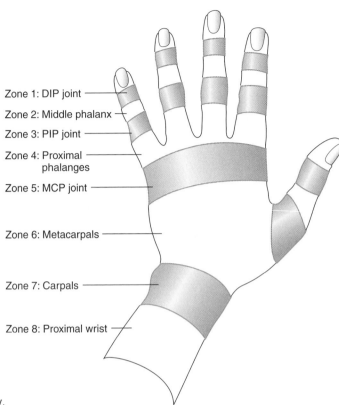

▲ **Figure 29–12.** Zones of extensor tendon injury.

demonstrate an avulsed chip fragment at the dorsum of the DIP joint. If the articular fracture involves more than 40% of the joint surface, referral to a hand specialist for open reduction is required. The extensor lag may not be present on the initial emergency department evaluation. Careful testing of extension at the DIP is important in identifying this problem. In many cases the patient is too uncomfortable to perform a good examination. If left untreated, a flexion deformity at the DIP joint will develop followed by hyperextension at the PIP joint (swan neck deformity) (Figures 29–14).

▶ Treatment

A. Open Mallet Injuries

Open injures are treated by tenorrhaphy and intramedullary fixation of the DIP joint by a hand surgeon. Give prophylactic antibiotics (see discussion of cellulitis, below).

B. Closed Mallet Injuries

Closed injuries may be treated by continuous dorsal external padded splint fixation of the DIP joint in full extension for 6–8 weeks. During splint changes, the joint should be held up in extension. Notify patients that any flexion at the DIP joint during the healing period will negate the healing that has already occurred and require another 6–8 weeks of treatment. The digit should be kept dry to prevent maceration of the skin.

▶ Disposition

These cases can have a poor outcome in the best of hands; therefore, have the patient follow-up with a hand surgeon.

3. Boutonniere Deformity

 ESSENTIALS OF DIAGNOSIS

▶ Suspect when trauma causes a painful, swollen PIP joint

▶ X-rays are usually normal

▶ Deformity is rarely clinically identifiable immediately after the event

Proximal

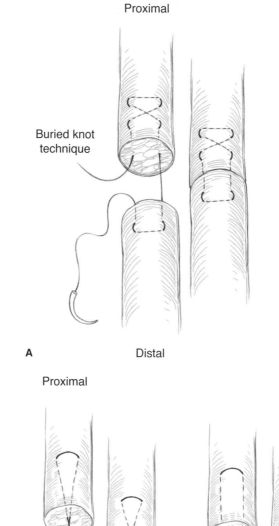

Buried knot
technique

A   Distal

Proximal

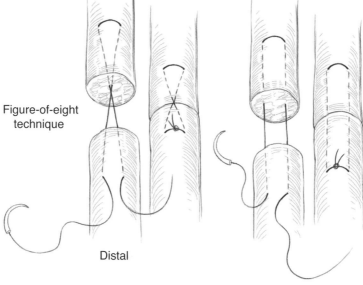

Figure-of-eight
technique

Distal

Horizontal mattress
technique

B

▲ **Figure 29–13.** Methods of tenorrhaphy. **A:** For large-caliber tendons. **B:** These suture techniques are best for thin tendons with limited separation of stumps (eg, digital extensors).

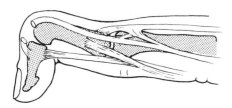

▲ **Figure 29–14.** Mallet finger with swan-neck deformity. Rupture, laceration, or avulsion of the insertion of the extensor mechanism results in mallet finger. (Modified and reproduced, with permission, from Way LW (editor): *Current Surgical Diagnosis & Treatment*, 9th ed. Appleton & Lange, 1991.)

▶ Clinical Findings

Early diagnosis of a closed MET (middle phalanx extensor tendon) rupture or avulsion is difficult before the boutonniere (buttonhole) deformity has occurred. High suspicion is needed when the patient presents with trauma and a painful, swollen PIP joint. Although uncommon, volar dislocations of the PIP joint can cause MET rupture. Unless a dislocation is present, radiographs are usually normal.

In boutonniere deformity, the distal joint is hyperextended and the PIP joint of the finger (the MP joint of the thumb) is flexed (Figures 29–15). Extensor hood integrity is lost at the apex of the PIP joint of the finger (MP joint of the thumb) as a result of laceration or blunt trauma to the dorsum of the joint. The deformity rarely manifests immediately after trauma and comes on insidiously as a result of gradual stretching of the injured hood. The underlying head of the bone protrudes through the hood, pushing aside the MET (extensor pollicis brevis of the thumb), which recedes, and the LETs (lateral extensor tendons) slip volarly to become flexors of the joint and hyperextensors of the distal joint.

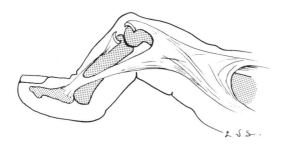

▲ **Figure 29–15.** Boutonniere deformity. Avulsion or laceration of the central extensor mechanism results in a flexion deformity at the PIP joint and hyperextension of the DIP joint—the boutonniere, or buttonhole, deformity. (Modified and reproduced, with permission, from Way LW (editor): *Current Surgical Diagnosis & Treatment*, 9th ed. Appleton & Lange, 1991.)

▶ Treatment

A. Open Injuries

Open injuries should be repaired (by a hand surgeon) as soon as possible with figure-of-eight nylon sutures and the joint splinted in full extension for 4 weeks with a palmar digital splint.

B. Closed Injuries

Closed injuries must be suspected if there is a history of a direct blow to the dorsum of the joint followed by swelling. Treatment consists of 4 weeks of PIP (thumb MP) splinting in extension to avoid boutonniere deformity, which rarely occurs if prompt treatment is provided.

Secondary reconstruction of this deformity is very difficult and may never restore full motion of the IP joints.

▶ Disposition

Open injuries should be irrigated and covered and the patient evaluated by a hand surgeon at once emergently. Patients with suspected closed MET injuries should get early referral to a hand surgeon. The hand should be splinted with the PIP joint in extension, leaving the MP and DIP joints mobile.

BONE AND JOINT INJURIES

Bone and joint injuries are discussed in more detail in Chapter 28, but a few general principles are emphasized here.

▶ Clinical Findings

If there is any question of bone or joint injury on X-ray, obtaining added views in other planes and identical views of the opposite extremity or a follow-up view in 7–10 days may resolve the issue.

▶ Treatment

A. Splinting

The wrist joint is the principal joint governing movement and comfort of an immobilized fracture. Therefore, it should be splinted initially. In addition, to splint one finger well, an adjacent finger should be splinted with it. The thumb may be immobilized alone. The preferred position should be that of wrist extension, functional finger flexion, and opposition of the thumb. The splint should be functional but applied in such a way that it can be loosened or removed if swelling or pain occurs. In addition, the splint should allow good visibility of the effected digit.

B. Stable Injuries

Stable dislocations or fractures can usually be treated in the emergency department by reduction and splinting, with appropriate anesthesia. Force should never be used. In lieu of force, open reduction is preferred.

C. Open or Unstable Injuries

Unstable closed injuries may include a dislocation that is not reducible by the EP, or one that spontaneously recurs after reduction. Open or unstable injuries require a specialist's skill. The patient should be given a temporary splint and dressing and referred to a hand surgeon for emergency follow-up care. Naturally, any structure with neurologic or vascular compromise requires prompt specialized intervention. Prophylactic antibiotics are indicated for open wounds.

▶ Disposition

Patients with closed, stable injuries should follow-up with an orthopedic surgeon or hand specialist in 2–3 days for assessment of comfort and integrity of the splint. Patients with open joint injuries, unstable injuries, or injuries that cannot be reduced easily must be referred early to a specialist experienced in hand surgery.

Hart RG, Fernandas FA, Kutz JE: Transthecal digital block: an underutilized technique in the ED. Am J Emerg Med 2005;23(3):340–342 [PMID: 15915410].

Perron AD et al: Orthopedic pitfalls in the emergency department: closed tendon injuries of the hand. Am J Emerg Med 2001;19:76 [PMID: 11146026].

INFECTIONS

Infections of the hand are frequently encountered in emergency departments. Nearly all infections result from neglect following trauma and are fostered by venous congestion and tissue edema.

Careful handling of tissue, elimination of dead space, immobilization and elevation of the arm immediately after injury, and avoidance of constriction by snug clothing or jewelry are far more important in preventing infection than any type of wound preparation or antibiotic prophylaxis. The objective of treatment of all infections is to reverse congestion and restore normal circulation. If there is a possibility of serious infection, immobilize the hand in a splint. Applying zinc oxide ointment next to the skin in the inner (core) dressing promotes drainage by preventing drying, caking, and sealing off of the wound.

All existing or potential infections should be monitored closely, for example, hourly or daily depending on the severity. Infections that may be treated in the emergency department include those of the nail folds, felons, simple abscesses, and cellulitis. Patients with other infections should be immediately referred.

1. Paronychia and Eponychia

ESSENTIALS OF DIAGNOSIS

▶ Swelling and collection of pus inside or around nail fold

▶ Consider X-ray to rule out foreign body or osteomyelitis

▶ Consider antibiotics if extensive cellulitis or lymphangitis is present

▶ Clinical Findings

Inflammation leading to a collection of pus inside the nail fold is seen after trauma (Figures 29–16A). If neglected, it may extend around the entire nail margin and cause a floating nail. The usual cause is *Staphylococcus aureus*. Cultures are rarely necessary. Chronic paronychia is found in patients with occupational exposure to moisture or cleaning solutions (ie, housekeepers or dishwashers) and is most often caused by *Candida albicans*.

An X-ray should be considered to rule out the presence of a foreign body or distal phalangeal osteomyelitis.

▶ Treatment

Treatment consists of simple incision, drainage, and elevation of the nail fold with a No. 11 scalpel at the site of maximum tenderness or pus (Figures 29–16B). Generally, there is no pain if an abscess is already pointing and no blood is drawn with the scalpel. If the scalpel causes any pain, administer a digital block anesthetic.

Antimicrobial agents are not indicated unless extensive cellulitis or lymphangitis is present. Chronic paronychia

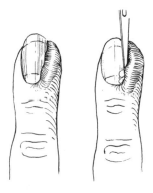

▲ **Figure 29–16.** Incision and drainage of paronychia. (Modified and reproduced, with permission, from Way LW (editor): *Current Surgical Diagnosis & Treatment*, 9th ed. Appleton & Lange, 1991.)

treatment may require nail removal, marsupialization of the eponychial fold, oral antibiotic, and topical antifungal ointment.

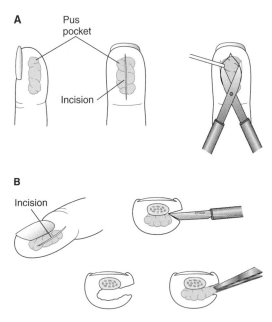

▶ **Disposition**

As with any hand infection, the patient should keep the hand elevated and follow up in 24–48 hours. A common complication is osteomyelitis of the distal phalanx. Chronic paronychia requires referral to a hand surgeon for possible marsupialization.

2. Herpetic Whitlow

ESSENTIALS OF DIAGNOSIS

▶ Collection of grouped vesicles with erythematous base on the fingertip

▶ Use of oral acyclovir in immunocompromised individuals

Herpetic whitlow is the most common viral infection of the hand, a self-limited herpes simplex viral infection of the distal finger. It classically presents as grouped vesicles with an erythematous base on the fingertip. Treatment is supportive; oral acyclovir is used in immunocompromised patients. These infections may be overlooked if not considered in the differential. Incision and drainage of herpetic bullae is contraindicated.

3. Felon

ESSENTIALS OF DIAGNOSIS

▶ Patient has a painful and swollen distal phalanx fat pad

▶ Staphylococcus aureus is the most common cause

▶ Most felons can be drained where the abscess points—usually mid pad—with a central longitudinal incision

▶ **Clinical Findings**

A felon is an abscess of the distal phalanx fat pad. *S. aureus* is the most common pathogen. The patient usually presents with a painful and swollen distal pulp space.

▶ **Treatment and Disposition**

Classic treatment of felons emphasized the need for early and complete incision through the septa via fishmouth

▲ **Figure 29–17.** Incision and drainage of felon. **A:** Central longitudinal incision—the recommended approach. **B:** Classic lateral or fishmouth incision, which has greater risk of complication.

incisions to provide adequate drainage and to relieve pressure (Figures 29–17). But complications include damage to nerves and blood vessels as well as unstable finger pads, and painful neuromas or anesthetic fingertips may result. Most felons can be drained where they point—usually in the mid pad—by a central longitudinal incision that does not cross the distal flexion crease. Felons can also be drained by a single lateral incision. The incision should be made along the ulnar aspect of digits II–IV and the radial aspects of digits I and V, avoiding pincher surfaces. The incision is started 0.5 cm distal to the DIP joint crease and dorsal to the neurovascular bundle of the fingertip. If the incision will be extensive, the digit must be anesthetized. These can be quite painful. Irrigate and loosely pack the wound, and then immobilize the finger. Treat empirically with antistaphylococcal oral antibiotics for 5 days and arrange follow-up in 1–3 days for wound care check.

4. Deep Fascial Space Infections

ESSENTIALS OF DIAGNOSIS

▶ All deep space abscesses require referral to a hand surgeon

▶ Antibiotics should be started in the emergency department

The four potential deep fascial space infections of the hand are the subfascial web space, the dorsal subaponeurotic space (collar button abscess), a midpalmar space abscess, and the thenar space. Deep space abscesses are frequently seeded with *S. aureus*, streptococci, and coliforms. All deep space infections require referral to a hand surgeon for operative exploration and drainage. Antibiotics should be initiated in the emergency department.

5. Cellulitis (Including Human and Animal Bites)

ESSENTIALS OF DIAGNOSIS

- ▶ A progressive cellulitis caused by Pasteurella multocida is easily seen in the first 24 hours
- ▶ Cellulitis due to other pathogens usually takes 2–3 days to become clinically evident
- ▶ Another pathogen, Capnocytophaga canimorsus, associated with animal bites, can cause overwhelming sepsis in immunocompromised individuals
- ▶ Have a high suspicion for closed-fist bite wound when caring for patient with open wound over the MP joint following an altercation. Patients with these seemingly small wounds often present later with significant infections.

▶ Treatment

A. Uncomplicated Cellulitis and Antibiotic Prophylaxis

Wounds with an increased risk of infection (ie, human or animal bites, crush wounds, or contaminated wounds) should have antibiotic coverage for *S. aureus* or *Streptococcus pyogenes*. Treatment recommendations include a first-generation cephalosporin such as cephalexin for oral use or cefazolin for intravenous use, or a penicillinase-resistant penicillin such as dicloxacillin for oral use or nafcillin or oxacillin for intravenous use. Trimethoprim–sulfamethoxazole (TMP–SMZ) or erythromycin may be effective in penicillin-allergic patients. Special consideration for polymicrobial coverage and possible admission are needed for diabetic patients and drug abusers.

B. Animal Bites

Infections caused by animal bites (ie, dog or cat) are often caused by *P. multocida*, which causes a rapidly progressive cellulitis, easily identifiable in 24 hours. Infections from other pathogens are not usually evident for 2–3 days. Another common pathogen, *C. canimorsus* (formerly known as DF-2), is a fastidious gram-negative rod that can cause overwhelming sepsis in immunocompromised individuals. Treatment for animal bites includes amoxicillin–clavulanate, clindamycin plus a fluoroquinolone in penicillin-allergic adults, or clindamycin plus TMP–SMZ in children. Do not close these wounds.

C. Human Bites

A wound over the MCP joint (especially of the dominant hand) is likely to represent a closed-fist bite wound sustained during an altercation. These wounds have a high likelihood for infection. Patients often present with infected "fight-bite" wounds several days after suffering a seemingly minor injury during a fight. Perform a thorough examination of these wounds, looking for injuries to the extensor tendon or joint capsule. Any violation of these structures mandates orthopedic consultation. Wounds that do not involve the joint capsule or the extensor tendon should be thoroughly irrigated and any devitalized tissue debrided.

The safest course of action is admission at the time of initial evaluation even without any signs of infection or tendon or joint involvement, though some support outpatient therapy with oral antibiotics and close follow-up. Infections from human bites may be those involving mixed anaerobes, streptococci, *S. aureus*, and *Eikenella corrodens* and should be treated in the hospital. Antibiotic treatment options include amoxicillin–sulbactam, cefoxitin, and ticarcillin–clavulanate. Penicillin-allergic patients may receive clindamycin plus TMP–SMZ or clindamycin plus fluoroquinolone. Prophylactic antibiotics for human bite wounds include amoxicillin–clavulanate or a second-generation cephalosporin. Given the propensity of these wounds to become infected, fight bites should never be sutured.

▶ Disposition

Hospitalization under the care of a hand specialist is required for severe cases (extensive cellulitis, involvement of tendons or joints, infections of the palmar space, systemic symptoms, or unusual pathogens) or if the patient is unreliable or unable to take oral antibiotics. Patients with cellulitis managed as outpatients should be seen every day and hospitalized if the process continues.

6. Suppurative Tenosynovitis

ESSENTIALS OF DIAGNOSIS

- ▶ Swelling, erythema, and tenderness along the tendon sheath
- ▶ Exquisite pain on passive movement of tendon
- ▶ Consider gonococcal infection in young adults without an open wound

▶ Clinical Findings

Suppurative tenosynovitis (nongonococcal) is characterized by swelling, erythema, and tenderness along the tendon sheath and, most important, exquisite pain on passive movement of the flexor tendon in the digit or the extensor tendon crossing the wrist. In flexor tenosynovitis, passive movement is achieved by holding the fingernail alone and prying it dorsally to extend the distal joint. The infection may have occurred because of an open wound contiguous to the involved tendon.

▶ Treatment and Disposition

Whenever there is inflammation with significant swelling, immediate hospitalization under the care of a hand specialist is required for open surgical drainage and parenteral antibiotic therapy. After obtaining appropriate specimens for culture, begin a cephalosporin (eg, cefazolin, 100 mg/kg/d in three divided doses) intravenously without waiting for the results of cultures. Immobilize the wrist and hand in a splint, and support the arm in a sling until operation can be performed.

7. Disseminated (Hematogenous) Gonococcal Infection

The diagnosis and treatment of gonococcal infection are discussed in Chapter 42. In young adults, tenosynovitis may be caused by gonococcal infection. The tenosynovitis is not associated with an open wound near the involved tendon sheath but is frequently associated with pustular skin lesions typical of gonococcal infection. Hospitalization for intravenous antibiotic therapy is usually indicated. In selected reliable patients whose diagnosis is confirmed, outpatient therapy with close follow-up may be possible. See Chapter 42 for recommended treatment.

Perron AD, Miller MD, Brady WJ: Orthopedic pitfalls in the ED: fight bite. Am J Emerg Med 2002;20(2):114 [PMID: 11880877].

MINOR CONSTRICTIVE PROBLEMS

▶ Clinical Findings

The three common constrictive problems described here are often seen in the emergency department.

A. Carpal Tunnel Syndrome (Compression of the Median Nerve)

Carpal tunnel syndrome is characterized by aching and numbness over the distribution of the median nerve (see Figures 29–9), with sparing of the small finger. These symptoms often awaken the patient from sleep and may be elicited by full flexion of the wrist for 30 seconds (Phalen maneuver).

Tapping over the median nerve at the wrist crease may feel like an electric shock (Tinel sign). Though unusual, patients with this nerve compression may present with rapid onset of acute edema and progressive loss of feeling after trauma, inflammation, or allergy, and it requires urgent consultation with a hand specialist.

B. Stenosing Flexor Tenosynovitis (Trigger Thumb or Trigger Finger)

Stenosing flexor tenosynovitis is characterized by local tenderness over the proximal tendon pulley at the MP joint, with pain referred to the PIP joint and a snapping when the finger or thumb goes through an active range of motion. Usually a history of repetitive strain is involved.

C. De Quervain's Tenosynovitis

De Quervain's tenosynovitis is characterized by pain and tenderness when tendons in the first dorsal compartment on the radial side of the wrist are actively or passively stretched; specifically, when the fist is clenched over the thumb while the wrist is put into marked ulnar deviation (Finkelstein's test).

▶ Treatment

A. Carpal Tunnel Syndrome

Initial treatment involves wrist splinting and the use of nonsteroidal anti-inflammatory drugs. Activity modification and therapeutic exercises may also improve symptoms. The next step in treatment is injection of the carpal canal using 1 mL of steroid and 2–3 mL of lidocaine. Oral steroids may also be of benefit; however, these treatments should not be offered in the ED setting. Patients with symptoms suggestive of Carpal Tunnel Syndrome require specialized follow-up, possible nerve conduction studies, and discussion of potential surgical options.

B. Flexor Tenosynovitis

Administration of nonsteroidal anti-inflammatory agents may be started in lieu of injection therapy. Steroids should not be injected if an infectious process is suspected. About 0.5 mL each of steroid and lidocaine should be injected into the synovial bursa through the tendon flexor pulley at the base of the digit. The finger should be splinted in extension.

C. De Quervain's Tenosynovitis

Nonsurgical treatment involves rest, splinting with a thumb spica splint, anti-inflammatory medications, stretching exercises, and corticosteroid injections. If injecting, use about 0.5 mL each of steroid and lidocaine at the radial styloid process but avoid the radial nerve. Steroid injections are not benign events and unless the EP is well trained and experienced, these procedures are best performed by a hand surgeon.

Disposition

Referral to a hand surgeon is advised because multiple injections or surgical release of the tight ligament or sheath may be required.

THERMAL INJURIES

See also Chapter 45.

1. First-Degree Burns

Clinical Findings and Treatment

Simple burns (redness without blistering) are treated with cold tap water rinse and analgesia. Comfort may be augmented by a soft nonirritating wrap to protect and immobilize the hand. Elevation and avoidance of constriction by snug garments are also advised.

Disposition

The patient should return or telephone for follow-up after 1–2 days.

2. Second-Degree Burns

Clinical Findings and Treatment

Blisters signify partial-thickness (second-degree) burns, which always retain cutaneous sensation even though they are variable in depth. Although this treatment is controversial, large blisters should be aspirated or un-roofed and debrided. Small blisters may be left intact. Silver sulfadiazine (Silvadene) cream may be applied topically. For sulfa-allergic patients, bacitracin or neomycin may be used instead. Second-degree burns may be dressed with a bulky dressing and the hand splinted in the position of function. Tetanus prophylaxis must be current (Chapter 30). In the case of burns caused by hot tar, the tar may be removed as described in Chapter 45.

Disposition

Patients with extensive burns or marked edema should be emergently referred to a hand specialist for evaluation and possible hospitalization. Patients with lesser involvement should be seen every 1–3 days for a dressing change, especially once blister debridement is started. Keep in mind that the thinner skin of a child's hand can more easily progress to second or third-degree injury, even in minor burns.

3. Third-Degree Burns

Clinical Findings and Treatment

Full-thickness (third-degree) burns require bulky, loose, sterile dressings with an anti-infective agent such as silver sulfadiazine. Appropriate elevation and splinting are also advised. Tetanus prophylaxis must be current (Chapter 30).

Disposition

If the burn is extensive (eg, >1–2 cm^2 [⅜–¾ in^2]) or is over the dorsum of a joint, refer the patient emergently to a hand specialist for decisions about the need for debridement and grafting.

4. Electrical Burns

(See also Chapter 46.) Burns from electricity are of two kinds: crossed circuit, producing arc heat; and conduction of high-voltage current within the tissues. Arc heat is often more frightening than extensively injurious to tissues. There is generally blackening of the skin owing to deposit of carbon. The burn may be anywhere from first-degree to third-degree in severity but is usually localized. The treatment of arc heat burns is the same as that of other thermal burns.

High-voltage conduction burns involve a point of entry and another point of exit. The deep tissues are often coagulated out of proportion to surface skin changes. Blood vessels and nerves are the pathways of conduction and therefore are most vulnerable. Immediate irreversible ischemia and paralysis are common. Such cases require hospitalization under the care of a hand specialist for urgent fasciotomy, where prophylactically indicated, and for observation for systemic effects of the electrical shock. Appropriate debridement (even amputation), grafting, and reconstruction will follow. Extremity destruction is sometimes overwhelming.

If the electrical conduction pathway within the body is not limited to the hand but also involves other areas, consideration should be given to possible myocardial injury. An electrocardiogram and cardiac isoenzymes (CK-MB and troponin) measurement should be obtained. Cardiac monitoring is necessary if myocardial injury is suspected.

5. Frostbite

(See also Chapter 46.) Exposure to cold may result in superficial or deep frostbite depending on the windchill factor and duration of exposure. Measures to prevent this vasoconstrictive disorder and the irreversible microvascular thrombotic events that lead to gangrene include the following: (1) avoiding exposure to wind, cold metal, snow, and ice by wearing protective gloves; (2) preserving the total body heat by wearing suitable clothing and head gear and avoiding sweat-producing physical effort or alcohol consumption; (3) ensuring adequate caloric intake, high in fat and carbohydrate; and (4) refraining from smoking.

Superficial frostbite is limited to the skin. It exists when the discomfort of fingers exposed to cold is replaced by numbness. Reversal by warming is urgently required and is usually heralded by a warm tingling sensation. Deep frostbite is signaled by pain and swelling of the entire hand, followed by extensive blister formation and dysesthesia. Deep frostbite requires hospitalization under the care of a hand specialist. Cryofibrinogenemia aggravates the problem and is worsened by the use of heparin, which facilitates precipitation of cryofibrinogen. Treatment consists of rest and warming the patient and the hands. Immersion in water at 37–40°C (98.6–104°F) for a short time (eg, 20 minutes) may be beneficial. Blisters must be debrided and dressed with sterile dressings. Sympathetic blockade should be considered.

Luce E: The acute and subacute management of the burned hand. Clin Plast Surg 2000;27(1):49 [PMID: 10665355].

Smith MA, Munster AM, Spence RJ: Burns of the hand and upper limb—a review. Burns 1998;24(6):493 [PMID: 9776087].

Mark Choi, BS et al: Pediatric hand burns: thermal, electrical, chemical. J Craniofac Surg 2009;20(4):1045–1048 [PMID: 19634213].

FOREIGN BODIES

Fishhooks, splinters, and other objects may have barbs or barb-like projections that prevent withdrawal from the wound in the normal retrograde way. Removal is possible by pushing the foreign body along the direction of entry and removing it via a counterincision where it presents under the tented skin. Nerve block or other anesthesia and tourniquet ischemia are necessary before extraction is attempted. Prophylactic antibiotics and tetanus immunization are often necessary.

Foreign bodies embedded in the hand may be difficult to locate and remove. The diagnosis is based on the history and examination, and X-rays are almost always useful in the case of glass or metal. Modalities such as computed tomography, magnetic resonance imaging, and ultrasound can be helpful in finding nonradiopaque foreign bodies. If immediate accessibility and easy removal seem possible, an attempt can be made to remove the foreign body using regional anesthesia, a tourniquet, and sterile technique with loupe magnification. Typically, however, the discoloration of tissues by blood precludes the immediate search for a foreign body, which will be found much more easily after 3–4 weeks when phagocytosis has cleared the blood. Before starting the procedure, tell the patient that if search and removal prove at all difficult (eg, longer than 10–15 minutes), the procedure will be abandoned and referral made to a hand specialist.

Consider leaving an entry wound open by inserting a loose drain, applying an appropriate dressing, and elevating and immobilizing the part. Give prophylactic local or systemic antibiotics and tetanus prophylaxis (Chapter 30). The patient can usually be assured that retrieval of small deep foreign bodies is not urgent, because they do not travel in the body, and that it is often contraindicated by the difficulty and risk of removal.

Blankstein A et al: Localization, detection and guided removal of soft tissue foreign bodies in the hands using sonography. Arch Orthop Trauma Surg 2000;120(9):514 [PMID: 11011671].

COMPLEX HAND INJURIES

▶ Classification

Complex injuries include the following: amputations, serious tendon injuries, nerve injuries, high-pressure injection injuries, closed compartment syndromes, mangling injuries, and gunshot wounds.

▶ Evaluation and Initial Management

In complex injuries, emphasis should be placed on early, rapid diagnosis and institution of supportive therapy. Many complex injuries require referral to a hand specialist urgently. In all cases, use conservative measures as outlined below.

A. Avoid Manipulation

Once the decision has been made to transfer or hospitalize the patient, the extremity should not be handled, probed, manipulated, or otherwise disturbed unless absolutely necessary. Foreign material that can be easily lifted out should be removed. Protect with a sterile dressing and, if necessary, a loosely applied splint pending definitive management.

B. Prepare for Possible Urgent Surgery

If there is a reasonable likelihood of surgery within 8–10 hours, give nothing by mouth. An intravenous infusion should be started in the uninjured limb and laboratory work ordered.

C. Give Antibiotics

In the case of open or penetrating wounds, antibiotics should be given parenterally (preferably intravenously in the uninjured extremity) as soon as possible; the earlier they are started, the more effective they are. Give cefazolin, 1–2 g intramuscularly or intravenously every 6–8 hours (adult dose) or 25–100 mg/kg/d intramuscularly or intravenously, divided every 4–8 hours (for children aged >1 month).

1. Amputations

▶ Clinical Findings

Amputations account for about 1% of hand injuries. The diagnosis of amputation is obvious on inspection of the part. Amputations are generally classified as partial (incompletely severed part) or complete.

Generally, tidy amputations at the level of the middle phalanx or the wrist or distal forearm have the best chance of functionally successful replantation. In the case of single-digit amputation, surgeons are much more inclined to favor replantation of a thumb than of a single finger. Discussions with the patient or relatives regarding the feasibility of replantation should be left to the hand surgeon.

▶ Treatment and Disposition

A. Replantation Possible

Place the amputated member in gauze moistened with saline and then place it in a sealed plastic bag or container that is maintained at 4°C (39.2°F) (eg, on wet ice). *Do not freeze the amputated part,* because this destroys its viability.

After starting appropriate supportive measures, if the treating facility is not capable of providing the microsurgical specialized care required for replantation, arrange promptly for referral to a capable facility. The treating physician must contact a microsurgical specialist at the hospital to which he or she would like to refer the patient in order to obtain the specialist's permission for transfer. Failure to do so could be considered a violation of the law (COBRA-EMTLA; see Chapter 5) and might subject the referring physician and hospital to significant financial penalties.

B. Replantation Impossible

If the amputated member is either not recovered or is clearly not salvageable, appropriate in-house or emergency department surgery should be undertaken to close the stump. Except for the simple fingertip pad amputation (discussed above), these injuries should almost always be referred to a hand specialist.

2. Flexor and Proximal Extensor Tendon Injuries

ESSENTIALS OF DIAGNOSIS

▶ First suspect that tendon injury may exist; impairment may not become evident until hours, days, or weeks later

▶ Check strength of digit against resistance

▶ Direct visualization and examination of open wound in sterile, bloodless field is indicated

▶ General Considerations

Almost all flexor tendon injuries, and those extensor injuries in which the proximal tendon has retracted out of reach, are considered complex injuries. Management of easily accessible extensor tendon injuries is discussed earlier in this chapter.

▶ Clinical Findings

A crucial step in the emergency management of any flexor or proximal extensor tendon injury is to suspect that it may exist and make the proper diagnosis. Impairment of a partially divided tendon (sometimes subtotally or even totally divided) may be functionally masked at the outset, only to become evident hours, days, or weeks later.

In open injuries, tendon lacerations can often be diagnosed by the abnormal stance of the involved part of the hand and almost always by careful functional examination. If the diagnosis is not obvious, but the location of the wound raises the possibility of tendon injury, direct examination of the wound is indicated. Visualization of flexors can be difficult anywhere, whereas visualization of extensors is difficult mainly when they lie proximal to the metacarpal necks.

Occasionally the emergency physician will see a closed profundus tendon rupture. These injuries are often referred to as "jersey finger" because it often occurs when a tackler grasps another's jersey and the jersey is ripped from the tackler's hand. Such an injury almost always follows sudden violent stretch of the flexor, after which the patient is unable to flex the distal phalanx.

▶ Treatment

Obtain immediate consultation with a hand specialist. Dress the wound after irrigation, and splint the wrist and hand. Remove jewelry and snug garments, and elevate the extremity until definitive treatment can be given. Flexor tendon repair may be delayed as long as 10 days without compromising the eventual outcome. However, early evaluation by a hand surgeon is advisable. If tendon repair is to be delayed, the wound should be sutured and appropriate antibiotics administered (eg, cefazolin, 1–2 g intravenously, followed by cephalexin, 500 mg orally four times daily for 3–5 days).

▶ Disposition

Visualization of a lacerated tendon sheath is a reason for referral unless the entire course of the tendon gliding beneath the laceration is observed to be intact. If in doubt, refer immediately, because neglected partial tendon lacerations can go on to rupture.

3. Nerve Injuries
▶ Clinical Findings

Early diagnosis is crucial. The cause and nature of injury, the symptoms, or the location and depth of a laceration may suggest possible nerve injury. If careful motor and sensory examination is performed (Figures 29–18 and 29–19), few significant nerve injuries will be missed.

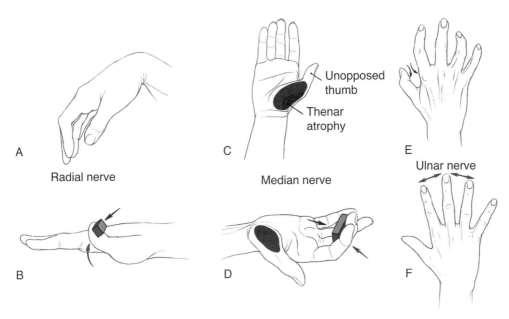

▲ **Figure 29–18.** Assessing nerve injury. **A:** Wrist drop in radial injury. **B:** Forceful extension of thumb tip is lost in radial nerve injury. **C:** "Ape hand" deformity in median nerve injury. **D:** Forceful flexion of tip of index finger is lost in high median nerve injury. **E** and **F:** Thumb web atrophy and clawing of ring and small fingers, and loss of abduction and adduction in ulnar nerve injury.

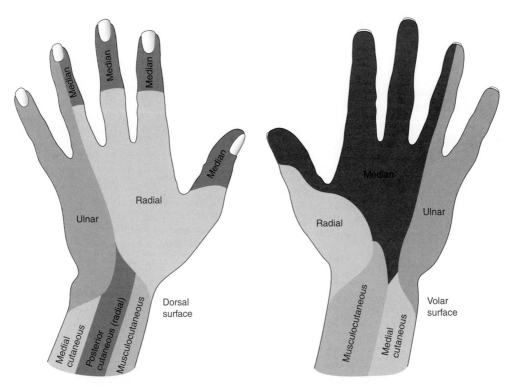

▲ **Figure 29–19.** Sensory distribution of the hand.

Treatment

Appropriate dressing and splinting should be applied when indicated and the patient warned about injury to anesthetized skin until definitive treatment can be given.

Disposition

Refer the patient to a hand surgeon, and determine when the patient is to be transferred for definitive care.

4. High-Pressure Injection Injuries

ESSENTIALS OF DIAGNOSIS

► Initial appearance of hand may show only pinpoint portal of entry and look deceptively normal
► Obtain an X-ray
► Ask about the type, amount, and velocity of the injected material

Clinical Findings

High-pressure jets of a variety of hot and cold fluids (eg, grease, water, plastics, organic solvents) and gases are widely used in industry. Accidental penetration of the skin through a pinpoint portal of entry may result in devastating damage, even though the initial (postinjection) appearance of the hand or other body part is usually deceptively normal. This is because the foreign material spreads instantly along tissue planes and is widely distributed in the hand or other part. Spread of material up a flexor tendon sheath after penetration of a digital pad is quite common. An X-ray should be obtained, because some injected materials are radiopaque (eg, lead-based paint). When a chemical, inflammatory, or thermal response becomes manifest 4–12 hours after injury, extensive ischemia and tissue necrosis may be seen. Important historical factors are the type, amount, and velocity of the injected material and the anatomic location. The type of material injected is the most important clue to the severity of the injury.

Treatment and Disposition

Give analgesics for pain if necessary, and splint the extremity in a sling for comfort. Digital blocks are contraindicated due to the possibility of increased tissue pressure and vascular compromise. Obtain X-rays.

Give nothing by mouth, and consult a hand surgeon immediately regarding referral. Prompt tetanus prophylaxis, systemic antibiotics, and decompressive surgery (eg, fasciotomy) must be arranged in most cases. Even so, the prognosis for maintaining circulation and salvaging function is often dismal.

5. Closed Compartment Syndromes

ESSENTIALS OF DIAGNOSIS

► History of progressive pain and rock-hard compartment
► Pain on passive movement
► Hypoesthesia or paralysis of the digits

General Considerations

A compartment syndrome (eg, congestion progressing to various degrees of ischemia) can occur in any space of the digit, hand, forearm, or arm. It may involve a single space (eg, extensor and flexor compartments of the forearm and intrinsic muscle compartments of the hand). Obstructed venous flow leads to microvascular stagnation and death of muscle, fat, and nerves. Compartment syndrome may result from external compression (eg, a tight cast, prolonged pressure against an extremity of a comatose patient) or from internal swelling (eg, from severe bleeding, crush injury, burn, fracture, allergy, or infectious inflammatory reaction). The fate of a neglected case in which surgical decompression has not been performed is late fibrosis and severe functional impairment.

Clinical Findings

The typical patient presents with a history of progressive severe pain (eg, throbbing) and a rock-hard compartment. When the whole forearm and hand are involved, there is hypoesthesia, reluctance or inability to move the digits, and pain on passive extension of flexed digits. Pain perception may be lost as pressure on the nerves destroys their conducting ability.

Treatment

Treatment is supportive until definitive surgical decompression can be performed. Support the limb in a sling, and give analgesics for pain. The affected hand should be reassessed frequently for signs of circulatory compromise. Pallor, reduced capillary refill, loss of doppler pulses and increasing pain should alert the physician to the need for fasciotomy. In the absence of prompt surgical care, bedside escharotomy along the dorsal interosseus muscle compartments of the hand may release significant subcutaneous pressure. The incision should reach down to the pliable or fatty tissues, and extend the length of the eschar. If the eschar involves the forearm, mid-lateral incisions may be performed. This procedure should only be performed in the ED if the wait for definitive decompression will lead to prolonged tissue ischemia.

▶ Disposition

Urgent hospitalization for surgical decompression under the care of a hand specialist is indicated.

6. Mangling Injuries

▶ Clinical Findings

Mangling injuries include gunshot and blast wounds, severe open crush wounds, severe bites by large animals, and a large variety of ripping or tearing injuries (ie, lawnmower- or snowblower-associated injuries). The common denominators are multitissue involvement, distortion, and significant wound contamination.

▶ Treatment

Rapid initiation of supportive measures; loose, bulky, sterile dressing and splinting; immediate administration of antibiotics (eg, cefazolin, 50–100 mg/kg/d intravenously or intramuscularly in 2–3 divided doses); and definitive surgical treatment are important to a successful outcome.

▶ Disposition

All such injuries require immediate hospitalization and referral to a hand specialist for operative debridement and repair.

Arellano A, Wegener E, Freeland A: Mutilating injuries to the hand: early amputation or repair and reconstruction. Orthopedics 1999;22(7):683 [PMID: 10418865].

Chin G et al: Snow blower injuries to the hand. Ann Plast Surg 1998;41(4):390 [PMID: 9788219].

Lewis HG et al: A 10-year review of high-pressure injection injuries to the hand. J Hand Surg [Br] 1998;23(4):479 [PMID: 9726548].

Martin C, Gonzalez del Pino J: Controversies in the treatment of fingertip amputations. Clin Orthop 1998;353:63 [PMID: 9728160].

Vasilevski D et al: High-pressure injection injuries to the hand. Am J Emerg Med 2000;18:820 [PMID: 11103737].

Feldmann, ME, et al: Early management of the burned pediatric hand. J Craniofac Surg 2008;19:4 [PMID: 19634213].

▼ SPECIAL EMERGENCY DEPARTMENT PROBLEMS

1. Removal of Rings

All rings, bracelets, wristwatches, and snug shirtsleeves and coat sleeves should be prophylactically removed whenever injury, surgery, infection, or other cause of acute swelling of any part of the hand exists. Failure to do so may lead to serious congestion and unnecessary complications.

A ring on a swollen finger can be removed in three ways:

1. Lubricate the skin with soap and carefully slip off the ring.

2. Wrap the digit snugly with a string from the distal tip to just below the ring, and in that way "milk" edema out of the digit so that the ring can be removed over the string.

3. Cut the ring with a commercial ring cutter, spread it with two pairs of pliers, and remove it. This is the preferred method when there is significant digital injury or swelling distal to the ring.

2. Snakebite

See Chapter 46 for treatment.

Wound Care

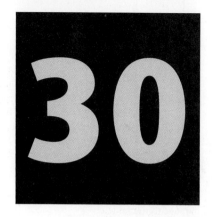

30

Thomas R. Jones, MD, MDiv, FAAEM[1]

EMERGENCY MANAGEMENT OF LIFE-THREATENING PROBLEMS

The "ABC's" of resuscitation must be addressed before wounds are evaluated. Open wounds are dramatic and often draw the attention of the emergency physician or resuscitation team away from more life-threatening injuries. It is rare that bleeding from even large tissue defects will immediately impact the patient's survival. Secure the airway, ensure adequate ventilation, and stabilize blood pressure prior to assessing wounds.

HEMOSTASIS

Direct Pressure

The simplest and most common method used to achieve hemostasis is direct pressure. A bulky dressing wrapped firmly with an elastic bandage will usually stop venous, capillary, and arteriolar hemorrhage. Most smaller arterial bleeding can be temporarily stopped with this method and larger bleeding vessels may be controlled with digital pressure. Large arteries may ultimately require vascular repair or suture ligation.

Suture Ligation

The decision to ligate an artery should be made cautiously; any uncertainty as to the impact on distal tissue perfusion should prompt consultation of the appropriate surgical specialist. Proximal extremity arterial injuries require emergency vascular surgery consultation.

Simple tying or suture ligation is indicated for most vessels more than 2 mm ($\frac{1}{16}$ in)in external diameter. To avoid excessive tissue trauma, one must precisely identify and clamp the vessel end prior to ligation. Severed arteries usually require only simple tying. Veins, however, do not hold ligatures well, and suture ligation is preferable. Suture ligation may be performed by passing the suture needle through a portion of the vessel wall and then circumferentially tying the vessel. This method prevents slippage of the ligature. *Caution:* Do not ligate arteries and veins en masse, because this may predispose to arteriovenous fistula formation. Absorbable sutures are preferred for tying and suture ligation in the acute wound. Synthetic absorbable sutures (polyglycolic acid [Dexon] and polyglactin

[1] This chapter is a revision of the revision by David A. Fritz, MD, FACEP, from the 6th edition.

[Vicryl]) are advantageous because of their low reactivity and high friction coefficients. Chromic catgut is also satisfactory.

▶ Tourniquets

Inflatable cuff tourniquets can be used for temporary hemostasis during wound exploration and repair but are not recommended for periods over 20–40 minutes. Inflate the pressure cuff on the extremity proximal to the wound until hemostasis is achieved. Take particular care to remove tourniquets after 15–20 minutes and before the procedure is completed to check for residual bleeding. A tourniquet inadvertently left in place may cause permanent ischemic damage to the limb.

▶ Epinephrine-containing Anesthetics

Epinephrine-containing local anesthetic agents such as lidocaine or bupivacaine are commonly used to control bleeding prior to wound repair. This can particularly be useful in highly vascular areas such as the scalp where bleeding can be difficult to control.

▶ Electrocautery

Surgical mono- and bipolar electrocautery units cause hemostasis through thermal coagulation of blood and tissue. The resulting tissue damage lessens the appeal of this technique. Disposable hand-operated electrocautery units are also available.

▶ Bleeding Scalp Wounds

Rarely, bleeding from a scalp wound cannot be stopped using direct pressure or by infiltration of epinephrine-containing anesthetic agents. This is particularly true when tissue maceration has occurred due to blunt trauma. In this instance, it may be necessary to place deeper 2-0 or 3-0 absorbable sutures after wound cleansing to close the tissue defect and place an external pressure dressing. If a significant hematoma forms, it may be necessary to reexplore the wound and place an external drain.

When time allows, a closure with a running, locking 2-0 or 3-0 nonabsorbable suture may provide the best hemostasis and wound closure simultaneously.

▶ Chemical Cautery

Silver nitrate and other caustics achieve hemostasis through tissue coagulation but are not recommended for wound hemostasis because of the amount of tissue necrosis they produce. American military forces are testing newer forms of powdered and gel adhesive procoagulants. Some of these generate high temperatures due to an exothermic chemical reaction, and reports of thermal tissue damage may limit utility in the civilian sector.

▼ WOUND ASSESSMENT

HISTORY

A detailed, thorough history is essential for assessing the extent of injury and for organizing appropriate wound management. Three basic questions are used to reconstruct the history of the injury.

A. When Did the Injury Occur?

The time of injury is important for determining the interval between injury and treatment. Most civilian injuries contain fewer than 10^5 bacteria per gram of tissue in the first 6 hours and are therefore relatively safe to close. Wound repair after 6 hours is dependent on many factors, including vascularity of the area, degree of contamination, and health status of the patient. The longer the wound has been present, the more likely an infection will occur after primary closure. As a rule, tissue resistance to infection is directly proportionate to blood supply. Facial lacerations may often be closed safely within 24 hours of injury, owing to the abundant blood supply in that area.

B. Where Did the Injury Occur?

What were the possible contaminants associated with the injury? Contact with feces, pus, saliva, or soil greatly increases the risk of infection and should be considered when deciding on timing of closure.

C. How Did the Injury Occur?

The potential damage to deeper structures can be estimated by review of the mechanism of injury. Any high-velocity-missile injury has the potential to damage deeper structures, and the wound tract should be assessed carefully. Blunt injuries may crush tissue and fracture underlying bone, leaving an open fracture, compartment syndrome, or arterial disruption.

TYPES OF INJURIES

A. Lacerations

Lacerations cause minimal tissue injury and are relatively resistant to infection.

B. Puncture Wounds

Puncture wounds may become infected, especially if they are contaminated or if a foreign body is present.

C. Stretch Injuries

Stretch injuries can produce damage to blood vessels, nerves, ligaments, or tendons, which is not visible superficially.

D. Compression or Crush Injuries

Compression or crush injuries result in the greatest amount of tissue necrosis. Hemorrhage into the soft tissues is common, resulting in ecchymosis and hematoma formation. The crushed tissue has a markedly impaired ability to heal and resist infection. Depending on location, these injuries are at high risk to develop compartment syndrome.

E. Bites

Bites are heavily contaminated and may require delayed closure.

EXAMINATION

Complications arising from wound care are a common basis for malpractice claims against emergency physicians. Inspection should be conducted in an emergency care or surgical facility where adequate lighting and equipment are available. Wound hemostasis must be achieved for proper evaluation of involved structures and to rule out foreign bodies. The extra time spent in preparing the proper environment for wound examination often decreases total procedure time by facilitating the repair. Sterile technique and gentle handling of tissues are mandatory to avoid additional tissue injury or contamination.

If deep injuries cannot be assessed adequately through the existing surface defect, consider extending the laceration by undermining the skin beyond the wound edges with a scalpel. Obtaining sufficient exposure of the wound may reveal tendon injuries, joint capsule penetration, or foreign bodies.

▶ Assess Type and Extent of Injury

In assessing the type and extent of injury, consider the following questions:

- Is there loss of function in the injured part?
- Are important underlying structures involved such as nerves, major blood vessels, ducts, ligaments, bones, or joints?
- What is the level of contamination in the wound?
- Are any foreign bodies present?
- What is the viability of the injured parts? Are any parts missing?

▶ Tissue Avulsion

The viability of an avulsion flap depends not only on the vascularity of the flap but also on the length versus base ratio, maceration of the tissue involved, and vascularity of the surrounding tissue. A long flap of badly macerated tissue with a narrow base will probably not survive and should be excised while a clean, short flap on the face will almost certainly heal uneventfully.

▶ Consider Location of Wound

A. Scalp

The blood supply to the scalp is excellent and wound infections rarely occur. The physician should examine scalp wounds carefully to ensure that the galea is not involved. Galeal lacerations should be cleaned and sutured with absorbable suture to prevent subgaleal hematoma formation and subsequent infection.

B. Face

Facial wounds can have dramatic effects on a patient's appearance; every effort should be made to minimize scarring and to prevent tissue loss. Debridement of facial tissue is rarely necessary and may cause distortion of features as the scar matures. Take special care with ear, eyelid, and nasal lacerations. Experienced emergency physicians maintain a low threshold for consulting their plastic surgery colleagues on complicated facial wounds.

C. Neck

Deep injuries to the neck frequently involve important underlying structures (Chapter 23). These complex anatomic areas cannot be extensively debrided without major functional or cosmetic loss. Wound evaluation and repair are often best done in the operating room by a maxillofacial, otolaryngology, or general surgeon.

D. Chest and Abdomen

Wounds of the chest and abdomen must be evaluated for possible communication with a body cavity as well as internal organ injury (Chapters 24 and 25).

E. Extremities

Hand injuries represent a significant proportion of emergency department patients and require special attention. Loss of function of even one digit can permanently impair a patient's ability to perform their vocation or avocation. Apparently minor puncture wounds may injure nerves, tendons, or arteries and cause significant impairment if not diagnosed during the initial presentation. Perform a complete neurovascular examination of every significant hand injury including function of the median, ulnar, and radial nerves (motor, light touch, and two-point discrimination); intrinsic hand muscles; extensor and both deep and superficial flexor tendons; radial and ulnar artery pulses; capillary refill; and wrist flexors and extensors.

Wounds on the plantar surface of the foot are particularly prone to infection. After thorough wound cleaning many emergency physicians will allow these wounds to heal without primary repair.

Table 30–1. Drugs Used for Local Anesthesia.[a]

	Cocaine	Procaine (Novocain)	Tetracaine[b] (Pontocaine)	Lidocaine (Xylocaine, Many Others)	Bupivacaine[b] (Marcaine, Sensorcaine)	Mepivacaine (Carbocaine)
Potency (compared to procaine)	3	1	10	2–3	9–12	1.5–2
Toxicity (compared to procaine)	4	1	10	1–1.5	4–6	1–1.5
Stability at sterilizing temperature	Unstable	Stable	Stable	Stable	Stable	Stable
Total maximum adult dose	100–200 mg	500 mg	50–100 mg	300 mg	175 mg	400 mg
Total maximum pediatric dose	—	—	—	4 mg/kg	—	5 mg/kg
Infiltration Concentration[c] Onset of action Duration	— — —	0.25–1% 5–15 min 45–60 min	0.05–0.1% 10–20 min 1.5–3 h	0.5–1% 3–5 min 30–60 min	0.25% 5–10 min 1.5–2 h	0.5% 5–10 min 1.25–2.5 h
Nerve block Concentration[c] Onset of action Duration	— — —	1–2% 5–15 min 45–60 min	0.1–0.2% 10–20 min 1.5–3 h	1–2% 5–10 min 1–1.5 h	0.25–0.5% 7–21 min 2–6 h	1–2% 5–10 min 1.25–2.5 h

[a]Addition of vasopressor prolongs duration by 25–50%; exercise care when used topically, to avoid excessive systemic absorption.
[b]Not recommended for children.
[c]0.5% solution = 5 mg/mL; 1% solution = 10 mg/mL; 2% solution = 20 mg/mL.

Prepare for Definitive Care

After initial assessment, cover the wound with a sterile dressing until definitive management, or further evaluation can be performed. Obtain any necessary X-rays only after the wound has been protected from the possibility of additional contamination. If considerable delay in definitive evaluation and management is anticipated, the wound should be cleaned, conservatively debrided, and temporarily closed or covered. Extensive wounds—or minor ones involving major structures—are best evaluated and managed in the operating room.

ANESTHESIA

Preliminary Examination

Perform a careful sensory and motor neurologic examination before administering anesthetic.

Choice of Agent

Local anesthetics have varying attributes with regard to safety, potency, duration of action, and effects on the local wound milieu (Table 30–1). Lidocaine is perhaps the safest local anesthetic, because allergic reactions are rare. The major problem with all local anesthetics is systemic absorption resulting in cardiovascular and central nervous system toxicity. For an adult, the maximum safe dose of 1% lidocaine without epinephrine is 5 mg/kg (do not exceed 300 mg) and for 1% lidocaine with epinephrine, 7 mg/kg (do not exceed 500 mg). For children, the safety and efficacy of lidocaine and mepivacaine are known; child safety and efficacy of the other drugs in Table 30–1 are not known.

Topical Anesthesia

Topical anesthesia is especially useful in the management of small wounds in children who do not tolerate local infiltration. A commonly used combination solution is LET (lidocaine, epinephrine, and tetracaine). TAC (tetracaine, adrenaline, and cocaine) has been largely abandoned due to risks of systemic toxicity and potential abuse. To apply the solution, soak a gauze pad in it and place the pad directly over the wound for 20 minutes. Do not use over mucous membranes or areas with end-arterial circulation (fingers, toes, nose, and penis). Anesthesia can often be judged by the appearance of blanching at the wound site. Use the minimal amount of anesthetic necessary.

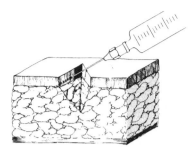

▲ **Figure 30–1.** Injection of local anesthetic for wound closure. (Reproduced, with permission, from Dunphy JE, Way LE (editors): *Current Surgical Diagnosis & Treatment.* 5th edn. Lange, Los Altos, CA, 1981.)

▶ Inhalation Anesthesia

Inhalation anesthesia with nitrous oxide administered by experienced personnel can be a useful adjunct, especially for children.

▶ Local Infiltration

Infiltration of a local anesthetic agent is performed gently near the edge of the wound or directly into the wound with a small (No. 25–30) needle (Figure 30–1). Pain associated with local infiltration is partly due to the stretching of sensitive nerve endings in the dermis and may also be due in part to the difference in acidity of some anesthetics (the pH of commercial preparations of lidocaine is 5–7). Associated pain can be reduced by using smaller amounts of more concentrated anesthetic solutions and slower infiltration rates or, in the case of lidocaine, by preparing it as a buffered solution (9 mL of 1% lidocaine, to which 1 mL of sodium bicarbonate solution, 44 mEq/50 mL, is added). Restrict the dose of anesthetic to the least amount that will provide adequate anesthesia. This is particularly true for facial lacerations, where infiltration distorts important landmarks and makes precise matching of wound edges difficult. Infiltration of anesthetic directly into the wound is less painful but may spread infection in heavily contaminated wounds.

Injecting a small skin wheal and then advancing slowly, pausing to let each increment of tissue become anesthetized, is a more time-consuming method but less painful to the patient.

▶ Regional Anesthesia

Regional anesthesia (sensory nerve blockage at a site proximal to the wound) is more technically challenging than local anesthesia, but it provides a larger anesthetic area and allows more extensive exploration and manipulation of the tissues. Because local wound anatomy is not distorted by regional block, more precise alignment of wound edges

is possible. Onset of anesthesia is a function of the type of agent used and how close to the nerves the agent is injected. The duration of anesthesia can be prolonged with epinephrine; however, epinephrine should not be used for digital nerve blocks. Regional anesthesia is particularly suitable for extremity injuries complicated by heavy contamination or in extensive injury requiring long operating times for repair. It is also used in patients who are not good candidates for general anesthesia.

A. Pitfalls of Regional Anesthesia

Pitfalls of regional anesthesia include difficulty in placing the anesthetic close to the supplying sensory nerve; loss of valuable time in waiting for it to take effect; and risk of permanent injury to the nerve from direct infiltration of anesthetic into the nerve.

▶ Common Regional Blocks for Hand Surgery

Several techniques for regional blocks in hand surgery are described below. Whatever the method used, a thorough understanding of anatomy is crucial. Avoid probing injections because of the risk of paresthesias. Attempt to infiltrate the anesthetic without penetrating the nerve sheath, because this may injure the nerve.

Use a 25- or 27-gauge needle; larger needles may cause significant nerve injury. Wait about 10 minutes for the full anesthetic effect in digital blocks and 20 minutes for wrist blocks.

A. Digital Block

The technique requires two separate needle sticks with four injections of 1 mL of 1% lidocaine next to the nerve bundle of all four digital nerves. The needle is first inserted dorsally to block the dorsal digital nerve and is then redirected without removal toward the volar nerve and the anesthetic is injected. The procedure is repeated on the opposite side of the digit.

B. Radial Nerve Block

The radial sensory nerve emerges beneath the brachioradialis tendon (Figure 30–2) about 6 cm (2 ⅜ in) above the Lister tubercle. Inject about 4 mL of lidocaine in a 2-cm (¾ in) wide band 4 cm (1 in) above the Lister tubercle.

C. Median Nerve Block

The median nerve at the wrist lies just radial and deep to the palmaris longus tendon and the transverse carpal ligament (Figure 30–3). The palmaris longus, when present, is easily identified by having the patient make a fist and flex the wrist. Insert the needle dorsally and distally between the palmaris longus and flexor carpi radialis, and inject 4 mL. The

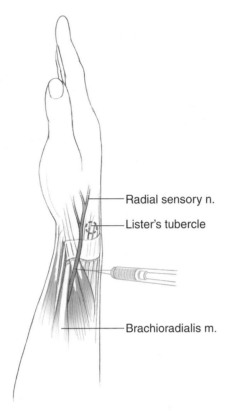

▲ **Figure 30–2.** Radial nerve block, in which anesthetic is injected in a 2-cm (¾ in) wide band 4 cm (1 ⁹⁄₁₆ in) proximal to the Lister tubercle on the radial aspect of the forearm.

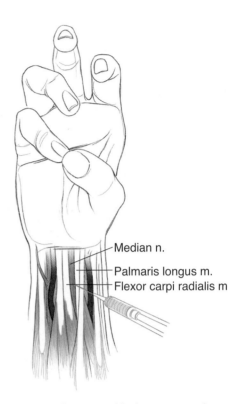

▲ **Figure 30–3.** Median nerve block. Inject anesthetic around the median nerve just proximal to the wrist. The nerve is located between the tendons and the palmaris longus and flexor carpi radialis.

lidocaine can be milked into the carpal tunnel to achieve the maximum blocking effect.

D. Ulnar Nerve Block

The ulnar nerve and artery course just dorsal to the flexor carpi ulnaris at the wrist (Figure 30–4). Avoid inadvertent injection of anesthetic into the artery by aspirating as the needle is advanced. Inject 2 mL on the ulnar side of the flexor carpi ulnaris. An additional 2 mL should be injected on the radial side to achieve a total block.

▶ Common Regional Blocks for Facial Surgery

A. Infraorbital Nerve Block

The infraorbital foramen can be easily palpated along the anterior maxilla and lies along a line drawn between the pupil and the maxillary canine. Inject about 1–2 mL as the needle is advanced from a lateral to a medial direction (Figure 30–5). Avoid penetrating the nerve by being careful not to enter the foramen. An intraoral approach may also

be used. Wait for symptoms of numbness of the upper lip. Infraorbital nerve block provides anesthesia of the cheek, upper lip, and parts of the nose.

B. Supraorbital Nerve Block

The exit of the supraorbital nerve from the orbit is readily identified by palpating the supraorbital notch. Inject a total of 1–2 mL of anesthetic about 0.5 cm (3/16 in) above the orbital rim (Figure 30–6). Advance the needle from a lateral to a medial direction, and avoid penetrating the nerve. If both supraorbital and infratrochlear blocks are needed, the wheal should be extended medially toward the midline. Supraorbital block is useful in anesthetizing the forehead.

CLEANING AND DEBRIDEMENT

▶ Hair Removal

Wounds in hairy areas are difficult to debride and suture, and hair in a wound acts as a foreign body, delaying healing,

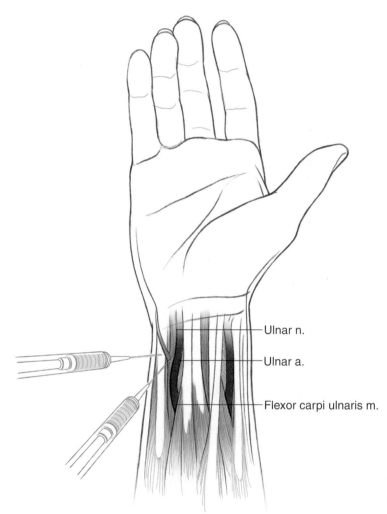

▲ **Figure 30–4.** Ulnar nerve block. Inject anesthetic around the ulnar nerve just proximal to the wrist on either side of the flexor carpi ulnaris.

Ulnar n.

Ulnar a.

Flexor carpi ulnaris m.

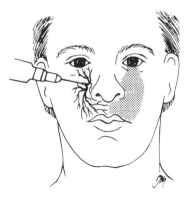

▲ **Figure 30–5.** Infraorbital nerve block. Intraoral or percutaneous injection around the palpable infraorbital foramina will result in anesthesia within the stippled area.

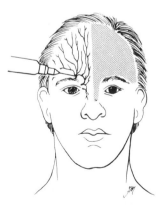

▲ **Figure 30–6.** Supraorbital nerve block. Inject anesthetic slightly superior to the orbital ridge at the supraorbital notch. Stippling shows area of anesthesia from ipsi-lateral injection.

and promoting infection. Shaving hair around wound edges facilitates management but invites wound infection if the infundibulum of the hair follicle is injured. Contamination can be minimized by clipping the hair 1–2 mm ($\frac{1}{16}$ in) above the level of the skin. Depilatory agents and special razors equipped with recessed blades also allow safe removal of hair without infundibular injury.

A method of scalp laceration repair using the native hair to tie wound edges together has been described and seems to have no increased risk of infection when compared to standard suture repair. Reports of the hair spontaneously untying have led some physicians to place a drop of skin adhesive to the hair after tying.

Caution: Eyebrow and eyelash hair should never be removed, since removal destroys critical landmarks and makes accurate alignment of wound edges difficult. Misalignments may cause notch or step-off deformities in the brow line. Eyebrow hair also regrows slowly, creating a cosmetic problem.

▶ Mechanical Cleansing

As an adjunct to surgical debridement, mechanical cleansing of the wound by irrigation or scrubbing is quite effective. Soaps and detergents should not be used in the open wound in conjunction with mechanical cleaning.

A. Irrigation

The most reliable and well-tested method of emergency wound cleaning is high-pressure irrigation with normal saline. Pressures of 7–11 lb/in^2 must be achieved to mechanically remove bacteria and particulate debris.

Numerous commercial devices are available for high-pressure irrigation, but the simplest and least expensive is syringe irrigation. A 35- or 50-mL syringe and a 19-gauge or blunt needle connected to a reservoir of irrigating fluid by a three-way stopcock are suitable. Commercial splash guards are also available, which attach to a syringe and allow for the requiredpressure while providing protection from bodily fluids.

Bulb syringe irrigation has been shown to be no more effective in preventing wound infection than no irrigation at all. Soaking wounds in saline does not remove bacteria and may allow for further contamination of the wound. The commonly used method of puncturing holes in the cap of a plastic liter bottle of saline and squeezing the contents into the wound does not achieve the necessary pressure to remove significant amounts of bacteria and should no longer be used.

Normal saline (or similar balanced crystalloid solution) is forcefully injected close to the wound surface and perpendicular to the surface of the skin. The amount of irrigant used depends on the size of the wound and the suspected extent of contamination.

Since large volume irrigation is preferred, when the wound can be placed under a faucet supplied by chlorinated city water, the wound may be irrigated in this fashion since studies have not shown an increased risk of infection as compared with sterile saline.

B. Mechanical Scrubbing

1. Sponge—Mechanical scrubbing of the wound surface is usually best performed with a highly porous sponge. Sponges routinely used for hand washing work well. Brushes and low-porosity sponges decrease the wound's resistance to infection.

2. Brush—"Abrasion tattooing," in which debris is embedded in the skin, requires vigorous scrubbing or dermabrasion to remove embedded debris. Soaps and detergents should not be used.

▶ Skin and Wound Cleansers

Cleanse the wound and surrounding skin to remove transient microflora, gross debris, coagulated blood, and the like.

A. Normal Saline

In most instances, simply washing the open wound with saline under pressure (see above) removes most of the surface bacteria.

B. Nonionic Surfactant

The nonionic surfactant Pluronic polyol F-68 has been shown to be effective as a wound cleansing agent without demonstrably impairing resistance to infection or wound healing.

C. Hydrogen Peroxide

The foaming action of hydrogen peroxide is frequently used to remove particulate debris and recently clotted blood from wounds. A dilute solution of hydrogen peroxide is very useful for removing dried blood and debris from around wound edges. Undiluted hydrogen peroxide should *not* be used directly in a wound due to risk of cytotoxicity.

D. Ionic Soaps and Detergents

Ionic soaps and detergents (eg, pHisoHex) should *not* be used for wound cleansing, because they are extremely irritating to tissues and increase the potential for infection if used directly on the wound. They may be used for cleansing of intact skin surrounding the wound, although they have not been shown to be superior to ordinary soap or other agents for this purpose. After application, they should be removed by thorough rinsing with water.

E. Skin Disinfectants and Antimicrobials

The use of 1% povidone-iodine to irrigate wounds is widely debated. It is effective as a skin disinfectant prior to surgery, but concentrated iodine is cytotoxic. There is probably no significant advantage or disadvantage to dilute povidone-iodine solution compared to normal saline. Irrigation of wounds with antibiotic solutions has been associated with a slightly decreased rate of wound infection but at a much greater cost.

▶ Debridement

Remove retained debris and devitalized tissue by surgical excision and mechanical cleansing. Surgical debridement consists of excising devitalized or severely contaminated tissues and irregular areas that interfere with wound closure. Use a stainless steel scalpel blade for debridement. Facial tissue should only be debrided by the appropriate surgical specialist.

A. Total Excision of the Wound

The simplest method of debridement is total excision of the wound, creating a surgically clean area. *Caution:* Total excision is appropriate only for wounds that do not involve specialized structures (eg, injuries of the abdominal wall and thighs). More selective debridement is indicated for wounds on the hand or face.

B. Selective Debridement

In most situations, it is best to mechanically cleanse the wound and then perform selective debridement of all grossly nonviable tissue. Signs of tissue necrosis include gray or black color and lack of bleeding when the tissue is incised. Remove all nonviable portions. Mangled, irregular wound edges imply severe local tissue injury and should be sharply debrided. If it appears that adequate debridement would prevent tension-free simple closure, consult an experienced surgeon for wound management.

Excision procedures on the face, particularly those on specialized structures, such as the ear or nose, require a conservative approach. The facial area has an abundant blood supply that enables tissues to survive on surprisingly small pedicles. In these cases, observation and expectant treatment are warranted. Obtain surgical consultation before performing any debridement of a specialized part.

WOUND CLOSURE

After the wound has been examined, anesthetized, cleaned and debrided, and reexamined, the physician must decide whether to close it. Primary wound closure is preferable because of faster healing, less scarring, improved hemostasis, and better aesthetic and functional results. All foreign bodies must be removed to minimize the chance of infection.

▶ Contraindications to Wound Closure

Several factors affect the risk of infection with wound closure and determine whether closure is justified.

A. Heavy Bacterial Colonization

A prolonged interval (more than 6 hours) between injury and attempted closure may be a contraindication to wound closure. In a generously vascularized area such as the face, wound closure may be attempted up to 24 hours after injury. Heavily contaminated wounds (eg, bites) should be left open. Active wound infection at the time of the emergency department visit contraindicates closure of the wound.

B. Major Tissue Defects

Closure is contraindicated if the wound cannot be closed without excessive tension.

C. Other Factors

Closure is contraindicated if there are retained foreign bodies, devitalized tissue, or tissue with borderline per-fusion.

▶ Primary Closure

The objectives of primary wound closure are (1) precise alignment of injured parts to facilitate rapid healing, return of function, and a good cosmetic result and (2) avoidance of tissue injury (eg, excessive electrocautery, strangulating sutures), hematoma formation, and wound tension.

A. Delayed Primary Closure

Contaminated wounds, if properly debrided, will gain resistance to infection if left open. After 48–96 hours, these wounds can then be closed with essentially no loss in wound healing time. Consider delayed primary closure in the case of wounds contaminated by feces, pus, foreign body, or saliva in the case of bite wounds. Crush and blast injuries and avulsion injuries are markedly susceptible to infection and necrosis and should also be considered for delayed closure.

After initial debridement, gently pack the wound with saline moistened fine-mesh gauze. This should be changed 1–3 times a day until closure of the wound. This method requires a dependable patient, and interim wound checks may be indicated. The wound should be examined for signs of infection at follow-up. If no infection is suspected, the wound can be closed in the same manner as in primary closure.

1. Suture Selection

All sutures represent foreign bodies in the wound. For this reason, use the smallest size and the least amount of suture that will achieve adequate tissue apposition.

The size and location of the wound and the desired precision of closure generally dictate the choice of needle and suture size. Generally, fine sutures are used in wounds (or their parts) requiring precise alignment; 5-0 and 6-0 sutures are preferred for closure of facial lacerations. Layered closure (fascia, dermis) of any wound allows placement of fine epidermal sutures anywhere on the body. The epidermis itself has little tensile strength, and sutures are placed in this layer only to achieve accurate alignment of wound edges.

Percutaneous closure of the epidermis and dermis in regions other than the face is best managed by the use of 3-0 or 4-0 suture material. Suture marks are the result of tension in the tied suture and the length of time the suture is left in place.

▶ Absorbable Sutures

Absorbable sutures are biodegraded and lose their tensile strength in 2–6 weeks.

A. Gut Sutures

Sutures derived from sheep submucosa or beef serosa are digested by proteolytic enzymes in the wound. They are more rapidly degraded in the presence of infection. The knot-holding ability of plain gut is rather inconsistent; chromic gut seems to be better in this regard.

1. Plain gut—Plain gut incites an intense inflammatory reaction in the wound and loses its tensile strength within 2 weeks.

2. Chromic gut—Treatment of gut with chromium salts decreases its tissue reactivity and prolongs its survival to about double that of plain gut. In some studies, however, it has been shown to potentiate infection more than the plain gut.

B. Synthetic Sutures

Polyglycolic acid (Dexon), polyglactin (Vicryl), and polydioxanone (PDS) produce minimal tissue reaction in the wound and are most commonly used for dermal and subcutaneous closures and vascular ligation.

1. Degradation—Polyglycolic acid and polyglactin are degraded by hydrolysis and lose 50% of their tensile strength in 14–20 days and about 90% by the fourth week (comparable to chromic catgut). Polydioxanone, a third-generation synthetic absorbable suture, loses 50% of its tensile strength in 5 weeks and 90% at 2 months.

2. Tying qualities—Although similar to silk in their handling characteristics, polyglycolic acid and polyglactin sutures do not hold knots quite as well. Polydioxanone looks, feels, and handles like monofilament nylon or polypropylene.

3. Use in acute wounds—Absorbable synthetic sutures are probably superior to gut sutures in acute wounds because of their low tissue reactivity and resistance to degradation in the presence of infection. The monofilament characteristics

of polydioxanone make it almost the ideal synthetic absorbable suture.

▶ Nonabsorbable Sutures

Nonabsorbable sutures are degraded very slowly or not at all in the tissues.

A. Silk

Silk sutures represent the most common type of natural fiber suture. Silk gradually loses its tensile strength and is classified as a slowly absorbable suture material. The tissue reactivity of silk is the greatest of all nonabsorbable sutures, and its use in acute wounds has generally been abandoned.

B. Synthetic Sutures

1. Dacron—Dacron is a polyester that elicits less tissue reaction than silk. Because of its high friction coefficient, it is as difficult to handle as a suture. The friction injury imposed on the tissues by Dacron can be overcome by coating it with Teflon.

2. Nylon—Nylon causes less tissue reactivity than Dacron, and its use in contaminated wounds results in lower wound infection rates. Monofilament nylon sutures lose approximately 20% of their tensile strength within a year after placement in a wound. The monofilament form of nylon is quite stiff and does not hold knots well. Multifilament nylon sutures completely lose their tensile strength in the wound after 6 months, but they are easier to tie than monofilament sutures.

3. Polypropylene and polyester—Polypropylene and polyester materials cause the least reactivity of all suture materials. They maintain their tensile strength indefinitely and are the suture material of choice for closure of contaminated wounds. These materials are used most commonly for fascia and skin closure. They are also advantageous in the repair of vascular, nerve, and tendon injuries. Because of their softer consistency, these materials generally hold knots better than does nylon.

2. Wound Tapes

Sutureless closure of the acute wound provides maximum resistance to infection. Various tape materials have been used and have resulted in significantly diminished wound infection rates compared to those in suture closure. Tape closure is most advantageous in the contaminated wound but is also useful in superficial clean and tidy wounds, wounds in children, and wounds in obese patients.

Tape closure is inferior to suture closure in maintaining precise wound edge alignment and eversion, requisites for cosmetically acceptable closure. However, tape closure is often used after early removal of sutures in order to minimize suture marks and to provide additional splinting of the wound until tensile strength is sufficient to resist local forces tending to pull the edges of the wound apart.

▶ Attributes of Wound Tapes

To be effective, skin tapes must be strong enough to support the wound edges in close apposition until sufficient healing has occurred. The tapes must have excellent skin adherence and should not macerate the underlying skin surface. Removing all moisture and using a defatting agent (eg, acetone) enhances adhesiveness to the skin, and tapes so applied will adhere for up to 2 weeks. Although tincture of benzoin is occasionally used to increase adhesiveness and may initially enhance tape adhesion, it is solubilized by skin oils and rapidly loses its effectiveness.

▶ Wound Tapes Over Deep Sutures

Suture closure in irregular lacerations and crush injuries allows for better approximation of skin edges than does tape closure. Moreover, tape only approximates the superficial portion of the wound, leaving the deeper wound layers more vulnerable to local biomechanical stresses and resulting in a weak, unsightly scar. In clean wounds, it is sometimes preferable to close the deeper layers with sutures and then approximate the superficial layers with tape.

3. Metallic Staples

Many types of disposable skin staple devices are available. The staple configurations vary but are primarily designed to approximate wound edges with minimal tissue trauma. Some staples project above the skin surface to avoid staple marks. As with wound tapes, precise epidermal alignment is difficult to achieve with a skin staple, and these devices should not be used for cosmetic skin closures. Because a stapled wound usually does not contain dermal sutures, its tensile strength depends on the presence of the staple, and this must be kept in mind when considering staple closure of wounds subjected to increased tension (eg, joint surfaces, mobile parts). If early removal of the staple is contemplated, the wound should be supported by skin tapes until the wound gains sufficient tensile strength to withstand local biomechanical forces. The time required varies from 1 to 2 weeks depending on the wound's location.

4. Tissue Adhesives

Cyanoacrylate tissue adhesives (Dermabond) are widely available. These adhesives polymerize rapidly when applied to tissues and form an adhesive layer on top of intact epithelium to hold the wound edges together. These adhesives cause an intense inflammatory reaction and should be used only on minor superficial lacerations. They should not be used near the eye, on mucous membranes or mucosal surfaces, on moist areas, or on areas with dense hair. Tissue adhesives should not be used for infected wounds.

Tissue adhesives are useful for minor wounds, those less than 5 cm in length and with separated wound edges less than 0.5 cm; they are most beneficial for wounds that would close spontaneously. Wounds greater than 5 cm in length and 0.5 cm in separation have increased tensile forces that may lead to poor wound edge approximation and a poor cosmetic outcome. Subcutaneous sutures may be useful in decreasing wound edge tension and may lead to a far better cosmetic result.

Preparation of wounds for closure with tissue adhesives is the same as that for sutures. Thoroughly cleanse the wound and control bleeding before applying tissue adhesive. Hold the wound edges together and slightly everted with tissue forceps. Apply the adhesive by lightly wiping the applicator tip in the direction of the long axis. Apply a few layers quickly and then hold the wound edges together for about 60 seconds to ensure adequate bonding. Once applied, tissue adhesives should not be covered with ointment, skin tapes, or dressing. If any adhesive is applied to unwanted areas, it can be removed with petroleum jelly or acetone (nail polish remover). Many tissue adhesives are commercially available, with many different applicator sizes and applicator tips. Also available are accessories to assist with the entire procedure, from wound cleansing devices to tissue forceps of various sizes and shapes for any size or shape wound.

Among the benefits of tissue adhesives is better cosmetic appearance, if used appropriately. The manufacturer of Dermabond states that the incidence of wound infection with this product is 3.6% and the incidence of dehiscence requiring retreatment is 2.2%; neither finding was statistically different on comparison with wounds closed with sutures.

5. Choice of Closure Technique

The choice of an appropriate material for wound closure is based on biologic and mechanical properties of the material and the characteristics of the wound. Decisions about layers to be closed are based on several factors, the most important of which are stress, dead space, and skin approximation.

▶ Fascia

In soft tissue wounds that do not involve the face, the strength of closure depends on the fascia. Because fascia heals slowly, the suture material should be capable of maintaining its strength for a long time. Synthetic nonabsorbable sutures are best for this purpose.

▶ Muscle and Fat

Muscle and fat do not hold sutures well, and closure is performed primarily to obliterate dead space. Dead space results from traumatic tissue loss, debridement, or gaping of subcutaneous layers. Suturing of dead space invariably produces additional tissue trauma and necrosis and is contraindicated in the closure of contaminated wounds. When such suturing is performed, it should be accomplished with the fewest possible loosely placed sutures. Chromic gut or one of the synthetic absorbable sutures should be used for this purpose.

▶ Skin

Skin closure may be accomplished by layers, full-thickness percutaneous sutures, skin tapes, or a combination of these methods. The type of skin closure method chosen depends on the forces tending to open the wound and how good a cosmetic result is desired. The width of the scar that will result from healing will be influenced by the local stresses of the surrounding tissues. The direction of maximum force of skin tension is usually parallel to the skin wrinkles. Wounds oriented in the same direction as local stresses are subjected to less tension during healing and consequently produce a less visible scar. Examples include transverse lacerations of the forehead and vertical lacerations of the upper lip. Wounds that cross lines of maximal skin stress will be subjected to increased tension during healing. These wounds frequently widen with time and have a tendency to form hypertrophic scars. Examples are transverse lacerations of the cheek and axial lacerations over the elbows.

The propensity of a scar to hypertrophy is also influenced by factors unrelated to its location or technique of closure. The tendency of children and adolescents to form hypertrophic scars is notorious and is probably influenced by elevated levels of growth hormone or other growth factors. Pregnant women have an increased incidence of hypertrophic scar formation that decreases with the resumption of normal menses after delivery; this tendency is often associated with a parallel increase in pigmentation coinciding with pregnancy. Some investigators have postulated that hypertrophic scars and pigmentation are under similar hormonal influences. An increased incidence of hypertrophic scar and keloid formation is also found in blacks and other dark-skinned races. These specific groups of patients will demonstrate an exaggerated scar formation response that can be controlled only by manipulation of the wound in ways beyond the technical aspects of closure. Not all patients in these groups will form hypertrophic scars, however, and it is impossible to predict which patients might, except perhaps in the case of patients who have a history of hypertrophic scar formation. In these patients, precise wound closure using fine suture materials and atraumatic technique may lessen the degree of hypertrophic scarring that might otherwise result. In the acute wound, however, primary consideration is given to the location and orientation of the wound and its method of closure.

6. Drainage of the Wound

Drains constitute foreign bodies, produce tissue necrosis, serve as conduits for bacterial contamination of the wound, and are not very effective in preventing hematoma formation. If sound principles of management have been carefully followed, drains are usually unnecessary in the acute wound. If oozing cannot be controlled, it is preferable to delay wound closure. Drains, however, may be effective in evacuating pus and necrotic exudates that might be found in heavily contaminated or already infected wounds.

POSTOPERATIVE WOUND CARE AND DRESSINGS

Postoperative wound care should provide an ideal environment for wound healing. This is accomplished primarily through the use of dressings. A dressing serves one or more of seven different functions: protection, immobilization, control of edema (compression), absorption, debridement, delivery of topical medications (antibiotics), and cosmetic appearance.

Wounds closed by percutaneous sutures are susceptible to surface bacterial invasion for the first 48 hours after closure. During this time, the wound should be protected with sterile dressings or frequent suture line care.

A. Dressing a Wound

If dressings are used, nonadherent materials (eg, Telfa, petrolatum-impregnated gauze) are favored because removal is easy and does not disturb sutures or coated wound edges.

Petrolatum-impregnated dressings have been shown to decrease the rate of epithelialization in partial-thickness wounds. For this reason, ointment-impregnated dressings (eg, bacitracin, polymyxin B sulfate, or nonadherent occlusive dressings) are preferred for this particular type of wound. Neomycin has a risk or allergy that rivals the rate of wound infection, and since a local allergic reaction and a wound infection have similar characteristics, neomycin use should be cautioned.

Occlusive or semiocclusive polyurethane, methacrylate, silicone polymer, or gel dressings provide excellent protection, and most do not alter the rate of normal epithelialization. If the wound contains residual necrotic debris or significant levels of bacterial contamination, however, the risk of wound infection is increased with these dressings.

B. Undressed Wounds

Suture line care without a dressing is commonly used for facial wounds and involves frequent meticulous cleansing with saline or dilute hydrogen peroxide solution. Cleansing removes the adherent coagulum from the suture–skin juncture, decreasing the likelihood of stitch abscess formation. After cleansing, the wound is dressed with an antibiotic cream or ointment (eg, bacitracin and polymyxin B sulfate).

C. Tape Dressings

Taped wounds are quite resistant to surface bacterial contamination. They usually require no protection other than that provided by the tape itself. These wounds should be checked frequently for wound drainage beneath the tape. Excessive drainage can cause maceration of the wound edge and thereby provide an excellent medium for bacterial proliferation.

▶ Immobilization

Immobilization of the wound enhances resistance to infection, reduces sheer forces, and may accelerate healing.

A. Materials

Immobilization is accomplished with splints, bulky dressings, skin tapes, or combinations of these methods.

B. Duration of Immobilization

Ideally, immobilization of the wound should be continued until it is no longer vulnerable to infection and has gained sufficient strength to withstand the stresses of motion and skin tension. Wounds become resistant to infection within a week, but development of maximal strength requires about 6 weeks. Protracted immobilization will defeat its possible advantages, for example, possibly producing permanent joint contractures in elderly persons or promoting formation of deep venous thrombi. The advantages of wound immobilization must be weighed against the undesirable consequences.

▶ Control of Edema

Edema slows tissue healing and increases pain. Edema increases in the first 48 hours postinjury and subsides over the next 5 days. The main methods of edema control are elevation of the wound and compression dressings.

A. Elevation

Elevation of the wound above the level of the heart is the simplest way to limit the amount of excess tissue fluid in the wound. Slings are generally not useful in this regard. Advise the patient to elevate the wound above the level of the shoulders while at rest. One simple way to achieve this is place a pillow on the chest while in the semirecumbent position and placing the arm and hand on top.

B. Compression Dressing

In certain situations, it is advantageous to "apply pressure over the wound along with elevation by using bulky pressure dressings."

Caution: Compression dressings should not be used in crush injuries or in injuries that tend to develop into compartment syndromes (eg, severe injuries of the forearm or leg). Continued pain or diminished sensitivity necessitates removal of the dressing and careful examination of the wound. Although these dressings are often used to absorb bloody oozing at the operative site, they should not be used as a substitute for diligent hemostasis.

Avoid constriction of proximal parts with these dressings, because venous and lymphatic congestion will occur as result of the tourniquet effect.

Bony prominences must be carefully padded, with generous use of bulk. To ensure uniform compression throughout and to avoid constriction and pressure-point injury, smooth, even wrapping that avoids lumps is necessary when compression dressing is applied.

In managing hand wounds, it is important to place 1 or 2 layers of gauze between the fingers to prevent maceration. The toes and fingertips should be exposed so that the physician can assess sensibility and capillary refill. Rolled gauze or bias-cut stockinet is preferred over elastic bandages, which are often too constricting. The finished dressing should be firm but not strangulating.

In extremity injuries, compression dressing should extend proximally from the most distal point. For example, a wound of the forearm requiring a compression dressing is managed by applying the dressing starting from the fingers to above the wound.

▶ Absorption

The absorptive capabilities of a dressing are used to remove bloody and serous ooze from the wound or drainage site.

A. Closed Wounds

In closed wounds, dry dressings are preferable, because moist ones will cause maceration of the skin and invite bacterial invasion.

B. Open Wounds

In open wounds, it is preferable to apply moist dressings to the open wound surface and back them with dry dressings to achieve a capillary effect. The exception to this principle is deep, tunnel-shaped wounds, where surface evaporation is limited, thus diminishing the capillary effect. These wounds are best managed by packing with dry gauze to achieve maximum absorption.

C. Materials

In all instances, absorptive dressings should be composed of fine-mesh gauze or spun fabric.

Caution: Absorbant dressing must be changed frequently to avoid the proliferation of toxin-producing bacteria.

Absorbant dressing have been associated with toxic shock syndrome.

▶ Debridement

Dressings are frequently used for mechanical debridement of the open wound. The traditional wet-to-dry method utilizes avulsion of adherent tissues to remove devitalized remnants from the wound surface. Unfortunately, this method does not discriminate between viable and nonviable elements and reinjures the wound with each dressing change. Although painful and detrimental to wound healing, this method is effective in removing fine tenacious material from the wound surface. It should be discontinued as soon as the desired effect has been achieved.

The technique is as follows: Several layers of moist gauze are applied to the wound surface and allowed to dry. After about 4 hours, the adherent dressing is removed. Moistening the dry dressing before removal to loosen the dressing and lessen the pain of removal (as may be done by a sympathetic hospital attendant) defeats the purpose.

▶ Delivery of Topical Antibiotics

The most common medicaments used in a dressing are antibacterials. Topical antibacterials are used to control bacteria that cannot be reached by systemic agents. They are *not* a substitute for adequate debridement.

A. Topical Antibacterial Agents

Mafenide (Sulfamylon) and silver sulfadiazine (Silvadene) are most effective in this regard. These agents are also useful in partial-thickness injuries or marginally viable tissues (eg, abrasions, burns, crush injuries). By decreasing the potential for bacterial invasion, they diminish the likelihood of infection and the resulting tissue necrosis.

B. Adverse Reactions

Use of these agents must be monitored closely, because excessive amounts may cause acid–base imbalances (mafenide) or leukopenia (silver sulfadiazine). Both agents retard wound epithelialization and should be discontinued when the necrotic debris has been removed and wound bacterial counts are fewer than 10^5 organisms per gram of tissue.

▶ Cosmetic Appearance

To the patient or casual observer, the sight of a wound is abhorrent and may be an occasion for adverse response. A dressing hides the wound and allows the patient to proceed with the process of rehabilitation without that distraction. In addition, a carefully applied, neat-appearing dressing reassures the patient that good wound care has been provided.

1. Potential Infections and Antimicrobials

Antimicrobials may be effective in preventing wound infection, particularly when the wound has fewer than 10^6 organisms per gram of tissue before treatment is started. Wounds with more than 10^6 organisms per gram of tissue often become infected despite antibiotic prophylaxis and should be left open. Systemic antibiotics, to be effective, must be started as soon as possible following injury, preferably within 4 hours. Topical antibiotics are commonly used to suppress bacterial growth, although their efficacy at preventing subsequent infection is probably low. The likelihood of wound infection must be judged by the mechanism of injury, the level of contamination, the adequacy of debridement, and the patient's general health status.

If adequate wound management must be delayed for any reason, then consider systemic antimicrobial prophylaxis.

Sharp, clean lacerations are markedly resistant to infection and in most instances will not require chemoprophylaxis. Open wounds, by virtue of their inflammatory response and resistance to bacterial dissemination, rarely become infected unless the initial level of contamination is great and cannot be reduced by cleansing and debridement. Furthermore, the fibrinous coagulum in these wounds limits the possible effectiveness of systemic antimicrobials on bacterial contaminants, thus making their use impractical.

Deep wounds or those that involve poorly vascularized structures such as bone, tendon, ligament, or fascia should be treated with systemic antibiotics prophylactically. Oral mucosal lacerations rarely require systemic antibiotic prophylaxis, because the infection rate is low and randomized trials have not demonstrated a benefit from such treatment. Grossly contaminated wounds such as those that come in contact with feces, pus, or saliva should not be closed. Systemic antimicrobial therapy is mandatory. The choice of drug is based on the suspected predominant pathogen (Table 30–2).

Table 30–2. Choice of Antimicrobials for Prevention of Infection in Specific Types of Wounds.[a]

Type of Wound	Antimicrobial of Choice	Alternative
Human bite	Amoxicillin/clavulanate 875/125 mg b.i.d.	Cefuroxime 250-500 mg b.i.d.
Animal bites	Amoxicillin/clavulanate 875/125 mg b.i.d.	Clindamycin 150-450 mg q.i.d. plus Ciprofloxacin 500 mg b.i.d.
Other wounds	Amoxicillin/clavulanate 875/125 mg b.i.d.	Clindamycin 150-450 mg q.i.d. or Cephalexin 500 mg q.i.d.

[a]These recommendations apply only to wounds *without* evidence of infection at the time of examination and should be given for 3-5 days.

Table 30-3. Guide to Tetanus Prophylaxis in Wound Management.

History of Tetanus Immunization (Doses)	Clean Minor Wounds		All Other Wounds	
	Td[a]/Tdap	TIG[a]	Td[a]/Tdap	TIG[a]
Uncertain or <3 doses	Yes	No	Yes	Yes
3 or more doses	No[b]	No	No[c]	No

[a]Td = Tetanus and diphtheria toxoids, adult type, for persons older than 7 years. DTP for children younger than 7 years. TIG = Tetanus immune globulin. Tdap (Tetanus, diphtheria and pertussis).
[b]Yes if it has been more than 10 years since last dose.
[c]Yes if it has been more than 5 years since last dose.

2. Tetanus Immunization Status

Tetanus has become rare in civilized countries due to emphasis on immunization. Tetanus is more likely to occur in IV drug abusers, immigrants, and older adults, particularly women. Table 30–3 shows the recommended tetanus immunization guidelines based on immunization history and wound type. Tetanus toxoid should be administered to anyone who has not received a booster within 10 years or who has not completed the primary series of three doses. Td (tetanus toxoid combined with adult-dose diphtheria toxoid) is preferable to tetanus toxoid alone. If passive immunization is required, human tetanus immune globulin is indicated. The recommended dose is 250 units intramuscularly. If both Td and tetanus immune globulin or antitoxin are given, they should be administered in separate sites using separate syringes.

3. Rabies Prophylaxis

▶ **Assess Risk of Rabies Exposure**

See Figure 30–7.

A. Species of Biting Animal

Carnivorous animals (especially skunks, foxes, badgers, bobcats, coyotes, raccoons, dogs, and cats) and bats are more likely to be infected and are vectors for rabies. Lagomorphs (rabbits and hares), Picas (chinchillas), and Rodents (squirrels, hamsters, guinea pigs, gerbils, chipmunks, rats, and mice) rarely transmit rabies in the United States.

B. Determine if Animal Is Rabid (if Possible)

(*Note*: Behavior is *not* a reliable sign of the rabid state.) If examination of the animal's brain for rabies is negative, it can be assumed that the animal's saliva did not contain rabies virus.

Healthy domestic dogs and cats should be observed for 10 days by a veterinarian. If signs of rabies develop, the animal should be killed and its brain examined for rabies virus at the local public health laboratory.

Stray or unwanted dogs and cats that cause bites should be euthanized immediately and the brain examined for rabies. Wild animals that cause bites should be sacrificed immediately and the brain examined for rabies.

C. Circumstances of Biting Incident

Unprovoked attacks are more likely to mean that the animal is rabid; unfortunately, it may be difficult to distinguish between normal defensive or territorial behavior. Bites from apparently healthy animals that are fighting or feeding or that have been picked up or petted should be considered provoked and so have a low likelihood of causing rabies.

D. Types of Exposure

Any penetration of skin by teeth is regarded as a bite. Nonbite exposure consists of contamination of scratches, abrasions, mucous membranes, or previous wounds with infected animal saliva. Finding a bat within a bedroom, regardless of presence or absence of bite marks or the proximity of the animal to humans, should be considered an exposure.

E. Rabies Immunization Status of Animal

Vaccines are effective for cats and dogs but are *not* effective in preventing rabies in other animals, especially wild animals that have been domesticated (eg, pet skunks and foxes).

F. Prevalence of Rabies in Region

Certain areas are devoid of rabies (eg, San Francisco, Alaska, and Great Britain). Some rural areas are considered at high risk for rabies (eg, Texas–Mexico border).

▶ **Management of Patients at High Risk**

Provide tetanus prophylaxis (see above), and give antibiotics if indicated (see above). Quickly administer appropriate postexposure rabies prophylaxis (see Figure 30–7 and Tables 30–4 and 30–5).

Act quickly! The sooner antirabies measures are instituted, the more effective they are.

A. Wound Care

This is the most important step. Wash the wound copiously with 20% green soap tincture and water. Quaternary ammonium compounds and alcohol are no longer recommended.

B. Passive Immunization

1. Rabies immune globulin USP—This neutralizing antibody should be given to all patients except those previously

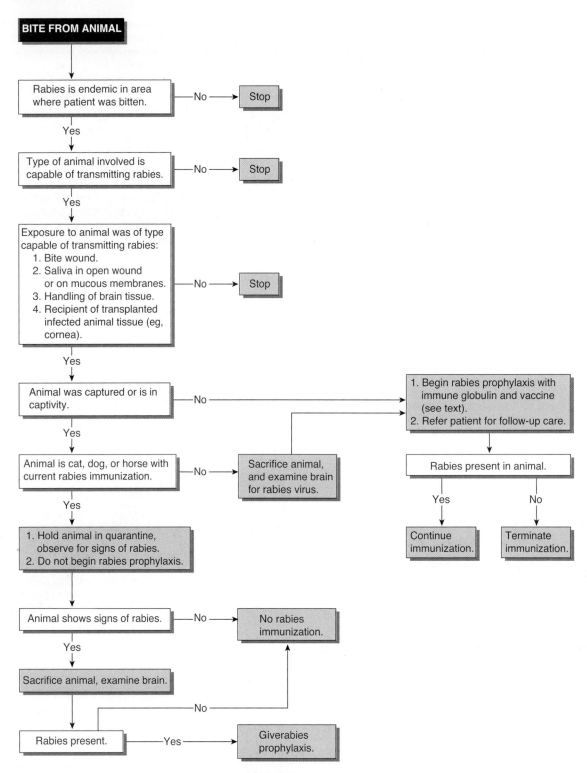

▲ **Figure 30–7.** Algorithm for management of possible rabies exposure.

Table 30–4. Rabies Postexposure Prophylaxis Guide.

Animal Species	Condition of Animal at Time of Attack	Treatment of Exposed Person[a]
Domestic Dog and cat	Healthy and available for 10 days of observation	None, unless animal develops rabies[b]
	Rabid or suspected rabid	RIG and HDCV[e]
	Unknown (escaped)	Consult public health officials. If treatment is indicated, give RIG and HDCV[c]
Wild Skunk, bat, fox, coyote, raccoon, bobcat, and other carnivores	Regard as rabid unless proved negative by laboratory tests[d]	RIG and HDCV[e]
Other Livestock, rodents, and Lagomorphs (rabbits and hares)	Consider individually. Local and state public health officials should be consulted on questions about the need for rabies prophylaxis. Bites of squirrels, hamsters, guinea pigs, gerbils, chipmunks, rats, mice, rabbits, and hares almost never call for antirabies prophylaxis	

These recommendations are only a guide. In applying them, take into account the species involved, the circumstances of the bite or other exposure, the vaccination status of the animal, and the presence of rabies in the region. Local or state public health officials should be consulted if questions arise about the need for rabies prophylaxis.

[a]All bites and wounds should immediately be thoroughly cleansed with soap and water. If antirabies treatment is indicated, both rabies immune globulin (RIG) and human diploid cell vaccine (HDCV) should be given as soon as possible, regardless of the interval from exposure.

[b]During the usual holding period of 10 days, begin treatment with RIG and HDCV at first sign of rabies in a dog or cat that has bitten someone. The symptomatic animal should be killed immediately and tested.

[c]If HDCV is not available, use purified chick embryo cell vaccine (PCECV). Local reactions to vaccines are common and do not contraindicate continuing treatment. Discontinue vaccine if fluorescent antibody tests of the animal are negative.

[d]The animal should be killed and tested as soon as possible. Holding for observation is not recommended.

[e]If RIG is not available, use antirabies serum, equine (ARS). Do not use more than the recommended dosage.

immunized who have documented antibody titers or those who have received preexposure human diploid cell rabies vaccine prophylaxis or a full course of human diploid cell rabies vaccine. Give 20 IU/kg at the onset of rabies therapy; rabies immune globulin can be given as late as the eighth day if necessary. The full dose of rabies immune globulin should be thoroughly infiltrated in and around the wound; any remaining rabies immune globulin should be injected intramuscularly at a site distant from vaccine administration. Because rabies immune globulin may partially suppress the antibody response to vaccine, no more than the recommended dose should be given.

Table 30–5. Rabies Postexposure Immunization Regimens.

	Postexposure		
Rabies Vaccine	Number of 1-mL Doses	Route of Administration	Intervals Between Doses
HDCV PCECV	4[a]	Intramuscular	Doses given on days 0, 3, 7, 14

Postexposure rabies prophylaxis for persons exposed to rabies consists of the immediate, thorough cleansing of all wounds with soap and water, administration of rabies immune globulin (RIG) and the initiation of either and human diploid cell vaccine (HDCV) or purified chick embryo cell vaccine (PCECV), according to the following schedule.

[a]An additional dose on day 28 should be given only to immunocompromised patients.

C. Active Immunization

Human diploid cell rabies vaccine is an inactivated virus vaccine prepared from rabies virus grown on human diploid fibroblasts. Give four 1-mL doses intramuscularly on specified days. The first dose is given as soon as possible after the bite; subsequent doses are given on days 3, 7, and 14. An alternative immunization is the chick embryo cell vaccine (PCECV) given at the same dose and schedule.

If preexposure human diploid cell rabies vaccine prophylaxis and adequate booster doses have been given (because of occupation as a veterinarian, for example), only two 1-mL intramuscular doses of human diploid cell rabies vaccine are needed, one as soon as possible after the bite and the other 3 days later.

Routine serologic testing after treatment with human diploid cell rabies vaccine is not necessary unless the patient is immunocompromised or is taking corticosteroids.

Table 30–6. Timing of Suture Removal.

Location	Time (Days)
Eyelid	3
Cheek	3–5
Nose, forehead, neck	5
Ear, scalp	5–7
Arm, leg, hand, foot	7–10+
Chest, back, abdomen	7–10+

Individuals taking steroids should discontinue the medication while receiving antirabies treatment.

4. Follow-up Care of the Wound

Patients must be given verbal and written instructions specifically describing wound care, how to recognize infection, and when to return for wound checks or suture removal.

5. Suture Removal

The timing of suture removal depends on many factors such as location; type of wound closure; presence of infection; and the patient's age, health, and compliance. Table 30–6 is a general guideline for suture removal in healthy adults with uncomplicated wounds. Modifications of these recommendations should be tailored to individual patients.

Kretsinger K, Broder KR, Cortese MM et al: Preventing tetanus, diphtheria, and pertussis among adults: use of tetanus toxoid, reduced diphtheria toxoid and acellular pertussis vaccine recommendations of the Advisory Committee on Immunization Practices (ACIP) and recommendation of ACIP, supported by the Healthcare Infection Control Practices Advisory Committee (HICPAC), for use of Tdap among health-care personnel. MMWR Recomm Rep 2006;55:1–37 [PMID: 17167397].

McManus J, Wedmore I, Schwartz RB (editors): *Emergency Department Wound Management.* Emerg Med Clin N Am 2007; 25:1–248.

Rupprecht CE, Briggs D, Brown CM, Franka R, Katz SL, Kerr HD, Lett SM, Levis R, Meltzer MI, Schaffner W, Cieslak PR; Centers for Disease Control and Prevention (CDC): Use of a reduced (4-dose) vaccine schedule for postexposure prophylaxis to prevent human rabies: recommendations of the advisory committee on immunization practices. MMWR Recomm Rep 2010;59:1–9 [PMID: 20300058].

Singer AJ et al: Closure of lacerations and incisions with octylcyanoacrylate: A multicenter randomized controlled trial. Surgery 2002;131:270 [PMID: 1189403].

Thompson WL et al: Peripheral nerve blocks and anesthesia of the hand. Mil Med 2002;167:478 [PMID: 12099083].

▼ EMERGENCY TREATMENT OF SPECIFIC TYPES OF WOUNDS

FACIAL LACERATIONS

See Chapter 23.

INTRAORAL LACERATIONS

Lacerations of the oral mucosa and tongue may not require closure if they are small. The rich blood supply promotes rapid healing, and cosmetic considerations are minimal. However, large or gaping wounds, through-and-through lacerations, and lacerations involving important deep structures, such as muscle or bone, require repair. In such wounds, after irrigation with saline, disrupted muscle should first be approximated with absorbable suture (eg, 5-0 Vicryl) and the mucosa closed with absorbable suture (eg, 5-0 chromic gut or Vicryl). It is best to use the minimum number of sutures that will allow approximation of the wound edges.

Through-and-through lacerations of the lip merit special attention:

1. Irrigate the wound thoroughly, inside and out. A dry gauze roll between the lip and teeth will help prevent recontamination of the irrigated wound.

2. Close the mucosal laceration with absorbable suture (eg, 5-0 chromic gut or Vicryl).

3. Irrigate the wound again from the outside. The sutured mucosa will prevent reentry of saliva.

4. If the orbicularis oris muscle is disrupted, approximate it with absorbable suture (eg, 5-0 Vicryl).

5. Close the external skin with interrupted sutures of 6-0 monofilament nylon. Take extreme care to line up the opposing vermilion borders of the lip.

6. Examine the adjacent teeth that produced the wound; they may be fractured or avulsed.

BLAST INJURIES

▶ Clinical Findings in Blast Injuries

Wounds resulting from high-velocity missiles and shotgun blasts are among the most severe wounds encountered in civilian practice. Extensive tissue destruction is incurred locally, with loss or disruption of the wound parts to form a cavity. Sites distant from the point of impact may be injured as a result of shock waves transmitted through tissues. The extent of injury of these complex wounds is difficult to assess.

▶ Treatment of Blast Injuries

Initial care is directed at hemostasis, cleansing, and minimal debridement. It is wise not to close the wound primarily.

Repeated staged exploration at first presentation and then again 24 hours and 48 hours apart is used to remove necrotic or devitalized tissues. Antibiotic prophylaxis is recommended. Cefazolin, 1 g intravenously every 8 hours, is satisfactory. The wound is then closed secondarily, with priority given to reestablishment of bony relationships, followed by soft tissue coverage.

▶ Disposition

Hospitalize these patients for management.

HIGH-PRESSURE INJECTION INJURIES

▶ General Considerations

High-pressure injection equipment is used in industry to force liquids such as paint, paint thinner, oil, or grease through a small nozzle under high pressure, sometimes at pressure exceeding several thousand psi. If the nozzle is held against or close to the skin, it is possible for the liquid stream to be injected through the skin and into the subcutaneous tissues.

▶ Clinical Findings

These injuries have the potential for severe sequelae usually resulting from direct trauma and intense inflammation incited by the injected liquid. The edema that develops from the resulting inflammation can lead to increased tissue compartment pressures and may lead to compartment syndrome. The type of injected material and amount and pressure velocity will determine the degree of inflammation and severity of injury.

Patients with these types of injuries usually have small puncture wounds that are usually isolated to the extremities. Patients often present with pain out of proportion to the appearance of the wound and, if early, often with only minimal swelling. Because the material is injected at great force, the distance it can be injected into the tissues from injection site can be significant.

▶ Treatment and Disposition

Carefully assess neurovascular function at the time of presentation and attempt appropriate pain control via parenteral analgesics. Avoid digital blocks because of the resulting increase in pressure. Parenteral antibiotics should also be initiated at first presentation, directed at normal skin flora (*Staphylococcus* and *Streptococcus*). Appropriate radiographs should be obtained because some materials are radiopaque and may demonstrate the extent of subcutaneous spread and may also show the presence of subcutaneous emphysema. Early consultation with a hand specialist or other surgical specialist for early surgical debridement and follow-up is recommended.

DEGLOVING INJURIES

▶ Clinical Findings

Separation of the skin and subcutaneous tissues from the underlying musculofascial planes constitutes a degloving injury. For flaps attached by a pedicle, the determinant of survival is their circulation.

▶ Treatment and Disposition

All but trivial degloving injuries require hospitalization and plastic surgical consultation is advisable.

AMPUTATIONS

Amputations of extremities and digits require careful prehospital care. The viability of the amputated part will depend on the degree of tissue damage, amount of ischemic time, and the ambient temperature. Reimplantation is usually possible with less than 6 hours of warm ischemic time. Cooler temperatures will prolong this window and cooling the amputated part correctly can extend this time to 24 hours in some instances. First responders should be trained to locate amputated parts, clean the parts with normal saline, and to wrap the part in saline-moistened (not wet) gauze. The part should then be placed in a waterproof plastic bag and the bag placed on ice for transport to the hospital. Amputated parts should *never* be placed directly into water or saline baths or in direct contact with ice. "Dry" ice should never be used to cool amputated parts as freezing of the tissue will occur.

The level of the amputation will affect the surgeon's decision to attempt reimplantation; physician-to-physician discussions are mandatory prior to transfer to a reimplantation center.

BITES

Most nonprimate mammalian bite wounds are minor, and only about 10% require suturing. The rare patient with major injuries sustained in an animal attack should be evaluated and receive treatment as any other patient with severe trauma.

Meticulous wound care is the cornerstone of therapy for bite wounds and is the most important factor in preventing infection. The wound should be cleansed, debrided, and copiously irrigated. Treat all bite wounds on the extremities aggressively, with antibiotics and elevation and immobilization of the affected part.

Routine cultures in the absence of infection need not be obtained, because there is no useful correlation between positive cultures and wounds that later develop clinical signs of infection. Antimicrobial prophylaxis (see Table 30–2) is recommended for all human and most cat bites but only for high-risk dog bites (below). The need for tetanus and rabies prophylaxis (Tables 30–3 and 30–4) should also be evaluated.

1. Dog Bites

Dog bites cause open wounds, often with tissue necrosis secondary to crush injury. Treat by prompt excisional debridement within 6 hours. If the extent of the wound or the length of time since injury precludes primary closure, the wounds should be irrigated, debrided, and left open or loosely sutured. Infection is unusual, and antimicrobial prophylaxis is not indicated in routine cases.

Dog bites associated with a high risk of infection are those of the hand, puncture wounds, and injuries more than 6–12 hours old. These wounds should be treated with vigorous local care and left unsutured. Antibiotic prophylaxis is recommended (Table 30–2). Low-risk bites do not require prophylactic antibiotics and may be sutured after appropriate wound care. Hospitalization is rarely indicated unless injuries are multiple or extensive or infection is present.

Infected bites should be cleansed and debrided and the affected limb immobilized and elevated. A parenteral dose of a first-generation cephalosporin should be administered in the emergency department and the patient discharged with oral antibiotics (same as those for prophylaxis, above) for 7–10 days. Patients should receive follow-up care within 1–2 days and be instructed to return earlier if their condition worsens. Hospitalize patients who have symptoms of sepsis.

Alcoholic patients and immunocompromised patients are at risk from rapidly overwhelming sepsis due to *Capnocytophaga canimorsus* after even minor dog bites.

2. Cat Bites

Cat bites cause deep puncture wounds with little crush injury and are associated with a high risk of infection, mainly with *Pasteurella multocida*. Wounds caused by cat claws are considered equivalent to bites. Treatment includes local cleansing, debridement, and prophylactic antibiotics for all significant bites. (Table 30–2).

Cat bite infections occurring within 24 hours are due to *P. multocida* and should be treated as mentioned above. Wounds becoming infected after 24 hours should be treated with a first-generation cephalosporin or amoxicillin/clavulante (see Dog Bites, above) for 7–10 days.

Hospitalization is rarely indicated unless infection is severe or involves the hand. Primary closure should not be performed except in low risk, cosmetically disfiguring facial bites.

3. Human Bites

▶ General Considerations

Adult human bites are more serious than dog or cat bites. They are characterized by crush and tear injuries and are commonly located over the knuckles or the dorsum of the hand, frequently involving the tendons or joints. Inoculation of large numbers of bacteria from dental plaque also occurs. (Bites by children appear to carry a low risk of infection because of fewer mouth bacteria and less biting force.) Despite their rather innocuous initial appearance, these wounds are extremely dangerous, because they are prone to severe necrotizing infection.

▶ Treatment and Disposition

Hospitalize patients with suspected tendon, joint, or cartilage involvement (eg, bites of the hand or ear) for vigorous irrigation, debridement, and parenteral antimicrobials (high-dose penicillin or clindamycin). Wounds of this type are never closed. Bites of other structures may be treated with vigorous irrigation and debridement in the emergency department, followed by antimicrobial prophylaxis (see Table 30–2). The injured part should be elevated, immobilized, and checked frequently to assess the possible spread of infection. The patient should be reexamined within 6–18 hours and subsequently at 1–2-day intervals for a week.

Signs of necrotizing infection are progressive erythema, blistering, and frank necrosis. If these signs are already present at the time of initial evaluation, hospitalization is indicated for wide debridement of the involved parts and parenteral antimicrobial therapy.

PUNCTURE WOUNDS

▶ General Considerations

Puncture wounds are at risk of becoming infected, especially if dirty, contaminated, or containing foreign materials. Wounds associated with penetration through the soles of shoes (especially sneakers) often contain particulate debris and are particularly susceptible to infection. If joint capsule or bone is penetrated, septic arthritis and osteomyelitis can occur. *Pseudomonas* species are common pathogens.

All puncture wounds should be probed gently with forceps or a long (6.5 cm or 2.5 in), 22-gauge needle for the presence of foreign bodies; control pain as needed with 1% lidocaine anesthetic. Obtain soft-tissue X-rays of all wounds for which the history or mechanism of injury suggests retention of a foreign body (eg, broken glass and flying piece of metal), even if results of the wound probe are negative.

▶ Treatment and Disposition

A. Wound Cleansing and Exploration

Irrigate the wound with normal saline under pressure and cleanse it with 1% povidone-iodine solution. Probe gently and remove foreign materials. Local infiltration with 1% lidocaine and slight enlargement of the wound may be necessary for adequate exploration. Extensive dissection in the emergency department to search for small or deeply embedded objects is not recommended.

B. Tetanus and Antibiotics Prophylaxis

Ensure that tetanus prophylaxis is up to date (see Table 30–3). Treat dirty or deep wounds, especially those with possible joint or bone involvement, with prophylactic antibiotics (Table 30–2). If penetration occurred through the sole of a sneaker (unless very superficial), consider prophylaxis against the high risk of *Pseudomonas* infection with antipseudomonal cephalosporin as a single parenteral dose (eg, ceftazidime, 1 g intramuscularly) or ciprofloxacin 500 mg BID for 3–5 days.

C. Elevation and Follow-up

Instruct patients to elevate any involved extremity and, in foot injuries, to bear no weight for 3–5 days. Except in the case of superficial punctures, patients should be reexamined in 5–7 days or earlier if increased pain, redness, red streaking, or pus is noted.

D. Osteomyelitis

Patients with pain persisting longer than 5–7 days or with an abnormal erythrocyte sedimentation rate may have osteomyelitis. In either case, obtain X-rays of the affected area and, if normal, consider referral for limited bone scan of the area. Refer patients with osteomyelitis to the specialist appropriate to the area of involvement.

E. Retained Foreign Bodies

Retained foreign bodies in critical areas (eg, eye) require urgent specialty consultation. Refer patients with possible retained foreign bodies in noncritical areas for outpatient surgical removal in 2–3 weeks.

Abubaker AO: Use of prophylactic antibiotics in preventing infection of traumatic injuries. Dent Clin North Am 2009;53: 707–715 [PMID: 19958907].

Dendle C, Looke D: Management of mammalian bites. Aust Fam Physician 2009;38:868–874 [PMID: 19893832].

Gonzalez R, Kasdan ML: High pressure injection injuries of the hand. Clin Occup Environ Med 2006;5:407–411 [PMID: 16647657].

Halaas GW. Management of foreign bodies in the skin. Am Fam Physician 2007;76:683–688 [PMID: 17894138].

Morrison WA, McCombe D: Digital replantation. Hand Clin 2007;23:1–12 [PMID: 17478248].

Nakamura Y, Daya M: Use of appropriate antimicrobials in wound management. Emerg Med Clin North Am 2007;25: 159–176 [PMID: 17400079].

Singer AJ, Dagum AB: Current management of acute cutaneous wounds. N Engl J Med 2008;359:1037–1046 [PMID: 18768947].

Soucacos PN: Indications and selection for digital amputation and replantation. J Hand Surg [Br] 2001;26:572 [PMID: 11884116].

Wolf SJ, Bebarta VS, Bonnett CJ, Pons PT, Cantrill SV: Blast injuries. Lancet. 2009;374:405–415 [PMID: 19631372].

Eye Emergencies

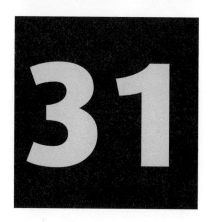

Robert D. Greenberg, MD, FACEP

Kimrey J. Daniel, MD

EMERGENCY EVALUATION OF IMPORTANT OCULAR SYMPTOMS

EVALUATION OF THE RED OR PAINFUL EYE

See Figure 31–1 and Table 31–1.

▶ History and Examination

Historical factors are important in determining the cause of ocular complaints. History, when correlated with characteristic ocular findings on focused physical examination, usually makes the diagnosis. History should include use of eye drops, previous episodes, onset of pain, contact lens use, systemic illnesses and findings, and associated symptoms.

The components of a complete eye examination include the following.

A. Visual Acuity

Visual acuity testing using a standard acuity chart (Snellen). An acute change in vision usually indicates disease of the eyeball globe or visual pathway. Pain and decreased acuity indicate corneal disease, acute angle-closure glaucoma, or iritis.

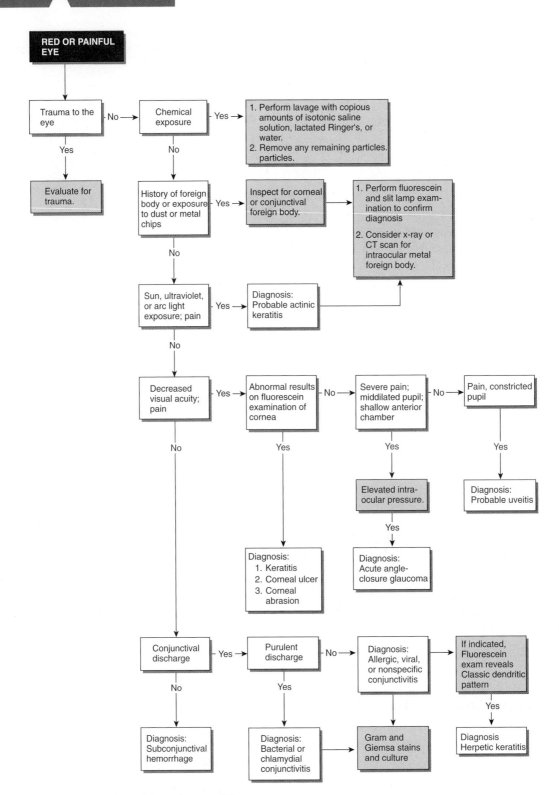

▲ **Figure 31–1.** Assessment of the red or painful eye.

Table 31–1. Differential Diagnosis of Nontraumatic Unilateral Redness and/or Eye Pain. The Most Helpful Findings are Shaded.

History and Clinical Findings	Conjunctivitis	Iritis	Acute Glaucoma	Corneal Infection (Bacterial Ulcer)	Corneal Erosion
Incidence	Extremely common	Common	Uncommon	Uncommon	Rare
Onset	Insidious	Insidious	Sudden	Slow	Sudden
Vision	Normal to slightly blurred	Slightly blurred	Markedly blurred	Usually blurred	Blurred
Pain	None to moderate	Moderate	Severe	Moderate to severe	Severe
Photophobia	None to mild	Severe	Minimal	Variable	Moderate
Nausea and vomiting	None	None	Occasional	None	None
Discharge	Moderate to copious	None	None	Watery	Watery
Ciliary injection	Absent	Present - perilimbal	Present	Present	Present
Conjunctival injection	Severe diffuse in fornices	Minimal	Minimal, diffuse	Moderate, diffuse	Mild to moderate
Cornea	Clear	Usually clear	Steamy	Locally hazy	Hazy
Stain with fluorescein	Absent	Absent	Absent	Present	Present
Hypopyon	Absent	Occasional	Absent	Occasional	Absent
Pupil size	Normal	Constricted	Middilated, fixed, and Irregular	Normal	Normal or constricted
Intraocular pressure	Normal	Normal	Elevated	Normal	Normal
Gram-stained smear	Variable; depending on cause	No organisms	No organisms	Organisms in scrapings from ulcers	No organisms
Pupilary light response	Normal	Poor	None	Normal	Poor to normal

B. Inspection

Inspection of the eye to include conjunctiva, cornea, sclera, lens, and pupil, external lids, lashes, lacrimal ducts, orbits, and periorbital areas for sign of trauma, infection, exudate, or irritation.

C. Pupillary Function

Check pupillary function for shape, symmetry, and reactivity to light and accommodation.

D. Extraocular Muscle Function

Extraocular muscle function for any signs of entrapment or palsy.

E. Visual Fields

Check for abnormalities in the visual fields; this is generally done in the emergency department by confrontation.

F. Fundoscopy

Direct fundoscopy is generally used to check the retina, optic disc, and retinal vessels.

G. Slit-Lamp Examination

Slit-lamp examination should be done before and after fluorescein staining to check for corneal abnormalities and examine the anterior chamber.

H. Intraocular Pressure

Intraocular pressure (IOP) can be tested with a Tono-Pen or Schiotz tonometer (described later in this chapter). Abnormally high pressure may be grossly estimated by palpation, ie, tactile tonometry.

I. Other Studies

Further diagnostic studies including blood tests, cultures, plain X-rays, bedside ultrasound, computed tomography (CT) scan, or magnetic resonance imaging (MRI) of the orbits may be needed to definitively establish a diagnosis.

▶ Disposition

Patients thought to have acute ocular conditions that may permanently decrease visual acuity (eg, acute angle-closure glaucoma) should have urgent ophthalmologic consultation. Patients with other conditions may receive treatment and be discharged with appropriate follow-up.

EVALUATION OF ACUTE UNILATERAL VISUAL LOSS

See Figure 31–2.

▶ Look for Trauma

Exclude trauma as a cause of visual loss. Both blunt and penetrating ocular injuries may result in blindness.

▶ History and Examination

Obtain a history from the patient (rate of onset of visual loss; whether it is unilateral or bilateral, painful or painless, with or without redness). Ophthalmologic examination should emphasize visual acuity and visual field testing.

A. Inability to Visualize Retina

Cloudy media will may completely obscure the retina (red reflex blunted or absent) or will make it impossible to visualize retinal landmarks such as the optic disc. Chronic causes of hazy media are common (eg, cataracts) and may complicate the evaluation of acute visual loss.

B. Abnormal Visual Fields

Grossly abnormal visual fields are usually caused by central nervous system disease and thus generally affect both eyes (not always to the same degree). The retinas are usually normal on ophthalmoscopic examination.

1. Hemianopia—Hemianopia is usually due to postchiasmal neurologic disorders (eg, tumor, aneurysm, migraine, stroke), in which case other acute neurologic lesions are present as well. Rarely, it is psychogenic functional in origin.

2. Central scotoma—A central scotoma indicates isolated macular involvement typical of retrobulbar neuritis and may or may not be associated with pain.

3. Tubular vision—Tubular vision not in conformity with the laws of optics is characteristic of psychogenic functional visual loss.

C. Abnormal Retina

An abnormal retina, usually in the eye with visual loss, is characteristic of several rare but serious conditions.

1. Central retinal artery occlusion—In central retinal artery occlusion, the fundus is usually pale with a cherry-red fovea. *This is a medical emergency* (see below).

2. Central retinal vein occlusion—Central retinal vein occlusion is associated with multiple widespread retinal hemorrhages.

3. Retinal hemorrhage—Retinal hemorrhage from other causes (eg, anticoagulation) may produce visual loss.

4. Retinal detachment—Retinal detachment produces visual loss preceded by visual flashes. If visual acuity is affected, detachment is large and may be easily visible on direct ophthalmoscopy; however, small detachments may require indirect ophthalmoscopy for visualization. Flashes of light may also occur in patients with migraine or as a result of posterior vitreous detachment.

▶ Differential Diagnosis

Causes of acute visual loss are listed and discussed below.

A. Acute Angle-closure Glaucoma

Acute angle-closure glaucoma causes corneal edema, but the more striking findings are eye pain; pupils fixed in mid position or dilated, often with irregular margins; a shallow anterior chamber angle (Figure 31–3); hyperemic conjunctiva; and significantly increased IOP. *Acute angle-closure glaucoma is a medical emergency* (see below).

B. Corneal Edema

Severe corneal edema of diverse causes (eg, abrasion, keratitis, postoperative) may cause visual loss with eye pain.

C. Hyphema

Hyphema is the presence of blood in the anterior chamber. This is generally traumatic in nature, although spontaneous hyphema may occur especially in patients on anticoagulant medications.

D. Vitreous Hemorrhage

Vitreous hemorrhage causes painless visual loss due to accumulation of blood in the posterior chamber. The anterior chamber is clear. The red reflex is often absent.

E. Endophthalmitis

Endophthalmitis (intraocular infection) is a rare condition usually associated with eye pain and decreased visual acuity. Eye examination will disclose pus in the anterior chamber (hypopyon) or vitreous. Systemic illnesses associated with endophthalmitis include ankylosing spondylitis, ulcerative colitis, other seronegative arthropathies, sarcoidosis, toxoplasmosis, tuberculosis, syphilis, and herpes zoster.

▶ Disposition

Patients with sudden visual loss due to ocular disease should have ophthalmologic consultation.

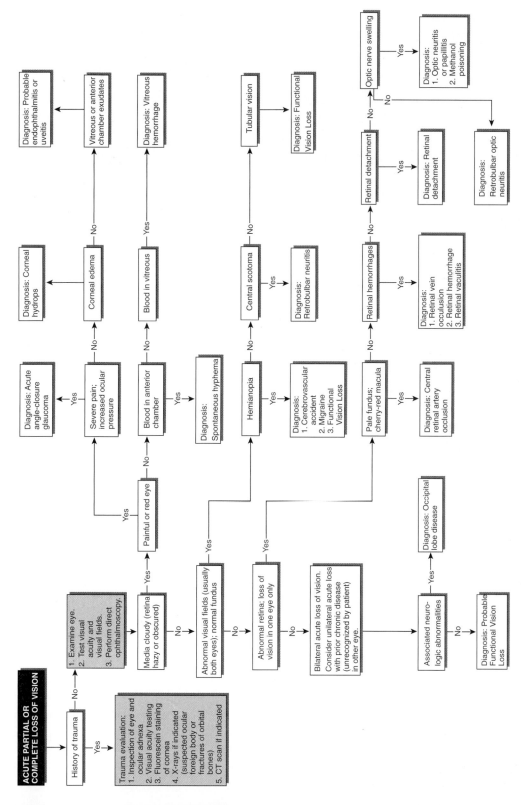

▲ **Figure 31–2.** Assessment of acute partial or complete loss of vision.

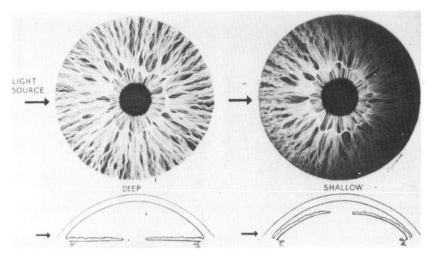

▲ **Figure 31–3.** Estimation of depth of anterior chamber by oblique illumination. (Courtesy of R. Shaffer.) (Reproduced, with permission, from Riordan-Eva P, Whitcher JP: *Vaughan & Asbury's General Ophthalmology*, 16th ed. McGraw-Hill, New York, 2004.)

OCULAR CONDITIONS REQUIRING IMMEDIATE TREATMENT

ACUTE ANGLE-CLOSURE GLAUCOMA

ESSENTIALS OF DIAGNOSIS

▶ Acute onset of moderate to severe, unilateral eye pain with associated nausea and vomiting

▶ Perilimbal eye redness with a mid-dilated, unreactive, irregular pupil

▶ Increased IOP confirms diagnosis

▶ General Considerations

Acute angle-closure glaucoma results from a sudden increase in IOP from blockage of the anterior chamber angle outflow channels by the iris root. This sudden rise in IOP causes intraocular vascular insufficiency that may lead to optic nerve or retinal ischemia and can cause permanent vision loss within hours. Prompt management is needed to minimize the likelihood of permanent vision loss.

▶ Clinical Findings

Acute angle-closure glaucoma is characterized by sudden onset of blurry vision, followed by severe pain, halos around lights, photophobia, frontal headache and nausea and vomiting. Other findings include a red eye with fixed or sluggish mid-dilated pupil, shallow anterior chamber, and hazy cornea. IOP will be greater than 30 mm Hg. Risk factors include myopia, hyperopia, shallow anterior chamber, narrow angle, and anterior placement of lens.

▶ Differential Diagnosis

(See Figure 31–2 and Table 31–1.) In iridocyclitis (iritis), IOP is normal and the pupil is small. In conjunctivitis, IOP is normal and the pupil is not affected. Corneal ulcer is diagnosed by fluorescein staining of the cornea.

▶ Treatment

Acute angle-closure glaucoma is an emergency. Timely treatment is important. Obtain ophthalmologic consultation for emergency management and reduce the IOP by one or more of the following means:

· Timolol, 0.5%, one drop in the affected eye

· Pilocarpine, 2% eye drops, two drops every 15 minutes for 2–3 hours

· Mannitol, 20%, 250–500 mL intravenously over 2–3 hours

· Acetazolamide, 500 mg orally or 250 mg intravenously

Glycerin, 1g/kg orally in cold 50% solution mixed with chilled lemon juice. Give sedation, antiemetics, and analgesics as necessary to control pain nausea and agitation.

▶ Disposition

Acute angle-closure glaucoma calls for urgent initiation of medical therapy and ophthalmologic consultation.

CENTRAL RETINAL ARTERY OCCLUSION

ESSENTIALS OF DIAGNOSIS

- ▶ Sudden, painless complete loss of vision in one eye
- ▶ Ophthalmoscopy demonstrates pallor of disc, retinal edema, cherry-red fovea, and "boxcar" appearance of retinal veins
- ▶ Treatment should be initiated immediately

▶ General Considerations

Central retinal artery occlusion is most commonly embolic in origin. Vision loss can occur in as little as 90 minutes from time of onset. Mitigating factors include occlusion time, cilioretinal artery patency, and cause of the occlusion.

▶ Clinical Findings

There is typically a history of sudden, complete, painless loss of vision in one eye, usually in an older person or others at risk for thromboembolic disease. Ophthalmoscopic examination discloses pallor of the optic disc, edema of the retina, cherry-red fovea, bloodless constricted arterioles that may be difficult to detect, and "boxcar" segmentation of blood in the retinal veins.

▶ Treatment

Central retinal artery occlusion is an emergency. Vision may be permanently lost in as short as 90 minutes, although visual recovery has occurred up to 3 days after occlusion. It is recommended that treatment be started if the patient is seen within 24 hours of symptom onset.

Treatment measures consist of ocular massage (moderate pressure for 10 seconds and release for 5 seconds), timolol ophthalmic, intravenous acetazolamide, or inhaled carbogen (oxygen–carbon dioxide mixture of 95% oxygen and 5% carbon dioxide). Other modalities to be considered by ophthalmology are direct infusion of thrombolytics in the ophthalmic artery or anterior chamber paracentesis. Hyperbaric treatment may be beneficial, if available.

▶ Disposition

Ophthalmologic consultation should be obtained on an emergency basis.

ORBITAL CELLULITIS

ESSENTIALS OF DIAGNOSIS

- ▶ Periorbital swelling and redness
- ▶ Painful, limited extraocular movement
- ▶ Intravenous antibiotics and admission

▶ General Considerations

Acute infection of the orbital tissues is generally caused by *Streptococcus pneumoniae*, other streptococci, *Staphylococcus aureus*, and (previously, chiefly in children) *Haemophilus influenzae*. Less frequently, certain fungi of the Phycomycetes group may cause orbital infections (rhinoorbitocerebral mucormycosis) in diabetics. Most causative organisms enter the orbit by direct extension from the paranasal sinuses (primarily ethmoid) or through the vascular channels draining the periorbital tissues. Rarely, infection may spread to the cavernous sinus or meninges.

▶ Clinical Findings

There may be a history of sinusitis or periorbital injury, pain in and around the eye, and possibly reduced visual acuity. Examination may demonstrate swelling and redness of the eyelids and periorbital tissues, chemosis of the conjunctiva, rapidly progressive exophthalmos, and ophthalmoplegia. Disc margins may be blurred, and fever is commonly present. Radiographic evaluation may demonstrate sinusitis with or without soft tissue orbital infiltration.

Patients with invasive infection due to the Phycomycetes group (*Mucor, Rhizopus,* and other genera) may present with rapidly progressive orbital cellulitis, often with cavernous sinus thrombosis. Diabetic and immunocompromised patients are at increased risk. Examination often reveals coexisting maxillary and/or ethmoid sinusitis and palatal or nasal mucosal ulceration.

▶ Treatment and Disposition

Obtain cultures of blood and periorbital tissue fluid. Obtain CT scan of the orbit to rule out orbital abscess and intracranial involvement. Patients should be admitted and appropriate broad-spectrum intravenous antibiotics started (ceftriaxone 1–2 g IV plus vancomycin 1 g IV or piperacillin/tazobactam 3.375 g IV). Obtain immediate ophthalmologic and or otolaryngologic (ENT) consultation. Patients with orbital phycomycosis are given intravenous amphotericin B and require surgical intervention for debridement of infected tissue. Neurosurgical consultation may be needed for any intracranial involvement.

CAVERNOUS SINUS THROMBOSIS

ESSENTIALS OF DIAGNOSIS

▸ Complication from facial or sinus infections

▸ Decreased vision associated with headache, nausea, fever, chills, and other signs of systemic infection

▸ Early administration of parenteral antibiotics

▸ General Considerations

Cavernous sinus thrombosis is usually associated with orbital and ocular signs and symptoms. The infection results from hematogenous spread from a distant site or from local extension from the throat, face, paranasal sinuses, or orbits. Cavernous sinus thrombosis starts as a unilateral infection and commonly spreads to involve the other cavernous sinus.

▸ Clinical Findings

The patient may complain of chills, headache, lethargy, nausea, pain, and decreased vision. Fever, vomiting, and other systemic signs of infection may be present. Ophthalmologic examination discloses unilateral or bilateral exophthalmos, absent pupillary reflexes, and papilledema. Involvement of the third, fourth, and sixth cranial nerves or of the ophthalmic branch of the fifth nerve leads to limitation of ocular movement and decrease in corneal sensation.

▸ Treatment and Disposition

Obtain blood cultures and start appropriate antibiotics (nafcillin, plus a third-generation cephalosporin). Consider vancomycin if methicillin-resistant *S. aureus* is suspected or prevalent. Obtain CT scan of the head and orbits. Seek ophthalmologic, neurologic, and medical consultation early. Although controversial, anticoagulation with heparin can be safely considered for patients with a deteriorating clinical condition after excluding intracranial hemorrhage radiologically.

ENDOPHTHALMITIS

ESSENTIALS OF DIAGNOSIS

▸ Pus in anterior chamber (hypopyon) is diagnostic

▸ Obtain emergency ophthalmology consultation for drainage and antibiotic treatment

▸ General Considerations

Endophthalmitis is an acute microbial infection confined within the globe. Infection involving the sclera as well as other intraocular structures is called panophthalmitis. Infections of the globe can be exogenous or endogenous. Exogenous infection results from penetrating injury or may follow intraocular surgery or a ruptured corneal ulcer. Endogenous infection by the hematogenous route is less common and may be accompanied by fever and chills.

▸ Clinical Findings

The patient complains of pain, blurred vision, and photophobia. Examination discloses redness and chemosis of the conjunctiva, swelling of the eyelid, hypopyon (pus in the anterior chamber), and cloudy media (fundus hazily seen, or absent red reflex).

▸ Treatment and Disposition

Send blood culture, obtain emergency ophthalmologic consultation, and give sedation and analgesics. The patient may have to undergo anterior chamber tap and vitreous aspiration (by an ophthalmologist). Send specimens obtained for staining with Giemsa and Gram stains and for cultures on appropriate media.

Check stained smears of ocular fluid, and if no organisms are seen, give empiric subconjunctival and systemic antibiotics (vancomycin and an aminoglycoside or third-generation cephalosporin) while results of culture are pending.

RETINAL DETACHMENT

ESSENTIALS OF DIAGNOSIS

▸ Painless decrease in vision

▸ History of flashes of light, then "curtain" in visual field

▸ Urgent consultation for surgical repair

▸ General Considerations

Detachment of the retina is actually separation of the neurosensory layer from the retinal pigment epithelium. Sub-retinal fluid accumulates under the neurosensory layer. Detachment may become bilateral in one-fourth of cases. Retinal detachment is more common in older people and in those who are highly myopic. Hereditary factors may also play a role. Three types of primary retinal detachment are recognized: (1) rhegmatogenous detachment (most common), from retinal holes or breaks; (2) exudative detachment, usually from inflammation; and (3) traction detachment, which occurs when vitreous bands pull on the retina.

Minimal to moderate trauma to the eye may cause retinal detachment, but in such cases predisposing factors such as changes in the vitreous, retina, and choroid play an important role in pathogenesis. Severe trauma may cause retinal tears and detachment even if there are no predisposing factors.

► Clinical Findings

The patient complains of painless decrease in vision and may give a history of flashes of lights or sparks. Loss of vision may be described as a curtain in front of the eye or as cloudy or smoky. Central vision may not be affected if the macular area is not involved; this frequently causes a delay in seeking treatment. Patients in whom the macula is detached present to the emergency department with sudden deterioration of vision.

IOP is normal or low. The detached retina appears gray, with white folds and globular bullae. Round holes or horseshoe-shaped tears may be seen by indirect ophthalmoscopy in the rhegmatogenous detachment. Vitreous bands or other changes may be seen in the traction type of detachment.

► Differential Diagnosis

Primary retinal detachment should be differentiated from detachment secondary to other causes, for example, from preeclampsia–eclampsia or tumors of the choroid.

► Treatment and Disposition

Arrange for referral to an ophthalmologist. If the macula is attached and central visual acuity is normal, urgent surgery, which is successful in about 80% of cases, may be indicated. If the macula is detached or threatened, operation should be scheduled on an urgent basis, because prolonged detachment of the macula results in permanent loss of central vision.

TOXIC CAUSES OF BLINDNESS

A wide variety of organic chemicals may lead to visual deterioration. Ingestion of chemicals that cause corneal or lenticular opacities usually leads to insidious onset of visual loss. Ingestion of compounds that cause damage to nervous tissue may lead to slow or rapid deterioration of vision. Exposure to toxic doses of methanol, halogenated hydrocarbons (eg, methyl chloride), arsenic, and lead may cause permanent visual damage. Acute or chronic administration of drugs such as ethambutol, chloramphenicol, quinine, and salicylates may also cause optic neuritis and loss of vision.

By far the most common toxic cause of blindness is methanol (methyl alcohol). Ingestion of only a few milliliters may cause permanent blindness. Acute methanol poisoning causes nausea, vomiting, and abdominal pain. Headache, dizziness, and delirium may occur. Loss of vision may be complete and sudden within a few hours after drinking methanol or may occasionally be noted about 3 days after exposure. Pupillary reflexes are sluggish. Ophthalmoscopic examination shows swelling and hyperemia of the optic nerve head, distention of the veins, and peripapillary edema of the retina.

Hospitalize the patient immediately. See Chapter 47 for details of evaluation and treatment.

Bagwell SH, Seupaul RA: Images in emergency medicine. Orbital cellulitis. Ann Emerg Med 2006;48:633,639 [PMID: 17052567].

Bertino JS: Impact of antibiotic resistance in the management of ocular infections: the role of current and future antibiotics. Clin Ophthalmol 2009;3:507–521 [PMID:19789660].

Canadian Ophthalmological Society: Assessment of the red eye. http://www.eyesite.ca/7modules/Module2/html/Mod2Sec1.html (last accessed on July 31, 2010).

Chuah JL, Ghosh YK, Richards D: Ocular ischemic syndrome: a medical emergency. Lancet 2006;367:1370 [PMID: 16631917].

Dargin JM, Lowenstein RA: The painful eye. Emerg Med Clin North Am 2008;26:199–216 [PMID: 18249263].

Naradzay J, Barish RA: Approach to ophthalmologic emergencies. Med Clin North Am 2006;90:305–328 [PMID: 16448877].

Vortmann M, Schneider JI: Acute monocular visual loss. Emerg Med Clin North Am 2008;26:73–96 [PMID: 18249258].

▼ NONTRAUMATIC OCULAR EMERGENCIES

ACUTE DACRYOCYSTITIS

ESSENTIALS OF DIAGNOSIS

► Swelling, redness, and tenderness over the lacrimal sac on the lateral, proximal aspect of the nose

► Warm compresses and systemic antibiotics for treatment

► General Considerations

Acute infection of the lacrimal sac occurs in children and adults as a complication of nasolacrimal duct obstruction. The most frequently encountered causative organism is *S pneumoniae*.

► Clinical Findings

The patient complains of pain. There may be a history of tearing and discharge. Examination discloses swelling, redness, and tenderness over the lacrimal sac (Figure 31–4).

Pus should be collected, for Gram-stained smear and culture, by applying pressure over the lacrimal sac.

► Treatment

Begin systemic antibiotics with cephalexin or amoxicillin–clavulanate. Topical antibiotic drops may also be used, but

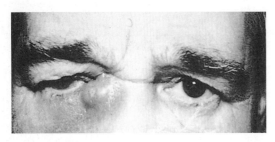

▲ **Figure 31–4.** Acute dacryocystitis. (Reproduced, with permission, from Riordan-Eva P, Whitcher JP, eds. Vaughan & Asbury's *General Ophthalmology*, 17th ed. New York, NY: McGraw-Hill; 2008.)

not alone. Use warm compresses 3–4 times daily. Consider incision and drainage of a pointing abscess.

 Disposition

The patient can be discharged to home care with a prescription for systemic antibiotics and instruction in how to apply warm local compresses. Consult an ophthalmologist for consideration of surgical correction. The patient should be seen again within 1–3 days.

ACUTE DACRYOADENITIS

> ### ESSENTIALS OF DIAGNOSIS
>
> ▶ Swelling, erythema, and pain at the lacrimal gland located at the temporal aspect of the upper eyelid

 Clinical Findings

Infection and inflammation of the lacrimal gland is characterized by swelling, pain, tenderness, and redness over the upper temporal aspect of the upper eyelid.

 Differential Diagnosis

Acute dacryoadenitis must be differentiated from viral infection (mumps), sarcoidosis, Sjögren's syndrome, tumors, leukemia, and lymphoma.

 Treatment

Purulent bacterial infections should be treated by incision and drainage of localized pus collections, antibiotics, warm compresses, and systemic analgesics. Viral dacryoadenitis (mumps) is treated conservatively.

 Disposition

The patient should be referred to an ophthalmologist for follow-up care in 2–3 days.

ACUTE HORDEOLUM (STYE)

 ### ESSENTIALS OF DIAGNOSIS

▶ Pain and redness with swelling over the eyelid

▶ Warm compresses and topical antibiotic three times daily

 General Considerations

Acute hordeolum is a common infection of the lid glands: the meibomian glands (internal hordeolum) and the glands of Zeis or Moll (external hordeolum). The most frequent causative organism is *S. aureus.*

 Clinical Findings

A stye is characterized by pain and redness with variable swelling over the eyelid. A large hordeolum may rarely be associated with swelling of the preauricular lymph node on the affected side, fever, and leukocytosis.

 Treatment

If pus is localized and pointing out to the skin or conjunctiva, a horizontal incision may be made through the skin or a vertical incision through the conjunctiva.

 Disposition

The patient can be discharged to continue treatment with warm compresses three times daily and topical antibiotic ointment (erythromycin 0.5% or gentamicin 0.3%) twice daily at home.

EYELID INFECTIONS (PRESEPTAL CELLULITIS)

> ### ESSENTIALS OF DIAGNOSIS
>
> ▶ Pain, tenderness, edema, and erythema around the eye
>
> ▶ No pain with ocular movement
>
> ▶ Antibiotic treatment and daily follow-up to ensure that the infection does not progress to orbital cellulitis

General Considerations

Preseptal cellulitis is an infectious process of the eyelid. Common causative organisms are *S. aureus*, streptococci, and *H. influenzae*. Viral causes should be considered if associated with a skin rash (eg, herpes zoster).

Clinical Findings

There is tenderness, erythema, and edema of the eyelid. No proptosis, pain with ocular movement, or restriction of extraocular motility is present. If any of these are present, consider orbital cellulitis.

Treatment

Give amoxicillin-clavulanate or cephalexin for 10 days. Antivirals may be considered if herpes zoster is suspected. Incision and drainage may be needed in more severe cases.

Disposition

The patient can be discharged with daily follow-up. If the patient fails antibiotics or has worsening symptoms, administer intravenous antibiotics and obtain ophthalmology or ENT consultation.

SPONTANEOUS SUBCONJUNCTIVAL HEMORRHAGE

ESSENTIALS OF DIAGNOSIS

▶ Painless collection of blood in the subconjunctival tissue
▶ Vision is not affected

General Considerations

Rupture of small subconjunctival vessel that occurs spontaneously or preceded by a bout of coughing, sneezing, or vomiting.

Clinical Findings

Bright red to dark maroon blood underneath the conjunctiva. Painless with no visual loss. Check for hypertension or coagulopathies with recurrent or bilateral hemorrhage.

Treatment and Disposition

The best treatment is observation, although many patients are very concerned and require extensive reassurance before leaving the emergency department. Consider using artificial tear drops or ointment if needed for protruding chemotic tissue.

CONJUNCTIVITIS

ESSENTIALS OF DIAGNOSIS

▶ Most frequent cause of red eye
▶ Purulent drainage and conjunctival hyperemia help with diagnosis

General Considerations

Conjunctivitis is the most frequent cause of red eye. It should be dealt with as an urgent medical problem until it is certain that the process is under control.

Causes of Acute Conjunctivitis

A. Infection

Acute conjunctivitis may be caused by bacterial, viral, parasitic, fungal, or chlamydial infection.

B. Chemical Irritation

Chemical irritations causing acute conjunctivitis include chlorine gas and tear gas.

C. Allergy

Allergic causes of acute conjunctivitis include vernal keratoconjunctivitis, hay fever, and other common allergens.

D. Skin Disorders

Skin disorders such as Stevens–Johnson syndrome, acne rosacea, Lyell disease, Kawasaki disease, and psoriasis may cause acute conjunctivitis.

E. Systemic Disorders

Sjögren's syndrome and vitamin A deficiency may cause acute conjunctivitis.

Clinical Findings

(See Table 31–2.) The patient complains of a "scratchy" sensation or pain, with conjunctival discharge. One or both eyes may be affected. Adherence of the eyelids upon awakening is common in bacterial conjunctivitis.

Examination discloses conjunctival hyperemia, purulent or mucopurulent discharge, and variable degrees of lid swelling. In appropriate cases, material may be taken from the conjunctival sac for smear (Gram and Giemsa stains) and culture on blood and chocolate agar. Viral cultures may also be indicated.

Table 31–2. Differential Diagnosis of Conjunctivitis.

Clinical Features	Bacterial	Chlamydial	Viral	Allergic	Irritant
Onset	Acute	Acute or subacute.	Acute or subacute	Recurrent	Acute
Pain	Moderate	Mild to moderate	Mild to moderate	None	None to mild
Discharge	Copious, purulent	Moderate, purulent	Moderate, seropurulent	Moderate, clear	Minimal, clear
Gram-stained smear	PMNs, bacteria	PMNs, monocytes, no bacteria	PMNs, monocytes, no bacteria	Eosinophils present	Negative
Routine culture	Usually *Staphylococcus aureus*, pneumococci	Negative	Negative	Negative	Negative
Special culture	...	*Chlamydia*	Adenoviruses; occasionally enteroviruses; rarely others	Negative	Negative
Preauricular adenopathy	Common	Common	Common	No	Rare

PMNs = polymorphonuclear neutrophils

Treatment

Prescribe topical sulfacetamide 10% eye drops, or ciprofloxacin 0.3% eye drops four times daily, and erythromycin or tetracycline ophthalmic ointment at bedtime for suspected bacterial conjunctivitis.

For suspected chlamydial infection (eg, history of urethritis), prescribe topical and systemic tetracycline or erythromycin. Give 0.5 g four times daily for 21 days (adult dose). Doxycycline, 100 mg twice daily, may be substituted for tetracycline. Consider treatment for gonorrhea.

Disposition

Discharge patients to home care with instructions to return for follow-up in 48–72 hours. Patients who do not respond to treatment should be referred to an ophthalmologist.

BACTERIAL CORNEAL ULCER

ESSENTIALS OF DIAGNOSIS

▶ Examination with fluorescein aids in diagnosis
▶ Antibiotic treatment and close follow-up are mandatory
▶ Common in contact lens wearers

General Considerations

Corneal infections may be due to bacteria, viruses, chlamydia, or fungi. The conjunctiva may or may not be involved. Bacterial corneal ulcers are serious, because rapid perforation of the cornea and loss of aqueous humor may occur; bacterial endophthalmitis may occur if bacterial ulcers are not properly treated.

Clinical Findings

The patient complains of pain and photophobia, blurring of vision, and eye irritation. Examination discloses conjunctival hyperemia and chemosis, corneal ulceration, or whitish–yellowish infiltration. The examination is facilitated by fluorescein staining and inspection with ultraviolet light. Hypopyon may be present. Scrapings from the cornea should be taken for culture and staining with Gram and Giemsa stains.

Differential Diagnosis

See Table 31–1.

Treatment and Disposition

Management of bacterial corneal infections causing corneal ulcers must be instituted as early as possible. Ophthalmologic consultation should be obtained urgently.

VIRAL KERATOCONJUNCTIVITIS

ESSENTIALS OF DIAGNOSIS

▶ Unilateral redness and pain with palpebral conjunctival follicles
▶ Adenovirus is most common; however, antibiotic eye drops are commonly used

▶ Clinical Findings

Viral keratoconjunctivitis is an acute conjunctivitis and keratitis caused most frequently by adenovirus (types 8 and 19). The patient complains of eye redness associated with tearing and moderate pain. The onset is often unilateral, and this eye is more severely affected. Photophobia may be intense and noted 5–14 days after onset. Examination discloses swelling of the eyelids and bulbar conjunctival hyperemia, with follicles and possibly a pseudomembrane noted over the palpebral conjunctiva. A tender preauricular lymph node can often be palpated. Subconjunctival hemorrhage may occur within 48 hours. Corneal epithelial keratitis accompanies the conjunctivitis, but subepithelial opacities are not seen until 5–14 days after onset of symptoms.

In adults, the disease is confined to the external eye. Children may have fever, pharyngitis, and diarrhea (pharyngoconjunctival fever). Staining of conjunctival scrapings with Giemsa stain demonstrates a predominantly mononuclear inflammatory reaction. When pseudomembranes occur, polymorphonuclear neutrophils may be seen. Culture for adenovirus is usually positive in the first 2 weeks after onset. Chlamydial conjunctivitis should always be considered in the differential diagnosis.

▶ Treatment

Treatment is symptomatic. Topical decongestants may be helpful. Dark glasses may relieve photophobia. If the diagnosis is uncertain, send material for bacterial culture, and start sulfacetamide, 10% eye drops four times daily, and tetracycline, 1% (10 mg/g) ointment twice daily, while awaiting laboratory results.

Since epidemics have been caused by iatrogenic spread of the viral agent, handwashing and other preventive measures are of utmost importance.

▶ Disposition

The patient should be discharged with follow-up in 2–3 days. Patients should take care to avoid spread of virus from ocular secretions to other family members and coworkers. Ideally, they should be off work until symptoms resolve.

ACUTE HYDROPS OF THE CORNEA

ESSENTIALS OF DIAGNOSIS

▶ Sudden, painless decrease in vision
▶ Unaffected eye shows keratoconus

▶ General Considerations

Acute hydrops of the cornea may occur in patients with keratoconus who develop rupture of Descemet's membrane, with resulting infiltration of the corneal stroma by aqueous humor. This may occur suddenly, resulting in corneal clouding.

▶ Clinical Findings

The typical presentation is of sudden, painless, marked decrease in visual acuity in a patient with keratoconus. There may be mild eye irritation, and the cornea is cloudy as a result of corneal edema. Bacterial or viral keratitis must be ruled out.

▶ Treatment

Hypertonic eye drops, for example, sodium chloride, 2% or 5% solution, should be instilled four times daily for 1 week. Apply a stream of hot air twice daily by hair dryer to speed dehydration of the cornea. Avoid rubbing the eye.

▶ Disposition

Refer the patient to an ophthalmologist within 24–72 hours.

HYPHEMA

ESSENTIALS OF DIAGNOSIS

▶ Sudden decrease in visual acuity
▶ Sitting the patient up can aid in the diagnosis, because blood will accumulate inferiorly
▶ Must check IOP

▶ General Considerations

Hyphema (blood in the anterior chamber) is usually caused by nonperforating trauma to the eye. In rare instances, hyphema may occur spontaneously as a complication of an ocular or systemic disorder or anticoagulation.

▶ Clinical Findings

Hyphema is characterized by sudden decrease in visual acuity. If the IOP is elevated, there may be pain in the eye with or without headache. The whole anterior chamber may be filled with blood, or a blood level may be seen. The conjunctiva may be hyperemic with perilimbal injection.

▶ Treatment

Elevate the patient's head 30°. Cover the affected eye with a shield. Ophthalmologic consultation is needed.

Recently, intracameral injection (performed by an ophthalmologist) of 25 µg of t-PA has been shown to expedite the resorption of blood clots in the anterior chamber. Aminocaproic acid can be used topically to stabilize the clot and decrease the rate of rebleeding.

▶ Disposition

Acute care and evaluation by an ophthalmologist is essential. Operative evacuation of nonabsorbed blood clots may be required. Recurrence of bleeding on the third to fifth days following injury is not uncommon. Patients with hyphema should have daily follow-up for 5 days and then as directed by the ophthalmologist.

UVEITIS (IRITIS AND IRIDOCYCLITIS)

ESSENTIALS OF DIAGNOSIS

▶ Photophobia, pain, and constricted pupil secondary to ciliary spasm

▶ Mydriatics are key to treatment

▶ General Considerations

The uvea consists of the iris, ciliary body, and choroid. Anterior uveitis is inflammation of the iris and ciliary body, or iridocyclitis. Inflammation of all three structures is called panuveitis.

▶ Clinical Findings

(See Table 31–1.) The patient complains of blurred vision, photophobia, and head or ocular pain. Ciliary injection may be present around the limbus, and conjunctival injection may be minimal. IOP may be elevated. There is no conjunctival discharge.

▶ Treatment

Instill a cycloplegic mydriatic agent, such as tropicamide or cyclopentolate, 1% eye drops, one drop every 8 hours. If IOP is elevated, give acetazolamide, 250 mg orally every 6 hours. Prednisolone acetate, 1% eye drops, five times daily may be indicated after ophthalmologic consultation.

▶ Disposition

Patients with uveitis should be seen the next day for follow-up care. Continuing care should be by an ophthalmologist. The cause of uveitis should be investigated.

VITREOUS HEMORRHAGE

ESSENTIALS OF DIAGNOSIS

▶ Sudden, painless loss of vision

▶ Patient complains of seeing "floaters"

▶ Secondary to trauma, retinal detachment, or diabetic retinopathy

▶ Urgent ophthalmology consultation is needed

▶ General Considerations

Spontaneous hemorrhage into the vitreous body may result from local factors in the eye (eg, retinal tears, tumors, inflammation, venous occlusion, retinal detachment) or from associated systemic disorders (eg, hematopoietic diseases, diabetes mellitus, hypertension) (Table 31–3). Blood in the vitreous body clots rapidly, and removal of red blood cells is retarded because of the network of collagen fibers and hyaluronic acid.

▶ Clinical Findings

Vitreous hemorrhage is characterized by sudden, painless loss or deterioration of vision in the affected eye. The eye is not red. The red reflex of the fundus is hazy, faint, or becomes black. Details of the retina and optic nerve are obscured by the cloudy vitreous.

▶ Treatment and Disposition

The patient should be evaluated urgently by an ophthalmologist. Partial or total vitrectomy may have to be considered later if absorption of blood does not occur or vitreous clouding occurs secondary to organization of the blood clot. Photocoagulation of the neovascular network (ie, new blood vessel formation, as occurs in diabetic or sickle cell retinopathy), when present, may be considered in some cases as a prophylactic measure.

Table 31–3. Some Known Causes of Spontaneous Vitreous Hemorrhage not Associated with Trauma.

Diabetic retinopathy
Retinal tear
Posterior vitreous detachment
Retinal vein occlusion
Retinal detachment
Sickle cell disease
Ocular toxocariasis
Hypertension

Recent studies have shown that intravitreal injection of 25 μg of t-PA may be considered in selected patients with traumatic vitreous hemorrhage.

RETINAL HEMORRHAGE

ESSENTIALS OF DIAGNOSIS

► Painless loss of vision occurs if the hemorrhage is in the macular area
► May be asymptomatic

▶ General Considerations

Retinal hemorrhage may be due to trauma, local ocular disease, or systemic disorders (Table 31–4). Hemorrhages may occur in superficial or deep layers of the retina or in the preretinal or subhyaloid space.

▶ Clinical Findings

The patient may complain of sudden decrease in vision when hemorrhage occurs in the macular or perimacular area. Small peripheral retinal hemorrhages cause no symptoms. Superficial retinal hemorrhages occurring in the nerve fiber layer are bright red and flame-shaped on ophthalmoscopic examination. Deep retinal hemorrhages are round and have a dark red color. Subhyaloid hemorrhage occurs in the space between the vitreous body and the internal limiting membrane and may have a boat-shaped appearance. A neovascular network may rupture and cause retinal or vitreous hemorrhage.

Table 31–4. Systemic Conditions Associated with Retinal Hemorrhage.

Hypertension
Atherosclerosis
Diabetes mellitus
Hemoglobinopathies (eg, sickle cell disease)
Anemia
Subacute infective endocarditis
Leukemia, lymphoma
Hyperviscosity syndromes
Cancer (rarely) (eg, breast, eye)
Giant cell arteritis, Takayasu arteritis
Infections (eg, cytomegalovirus)
Autoimmune disease (eg, lupus erythematosus.
   polyarteritis nodosa)
Intracranial tumor
Anticoagulation

▶ Treatment and Disposition

There is no specific treatment. The patient should be referred to an ophthalmologist for further care and to prevent recurrences.

CENTRAL RETINAL VEIN OCCLUSION

ESSENTIALS OF DIAGNOSIS

► Unilateral, painless loss of vision
► Often in elderly with glaucoma or hypertension

▶ General Considerations

Central retinal vein occlusion occurs most frequently in elderly patients with glaucoma or hypertension. The incidence is also increased in diabetes mellitus, autoimmune diseases, Waldenström macroglobulinemia, cryoglobulinemia, sickle cell disease, polycythemia vera, and leukemia.

▶ Clinical Findings

The patient complains of sudden painless unilateral loss of vision. Ophthalmoscopy reveals dilated and tortuous veins, retinal and macular edema, multiple or diffuse retinal hemorrhages, and attenuated arterioles.

▶ Treatment and Disposition

There is no specific therapy. Refer the patient to an ophthalmologist for assessment of possible glaucoma or associated systemic disease. If local predisposing factors such as glaucoma are ruled out, patients with occlusion should have a complete medical evaluation.

OPTIC NEURITIS

ESSENTIALS OF DIAGNOSIS

► Painful unilaterally, especially with movement
► Afferent pupillary defect
► Many causes: case should be discussed with ophthalmologist or neurologist

▶ General Considerations

Optic neuritis may be due to a variety of causes, including demyelinating diseases; systemic infections; nutritional and metabolic disorders; exposure to toxic substances (eg, arsenic, methanol, lead, tobacco); vascular insufficiency; and local extension of infection from intraocular structures, sinuses, or meninges. Optic neuritis includes retrobulbar neuritis (inflammation of the optic nerve posterior to the globe), in which there are by definition no ophthalmoscopic findings.

▶ Clinical Findings

Typical age of presentation is 25–40 years and females are represented twice as often as males. The patient complains of rapidly decreased vision in one (or rarely both) eyes and sometimes pain on moving the eye. Loss of central vision, tenderness in the eye, and perception of color as dull may also be present. Uhtoff phenomenon (decreased vision with heat or exercise) may be present. The pupillary reflex is sluggish. Ophthalmoscopic examination in optic neuritis shows hyperemia of the optic nerve head (may not be present in retrobulbar neuritis), congestion of the large veins, blurring of the disc margin, peripapillary retinal edema, and flame-shaped hemorrhages near the optic nerve head. Visual field testing discloses a central scotoma.

▶ Treatment and Disposition

Treatment depends on the cause. Intravenous corticosteroids may be helpful in cases associated with demyelinating disease. The patient should be referred to an ophthalmologist or neurologist for further care within 1 or 2 days.

Dargin JM, Lowenstein RA: The painful eye. Emerg Med Clin North Am 2008;26:199–216 [PMID: 18249263].

eMedicine Ophthalmology. , Omaha, NE (last accessed on March 23, 2010).

German CA, Baumann MR, Hamzavi S: Ophthalmic diagnosis in the ED: optic neuritis. Am J Emerg Med 2007;25:834–837 [PMID: 17870491].

Khor WB, Aung T, Saw SM, Wong TY et al: An outbreak of Fusarium keratitis associated with contact lens wear in Singapore. JAMA 2006;295:2867–2873 [PMID: 16804153].

Sethuraman U, Kamat D: The red eye: Evaluation and management. Clin Pediatr 2000;48:588–600 [PMID:19357422].

▼ OCULAR BURNS AND TRAUMA

OCULAR BURNS

ESSENTIALS OF DIAGNOSIS

▶ History and physical examination

▶ Copious irrigation with normal saline, lactated Ringer's, or water after topical anesthetic is placed

▶ Check pH after irrigation; should be 6.8–7.4

▶ General Considerations

Apart from the history, the diagnosis of burns is usually based on the presence of swollen eyelids with marked conjunctival hyperemia and chemosis. The limbus may show patchy balanced areas with conjunctival sloughing, especially in the interpalpebral area. There is usually corneal haze and diffuse edema, with wide areas of epithelial cell loss and corneal ulcerations. Corneal ulcerations can be better visualized with blue light following instillation of fluorescein.

ALKALI BURNS

▶ Clinical Findings

Alkali burns (especially particulate alkali such as lime) are very serious, because even after apparent removal of the offending agent, tiny particles may remain lodged within the cul-de-sac and cause progressive damage to the eye.

▶ Treatment

Instill a topical anesthetic *immediately* (proparacaine, 0.5%; or tetracaine, 0.5%), and then copiously irrigate the eye with 2–3 L isotonic saline solution, water, or lactated Ringer's solution. A lid retractor may be useful.

Double eversion of the eyelids should be performed to look for and remove material lodged in the cul-de-sac. Solid particles of alkali should be removed with forceps or a moist cotton swab. After particles have been removed, irrigate again. *Do not attempt to neutralize the alkali with acid, because the exothermic reaction may cause further injury.*

Instill topical mydriatic, cycloplegic eye drops, and antibiotic ointment. After irrigation, the pH of the eye should be checked and the range should be 6.8–7.4. If the pH is still high, continue with irrigation. Parenteral narcotic analgesia is often required for pain relief. If IOP is elevated, begin treatment with acetazolamide.

▶ Disposition

Obtain ophthalmologic consultation.

ACID BURNS

▶ Clinical Findings

Acid burns as a rule cause damage more rapidly but are generally less serious than alkali burns, because they do not cause progressive destruction of ocular tissues (as do alkali burns).

▶ Treatment

Immediately after exposure, irrigate the eyes copiously with sterile isotonic saline solution, lactated Ringer's, or tap water. Topical anesthetic (proparacaine, 0.5%) may be instilled to minimize pain during irrigation. Do not attempt to neutralize the acid with alkali.

Parenteral or oral narcotic analgesics may be necessary. Patch the eye if corneal defects are present.

Disposition

Obtain ophthalmologic consultation.

THERMAL BURNS

Clinical Findings

Injury due to thermal burns of the eyelids, cornea, and conjunctiva may range from minimal to extensive. Superficial corneal burns have a good prognosis, though corneal ulcers may occur as a result of loss of corneal epithelium.

Thermal burns of the skin of the eyelids may be first, second, or third degree. Conjunctival hyperemia is noted. The cornea may show diffuse necrosis of the exposed corneal epithelium in the interpalpebral area. Corneal haze due to corneal edema is frequently seen in thermal burns of the cornea and may lead to decrease in vision.

Treatment

The treatment of ocular burns is similar to the treatment of burns occurring elsewhere on the body (Chapter 45). Provide systemic analgesia. Instill proparacaine, 0.5%, or tetracaine, 0.5%, to minimize pain during manipulation. In cases of corneal burns, instill a mydriatic agent.

Disposition

Obtain ophthalmologic consultation.

BURNS DUE TO ULTRAVIOLET RADIATION

Destruction of the corneal epithelium by ultraviolet light is known as actinic keratitis, snow blindness, and welder's arc burn (flash burn), depending on the source of ultraviolet radiation.

Clinical Findings

The patient complains of pain, extreme photophobia and gives a history of exposure to ultraviolet light 6–12 hours earlier (eg, skiing, welding, or tanning). Examination discloses tearing, conjunctival hyperemia, and corneal haziness. There may be a superficial punctate staining of the cornea seen with fluorescein and with magnification (eg, slit lamp).

Treatment

Topical anesthetic should be instilled during the eye examination only. Do not give the patient a topical anesthetic to use at home. Instill a mydriatic agent and an antibiotic ointment. Recovery occurs within 12–36 hours. Provide systemic analgesics for pain.

Disposition

Twenty-four hour follow-up should be arranged.

MECHANICAL TRAUMA TO THE EYE

 ESSENTIALS OF DIAGNOSIS

▶ History is key to diagnosis
▶ Careful examination is needed
▶ Can be complicated by other injuries

General Considerations

Ocular trauma may be classified as penetrating or nonpenetrating. Trauma can lead to serious damage and loss of vision. Eye injuries are common in spite of the protection afforded by the bony orbit and the cushioning effect of orbital fat. Prevention and occupational safety measures should be stressed.

Evaluation

Obtain a history of the injury from the patient or witness. Measure and record visual acuity with and without correction. Inspect the eyelids, conjunctiva, cornea, anterior chamber, pupils, lens, vitreous, and fundus for breaks in tissue and hemorrhage. Search for corneal lesions (eg, abrasion) by instilling fluorescein dye and examining the eye using a light with a light-blue filter.

X-ray examination or CT scan may be indicated to rule out radiopaque foreign bodies and to look for fractures of orbital bones.

Treatment and Disposition

Consult an ophthalmologist immediately for patients with sight-threatening injuries. Avoid causing further damage by manipulation. For more detailed discussion of Treatment and Disposition, see under the specific type of injury.

For severe pain, photophobia, or foreign body sensation, instill a topical anesthetic (eg, proparacaine, 0.5%, one or two drops once or twice). Systemic analgesics may be required. Cover the eye with an eye shield.

PENETRATING OR PERFORATING INJURIES

General Considerations

Penetrating or perforating ocular injuries require immediate careful attention and prompt surgical intervention to prevent possible loss of the eye and to preserve vision.

Many facial injuries, especially those occurring in automobile accidents, are associated with penetrating ocular trauma. Some injuries may be concealed and inapparent because of eyelid swelling or because the patient's other life-threatening injuries have (appropriately) dominated the attentions of the emergency department team. Such injuries, if not promptly attended to, may lead to loss of vision. Unfortunately, impaired or unconscious patients may have occult or untreated injuries as a cooperative patient is needed for an appropriate eye examination.

▶ Evaluation

Obtain and record a description of how the injury occurred. Examine the eye and ocular adnexa, including vision testing if the patient's condition permits. Do not apply pressure on the globe. In the appropriate setting, CT scan is indicated to rule out intraocular radiopaque foreign body and to look for fractures of orbital bones.

▶ Clinical Findings

Penetrating injuries are those that cause disruption of the outer coats of the eye (sclera, cornea) without interrupting the anatomic continuity of that layer, thus preventing prolapse or loss of ocular contents. Perforating injuries are those resulting in complete anatomic disruption (laceration) of the sclera or cornea. Such wounds may or may not be associated with prolapse of uveal structures. Wounds of the sclera or cornea are often associated with intraocular or intraorbital foreign bodies.

▶ Treatment

The objectives of emergency management of ocular penetrating or perforating injuries are to relieve pain, preserve or restore vision, and achieve a good cosmetic result. Relieve pain with systemic analgesia, as needed. A sedative may be required. Cover the eye with an eye shield. Patch the uninjured eye also to minimize ocular movements. Do not manipulate the eye, instill eye drops, or apply antibiotic treatment.

Give tetanus prophylaxis, if needed (Chapter 30). Prohibit oral intake until the patient is examined by an ophthalmologist, since urgent surgery may be required. Provide hydration with intravenous fluids.

Give parenteral antibiotics directed against gram-negative and gram-positive organisms. Give antiemetic agents to prevent further injury from IOP increase.

▶ Disposition

The patient should be seen on an emergency basis by an ophthalmologist for management of severe injuries, investigation of intraocular foreign bodies, and immediate surgical repair as required. Prompt repair of uveal prolapse decreases the risk of sympathetic ophthalmia in the uninjured eye. Delay in management of corneal lacerations may increase the risk of surgical and postoperative complications.

BLUNT TRAUMA TO THE EYE, ADNEXA, AND ORBIT

Contusions of the eyeball and ocular adnexa result from blunt trauma. The outcome of such an injury cannot always be determined, and the extent of damage may not be obvious upon superficial examination. Careful eye examination is needed, along with X-ray examination or CT scan when indicated.

▶ Types of Injury

A. Eyelids

Check the eyelids for ecchymosis, swelling, laceration, and abrasions.

B. Conjunctiva

Check the conjunctiva for subconjunctival hemorrhages or laceration of the conjunctiva.

C. Cornea

Check the cornea for abrasion, edema, laceration, or rupture.

D. Anterior Chamber

Check the anterior chamber for hyphema, recession of angle, or secondary glaucoma.

E. Iris

Check the iris for iridodialysis, iridoplegia, rupture of iris sphincter, iris prolapse through corneal or scleral lacerations, or iris atrophy.

F. Ciliary Body

Check the ciliary body for hyposecretion of aqueous humor or for ciliary body prolapse through scleral lacerations.

G. Lens

Check the lens for dislocation or cataract.

H. Vitreous

Check the vitreous for hemorrhage or prolapse.

I. Ciliary Muscle

Check the ciliary muscle for paralysis or spasm.

▶ Treatment and Disposition

Injury severe enough to cause intraocular hemorrhage (eg, vitreous hemorrhage or hyphema) involves the danger of delayed secondary hemorrhage from a damaged uveal vessel, which may cause intractable glaucoma and permanent damage to the globe. In such cases, ophthalmologic consultation is necessary to rule out other eye injuries.

Except for rupture of the globe itself, contusions do not usually require immediate definitive treatment. Apply an eye shield if the globe has been perforated and consult an ophthalmologist.

1. Ecchymosis of the Eyelids (Black Eye)

▶ Clinical Findings

Blood in the periorbital tissues may occur from direct trauma or a blow to adjacent areas. The loose subcutaneous tissue around the eye permits blood to spread extensively. The diagnosis is usually obvious. Always rule out trauma to the eye itself (hyphema, blowout fracture, or retinal detachment).

▶ Treatment

Apply cold compresses to decrease swelling and help stop bleeding. Exclude more serious ocular injury by careful examination.

▶ Disposition

If the eye itself is uninjured, no follow-up contact is necessary.

2. Lacerations of the Eyelids

▶ Clinical Findings

Lacerations or other wounds of the eyelids may be associated with serious ocular injuries not apparent at first examination. These could include injury to the lacrimal system, levator muscle, or optic nerve. A meticulous search for such injuries is indicated in every patient with eyelid lacerations.

▶ Treatment and Disposition

Patients with lacerations of the eyelids require suturing and an extensive eye evaluation. Lacerations involving the tarsal plate, the upper eyelid levator mechanism, medial canthal area, and all through and through should be repaired by an ophthalmologist.

3. Orbital Hemorrhage

▶ Clinical Findings

Exophthalmos and subconjunctival hemorrhage in a patient with a history of blunt trauma to the face suggest rupture of orbital blood vessels. There may be conjunctival chemosis or ecchymosis of the eyelids.

▶ Treatment and Disposition

Apply cold compresses, and obtain urgent ophthalmologic consultation.

4. Fracture of the Ethmoid Bone

The ethmoid bone is part of the medial wall of the orbit. Fracture of the ethmoid bone most frequently occurs with blunt trauma to the orbit.

▶ Clinical Findings

Fracture of the ethmoid bone is most commonly manifested by subcutaneous emphysema of the eyelids. There may or may not be ecchymosis of the eyelids. Imaging reveals air in the orbit. Fractures of other orbital bones should be ruled out by radiography.

▶ Treatment

Fractures of the ethmoid bone usually do not require operative reduction. Provide analgesia as needed. Apply cold compresses. Give systemic antibiotic. Instruct the patient to avoid sneezing or blowing the nose.

▶ Disposition

Refer the patient to an ophthalmologist or facial surgeon within 1 or 2 days.

5. Blowout Fractures of the Floor of the Orbit

▶ Clinical Findings

Blowout fracture may be associated with enophthalmos and hypotropia (visual axis of the injured eye is displaced downward in comparison to that of the sound eye), diplopia in the primary position or in upward gaze, limitation of ocular movement in upward gaze, and decreased or absent sensation over the maxilla. CT scan of the orbit shows orbital floor displacement.

▶ Treatment

Provide analgesia as needed. Apply a topical antibiotic ointment such as gentamicin, 0.3%. Apply cold compresses and a sterile eye patch.

▶ Disposition

Seek early consultation with an ophthalmologist or other facial surgeon.

6. Corneal Abrasions

 ESSENTIALS OF DIAGNOSIS

- ▶ Pain, photophobia, blurry vision
- ▶ Uptake of fluorescein stain is key to diagnosis
- ▶ Always rule out globe perforation

▶ Clinical Findings

The patient complains of pain, photophobia, and blurring of vision. There is usually a history of trivial trauma. Patients with severe pain and blepharospasm may require proparacaine, 0.5%, instilled in the eye to facilitate eye examination. In severe cases, the eye is red and the corneal surface is irregular and loses its normal luster. Staining with fluorescein reveals a defect in the corneal epithelium. Rule out infection or perforation of the globe as necessary.

▶ Treatment

Irrigate the eye gently with sterile saline solution if needed to remove debris and loose foreign bodies. In severe cases, instill tropicamide to relax the ciliary muscle and relieve pain. Instill ophthalmic antibiotic ointment. *Caution:* Do not use ointment containing corticosteroids. Consider nonsteroidal antiinflammatory ophthalmic drops for pain control. Provide systemic analgesia as needed. Never give the patient topical anesthetics, which may lead to irreversible corneal damage.

▶ Disposition

Refer patients for daily outpatient follow-up care. Ophthalmologic consultation should be obtained for corneal abrasions that fail to resolve in 48–72 hours.

7. Corneal and Conjunctival Foreign Bodies

ESSENTIALS OF DIAGNOSIS

- ▶ Pain, foreign body sensation
- ▶ Examine using fluorescein stain; make sure to look under lids
- ▶ May need to rule out intraocular foreign body

▶ Clinical Findings

There may be a history of working with high-speed tempered steel tools (eg, drilling), or there may be no history of trauma to the eye and the patient may even be unaware of a foreign body in the eye. In most cases, however, the patient complains of a foreign body sensation in the eye or under the eyelid, or just irritation in the eye. A corneal foreign body can be seen with the aid of a loupe and well-focused diffuse light or slit lamp. Conjunctival foreign bodies often become embedded in the conjunctiva under the upper eyelid. The lid must be everted to facilitate inspection and removal.

Fluorescein should be instilled to visualize minute foreign bodies not readily visible with the naked eye, loupe, or slit lamp. Rule out intraocular foreign body with soft tissue X-ray or CT scan as indicated.

▶ Treatment

Some loose foreign bodies can be removed with a moist cotton swab. Foreign bodies superficially embedded can be removed with the tip of a hypodermic needle or blunt spud.

Anesthetize the cornea first with proparacaine or tetracaine solution, 0.5%. Instill ophthalmic antibiotic ointment (gentamicin, 0.3%; or sulfacetamide, 10%) or eye drops after the foreign body has been successfully removed.

▶ Disposition

The patient should be seen again in 24 hours unless they have no symptoms or changes in vision. Referral to an ophthalmologist may be indicated for deep corneal foreign bodies or large foreign bodies within the visual axis.

8. Traumatic Lens Dislocation and Cataract Formation

▶ Clinical findings

Lens dislocation following blunt trauma to the eye may present with double vision in one eye (rarely both), blurred vision, and distortion. A tremor of the iris after rapid eye movements may also be present. The lens may be visualized by ophthalmoscopy or imaging with CT scan. History and physical are critical to diagnosis. Lens dislocation may also be associated with medical disorders, such as Marfan syndrome, homocystinuria, or spherophakia. Lens dislocation becomes an emergency if the subluxed lens (anterior subluxation) obstructs aqueous flow, leading to acute glaucoma. If the lens capsule is disrupted, the stroma of the lens may swell and become cloudy, also leading to acute glaucoma and development of cataracts. These may also be present after lightning strike or electrical injury.

▶ Treatment

Patients with lens dislocation should be referred to an ophthalmologist for surgical repair, with emergent referral for increased IOP. There is no treatment for traumatic cataracts.

▶ Disposition

Emergent ophthalmology referral for dislocation associated with increased IOP, otherwise timely referral to ophthalmologist is sufficient.

Allman KJ, Smiddy WE, Banta J et al: Ocular trauma and visual outcome secondary to paintball projectiles. Am J Ophthalmol 2009;147:239–242 [PMID: 18835471].

Bord SP, Linden J: Trauma to the globe and orbit. Emerg Med Clin North Am 2008;26:97–123 [PMID: 18249259].

Burger BM, Kelty PJ, Bowie EM: Ocular nail gun injuries: epidemiology and visual outcomes. J Trauma 2009;67:1320–1322 [PMID: 20009684].

Hahn B, Kass D, McCarroll N: Elderly woman with eye pain: ectopia lentis. Ann Emerg Med 2008;52:474,481 [PMID: 18809110].

McGwin G, Jr, Owsley C: Incidence of emergency department-treated eye injury in the United States. Arch Ophthalmol 2005;123:662–666 [PMID: 15883286].

Naradzay J, Barish RA: Approach to ophthalmologic emergencies. Med Clin North Am 2006;90:305–328 [PMID: 16448877].

Ng W, Chehade M: Taser penetrating ocular injury. Am J Ophthalmol 2005;139:713–715 [PMID: 15808172].

Pokhrel PK, Loftus SA: Ocular emergencies. Am Fam Physician 2007;76:829–836 [PMID: 17910297].

Soparkar CN, Patrinely JR: The eye examination in facial trauma for the plastic surgeon. Plast Reconstr Surg 2007;120:49S–56S [PMID: 18090728].

Steinberg DA, Leslie CL: Traumatic dislocation of the crystalline lens. J Trauma 2005;58:213–214 [PMID: 15674178].

▼ EQUIPMENT AND SUPPLIES

▶ Basic Equipment

A great many specialized instruments have been devised for the investigation of eye disorders. Most emergency conditions can be diagnosed with the aid of a few relatively simple instruments. The following should be available in the emergency department:

- Hand held flashlight with fresh batteries
- Slit lamp
- Ophthalmoscope (preferably with a blue filter lens)
- Visual acuity chart (Snellen)
- Tonometer
- Pinhole and occluder
- Eye shield (plastic or metal) and tape

▶ Basic Medications

See Table 31–5.

A. Local Anesthetics

Proparacaine, 0.5%, or tetracaine, 0.5%, may be used. These medications have white caps on the bottles.

B. Dyes

Fluorescein papers or drops should be available.

C. Mydriatics

These medications have red caps on the bottles. Tropicamide ophthalmic solution, 0.5% or 1%, is a satisfactory mydriatic when the examiner wishes to obtain a clear view of the lens, vitreous, or ocular fundus. It may also be used for short-term relief for ciliary spasm.

D. Miotics

Miotic drops have green caps. The miotic agent pilocarpine, 1% or 2%, should be on hand.

E. Antibacterial Agents

Antibacterial agents include tetracycline, 1% ophthalmic ointment; polymyxin B-bacitracin ophthalmic ointment; sulfacetamide, 10% ophthalmic solution or ointment; erythromycin, 0.5% ointment; ciprofloxacin, 0.3% drops; and polymyxin B trimethoprim solution or gentamicin, 0.3% ointment.

▼ COMMON TECHNIQUES FOR TREATMENT OF OCULAR DISORDERS

▶ Eversion of the Upper Eyelid

The patient is instructed to look down. Grasp the eyelashes at the outer margin of the lid with the thumb and forefinger of one hand, and gently and slowly draw the lid downward and outward. Using a cotton swab, press against the upper edge of the tarsus over the center of the lid while turning the lid margin rapidly outward and upward over the applicator. With the lashes thus held against the upper orbital rim, the exposed palpebral conjunctiva can be inspected closely. After the examination is completed and the foreign body removed (if possible), when the patient looks up, the lid returns to its normal position.

▶ Eye drops

The patient should sit with both eyes open and looking up. Pull down slightly on the lower lid, and place two drops in the lower cul-de-sac. The patient is then asked to look down while finger contact on the lower lid is maintained. Do not let the patient squeeze the eye shut. Do not touch the eye or the eyelid with the applicator; likewise, do not instill eye drops with the dropper held far away from the eye.

▶ Ointments

Ointments are instilled in the same way as liquids. While the patient is looking up, lift out the lower lid to trap the medication in the conjunctival sac.

▶ Warm Compresses

Use a clean towel or washcloth soaked in warm tap water well below the temperature that will burn the thin skin covering the eyelids. Warm compresses are usually applied to the area for 15 minutes four times daily. The therapeutic rational is to increase blood flow to the affected area and decrease pain and inflammation.

▶ Removal of Superficial Corneal Foreign Body

The main considerations are good illumination, magnification, anesthesia, proper positioning of the patient, and

Table 31–5. Commonly Used Ophthalmic Medications.

Medication	Indication	Dosage, Forms, and Duration
Antimicrobials		
Bacitracin Bacitracin and polymyxin B (Polysporin)	Gram-positive organisms	Ophthalmic ointment: place ointment four times daily for 7–10 days
Chloramphenicol (Chloroptic)	Gram-positive and gram-negative organisms	0.5% solution, 1% ointment: 1–2 drops or place ointment 3–6 times daily for 7–10 days
Ciprofloxacin (Ciloxan) Norfloxacin (Chibroxin) Ofloxacin (Ocuflox)	Gram-positive and gram-negative organisms	0.3% solutions for conjunctivitis: 1–2 drops every 2 hours for 2 days, then every 4 hours for 5 days For ulcer, two drops every 15 minutes for 6 hours, then two drops every 30 minutes for the next 18 hours; day 2, use two drops every hour; days 3–14, use two drops every 4 hours
Erythromycin (Ilotycin)	Gram-positive organisms, *Chlamydia*	0.5 % ointment 4 times a day for 5–7 days
Gentamicin (Genoptic, Garamycin) Tobramycin (Tobrex) Neomycin with bacitracin and polymyxin B (Neosporin)	Gram-positive and gram-negative organisms; covers *Pseudomonas*	Gentamicin and tobramycin as 0.3% solution and 0.3% ointment Neomycin, 1–2 drops every 2–4 hours 10 days; for ointment, use 2–4 hours for 7–10 days
Polymyxin B & trimethoprim (Polytrim)	Gram-positive organisms	Ophthalmic solution: one drop every 3 hours for 7–10 days
Sulfacetamide sodium (Bleph-10, Sulamyd)	Gram-positive and gram-negative organisms; does not cover *Pseudomonas*	10%, 15%, 30% solutions: two drops every 2–3 hours for 7–10 days 10% ointment; place ointment every 3–4 hours for 7–10 days
Trifluridine (Viroptic)	Herpes	1% solution: one drop every 2 hours while awake with maximum nine drops per day; after reepithelialization, decrease to one drop every 4 hours for 7 days
Mydriatics		
Atropine sulfate	Dilation, uveitis, cycloplegia	0.25–2% solution; lasts 2 weeks
Cyclopentolate (Cyclogyl)	Dilation, cycloplegia	2–5% solution; lasts 48 hours
Phenylephrine (Neosynephreine)[a]	Dilation, no cycloplegia	2.5–10% solution; lasts 2–3 hours
Scopolamine (Hyoscine)	Dilation, cycloplegia	0.25% solution; lasts 7 days
Anesthetics[b]		
Proparacaine (Ophthetic Alcaine)	Local anesthesia	0.5% solution
Tetracaine (Pontocaine)	Local anesthesia	0.5% solution

[a]Cardiac patients should not use phenylephrine.
[b]Anesthetics should not be prescribed for unsupervised use.

sterile technique. The patient's visual acuity should be recorded first.

The patient may be sitting or supine. A loupe should be used unless a slit lamp is available. An assistant should direct a strong flashlight into the eye at an oblique angle. The examiner may then see the corneal foreign body and remove it with a moist cotton swab. If this is not successful, the foreign body may be removed with a metal spud while the lids are held apart with the other hand to prevent blinking. An antibacterial ointment may be instilled after the foreign body has been removed.

Home Medication

At home, the same techniques should be used as described above except that drops should be instilled with the patient lying supine. Experienced patients (eg, those with glaucoma) are usually quite skillful in self-administration of eye drops.

Tonometry

Tonometry is the determination of IOP using a special instrument that measures the amount of corneal indentation produced by a given weight. Tonometry readings should be taken on any patient suspected of having increased IOP.

A. Precautions

Tonometry should be done with great caution on patients with corneal ulcers. It is extremely important to clean the tonometer before each use by carefully wiping the footplate with a cotton swab moistened with sterile solution (be sure it is dry before using) and to sterilize the instrument. Corneal abrasions are rarely caused by tonometry. Epidemic keratoconjunctivitis can be spread by tonometry, and this can be prevented if the tonometer is cleaned before each use and the principle of handwashing between patients is meticulously observed. Disposable covers are also available for some tonometers.

B. Technique

Anesthetic solution (tetracaine, 0.5%; or proparacaine, 0.5%) is instilled into each eye. The patient lies supine and is asked to stare at a spot on the ceiling with both eyes or at a finger held directly in the line of gaze overhead. The lids are held open without applying pressure on the globe. The tonometer is then placed on the corneal surface of each eye and the scale reading taken from the tonometer. The IOP is determined by referring to a chart that converts the scale reading to millimeters of mercury for a Schiotz tonometer or by digital readout on the electronic devices. Normal IOP is 12–20 mm Hg.

C. Interpretation of Abnormalities

If the IOP is 20 mm Hg or more, further investigation is indicated to determine whether glaucoma is present.

Corneal Staining

Corneal staining consists of instillation of fluorescein into the conjunctival sac to outline irregularities of the corneal surface. Staining is indicated in corneal trauma or other corneal disorders (eg, herpes simplex keratitis) when examination with a loupe or slit lamp in the absence of a stain has not been satisfactory.

A. Precautions

Because the corneal epithelium—the chief barrier to corneal infection—is usually interrupted when corneal staining is indicated, be certain that whatever dye is used (particularly fluorescein) is sterile.

B. Equipment and Materials

Note: Fluorescein must be sterile. Fluorescein papers or sterile individual dropper units are safest. Fluorescein solution from a dropper bottle may be used, but there is a substantial risk of contamination.

C. Technique

The individually wrapped fluorescein paper is wetted with sterile saline or touched to the wet conjunctiva so that a thin film of fluorescein spreads over the corneal surface. Any irregularity in the cornea is stained by the fluorescein and is thus more easily visualized using a light with a blue filter.

D. Normal and Abnormal Findings

If there is no superficial corneal irregularity, a uniform film of dye covers the cornea. If the corneal surface has been altered, the affected area absorbs more of the dye and will stain a deeper green.

Estimation of Anterior Chamber Depth

(See Figure 31–3.) Using a hand flashlight, shine the light obliquely and parallel to the plane of the iris across the cornea and anterior chamber. A normal anterior chamber will be fully illuminated. With a shallow anterior chamber (as in angle-closure glaucoma), the anteriorly displaced iris will cast a shadow.

▼ COMMON PITFALLS TO BE AVOIDED IN THE MANAGEMENT OF OCULAR DISORDERS

Dangers in the Use of Local Anesthetics

Unsupervised self-administration of local anesthetics is dangerous, as the patient may further injure an anesthetized eye without knowing it. Furthermore, most anesthetics delay healing. This is particularly true of butacaine, which also elicits a high incidence of allergic responses. Therefore, patients should not be given local anesthetics to take home. Eye pain should be controlled by systemic analgesics.

Errors in Diagnosis

The most common mistaken ophthalmologic diagnosis is conjunctivitis when the correct diagnosis should be iritis (anterior uveitis), glaucoma, or corneal ulcer (especially herpes simplex ulcer). The differentiation between iritis and acute glaucoma may be difficult also.

Misuse of Atropine

Atropine must never be used in routine diagnosis. It causes cycloplegia (paralysis of the ciliary muscle) of about 14 days' duration and can precipitate an attack of glaucoma if the patient has a narrow anterior chamber angle.

▶ Dangers of Local Corticosteroid Therapy

Local ophthalmologic corticosteroid preparations (eg, prednisolone) are often used for their anti-inflammatory effect on the conjunctiva, cornea, and iris. Although a patient with conjunctivitis, corneal inflammation, or iritis can be made more comfortable with topical corticosteroids, it must be stressed that the corticosteroids are associated with four very serious complications when used in the eye: herpes simplex keratitis, open-angle glaucoma, cataract formation, and fungal infection.

Corticosteroids should not be used unless specifically indicated (eg, in iritis, certain types of keratitis, and acute allergic disorders), and patients using prescribed topical corticosteroids should always see an ophthalmologist for follow-up examination.

▶ Overtreatment

Some patients with chronic conjunctivitis or keratitis may be made worse by overtreatment with topical medications. These patients should be evaluated by an ophthalmologist.

Emergency Disorders of the Ear, Nose, Sinuses, Oropharynx, & Mouth

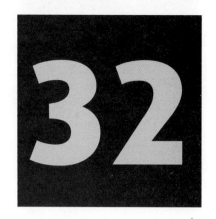

Timothy C. Stallard, MD

immediate Management of Potentially
Harmful Disorders
    Ear Pain
    Hearing Loss
    Vertigo
    Epistaxis
    Nasal Obstruction
    Sore Throat
    Tooth Fracture
    Tooth Subluxation or Avulsion
    Postextraction Tooth Hemorrhage
Management of Specific Disorders
    Disorders of the Ear
    Cerumen Impaction

Frostbite
Chronic (Suppurative) Otitis Media
Disorders of the Sinuses (Sinusitis)
Disorders of the Oropharynx
Peritonsillitis (Peritonsillar Cellulitis and Abscess)
Epiglottitis
Croup
Disorders of the Mouth
Tooth Anatomy
Tooth Pain
TMJ Pain
TMJ Dislocation

IMMEDIATE MANAGEMENT OF POTENTIALLY HARMFUL DISORDERS

EAR PAIN

The complaint of ear pain is more common among children than adults and usually relates to an infectious process. Though some conditions are serious, patients with most ear pain conditions can receive treatment and be discharged by the emergency physician without consultation (Table 32–1).

▶ Clinical Findings

A. History

Ask patients about history of trauma, surgery, or recurrent infections involving the ear. Also ask about specific symptoms (eg, recent fever, upper respiratory infection, or canal discharge) and pain quality (eg, pain, pressure, itching, or "buzzing" sounds). Have the patient identify the exact location of the pain. A narrow differential diagnosis can be explored based on these historical characteristics.

B. Physical Examination

Visually inspect the external ear, external canal orifice, and surrounding structures. Palpate the area surrounding the ear to identify lymph nodes or a bony prominence. Tender nodes are common in infections of the middle and external ear. Pain, swelling, and erythema at the mastoid process should prompt the clinician to consider mastoiditis. Next, view the canal and tympanic membrane. Make careful note of the appearance of the tympanic membrane regarding color, reflectivity, visibility of landmarks, and presence of fluid, air bubbles behind the membrane, or perforations. Check tympanic membrane motility by insufflation. Compare to the normal ear. If the ear examination is normal, look to the upper teeth and temporomandibular joint as possible causes.

Table 32–1. Diagnosis and Treatment of Ear Pain.

Diagnosis	Diagnostic Clues	Treatment	Comments
Acute mastoiditis	Fever or chills, pain, swelling, and erythema at mastoid process; typically an extension of acute otitis media; normal canal and findings of concurrent otitis media	ENT consultation, admission, IV antibiotics, possible necessity for surgical intervention; Cefotaxime, 1 g IV q 24 h, or ceftriaxone, 1–2 g IV q 24 h	Relatively rare; usually *S. pneumoniae, S pyogenes, S. aureus;* if it develops after resolved otitis media: acute coalescent mastoiditis
Bullous myringitis	Severe ear pain, TM bullae on TM surface, with surrounding erythema; middle ear space not affected	Erythromycin (EES, adult: 400 mg q.i.d.; child: 10 mg/kg q.i.d.), doxycycline, azithromycin	*Mycoplasma* (or viral)
Chondritis, perichondritis	Pain or swelling to the external (cartilaginous) ear; recent ear trauma; warm, erythematous, tender auricle, pinna skin; evidence of recent trauma or piercing; if ear is deformed, suspect chondritis (cartilage infection)	Remove foreign bodies, irrigate wounds; warm soaks and oral cephalexin; outpatient ENT follow-up; if evidence of cartilage involvement, ENT consultation, admission, IV antibiotics	
Foreign body	Usually young child, witnessed insertion; foreign body in canal	Removal is typically uncomfortable; tailor method to the characteristics of the foreign body (Frazier suction, alligator forceps, curette); prep with topical anesthetic; children may require restraint or sedation	If canal trauma is present, treat as for otitis externa, outpatient follow-up
Infected sebaceous cyst	Pain in canal; no discharge; erythematous, cystic canal surface; pain with pinna traction	Incise and drain cysts; cephalexin or dicloxacillin; outpatient ENT follow-up	May prevent recurrence with selenium sulfide (Selsun) or ketoconazole/steroid shampoo
Insect in canal	Buzzing or movement sensation; insect in canal or on TM catheter; flush out when patient is calm	Immobilization will relieve the discomfort; instill mineral oil in the canal with a syringe and flexible tip	Alternatively, may remove a large insect with narrow alligator forceps through the otoscope
Otitis externa (swimmer's ear)	Common in regular swimmers; ear pain, itching. Purulent discharge, erythematous canal, pain with pinna traction; canal may be occluded by wall edema; normal hearing unless canal is occluded	Place a cotton wick through an obstructed or near-obstructed canal; treat with topical steroid and antibiotic preparations: hydrocortisone-polymyxin neomycin (Cortisporin Otic), 4 drops q.i.d., or hydrocortisone-ciprofloxacin (Cipro HC Otic), 3 drops b.i.d.	Typically *Pseudomonas;* outpatient follow-up within 3 days; reduce recurrence risk with drying rubbing alcohol drops following water exposure; consider malignant variant in diabetic, immunocompromised, or elderly patients
Otitis externa (malignant)	Elderly, immunocompromised, or diabetic patient with findings of otitis externa; physical findings as above	ENT consultation, admission, IV antibiotics (imipenem-cilastatin, 500 mg IV q 6 h; ciprofloxacin, 400 mg IV q 12 h or 750 mg PO q 12 h)	*Pseudomonas* can cause rapidly progressing, necrotizing disease among vulnerable patients; outpatient treatment may be acceptable in early disease; CT scan if mastoid osteomyelitis is suspected
Serous/secretory otitis media	Preceding upper respiratory infection or otitis media; unilateral hearing loss, pain, pressure, or bubbling sound (all of variable severity); normal canal; TM not erythematous, but decreased motility and light reflex; landmarks visible; air–fluid levels behind TM	Decongestant for 14 days	Not infectious; relates to eustachian canal obstruction; obtain ENT evaluation if it does not resolve in 2 weeks; some clinicians rous (mobile fluid) from secretory (thick, nonmotile fluid) otitis, but treatment is the same

(continued)

Table 32–1. Diagnosis and Treatment of Ear Pain. (*Continued*)

Diagnosis	Diagnostic Clues	Treatment	Comments
Suppurative otitis media	Common in children; preceding upper respiratory infection; may lead to TM rupture (severe pain followed by rapid, spontaneous relief); normal canal; TM is erythematous, dull light reflex, limited motility (most specific), landmarks not visible; compare to other side; make note of TM rupture, if present; decreased hearing on affected side	Amoxicillin (adults: 500 mg t.i.d. × 10 d; children: 15 mg/kg t.i.d. × 10 d); if child has had abscess in past month, high-dose amoxicillin (30 mg/kg t.i.d. × 10 d); if recent treatment failure, amoxicillin-clavulanate (Augmentin, 25–30 mg/kg t.i.d. × 10 d); other options, trimethoprim-sulfamethoxazole, cefuroxime, ceftriaxone IM	Typical organisms: *S. pneumonia, H. influenzae* (children); ruptured TM will require follow-up every 2–4 weeks to ensure healing

TM, tympanic membrane.

C. Other Studies

If history and physical examination suggest mastoiditis, computed tomography (CT) scan should be obtained.

▶ Treatment

Each condition requires a specific treatment (see Table 32–1).

HEARING LOSS

Sudden hearing loss is a deficit of less than 3 days duration and may be partial or complete. Diagnoses can be categorized as conductive (mechanical cause) or sensorineural (inner ear or cochlear nerve-central nervous system cause). Medication-related hearing loss is usually dose and duration related. Many potential causes must be considered (Table 32–2).

▶ Clinical Findings

A. History

The patient's account of precipitating events (trauma or recent activities) and the duration of symptom onset (seconds, hours, days) should help narrow the focus on possible causes. Unilateral deafness should increase the suspicion for a structural process (conductive or acoustic neuroma), whereas bilateral symptoms would suggest a systemic (metabolic or drug related) problem. Take a careful medication history. Severity (partial vs complete loss of hearing) also should be assessed. Finally, the presence of tinnitus, vertigo, or other neurologic symptoms should alert the clinician to the likelihood of a sensorineural cause.

B. Physical Examination

Look at the canals and tympanic membranes to rule out foreign body obstruction, infection, or injury. The cranial nerves should be examined. Weber and Rinne tests are useful for differentiating between conductive and sensorineural causes only in cases with unilateral hearing loss. The Webber test is performed by placing a vibrating 512-Hz tuning fork on the midparietal head (Figure 32–1). Sound should be heard equally on both sides. The Rinne test is performed by placing the base of a vibrating fork on the mastoid process. When the patient can no longer hear the sound, it is quickly moved off the bone and the tines placed at the ear canal

Table 32–2. Causes of Sudden Hearing Loss.

Conductive
  Foreign body or mass (U)
  Otitis externa with obstruction (U)
  Otitis media (U)
  Otosclerosis (U)
  Tympanic membrane rupture (U)
Infectious
  Herpes (simplex, zoster) (B)
  Mononucleosis (Epstein-Barr virus, cytomegalovirus) (B) Mumps (B)
  Syphilis (B)
Hematologic
  Berger disease (B)
  Leukemia (B)
  Polycythemia (B)
  Sickle cell anemia (B)
Metabolic
  Diabetes mellitus (B)
  Hyperlipidemia (B)
Medication
  Aminoglycosides (B)
  Loop diuretics (B)
  Salicylates (B)
Other
  Acoustic neuroma (U)
  Acoustic trauma (loud noise) (U or B)
  Meniere disease (U or B)

Note: All are sensorineural except in the conductive category. U, unilateral; B, bilateral (typically).

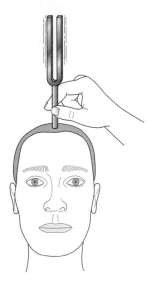

▲ **Figure 32–1.** In the Webber test, vibrations are louder on the side with a conductive deficit.

(Figure 32–2). Repeat on each side. The patient should be able to hear the vibration in the air after the fork is removed from the bone. In sensorineural hearing loss, the Rinne test will be normal bilaterally and the Webber test will lateralize to the unaffected side. In conductive hearing loss, the Webber test will lateralize to the affected side and the Rinne test will also be abnormal on that side.

C. Other Studies

Bloodwork is helpful if infectious or metabolic causes are being considered. CT or magnetic resonance imaging (MRI) scan is appropriate for a suspected acoustic neuroma.

▶ Treatment

Treatment should be directed toward the underlying disorder. Rapid follow-up by the appropriate provider (ie, otolaryngologist and neurologist) is recommended.

VERTIGO

True vertigo is a sense of motion when one is stationary. It is typically described as feeling the world spin. It can be quite disconcerting to patients, some of whom present in dramatic discomfort.

▶ Clinical Findings

A. History

The most important determination is between central (central nervous system) and peripheral (relating to the eighth cranial nerve or the inner ear apparatus) causes. This classification usually can be resolved on the basis of history alone (Table 32–3). Symptoms that are severe, of sudden onset, and related to head movement are typically caused by a peripheral disorder. Ask about recent use of potentially vestibulotoxic drugs such as aminoglycosides, vancomycin, phenytoin, quinidine, and minocycline. Caffeine, nicotine, and alcohol are known to exacerbate symptoms. Head trauma can occasionally lead to semichronic symptoms (lasting months to years). Specific causes of peripheral vertigo are described in Table 32–4.

B. Physical Examination

Examine the ear canal, tympanic membrane, cranial nerves, and cerebellar function. All patients with vertigo may have difficulty with the tandem walk exercise, but the presence of focal cerebellar examination findings (rapid alternating movements, heel-shin slide, or finger-to-nose pointing tests)

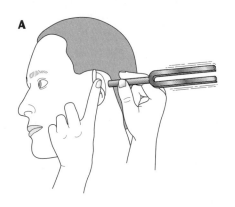

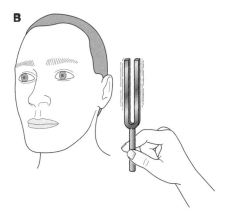

▲ **Figure 32–2.** **A.** Bone vibration that is longer than air vibration indicates a conductive problem. **B.** In a sensorineural deficit, air conduction is significantly longer than bone conduction.

Table 32–3. Central Versus Peripheral Vertigo.

Symptom or Examination Finding	Peripheral Causes	Central Causes
Duration of onset	Minutes to hours	Weeks to months
Intensity	Severe	Moderate
Nausea, vomiting	Typical	Often absent
Relation to head movement	Movement exacerbates symptoms	Often symptoms unrelated to movement
Patient age	Any; often young	Usually elderly
Nystagmus	Always horizontal or rotatory; worse with head movements and fatigues over 5-30 seconds	Presence is variable; may be vertical or horizontal with no fatigue
Cranial nerve or cerebellar deficits	Absent	Often present (especially ataxia-usually with slow onset; sudden onset suggests cerebellar hemorrhage)
Hearing	Often decreased (unilateral) or with tinnitus	Usually normal
Causes	Meniere's disease Labyrinthitis (viral or bacterial) (Benign) positional vertigo Canal foreign body or otitis media Acoustic neuroma	Drugs Cerebellar mass or stroke Encephalitis or brain abscess Vertebral basilar artery insufficiency Temporal lobe epilepsy Multiple sclerosis

should raise suspicion for a central cause. Identifying nystagmus, especially with head movement can help narrow the differential diagnosis. The Dix-Hallpike test can help elicit the vertigo symptoms and nystagmus if they are not present at rest. In this test, the examiner places a hand on the patient's occiput, and the patient is rapidly reclined from an upright position onto a flat surface. The head should extend off the back edge so that the neck can be somewhat hyperextended. The test can be repeated with the head rotated to each side. A positive result occurs with acute worsening of the vertigo or production of nystagmus. Nystagmus relating to a peripheral cause typically starts in 1–3 seconds and diminishes over

Table 32–4. Causes of Peripheral Vertigo.

Condition	Diagnosis	Comments
Acoustic neuroma	Gradual (days to weeks) onset, unilateral hearing loss and tinnitus; initially mimics vestibular neuronitis, but symptoms worsen over weeks as tumor progresses centrally; central signs and symptoms (decreased corneal reflex, ataxia) later in course; diagnosis by CT scan	Schwann cell tumor; recovery correlated with early surgery
Benign paroxysmal (positional) vertigo	Symptoms and nystagmus associated with head movement—often subsiding gradually several minutes after movement	Most common cause of peripheral vertigo; typically no specific cause
Ménière disease (paroxysmal labyrinthine vertigo)	Associated with unilateral hearing loss and tinnitus; vertigo with sudden onset and short (1-24 h) duration; intense, recurrent, associated with vomiting and distress; ear pressure; nystagmus during the attacks, not between or positional	Sometimes associated with high salt intake; may improve with low-sodium diet
Suppurative labyrinthitis	Prominent hearing loss and vertigo; temporally related to recent bacterial infection of middle or inner ear; diagnosis by CT scan	CT scan to evaluate for mastoiditis; requires inpatient treatment with intravenous antibiotics or surgery
Vestibular neuronitis	Symptom onset over 1-2 hours; nystagmus and discomfort associated with head movement; nohearingloss	Lasts 3-7 days, but mild symptoms may persist for weeks; thought to be related to viral labyrinthitis

ovement. Nystagmus from a cen-
extinguish.

scan or MRI) is warranted for patients with
a suspected central cause or elderly patients with equivocal
findings. MRI provides superior resolution of the cerebellum, though CT scan will typically rule out large lesions.

▶ Treatment

Patients with prolonged nausea and poor fluid intake will
often require intravenous hydration. Pharmacotherapy is
more successful in peripheral-type vertigo. It is directed
at relief of symptoms and does not affect the duration of
the illness. The first-line agent is oral meclizine (25–50 mg
every 8–12 hours), but patients unable to manage oral
fluids are better off with intravenous normal saline and
diazepam (5–10 mg intravenously, 2–4 mg intravenously
for the elderly). In general, drugs with anticholinergic
effects are useful. These include diphenhydramine (50 mg
intramuscularly or orally every 6–8 hours), dimenhydrinate
(50–100 mg intramuscularly or orally every 4 hours), cycliz-
ine (50 mg orally every 6 hours), and promethazine (25 mg
orally, rectally, or intravenously every 6–8 hours). Patients
with peripheral vertigo can be discharged after moderate
improvement of symptoms and ability to take oral liquids.
Some patients may need to be admitted to hospital for severe
symptoms or inability to maintain oral intake. Depending on
the cause, symptoms are likely to last several hours to 1 week
but may persist for 4–5 weeks. Many patients with central
vertigo will require inpatient management targeted at the
underlying cause, though those who are comfortable after
treatment and have firm follow-up can be discharged.

A particle repositioning (Epley) maneuver may be
attempted if positional vertigo is suspected. It is based on
the belief that moving the canalith to the utricle area of the
inner ear will prevent it from stimulating the sensory mechanism. All motions should be done slowly such that each full
cycle of the maneuver takes 2 minutes. First, perform the
Dix-Hallpike test. Then place the patient in a sitting position,
turn the head 45° toward the affected side, lay the patient
down, and allow the head to extend 45° beyond neutral while
hanging off the top edge of the bed. Rotate the extended head
to the midline and then 90° away from the affected side (as
determined by the fast component of the nystagmus). Then
flex the neck to neutral, sit the patient up, and rotate the
head back to midline. The maneuver often must be repeated
several times to be successful.

EPISTAXIS

Most episodes of epistaxis do not result in significant blood
loss, are not life-threatening, and can be managed with minimally invasive measures. However, the clinician should begin
with an assessment of hemodynamic stability and provide

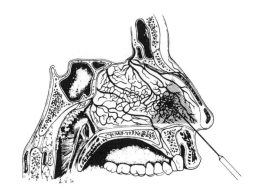

▲**Figure 32–3.** Cauterization of bleeding at the Kiesselbach
plexus.

support (intravenous fluids or blood products) when appropriate. The typical bleeding site is the Kiesselbach area of the
anteromedial nostril, an area at risk due to the anastomoses
of three separate arteries (Figure 32–3). Though predominantly due to trauma or environmental exposure, epistaxis
can rarely be the first symptom of a growing nasal or sinus
malignancy.

▶ Clinical Findings

A. History

Many patients will be predisposed to bleeding, due to warfarin, platelet-inhibiting medications, renal failure, or hemophilia. Initial history should be directed toward medications
as well as easy bruising or bleeding. In cold seasons, the dry
conditions created by heated indoor air can dehydrate the
airways, predisposing the nasal mucosa to cracking. The
repeated blowing and wiping of a nose in the setting of
upper respiratory infection or allergic rhinitis can abrade
and injure the mucosal surface as can blunt trauma and nose
picking. The possibility of pregnancy should be assessed
since the incidence of epistaxis is increased and the choice of
pharmacologic agents may be changed by this knowledge.

B. Physical Examination

Hemodynamically stable patients are best examined sitting
upright. In this position, most blood will exit the anterior
nose and ingestion or aspiration will be minimized. If the
bleeding is active, the patient should be told to clear each
nostril of clots and then pinch the entire cartilaginous
portion of the nose for 15 minutes continuously. This is
sometimes all that is required to stop the bleeding (however,
the nose should always be reexamined to confirm hemostasis). During this time, the clinician should don protective
clothing and eyewear and set up adequate lighting, a nasal
speculum, and a suction device. The predominant side of
the epistaxis should be noted. Bilateral bleeding suggests a
posterior source. All mucosal surfaces of the nose should be

examined for bleeding and the integrity of the septum confirmed. Observe the posterior oropharynx for 10–15 seconds to confirm whether fresh blood is flowing down the back wall. Bilateral bleeding suggests a posterior source as does a large amount of fresh blood in the oropharynx and little in the anterior nose.

▶ Treatment

A. Anterior Epistaxis

Epistaxis from an anterior source can usually be controlled. In general, minimally invasive and technically simple methods are preferred, but refractory bleeding requires escalation to more invasive procedures. Some patients may benefit from gentle opiate or benzodiazepine sedation. While using the suction device to keep the field clear of blood, apply 1% phenylephrine, 4% cocaine, or 2% lidocaine-epinephrine solution with a cotton swab or pledget for vasoconstriction and local anesthesia. Alternatively these solutions may be sprayed onto the mucosal surface. When the bleeding site can be visualized, simple cautery with silver nitrate is often all that is required (see Figure 32–3). Exercise care to use only unilateral, brief applications. Roll the tip a short distance from above and over the bleeding site to prevent interference from blood flowing downward.

Bleeding that persists should be treated with packing. Several options are available. Cotton pledgets soaked with vasoconstrictive agents such as phenylephrine or lidocaine-epinephrine can be placed in the inferior nostril via narrow forceps and successively pushed superiorly until the nostril is packed. Commercial nasal tampons are simple to place (Figure 32–4A). They are inserted blindly along the inferior (floor) surface of the nostril and then expanded with the application of saline or 1:1 dilutions of the vasoconstricting agent. Take care not to injure the lateral turbinates. As the material expands, pressure is uniformly applied to the inner walls, tamponading bleeding. Procoagulant products (Surgicel, Gelfoam) may be used alone or in conjunction with other materials to augment the hemostatic effect.

If none of these methods is successful, a formal anterior pack with petroleum jelly gauze strip material may be necessary. It is placed in a similar fashion to the pledgets: the end of a continuous strip is placed inferiorly and far back in the nose, then pushed up to tamponade the upper surfaces and make room for successive strips. The nostril must be fairly tightly packed, and most clinicians repeat the procedure on the other side if bleeding persists. Many authors suggest that patients with nasal packs should receive prophylaxis against bacterial sinusitis: amoxicillin–clavulanate, 875 mg twice daily for adults, 40 mg/kg/d divided two to three times daily for children. More study is needed, but some studies indicate antibiotics may not be needed in these patients. Packing material should be removed in 3–5 days. Patients with anterior packs can be discharged to home.

B. Posterior Epistaxis

Posterior bleeding more typically arises from an arterial source and will not respond to the methods described above. Treatment of this entity usually requires the use of a nasal balloon device (Epistat, Nasostat) (Figure 32–4B). In addition to a posterior balloon, the specialized devices have an anterior tamponade apparatus (balloon or expanding tampon) that can be inflated or expanded independently. To prevent ischemia of the anterior nasal mucosa, the anterior portion is intended to exert less pressure than the posterior balloon. Insert it into the nostril such that the balloon is in the posterior portion of the nose. Then inflate the posterior balloon with saline until the point of discomfort. Properly placed, the posterior balloon may be all that is required to stop the bleeding. Usually, though, the anterior nose should be packed as well. Most patients with posterior packs should be admitted for airway observation, prophylactic antibiotics, and ENT consultation.

NASAL OBSTRUCTION

Most patients who present to the emergency department will have an acute obstruction (foreign body, trauma). Rarely, the problem is a complication of a chronic obstructive condition, such as an infection relating to a tumor or deviated septum.

▶ Clinical Findings

A. History

Ask the patient how long the symptoms have been present and whether there were any precipitating events. In children, the most common cause of obstruction is a foreign body, often a colorful bead or a piece of food, and the history and diagnosis will be straightforward. Patients should also be queried regarding presence of a discharge. Purulent or foul-smelling discharge suggests an established organic foreign body. Nearly all cases of nasal obstruction will involve one side, negating the risk of airway compromise and allowing for outpatient workup of cases that defy emergency department management.

B. Physical Examination

Look into each nostril with the otoscope or a nasal speculum. Most conditions can be characterized and treatment initiated based on direct inspection (Table 32–5).

SORE THROAT

Many conditions lead to the common symptom of throat pain, and although most are relatively benign, several can result in airway compromise and require heroic interventions. The patient who presents with drooling, severe difficulty in swallowing, stridor, or difficulty moving air should be examined in a setting where airway equipment is

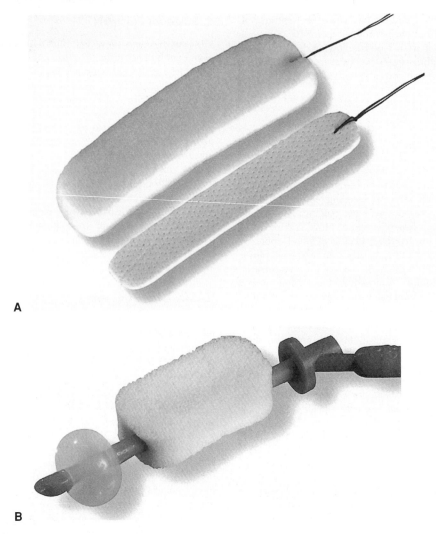

A

B

▲ **Figure 32–4.** The Xomed Merocel Pope (A) and Epistat II (B) products.

close by. The evaluation of persons with obstructive airway symptoms requires balancing the need for examination and imaging studies with their safety, because certain conditions may worsen with time. In some cases, it may be prudent for a person skilled in airway management to be present while ancillary tests such as X-rays are obtained. In general, children with these symptoms should remain with the parent and any source of excessive stimulation such as lab draws or intravenous lines should be avoided.

▶ Clinical Findings

A. History

In children, a careful immunization history may help identify those at risk for *Haemophilus influenzae* type B (Hib)

infections. Although the incidence of pediatric epiglottitis has fallen dramatically as a result of the Hib vaccine, it is not zero. The rapid development of severe symptoms requires a prompt workup and treatment. The presence of associated odynophagia (pain with swallowing) or dysphagia (difficulty swallowing) should prompt the examiner to consider imaging the neck. Fever, cough, or sputum should prompt consideration of other infectious causes. Diffuse symptoms (eg, headache, body aches, chest and joint pains, diarrhea) suggest a viral source.

B. Physical Examination

Patients with significant airway swelling and compromise (epiglottitis, abscesses) voluntarily sit straight up with the

Table 32–5. Diagnosis and Treatment of Nasal Obstruction.

Diagnosis	Diagnostic Clues	Treatment
Abscess	Red, tender, fluctuant mass	Incise, drain, place temporary wick, or pack inside to prevent recurrence
Choanal atresia	Neonates only; nasal tube will be difficult to pass on affected side	ENT consultation in emergency department
Deviated septum	Chronic symptoms, though may be acutely worsened by local or sinus infection; outpatient CT scan will demonstrate extent	Treat sinusitis, if present; ENT referral
Foreign body	Typically infants, small children; objects evident by inspection of the nostril; purulent discharge may indicate concurrent sinusitis	Remove with forceps, Shukneckt suction device, have parent blow forcefully in patients mouth while occluding the normal nostril
Hematoma	Usually recent history of trauma; mass is anterior, usually on septum; examine by transilluminating the septum with bright light	Incise, drain completely, pack loosely to ensure that mucosal layer is in contact with underlying cartilage
Polyps	Usually painless, small; cause minimal obstruction; may be directly visible through nostrils	ENT referral
Rhinitis (allergic, viral)	Clear discharge, bilateral symptoms; allergic rhinitis is usually seasonal or related to environment change or pet exposure; often with eye involvement; viral rhinitis has concurrent upper respiratory symptoms	Symptomatic: decongestants, antihistamines
Tumor	Gradually progressive symptoms to critical point of emergency department presentation; discharge may be blood streaked; mass is nonfluctuant	ENT referral; emergency department ENT consultation if bilateral

neck slightly extended. Such a general appearance is ominous. Examine the floor of the mouth, looking for focal elevations and tongue displacement. Look at the gingiva for evidence of abscess.

Examine the uvula, tonsillar pillars, and entrance of the oropharynx for swelling, exudate, or erythema. Asymmetry should increase the suspicion for an abscess (Figure 32–5). Examine the anterior neck for lymphadenopathy, masses, or asymmetry. Palpate the larynx for tenderness, particularly if the remainder of the physical examination is unimpressive.

C. Other Studies

Lateral and anteroposterior soft tissue neck X-rays can be useful for identifying epiglottis or retropharyngeal abscesses (Figure 32-6), but they do not reliably rule out these processes. These tests should not be done initially in the unstable patient as described above. Stable patients will benefit from intravenous contrast CT scan to delineate the exact location and extent of any mass or abscess.

▶ Treatment

Each condition requires specific treatment (Table 32–6). Simple pharyngitis is by far the most common cause of sore throat among children and adults, and viral infections

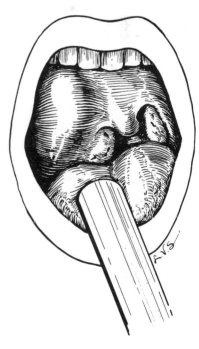

▲ **Figure 32–5.** Asymmetric tonsillar pillar swelling and uvular displacement are typical of peritonsillitis.

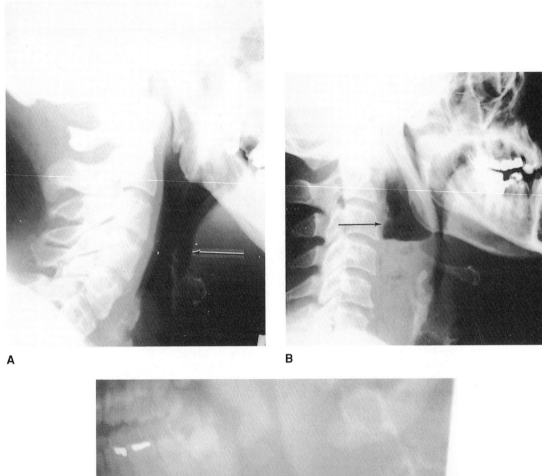

A

B

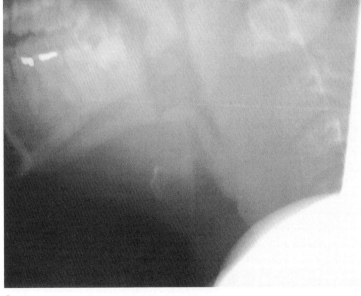

C

▲ **Figure 32–6.** Soft-tissue lateral X-rays. **A:** A normal soft tissue lateral X-ray demonstrating no enlargement of the epiglottis or tissues between the airway and cervical vertebrae. **B:** Retropharyngeal abscess in an adult. The airway is displaced anteriorly by a mass that contains an air–fluid level. **C:** Epiglottitis in a child. The epiglottis is enlarged and has a "thumbprint" shape.

Table 32–6. Diagnosis and Treatment of Sore Throat.

Diagnosis	Diagnostic Clues	Treatment	Comments
Allergic reaction	Often history of recent food intake; may progress over 5–30 minutes, when severe; quality of voice may help identify location of the swelling (hoarse: supraglottic airway; muffled or nasal: oropharynx); edematous mucosa (uvula, soft palate) may be visible by direct oropharynx inspection	Epinephrine, 0.3 mg SQ; diphenhydramine, 50 mg IM; methylprednisolone, 125 mg IV/IM; histamine blockers (famotidine, ranitidine) are controversial; intubate if severe obstruction is present	Multiple possible routes of antigen entry, though most are ingestion or inhalation; may be accompanied by hives or anaphylaxis; throat pain may be the minor complaint
Anaerobic pharyngitis (Vincent angina)	May involve mouth and pharynx, associated with poor oral hygiene; mucosal ulceration, pseudomembranes, foul breath	Hydrogen peroxide rinses and oral penicillin or doxycycline	Clinical diagnosis
Bacterial Common; pharyngitis	Fever; sore throat without cough; bilateral tonsillar swelling; and white, tender cervical lymphadenopathy; often difficult to differentiate from viral pharyngitis on clinical grounds; culture	Although streptococci predominate in children, other organisms (*Mycoplasma, Chlamydia*) may cause some adult illness; benzathine penicillin, 1.2 million units IM (300,000–600,000 units if <27 kg) affords good compliance	Consider epiglottitis; uncommonly causes airway obstruction, but admit patient if oral secretions are difficult to control; penicillin has a 10–20% failure rate; use erythromycin or equivalent if treatment failure; untreated group A streptococcal infection is associated with acute rheumatic fever
Diphtheria	Ill appearing; fever, dysphagia common; prominent gray pseudomembrane over tonsillar pillars; diphtheria culture of throat swabs	Give antitoxin, observe for allergic reaction; erythromycin or penicillin; admit with respiratory isolation	Uncommon in United States; occasional toxic systemic sequelae
Epiglottitis	Fever, voice hoarseness, severe pain, worse with swallowing; drooling and sniffing position when swelling is severe; condition is now as or more prevalent in adults, who may have less acute presentations; useful studies: soft tissue neck X-ray (enlarged epiglottis—"thumbprint" sign), fiberoptic laryngoscopy (red, swollen only at bedside in stable adults)	Immediate airway intervention in unstable patients or ENT consultation and operating room intubation in less acute children; consider blood cultures and early IV antibiotics (ceftriaxone, 50 mg/kg IV q 12 h); all patients need admission coverage	Routine use of the *H. influenzae* vaccine has sharply decreased the incidence among children; epiglottitis in a vaccinated individual should prompt consideration of an antibiotic with *S. aureus* and streptococci
Gonococcal, chlamydial pharyngitis	Variable exudate, symptoms sometimes mild; culture of DNA testing of oropharyngeal swabs; requires genital examination and testing; test sex contacts	Similar to genital infections, though more failures occur with oral form; ceftriaxone, 125 mg IM × 1 dose, and doxycycline, 100 mg q 12 h × 10 d	Results from orogenital contact; symptoms may be mild and chronic
Herpes pharyngitis	Vesicles in oropharynx and mouth, exudate, fever; laboratory examination of lesion scrapings permits confirmation	Acyclovir, famciclovir, or valacyclovir are indicated in immunocompromised patients and may shorten the course for others	Typically history of orogenital contact
Infectious mononucleosis	Fever, pale exudates on tonsillar pillars; generalized lymphadenopathy, splenomegaly; monospot and liver function tests; blood count differential: atypical mononuclear cells	Supportive care; consider steroids, IV fluids, and admission for patients with severe swelling and dehydration	Typically aged 15–30 years

(continued)

Table 32–6. Diagnosis and Treatment of Sore Throat. (*Continued*)

Diagnosis	Diagnostic Clues	Treatment	Comments
Ludwig angina	Fever, dysphagia, mouth floor and neck swelling, pain; often associated with voice change; typically follows poor dental care or recent lower molar extraction; elevation and firm, tender floor of mouth-often unilateral; trismus and firm, tender upper neck often present; CT scan most useful to confirm diagnosis in stable patients	Position patient upright and protect airway as dictated by clinical appearance; when indicated, fiberoptic intubation is preferred; IV antibiotics for polymicrobial and anaerobic flora: ticarcillin-clavulanate or piperacillin–tazobactam with clindamycin or metronidazole; all patients need admission	Surgery is required for patients who do not respond to antibiotics; dental examination and removal of affected teeth; high aspiration complication rate
Peritonsillar cellulitis and abscess	Most common deep-space infection in throat; a progression of bacterial tonsillitis; most common in young adults; fever, difficulty and pain with swallowing, "hot potato" voice, and foul-smelling breath; trismus is typical, and the examination reveals unilateral soft palate swelling and uvular deviation; consider CT scan	Typically responds to incision and drainage, though multiple (3-4) punctures with an 18-gauge needle and aspiration have been advocated; penicillin and clindamycin; patients with mild cases and no airway compromise can be discharged with ENT follow-up	To prevent uncontrolled rupture, use only gentle intraoral pressure on the peritonsillar mass; the carotid artery is 2.5 cm posterior and lateral to the peritonsillar tissue; avoid deep penetration of the abscess with sharp instruments
Retropharyngeal, prevertebral abscess	Mainly affects children aged <6 years; fever, pain, and difficult swallowing; voice change (described as a "duck quack" sound); stridor if severe; pain with forced side-to-side movement of the thyroid cartilage; lateral neck X-rays demonstrate anterior displacement of trachea by diffuse soft tissue mass; CT scan with IV contrast if plain X-rays not definitive	Stabilize airway, ENT consultation, IV antibiotics to cover mixed oral and anaerobic infection (see Ludwig angina), admission. Large abscesses will require incision and drainage	Abscess may rupture into mediastinal or pleural spaces; presence of trismus and a tender, firm swelling in the anterior neck triangle should increase suspicion for parapharyngeal abscess

predominate (90%). Recent investigations suggest that differentiating bacterial from viral causes is difficult to accomplish by appearance alone. Untreated group A streptococcal infections have been associated with acute rheumatic fever and valvular heart disease.

The broad application of antibiotics will inevitably lead to emergence of resistant strains. The combination of throat pain, fever, tender anterior cervical lymph nodes, and the absence of a cough suggest streptococcal infection and might reasonably be treated immediately. Otherwise, many clinicians rely on rapid streptococcal tests or culture to determine which patients need antibiotics. This approach requires a reliable follow-up mechanism to be successful. Anxious parents can usually be convinced of the wisdom of this strategy because it avoids unnecessary antibiotics and the occasional allergic reaction.

Consideration should be given to the use of steroids in patients with significant odynophagia or dysphagia. Among sicker children and adults, the need for admission will depend on serial assessment of breathing comfort and ability to take oral liquids and maintain hydration.

TOOTH FRACTURE

Tooth fractures are graded by the Ellis classification system (Figure 32–7). Fractures of the enamel alone (Ellis class I) require no urgent treatment (save gentle smoothing of any rough edges with sandpaper). An office dentist can fill in the defect later to satisfy cosmetic needs, but there is no risk of long-term damage to the tooth. Class II fractures are deeper and expose the dentin. A patch of yellow in the middle of the tooth defect characterizes such injuries. The dentin is vulnerable to bacteria, and prompt covering is essential for long-term preservation of the tooth. The wound should be irrigated with sterile saline, dried, and covered with calcium hydroxide paste, foil, or equivalent dressing. Because the permanent teeth in children have relatively thin dentin layers, bacterial penetration to the pulp is a greater risk in Ellis II fractures and dental consultation is appropriate if readily available.

Identification of blood or a pink spot in the defect indicates exposure of the pulp and an Ellis class III injury. Typically, this portion of the tooth is quite sensitive, making most class III fractures quite painful. Treatment is the same

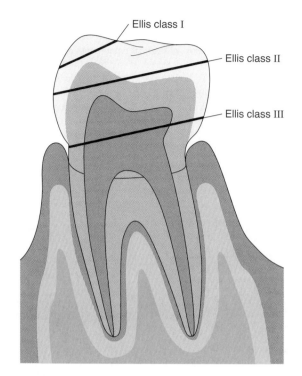

▲ Figure 32–7. The Ellis tooth fracture classification system.

as an Ellis class II injury with dental consultation within 24 hours. Consider applying a local anesthetic block for management of pain.

TOOTH SUBLUXATION OR AVULSION

Subluxation is a traumatic injury and results in a tooth that is, to varying degrees, loose in the socket. The subluxed or avulsed tooth should be identified as primary (deciduous) or secondary. Primary teeth require no treatment other than removal if significantly subluxed to prevent ankylosis to the alveolar bone or aspiration. Gentle pressure by grasping the tooth with a sterile gauze dressing will demonstrate the degree of subluxation. Patients with minimal laxity (up to 2 mm at tip) can be discharged with advice to eat only liquid or soft foods and follow-up with a dentist. Moderate mobility (more than 2 mm) or teeth that appear partly extruded from the socket depth will require socket reseating and a splint to prevent further injury to the vascular supply and fibrous cementum connections with the underlying alveolar bone. Immobilizing the tooth will maximize its long-term viability. Various materials are available for this purpose. If the emergency physician has access to these materials, he or she may apply the splint and discharge the patient with dental follow-up. At the very least, a foil-like material can be pressed over the loose tooth and its neighbors to anchor it.

Total avulsion is a somewhat more urgent matter, because the chance for tooth survival falls with every minute it is out of the socket. If the tooth cannot be found, the possibility of tracheal aspiration should be investigated. Hanks Balanced Salt Solution (HBSS) is the perfect storage and transportation medium. Milk, saliva, and normal saline are less ideal options. Plain water or dry surfaces are to be avoided. Dry teeth will benefit from a brief soak in HBSS or normal saline, but there should be little delay before replanting them directly into the socket. This procedure cannot wait for the dental consultant and can be done by the first clinician to make contact with the patient.

When handling the tooth, touch only the crown (enamel) surface of the tooth. Do not scrub or manually clean the root as this may cause damage to the cementum, which is very fragile. After irrigation with HBSS or saline, place the tooth firmly into the socket. Compare the shape of mirror-image teeth on the other side of the mouth to clarify proper orientation if multiple teeth are out. Splinting (see above) will ensure that the tooth remains securely in place. This may require consulting the dentist. A short course (5 days) of prophylactic antibiotics should be given and dental follow-up arranged.

POSTEXTRACTION TOOTH HEMORRHAGE

Bleeding from the site of a recently extracted tooth may result from the simple dislodgment of clot from the base of the socket or may be a sign of an underlying coagulopathy. Patients should be asked about a history of hemophilia or use of antiplatelet or anticoagulant drugs. Laboratory testing may be necessary to evaluate the coagulation status. Initial management should entail placing rolled cotton gauze in the socket and asking the patient to bite down for 20 minutes. As an adjunct, lidocaine–epinephrine can be injected into the gingiva at the bleeding site prior to gauze pressure. Bleeding that does not respond to these measures will require dental consultation for revision of the socket.

Bagai A, Thavendiranathan P, Detsky AS: Does this patient have hearing impairment? JAMA 2006;295: 416–428 [PMID: 16434632].

Bhattacharyya N, Baugh RF, Orvidas L, Barrs D, Bronston LJ, Cass S, Chalian AA, Desmond AL, Earll JM, Fife TD, Fuller DC, Judge JO, Mann NR, Rosenfeld RM, Schuring LT, Steiner RW, Whitney SL, Haidari J, American Academy of Otolaryngology-Head and Neck Surgery Foundation. Clinical practice guideline: benign paroxysmal positional vertigo. Otolaryngol Head Neck Surg 2008;139:S47–S81 [PMID: 18973840].

Biswas D, Mal RK: Are systemic prophylactic antibiotics indicated with anterior nasal packing for spontaneous epistaxis? Acta Otolaryngol 2009;129:179–181 [PMID: 18607977].

Chu YH, Lee JC: Images in medicine. Unilateral epistaxis. N Engl J Med 2009;361: e14 [PMID:19710479].

Elias H, Baur DA: Management of trauma to supporting dental structures. Dent Clin North Am 2009;53:675–689 [PMID: 19958905].

Ho EC, Chan JY: Front-line epistaxis management: let's not forget the basics. J Laryngol Otol 2008;122:696–699 [PMID:18384699].

Korb K, Scherer M, Chenot JF: Steroids as adjuvant therapy for acute pharyngitis in ambulatory patients: a systematic review. Ann Fam Med 2010;8:58–63 [PMID: 20065280].

Leong SC, Roe RJ, Karkanevatos A: No frills management of epistaxis. Emerg Med J 2005;22:470–472 [PMID: 15983079].

Neuhauser HK, Lempert T: Vertigo: epidemiologic aspects. Semin Neurol 2009;29:473–481 [PMID: 19834858].

Robertson KA, Volmink JA, Mayosi BM: Antibiotics for the primary prevention of acute rheumatic fever: a meta-analysis. BMC Cardiovasc Disord 2005;5:11 [PMID:15927077].

van den Aardweg MT, Rovers MM, de Ru JA, Albers FW, Schilder AG: A systematic review of diagnostic criteria for acute mastoiditis in children. Otol Neurotol 2008;29:751–757 [PMID: 18617870].

MANAGEMENT OF SPECIFIC DISORDERS

DISORDERS OF THE EAR

Please refer to the Immediate Management section and Table 32–1 for discussion of the following conditions: otitis externa, malignant otitis externa, foreign body or insect in canal, infected sebaceous cyst, chondritis, perichondritis, suppurative and serous otitis media, bullous myringitis, and acute mastoiditis.

CERUMEN IMPACTION

ESSENTIALS OF DIAGNOSIS

► Readily apparent by direct otoscope inspection

▶ Clinical Findings

The walls of the ear canal possess a secretory mechanism that results in a coating of the familiar waxy substance—cerumen. Over months, this material can collect and result in canal obstruction. Rarely does the material need to be removed on an emergency basis, but its presence can lead to mild pressure, vertigo, or hearing loss symptoms, and it may obscure inspection of the tympanic membrane.

▶ Treatment

Two methods are available for evacuation: blunt removal and irrigation. Blunt removal entails use of a plastic curette, and care must be taken not to puncture the tympanic membrane or injure the walls of the canal. Large, hard impactions may defy easy removal by this method and are better

suited to removal by irrigation. Blunt removal should be discontinued if it becomes clear that the drum is perforated. For irrigation, a warm solution of equal parts 3% hydrogen peroxide and water is directed at the mass with a flexible catheter. Cut the catheter of a butterfly needle and attach the remaining tubing to a 30-cc syringe. The flexible tubing can be inserted directly into the canal by the patient or clinician with little risk of injuring the walls or tympanic membrane. Repeated emergency department irrigation at 15-minute intervals will remove all but the hardest masses. If this method does not work, continued home treatments will soften and clear the remaining obstruction within a few days. Care should be taken with either method in elderly or diabetic patients because canal trauma may predispose the patient to malignant otitis externa.

FROSTBITE

ESSENTIALS OF DIAGNOSIS

► Protruding appendages (ie, nose, ears, fingers, toes) are affected most often
► Pale color, insensate
► Injury borders may not be apparent for several hours

▶ Clinical Findings

The nose and auricle are particularly vulnerable to injury from cold exposure. Superficial skin injuries are red and tender in the emergency department, but moderate and severe cases will appear pale and lack sensation prior to warming. Pain may not develop until later. After warming, the skin appearance will provide clues to the severity and extent of the damage. Inspect the lips, nose, and auricle regarding shape and contours, sensation, edema, skin color, and lesions. It may be helpful to draw a diagram showing the borders of injury. The distal edges of the auricle and tip of the nose are typically the first to be affected by cold exposure, with injury progressing proximally after prolonged exposure.

▶ Grading the Injury

Accurate grading of cold exposure injuries can be attempted 1–2 hours after rewarming, but serious cases may require 1–2 days of observation for full assessment. Frostnip is a mild form of injury, characterized by pain, pallor, and numbness and resolves with no permanent injury after rewarming. Frostbite is graded in four levels of severity:

1. First-degree injuries demonstrate hyperemia and edema, with eventual return of most sensation.

2. Second-degree injuries are similar to first-degree injuries but involve blisters. Recovery of sensation is variable.

3. Third-degree injuries exhibit deeper skin and cartilaginous tissue damage, with smaller, hemorrhagic blisters. There is significant permanent sensory deficit.

4. Fourth-degree injuries remain pale, insensate, develop no blisters, and have permanent skin and cartilage breakdown. There is eventual full-thickness necrosis and deformity.

▶ Treatment

Patients should be assessed for systemic cold injury and receive treatment for core hypothermia if necessary. The injured areas should not be rewarmed until there is no chance of refreezing. Structures of the face may be gently rewarmed using warm saline soaked gauze. The ear should be covered (usually with a head wrap) with care taken to preserve the inherent shape and projection of the pinna. Gauze padding may be loosely placed in and behind the ear to preserve its shape until it has healed. The full extent of injury may take days to become apparent, and hospitalization for wound care is appropriate for severe (third or fourth-degree) injuries. No attempt should be made to excise injured tissue in the first 2 days since some tissues that initially seem nonviable will survive with time. Update the tetanus toxoid. Recovered areas will remain abnormally cold sensitive and prone to injury, because the tissues rarely heal completely. Encourage patients to avoid future cold exposure.

CHRONIC (SUPPURATIVE) OTITIS MEDIA

ESSENTIALS OF DIAGNOSIS

▶ Persistent ear pain and discharge despite antibiotics

Chronic otitis media refers to persistent infection of fluid behind the tympanic membrane of several weeks or more. There may be varying degrees of discharge. Ordinary ruptures of the tympanic membrane heal in 1–2 weeks, and persistent defects should prompt close scrutiny. Accumulations of keratin result in formation of a cholesteatoma, which can contribute to injury to the bony structures of the middle ear. Persistent infections of the middle ear have an infrequent association with meningitis as well as mastoiditis. CT scan will reveal the latter condition, and clinical judgment should be used to determine which patients need a lumbar puncture. Management of mastoiditis is usually surgical.

Infections limited to the middle ear should be treated with antibiotics (see Table 32–1) and prompt outpatient ENT evaluation.

DISORDERS OF THE SINUSES (SINUSITIS)

ESSENTIALS OF DIAGNOSIS

▶ Midface pain associated with fever and purulent nasal discharge
▶ Often recurrent

▶ General Considerations

The paranasal sinuses (maxillary, frontal, ethmoid, and sphenoid) are ordinarily air filled and communicate with the nasal passages through small ostia. Most cases of sinusitis occur in the setting of functional or anatomic obstruction, inflammation, and impaired drainage. While most are viral, some will have an element of bacterial overgrowth. Chronic sinusitis occurs with infections that persist for more than 3 months—often in a setting of irreversible obstruction or resistant bacteria and may require surgical drainage.

▶ Clinical Findings

A. History

Sinusitis universally causes pain and pressure to the upper face, which may be perceived as a frontal headache. Fever, chills, and nasal discharge are common. Maxillary sinusitis commonly causes pain in the upper teeth. Symptoms typically worsen over 1–3 days and may follow an upper respiratory infection. Some patients with structural anomalies are predisposed to these infections and may give a history of similar previous episodes.

B. Physical Examination

Fever may be present. Examine the patient for signs and type of nasal discharge. Classically, pressure or gentle tapping over the affected sinus will reveal tenderness on one side. The maxillary sinus is most often affected and can be examined by applying bilateral thumb pressure to the inferior aspect of the zygotic prominence above the corners of the mouth. Transillumination of the maxillary sinus can be accomplished in a darkened room by placing the otoscope light source directly against the zygoma and observing transmission of light through the anterior hard palate. The presence of purulent fluid in the maxillary sinus will decrease the transmission of light on one side.

C. Other Studies

Plain sinus X-rays may reveal the presence of large sinus fluid collections (Figure 32–8A and B), but CT scan is the most sensitive test and will reveal anatomic anomalies such as small tumors or a deviated septum (Figure 32–8C). Radiographic studies are not necessary unless the diagnosis is in doubt.

▶ Treatment

Culturing the sinus fluid directly is not practical in the emergency department. If bacterial infection is strongly suspected by the presence of prolonged fever, empiric antimicrobial therapy should cover *H. influenzae, Moraxella catarrhalis,* and gram-positive bacteria. Amoxicillin–clavulanate, 875 mg twice daily, covers β-lactamase-resistant strains and the mixed flora typical of these infections. Trimethoprim/sulfamethoxazole and cefuroxime are alternatives for penicillin-allergic patients. Short course therapy has been shown to be as effective as long term therapy for these patients.

Nasal decongestant pills and sprays can sometimes reduce swelling around the sinus ostia and promote drainage. Steroids should be considered to relieve inflammation in these patients as well. Often the infection in the sinus is related to a mass (tumor, polyp, deviated septum, turbinate anomaly) or inadequate drainage. Patients should be referred to an otolaryngologist for persistent or recurrent episodes.

Chronic sinusitis has been associated with *Staphylococcus aureus* infections, but lasting resolution will often follow only surgical drainage and correction of the anatomic obstruction. Immunocompromised persons are at risk for *Pseudomonas aeruginosa* and fungal infections.

▶ Complications

Several conditions related to sinus infection have been described. Direct extension of the infection to surrounding tissues can lead to frontal osteomyelitis, facial cellulitis, periorbital cellulitis, or periorbital abscess. For this reason, high fever, ocular movement problems, exophthalmos, diplopia, facial skin swelling, erythema, or extreme tenderness should be studied by CT scan. Intracranial extension can lead to meningitis, cavernous sinus thrombosis, brain abscess, or subdural empyema. Therefore, prominence of a headache or neurologic findings should prompt examination with CT scan or lumbar puncture.

DISORDERS OF THE OROPHARYNX

Please refer to the Immediate Management section and Table 32–6 for discussion of epiglottitis, Ludwig's angina, and other causes of throat pain. What follows is a more detailed discussion regarding the pathophysiology and treatment of airway deep space infections.

PERITONSILLITIS (PERITONSILLAR CELLULITIS AND ABSCESS)

ESSENTIALS OF DIAGNOSIS

▶ Extensive swelling does not typically obstruct the airway
▶ "Hot potato" voice
▶ Fever, severe pain
▶ Systemic dehydration typical

▶ General Considerations

Peritonsillitis, peritonsillar cellulitis, and abscess (also known collectively as *quinsy*) are extensions of mixed-flora bacterial infections of the tonsils. The differentiation between cellulitis and abscess is difficult to make on clinical grounds and is determined by identification of an abscess by intravenous contrast CT scan or more commonly by drainage of pus after aspirating or incising the mass. Some have utilized bedside ultrasound to confirm the presence of abscess. See Table 32–6 for a review of typical symptoms and a differential diagnosis. These patients will all commonly have some level of trismus or difficulty opening the mouth. Once the diagnosis is made, most peritonsillar masses should be treated with intravenous antibiotics and a drainage procedure in the emergency department.

▶ Drainage Procedure

A. Preparation

First, make certain that the patient does not have obstructive airway issues. Patients with impending airway collapse should receive an emergency artificial airway prior to decompression of the mass. The patient should be placed sitting upright with support for the occiput. The upright position makes handling of oral secretions easier, and the occipital support helps the patient relax and restricts movement during the procedure. The tonsillar mass should be palpated gently with a cotton swab to confirm fluctuance. Bedside ultrasound using a high frequency transducer may be used at this time as well. A pulsatile mass should prompt the clinician to order an intravenous contrast enhanced CT scan to confirm the diagnosis and rule out the possibility of carotid artery aneurysm. For the drainage procedure to be successful, patients must not have extreme trismus and they should be cooperative and well anesthetized. Patients will generally be more cooperative when premedicated with a moderate dose of an opiate analgesic. Next, use a topical anesthetic spray such as benzocaine–tetracaine, followed by an injection of 1–2 mL of 2% lidocaine–epinephrine into

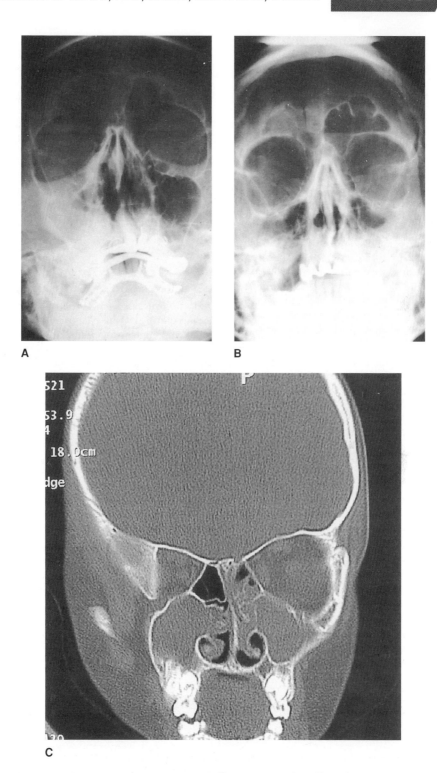

▲ **Figure 32–8.** Sinus imaging. **A:** Frontal sinusitis. **B:** Maxillary sinusitis. The affected air spaces are opacified due to being filled with fluid. **C:** CT scan demonstrating bilateral maxillary sinus and one ethmoid sinus opacification consistent with sinusitis.

the mucosal layer over the abscess. Frazier suction should be made ready for control of secretions and any pus or blood that results from the procedure.

B. Needle Drainage

Place an 18-gauge needle on a 10-mL syringe. The tip of the plastic needle cap should be cut off such that when placed back on the needle, 0.5 cm of the needle protrudes beyond the end. This will prevent accidental deep penetration of the mass. Insert the needle on an axis level with the tongue into the superior pole of the peritonsillar mass (the most common site for fluid) and aspirate (Figure 32–9). Remove and culture as much fluid as possible. Next, aspirate from the middle pole, and then the inferior pole. Take care to avoid directing the needle in a lateral direction so as to avoid puncturing the carotid artery. Because the needle may have missed the pocket of fluid, or the fluid may have been too thick to flow through the needle, a negative aspirate procedure does not rule out an abscess.

C. Open Drainage

Though many clinicians advocate needle aspiration (with antibiotics) as a safer and more comfortable method, incision and drainage with a scalpel blade appear to minimize recurrence risk. After anesthetizing the upper pole of the mass (see Figure 32–9), tape should be wrapped around the proximal aspect of the blade to prevent it from being inserted deeper than 0.5 cm. A single stab of depth 0.5 cm is made into the superior pole and extended no more than 0.5 cm in an inferolateral direction, being careful to avoid the carotid artery. Place the suction device tip into the incised area to remove any pus. Any bleeding that develops will usually resolve after the patient gargles with diluted hydrogen peroxide or salt water.

Patients should be observed for at least 1 hour following the procedure. Most are dehydrated and will benefit from intravenous fluids. Those able to take oral fluids and medications can be discharged with oral antibiotics. The preferred regimen is penicillin, 2–4 million units intravenously followed by 500 mg orally four times daily, or cephalosporins (eg, cefazolin 1 g intravenously, followed by cephalexin 500 mg four times daily for 10 days). Most patients will need oral nonsteroidal antiinflammatory agents and opiate analgesics for pain control. ENT follow-up in 2–3 days should be arranged. Patients with high fever, those unable to take oral fluids, and immunocompromised patients should be admitted for intravenous fluids and antibiotics. Some authors have advocated admitting patients with negative aspirates as well, for intravenous antibiotics and close observation.

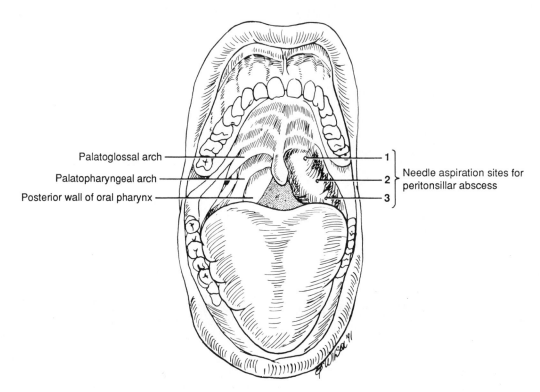

▲ **Figure 32–9.** Needle drainage sites for peritonsillar abscess.

EPIGLOTTITIS

ESSENTIALS OF DIAGNOSIS

▶ Fever, throat pain, swallowing pain

▶ Decreased prevalence in children

▶ Adults appear nontoxic

▶ Definitive diagnosis by endoscopy

Due to widespread use of the Hib vaccine, epiglottitis is now more common among adults than children. Children with epiglottitis have high fever and varying levels of toxicity by appearance (see Table 32–6). In children suspected of having epiglottitis, every attempt should be made to keep the child calm. No intravenous sticks should be attempted and the child should remain with the parent. A skilled pediatric airway specialist must be called (this may be the emergency physician, otolaryngologist, or anesthesiologist) and should remain with the patient. If patient stability permits, this clinician can accompany the child and parent while a lateral soft tissue neck X-ray is obtained. This may demonstrate the enlarged epiglottis (see Figure 32–6C), but a normal X-ray does not rule out the diagnosis. If the patient is toxic appearing or the diagnosis uncertain, the patient should be accompanied to the operating room where laryngoscopy and endotracheal intubation can be accomplished in a setting where a surgical airway can be easily done if needed. All pediatric patients found to have epiglottitis should ultimately be intubated for airway protection.

Adults with epiglottitis usually present with 2–3 days of steadily worsening throat pain, difficulty swallowing, and fever. The potential for rapid loss of airway patency is lower among adults than children, and most patients can have X-ray and emergency department flexible fiberoptic laryngoscopy without concern for rapid airway collapse. Those with epiglottitis should be admitted and receive intravenous antibiotics and fluids.

CROUP

ESSENTIALS OF DIAGNOSIS

▶ Associated with a recent upper respiratory infection

▶ "Barking" cough

▶ Often quick resolution

▶ General Considerations

Croup (laryngotracheobronchitis) is exclusively a disease of children, affecting mainly those aged from 6 months to 3 years. It is the most common cause of stridor among young children presenting to the emergency department. Unlike the supraglottic swelling of epiglottitis, croup leads to obstruction of the subglottic trachea (below the cords, mainly at the level of the cricoid cartilage).

▶ Clinical Findings

A. History

The predominant cause is parainfluenza virus, and its peak incidence is in fall and winter. The children are typically brought in at night, having recently developed a barking cough preceded by 2–3 days of a viral-type respiratory infection. The stridorous breathing is noisy and high pitched, a result of air traveling through a severely narrowed upper airway. Frequently, the symptoms will have improved by the time of arrival at the emergency department—possibly related to cool humid night air. Because an aspirated airway foreign body could mimic the symptoms of croup, parents should be questioned regarding this possibility.

B. Physical Examination

Children with croup usually appear nontoxic. When present, fever is usually low grade, reflecting an underlying viral infection. With exertion or crying, rapid air movement through the small subglottic aperture becomes difficult and respiratory distress worsens. Because the lungs are not affected, the oxygen saturation is typically normal except in extreme case when the narrowing becomes severe. Older children may have a barking cough or hoarseness. Oropharyngeal examination is normal or may reveal the bilateral nonspecific erythema and swelling associated with a viral upper respiratory infection. Any unilateral swelling or tonsillar exudates should prompt consideration of bacterial surface or closed-space infections. Transmitted airway noise may obscure auscultation of lung sounds, which are normal in croup. The patient should be examined for mental state, oxygenation, and use of accessory muscles.

C. Other Studies

An anteroposterior soft tissue neck X-ray will demonstrate the steeple sign of upper tracheal narrowing (Figure 32–10A and B). The serum white blood count may be elevated, but this is not specific for croup and has little value for differentiating croup from other processes.

▶ Treatment

Consideration should be given to the stability of the patient's airway. Croup rarely leads to complete airway obstruction except in the very young (<6 months), and mild epiglottitis

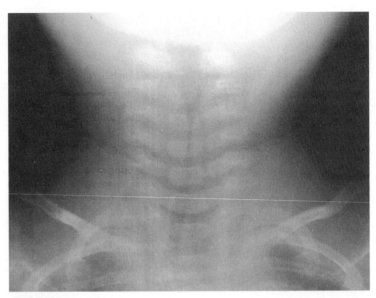

A

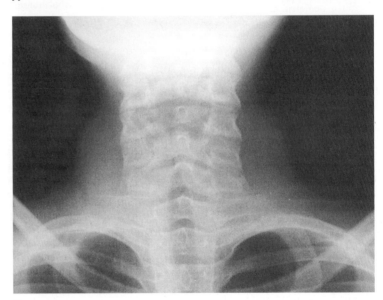

B

▲ **Figure 32-10.** The "steeple" sign of croup in a 1-year-old (**A**) and a 12-year-old (**B**).

can present with symptoms similar to croup (see Epiglottitis section above). The initial therapy is nebulized saline, which can be delivered by face mask or by having the parent direct the mist at the child's mouth. Nebulized racemic epinephrine should be used for patients who exhibit resting stridor: place 10 drops of 2.25% solution and 2–3 mL of saline in a nebulizer. The treatment may be repeated every 20–30 minutes. The child should be observed for 2–3 hours after the last treatment to assure that a rebound in symptoms does not occur. Dexamethasone, 0.6 mg/kg intramuscularly or

orally, is a useful adjunct for croup. Serial clinical evaluations of patient comfort will help identify the small percentage of children who will require admission for observation and further therapy. The majority of patients may be discharged with steroids for several days and outpatient follow-up.

DISORDERS OF THE MOUTH

Though myriad disorders involve the teeth and periodontal tissues, patients typically present to the emergency

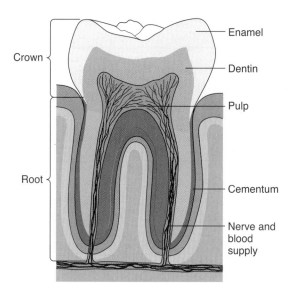

▲ Figure 32–11. Tooth anatomy.

department with acute processes in the mouth such as pain. Careful examination of the mouth is the key to correct diagnosis.

TOOTH ANATOMY

Teeth consist of a central pulp tissue, which is innervated by pain fibers and produces dentin (Figure 32–11). The dentin surrounds the pulp, makes up the bulk of the tooth mass, and is coated with enamel—a hard material that forms the outer surface of the tooth. The tooth surface of the root portion comprises cementum, which is less dense than enamel and not designed to withstand exposure to mouth flora and acids. Each tooth is embedded in periodontium, which consists of a bony support (alveolar bone) that is contiguous with underlying mandible and maxilla. The gingiva is the highly vascular mucosal tissue (gums) that covers the alveolar bone.

TOOTH PAIN

See Table 32–7.

ESSENTIALS OF DIAGNOSIS

▶ Commonly associated with prior tooth injury or cavity
▶ Differentiate simple infection from abscess

▶ Clinical Findings

A. History

Duration and rate of pain onset may be useful clues to a subacute process, whereas recent trauma or dental instrumentation would suggest a noninfectious problem. The location and distribution of the pain should be ascertained. Pain that worsens with chewing implicates a local tooth problem.

B. Physical Examination

The focus of the examination should be the area said to be painful. Tap on suspect teeth with a tongue blade—this will elicit tenderness from infections inside the tooth (pulpitis) and at the tooth root (periapical abscesses). A high degree of tenderness suggests the latter. A thorough viewing of the tooth and surrounding periodontium from all sides (use a warmed mirror to look at the lingual aspect) may demonstrate the cavity or any swelling. Focal erythema, swelling, and fluctuance would suggest a periodontal abscess. Examine the gingiva for ulcerations and pseudomembranes (acute necrotizing ulcerative gingivitis). The presence of blood can indicate poor periodontal health or may have resulted from recent trauma or instrumentation. Examine the tongue and floor of the mouth. Extension of dental infections into the soft tissues of the mandible can lead to Ludwig's angina, characterized by a firm, boardlike mouth floor and tongue elevation (see Table 32–6).

C. Other Studies

CT of the head and neck may be used to define the extent of the infection and rule out other severe diseases.

▶ Treatment

Because most conditions are best treated definitively in a fully equipped dental office, oral analgesics and discharge with dental follow-up are usually indicated. Most patients benefit from antiinflammatory agents such as ibuprofen or naproxen, or oral opiate analgesics such as codeine or hydrocodone as an adjunct. Care should be taken not to promote narcotic drug abuse, since dental pain is a favored complaint of drug seekers.

Application of a tooth block with a long-acting local anesthetic can provide hours of relief for those with severe pain and can reduce the reliance on oral analgesics.

Most painful tooth conditions also require therapy with an antibiotic. Oral penicillin, 500 mg four times daily, is the treatment of choice for typical tooth and periodontal infections, but immunocompromised patients and those with high fever or severe illness should have parenteral penicillin, 15–20 million units/d, or a cephalosporin as well as clindamycin for anaerobic (mainly *Bacteroides fragilis*) coverage. Amoxicillin–clavulanate is a single oral agent that covers these organisms.

Table 32–7. Diagnosis and Treatment of Tooth Pain.

Diagnosis	Diagnostic Clues	Treatment	Comments
Acute necrotizing ulcerative gingivitis (trench mouth)	Diffuse gingival pain, tenderness; may be accompanied by fever; gingival tissues are ulcerated and may be covered with a gray pseudomembrane; mouth has a foul odor	Requires meticulous oral hygiene: saltwater or hydrogen peroxide rinses, frequent brushing; topical and systemic oral analgesics, oral antibiotics, dental follow-up	Represents an infection of the gingiva by native mouth flora; more common in immunocompromised persons but mostly associated with poor oral hygiene
Aphthous stomatitis	Formation of small (2–3 mm) white plaques on mucosal surfaces of the mouth; tender to touch, may bleed if scraped; surrounding erythema suggests secondary infection	Topical analgesics and oral rinses (hydrogen peroxide); oral antibiotics for superinfected lesions	Onset often relates to stress or poor nutrition
Periapical abscess	Signs and symptoms of simple caries but with fever and extreme sensitivity to tooth percussion; panorex film to demonstrate abscesses	Incision and drainage, usually by a dental consultant; intravenous antibiotics in the emergency department, followed by oral antibiotics at home	Extension of the pulp infection into the root and periodontium, with resultant formation of an abscess
Periodontal abscess	Focal gingival swelling, erythema, fluctuance; tender to pressure	Incision and drainage; procedure is simpler than for a periapical abscess, because pocket is superficial; anesthetize with lidocaine–epinephrine prior to stab incision	Advisable to suture a small piece of Pen-rose drain or iodoform tape into the cavity to keep open for 2–3 days (until follow-up)
Postextraction pain	Pain immediately following removal of a tooth; rarely, pain will develop 3 days following the procedure, and examination of the socket reveals the foul odor and localized erythema consistent with a periodontal socket infection	For immediate pain: oral analgesics; socket infections require opiate analgesics or tooth block; the socket should be irrigated and oral antibiotics given; dental consultation is preferable, as the socket can be packed with dental paste for prompt pain relief	If dental consultation is not available in the emergency department, patients with socket infection should be referred to the dentist for prompt follow-up
Pulpitis	Poor dental care (by patient history or examination of mouth); defect in tooth enamel may be visible; no fever; pain localized to 1–2 teeth, which are tender to tapping	Oral analgesics, antibiotics; consider tooth block (see text)	Prompt (1–2 d) dental follow-up: tooth may need removal; simple caries are painless; presence of pain implies extension of the defect into pulp, with resultant inflammation
Root canal pain	Pain in a tooth following a root canal procedure; tender with pressure and chewing; tooth may appear to sit higher above the gingival ridge than appropriate	Dental consultation; build-up of gas or fluid at the tooth apex may require release	Pain may respond poorly to systemic or tooth block analgesia
Subluxation or avulsion	Loose (subluxation) or absent (avulsion) tooth	Replace, splint (see text)	Tooth survival correlates with subluxation severity and time the tooth is out of the socket
Tooth eruption	Infants aged 6 months to 3 years: primary teeth; associated with low-grade fever and (infrequently) diarrhea; secondary teeth begin to appear at age 5 years; third (wisdom) molars can become impacted, causing inflammation and pain with chewing; occasional periodontal abscess	Treat dehydration, if present; in infants and children: topical anesthetics, oral ibuprofen; for third molar impaction, drain abscess (if present), oral analgesics, antibiotics	Third molars may require removal, and these patients should be referred for prompt dental follow-up
Tooth fracture	History of a blow to the mandible or recent dental procedure or hardware; pain with chewing; fissure in tooth may be visible	Oral analgesics. Cover exposed dentin or pulp.	Need prompt dental follow-up

TMJ PAIN

TMJ pain (also broadly labeled temporomandibular disorder) is an inflammatory process of the temporomandibular joint, which often relates to overuse, trauma, or various arthritides.

▶ Clinical Findings

The joint area is tender to pressure on one or both sides, and pain is elicited with biting down on a tongue blade and mandible manipulation. The examiner can grip the chin and lower incisors and gently rock the mandible from side to side to elicit TMJ tenderness. Except in cases of recent trauma, X-ray images are rarely indicated in the acute setting.

▶ Treatment and Disposition

The usual therapy is for the patient to reduce the forceful use of the joint by avoiding hard foods and to use antiinflammatory medications for 1–2 weeks. Follow-up with a dental professional for persistent pain is recommended, at which point chewing and biting habits can be explored. Occasionally, corrective appliances are used to promote correct positioning and use of the jaw.

TMJ DISLOCATION

ESSENTIALS OF DIAGNOSIS

- ▶ Inability to close mouth
- ▶ Sudden onset, associated with a "click"

Typically the patient gives a history of wide mouth opening (typically a yawn or laughter) followed by an inability to close the mouth after feeling a click. They present with mouth open, are unable to speak clearly, and are sometimes distressed due to masseter spasm and pain. If the examination reveals deviation of the mandible to one side, the dislocation may be unilateral.

Reduction of the dislocation is relatively easy. Premedication with benzodiazepines for relaxation of masseter spasm and sedation is very helpful. The patient sits on a stretcher with the back up to support the head. Several advise a trial at extraoral reduction before the intraoral approach. To accomplish this, the clinician grasps the coronoid process and the anterior surface of the angle of the mandible through the cheek and applies steady downward and backward pressure. If not successful, the intraoral approach can be tried. The clinician faces the patient, and after padding the thumbs with layers of gauze to prevent injury, places them on the posterior lower molars and grips the underside of the mandible angle with the fingers. Steady, firm downward pressure is applied onto the rear molars. Successful reduction is characterized by a sudden snapping of the mandible back into place, which can put the examiner's digits at risk of a bite injury if he or she is not prepared. The patient will have immediate relief. Patients who sustain this injury are at increased risk for developing it again and should be warned to avoid wide mouth openings in the future.

Ardehali MM, Kouhi A, Meighani A, Rad FM, Emami H: Temporomandibular joint dislocation reduction technique: a new external method vs the traditional. Ann Plast Surg 2009;63:176–178 [PMID: 19542876].

Brook I: Current management of upper respiratory tract and head and neck infections. Eur Arch Otorhinolaryngol 2009;266:315–323 [PMID: 18985371].

Chan Y, Kuhn FA: An update on the classifications, diagnosis, and treatment of rhinosinusitis. Curr Opin Otolaryngol Head Neck Surg 2009;17:204–208 [PMID:19346944].

D'Agostino J: Pediatric airway nightmares. Emerg Med Clin North Am 2010;28:119–126 [PMID: 19945602].

Falagas ME, Karageorgopoulos DE, Grammatikos AP, Matthaiou DK: Effectiveness and safety of short vs long duration of antibiotic therapy for acute bacterial sinusitis: a meta-analysis of randomized trials. Br J Clin Pharmacol 2009;67:161–171 [PMID: 19154447].

Jurkovich GJ: Environmental cold-induced injury. Surg Clin North Am 2007;87:247–267 [PMID: 17127131].

Marom T, Cinamon U, Itskoviz D, Roth Y: Changing trends of peritonsillar abscess. Am J Otolaryngol 2010;31:162–167 [PMID: 20015734].

Mazza D, Wilkinson F, Turner T, Harris C, Health for kids guideline development group: evidence based guideline for the management of croup. Aust Fam Physician 2008;37:14–20 [PMID: 19142265].

Mohr WJ, Jenabzadeh K, Ahrenholz DH: Cold injury. Hand Clin 2009;25:481–496 [PMID: 19801122].

Nentwich L, Ulrich AS: High-risk chief complaints II: disorders of the head and neck. Emerg Med Clin North Am 2009;27:713–746 [PMID: 19932402].

Nguyen DH, Martin JT: Common dental infections in the primary care setting. Am Fam Physician 2008;77:797–802 [PMID: 18386594].

Ramakrishnan K, Sparks RA, Berryhill WE: Diagnosis and treatment of otitis media. Am Fam Physician 2007;76:1650–1658 [PMID: 18092706].

Ramirez-Schrempp D, Dorfman DH, Baker WE, Liteplo AS: Ultrasound soft-tissue applications in the pediatric emergency department: to drain or not to drain? Pediatr Emerg Care 2009;25:44–48 [PMID: 19148015].

Roland PS, Smith TL, Schwartz SR, Rosenfeld RM, Ballachanda B, Earll JM, Fayad J, Harlor AD Jr, Hirsch BE, Jones SS, Krouse HJ, Magit A, Nelson C, Stutz DR, Wetmore S: Clinical practice guideline: cerumen impaction. Otolaryngol Head Neck Surg 2008;139:S1–S21 [PMID: 18707628].

Sidebottom AJ: Current thinking in temporomandibular joint management. Br J Oral Maxillofac Surg 2009;47:91–94 [PMID: 19155105].

Siegel RM: Acute otitis media guidelines, antibiotic use, and shared medical decision-making. Pediatrics 2010;125:384–386 [PMID: 20100752].

Smith JA, Danner CJ: Complications of chronic otitis media and cholesteatoma. Otolaryngol Clin North Am 2006;39:1237–1255 [PMID: 17097444].

Vergison A, Dagan R, Arguedas A, Bonhoeffer J, Cohen R, Dhooge I, Hoberman A, Liese J, Marchisio P, Palmu AA, Ray GT, Sanders EA, Simões EA, Uhari M, van Eldere J, Pelton SI: Otitis media and its consequences: beyond the earache. Lancet Infect Dis 2010;10:195–203 [PMID: 20185098].

Vissers RJ, Gibbs MA: The high-risk airway. Emerg Med Clin North Am 2010;28:203–217 [PMID: 19945607].

Pulmonary Emergencies

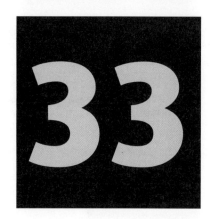

David A. Smith, MD

ASTHMA AND CHRONIC OBSTRUCTIVE PULMONARY DISEASE

See also Chapter 13.

 ESSENTIALS OF DIAGNOSIS

Asthma

► Cough, wheezing, chest tightness, often worse at night

► Physical examination:Prolonged expiratory phaseor bilateral wheezing, tachypnea, tachycardia, hypoxia

► Reversible with bronchodilators

Chronic Obstructive Pulmonary Disease

► Smoker with chronic productive cough complains of dyspnea

► Increased sputum production, bilateral wheezing, rales, and rhonchi

▶ General Considerations

Obstructive lung disease is classified into two categories: asthma and chronic obstructive pulmonary disease (COPD). Patients with asthma have disease that is episodic and reversible to a significant degree. Between acute attacks these patients may have relatively normal lung function. However, patients who have persistent inflammation may develop over time permanent changes that contribute to a decline in functional capacity. Patients with COPD have significant fixed airway obstruction that remains at baseline even when the patient's illness is under optimal control. In addition to the concept of reversibility, there are other characteristics that distinguish these two groups. Asthmatic patients tend to be younger and more likely to have allergic triggers and conditions. A family history is common. Patients with COPD usually have a long history of cigarette smoking and more significant permanent lung injury and chest remodeling. Associated right heart failure does not occur in asthma but is common in advanced cases of COPD.

Many conditions commonly associated with asthma and COPD exacerbations are listed in Table 33–1. Some of these

Table 33–1. Common Precipitating Factors in Acute Asthma and Exacerbations of Chronic Obstructive Pulmonary Disease.

Infection (especially upper respiratory tract viral infections)
Drugs (aspirin, nonsteroidal anti-inflammatory agents, food coloring, β-blockers)
Exercise
Emotional stress
Inhaled irritants (eg, air pollution, cigarette smoke)
Occupational exposure to dusts, gases, etc
Aeroallergens (pollens, grasses, molds, animal dander)
Gastroesophageal reflux disease
Weather changes (especially cold)
Menses (catamenial asthma)

conditions are treatable, and the clinician should ask about them specifically while taking the patient's history.

There are two varieties of COPD: chronic bronchitis and emphysema. Chronic bronchitis is characterized by chronic cough and sputum production and is almost invariably associated with prolonged and heavy cigarette smoking. Such patients usually have increased lung volumes and a barrel-shaped chest with increased lung markings on chest X-ray. In advanced cases they may have cyanosis and peripheral edema due to right heart failure. Patients with emphysema on the other hand are typically thin without cyanosis and breathe through pursed lips. Accessory muscle use is more prominent. The chest X-ray usually shows a paucity of lung markings reflecting tissue destruction. Some patients with emphysema have genetic factors (α_1-antitrypsin deficiency) as the basis of their illness, but most have a long history of cigarette smoking.

▶ Clinical Findings

A. Asthma

1. History—Most asthmatic patients present with exacerbations of known disease with shortness of breath and cough. They frequently complain of tightness in the chest. Those with significant chest pain, fever, or purulent sputum may have associated pneumonia. Acute attacks are frequently precipitated by upper respiratory infection, exercise, or inhaled allergens.

2. Physical examination—Most patients are wheezing and coughing with respiratory distress. Tremor and tachycardia are common due to a combination of sympathomimetic therapy and the stress of the illness. Mild degrees of hypoxia are common. Dehydration due to inadequate oral intake or vomiting is almost always present. Tachypnea and sometimes fever increase insensible losses. Thick and tenacious secretions tend to cause mucous plugging and significantly contribute to impaired gas exchange.

Patients with moderate distress typically prefer to sit up and frequently are agitated, tachycardic, and tachypneic with accessory muscle use. Patients with severe distress may be hypoxic even with supplemental oxygen or have marked abnormalities of vital signs. Those with alteration of mental status, CO_2 retention, or who begin to tire are in danger of respiratory arrest.

B. Chronic Bronchitis and Emphysema

1. History—COPD is a chronic disease and baseline functional limitations are characteristic of the illness. The presentation of an acute exacerbation is increased shortness of breath, wheezing, and cough that becomes progressively worse over several days. An increase in sputum production is frequently seen, especially in patients with chronic bronchitis. Activity tolerance becomes more limited in these patients. Most are dyspneic at rest when they present to the emergency department.

2. Physical examination

A. EMPHYSEMA—Patients with emphysema have diminished breath sounds due to the loss of lung parenchyma. Patients with advanced disease are usually thin and appear uncomfortable even at baseline with obvious use of accessory muscles. These patients may be described as "pink puffers" because they are generally not cyanotic or significantly hypoxic and breathe through pursed lips.

B. CHRONIC BRONCHITIS—In addition to wheezing and prolonged expiration, patients with chronic bronchitis usually have a few course rales and prominent rhonchi. Heart tones are usually distant because of a barrel shape to the chest and the loss of pulmonary parenchyma that transmits sound. They frequently are moderately obese. Peripheral edema may be due to right heart failure associated with advanced disease. Patients with chronic bronchitis are not as uncomfortable in appearance as those with emphysema and frequently have minimal symptoms in the face of pronounced CO_2 retention and hypoxia. These patients are sometimes referred to as "blue bloaters," because of the frequent occurrence of cyanosis and edema.

▶ Evaluation

A. Medical History

In addition to standard medical history, the use of oxygen at home is important. Patients who have required ICU care or intubation are at greater risk for severe disease. Continued smoking contributes more than any other factor to the increased risk of illness and death.

B. Laboratory and Other Findings

1. Pulse Oximetry—Pulse oximetry usually gives better information regarding oxygenation than do blood gases because it is available in real time. An accurate reading depends on good blood flow and a thin body part to attach the device. When a good arterial waveform is visible on the monitor the readings are very accurate and reliable.

2. Blood gases—The assessment of alveolar ventilation and respiratory acidosis are best evaluated with blood gas analysis. Many patients with COPD but particularly those on home oxygen have a chronic respiratory acidosis (elevated PCO_2) with metabolic compensation (increased total CO_2, or bicarbonate). A low pH is indicative of acute decompensation. Comparing values from previous measurements is helpful in assessing the significance of these abnormalities.

3. Chest X-ray—Most patients with mild asthma will not need a chest X-ray unless pneumonia or pneumothorax is suspected. Patients with COPD or advanced age are more likely to have important findings on chest X-ray. Congestive heart failure, pleural effusions along with lung cancer, and associated complications are important diagnoses that may be made or suspected with plain images of the chest. If pulmonary embolism (PE) is suspected, then CT scanning with contrast is necessary.

4. Peak expiratory flow measurement—Peak expiratory flow (PEF) measurements are a practical way of following the severity of illness and response to therapy in patients with asthma. The values should be compared with predicted peak flow values, which are based on age, sex, and height.

5. Electrocardiogram—Most patients with significant respiratory distress or abnormal vital signs should be placed on a cardiac monitor and the cardiac rhythm determined. The electrocardiogram provides additional information where the rhythm is not easily determined from a single lead monitor or if cardiac ischemia is suspected.

6. CBC and Electrolytes—Some patients with COPD are polycythemic due to chronic hypoxia. Metabolic compensation from chronic CO_2 retention is usually evident from venous electrolytes in the form of an elevated bicarbonate as reflected in the total CO_2.

7. Microscopic examination of sputum—Sputum examination is primarily useful in selected patients when adequate specimens are available and pneumonia is suspected. They also can be useful in the diagnostic evaluation when atypical pathogens such as mycobacteria or *Legionella* species are suspected.

8. Drug levels—Theophylline is no longer commonly used. Patients who do take theophylline may be toxic and drug levels are indicated if toxicity is suspected.

Differential Diagnosis

A. Adults

Most patients with COPD present with a long history of previous exacerbations similar to the present episode.

The diagnostic challenge is usually in the identification or exclusion of associated conditions including congestive heart failure, PE, pneumothorax, and cancer of the lung. Most patients are elderly and at risk for all these illnesses. In many cases, the reason for dyspnea may be multifactorial. Patients with fever may have pneumonia or another type of infection. If chest pain is present, associated cardiac disease must be considered. Other pulmonary pathology such as pneumothorax may be present. It cannot be stressed too strongly that many patients who present with wheezing actually have acute heart failure as the primary reason for dyspnea. Impressively elevated blood pressure is a valuable clue to the presence of associated acute heart failure.

B. Children

Respiratory syncytial virus infection is a significant cause of wheezing and respiratory distress in young children. Rapid testing for these infections helps to identify these patients but usually does not change therapy. The test is used to determine the need for respiratory isolation if the patient requires hospitalization. Most children may be given a diagnosis of reactive airway disease and treated in a similar manner. Foreign body aspiration typically presents with the acute onset of wheezing and respiratory distress in a crawler or young toddler.

Treatment

Asthma by definition should be largely reversible with treatment. Patients with COPD have fixed obstruction but do have episodes when symptoms are exaggerated and can be improved with therapy.

1. Provide supplemental oxygen

A. Oxygen therapy—Most patients with mild asthma can be treated with nasal cannula oxygen at 2–4 L/min. Patients whose saturations fall below 90% require higher concentrations by mask. Patients who are anxious, hypoxic, and struggling to breathe should receive high concentrations of oxygen as necessary to achieve adequate oxygen saturations. A nonrebreather mask with an oxygen reservoir can be used to deliver nearly a 100% inspired oxygen concentration if necessary.

B. CO_2 narcosis—Some patients with advanced COPD, especially those maintained on oxygen at home, may develop CO_2 narcosis if high concentrations of oxygen are used. Such patients develop an altered mental status when their hypoxic ventilatory drive is removed, CO_2 levels rise, and a respiratory acidosis develops. Most of the time, this is seen when a patient not short of breath is treated with oxygen for another reason such as chest pain.

2. Hydration—Patients are usually in need of intravenous fluids. This is particularly true of asthmatics and an aspect of treatment that is frequently neglected. Young adults with asthma and without cardiac disease should receive 1–2 L of normal saline over the first hour or two and at 500 cc/h thereafter. Children should be treated with 20 cc/kg of saline as a bolus.

Patients with COPD are usually older and may have associated cardiac disease; therefore, caution is indicated in these patients to avoid fluid overload. A fluid bolus of 250–500 cc of saline is typically appropriate in an elderly patient or someone with known heart disease.

3. Respiratory support—If patients begin to tire or show signs that failure of ventilation is developing, they should be supported mechanically.

A. BiPAP—The technology of noninvasive treatment with Bilevel (BiPAP) support has improved over the last several years. Many patients who otherwise would require intubation can be supported noninvasively and avoid the risks of an artificial airway. An initial setting of 10 cm H_2O of inspiratory pressure and 5 cm H_2O of expiratory pressure is usually an appropriate initial setting for BiPAP support for either asthma or COPD.

B. INTUBATION—If a patient cannot manage their airway either because of confusion, lethargy, or agitation, then they will require an artificial airway (see Chapter 7). Patients may also require intubation because of excessive secretions or a need for frequent suctioning. Controlled rapid sequence intubation is preferable to crash intubation which may be required if the patient suddenly deteriorates. Larger endotracheal tubes facilitate suctioning and bronchoscopy and should be used if possible. Low tidal volume ventilation (Table 33–2) helps to decrease overdistention, air trapping, and resultant barotrauma. Measurement of blood gases is

Table 33–2. Settings for Low Tidal Volume Ventilation.

Tidal Volume	6 mL per kilogram of predicted, not actual, body weight
Predicted Body Weight in Men = 50.0 + 0.91 (height in centimeters − 152.4)	
Predicted Body Weight in Women = 45.5 + 0.91 (height in centimeters − 152.4)	
Initial Respiratory Rate	18 to 22 breaths per minute
Partial pressure of carbon dioxide P_{CO_2}	Less than 80 mm Hg
Plateau airway pressure	30 cm of water or less
Target arterial oxyhemoglobin saturation	Greater than 90%

important in guiding therapy when positive pressure support of any kind is used.

4. β-Adrenergic agonists—These medications are the mainstay of treatment for asthma and COPD. The ones most commonly used are the short-acting β_2-selective agents. These agents cause rapid relaxation of bronchial smooth muscles, resulting in bronchodilation, and reducing airflow obstruction. Albuterol, levalbuterol (the R-isomer of albuterol), and metaproterenol are used most often. Inhalation, through metered-dose inhalers (MDIs) or nebulizers, has been shown to be faster and to deliver higher concentrations of medication to the lungs with fewer systemic side effects than oral preparations. However, MDIs require coordination and a cooperative, alert patient who can hold his or her breath for 5–10 seconds. Therefore, passive nebulized β_2-agonists are more often used in moderate and severe exacerbations. For mild disease, albuterol MDI dosing is 4–6 puffs every 20 minutes (up to 4 hours), and nebulized solutions should be given at 2.5 mg every 20–30 minutes. Patients who are severely ill may receive 5 mg every 20–30 minutes or a continuous treatment for an hour or more. Attention to monitoring the patient for tachycardia and for signs of respiratory failure should be continued and not neglected in patients on continuous treatment.

5. Anticholinergics—Ipratropium nebulized solution, 0.5 mg every 20–30 minutes, can be used. This is frequently mixed with albuterol and given every 20–30 minutes. Hospitalized patients may be scheduled every 4–6 hours.

6. Systemic corticosteroids—Steroids are well known to inhibit both inflammatory cell recruitment and the release of inflammatory mediators into the airways. Many patients with moderate to severe obstructive airway disease take chronic steroids. Although steroids do not initially change emergency department management, these medications are crucial to reduce the rate of relapse in moderate to severe exacerbations. They can also be helpful in mild attacks if the patient is not responding well to initial bronchodilator treatments. Consider steroids if the patient is taking oral or inhaled steroids, has had prolonged symptoms, or recently completed a steroid taper. Patients who are severely ill should receive steroids. Steroid doses for adults are prednisone, 40–60 mg orally, or methylprednisolone, 60–125 mg intramuscularly or intravenously. Dosing for children includes prednisone, 2 mg/kg orally, or methylprednisolone 0.5–2 mg/kg intravenously. Discharge the patient to home with a steroid burst (adults: prednisone, 40 mg/d; children: 1 mg/kg, for 3–5 days) or taper (10–14 days) depending on severity.

7. Antibiotics—Antibiotics are typically not indicated for mild asthma unless evidence of infection is present on physical examination or chest X-ray. Patients with an acute

~~exacerbation of COPD~~, presenting with worsening dyspnea and increased cough and sputum production, ~~usually benefit from antibiotics.~~ Patients who have associated pneumonia should be treated with antibiotics. (See Pneumonia & Bronchitis, below.)

A. Other Known Treatment Modalities

1. Magnesium sulfate—Magnesium has a direct relaxing effect on bronchial smooth muscle and also helps to stabilize many inflammatory mediators. For patients with severe asthma, magnesium (in conjunction with ongoing treatment) may help improve airway obstruction and avoid intubation. The dosing is 2–3 g intravenously, infused at 1 g/min, with close monitoring of blood pressure. The infusion should stop if hypotension, respiratory depression, or decreased deep tendon reflexes occurs.

2. Methylxanthines—Theophylline (oral) or aminophylline (intravenous) are moderately effective bronchodilators. However, toxicity, particularly vomiting and resulting dehydration, is a particular problem. ~~These medications are no longer recommended for the treatment of acute exacerbations of asthma or COPD~~.

3. Ketamine—Ketamine has been shown to be a significant bronchodilator and can be used to facilitate intubation of severely agitated patients with refractory disease (status asthmaticus). Usual anesthetic induction dose is 1–2 mg/kg intravenously or 4 mg/kg intramuscularly.

▶ Disposition

A. Asthma

Asthma patients who demonstrate a good response (PEF > 70% of predicted) and whose symptoms have resolved can be discharged home. Those with an incomplete response to treatment (PEF, 50–70% of predicted), with improved symptoms, and no hypoxia can be discharged if close follow-up and correct use of inhalers can be demonstrated. Most patients that have returned to the emergency department within 3 days should be admitted for continued treatment in the hospital.

B. Acute Exacerbations of COPD

Acute exacerbations of COPD are ~~more difficult and resolve slower than acute exacerbations of asthma. Most patients with COPD will require admission.~~ Some patients will have significant comorbidities such as pneumonia or associated heart failure. Some are severely ill and require ICU care. Many patients are elderly and social issues such as the availability of home health care, and assistance with the activities of daily living make treatment outside the hospital impractical.

Garpestad E, Brennan J, Hill NS: Noninvasive ventilation for critical care. Chest 2007;132:711–720 [PMID: 17699147].

Holley AD, Boots RJ: Review article: management of acute severe and near-fatal asthma. Emerg Med Australas 2009;21(4): 259–268 [PMID: 19682010].

Krishnan JA, Davis SQ, Naureckas ET, Gibson P et al: An umbrella review: corticosteroid therapy for adults with acute asthma. Am J Med 2009;122:977–991 [PMID: 19854321].

Peters SG: Continuous bronchodilator therapy. Chest 2007; 131(1):286–289 [PMID: 17218588].

▼ PULMONARY VASCULAR DISEASES

ACUTE PULMONARY EMBOLISM

 ESSENTIALS OF DIAGNOSIS

- ▶ Acute onset of dyspnea, pleuritic chest pain, tachypnea, tachycardia
- ▶ Hypoxemia with widened A-a gradient
- ▶ Pulmonary angiogram is gold standard

▶ General Considerations

A variety of clinical conditions may cause clots to form in the venous system that when dislodged will cause pulmonary emboli (Table 33–3). Venous thrombosis may

Table 33–3. Conditions that Predispose to Pulmonary Embolization.

Venous stasis
Prolonged immobility (eg, bed rest, stroke)
Chronic obstructive pulmonary disease
Congestive heart failure
Venous endothelial damage
Surgery within past 3 months
Fractures of long bones or hip
Burns
Lower extremity trauma
Hypercoagulability
Malignant neoplastic disease
Use of oral contraceptives
Marked obesity
Protein C or S deficiency
Antithrombin III deficiency
Presence of factor V Leiden
Previous history of deep venous thrombosis or pulmonary embolism

result from a generalized hypercoagulable state, venous endothelial injury, or local stasis (Virchow triad). Clots that cause clinically significant pulmonary emboli form most commonly in the iliofemoral and pelvic venous beds. Pulmonary embolization, from veins of the upper extremities or distal lower extremities, is unusual and rarely clinically significant.

When embolization occurs, the manifestations depend on the size of the embolism, the patient's underlying cardiorespiratory status, and whether subsequent infarction of pulmonary tissue occurs. With small to medium sized emboli, obstruction of a localized portion of the pulmonary vascular tree causes local atelectasis with resulting ventilation–perfusion (V/Q) abnormalities and hypoxemia. Reflex hyperventilation with resultant hypocapnia and tachycardia also occurs. With massive embolization (obstructing over 60% of the vascular bed), acute pulmonary hypertension, right heart strain, systemic hypotension, and shock may also occur. Pulmonary emboli may also present with sudden cardiovascular collapse and death.

▶ Clinical Findings

A. Symptoms and Signs

The illness often begins abruptly, and a predisposing underlying condition is almost always present. Dyspnea and chest pain are the usual presenting symptoms. Tachycardia and hypoxia are the most common clinical signs. Fever, hypotension, cyanosis, pleural friction rub, and pulmonary consolidation may be the result of PE but are usually the result of other illnesses when they occur.

B. Laboratory and Other Findings

1. Chest X-ray—The chest X-ray is abnormal in most patients with pulmonary embolization with infarction but the abnormalities are often nonspecific (eg, atelectasis, pleural effusions, small infiltrates). The Westermark sign (dilated pulmonary vasculature proximal to embolus with oligemia distal) and Hampton's Hump (a pleural-based density with a rounded border facing the hilum) are more suggestive though uncommon findings with pulmonary emboli.

2. Electrocardiogram—The electrocardiogram is often abnormal, usually demonstrating tachycardia or diffuse nonspecific ST-T abnormalities. The classic finding of acute right heart strain (S1/Q3/T3; T-wave inversion in leads V1–V3) is more specific but somewhat uncommon.

3. Arterial blood gases—A clinically significant PE is usually but not always associated with hypoxemia (oxygen saturation < 90%; Po_2 < 80 mm Hg). Hyperventilation and hypocapnia are also common findings. An arterial puncture is required to measure the arterial Pco_2 and calculate an alveolar-arterial oxygen gradient (A-a gradient). The

value of the A-a gradient over the more easily measured oxygen saturation by pulse oximetry is minimal. Most of the time the additional time, discomfort and expense is not justified by any additional discriminatory ability of the A-a gradient.

4. D-dimer—The serum levels of the D-dimer (a degradation product of crosslinked fibrin) have been shown to be a highly sensitive (95%) screening examination for the formation of acute thrombus. The test is nearly always positive in patients with recent trauma or surgery or any process that produces bleeding and requires hemostasis. In patients who are at low risk for PE (low pretest probability) a negative test can be helpful in ruling out PE. Patients who are not at low risk should undergo a more definitive test such as CT scanning.

5. Geneva score—The Geneva score is a clinical decision tool that can be used in the diagnostic evaluation of patients with suspected PE. The original score was revised to preclude the need for arterial blood gasses. The revised and simplified Geneva score (Table 33–4) has the same diagnostic utility as the original score and its calculation is more reliable. A simplified score of 0-2 indicates the patient is unlikely to have a PE and when combined with a normal D-dimer test, the clinical probability of a PE is 3% or less.

C. Diagnostic Imaging

1. Contrast-enhanced CT scan—Contrast-enhanced CT scan allows for rapid evaluation and is accurate but requires intravenous contrast enhancement and expert radiographic

Table 33–4. Simplified Revised Geneva Score.

Variable	Score[a]
Age greater than 65 years	1
Previous DVT or PE	1
Surgery (under general anesthesia) or fracture (of lower limbs) within 1 month.	1
Active malignant condition (solid or hematologic, currently active or considered cured < 1 year	1
Unilateral lower-limb pain	1
Hemoptysis	1
Heart rate 75-94	
Heart rate greater than or equal to 95	1
Pain on lower-limb deep venous palpation and unilateral edema	1

[a]A score of 0–2 are unlikely to have a PE and when combined with a normal d-dimer test, the clinical probability of a PE is 3% or less.

interpretation. The technology has improved in recent years and now includes automated bolus injection and fast, high-resolution, multislice CT scanners. CT scanning also provides a wealth of information regarding other chest pathologies, such as pneumonia, pleural effusion, masses, and vascular pathology, such as aneurysms. Contrast allergy is sometimes an issue. Pretreatment with steroids and antihistamines can be done if a contrast allergy is suspected and the study is necessary.

2. Ventilation–perfusion radionuclide lung scan (V/Q scan)—V/Q scanning has been replaced with contrast-enhanced CT scanning except in cases of contrast allergy. A normal perfusion scan essentially excludes significant embolization. In many patients the perfusion scan will not be normal (most commonly with COPD) and the ventilation scan is used to look for areas of mismatched ventilation and perfusion. A high-probability V/Q scan is defined as a large perfusion defect in areas of normal ventilation and is highly specific (but insensitive) for acute pulmonary emboli. An indeterminate V/Q scan (also reported as nondiagnostic, low probability, or intermediate probability) is more difficult to use clinically.

3. Venous Doppler ultrasound—Doppler ultrasound is a noninvasive test used in the diagnosis of deep venous thrombosis. The test is sensitive and specific. A positive venous Doppler lends supportive evidence that the patient has thrombosis; however, thrombosis can occur without embolization. Many patients with significant pulmonary emboli are asymptomatic in their lower extremities and have negative lower extremity Doppler studies.

4. Pulmonary angiogram—The diagnostic accuracy of pulmonary angiography is considered to be the best of any procedure available. Frequently, CT images are convincing enough to be considered pathognomonic and in that case angiography does not offer a diagnostic advantage. Angiography requires right heart catheterization, which is usually done only as part of thrombolytic treatment for patients hemodynamically compromised by the size of the embolus.

▶ Treatment

A. Hemodynamic Support

Correct hypoxemia with supplemental oxygen. Patients with large emboli may be hypotensive and require resuscitation with intravenous fluids. Pressors and positive pressure ventilation are poorly tolerated and should be avoided unless absolutely necessary.

B. Anticoagulation Therapy

Anticoagulation is the standard treatment and should be administered as soon as the diagnosis of pulmonary embolization is made. If a delay in diagnosis is anticipated and there are no contraindications, patients may be treated presumptively. This most often occurs when CT scanning is not available and the patient must be transferred to another institution or held overnight.

The usual dose of unfractionated heparin (UFH) is an initial 80 IU/kg bolus followed by 18 IU/kg/h infusion. Many institutions have protocols for heparinization and the use of one is recommended. Low-molecular weight heparin (LMWH) (enoxaparin 1 mg/kg SC q 12 hours or dalteparin 200 units /kg/day SC divided qd to BID) and fondaparinux(a factor X_a inhibitor) 7.5 mg SC qd are as effective and safe as UFH and are more convenient. Compared with UFH, LMWH and fondaparinux are more expensive medications but may reduce the total hospital cost and length of stay.

C. Thrombolytic Therapy

Although anticoagulation is sufficient treatment for most patients with pulmonary emboli, a few patients who present with hemodynamic compromise may benefit from thrombolytic therapy via a pulmonary artery catheter. Peripherally administered thrombolytic treatment has not been shown to be of value.

D. Surgical Treatment

A transvenous catheter embolectomy or open surgical embolectomy may be a lifesaving maneuver in a patient with massive emboli and refractory hypotension. The usual indication for a vena cava filter is the failure of anticoagulation to prevent thromboembolism.

▶ Disposition

Hospitalize all patients for continued anticoagulation and supportive care. Patients with hemodynamic impairment, or those receiving thrombolytics, should be monitored in the ICU. Patients in whom PE is strongly suspected should be hospitalized for anticoagulation (if no contraindications are present) until a definitive diagnosis can be made.

Adam SS, Key NS, Greenberg CS: D-dimer antigen: current concepts and future prospects. Blood 2009;113:2878–2887 [PMID: 19008457].

Costantino MM, Randall G, Gosselin M, Brandt M, Spinning K, Vegas CD: CT angiography in the evaluation of acute pulmonary embolus. Am J Roentgenol 2008;191:471–474 [PMID: 18647919].

Klok FA, Mos IC, Nijkeuter M, Righini M et al: Simplification of the revised Geneva score for assessing clinical probability of pulmonary embolism. Arch Intern Med 2008;168:2131–2136 [PMID: 18955643].

Tapson VF: Acute pulmonary embolism. N Engl J Med 2008;358:1037–1052 [PMID: 18322285].

HEMOPTYSIS

▶ General Considerations

The most common cause of hemoptysis, bronchitis, is primarily a diagnosis of exclusion. The more significant causes such as cancer, tuberculosis, and autoimmune disorders such as Goodpasture's syndrome are uncommon but still deserve consideration in the patient who admits to coughing up blood. A list of conditions that cause hemoptysis is discussed in Table 33–5. Massive hemoptysis is defined in terms of volume as 200–600 cc in 24 hours. This broad range is in part a manifestation of the difficulty of measuring the volume of expectorated blood. Many patients with life-threatening hemopysis are elderly and have associated co-morbid conditions.

▶ Clinical Findings

A. History

Hemoptysis is the coughing of blood. This needs to be clearly differentiated from the vomiting of blood (hematemesis) as the diagnostic approach is different. If a patient complains of spitting blood, this may mean that the blood is not being coughed into the oropharynx. The blood may be from the mouth, nose, or nasopharynx and not of tracheobronchial origin. It is important to clarify a history of spitting blood.

B. Physical Examination

The vital signs are important as is the presence of pallor or cyanosis. Physical findings in the chest are generally nonspecific but may indicate the presence of effusions, pulmonary masses, or airspace disease such as that due to bloody fluids in the alveoli. The heart examination may be abnormal due to the presence of a cardiovascular cause of hemoptysis such as mitral stenosis.

C. Laboratory Evaluation

Patients who appear pale or report significant blood loss should be evaluated for anemia. Coagulation studies should be obtained on patients who take warfarin or have liver disease and blood gases on patients in severe respiratory distress.

D. Imaging

A chest X-ray is an important study in patients with hemoptysis. CT scanning of the chest should be considered in the diagnostic evaluation if the initial plain film is abnormal and nondiagnostic. Angiography may be necessary if bleeding is massive and offers the possibility of treatment via embolization.

▶ Treatment

Treatment of hemoptysis in the emergency department usually is limited to general supportive care. An upright position is preferred. If the patient must be recumbent they should be positioned with the radiographically normal (presumably nonbleeding) lung up. If intubation is necessary large-bore endotracheal tubes (greater than 7.5) are helpful in facilitating fiberoptic bronchoscopy.

A. Bronchoscopy

Rigid bronchoscopy and selective intubation of the nonbleeding lung should be considered if bleeding is massive. The use of a double-lumen tube may be preferable but is technically more challenging. Endobronchial therapy during bronchoscopy may be successful in controlling the bleeding.

B. Interventional Radiology

Ninety per cent of massive hemoptysis is due to bleeding from the bronchial rather than the pulmonary circulation. Selective embolization of the involved bronchial arterial segment is effective in controlling the bleeding in about 90% of patients. The major risk of this technique is spinal cord ischemia, which may be minimized by

Table 33–5. Conditions Causing Hemoptysis.

Pulmonary hemoptysis
  Pulmonary parenchymal disease
    Bronchitis
    Bronchiectasis
    Tuberculosis
    Lung abscess
    Pneumonia
    Fungal infection of old cavities (eg, aspergilloma)
    Lung parasites (ascariasis, schistosomiasis, etc)
    Pulmonary neoplasms
    Pulmonary infarction
    Trauma
    Arteriovenous malformations
    Pulmonary vasculitis
    Goodpasture's syndrome
  Extrapulmonary disease
    Thrombocytopenia
    Other coagulopathies
    Heart failure
    Mitral stenosis
Nonpulmonary hemoptysis
  Aspiration of blood from nasal, oropharyngeal, gastrointestinal, or other bleeding site
Pseudohemoptysis
  Production of red-tinged sputum not due to blood

selective techniques that avoid embolization of the anterior spinal artery.

C. Surgical Treatment

Surgical resection of the involved lobe or pulmonary segment may be necessary but depends on a localized site of bleeding. The patient must have adequate pulmonary reserve, have focal disease, and be an acceptable surgical candidate.

▶ Disposition

Massive hemoptysis requires ICU admission and a team approach involving the pulmonologist, interventional radiologist, and the thoracic surgeon. Most patients with minimal degrees of hemoptysis due to bronchitis can be managed as outpatients. Patients who are suspected of having pulmonary tuberculosis should be isolated and treated presumptively until definitive studies can be completed.

Bidwell JL, Pachner RW: Hemoptysis: diagnosis and management. Am Fam Physician 2005;72:1253–1260 [PMID: 16225028].

Van Den Berg JC: Bronchial artery embolization. In Golzarian J, Sun S, Sharafuddin MJ (editors). *Vascular embolotherapy: A comprehensive approach.* Volume 1 General Principles, Chest, Abdomen, and Great Vessels. New York, NY: Springer; 2006: 263–278.

PULMONARY ARTERIAL HYPERTENSION (PAH)

▶ General Considerations

ESSENTIALS OF DIAGNOSIS

▶ Exertional shortness of breath or syncope

▶ Absence of congestive changes on chest X-ray

▶ Loud pulmonic closure, P2

Pulmonary hypertension may be secondary to another lung disorder such as COPD, left-sided heart disease, or recurrent pulmonary thrombo-embolic disease. Pulmonary arterial hypertension (PAH) is a diagnosis category that is not a secondary result of the aformentioned causes but does include familial types and those associated with collagen vascular diseases such as scleroderma, HIV infection, and toxic exposures. Anatomically this disorder is characterized by the remodeling of the pulmonary circulation with occlusion

of the lumen in the medium-sized and small pulmonary arteries. The afterload of the right ventricle increases as this occurs which causes an obstruction to flow in the pulmonary arterial tree and increases the pressure as the right ventricle attempts to compensate.

▶ Clinical Findings

A. Symptoms and Signs

Common symptoms are shortness of breath especially with exertion. Exertional syncope may also be a presenting complaint. Pulmonary venous hypertension from congestive heart failure causes shortness of breath while lying flat while PAH typically does not. A loud pulmonic closure, P2 may be present on auscultation. Peripheral edema may occur.

B. Imaging and Laboratory Findings

PAH, may be suspected, may be identified with echocardiography but diagnosis requires measurements of pressure and flow with a Swan-Ganz catheter. Pulmonary artery wedge pressure should be less than 15 mm Hg and the pulmonary artery pressure greater than 25 mm Hg to make the diagnosis.

▶ Treatment and Disposition

A. Phosphodiesterase Type 5 Inhibitors

Phosphodiesterase type 5 inhibitors were first developed to treat erectile dysfunction but also are effective in patients with PAH who have symptoms that are mild to moderately severe. Sildenafil is marketed as Revatio(TM) when used to treat PAH instead of Viagra(TM), and tadalafil is marketed as Adciraca(TM) instead Cialis(TM) for this indication.

B. Prostaglandins

In severe disease epoprostenol (synthetic prostacyclin, marketed as Flolan(TM)) is indicated. Since the drug lasts only 3–5 minutes it must be administered by continuous infusion via a central venous catheter. These patients may be seen in emergency situations with complications from the indwelling catheter but the major issue is that the interruption of the infusion may cause rapid reversal of symptoms. This can be life threatening. Immediate consultation with the patient's pulmonologist should be obtained if this is suspected.

Humbert M: Update in pulmonary hypertension 2008. Am J Respir Crit Care Med 2009;179:650–656 [PMID: 19351872].

▼ PLEURAL AND MEDISTINAL CONDITIONS

PNEUMOTHORAX

See also Chapters 13 and 24.

ESSENTIALS OF DIAGNOSIS

Pneumothorax

► Pleuritic chest pain

► Acute-onset dyspnea

► Decreased breath sounds on affected side

► Evidence of lung collapse on chest X-ray

Tension Pneumothorax

► Displaced PMI

► Shift of the trachea

► Jugular venous distension

▶ General Considerations

Pneumothorax is the abnormal collection of air within the pleural space. This condition may be classified as either spontaneous (primary or secondary), traumatic, or iatrogenic. Pneumothorax may also be either simple or under tension and further classified as either primary (not associated with underlying lung disease) or secondary to some other disease in the lung.

Primary spontaneous pneumothoraces occur in patients without clinically apparent lung disease (often young, tall men, aged 20–40 years, who usually smoke). Secondary pneumothoraces are a complication of preexisting underlying pulmonary disease such as COPD, pneumonia particularly Pneumocystis jirovecii pneumonia, cystic fibrosis, asthma, or tuberculosis. Traumatic pneumothoraces are due to either blunt or penetrating chest trauma. Iatrogenic pneumothorax may occur during subclavian line placement, thoracentesis, or following lung or pleural biopsy. Pneumothorax may also result from barotrauma during positive pressure ventilation.

▶ Clinical Findings

A. Symptoms and Signs

Patients usually present with pleuritic chest pain but may also have tachypnea and shortness of breath. Breath sounds are diminished on the affected side. Pneumothorax under tension may cause severe respiratory compromise and cardiovascular collapse. Other clinical findings include tracheal deviation and displacement of the point of maximal impulse (PMI) to the opposite side.

B. Imaging and Laboratory Findings

Plain chest X-ray (frontal view) is usually diagnostic. Expiratory films may demonstrate small pneumothoraces that are not visible on inspiratory films. Chest CT will often be helpful in identifying associated pathology, such as pneumocystis pneumonia or differentiating pneumothorax from emphysematous blebs in patients with COPD.

▶ Treatment and Disposition

A. Primary Spontaneous Pneumothorax

A small pneumothorax will usually resolve without treatment. Supplemental oxygen increases the rate of reabsorption slightly and is appropriate during a short period of observation in the emergency department. Patients may also be treated with small-bore catheter attached to a Heimlich valve. Patients with Heimlich valves may be candidates for outpatient treatment provided adequate follow-up arrangements can be made. If the pneumothorax fails to re-expand then a 24F–28F standard chest tube attached to water seal will be required.

B. Secondary Spontaneous Pneumothorax

Patients with secondary pneumothorax in general, will require standard chest tube drainage with a water seal device and admission to the hospital. The underlying illness often requires additional intervention such as antibiotics, surgery, or additional diagnostic evaluation.

C. Traumatic Pneumothorax

Most patients with traumatic pneumothorax have associated hemothorax that requires large chest tubes and water seal drainage with suction. The initial tube when hemothorax is suspected should be 32F or larger. The frequent use of chest CT in trauma patients has resulted in some small pneumothoraces being identified. Some of these patients may be placed under observation without chest tubes if positive pressure ventilation is not required.

D. Tension Pneumothorax

Tension pneumothorax is produced if air continues to enter the pleural space with a valve preventing its exit. This is most common in patients with traumatic pneumothorax. Patients with tension pneumothorax should be treated with immediate decompression and not wait for radiographic confirmation. The best approach, if time permits, is tube thoracostomy. If the patient is in extremis, then needle decompression may be performed with a 14–16-gauge needle inserted in the second intercostal space at the midclavicular line. Such patients will subsequently need tube thoracostomy drainage to a water seal device.

Zehtabchi S, Rios CL: Management of emergency department patients with primary spontaneous pneumothorax: needle aspiration or tube thoracostomy? Ann Emerg Med 2008;51:91–100 [PMID: 18166436].

Caceres M, Ali SZ, Braud R et al: Spontaneous pneumomediastinum: a comparative study and review of the literature. Ann Thorac Surg 2008;86:962–966 [PMID: 18721592].

PNEUMOMEDIASTINUM

▶ General Considerations

Pneumomediastinum is gas in the mediastinum outside the lumen of the esophagus or airways of the tracheobronchial tree. This occurs most commonly from ruptured aveoli when the gas dissects centrally along the bronchovascular interstitial sheaths. This is common in asthmatics but also occurs in blunt trauma and occasionally with forceful coughing. Pneumomedistinum also occurs in patients that Valsalva while smoking illicit substances such as crack cocaine. In such situations, pneumomedistinum is benign and the clinician's attention is appropriately focused on the underlying condition. Gas can enter the mediastinum from lacerations of the GI tract particularly the esophagus or from air containing structures in the head or neck. Air may dissect into the medistinum from ruptured retroperotneal structures in the abdomen including the rectum or from a perforated diverticulum.

▶ Clinical Findings

The only specific physical sign of pneumomedistinum is Hamman's crunch, a crunching sound heard over the heart on auscultation of the chest. Otherwise pneumomedistinum is essentially a radiologic diagnosis identified by lucent streaks of gas that outline mediastinal structures. These include the medistinal pleura, the trachea and its branches or the pulmonary artery or aorta. Sometimes pneumomediastinum is more obvious on the lateral than on the frontal view of the chest. Mediastinal gas may also be seen outlining the superior surface of the diaphragm and separating it from the heart. Boerhaave's syndrome is rupture of the esophageal wall due to vomiting. The typical patient develops severe retrosternal chest pain after retching and vomiting often in the setting of heavy alcohol use.

▶ Treatment and Disposition

The treatment of pneumomedistinum is always directed at the underlying disorder whether it be asthma, trauma, or drug abuse. Esophageal rupture as in Boerhaave's syndrome is a fatal disorder without prompt thoracotomy, esophageal repair and wide medistinal drainage. Tracheobronchial rupture must be recognized quickly because continued attempts to ventilate the lungs may force additional air into the medistinum with resultant compression and displacement of other medistinal structures.

PLEURAL EFFUSION

ESSENTIALS OF DIAGNOSIS

- ▶ Pleuritic chest pain, dyspnea with or without fever, cough
- ▶ Decreased breath sounds, decreased tactile fremitus on affected side
- ▶ Thoracentesis is definitive diagnostic and often therapeutic procedure

▶ General Considerations

Pleural effusions are an abnormal collection of fluid between the parietal and visceral pleura as a result of a local disease process or inflammation. Normally 5–15 mL of serous fluid is present in the pleural space. An effusion can be classified as either an exudate or transudate to help in differential diagnosis. Exudative fluid analysis reveals (1) pleural fluid protein to serum protein ratio greater than 0.5, (2) pleural fluid lactate dehydrogenase (LDH) to serum LDH ratio greater than 0.6, and (3) pleural fluid LDH greater than two-third of the upper limit of normal serum LDH. Exudates are associated with direct disease of the pleura itself usually from infection, inflammation, or malignancy. Transudates do not have the above-mentioned characteristics and are most commonly caused by congestive heart failure, cirrhosis with ascites, or nephrotic syndrome. Every patient with a newly diagnosed pleural effusion requires prompt evaluation to determine the cause so that early and appropriate therapy can be given.

▶ Clinical Findings

A. Symptoms and Signs

The patient may complain of pleuritic or nonpleuritic chest pain or dyspnea. Chest examination discloses dullness, decreased breath sounds, and decreased tactile fremitus on the involved side. Large effusions may cause hypoxia and respiratory distress by compressing adjacent lung tissue and limiting expansion of the remaining lung.

B. Imaging

Upright posteroanterior and lateral chest X-ray can demonstrate pleural fluid in most cases if more than 250 mL of fluid is present (eg, blunting of costophrenic angles). Decubitus films are useful to demonstrate the presence of free flowing pleural fluid suitable for removal by thoracentesis. CT scanning of the chest can be helpful to identify small effusions and identify associated pathology such as pneumonia, tumors, or pulmonary emboli.

Treatment

A. Oxygen

If dyspnea is present, obtain pulse oximetry or blood gas measurements, and begin supplemental oxygen by mask or nasal cannula.

B. Thoracentesis

If the chest X-ray shows a large fluid accumulation (ie, most of one hemithorax), and the patient is in respiratory distress, thoracentesis with removal of fluid should be considered for relief of symptoms. Reexpansion pulmonary edema rarely occurs but is a risk of this procedure and should be treated in similar fashion to acute cardiogenic pulmonary edema if it occurs. Recovered fluid should be sent for cell counts, protein, LDH, glucose, and pH. Pleural fluid cytology should be considered if undiagnosed malignancy is a consideration. If the patient is not in distress, thoracentesis may be deferred until after hospital admission.

C. Empyema

Infection of a pleural effusion is an empyema, literally a purulent effusion. In addition to antibiotic therapy, an empyema will require chest tube drainage if the fluid is grossly purulent or the gram stain is positive. Drainage is also indicated if the pH is < 7.0. If the pH is between 7.0 and 7.2 the management of the effusion should be individualized and repeat thoracentesis considered in 24 to 48 hours.

Disposition

All patients with unexplained pleural fluid accumulations should be hospitalized for diagnosis and treatment. Stable patients with recurrent fluid of known cause (eg, metastatic cancer or heart failure) should be referred to their regular source of medical care or given treatment in the emergency department (eg, by thoracentesis) and discharged unless the underlying illness requires hospitalization.

Feller-Kopman D, Berkowitz D, Boiselle P, Ernst A: Large-volume thoracentesis and the risk of reexpansion pulmonary edema. Ann Thorac Surg 2007;84:1656–1661 [PMID: 17954079].

Porcel JM, Light RW: Diagnostic approach to pleural effusion in adults. Am Fam Physician 2006;73:1211–1220 [PMID: 16623208].

▼ PULMONARY INFECTION

PNEUMONIA AND BRONCHITIS

ESSENTIALS OF DIAGNOSIS

Pneumonia
▶ Fever, productive cough, dyspnea, pleuritic chest pain
▶ Rales, rhonchi, wheezing, or hemoptysis
▶ Decreased breath sounds or dullness to percussion over affected lobe
▶ Infiltrate on chest radiograph

Bronchitis
▶ Cough associated with midline chest pain or burning
▶ Fever, dyspnea

General Considerations

Bronchitis is an inflammatory condition involving the tracheobronchial tree. The diagnosis of pneumonia implies the additional involvement of the pulmonary parenchyma and aveoli. The primary clinical difference between these two entities is the presence of an infiltrate on the chest X-ray in the case of pneumonia. Bronchitis in a patient without underlying lung disease should not cause hypoxia but pneumonia may if the consolidation of the pulmonary parenchyma is large. Fever may be present in both conditions but is more prominent in pneumonia.

Clinical Findings

A. Acute Bronchitis

Patients complain of cough, fever, and constitutional symptoms. The cough is initially dry but can become productive and is often associated with a midline chest pain or burning. Hemoptysis in small amounts is sometimes present. Rhonchi that clear with coughing is a characteristic finding. The presence of rales is more characteristic of pneumonic consolidation or other condition involving the pulmonary parenchyma such as pulmonary fibrosis. Laboratory tests are not helpful in making the diagnosis. Chest X-ray will show no evidence of infiltrate and is not indicated unless patients are dyspneic, hypoxic, or have significant comorbidities (eg, COPD, dementia). Cigarette smoking is a cause or contributing factor in many cases.

B. Pneumonia

1. Symptoms and signs—Patients present with fever, dyspnea, cough, pleuritic chest pain, and increased sputum production Auscultation of the chest may reveal rales or rhonchi. There may be areas of dullness to percussion over an infiltrate. Bronchial breath sounds are a classic finding over a dense infiltrate that abuts the pleura.

2. Cultures and serologic testing—The results of blood cultures direct the therapy in only a minority of cases but are an important quality measure in patients admitted to the hospital. They should be obtained before antibiotics are given. Sputum gram stain and culture are needed only if an atypical cause is suspected.

3. Laboratory evaluation—Some helpful tests include pulse oximetry and blood gas measurements, white cell count, hemoglobin and hematocrit (anemia), and a basic metabolic panel (dehydration, renal insufficiency). Screening for HIV, tuberculosis, *Legionella*, and *Mycoplasma* are appropriate for patients at risk for these diseases.

▶ Treatment

A. Acute Bronchitis

Intravenous fluids should be given to patients who are significantly dehydrated and unable to tolerate oral fluids. Otherwise, treatment with antipyretics and cough suppressants are sufficient in uncomplicated cases. β-Adrenergic MDIs (albuterol) may improve symptoms even if wheezing is not present. Antibiotics are not recommended because the primary cause is likely viral. Many patients are smokers and need to be counseled regarding cessation.

B. Pneumonia

1. Community acquired pneumonia (CAP)—Outpatient antibiotic therapy for CAP is typically a macrolide antibiotic such as azithromycin or an extended spectrum fluoroquinolone such as levofloxacin. Doxycycline is an acceptable alternative. Each should be given for 7–10 days (except azithromycin, which is used for only 5 days). Patients who require admission should be started on (1) an extended spectrum fluoroquinolone or (2) a macrolide plus a β-lactam/β-lactamase inhibitor.

2. Health care associated pneumonia (HCAP)—Patients who have a history of recent exposure to high risk area of the health care system (Table 33–6) fall into the category of HCAP. Pneumonia in this case is more likely to be caused by organisms such as hospital acquired methicillin-resistant Staphylococcus aureus (HA-MRSA) or Pseudomonas aeruginosa. Prompt administration of antibiotic therapy

Table 33–6. Risk Factors for Health Care Associated Pneumonia.

Hospitalization in an acute care hospital for two or more days in the last 90 days
Residence in a nursing home or long-term care facility in the last 90 days
Receiving outpatient intravenous therapy (like antibiotics or chemotherapy) within the past 30 days
Receiving home wound care within the past 30 days
Attending a hospital clinic or dialysis center in the last 30 days
Having a family member with known multidrug resistant pathogens

is important with a goal of within 6 hours of presentation to the emergency department. The selection of antibiotics is institution dependent but should adhere to published guidelines. As a general rule treatment requires combination therapy using an antipseudomonal cephalosporin, β-lactam, carbapenem or monobactam(aztreonam) plus an antipseudomonal fluoroquinolone or aminoglycoside plus an agent such as linezolid or vancomycin to cover MRSA.

▶ Disposition

Patients should be hospitalized if they require oxygen or are unable to tolerate oral antibiotics. Vomiting or inability to maintain adequate oral intake of fluids with the need for intravenous fluids is another appropriate indication for hospital admission. Various severity indices such as the pneumonia severity score (PORT score) or CURB-65 score have been developed to predict morbidity and mortality in patients with pneumonia. These were not developed to predict the need for hospitalization but the elements that they enumerate such as advanced age, significant comorbidities, alteration of vital signs or alteration of mental status should be considered in the decision to hospitalize patients with pneumonia. Patients who require hemodynamic monitoring or blood pressure support with catacholamines will require ICU admission.

Kanwar M, Brar N, Khatib R, Fakih MG: Misdiagnosis of community-acquired pneumonia and inappropriate utilization of antibiotics: side effects of the 4-h antibiotic administration rule. Chest 2007;131:1865–1869 [PMID: 17400668].

Lutfiyya MN, Henley E, Chang LF, Reyburn SW: Diagnosis and treatment of community-acquired pneumonia. Am Fam Physician 2006;73:442–450 [PMID: 16477891].

Menendez R, Torres A: Treatment failure in community-acquired pneumonia. Chest 2007;132:1348–1355 [PMID: 17934120].

PULMONARY TUBERCULOSIS

ESSENTIALS OF DIAGNOSIS

▶ Fever, weight loss, hemoptysis, night sweats

▶ Chest X-ray notes hilar adenopathy with parenchymal infiltrates, often upper lobes or apical

▶ Positive purified protein derivative (PPD) skin test with positive acid-fast bacilli on sputum smear

▶ Sputum culture for Mycobacterium tuberculosis is definitive diagnosis

▶ General Considerations

Pulmonary infection is caused when susceptible individuals inhale aerosolized droplets infected with Mycobacterium tuberculosis. This disease was reestablished as a major concern in the United States in the mid-1980s when the incidence rose sharply. The major causes for this resurgence has been the HIV epidemic, immigration of people with undiagnosed tuberculosis from high-risk countries in Asia, Africa, and Latin America, previously established suboptimal antimicrobial regimens, and patient noncompliance. The goal in the emergency department is early diagnosis, treatment, and referral for these patients and to protect hospital staff via early patient isolation.

▶ Clinical Findings

Tuberculosis should be considered in patients who present with pneumonia or cough and are members of one of the previously mentioned high risk groups.

A. Symptoms and Signs

The most common symptom that will call attention to the diagnosis of tuberculosis is a prolonged cough (more than 3 weeks) especially if bloody. Fever is also common, especially during the day with resolution at night. Night sweats are a typical complaint. Fatigue, malaise, and weight loss with anorexia are common. Patients frequently will appear chronically ill. Chest examination may be normal or rales may be present.

B. X-ray Findings

Primary tuberculosis may appear on chest X-ray as parenchymal consolidation, atelectasis, pleural effusion possibly with paratracheal lymphadenopathy. A calcified Ghon complex is evidence of healed primary infection.

Reactivation tuberculosis often has a predilection for the upper lobes. Immunocompromised patients, especially HIV patients, may present with a myriad of findings on the chest X-ray.

C. Laboratory Findings

1. Cultures and serologic testing—Tuberculosis is often identified with serologic tests that use nucleic acid amplication with a polymerase chain reaction for the detection of bacterial DNA (PCR tests). Sputum cultures require several weeks but are important because of the emergence of multidrug-resistant tuberculosis. Treatment will depend on susceptibility results. Definitive diagnosis in the emergency department is essentially impossible. For this reason, individuals who are suspected of having the disease should be placed on respiratory isolation to protect the health care workers that come into contact with the patient.

2. Tuberculosis skin testing—If a patient is suspected of having tuberculosis, an intradermal purified protein derivative (PPD) skin test can be administered. This test is not completed and read until 48–72 hours after administration so appropriate follow-up to evaluate the patient will need to be arranged. A positive test (varying diameters of circumferential skin induration depending on risk factors for the disease) indicates previous infection or active infection. Positive PPD tests should be followed with chest X-ray to evaluate for new or active disease. Severely immunocompromised patients or HIV patients may be anergic so skin testing may be unreliable.

▶ Treatment

A. Confirmed or Suspected Tuberculosis

The treatment of active tuberculosis has been complicated by the emergence of drug-resistant organisms. Patients will require multidrug therapy if they are found to have active disease. Multidrug-resistant tuberculosis is defined as resistance to the two most effective first-line TB drugs: rifampicin and isoniazid. Extensively drug-resistant TB is also resistant to three or more of the six classes of second-line drugs.

B. Latent Tuberculosis

Latent tuberculosis occurs when patients have positive skin tests but negative chest X-ray and no clinical disease. These patients are at risk of reactivation tuberculosis and are generally treated with 9 months of isoniazid. Tuberculosis is still rare in the United States except in patients who are members of identified high risk groups. Patients at very low risk for tuberculosis should not be screened with skin testing because the problems associated with treating patients with false positive skin tests outweigh the potential benefit.

C. Reporting Requirements

The local health department must be informed of all cases of tuberculosis to ensure adequate care, availability of treatment resources, and compliance with therapy.

D. Disposition

Most patients with active disease are usually admitted with respiratory isolation for full workup and evaluation. The routine screening with skin testing for patients thought to be at risk can be utilized provided that the appropriate follow-up can be arranged. Intradermal skin tests will need to be read at 48 to 72 hours

Jacob JT, Mehta AK, Leonard MK: Acute forms of tuberculosis in adults. Am J Med 2009;122:12–17 [PMID: 19114163].

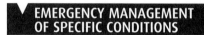

EMERGENCY MANAGEMENT OF SPECIFIC CONDITIONS

PULMONARY ASPIRATION SYNDROME

ESSENTIALS OF DIAGNOSIS

► High-risk patients with alteration of mental status
► Immediate respiratory difficulty due to chemical burn with, hypoxemia, rales, and wheezing
► Pulmonary infiltration either diffusely or in dependent areas of the lungs

▶ General Considerations

A. Pulmonary Aspiration Syndrome

Aspiration of gastric contents will produce a chemical pneumonitis (Pulmonary Aspiration Syndrome) similar to that caused by any irritant that is inhaled or aspirated in significant quantities. Mechanical obstruction by aspirated food particles will further impair gas exchange. Pulmonary infection is not a part of the initial lung injury but may subsequently develop as a result of it. Pulmonary aspiration is a frequent cause or contributor to the development of the acute respiratory distress syndrome (ARDS).

B. Aspiration Pneumonia

Aspiration of oropharyngeal secretions is typically chronic and may cause a bacterial pneumonia characterized as aspiration pneumonia. The chest X-ray usually shows consolidation in the lung segments which were dependent at the time of aspiration. If the patient was supine the posterior segments of upper or apical segments of lower lobes are involved. The basal segments of lower lobes particularly the right lower lobe are involved if the patient was upright. In individuals with poor dental hygiene and large amounts of dental plaque this commonly results in anaerobic lung abscess.

▶ Clinical Findings

Pulmonary aspiration syndrome occurring in the hospital may occur during anesthesia, cardiopulmonary resuscitation, or other procedures. Community-acquired cases are usually associated with trauma causing an alteration of mental status, drug overdose (including pronounced alcohol intoxication) or seizures. Sometimes vomiting and aspiration is a witnessed event. Within minutes to hours after aspiration, the patient develops productive cough; dyspnea; fever; leukocytosis; and rales on chest auscultation. Chest X-ray shows pulmonary infiltrates which are generally diffuse, although dependent segments of the lung (especially the right lower lobe) are more commonly involved. Food particles may be present on gross examination of sputum. The condition should be considered at least initially to be an inflammatory process in the lung not an infectious one.

▶ Treatment

Provide respiratory support (eg, supplemental oxygen) as necessary on the basis of arterial blood gas measurements (or pulse oximetry) and clinical findings. If the patient has significant dyspnea or respiratory distress, immediately establish airway control with intubation and mechanical ventilation. Witnessed aspirations should be treated by prompt oropharyngeal and tracheal suctioning. Acute obstruction of the upper airway should be treated immediately with the Heimlich maneuver. Retained, aspirated foreign bodies (greatest risk in children) often necessitate bronchoscopy for final diagnosis and removal. Corticosteroids have not been demonstrated to be helpful and may increase susceptibility to infection. Antibiotics for aspiration pneumonia should be given if infection occurs and not for prophylaxis following an episode of aspiration.

▶ Disposition

All patients should be hospitalized for observation and treatment.

Johnson J, Hirsch CS: Aspiration pneumonia. Recognizing and managing a potentially growing disorder. Postgrad Med 2003;113:99–102,105–106,111–112 [PMID: 12647477].

ACUTE LUNG INJURY AND ACUTE RESPIRATORY DISTRESS SYNDROME

ESSENTIALS OF DIAGNOSIS

- ▶ Recent known exposure to high-risk systemic or pulmonary etiologic agent
- ▶ Acute-onset of impaired gas exchange with a gradient between the inspired and arterial PO_2 (Pao_2/FiO_2 < 300 for acute lung injury and Pao_2/FiO_2 < 200 for ARDS)
- ▶ No chemical evidence of cardiogenic or volume overload pulmonary edema (pulmonary capillary wedge pressures < 18 mm Hg)
- ▶ Chest X-ray shows diffuse bilateral infiltrates

▶ General Considerations

Acute lung injury is defined as the acute onset of impaired gas exchange with a widened gradient between inspired and arterial PO_2 (Pao_2/FiO_2 < 300) and the presence of bilateral alveolar or interstitial infiltrates and the absence of congestive heart failure. The ARDS is used in acute lung injury when the impairment of oxygenation is severe (PaO_2/FiO_2 < 200). These conditions are characterized by diffuse alveolar damage and increased permeability of the alveolar–capillary membrane. Edema fluid and plasma proteins leak from the vasculature into the alveolar spaces. The primary result of this is impaired gas exchange principally involving oxygen. Any process that causes diffuse alveolar damage may cause this syndrome. Common causes presenting the emergency department are sepsis with or without a pulmonary focus, trauma, pulmonary aspiration syndrome, and thermal or chemical inhalation injury to the lung. Severe systemic illnesses such as pancreatitis and burns may cause this syndrome as can multiple blood transfusions. It is important to avoid overzealous fluid administration in these patients as this may aggravate the exudation of fluid into the alveoli. Over distension of the lung during positive pressure ventilation may also aggravate the injury to the lung particularly in children.

▶ Clinical Findings

A. Symptoms and Signs

The symptoms of the underlying illness are complicated by the impairment of oxygenation. If hypoxia is uncorrected then this may contribute impairment of essential metabolic functions such as the maintenance of cardiac output. The chest X-ray will also demonstrate the opacity caused by the

increase of fluids in the alveoli. Rales are the primary physical findings on auscultation of the chest. Heavy wet lungs increase the work of breathing and will increase the patients sense of dyspnea and malaise and make ventilation more difficult in the intubated patient.

B. Imaging and Laboratory Findings

Chest imaging always shows extensive infiltration depending on the inciting event. Most often opacity is diffuse and bilateral. Other processes such as pleural effusions and fractured ribs in trauma patients are common. The presence of pneumonia or PE may be present and very difficult to ascertain. If hypoxia is uncorrected then this will contribute to anaerobic metabolism and a lactic acidosis. Carbon dioxide exchange is much less affected and the PCO_2 may be normal or a respiratory alkalosis may develop as ventilation is increased to attempt to compensate for hypoxemia. Pulmonary artery occlusion pressures (pulmonary capillary wedge pressures) less than or equal to 18 mm Hg are consistent with acute lung injury and not fluid overload. All these patients are significantly stressed by their illness and the WBC count will usually be greatly elevated even in the absence of infection.

▶ Treatment

A. Provide Respiratory Support

1. Supplemental oxygen—Provide high initial oxygen concentration (FiO_2 = 50–100%), continue to monitor oxygen saturation with pulse oximetry, and titrate to the lowest FiO_2 to keep oxygen saturation greater than 90%.

2. Intubation and mechanical ventilation—Use low tidal volumes and permissive hypercapnia to limit peak airway pressures (Table 33–2).

B. Maintain Circulation

Avoid both dehydration and vigorous hydration. Central venous pressure monitoring is indicated and the CVP pressure should be kept between 8 and 12 mm Hg.

C. Treat Underlying Clinical Cause

Prompt evaluation with rapid identification of the underlying cause is paramount for the survival of these patients. Specific treatment for the inciting disorder (most commonly sepsis) should begin as soon as possible in the emergency department.

▶ Disposition

Hospitalize all patients who meet the criteria for ARDS severe (PaO_2/FiO_2 < 300) in the ICU. Almost all these patients will require intubation. Mild forms of acute lung injury often progress despite appropriate therapy and worsening of oxygenation should be anticipated.

Malhotra A: Low-tidal-volume ventilation in the acute respiratory distress syndrome. N Engl J Med 2007;357:1113–1120 [PMID: 17855672].

CYSTIC FIBROSIS

▶ Clinical Findings

Cystic fibrosis is an autosomal recessive disease, which causes thick and viscous mucus with subsequent obstruction and damage to organs with exocrine function. Patients will have a history of chronic lung disease with a gradual decline in pulmonary function, pancreatic insufficiency, and gastrointestinal complaints. Most symptoms of disease and many complications develop at an early age (2–20 years). Pulmonary disease is characterized by chronic infections with multiple organisms, with periodic acute exacerbations with increased sputum production and cough. Staphylococcus aureus and Haemophilus influenza are prevalent during childhood. Most patients eventually develop chronic infection with Pseudomonas aeruginosa or other virulent gram-negative organisms.

▶ Treatment

A. Pulmonary Infections

Antibiotic therapy is used to treat acute exacerbations of lung disease, either orally, parenterally, or via inhalation. Maintenance therapy with macrolide antibiotics particularly azithromycin has been shown to improve pulmonary function and reduce the number of respiratory exacerbations.

B. Other Therapy

Short-acting inhaled β-2-adrenergic receptor agonists are helpful especially in patients known to respond to them. Additional treatments include DNase I (dornase alfa) and hypertonic saline via nebulizer. High-dose ibuprofen is helpful in children and young adolescents with good lung function. Severe cystic fibrosis lung disease is a common indication for lung transplantation.

▶ Disposition

Patient with cystic fibrosis are best treated in close consultation with the patient's pulmonologist. Hospitalization is a particular problem in these patients because of the problem of antibiotic resistance in the hospital environment.

INTERSTITIAL PULMONARY DISEASE

▶ General Considerations

A variety of conditions may produce diffuse progressive pulmonary interstitial inflammation and fibrosis, including drugs, pneumoconiosis, collagen diseases, sarcoidosis, organic and inorganic dusts, and illnesses of unknown cause with pathologic features involving chiefly the lungs (eg, idiopathic interstitial fibrosis). Most of these illnesses are relatively uncommon. The principal feature of all of them is that dyspnea begins gradually and seldom occurs acutely without a background of increasing shortness of breath. When dyspnea of acute onset does occur, it is often due to inter-current illness (eg, pulmonary infection). Patients also have pulmonary function tests that demonstrate restrictive lung dysfunction and impaired gas exchange.

▶ Clinical Findings

Many patients with interstitial pulmonary disease will know their diagnosis; if not, it can seldom be made with certainty in the emergency department setting, because lung biopsy or bronchoalveolar lavage is often required.

A. Symptoms and Signs

Gradually increasing dyspnea, especially on exertion, is the only reliable symptom. Chest pain, cough, sputum production, and other symptoms may occur but are inconsistent. Physical findings are variable, but dry crackles (rales) at the bases of the lungs are common. Cyanosis and clubbing may be present as well.

B. Imaging

Chest X-ray usually shows interstitial infiltrates. Prior chest X-rays are helpful to identify chronic interstitial disease (interstitial fibrosis). CT scan of the chest is also helpful in assessing these patients. Other changes may be present depending on the disease process (eg, hilar adenopathy in sarcoidosis, conglomerate fibrosis in silicosis).

▶ Treatment and Disposition

Provide respiratory support as needed, and treat inter-current disease (eg, infection). Hospitalize patients with respiratory failure or recent marked worsening of symptoms or those in whom acute infection is suspected. Refer all patients not already under care to a pulmonary disease specialist. Early lung transplantation offers a surgical therapeutic option for selected patients.

Lynch DA, Travis WD, Müller NL et al: Idiopathic interstitial pneumonias: CT features. Radiology 2005;236:10–21 [PMID: 15987960].

Ryu JH, Daniels CE, Hartman TE, Yi ES: Diagnosis of interstitial lung diseases. Mayo Clin Proc 2007;82:976–986 [PMID: 17673067].

Cardiac Emergencies

Sameer Desai, MD

► Immediate Management

Cardiac disease is usually manifested by symptoms of chest pain, dyspnea or respiratory distress, cardiac arrest or syncope, or shock. Because these symptoms are so commonly encountered in the emergency department and they may result from disease in many organs other than the heart, they are discussed separately (Chapters 9, 10, 11, 13, and 14). Because almost any cardiac disease is at least potentially life-threatening, no attempt has been made in this chapter to categorize disorders on the basis of severity or to assign priorities in treatment.

▼ ACUTE CORONARY SYNDROME

Acute coronary syndrome (ACS) refers to a spectrum of conditions that develop from blood flow that is insufficient to meet the metabolic needs of the myocardium. Patients with an acute coronary syndrome exist on a clinical continuum from unstable angina to non-ST-segment elevation myocardial infarction to ST segment elevation myocardial infarction.

ACUTE MYOCARDIAL INFARCTION (CORONARY OCCLUSION)

Myocardial infarction results when arterial blood flow to the myocardium is suddenly decreased or interrupted. It is usually due to atherosclerotic coronary artery disease with plaque rupture and sudden occlusion by thrombus; vasculitis or emboli are less common causes. Complete occlusion, most often with thrombus, is found in 80–90% of patients with chest pain and ST segment elevation who are studied by coronary angioplasty within several hours of onset. Occasionally, patients dying of myocardial infarction are found to have nonoccluded coronary arteries, and infarction in such cases is presumably due to spasm of a coronary artery or thrombosis with complete lysis. Cocaine use has been associated with acute myocardial infarction, probably as a result of coronary spasm with or without intravascular thrombus formation. In myocardial infarction, severely ischemic and infarcted muscle contracts and relaxes poorly or not at all; if infarction is extensive, decreased cardiac output with heart failure or shock may result. After myocardial infarction, the ventricle may become aneurysmal or may even rupture. If conducting tissue is ischemic or infarcted, conduction abnormalities may occur. The infarcted endocardium attracts platelets and fibrin that may form mural clots, which can subsequently embolize. During acute myocardial infarction, the myocardium can become electrically unstable, resulting in arrhythmias that are frequently life-threatening.

Upon occlusion of a coronary artery, necrosis occurs in a time-dependent course, proceeding from endocardium to epicardium, generally over 4–6 hours. When residual perfusion by collateral vessels is present or lysis or thrombus occurs—either spontaneously or as a result of therapy—there will be salvage of myocardium. The earlier the reperfusion, the more myocardium is salvaged.

▶ Clinical Findings

A. Symptoms and Signs

Most patients with myocardial infarction have chest discomfort that is typically substernal and may radiate to the neck or left arm. However, pain can occur in atypical areas such as the right arm, shoulders, back, or epigastrium. The pain is classically oppressive or squeezing in character and may be associated with shortness of breath, dizziness, syncope or pre-syncope, anxiety, restlessness, nausea and vomiting, abdominal bloating, dyspnea, and diaphoresis. Patients' descriptions of "pain" and symptoms can vary greatly. Symptoms frequently begin at rest, worsens gradually, and persist for hours. Occasionally, myocardial infarction is painless—especially in elderly or diabetic patients—and is manifested by the acute onset of left heart failure, hypotension, or cardiac arrhythmias. Up to 25% of patients with an acute myocardial infarction may not develop any significant symptoms that would prompt the patient to seek medical attention.

Physical findings vary, and none are specific or diagnostic of myocardial infarction. An S_4 gallop or at times an S_3 gallop may be present. Occasionally, an apical systolic murmur or mitral insufficiency due to papillary muscle and left ventricular dysfunction is present. In patients with uncomplicated myocardial infarction, there may be no abnormal findings on physical examination. When cardiopulmonary physical findings are present, they tend to reflect the presence of complications (see below).

B. Electrocardiographic Findings

The electrocardiogram (ECG) can show signs of infarction (eg, hyperacute T waves, flipped T- waves, elevated ST segments, ST segment elevation myocardial infarction, and abnormal Q waves) in about half of patients. In the remainder, the initial ECG shows only nonspecific ST or T wave changes, or may be normal. It is important to try to compare EKG findings with previous ECG's to assess for changes.

Note: A normal ECG *does not* rule out the possibility of myocardial infarction or ACS. Continuous ST segment monitoring or serial ECGs and serial laboratory testing provide additional information and may demonstrate an evolving acute coronary syndrome in patients with initially nondiagnostic ECGs.

C. Laboratory Findings

CK-MB is found not only in the myocardium but also in brain and skeletal muscle, it is less specific for a myocardial ischemic event than some other markers. The CK-MB serum level elevates usually within 4–6 hours after the onset of an acute myocardial infarction and peaks within 12–24 hours. Levels return to baseline generally within 2–3 days of an acute myocardial infarction. Within 6 hours of an acute myocardial infarction, the sensitivity and specificity of elevations in the serum CK-MB levels are 17–62% and 92–100%, respectively. Many clinicians do not order CK-MB levels any longer because of the superior sensitivity and specificity of the cardiac troponin marker.

Troponin is a complex of three specific proteins found in striated muscle. Two of the subunits, cardiac troponin T (cTnt) and I (cTni), are useful as clinical markers of myocardial injury. Because these cardiac proteins are genetically unique, cTnt and cTni are the most cardiac-specific biochemical markers. With recent improvements in the assay, microinfarctions are diagnosed when elevations in cTnt or cTni occur without elevations in the CK-MB levels. After an acute myocardial infarction, cardiac troponin serum levels generally elevate within 2–6 hours, peak at 12–24 hours, and may stay elevated for 7–10 days. The sensitivities of elevations of cTnt and cTni within 6 hours of an acute myocardial infarction are 50–59 and 6–44%, respectively. The specificities of elevations of cTnt and cTni within 6 hours of an acute myocardial infarction are 74–96 and 93–99%, respectively.

One of the first cardiac markers used clinically, myoglobin, is still used by some today. Myoglobin is the most sensitive early marker of cardiac injury although it has very poor specificity. After an acute myocardial infarction, elevation occurs within 1–3 hours, levels peak within 4–12 hours, and levels remain elevated for 12–36 hours. The sensitivity of myoglobin for detecting myocardial infarction within 6 hours of symptom onset is considered very good at 55–100%. Some believe that because myoglobin is released in a noncontinuous manner and is very nonspecific, it is less helpful than other markers and should not be included in the standard evaluation for myocardial ischemia.

▶ Differential Diagnosis

For a complete differential diagnosis of chest pain, see Chapter 14. Aortic dissection, aneurysm, pericarditis, and gastrointestinal disorders (eg, peptic ulcer disease and pancreatitis) must be clinically excluded in patients being considered for thrombolytic therapy.

Note: The diagnosis of myocardial infarction is suggested by the history, and a decision to admit the patient to the coronary care unit immediately should be based on this information alone. No amount of laboratory data obtained in the emergency department will definitely rule out ACS. Further testing such as stress test, echocardiogram, and cardiac catheterization are needed to further assess for cardiac disease. In some institutions, once acute myocardial infarction is ruled out in low risk patients, patients are referred for early stress testing. If timely referral is unavailable, then these patients are best served by admission for stress testing. Though AMI can be ruled out with serial troponins and serial ECGs, unstable angina cannot be excluded without further evaluation. Patients discharged without stress testing should be advised to take a baby aspirin and avoid exertion until evaluation is completed.

▶ **Treatment**

Patients experiencing acute coronary syndromes should receive aggressive treatment with the goal of rapidly reperfusing ischemic myocardium. The two methods currently available are pharmacologic thrombolysis via plasminogen activators and percutaneous coronary intervention (PCI). The effectiveness of either modality in reducing mortality and myocardial damage depends on how early it is given after the onset of symptoms.

A. Immediate Measures

Upon arrival, a patient being evaluated for ACS should be placed on cardiac monitor, given oxygen via nasal canula or mask and have 2 peripheral IV's placed.

Aspirin is the first and most important medication given to ACS patients early in their course. 162–325 mg nonenteric, and chewed is most effective. If contraindicated, use 300 mg clopidogrel. Coumadin use is not a contraindication to single aspirin dose, and does not substitute for aspirin as mechanism of action is different. NSAIDS should not be used to treat chest pain thought to be cardiac in origin.

A12 lead ECG should be obtained as rapidly as possible, ideally within 10 minutes of arrival.

If chest pain is present, give nitroglycerin, 0.4 mg sublingually or one spray delivered to the oral mucosa. Repeat if no effect occurs in 5 minutes. If chest pain returns or continues and systolic blood pressure is above 100 mm Hg, start intravenous nitroglycerin at 10 μg/min and increase by 5 μg/min every 3–5 minutes until systolic blood pressure falls by 10% or chest pain is relieved. The systolic blood pressure should not drop below 90 mm Hg.

Morphine may be still be used for analgesia, particularly for STEMI patients. However for UA/NSTEMI patients it may have increased adverse effects.

Current AHA guidelines recommend beta blockers be initiated within 24 hours of presentation. IV beta blockers are not useful if being used to reduce blood pressure. Contraindications to giving beta blockers include CHF, bradycardia, conduction blocks and hypotension. Also be aware of higher risks if given in elderly, patients with suspected cocaine use, and COPD/asthma patients.

B. Additional Measures

Establish a laboratory test database including complete blood count (CBC) with differential, serum creatinine and electrolyte measurements, blood urea nitrogen determinations, enzyme levels (cTni or cTnt). Platelet count, prothrombin time, partial thromboplastin time, and blood for typing (and cross-matching if needed) should be obtained for patients to be given thrombolytic therapy. Monitor urine output.

C. Option 1: Thrombolytic Therapy

If a patient experiences an acute ST segment elevation myocardial infarction and no contraindications are present, pharmacologic revascularization is indicated especially if PCI is unavailable for more than 90 minutes. Many thrombolytic agents are available, including streptokinase, anistreplase (APSAC), alteplase (tissue plasminogen activator: t-PA), reteplase (r-PA), and tenecteplase (TNK). Thrombolytics should be initiated in the emergency department because the benefit of pharmacologic thrombolysis decreases with each passing hour after myocardial infarction. Some patients with myocardial infarction may benefit from thrombolytics up to 12 hours after the onset of chest pain, although 6 hours is generally considered the cutoff. Alteplase administration over 90 minutes improved survival when compared to streptokinase or 3-hour alteplase infusion. Even though intracranial bleeding events increased, alteplase demonstrated a long-term survival advantage presumably secondary to earlier thrombolysis and reperfusion of thrombosed coronary arteries. Compared to alteplase, TNK may offer advantages of a single bolus administration and fewer intracranial hemorrhage complications. Intracranial hemorrhage is the most devastating complication of thrombolytic therapy, occurring in 0.5–3.3% of patients.

1. Indications—The indications for pharmacologic revascularization are as follows:

- ST segment elevation of at least 0.1 mV in two or more contiguous leads (II, III, aVF or V1–V6, I, aVL) suggests acute injury in the absence of left bundle branch block. An acute true posterior myocardial infarction (with ST depression in leads V1–V4) is also an indication for thrombolysis. Patients with ongoing chest pain and a new (or not known to be old) left bundle branch block should also be considered for pharmacologic reperfusion.

- Both chest pain and ST elevation are not relieved by two to three sublingual nitroglycerin tablets.

- Patient is alert and oriented, or a family member or friend familiar with the patient's medical history is present.

- No contraindications to thrombolytic therapy or anticoagulation therapy are present (see below).

2. Contraindications—

A. **ABSOLUTE CONTRAINDICATIONS**—Absolute contraindications are as follows:

- History of any hemorrhagic cerebrovascular event (stroke, arteriovenous malformation, or aneurysm) or any nonhemorrhagic cerebrovascular event or transient ischemic attack (within the last year)

- Any intracranial neoplasm

- Active, internal bleeding (eg, serious gastrointestinal bleeding) excluding menses

- Suspected aortic dissection

B. **RELATIVE CONTRAINDICATIONS**—In the following conditions, the risks associated with thrombolytic therapy may be increased, and clinical judgment should be used in evaluating expected benefits:

- Recent (within 10 days) puncture of a noncompressible blood vessel

- Poorly controlled hypertension of several years' duration or severe, uncontrolled arterial hypertension (diastolic blood pressure greater than 110 mm Hg or systolic blood pressure greater than 180 mm Hg)

- Diabetic hemorrhagic retinopathy or hemorrhagic ophthalmic condition

- Current treatment with an anticoagulant with international normalized ratio greater than two to three or other bleeding diathesis

- Pregnancy

- Any other condition associated with a predisposition to bleeding (eg, ulcerative colitis, active peptic ulcer disease, polycystic kidneys, gastrointestinal arteriovenous malformation, vascular tumors) or bleeding within 4 weeks

- Prolonged (>5 minutes) or traumatic external cardiac compression or traumatic endotracheal intubation

- History of nonhemorrhagic cerebrovascular accident beyond 1 year

- Recent (within 4 weeks) trauma or major surgery at a noncompressible site (eg, coronary artery bypass surgery, organ biopsy, intra-abdominal surgery, or obstetric delivery)

3. Dosages—If indicated, the dosage regimens recommended are as follows:

A. **STREPTOKINASE**—The recommended dosage is 1.5 million units in 250 mL of 5% dextrose in water, given intravenously over 1 hour. Because of the risk of serious allergic reactions, streptokinase is contraindicated in patients who have ever received streptokinase previously.

B. **ALTEPLASE**—The recommended dosage is 15 mg intravenous bolus followed by 0.75 mg/kg (maximum 50 mg) intravenous infusion over 30 minutes and then 0.5 mg/kg (maximum 35 mg) over 60 minutes. Alteplase has a very short half-life (5 minutes); therefore, unfractionated heparin must be used to prevent reocclusion. Heparin should be started as a bolus of 60 units/kg at the start of the alteplase infusion followed by a maintenance dose of 12 units/kg. The reduction in mortality with alteplase thrombolysis (if used within 6 hours of symptom onset) is 23–30%, which translates into a number needed to treat of between 3 and 5 patients.

C. **ANISOYLATED PLASMINOGEN STREPTOKINASE ACTIVATOR COMPLEX (APSAC)**—The recommended dosage is 30 mg intravenously infused slowly over 5 minutes. Because of the risk of serious allergic reaction, patients who have received streptokinase or APSAC previously cannot be given the drug again.

D. **UROKINASE**—The recommended dosage is a loading dose of 0.5 million units over a 10-minute period. This is followed by infusion doses of 1.6–4.5 million units over 18–24 hours.

E. **RETEPLASE**—r-PA, a variation of t-PA, has a half-life of 13–16 minutes and is simpler to administer than t-PA. The dose is two 10-unit intravenous boluses over 2 minutes, with 30 minutes between each dose.

F. **TENECTEPLASE**—TNK is a third-generation variation of t-PA. It has improved fibrin specificity and a longer half-life, allowing single bolus administration. The dose is based on weight, ranging from 30 to 50 mg rapid bolus. Overall mortality compared to t-PA was equal; however, in patients presenting later in the course of an acute myocardial infarction, those given TNK had fewer episodes of nonintracranial bleeding.

Excellent evidence indicates that myocardial reperfusion salvages myocardium—resulting in better ventricular function than conventional management—and improves survival if reperfusion occurs within 6 hours after the onset of symptoms of myocardial infarction. Thrombolytic therapy may be beneficial in patients with persistent chest pain for up to 24 hours after onset of symptoms. t-PA results in a higher percentage of vessel patency (60–80%) than does streptokinase (30–60%) within the first hour with an associated improvement in survival.

4. Heparin—Heparin or anti-coagulant such as enoxaparin, or fondaparinux should be used in conjunction with any thrombin-specific thrombolytic agent such as alteplase. Because of the systemic fibrinolysis achieved by streptokinase or APSAC, anticoagulation with heparin is not indicated. Intravenous heparin, 60 units/kg bolus followed by 12 units/kg/h, should be given in a separate line while alteplase is infusing because of the short half-life of alteplase and the danger of recurring thrombosis. Anti-coagulation should be continued for 48 hours or longer.

5. Monitoring—Transfer patients given thrombolytic therapy to an intensive care unit as soon as possible after initiation of treatment. Monitor the following:

- blood pressure every 15 minutes during infusion and every 30–60 minutes thereafter
- ECG rhythm strip for reperfusion arrhythmias and ST segment changes
- bleeding complications and changes in neurologic status; avoid venous or arterial punctures and unnecessary trauma
- 12-lead ECG 4 hours after the start of therapy and as needed (eg, for recurrence of chest pain)
- cTni or cTnt 4 hours after initiation of treatment and at 4-hour intervals for 24 hours

D. Option 2: Percutaneous Coronary Intervention

Formerly termed angioplasty, PCI involves cardiac catheterization and various techniques to assess and restore vessel patency on an emergency basis. Coronary artery stenting has become the procedure of choice. When performed early in the course of an acute myocardial infarction, PCI has demonstrated improved survival rates over pharmacologic thrombolysis. Increased rates of normal flow and decreased rates of reocclusion in the infarct-related artery are much more likely when PCI is chosen over pharmacologic thrombolysis. In addition, early definition of coronary anatomy can be used to tailor therapy and improve risk stratification. One study comparing PCI with t-PA found a reduction in mortality of 4% with PCI. Major complications associated with thrombolytics such as intracranial bleeding do not occur with PCI. In patients with contraindications to thrombolytics, PCI is the only option available to restore perfusion and salvage myocardium. Rescue PCI is useful for patients who have received thrombolytics but whose chest pain or ST segment elevation has failed to resolve (50% decrease in ST elevation in 90 min after fibrinolysis begins). Unfortunately, PCI is not widely available; fewer than 18% of US hospitals are equipped to perform the procedure. If the time to PCI is expected to exceed 90 minutes for a patient with a ST segment elevation myocardial infarction, thrombolytics should be strongly considered in order to salvage as much myocardium as possible.

Facilitated PCI, as defined by administration of a fibrinolytic agent at partial or full dosing, with PCI performed immediately after is not currently recommended. This differs from rescue PCI as defined by PCI performed after fibrinolysis failure.

▶ Disposition

Hospitalize all patients with clinical histories suggesting myocardial infarction. For patients with ST segment elevation MI, ideally, a hospital capable of performing PCI will have a mechanism in place that allows an emergency physician to directly activate the cardiac catheterization laboratory so as to get the patient to definitive treatment as rapidly as possible. Patients with suspected myocardial infarction and normal initial ECGs and initial cardiac enzymes may be admitted to a monitored intermediate care unit.

COMPLICATIONS OF MYOCARDIAL INFARCTION

About 10–15% of patients reaching the hospital with myocardial infarction die during hospitalization. One or more complications occur in over half of all patients with myocardial infarction.

1. Shock (Cardiogenic Shock)

Shock complicating myocardial infarction occurs in 7–8% of patients and may be caused by extensive myocardial infarction with decreased cardiac output (most common), inappropriate reflex peripheral vasodilatation, arrhythmias, hypovolemia, right ventricular infarction, and mechanical complications such as ruptured ventricular septum and severe mitral regurgitation. Free-wall myocardial rupture results in tamponade and shock. The mortality rate is as high as 70–80% among patients with cardiogenic shock as a complication of acute myocardial infarction.

▶ Clinical Findings

Hypotension accompanied by confusion, obtundation or restlessness, cool skin, oliguria, and metabolic acidosis suggests shock. Mild to moderate hypotension alone is common in myocardial infarction and does not itself indicate shock. Shock in myocardial infarction may be due to many causes (see Table 11–1), which may be difficult to differentiate noninvasively (Table 34–1).

▶ Treatment

Use any or all of the measures discussed here as necessary (see also Chapter 11).

A. Airway Management

Give oxygen by mask or nasal cannula. Patients in shock with respiratory failure require endotracheal intubation.

B. Venous Pressure Monitoring

Consider monitoring central pressure with a Swan-Ganz pulmonary artery catheter (or, far less desirably, a central venous pressure catheter, since in acute myocardial infarction, left ventricular filling pressure can be markedly elevated with normal right ventricular filling pressure, and vice versa). Use an arterial line to measure blood pressure.

Table 34–1. Differential Diagnosis by Hemodynamics of Heart Failure and Hypotension After Myocardial Infarction.

Arterial Pressure	Central Venous Pressure	Pulmonary Arterial Wedge Pressre	Stroke Volume Index	Diagnosis	Treatment
→	→ or ↑	↑	→ or ↓	Heart failure	Diuretics; preload and afterload reduction
→ or ↓	→ or ↓	↓	↓	Hypovolemia	Saline volume loading
→ or ↓	↑	→ or ↓	→ or ↓	Pulmonary embolism Right ventricular myocardial infarction	Ventilation/perfusion scan; saline or dextran; volume loading; no diuretics
↓	→ or ↑	↑	↓	Cardiogenic shock	Inotropic agents; diuretics; preload and afterload reduction if arterial pressure can be maintained; counterpulsation

→ = Normal; ↓ = decreased or low; ↑ = elevated or high.

C. Other Measures

Give a fluid challenge (200 mL of saline intravenously over 20 minutes) if the patient is not in congestive heart failure (ie, no rales and no pulmonary edema on chest X-ray). Repeat as needed if congestive heart failure does not develop. Correct arrhythmias (see below). Insert a Foley catheter, and measure urine output hourly.

D. Drug Therapy

Give dopamine (or dobutamine), 2.5–20 mg/kg/min by continuous intravenous infusion. Use the smallest effective dose, guided by hemodynamic response. When shock is caused by inappropriate vasodilatation (rare), α-adrenergic drugs such as norepinephrine are useful.

E. Percutaneous Coronary Intervention

Evidence indicates that acute revascularization by PCI might be particularly effective in patients who develop cardiogenic shock early (within 3–6 hours) after onset of myocardial infarction. PCI acutely should be seriously considered in such patients because thrombolytics are ineffective in cardiogenic shock associated with an acute myocardial infarction. An intra-aortic balloon pump (IABP) can also be placed, typically in the cath lab. IABP counterpulsation can increase cardiac output and improve both coronary and systemic perfusion. IABP counterpulsation is contraindicated in patients with aortic valve disease or those with aortic dissection.

▶ Disposition

All patients with cardiogenic shock must be hospitalized, preferably in an intensive care unit. Therapy is directed at the likely causes of shock.

2. Congestive Heart Failure

Congestive heart failure is caused by extensive myocardial infarction, volume overload, arrhythmias, acute mitral regurgitation, or ventricular septal rupture.

▶ Clinical Findings

Symptoms and signs of congestive heart failure include dyspnea, anxiety, tachypnea, tachycardia, pulmonary rales or frank pulmonary edema, jugular venous distention, hypoxemia, and typical findings on chest X-ray (cardiomegaly, pulmonary vascular plethora, Kerley B lines, pleural effusion, or pulmonary infiltrates consistent with pulmonary edema). Wheezing may also be a sign of congestive heart failure (cardiac asthma). Suspect right ventricular infarction in inferior myocardial infarction if signs of right heart failure (right ventricular gallops, elevated central venous pressure, hepatomegaly, peripheral edema) are prominent in the absence of signs of left heart failure (dyspnea, rales, pulmonary congestion on chest X-ray).

▶ Treatment

A. Airway Management

Give oxygen by mask or nasal cannula. Treat respiratory failure if present.

B. Drug Therapy

1. Nitroglycerin—Give NTG either sublingual or spray, followed by IV infusion. NTG will decrease preload as well as afterload. In patients with inferior or right ventricular acute myocardial infarction, nitrates are relatively contraindicated because they may precipitate profound hypotension. Hypotension related to nitrates is treated with reduction or discontinuation of the infusion depending on the degree of symptomatic hypotension. Intravascular volume expansion with intravenous fluid infusions will often quickly correct hypotension.

2. Furosemide—Give furosemide as an intravenous bolus of at least the patient's normal total daily dose. If the patient is not already taking furosemide, administer a 40-mg intravenous bolus initially, and observe the diuretic response by monitoring the patient's symptoms and urine output.

Diuretics are contraindicated if right ventricular infarction is suspected.

3. ACE or ARB inhibitors can be used to decrease afterload.

4. Noninvassive positive pressure ventilation (CPAP/Bipap) has been shown to decrease need for intubation. Alveoli are kept open with positive pressure and work of the heart is reduced.

▶ Disposition

Treatment of congestive heart failure in the emergency department is directed at reducing the intravascular volume through diuretics or vasodilation. Patients with respiratory failure may require intubation in the emergency department. Hemodynamic monitoring with a pulmonary artery catheter may assist in assessing volume status. In the setting of an acute myocardial infarction, patients with congestive heart failure should be closely monitored in an intensive care unit.

3. Acute Mitral Regurgitation and Ventricular Septal Rupture

Mechanical failure of infarcted tissue (eg, rupture of the ventricular septum or of papillary muscle supporting the chordae tendineae) is a common cause of acute mitral regurgitation and ventricular septal rupture. Minimal-to-moderate mitral regurgitation is common after myocardial infarction as a result of papillary muscle and left ventricular wall dysfunction. Severe degrees of mitral regurgitation can result from marked ischemia with little or no infarction and can be completely reversed with revascularization.

▶ Clinical Findings

Abrupt, severe congestive heart failure with pansystolic regurgitation murmur suggests acute mitral regurgitation or ventricular septal rupture. Echocardiography to detect mitral regurgitation or the abnormal velocity jet of a ventricular septal defect can establish the diagnosis.

▶ Treatment

A. Immediate Measures

Treat heart failure with diuretics, morphine, and nitroglycerin.

Obtain urgent cardiologic and cardiac surgical consultation. IABP is a useful temporizing measure while the patient is being prepared for surgery.

B. Follow-Up Measures

The only life-saving treatment for most patients is emergency cardiac catheterization followed by surgery.

▶ Disposition

Hospitalize all patients in a critical care unit for treatment and surgery.

4. Myocardial Rupture

The chief cause of myocardial rupture is mechanical failure of an infarcted ventricular wall.

▶ Clinical Findings

Myocardial rupture is an uncommon cause of sudden death during acute myocardial infarction; it is responsible for only about 5% of deaths. Myocardial rupture is suggested by abrupt onset of hypotension with increased venous pressure (ie, cardiac tamponade). Pulseless electrical activity often occurs.

▶ Treatment and Disposition

If echocardiography or bedside emergency ultrasound demonstrates a pericardial effusion, pericardiocentesis is indicated and can be performed under ultrasound guidance (Chapter 6). When emergent ultrasound is not available to assess a patient for possible pericardial tamponade, blind pericardiocentesis may be life saving.

Obtain emergency cardiac surgical consultation for immediate cardiac surgery. This is successful in the few cases in which rupture has been minimal with slow intrapericardial hemorrhage.

5. Systemic or Pulmonary Embolization

See also Chapter 33.

Systemic or pulmonary embolization is commonly caused by intracardiac mural thrombosis or phlebothrombosis.

▶ Clinical Findings

The most common findings in pulmonary embolism are sudden unexplained dyspnea and tachycardia. Occasionally, pleuritic pain, signs of right heart strain, or abnormal chest X-ray may occur. Patients at greatest risk are those with thrombus visualized in the left or right ventricle by two-dimensional echocardiography. The diagnosis may be confirmed by computed tomography (CT) scan of the chest, lung scan, or arteriography (Chapter 33). Systemic embolization is suspected when symptoms and signs of arterial occlusion occur. The clinical picture depends on the artery occluded, for example, flank pain and hematuria with renal artery embolism; pallor, pain, and loss of pulse with brachial or femoral artery embolism; stroke with cerebral artery embolism.

▶ Treatment and Disposition

Give oxygen, draw blood for determination of prothrombin and partial thromboplastin times, and then begin systemic anticoagulation with heparin, 80 units/kg bolus followed by 18 units/kg/h infusion, or a low-molecular-weight heparin such as enoxaparin, 1 mg/kg subcutaneous administration every 12 hours. Pericarditis is a relative contraindication to anticoagulation because of the risk of bleeding into the pericardial sac, with resulting cardiac tamponade. Heparin is also contraindicated in patients with recent stroke, active duodenal ulcer, or active bleeding that cannot be controlled by direct pressure. Even though it does not cross the placenta, heparin must be used with caution in pregnant patients, especially during the third trimester. (Acute myocardial infarction during pregnancy is quite rare.)

With a massive pulmonary embolism with right heart failure or shock, intravenous fibrinolysis with streptokinase, urokinase, or t-PA has been recommended in doses similar to those given for acute myocardial infarction. Occasionally, mechanical disruption of the embolic thrombus by a catheter has been life saving.

Seek appropriate surgical consultation (with a thoracic, general, or vascular surgeon) for patients with persistent hypotension, contraindications to thrombolytic therapy, or systemic embolization who may benefit from surgical intervention (eg, angioplasty and embolectomy for a pulseless and ischemic extremity).

Patients who have received TPA or have hemodynamic instability should be hospitalized in an intensive care unit.

6. Pericarditis

When transmural myocardial infarction causes pericardial inflammation over the area of necrosis, pericarditis may occur within the first week. Pericarditis occurring more than 1 week after myocardial infarction may be the result of Dressler syndrome, an autoimmune reaction.

▶ Clinical Findings

Pericarditis usually does not appear until 2–3 days after the onset of myocardial infarction. The appearance of a friction rub is often the only manifestation; pain and ECG changes are often absent. Frequently, a small pericardial effusion may be detected by echocardiography. If a pericardial friction rub is heard in the first 24 hours after onset, suspect pericarditis as a primary diagnosis rather than as being due to acute myocardial infarction. Early ECG signs of pericarditis include diffuse ST segment elevation (with a concave upslope and indistinct J point) and diffuse PR segment depression (except in AVR, where the PR segment is elevated).

▶ Treatment

Treat pain with a nonsteroidal anti-inflammatory agent such as indomethacin, 25–50 mg orally three times a day. If pain is severe, give morphine, 2–4 mg intravenously every 5–10 minutes, and repeat as necessary.

▶ Disposition

Hospitalize the patient in a coronary care unit for pain control and monitoring for possible cardiac tamponade (rare).

ANGINA PECTORIS

▶ General Considerations

Myocardial ischemia (with attendant angina pectoris) results from an imbalance between myocardial oxygen supply and demand. Clinical findings vary depending on the severity of ischemia and on the frequency, duration, and rapidity of onset of ischemic episodes. If the demand for myocardial blood flow exceeds the capacity of the obstructed coronary arterial tree to supply it, the discomfort (angina pectoris) lasts until the excessive demand for coronary flow is reduced.

Discomfort is more intense and lasts longer when coronary blood flow decreases markedly, as occurs with sudden marked increase in coronary artery obstruction resulting from abrupt development of thrombus over an atherosclerotic plaque, embolization to a coronary artery, or sudden occlusion by coronary artery spasm. If myocardial necrosis then occurs, the condition is termed myocardial infarction; otherwise, the episode is one of acute coronary insufficiency, or preinfarction angina.

If obstruction is so severe that coronary blood flow is barely adequate to meet resting demands, even small increases in myocardial oxygen demand may cause angina. In addition, small aggregations of platelets on a ruptured plaque, spasm, or increased vasomotor tone can cause minor changes in the caliber of the severely obstructed coronary artery and precipitate angina.

Myocardial ischemia can exist in the absence of any chest discomfort. In patients with severe ischemia, 24-hour ECG monitoring shows that 80% of the episodes of ST segment depression lasting for a minute or more are present without angina (so-called silent ischemia). Painless myocardial infarction is not unusual in elderly or diabetic patients.

▶ Clinical Findings

A. Stable Angina (Angina of Effort)

By definition, the pattern of discomfort, its frequency of occurrence, and precipitating factors have remained the same for 3 or more months.

Discomfort is usually substernal but may originate in other areas (eg, elbow, forearm, shoulder, neck interscapular region, or jaw), although substernal discomfort eventually occurs. It is usually precipitated by activities that increase myocardial oxygen consumption (eg, exercise, eating, or emotional upset), lasts longer than 1 minute and usually less than 15 minutes, and is usually relieved by rest or nitroglycerin. Pain that meets these criteria usually indicates the presence of fixed coronary obstruction. The most important feature suggesting the diagnosis of angina pectoris is discomfort precipitated by exercise or emotion.

B. Unstable Angina

Anginal pain that begins in a patient previously free of pain (ie, pain of less than 1 month's duration) is called new-onset angina. Unstable angina is that which has changed in pattern, becoming more frequent (crescendo angina) and longer lasting. It is precipitated by a lesser degree of activity and may respond less to rest and nitroglycerin than does stable angina. Angina that occurs at rest without any obvious precipitating factor (rest angina) is the most serious form of unstable angina.

Sudden changes in angina not associated with increased myocardial oxygen demand (eg, increased blood pressure or heart rate) are presumed to be caused by a change in the anatomy of the coronary artery, for example, new vessel obstruction caused by progression of heart disease, development of thrombus, or other factors such as platelet aggregation or coronary spasm.

C. Atypical Angina, or Prinzmetal (Variant) Angina

Prinzmetal angina occurs as a result of a sudden, reversible, severe coronary artery obstruction (coronary artery spasm). It may occur in patients with fixed atherosclerotic coronary lesions and less often in those with minimal or no fixed coronary obstruction. Chest discomfort usually occurs without a precipitating cause. It frequently occurs at rest or awakens the patient at night. The discomfort frequently lasts longer than the usual episode of angina and is often accompanied by ST segment elevation (current of injury) that is transient and reversed in minutes after administration of nitroglycerin. With lesser degrees of spasm, ST segment depression may occur. Ventricular ectopy and ventricular tachyarrhythmias may also occur.

▶ Differential Diagnosis

See Chapter 14.

▶ Treatment and Disposition

A. Stable Angina

Nitroglycerin, 0.4 mg sublingually, is the drug of choice when pain starts. It may also be taken prophylactically several minutes before activities that regularly precipitate angina. Pain is usually relieved in 1–2 minutes. Nitroglycerin tablets deteriorate in about 6 months; headache and sublingual tingling are common side effects of active tablets.

Current recommendations for patients who have previously been prescribed NTG for angina, is to take one dose, and if not improving after 5 minutes, to call 911 before taking any more. If pain is improved, NTG can be repeated every 5 minutes up to 3 doses, and then 911 called only if pain not resolved.

B. Unstable Angina, Rest Angina, and Prinzmetal Angina

1. Immediate measures—Give oxygen by mask or nasal cannula. Hospitalize the patient immediately in the coronary care unit and obtain daily ECGs and myocardial enzyme determinations (cTni or cTnt) to detect possible myocardial infarction.

2. Aspirin—Start nonenteric-coated aspirin, 160–325 mg orally. Aspirin has been shown to reduce the incidence of myocardial infarction and death by about 50%.

3. Nitroglycerin—Apply nitroglycerin paste, 1.25 cm (½ in), to the skin under an occlusive dressing every 4 hours, or transdermal nitroglycerin patches may be substituted. Topical nitroglycerin can be used if the patient is pain free. If the pain persists, an intravenous infusion of nitroglycerin is indicated at an initial rate of 10 μg/min.

4. β-Blockers—Add a β-adrenergic blocking agent (eg, metoprolol, 25 mg orally) unless contraindicated (heart rate less than 60 beats/min, atrioventricular block, severe asthma, or chronic obstructive pulmonary disease). Calcium channel blockers are usually used for long-term treatment of patients with vasospastic or Prinzmetals angina. Beta blocker use is recommened in first 24 hours of unstable angina.

5. Morphine—Give morphine, 2–3 mg intravenously every 5–10 minutes, to relieve prolonged pain. Monitor blood pressure. Morphine's use in cardiac chest pain, particularly NSTEMI has been diminished as some observational studies showed worsened outcomes. Do not use NSAIDS for suspected cardiac chest pain as they have been shown to increase mortality.

6. Anticoagulation—Antiocoagulation may also be helpful in these patients. Use unfractionated heparin at 80 units/kg intravenous bolus followed by 18 units/kg/h intravenous infusion or a low-molecular-weight heparin such as enoxaparin, 1 mg/kg administered subcutaneously every 12 hours. In the SYNERGY trial in which enoxaparin and unfractionated heparin were compared, the primary end point of death or myocardial infarction at 30 days was statistically similar although bleeding complications were slightly more common in the enoxaparin group. Other drugs that are currently being studies and now used include fondaparinux and bivalirudin.

7. Other drug therapies—Glycoprotein IIB/IIIA receptor antagonists such as abciximab and the newer agents tirofiban and eptifibatide are approved for use in patients with acute coronary syndrome. These agents block platelet binding at the receptor site that cross-links fibrinogen to the platelets. Although these agents have shown promise when used in conjunction with PCI, their role in unstable angina is still being defined. In the future, there may be a role for combining these agents with lower dose fibrinolytics to improve reperfusion while curtailing bleeding complications.

8. Percutaneous coronary intervention—If pain continues despite treatment, consider PCI. If acute myocardial infarction has occurred and pain continues despite optimal medical management or thrombolytics, PCI must be considered. Percutaneous aortic balloon counterpulsation may also be useful in patients with cardiogenic shock.

ACC/AHA 2007 Guidelines for the Management of Patients With Unstable Angina/Non-ST-Elevation Myocardial Infarction—Executive Summary: A Report of the American College of Cardiology/American Heart Association Task Force on Practice Guidelines (Writing Committee to Revise the 2002 Guidelines for the Management of Patients With Unstable Angina/Non-ST-Elevation Myocardial Infarction) *Developed in Collaboration with the American College of Emergency Physicians, the Society for Cardiovascular Angiography and Interventions, and the Society of Thoracic Surgeons* Endorsed by the American Association of Cardiovascular and Pulmonary Rehabilitation and the Society for Academic Emergency Medicine. J Am Coll Cardiol 2007;50(7):e1-e157 657–668 [PMID: 17692738].

ACC/AHA 2005 guideline update for the diagnosis and management of chronic heart failure in the adult: a report of the American College of Cardiology/American Heart Association Task Force on Practice Guidelines (Writing Committee to Update the 2001 Guidelines for the Evaluation and Management of Heart Failure). J Am Coll Cardiol 2005;46(6):e1–82 [PMID: 16168273].

ACC/AHA/SCAI 2005 Guideline Update for Percutaneous Intervention—summary article: a report of the American College of Cardiology/American Heart Association Task Force on Practice Guidelines (ACC/AHA/SCAI Writing Committee to Update the 2001 Guidelines for Percutaneous Coronary Intervention). Circulation 2006;113(1):156–175 [PMID: 16391169].

Antman EM: Decision making with cardiac troponin tests. N Engl J Med 2002;346:2079 [PMID: 12087146].

Diop D, Aghababian RV: Definition, classification, and pathophysiology of acute coronary ischemic syndromes. Emerg Med Clin North Am 2001;19:259 [PMID: 11373977].

Karras DJ, Kane DL: Serum markers in the emergency department diagnosis of acute myocardial infarction. Emerg Med Clin North Am 2001;19:321 [PMID: 11373981].

Lee TH, Goldman L: Evaluation of the patient with acute chest pain. N Engl J Med 2000;342:1187 [PMID: 10770985].

Llevadot J, Giugliano RP, Antman EM: Bolus fibrinolytic therapy in acute myocardial infarction. JAMA 2001;286:442 [PMID: 11466123].

McPherson JA, Gibson RS: Reperfusion therapy for acute myocardial infarction. Emerg Med Clin North Am 2001;19:433 [PMID: 11373988].

Mishra PK: Variations in presentation and various options in management of variant angina. Eur J Cardiothorac Surg 2006;29:748–759 [PMID: 16481189].

Shannon AW, Harrigan RA: General pharmacologic treatment of acute myocardial infarction. Emerg Med Clin North Am 2001;19:417 [PMID: 11373987].

SYNERGY Executive Committee: Superior Yield of the New strategy of Enoxaparin, Revascularization and Glycoprotein IIb/IIIa inhibitors. Am Heart J 2002;143;952–960 [PMID: 12075248].

Heart failure is the expected outcome of many cardiac diseases. It is the reason for at least 20% of all hospital admissions for patients older than 65 years of age. The basic abnormality is inability of the heart to maintain cardiac output sufficient to meet systemic demands. Compensatory mechanisms include (1) dilatation of the ventricle to maintain normal stroke volume (Frank-Starling mechanism); (2) retention of sodium and water by the kidneys to maintain intravascular volume; (3) increased activity of the sympathetic nervous system, leading to tachycardia and increased systemic vascular resistance; and (4) increased serum renin and angiotensin, which stimulate aldosterone output and cause retention of sodium and water as well as increased systemic vascular resistance. Cardiac output is usually maintained at normal levels or below, but at the expense of increased ventricular volume and filling pressure. The increased ventricular filling or diastolic pressures result in increased pulmonary or systemic venous pressures, with consequent pulmonary or peripheral edema. Tissue and organ dysfunction may result from increased venous pressure, decreased cardiac output, and edema.

Recently, it has been recognized that in 20–50% of patients with heart failure, systolic function is preserved but the primary cause may be diastolic dysfunction in which the ventricle appears to be noncompliant; therefore, even with normal diastolic volumes the high filling pressure results in pulmonary congestion. This type of heart failure is seen in hypertension, especially in elderly patients, in hypertrophic cardiomyopathy, and in myocardial ischemia. In many patients, both systolic and diastolic dysfunction are present. An echocardiographic Doppler study should be performed in all patients with congestive heart failure to help determine the cause of the failure and the degree of systolic and diastolic dysfunction. The echocardiographic Doppler study need not be done in the emergency department.

Although the distinction between mild to moderate heart failure and severe heart failure is not absolute, it has practical therapeutic implications.

SEVERE HEART FAILURE, INCLUDING PULMONARY EDEMA

▶ Clinical Findings

A. Symptoms and Signs

Frank pulmonary edema may occur with severe left heart failure. Patients experience dyspnea at rest (Chapter 13) and in severe cases may be cyanotic and cough up frothy sputum. Peripheral edema may or may not be present; edema may be severe (anasarca) in severe right heart failure. Pulmonary edema may be accompanied by wheezing, and a loud S_3 sound is usually present. Loud rhonchi and rales may interfere with more detailed evaluation.

B. X-ray Findings

Chest X-ray may show pulmonary edema, pleural effusions, or cardiomegaly.

C. Laboratory Findings

Arterial blood gas measurements show hypoxemia; pH and Pco_2 vary, but hypocapnia and metabolic acidosis are common. With exhaustion, hypercapnia may occur, in which case intubation and mechanical ventilation are required. Recently, the serum level of a neuropeptide, brain-type natriuretic peptide (BNP), has been used clinically as a good marker for congestive heart failure. BNP is released from the ventricular myocardium in response to increases in ventricular wall tension. Above a BNP cutoff level of 100 pg/mL, the sensitivity and specificity are 90 and 76%, respectively, for differentiating congestive heart failure from other causes of dyspnea.

D. Electrocardiographic Findings

Sinus tachycardia is common in patients with severe heart failure. In patients with hypertensive heart disease, left ventricular hypertrophy may be evident. In addition, obtain an ECG to detect the presence of ischemia.

Of paramount importance is the establishment of the cause of the heart failure. Specific causes have specific therapies, for example, valve replacement for pulmonary edema from severe aortic stenosis, or lowering of blood pressure for hypertension.

Note: Acute myocardial infarction or ischemia must be considered in all patients with sudden onset of congestive heart failure.

▶ Treatment

A. Oxygenation and Venous Access

Begin oxygen by mask or nasal cannula. Insert a peripheral intravenous catheter and give 0.9% normal saline by microdrip infusion to keep the catheter patent or insert a saline lock catheter.

B. Nitroglycerin

Nitroglycerin, being a potent vasodilator, is useful in severe congestive heart failure because it reduces preload and afterload. The dose is 10 μg/min initially. Severe hypotension can develop, especially in the setting of an acute inferior or right ventricular infarction.

C. Furosemide

If the patient is not already taking oral furosemide, 40 mg intravenously is a common initial dose. For patients already taking oral furosemide, administer at least the daily dose as an intravenous bolus. If the patient fails to respond in 10 minutes, repeat the dose once.

D. Noninvasive Postitive Pressure Ventilation (NIPPV)

Noninvasive positive pressure ventilation (CPAP/Bipap) has been shown to decrease need for intubation. Alveoli are kept open with positive pressure and work of the heart is reduced.

ACE or ARB inhibitors can be used to decrease afterload.

E. Nitroprusside

If the cause of severe congestive heart failure is directly related to hypertensive emergency, administer nitroprusside, 2–20 μg/kg/min as a continuous infusion. While the patient is monitored carefully (arterial pressure monitor is recommended), the dose can be titrated to achieve the desired blood pressure.

F. Nesiritide

No longer used due to studies showing increased mortality. It still may play a role in some patients who are resistant to other treatment, however cardiologist consultation should be considered prior to initiating medication.

▶ Disposition

Hospitalize all patients with severe heart failure. Search for the reason behind the recurrent pulmonary edema, for example, noncompliance with regard to prescribed diet and medications, paroxysmal arrhythmias, institution of a medication with a negative inotropic effect, pulmonary emboli, or complicating disease.

MILD TO MODERATE HEART FAILURE

▶ Clinical Findings

A. Symptoms and Signs

Nocturnal cough or dyspnea, orthopnea, dyspnea on exertion, and ankle swelling are common. The patient is not in distress at rest. Cardiomegaly is almost always found and is usually associated with some symptoms or signs of underlying cardiac disease (eg, angina or findings characteristic of aortic stenosis). Other important signs include increased venous pressure, hepatojugular reflux, pulmonary rales or pleural effusion, sacral or peripheral edema, and S_3 gallop.

Because hypertension is one of the most common causes of heart failure, record the blood pressure reading in both arms with the patient supine and sitting.

B. X-ray Findings

Chest X-ray may demonstrate cardiomegaly and pulmonary congestion.

C. Electrocardiographic Findings

Although there are no specific ECG manifestations of heart failure, it is nonetheless helpful to obtain an ECG.

D. Laboratory Findings

Obtain serum electrolyte determinations, renal function tests, and blood urea nitrogen and serum creatinine measurements. When renal blood flow is decreased, a rise in blood urea nitrogen out of proportion to the rise in serum creatinine is common (prerenal azotemia). Recently, measurement of serum BNP (as mentioned in the previous section) has been shown to improve accuracy in the diagnosis of congestive heart failure.

▶ Treatment

Provide the patient with instructions for a low-sodium (1–2 g/d) diet. Prescribe a diuretic. A thiazide diuretic (eg, hydrochlorothiazide, 25 mg orally twice daily with potassium supplementation) should be sufficient initial therapy for most patients. Control hypertension if present (see below).

▶ Disposition

By definition, hospitalization is not required for patients with mild heart failure per se, although it may be prudent to hospitalize some patients (eg, unreliable patients, those with other underlying illnesses or new-onset symptoms). All patients should be referred for long-term care and should be seen again within 1 week after their visit to the emergency department. Most of these patients will be candidates for medical therapy with angiotensin-converting enzyme inhibitors (eg, captopril or enalapril) and β-blockers. These agents have been shown to improve symptoms in patients with moderate congestive heart failure.

ACC/AHA 2005 guideline update for the diagnosis and management of chronic heart failure in the adult: a report of the American College of Cardiology/American Heart Association Task Force on Practice Guidelines (Writing Committee to Update the 2001 Guidelines for the Evaluation and Management of Heart Failure). J Am Coll Cardiol 2005;46(6):e1–e82 [PMID: 16168273].

Collins SP, Hinckley WR, Storrow AB: Critical review and recommendations for nesiritide use in the emergency department. J Emerg Med 2005;29(3):317–329 [PMID: 16183453].

Colucci WS et al: Intravenous nesiritide in the treatment of decompensated congestive heart failure: Nesiritide Study Group. N Engl J Med 2000;343:246 [PMID: 10911006].

Hiestand B, Abraham WT: Safety and efficacy of nesiritide for acute decompensated heart failure: recent literature and upcoming trials.: Curr Cardiol Rep 2007;9(3):182–186 [PMID: 17470330].

Jessup M, Brozena S. Heart failure. N Engl J Med 2003;15;348,2007–2018 [PMID: 12748317].

Panacek EA, Kirk JD. Role of noninvasive ventilation in the management of acutely decompensated heart failure. Rev Cardiovasc Med 2002;3 Suppl 4:S35–S40 [PMID: 12439429].

▼ HYPERTENSION AND HYPERTENSIVE CRISIS

▶ Clinical Findings

The emergency physician evaluates patients with elevated blood pressures on a daily basis. The urge exists to treat all abnormal vital signs. Emergency physicians should avoid reflexively treating all elevated blood pressures without considering the patient in light of the clinical setting. For example, a patient experiencing pain or anxiety may be hypertensive in the emergency department simply as an adrenergic reflex. Aggressive treatment of asymptomatic hypertension in the emergency department may not be benign because it may lead to hypoperfusion and precipitate cerebrovascular ischemic events. When hypertension acutely causes symptoms, the organs most commonly affected include the brain, heart, and kidneys. Two categories of hypertension seen in emergency department patients merit further discussion: hypertensive urgency and hypertensive emergency. It is preferable not to use specific numbers to define these as they are relative to each patient.

A. Hypertensive Urgency

Hypertensive urgency is classically defined as a severely elevated blood pressure in a patient with no symptoms, signs, or laboratory findings of end-organ damage. Typical screening studies include serum creatinine (acute elevation), urinalysis (proteinuria, red blood cells, or red cell casts), chest X-ray (pulmonary edema or thoracic aortic dissection), and ECG (cardiac ischemia). These patients are however at risk for end organ damage if elevated blood pressure continues.

B. Hypertensive Emergency

Hypertensive emergency occurs when elevated blood pressure is responsible for symptoms, signs, or laboratory evidence of end-organ damage, such as mental status changes (hypertensive encephalopathy), intracranial hemorrhage, retinopathy, aortic dissection, cardiac ischemia or congestive heart failure, or acute renal failure.

▶ Treatment

A. Categories of Management

1. Hypertensive urgency—If history, physical examination, and screening tests do not reveal any end-organ damage, blood pressure should be controlled within 24–48 hours. Reliable patients can be discharged home with rapid follow-up with a primary-care physician for blood pressure recheck and initiation or adjustment of antihypertensive therapy if blood pressure remains elevated. If therapy is used, oral agents are appropriate. Clonidine, 0.2 mg by mouth followed by 0.1 mg every hour until the blood pressure is adequately controlled; captopril, 12.5–25 mg by mouth; or oral labetalol, 200–400 mg, may be used. If patient is discharged on medication, first line is typically HCTZ at a dose of 12.5–25 mg daily. Patient still needs to have urgent follow up as medications will likely need to be titrated.

2. Hypertensive emergency—Treatment involves rapid but controlled reduction in blood pressure using intravenous medications. The goal is to reduce the mean blood pressure by 25% within 1 hour of presentation. If the initial reduction is well tolerated by the patient, reduction to normal levels can be achieved over the ensuing 24 hours.

B. Drugs Used to Treat Hypertensive Emergencies

Caution: Avoid rapid, severe drops in blood pressure, because watershed cerebral infarction can occur. Blood pressure should be lowered gradually to the 160–180 mm Hg range acutely and then lowered further only gradually over a period of days with oral therapy.

1. Nitroprusside—Nitroprusside is a potent vasodilator. Give by continuous intravenous infusion at a rate of 2–20 μg/kg/min. This drug lowers blood pressure in seconds; stopping the infusion results in rapid return of blood pressure to the previous level. Hospitalization in an intensive care unit and intra-arterial pressure monitoring are usually required. Whenever nitroprusside is administered, it is advisable to monitor the blood pressure with an intra-arterial pressure catheter to avoid overshooting the titration and causing hypoperfusion.

2. Labetalol—Labetalol is a combination α- and β-blocker useful in hypertensive emergency. The dose is 20 mg intravenously over 2 minutes. IV drip can then be started and titrated. It is useful in pregnancy, as well as patients with intracranial pathology such as hemorrhage or stroke.

3. Hydralazine—Hydralazine is a vasodilator used mainly in pregnancy because it also increases uterine blood flow. The dose is 10–40 mg intravenously every 15–30 minutes. If a continuous infusion is required, the dose is 1.5–5.0 μg/kg/min.

4. Fenoldopam—Fenoldopam is particularly useful in patients with renal insufficiency or failure as an alternative to nitroprusside, which has been associated with cyanide toxicity. The initial dose is 0.1–1.6 μg/kg/min.

5. Enalaprilat—Enalaprilat is an intravenous angiotensin-converting enzyme inhibitor. It is useful in congestive heart failure or for stroke patients as an alternative to nitroprusside. The dose is 1.25–5.0 mg per dose over 5 minutes every 6 hours.

6. Nicardipine—Nicardipine is an IV calcium channel blocker. It is particularly useful in subarachnoid hemorrhage and ischemic stroke patients as cerebral perfusion is spared.

The initial dose is 5 mg/h and increased by 2.5 mg/h every 5 minutes (for rapid titration) to every 15 minutes (for gradual titration) up to a maximum of 15 mg/h.

7. Esmolol—Esmolol is a IV beta1 blocker. It is useful in situations such as aortic dissections. It is titratable and short acting. The loading dose: 500 mcg/kg over 1 minute; followed with a 50 mcg/kg/minute infusion for 4 minutes; if the response is inadequate the infusion is increased in 50 mcg/kg/min increments (no more frequently than 4 minute intervals) to a maximum of 200 mcg/kg/minute.

Patients with hypertensive crisis require immediate hospitalization. Patients with hypertensive urgency should be referred to a primary-care physician within 12–24 hours. Evidence-based recommendations do not exist for the optimal timing and degree of blood pressure control in hypertensive urgency patients.

McCowan, C: Hypertensive emergencies. Available at: http://emedicine.medscape.com/article/758544-overview [Accessed on March 2010].

Cherney D, Straus S: Management of patients with hypertensive urgencies and emergencies. J Gen Intern Med 2002;17:937 [PMID: 12472930].

Vidt DG: Emergency room management of hypertensive urgencies and emergencies. J Clin Hypertens 2001;17:158 [PMID: 11416701].

▼ PERICARDITIS, PERICARDIAL EFFUSION, AND CARDIAC TAMPONADE

PERICARDITIS AND PERICARDIAL EFFUSION

▶ General Considerations

Acute pericarditis may result from viral or bacterial infections (including tuberculosis), collagen vascular diseases (especially rheumatic fever and disseminated lupus erythematosus), uremia, penetrating and nonpenetrating trauma, or myocardial infarction, and it may develop after pericardiotomy or irradiation of the mediastinum. It also may be associated with neoplasm (especially lymphomas such as Hodgkin disease). Pericarditis may also develop from annular or myocardial abscesses due to infective endocarditis. Pericardial effusion, and even cardiac tamponade, may develop in patients with acquired immunodeficiency syndrome (AIDS). Occasionally, drugs such as hydralazine or procainamide can cause an immune-response pericarditis. Varying degrees of myocarditis usually accompany pericarditis and account for the ECG changes. It is important to make an accurate etiologic diagnosis of pericarditis, if possible, because the specific cause may dictate the type of treatment required.

Clinical Findings

A. Symptoms and Signs

Fever and symptoms of the underlying disease may be present. Acute pericarditis usually causes persistent anterior chest pain that is frequently made worse by lying down and made better by sitting up and leaning forward. A pleuritic component is common. Radiation of pain to the neck, left shoulder, or arm occurs frequently.

1. Pericardial friction rub—Present in 85% of patients with pericarditis, the pericardial friction rub is the most common and most important diagnostic finding. The pericardial friction rub may have one, two, or three components corresponding to atrial systole, the rapid ventricular filling phase, and ventricular systole. The rub is frequently accentuated by having the patient breathe deeply, lean forward or resting on elbows and knees. A pericardial rub is absent in some cases, however.

2. Pleural friction rub—A pleural friction rub may be present as well.

3. Pericardial effusion—Pericardial effusion is rarely revealed on physical examination and is usually suspected on chest X-ray and confirmed by echocardiogram. With large effusions, heart sounds may be diminished, and pulmonary consolidation, rales at the base of the left lung, and dullness to percussion below the left scapula (Ewart's sign) may be present. Pericardial rub may lessen or disappear as pericardial effusion develops or may persist in the face of a large effusion. A rapidly accumulating effusion may cause cardiac tamponade (see below).

B. ECG, Radiographic, and Other Studies

1. Electrocardiogram—The ECG is usually abnormal in pericarditis, but the most common findings are nonspecific ST and T wave abnormalities. Initially, changes relatively specific for pericarditis are ST segment elevation in many leads (usually I, II, aVF, and V2–V6), with preservation of the normal concavity of the ST segment. Return of ST segments to the baseline on the ECG in a few days is followed by symmetric T wave inversion. Occasionally, the J junction elevation of ST segments seen as a normal variant may be confused with the ECG changes of pericarditis; however, in the normal variant, these changes do not evolve further. In pericarditis, moreover, the ST segment elevation is usually 25% or more of the T wave height in leads V5 or V6. Depression of the PR segment is highly indicative of pericarditis. The PR segment depression is seen in multiple leads in pericarditis with the exception of AVR in which the PR segment is elevated.

2. X-rays—No chest X-ray changes are specific for pericarditis. In some patients, hypoventilation resulting from pleuritic pain may be sufficiently severe to cause atelectasis.

The chest X-ray is also an insensitive indicator of pericardial effusion, especially in the case of rapidly developing effusions that only minimally distend the pericardial sac. An enlarged cardiac silhouette with a "waterflask" contour may be seen in the case of large effusions that have developed gradually. At times, the presence of pericardial fluid may be suspected if a radiolucent line representing epicardial fat is seen on the lateral chest X-ray well inside the cardiac silhouette and separated from the sternum by pericardial fluid.

3. Echocardiography—Echocardiography is the most sensitive and specific noninvasive test for pericardial fluid and should be performed in all cases of suspected pericardial effusion or pericarditis.

4. Laboratory Studies—Draw blood for CBC, serum electrolyte measurements, renal function tests, systemic markers of inflammation such as erthrocyte sedimentation rate, C-reactive protein, and cardiac markers such as troponin.

Treatment

Begin ECG monitoring. Monitor blood pressure every 5–15 minutes. In patients with hemodynamic instability, insert a central venous pressure catheter (Chapter 7) and monitor central venous pressure to detect signs of possible cardiac tamponade (Table 34–2).

Relieve pain with morphine, 2–4 mg intravenously every 5–10 minutes, until pain is relieved; repeat as needed. Obtain an echocardiogram as soon as possible to look for signs of pericardial effusion. Consider consultation with a cardiologist. Consider pericardiocentesis (Chapter 7) to aid in etiologic diagnosis, especially if signs of infection (eg, fever) are present, suggesting pyogenic pericarditis or possible malignant pericarditis. If indicated, pericardiocentesis should be performed in an intensive care unit, cardiac catheterization lab with fluoroscopic guidance, or in the operating room. Pericardiocentesis in the emergency department should be done only to relieve decompensated cardiac tamponade and not to assist in etiologic diagnosis.

Disposition

Hospitalization of most patients with acute pericarditis is usually unnecessary. This is especially true of young patients with pericarditis who are hemodynamically stable with normal laboratory tests, and who are reliable with close follow-up available in 1–3 days. Admission is required in high-risk patients with pericarditis. These patients include those with a temperature above 38°C, a subacute onset, an immunosuppressed state, pericarditis associated with trauma, a history of oral anticoagulant therapy, clinical or serologic evidence of myocardial involvement (eg, elevation of cardiac isoenzymes), a large pericardial effusion (eg, more than 20 mm of echo-free space around the heart on ultrasound), or cardiac tamponade.

Table 34–2. Classification of Cardiac Tamponade.

	Blood Pressure	Heart Rate	Pulsus Paradoxus[a]	Central Venous Pressures
Normal hemodynamics (i.e., pericardial effusion without cardiac tamponade)	Normal	Normal to increased	Not present (≤10 mm Hg)	Normal
Compensated cardiac tamponade	Normal	Normal to increased	Present (>10 mm Hg)	Increased
Decompensated cardiac tamponade	Decreased; shock may be present	Increased	Present (>10 mm Hg)	Increased

[a]Normal is defined as ≤10 mm Hg.

CARDIAC TAMPONADE

▶ General Considerations

Accumulation of fluid in the pericardial space faster than the pericardium can accommodate it by distention results in compression of the heart, or cardiac tamponade. Pathophysiologic changes similar to tamponade may also result from constrictive pericarditis, although they are much more slowly progressive than tamponade resulting from rapidly accumulating pericardial fluid. The principal result of the cardiac tamponade is reduced diastolic filling of the ventricles, with resulting reduced cardiac output. Ultimately, shock and death supervene.

▶ Clinical Findings

A. Symptoms and Signs

1. Coexisting or antecedent findings—There may be coexisting or antecedent signs or symptoms of pericarditis or pericardial effusion or of the disease process causing effusion. However, some patients develop cardiac tamponade without coexisting findings.

2. Tachycardia and hypotension—If cardiac tamponade progresses so that central venous pressure rises higher than 18 mm Hg, right ventricular filing decreases, causing subsequent decreases first in right ventricular and then in left ventricular stroke volume. Reflex tachycardia and increased systemic vascular resistance result to support systemic blood pressure. As cardiac tamponade worsens, these compensations fail, resulting in a sharp drop in cardiac output and blood pressure (decompensated cardiac tamponade). Because death follows rapidly if decompensated tamponade is not relieved, even slight hypotension or tachycardia occurring in patients with suspected pericardial effusion must be carefully monitored.

3. Pulsus paradoxus—In the normal healthy individual, systolic blood pressure drops no more than 8–10 mm Hg on normal inspiration. This change is exaggerated in cardiac tamponade, and palpable pulse volume may also decrease on inspiration. Pulsus paradoxus is very sensitive but nonspecific for cardiac tamponade resulting from pericardial effusion but is less common in tamponade associated with constrictive pericarditis.

4. Kussmaul's sign—During inspiration in cardiac tamponade, there may be an increase in estimated central venous pressure (eg, by observation of jugular venous pulsation) rather than the normal decrease.

B. X-ray and Other Findings

1. Echocardiography—Echocardiography is the most sensitive and specific noninvasive test for the presence of pericardial fluid and should be performed as soon as possible in all patients with suspected cardiac tamponade. With cardiac tamponade, there is marked swinging of the heart and collapse of the right atrial and ventricular chamber on expiration. In addition, diastolic collapse of the right ventricle is diagnostic of pericardial tamponade.

2. X-rays—Findings on chest X-ray usually are not helpful in the diagnosis of cardiac tamponade. A sudden marked increase in apparent heart size should suggest the possibility of pericardial effusion. When cardiomegaly is present in the setting of pericarditis, it usually indicates a substantial pericardial effusion of more than 250 mL.

3. Electrocardiogram—In cardiac tamponade, the ECG may show electrical alternans either of the QRS complex alone or of the entire complex (P, QRS, and T waves). This finding is rare in pericardial effusion without tamponade. Low voltage QRS (less than 5 mm or 0.5 mV in the limb leads) is finding of pericardial effusion which is often present in patients with tamponade physiology.

C. Classification of Cardiac Tamponade

The severity of cardiac tamponade may be classified as set forth in Table 34–2.

▶ Treatment

A. Decompensated Cardiac Tamponade

Note: Decompensated cardiac tamponade is an immediate threat to life and requires emergency treatment.

1. Oxygenation and blood pressure support—Give oxygen by mask or nasal cannula. Insert a large-bore (≥16-gauge) peripheral intravenous catheter, and infuse crystalloid solution to support blood pressure. In an adult, give 300–500 mL in 10–20 minutes, and then continue the infusion based on the blood pressure response.

2. Dopamine—Give dopamine, 2–20 μg/kg/min intravenously. Adjust dosage based on the blood pressure.

3. Pericardiocentesis—If available, emergent echocardiography or emergent bedside sonography in the emergency department can be diagnostic. In addition, pericardiocentesis can be performed under ultrasound guidance (Chapter 6). If ultrasound is not available and the patient is in extremis, blind pericardiocentesis can be life saving.

B. Compensated Cardiac Tamponade

Give oxygen, as described above. Monitor blood pressure every 5–15 minutes. Start continuous ECG monitoring. Insert a central venous pressure catheter and monitor central venous pressure.

Insert a large-bore (≥16-gauge) peripheral intravenous catheter and keep it patent with crystalloid solution. Confirm the presence of pericardial fluid or (rarely) pericardial thickening by bedside emergency ultrasound or echocardiography within 1 hour.

Caution: Do not administer diuretics or preload reduction (eg, nitrates) to control venous plethora (hypotension will result). Treatment of the pericardial tamponade is recommended before administering any general anesthetic. Anesthesia will cause withdrawal of sympathetic support to the heart and venous bed and will result in severe hypotension.

▶ Disposition

Hospitalize all patients with suspected or documented cardiac tamponade, preferably in an intensive care unit, and obtain urgent cardiologic and cardiothoracic surgical consultation.

Bogolioubov A et al: Circulatory shock. Crit Care Clin 2001;17:697 [PMID: 11525054].

Lange RA, Hillis LD: Clinical practice. Acute Pericarditis. N Engl J Med 2004;351(21):2195–2202 [PMID: 15548780].

Goyle KK, Walling AD: Diagnosing pericarditis. Am Fam Physician 2002;66:1695 [PMID: 12449268].

Soler-Soler J et al: Management of pericardial effusion. Heart 2001;86(2):235 [PMID: 11454853].

▼ MYOCARDITIS AND CARDIOMYOPATHY

Many diseases affecting the myocardial muscle have heart failure as their ultimate outcome. Secondary cardiomyopathies may be classified as shown in Table 34–3.

In most patients, the cause is unknown. The most common cause of acute myocardial injury and heart failure is coronary artery disease with ischemia or infarction, and this diagnostic possibility must be considered in every patient who has sudden onset of congestive heart failure. Infectious causes of myocarditis include viruses (mainly enteroviruses,

Table 34–3. Classification of Causes of Secondary Cardiomyopathy, with Examples.

Infectious
  Viral disease (coxsackie B and arbovirus infections, poliomyelitis)
  Bacterial disease (diphtheria)
  Parasitic disease (Chagas disease)
  Rickettsial disease (scrub typhus)
Immunologic
  Rheumatic fever
  Systemic lupus erythematosus
Toxic
  Alcohol
  Emetine
  Doxorubicin
Muscular
  Pseudohypertrophic muscular dystrophy
Metabolic
  Hyperthyroidism
  Hypothyroidism
  Beriberi
  Glycogen storage disease
Infiltrative
  Amyloidosis
  Hemochromatosis
Neoplastic
  Lymphoma
Physical
  Hyperthermia
Peripartum

especially coxsackievirus B), bacteria, protozoa (*Trypanosoma cruzi* and *Borrelia burgdorferi*), and parasites (*Trichinella*).

▶ Clinical Findings

Symptoms and signs may mimic those of almost any form of heart disease. Chest pain is common. Mild myocarditis or cardiomyopathy is frequently asymptomatic; severe cases are associated with heart failure, arrhythmias, and systemic embolization. Manifestations of the underlying disease (eg, Chagas' disease) may be prominent. Most patients with biopsy-proven myocarditis report a recent viral prodrome preceding cardiovascular symptoms.

ECG abnormalities are often present, although the changes are frequently nonspecific. A pattern characteristic of left ventricular hypertrophy may be present. Flat or inverted T waves are most common, often with low-voltage QRS complexes. Intraventricular conduction defects and bundle branch block, especially left bundle branch block, are also common. An echocardiogram is useful to detect wall motion abnormalities or a pericardial effusion. Chest radiographs can be normal or can show evidence of congestive heart failure with pulmonary edema or cardiomegaly.

In acute myocarditis, cardiac enzymes (CK-MB, cTni, or cTnt) may be elevated. Endomyocardial biopsy is diagnostic.

Treatment

Bed rest is widely recommended, and there is some evidence supporting its benefits. If the cause of the disease is known (eg, trichinosis, acute rheumatic fever), begin therapy recommended for the underlying disease. Complications of myocarditis include chest pain, arrhythmias, embolization, and heart failure; these should be treated appropriately.

Disposition

Hospitalization is indicated unless the condition is chronic and stable.

AORTIC ANEURYSMS AND DISSECTIONS

See Chapter 40.

CONGENITAL HEART DISEASE

The differential diagnosis of congenital heart disease is beyond the scope of this book. The general principles of management are outlined below as a guide for emergency physicians.

Classification

Classification of congenital heart disease is based on the hemodynamic effects produced or on specific anatomic abnormalities:

- Left-to-right shunts—Interatrial septal defect, interventricular septal defect, patent ductus arteriosus
- Right-to-left shunts—Cyanotic heart disease (eg, transposition of the great vessels, tetralogy of Fallot, pulmonary atresia, tricuspid atresia)
- Valvular stenosis, hypoplasia, and atresia—Pulmonary valve and aortic valve stenosis, tricuspid atresia, pulmonary atresia, mitral and aortic atresia
- Abnormalities of position—Dextrocardia, transposition of the great vessels, corrected transposition
- Abnormalities of great vessels—Coarctation of the aorta, patent ductus arteriosus, arterial rings

Obviously, individual lesions may combine attributes from two or more categories. For example, tricuspid atresia is both a right-to-left shunt (owing to interatrial communication) and an atretic lesion.

Pathophysiology

Large left-to-right shunts cause increased blood flow through the lungs and volume overload of one or both ventricles. Right-to-left shunts cause systemic venous return to bypass the lungs and go directly into the arterial circulation. The resulting arterial desaturation (if severe with 3–5 g/dL desaturated hemoglobin) may cause central cyanosis.

Valvular obstruction (aortic or pulmonary stenosis) and aortic obstruction (coarctation of the aorta) cause afterload abnormalities of the involved ventricles. Vascular rings around the trachea and esophagus cause symptoms resulting from obstruction (eg, dyspnea, cough, dysphagia).

CYANOSIS

All infants (under age 1 year) who have cyanotic heart disease are at risk for potential serious illness with sudden life-threatening complications. Lesions producing right-to-left shunts are frequently undetected until after the newborn period, because pulmonary blood flow is maintained by a patent ductus arteriosus. When the ductus arteriosus begins to close, cyanosis becomes manifest. If the ductus arteriosus is the major source of pulmonary blood flow—as may be the case in pulmonary atresia—the patient may become markedly cyanotic and die rapidly after the ductus arteriosus closes.

No matter how well these children do or how asymptomatic they appear, their entire ability to oxygenate blood may depend on the presence of a patent ductus arteriosus, which may close unpredictably at any time.

Clinical Findings

Cyanosis is most apparent in highly vascularized areas with superficial capillaries, for example, lips, oral and conjunctival mucosa, and nail beds. With more severe hypoxemia and desaturation, other areas of skin may appear cyanotic. The diagnosis may be confirmed by arterial blood Po_2 measurements.

Treatment and Disposition

For neonates in extremis with shock or severe cyanosis related to suspected congenital heart disease, presume that the cause of decompensation is related to closure of the patent ductus arteriosus in the setting of a ductal-dependent lesion. Treatment to prevent closure is an intravenous infusion of Prostaglan E1 (PGE1) at 0.05–0.1 μg/kg/min. Strongly consider intubation as apnea is a side effect of the infusion in 10% of patients. All infants with cyanosis (intermittent or constant) should be hospitalized for immediate evaluation by a pediatric cardiologist, because emergency catheterization and angiocardiography may be necessary. Frequently, definitive diagnosis can be made by two-dimensional echocardiography, with and without Doppler ultrasound.

Older children with stable cyanotic heart disease do not require emergency hospitalization but should be referred for evaluation. If other signs of cardiac disease are present (eg, heart failure, arrhythmias), hospitalization or treatment is indicated as appropriate.

ANOXIC SPELLS

▶ Clinical Findings

Anoxic spells are common in patients with cyanotic heart disease and usually start after the infant is aged 3 months or older. They rarely occur after age 4–5 years. The spells frequently start with the infant becoming fussy and developing increasing cyanosis and tachypnea. The infant then suddenly goes limp. These spells often occur in the morning after a good night's rest or when the child becomes more active, usually during feeding or straining at stool, and they are associated with sudden marked increases in right-to-left shunting.

▶ Treatment

Place the child in the knee-chest position, and quickly give morphine, 0.2 mg/kg intramuscularly or subcutaneously. Give 100% oxygen by face mask, and be prepared to perform immediate intubation. If pH is 7.1 or lower, give sodium bicarbonate, 1–2 mEq/kg, intravenously to correct acidosis. If hypoglycemia is present or suspected, give 10% glucose solution intravenously at a rate of 5–10 mL/kg/h, and monitor blood glucose concentration.

In children with anoxic spells and tetralogy of Fallot, propranolol, 0.01 mg/kg slowly intravenously, has been helpful. The dose may be repeated in 5 minutes.

▶ Disposition

An unexplained episode of syncope, "limp spell," or convulsions in any child with known cyanotic heart disease should suggest anoxic spells. The child should be hospitalized immediately.

HEART FAILURE

Congestive heart failure in infancy is usually associated with large left-to-right shunts at the ventricular level (eg, ventricular septal defect) or arterial level (eg, patent ductus arteriosus). It may also be associated with obstructive lesions such as aortic stenosis, aortic or mitral atresia, and coarctation of the aorta. Rarely, the cause can be anomalous origin of the left coronary artery from the pulmonary artery. Congestive heart failure may occur in the infant with atrial tachycardia or atrial flutter with rapid ventricular response, with or without preexcitation syndromes. Underlying heart disease need not be present.

▶ Clinical Findings

Congestive heart failure in infants is manifested by dyspnea on exertion just as it is in adults. Because the most common strenuous activity in which an infant engages is feeding, an infant with congestive heart failure will have to stop and breathe at the end of each swallow. Difficulty in taking the entire bottle in the usual 15–20 minutes may therefore be the principal manifestation of heart failure. In addition, the baby may be sluggish and fussy and have a weak cry.

Physical findings in these infants are those of the underlying lesion as well as those associated with congestive heart failure.

A. Aortic Murmurs

In aortic murmurs (eg, pulmonary stenosis and coarctation of the aorta), systolic ejection murmurs are heard. They are frequently accompanied by ejection clicks. Patent ductus arteriosus or aortopulmonary windows are associated with continuous murmurs heard at the base of the heart. If stenosis is severe or if cardiac output is severely decreased, the murmur may not be loud.

B. Tachypnea and Tachycardia

Tachypnea and tachycardia are usually present.

C. Sweating

Because of the increased activity of the sympathetic nervous system in children with congestive heart failure, profuse sweating is common.

D. Biventricular Failure

Isolated left heart failure is unusual in infants. Biventricular failure with ventricular gallops, rales, hepatomegaly, and edema is more common.

E. Venous Distention

Because of the short neck in infants, venous distention frequently cannot be detected.

F. Hepatomegaly

Hepatomegaly may develop within a few hours after the onset of congestive heart failure and may resolve just as quickly with therapy.

▶ Disposition
A. Immediate Hospitalization

Any infant or child with newly diagnosed congestive heart failure—especially if it is associated with a systolic ejection murmur—must be hospitalized for immediate evaluation. The murmur may be due to aortic stenosis, pulmonary stenosis, or coarctation of the aorta, each of which requires prompt diagnosis and treatment.

B. Outpatient Care

Children with mild congestive heart failure due to stable, previously diagnosed congenital heart disease may be managed on an outpatient basis. Diuretics and digitalis (in older infants and children) are frequently effective.

PULMONARY HYPERTENSION

The child with a large ventricular septal defect or patent ductus arteriosus can develop significant irreversible changes in the pulmonary vascular bed within 2 years and must therefore be evaluated as soon as the problem is discovered.

Linear growth and weight gain may be slow. After age 2 years, compensatory mechanisms that decrease the size of the left-to-right shunt are frequent, for example, increased pulmonary vascular resistance, decreased pulmonary blood flow because of decreasing size of the ventricular septal defect, or development of infundibular pulmonary stenosis because of hypertrophy of the crista supraventricularis.

Prompt referral to a pediatric cardiologist is indicated if previously undiagnosed ventricular septal defect or patent ductus arteriosus is detected.

COARCTATION OF THE AORTA

The diagnosis of coarctation of the aorta is made by finding femoral pulses that are decreased or absent when compared to brachial pulses. If femoral pulses are present but faint, blood pressure taken with a cuff of the appropriate size in the upper and lower extremities should show lower blood pressure in the legs than in the arm if coarctation of the aorta exists. Prompt referral to a cardiologist is indicated.

Colletti JE, Homme JL, Woodridge DP: Unsuspected neonatal killers in emergency medicine. Emerg Med Clin North Am 2004;22(4):929–960 [PMID: 15474777] (Review).

Woods WA, McCulloch MA: Cardiovascular emergencies in the pediatric patient. Emerg Med Clin North Am 2005;23(4):1233–1249. [PMID: 16199347] (Review).

Cardiac Arrhythmias

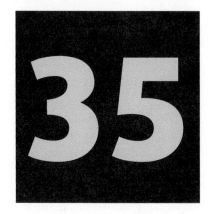

Joseph Heidenreich, MD

Patients with cardiac arrhythmias often present to the emergency department. The patient's clinical presentation determines the urgency with which the assessment and management should proceed. Patients with serious signs and symptoms (ie, shock, hypotension, congestive heart failure (CHF), severe shortness of breath, altered level of consciousness, ischemic chest pain, or acute myocardial infarction) require immediate treatment. With stable patients, more time is afforded for review of the 12-lead electrocardiogram (ECG) and rhythm strip to diagnose the cardiac arrhythmia. Review of available prior ECGs may also assist in arrhythmia diagnosis.

ELEVEN HELPFUL HINTS FOR EMERGENCY DEPARTMENT ARRHYTHMIAS

1. Obtain as much information as available. Always look at all 12 leads and be sure of name, date, age, correct lead placement, and standardization.

2. Know what each lead looks like normally (Figure 35–1); eg, lead I (and usually lead II and aVF) should look like the textbook PQRST except no Q wave. In lead I, the P, QRS, and T should all be upright, the intervals should be normal and the PR and ST baselines should be isoelectric.

3. A regular tachycardia with a rate close to 150 should prompt a search for atrial flutter.

4. Precise diagnosis of wide complex tachycardias (WCTs) can be difficult. If ventricular rate is irregular consider atrial fibrillation (AF) or atrial flutter with variable conduction and underlying bundle branch block (BBB).

5. Do not rely on computer readings. They may or may not be correct.

6. Single-lead rhythm strips may not have enough information. If time permits, always obtain a 12-lead ECG.

7. You cannot have too many ECGs. Serial ECGs are important. Sinus tachycardia rates tend to change over time.

8. Arrhythmias are common in acute ST elevation myocardial infarctions.

9. Tachyarrhythmias are divided into narrow or wide QRS width and then into regular or irregular.

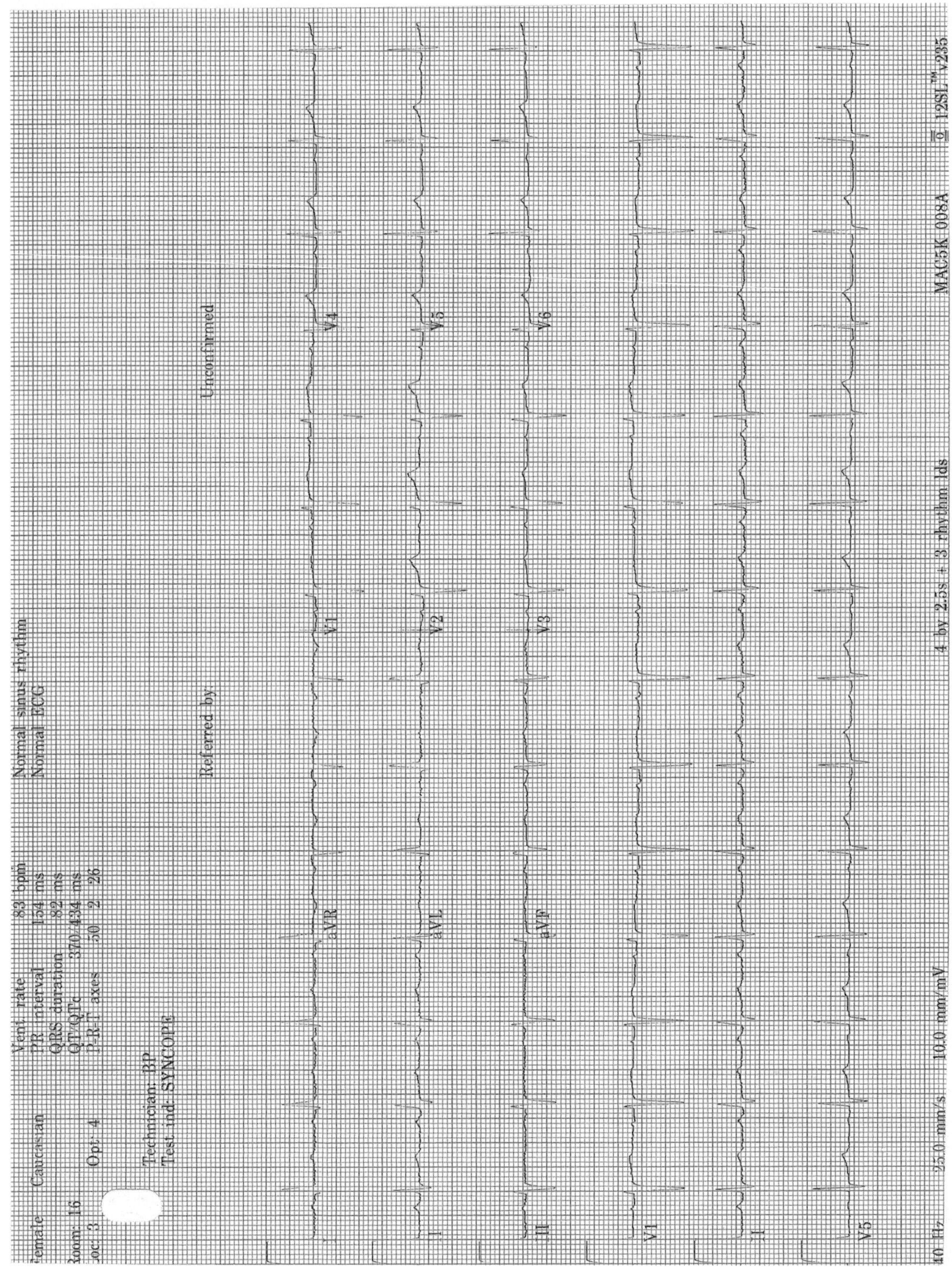

▲ **Figure 35–1.** Normal ECG.

10. Arrhythmia classifications and terminologies can be confusing and they change as new information becomes available.

11. If the heart rhythm is slow and the patient is hypotensive with signs of poor perfusion, assume transthoracic or transvenous pacing will be needed.

A NOTE ON CARDIOVERSION AND DEFIBRILLATION

No consensus exists on correct pad positioning and current ACLS guidelines endorse both the conventional or sternal apical positioning (one pad on the superior–anterior right chest just below the level of the clavicle and one pad on the inferolateral left chest) and the anteroposterior (the anterior pad as in the conventional method and the posterior pad on the right or left upper back). However, some authors feel that anteroposterior placement with the anterior pad over the right atrium and the posterior pad at the tip of the left scapula optimizes cardioversion of atrial tachyarrhythmias while placement of the anterior pad over the ventricles and posterior pad again at the tip of the left scapula works well for ventricular arrhythmias.

All currently manufactured defibrillators use biphasic waveforms so unless you are using an older machine, the energy setting will range from 0 Joules (J) to 200 J. All energy doses mentioned in this chapter will be for biphasic defibrillators. In addition to disease-specific energy recommendations, there are device-specific recommendations for the different biphasic defibrillator models for first shock energy dose in some situations. Notably, in ventricular fibrillation (VF) or pulseless ventricular tachycardia (VT) the initial shock is 120 for devices using a rectilinear waveform and 150–200 J for devices using a truncated exponential waveform ranging from 120 to 200 J. ACLS guidelines recommend that IF THE OPERATOR IS UNSURE of device-specific recommendations then the defibrillator's highest energy level should be used in this setting; this will be 200 J for all biphasic units and 360 J if you happen to still have a monophasic unit. The bottom line is that if you are uncertain on the energy dose in any emergent situation where electricity is required for an adult your best bet is turn the energy up as high as it will go as even maximal doses of energy are felt to be relatively safe.

▼ TACHYARRHYTHMIAS

Immediate synchronized cardioversion should be performed on all unstable patients with tachydsrythmias. The specific arrhythmia diagnosis (supraventricular or ventricular) does not need to be made immediately because initial management is the same. Patients with polymorphic ventricular tachycardia (PMVT) of 30 seconds or more and all unstable patients should be treated with immediate defibrillation.

In stable patients, the initial medical management will be guided by the underlying rhythm and a detailed history and physical examination. In recent years, the more traditional approach to categorize patients as either stable or unstable has been modified. Hemodynamically stable patients can be further subdivided into those with preserved or impaired cardiac function. Findings of impaired cardiac function in a patient who is otherwise stable may alter the pharmacologic treatment.

SUPRAVENTRICULAR ARRHYTHMIAS

1. Sinus Tachycardia

▶ **Clinical Findings**

(See Appendix, Figure 35–3.) Sinus tachycardia occurs when the sinus rate is faster than 100 beats/min. Usually the rate is 101–160 beats/min. Young, healthy adults can accelerate their heart rate up to 180–200 beats/min, particularly during exercise. Young children have been noted to have sinus rates up to 220 beats/min. Sinus tachycardia should not be viewed as a primary arrhythmia but more as a response to an underlying illness or condition. It is often normal in infancy and early childhood but can occur as a result of a number of conditions including pain, fever, stress, hyperadrenergic states, anemia, hypovolemia, hypoxia, myocardial ischemia, pulmonary edema, shock, and hyperthyroidism. Certain medications and illicit drugs can also cause tachycardia. The P wave in sinus tachycardia should have a positive axis in the frontal plane, ie, the P wave should be positive in lead I and aVF.

▶ **Treatment and Disposition**

The treatment of sinus tachycardia is directed at the underlying cause. This may include correction of dehydration with intravenous fluids, analgesic or antipyretic administration, or supplemental oxygen to correct hypoxia. Treatment aimed at correcting the heart rate rather than the underlying condition may be harmful if the tachycardia is compensatory and is supporting the cardiac output. Gradual slowing of the heart rate with treatment of the underlying condition or during carotid sinus massage may help to differentiate sinus tachycardia from other supraventricular arrhythmias. Adenosine administration with a 12-lead rhythm strip is helpful in differentiating from other causes of tachyarrhythmias. Further management, including the need for hospitalization, depends on the underlying condition.

2. Paroxysmal Supraventricular Tachycardia

▶ **Clinical Findings**

(See Appendix, Figures 35–6 to 35–11.) Paroxysmal supraventricular tachycardia (PSVT) is a general term that refers to a number of tachyarrhythmias that arise from above the bifurcation of the His bundle. Approximately 90% of these arrhythmias occur as a result of a reentrant mechanism; the remaining 10% occur as a result of increased automaticity.

Atrioventricular nodal reentrant tachycardia (AVNRT) is the most common form of PSVT, accounting for 50–60% of cases. The heart rate is usually 180–200 beats/min and is characterized by sudden onset and sudden termination. Because the reentrant mechanism occurs within the AV node itself, virtually simultaneous excitation of the atria and ventricles occurs. As a result, the P waves occur concurrent with the QRS complexes and are difficult to visualize on the ECG. Often, patients with AVNRT do not have underlying heart disease. Common precipitating factors include alcohol, caffeine, and sympathomimetic amines. Patients with AVNRT usually present in their third or fourth decade of life, and the majority (approximately 70%) are female.

Atrioventricular reciprocating tachycardia (AVRT) accounts for 30% of PSVT. In most cases, the impulse travels down the AV node and follows a retrograde path up the accessory bypass tract. Because activation of the ventricles occurs through normal conduction pathways, the accessory pathway is concealed, and the QRS morphology is normal. Consider AVRT if the heart rate is faster than 200 beats/min or if P waves are seen following the QRS complex.

Sinus node reentry and intraatrial reentry are uncommon causes of PSVT, accounting for approximately 5% of cases. In these arrhythmias, the heart rate is usually 130–140 beats/min. More often, patients with these arrhythmias have underlying heart disease.

Automatic atrial tachycardia is another uncommon arrhythmia, accounting for less than 5% of cases of PSVT. The heart rate is usually 160–250 beats/min but may be as slow as 140 beats/min. In this case, the underlying mechanism is increased automaticity rather than reentry. Automatic atrial tachycardia is commonly associated with underlying heart disease. This arrhythmia is difficult to treat and may be refractory to standard measures including cardioversion.

PSVT can be classified as AV nodal dependent or independent. This strategy may prove useful in formulating treatment options. AVNRT and AVRT are AV nodal dependent, meaning that the AV node is involved in the reentrant circuit. For these rhythms, pharmacologic management is designed to decrease conduction through the AV node.

▶ Treatment

A. Unstable Patients

Patients with PSVT who are hemodynamically unstable require immediate synchronized DC cardioversion. Current recommendations are to start with low-energy levels (50–100 J) and then to increase the initial dose by 50 J as needed until sinus rhythm is restored. If clinical circumstances permit, administer intravenous sedatives. Avoid the common error of delaying emergency cardioversion to perform other patient care activities. If immediate cardioversion is unavailable, physical maneuvers that cause vagal stimulation can be attempted.

Adenosine, β-blocker, or calcium channel blocker may be administered.

B. Stable patients

Tachycardia associated with PSVT is usually well tolerated unless the patient has underlying heart disease or left ventricular dysfunction.

1. Physical maneuvers—In stable patients, physical maneuvers causing vagal stimulation can be attempted prior to medication administration. Maneuvers that stimulate the vagus nerve such as the Valsalva maneuver (expiration against a closed glottis), Mueller maneuver (deep inspiration against a closed glottis), cold water facial immersion, and carotid sinus massage are at times effective in terminating PSVT that results from AV nodal and sinoatrial (SA) nodal dependent mechanisms. Perform carotid sinus massage only after auscultation for carotid bruits.

2. Pharmacologic treatment—If vagal stimulation is contraindicated or ineffective, adenosine is considered first-line medical therapy for conversion of PSVT. In general, pharmacologic agents with AV nodal blocking properties such as adenosine, β-blockers, calcium channel blockers, and digoxin are used for the acute management and prevention of AV nodal dependent PSVT. Other antiarrhythmic agents, such as procainamide and amiodarone, which exert effects at various levels of the cardiac conduction system are used for the management and prevention of AV nodal independent PSVT. Antiarrhythmic medications may be considered for conversion of PSVT when AV nodal blocking agents are unsuccessful.

A. ADENOSINE—Adenosine is an endogenous nucleoside that slows conduction through the AV node and is successful in terminating more than 90% of PSVTs resulting from AV nodal reentry mechanisms (AVNRT and AVRT). Adenosine may also be effective in terminating sinus node reentry tachycardia but is usually ineffective in terminating automatic atrial tachycardia. Often adenosine will cause a transient AV block, briefly exposing the underlying atrial activity. Administration of a medication with more prolonged effect on the AV node (β-blockers or calcium channel blockers) may provide a more sustained reduction in ventricular rate.

Administer adenosine rapidly, and follow each dose immediately with a 20-cc saline flush. Although current recommendations are to administer an initial intravenous dose of 6 mg over 1–3 seconds repeated at 2 and 4 minutes with 12-mg doses if this does not terminate the PSVT, many clinicians choose to forgo the initial 6-mg dose and will increase the dose to 18-mg if the 12-mg dose does not produce AV blockade. The 18-mg dose has been shown to be both safe and effective. Common side effects include unexplainable feeling of impending doom, facial flushing, hyperventilation, dyspnea, and chest pain. These side effects are often transient owing to the short half-life of adenosine (less than 5 seconds). Prewarning to the patient of these symptoms is helpful. The effects of adenosine are antagonized by caffeine and theophylline and potentiated by dipyridamole and carbamazepine. Heart transplant patients may be overly sensitive to the effects of adenosine; if necessary, use smaller doses. Because adenosine can provoke bronchospasm, use caution if it is being administered to patients with a history of reactive airway disease.

Adenosine can also be administered to a stable patient with a wide QRS complex tachycardia suspected to be supraventricular in origin. Adenosine is preferred over calcium channel blockers in patients with hypotension or impaired cardiac function and in patients concomitantly receiving β-adrenergic blocking agents.

B. β-BLOCKING AGENTS—β-blockers such as metoprolol or esmolol slow SA node impulse formation and slow conduction through the AV node. These medications should be used with caution in patients with a history of severe reactive airway disease and CHF.

Metoprolol is an alternative to calcium channel blockers, and is administered intravenously at a dose of 5 mg every 5 minutes for three doses. Esmolol is an ultrashort-acting β_1-selective β-blocker that has the advantage of a brief half-life (~10 minutes) and a rapid onset of action. Administer a loading dose of 0.5 mg/kg over 1 minute. This is followed by a maintenance infusion of 50 μg/kg/min. If the response is inadequate, another dose of 0.5 mg/kg can be administered after 4 minutes and the maintenance infusion increased to 100 μg/kg/min. When heart rate control is achieved, reduce the maintenance infusion to 25 μg/kg/min.

C. CALCIUM CHANNEL BLOCKERS—Calcium channel blockers such as diltiazem or verapamil are effective in converting PSVT to sinus rhythm. The efficacy of diltiazem and verapamil in terms of conversion rates, rapidity of response, and safety profile appear similar. These medications decrease SA and AV node conduction and cause prolongation of the AV node refractory period. Calcium channel blockers also decrease myocardial contractility and peripheral vascular resistance. Use calcium channel blockers with caution in patients with left ventricular dysfunction or CHF. Avoid these medications in patients with WCT of unknown origin, ventricular tachycardia (VT), or tachycardia with ventricular preexcitation. Hypotension is the most concerning side effect of intravenous administration and occurs in 10–15% of patients.

Verapamil—The initial dose of verapamil is 5–10 mg administered intravenously over 1–2 minutes. Additional doses of 5–10 mg can be administered every 15 minutes as needed until the desired effect is achieved or a total of 30 mg has been administered.

Diltiazem—The initial dose of diltiazem is 0.25 mg/kg administered intravenously over 2 minutes (20 mg for the average adult). If necessary, a dose of 0.35 mg/kg can be administered in 15 minutes. After conversion, a maintenance infusion can be started at 5–10 mg/h and can be increased to a maximum of 15 mg/h if needed.

The choice between β-blockers and calcium channel blockers depends on multiple factors, but both should not be given intravenously to the same patient. Both have rapid onset (minutes) and both should be used with caution in severe COPD and severe CHF. Medication that the patient is currently taking and physician preference are considerations. In patients with hyperthyroidism and congenital heart disease, β-blockers are the best choice.

D. DIGOXIN—Digoxin administration will increase vagal tone while reducing sympathetic activity. As a result, conduction through the AV node is slowed. Digoxin may be administered as an intravenous bolus dose of 0.5 mg. Additional doses of 0.25 mg may be given as needed every 4–6 hours, with a total dose not to exceed 1.25 mg in 24 hours. The immediate benefit of digoxin is lessened by its slow onset of action. When used in combination, digoxin may allow for lower doses of subsequently administered antiarrhythmic agents. Avoid digoxin in patients with AF with ventricular preexcitation.

E. AMIODARONE—Amiodarone is a class III antiarrhythmic agent with sodium- and potassium-channel blocking properties and β-blocking and calcium channel blocking properties. By virtue of its β-blocking and calcium channel blocking properties, amiodarone slows conduction through the AV node. In patients with impaired cardiac function or CHF, treatment options narrow. Amiodarone has a solid safety profile and may be an effective alternative agent in this situation. Amiodarone can be administered as a slow intravenous infusion of 150 mg over 10 minutes. This is followed by a maintenance infusion of 1 mg/min for 6 hours and then 0.5 mg/min. Additional bolus doses of 150 mg can be repeated as needed for resistant or recurrent PSVT up to a total daily dose of 2 g.

F. PROCAINAMIDE—Procainamide is a class IA antiarrhythmic agent with sodium channel blocking properties. Procainamide will slow conduction through both the AV node and, if present, an accessory bypass tract. Procainamide can be considered for patients with PSVT refractory to AV nodal blocking agents. The recommended loading dose of procainamide is 17 mg/kg administered as a slow intravenous infusion at a rate of 20–30 mg/min (1 g for an average adult). Stop the initial infusion if the arrhythmia is suppressed, hypotension develops, or the QRS complex widens by more than 50% of its original duration. After arrhythmia suppression, start a maintenance infusion at 1–4 mg/min.

▶ Disposition

Hospitalization should be considered for patients in PSVT with accompanying serious signs and symptoms, patients requiring emergency cardioversion, patients in PSVT with ventricular preexcitation, and patients with arrhythmias refractory to standard treatment. Outpatient follow-up care should be provided for the otherwise healthy patient with a transient episode of PSVT converted to sinus rhythm in the emergency department.

3. Atrial Fibrillation

▶ Clinical Findings

(See Appendix, Figures 35–12 and 35–13.) In AF, the atrial rate is disorganized and is 300–600 beats/min. AF is characterized by an irregularly irregular ventricular rate with the absence of discernible P waves.

AF is the most common sustained cardiac arrhythmia in adults. It is estimated that AF affects more than 2 million persons in the United States; its prevalence increases with age, approaching 10% in those older than 80 years. AF can occur in the absence of underlying heart disease or may be associated with a number of conditions, including chronic hypertension, valvular disease, cardiomyopathy, myocardial ischemia, myocarditis, pericarditis, or congenital heart disease. AF may also occur in the presence of other systemic disorders, including hyperthyroidism, pulmonary embolism, hypoxia, and excess consumption of alcohol or caffeine.

Patients with nonvalvular AF have approximately a 5% annual incidence of stroke as a result of a thromboembolic event. This risk increases fourfold in patients with mitral stenosis and increases dramatically in older patients, approaching 30% in patients aged 80–89 years.

▶ Treatment

Acute management of AF includes ventricular rate control and prevention of thromboembolic complications. Additional management considerations include restoration and maintenance of sinus rhythm.

A. Unstable Patients

Patients in AF with a rapid ventricular response who are hemodynamically unstable require immediate synchronized DC cardioversion. Recommendations are to start between 100 and 200 J biphasic and then to increase the dose in stepwise fashion as needed until sinus rhythm is restored.

B. Stable Patients

In stable patients with a rapid ventricular response, the initial goal is rate control. This can usually be achieved with β-blockers, calcium channel blockers, or digoxin. β-blockers

may prove most helpful in patients with hyperthyroidism but are relatively contraindicated in patients with acute decompensated CHF. Diltiazem and verapamil can often slow the ventricular rate and have the added benefit of antianginal effects and blood pressure control in hypertensive patients. In more than 90% of patients, a reduction in heart rate of at least 20% is noted. Diltiazem appears to be safe for use in patients with mild CHF. Digoxin can also help control the ventricular rate in patients with AF and may be useful in patients with left ventricular dysfunction. Its slower onset of action as compared to other agents makes it less useful for acute rate control. In patients with mild to moderate CHF, the administration of amiodarone may prove useful. Intravenous amiodarone can also be considered an alternative agent for rate control when the above agents fail. The specific medication choice will often be dictated by the urgency of the situation, the medication profile, physician preference, and the patient's underlying condition.

1. Anticoagulants—Prophylactic anticoagulation with warfarin has been shown to significantly reduce the incidence of stroke in patients with AF. If new-onset AF is of undetermined duration or greater than 48 hours duration, initiation of anticoagulation is necessary. Current recommendations include anticoagulation for 3 weeks, followed by elective cardioversion and then continued outpatient anticoagulation for four more weeks. An alternative strategy is initial anticoagulation with unfractionated or low-molecular-weight heparin followed by transesophageal echocardiography to evaluate the left atrial appendage for the presence of clot. If no clot is identified, the patient may safely undergo cardioversion, followed by anticoagulation for 4 weeks. If a left atrial appendage clot is identified by transesophageal echocardiography, recommendations include anticoagulation for 3 weeks, followed by cardioversion and then continued anticoagulation for four additional weeks. In patients with AF of less than 48 hours duration, anticoagulation is not recommended.

2. Antiarrhythmics—Various antiarrhythmic agents, including amiodarone, procainamide, and sotalol (class III), are used to chemically convert AF. Pharmacologic or electrical cardioversion may be considered in selected stable emergency department patients with AF of less than 48 hours duration. Remodeling, both anatomically and electrically, occurs soon after the onset of AF. Postponing cardioversion could lead to an increased resistance to attempts at conversion.

▶ Disposition

Patients with chronic rate-controlled AF do not require hospital admission. In patients with new-onset AF, hospitalization is often required for ventricular rate control, initiation of anticoagulation, and sometimes for initiation of antiarrhythmic therapy. If a patient presents with thromboembolic complications, hospital admission will also be necessary.

4. Atrial Flutter

▶ Clinical Findings

(See Appendix, Figure 35–14) In atrial flutter, the atrial rate is usually 250–350 beats/min. It is the most common underdiagnosed tachyarrhythmia. Sawtooth flutter waves may sometimes be seen on ECG, but should not be relied upon. Typically, atrial flutter will present with 2:1 AV conduction. For this reason, it is important to consider atrial flutter in the differential diagnosis of a regular tachycardia at approximately 150 beats/min, even in the absence of flutter waves. Atrial flutter is most commonly identified as negative waves in II, III, and aVF with positive flutter waves in lead V1.

If atrial flutter is suspected, several options are available to better identify atrial activity. Vagal maneuvers or administration of adenosine with a 12-lead rhythm strip may unmask flutter waves.

▶ Treatment

Acute management of atrial flutter includes ventricular rate control and prevention of thromboembolic complications. Additional management considerations include restoration and maintenance of sinus rhythm.

A. Unstable Patients

Patients in atrial flutter with a rapid ventricular response who are hemodynamically unstable require immediate synchronized DC cardioversion. Current recommendations are to start with between 50 and 100 J biphasic and then increase the energy dose in stepwise fashion as needed until sinus rhythm is restored.

B. Stable Patients

In stable patients with a rapid ventricular response, the initial goal is rate control. Adequate heart rate control can be achieved with the administration of either β-blockers or calcium channel blockers. Digoxin is often less effective acutely because of its slow onset of action. Amiodarone and diltiazem are alternatives for rate control in the stable patient with impaired cardiac function or CHF.

The stroke risk for patients in atrial flutter is less than that of AF. The same anticoagulation guidelines exist for atrial flutter as in AF.

▶ Disposition

Patients with chronic rate-controlled atrial flutter do not require hospital admission. In patients with new-onset atrial flutter, hospitalization is often required for ventricular rate control, initiation of anticoagulation, and sometimes for initiation of antiarrhythmic therapy.

5. Multifocal Atrial Tachycardia

▶ Clinical Findings

(See Appendix, Figure 35–15) In multifocal atrial tachycardia (MAT) the heart rate is typically 100–130 beats/min. The characteristic ECG finding is at least three different P wave morphologies. The rhythm often appears irregular and can at times be confused with AF. Varying PR intervals may also be noted. When the rate is slower than 100 beats/min, the term wandering atrial pacemaker is applied. Unless underlying aberrant conduction is present, the QRS complexes are narrow. Severe underlying chronic obstructive pulmonary disease accounts for approximately 60–85% of cases. Theophylline and digoxin levels should be checked since toxicity of these drugs can cause MAT.

▶ Treatment

The initial treatment of MAT is directed at correcting the underlying cause. As with AF, the initial goal of therapy is to achieve heart rate control. Because MAT does not respond to electrical cardioversion, pharmacologic intervention may be required.

Magnesium may be effective in converting MAT and can be administered as a 2 g intravenous bolus over 1 minute. This is followed by a 2 g/h infusion for 5 hours. Magnesium can still be effective if serum magnesium levels are in the normal range. Potassium repletion may be helpful in patients who are hypokalemic.

Amiodarone, digoxin, or diltiazem may be considered as alternative agents for rate control, especially when the patient exhibits findings of CHF.

▶ Disposition

Patients may require hospitalization for MAT if the heart rate is difficult to control or for further management of the underlying condition.

6. Preexcitation Arrhythmias

▶ Clinical Findings

(See Appendix, Figures 35–11 and 35–13) Patients with Wolff-Parkinson-White (WPW) syndrome have an accessory pathway. Anatomical location varies and the pathways can be AV (Kent), atrio-His (James), intranodal, and nodoventricular (Mahain). On the ECG, a short PR interval (less than 120 ms) and the presence of a δ wave (initial upward slurring of the QRS complex) signify ventricular preexcitation.

A variety of arrhythmias may occur in patients with WPW syndrome; approximately 70% is orthodromic AVRT. In this case, the cardiac impulse travels down the AV node (antegrade conduction) and stimulates the ventricles through the normal conduction pathways. The accessory

AV bypass tract serves as the retrograde limb of the circuit. In the absence of aberrant ventricular conduction or a fixed BBB, the morphology of the QRS complex is narrow without evidence of ventricular preexcitation (absent δ wave). The bypass pathway is considered concealed if the short PR and δ wave are not present on the baseline ECG.

Rarely, antidromic AVRT occurs whereby the accessory AV pathway acts as the antegrade limb of the circuit and the AV node as the retrograde limb. Antidromic AVRT will produce a wide QRS complex tachycardia and may masquerade as VT. The tachycardia may be extremely rapid (with ventricular rate 220–300), leading to ventricular fibrillation (VF) as a result of an R-on-T phenomenon.

AF is the second most common arrhythmia associated with WPW syndrome. AF with ventricular preexcitation has a high potential to precipitate hemodynamic compromise. AF with a rapid ventricular rate is characterized by an irregular tachycardia and a wide QRS complex resulting from ventricular preexcitation.

▶ Treatment

Patients with orthodromic AVRT who are hemodynamically unstable require immediate synchronized DC cardioversion. Current recommendations are to start between 50 J and 100 J biphasic and then to increase the initial dose in stepwise fashion as needed until sinus rhythm is restored. In patients with known WPW syndrome presenting with a narrow complex regular tachycardia, orthodromic AVRT can be assumed. In stable patients, the medical treatment will be the same as in AVNRT. Pharmacologic treatment with adenosine, β-adrenergic blocking agents, or calcium channel blockers can be administered as deemed necessary and appropriate for the individual case. In general, the treatment of orthodromic AVRT with AV nodal blocking agents is safe. The risk of enhancing antegrade conduction down the bypass tract is very low.

Treatment of AF with ventricular preexcitation (antidromic AVRT) is different from that of orthodromic AVRT. If the patient is hemodynamically unstable, immediate synchronized DC cardioversion starting at 100–200 J is warranted. The use of AV nodal blocking agents, specifically β-blockers, calcium channel blockers, and digoxin, is contraindicated. If conduction through the AV node is slowed, conduction down the accessory pathway may be enhanced, possibly degenerating to VF. Because procainamide will slow conduction through both the AV node and the accessory pathway, it is the medication of choice when AF with a rapid ventricular response is associated with ventricular preexcitation. Procainamide is also the medication of choice in antidromic AVRT. Amiodarone can be used as an alternative agent in treating AF with ventricular preexcitation and findings of CHF.

▶ Disposition

Hospitalization is not required for patients who are asymptomatic with evidence of ventricular preexcitation on the ECG

(sinus rhythm, short PR, and a δ wave). Consider hospitalizing patients who have serious signs and symptoms or those requiring cardioversion. In addition, hospitalization is recommended for patients with AF and ventricular preexcitation or antidromic AVRT. Patients who present with stable orthodromic AVRT may be discharged with close outpatient follow-up after pharmacologic conversion in the emergency department.

2005 American Heart Association Guidelines for Cardiopulmonary Resuscitation and Emergency Cardiovascular Care. Circulation 2005;112:IV35–IV46 [PMID: 16314375].

Delacrétaz E: Clinical practice. Supraventricular tachycardia. N Engl J Med 2006;354:1039–1051 [PMID: 16525141].

Innes JA: Review article: Adenosine use in the emergency department. Emerg Med Australas 2008;20:209–215 [PMID: 18549383].

Raghavan AV et al: Management of atrial fibrillation in the emergency department. Emerg Med Clin North Am 2005;23: 1127–1139 [PMID: 16199341].

Stahmer SA, Cowan R: Tachydysrhythmias. Emerg Med Clin North Am 2006;24:11–40 [PMID: 16308111].

Sulke N, Sayers F, Lip GY: Rhythm control and cardioversion. Heart 2007;93(1):29–34 [PMID: 16963490].

Watson T, Shanstila E, Lip GY: Modern management of atrial fibrillation. Clin Med 2007;7:28–34 [PMID: 17348571].

▼ VENTRICULAR ARRHYTHMIAS

1. Ventricular Tachycardia

▶ Clinical Findings

(See Appendix, Figures 35–16 and 35–17) Ventricular tachycardia is the most common cause of wide QRS complex tachycardia. The term VT is used when six or more consecutive ventricular beats occur. The ventricular rate is usually 150–220 beats/min, although rates slower than 120 beats/min may occur. Nonsustained VT is characterized by an episode lasting less than 30 seconds. Sustained VT is characterized by an episode lasting longer than 30 seconds, associated with hemodynamic compromise, or requiring therapeutic intervention for termination. WCT refers to a regular tachycardia with a QRS complex greater than 0.12 seconds (120 ms) in duration. WCT most often occurs as a result of either VT or SVT with aberrant conduction (underlying or rate-dependent BBB).

In more than 75% of patients presenting in the emergency department with regular WCT, the underlying arrhythmia is VT. The presence of structural heart disease, coronary artery disease, prior myocardial infarction, or CHF strongly suggests VT. Certain ECG findings favor VT over SVT with aberrant conduction. These findings include a QRS complex wider than 160 ms, the presence of fusion beats, and evidence of AV dissociation. AV dissociation occurs in about 20% of patients with VT and confirms the diagnosis (this is usually seen with ventricular rates less than 150). A common clinical error that must be avoided is to assume that

WCT is SVT with aberrant conduction. All cases of WCT of unknown origin should be managed as VT.

Electrical storm is a somewhat rare but well described entity that consists of recurrent ventricular tahchycardia, usually with an implanted defrillator that discharges repeatedly. Patients with this condition have a high mortality and will likely need sedation as well as sympathetic blockade to control the recurrent dysrhythmias. Anti-arrhythmics use is usually required and IV amiodarone is the drug of choice.

Ten Tips for the Diagnosis of Regular WCT

1. A WCT is most likely VT.
2. Consider toxicity—always think of hyperkalemia, tricyclic antidepressants, and digoxin. Treatment is different and cardioversion is not helpful.
3. If unstable, treat immediately with cardioversion.
4. Ask two questions: Prior MI? Tachycardia new since MI? Answering yes increases likelihood of VT to >90%.
5. Twelve-lead ECG is always best, if possible, before, during, and after treatment. Save all tracings.
6. Old ECGs are invaluable when looking for similar BBB patterns.
7. There are many algorithms for determining VT (vs SVT with BBB, aberrancy) and none are 100% accurate. The rules are difficult to remember and interpret. VT is likely if the following are identified:
   (a) RS absent in all precordial leads (seen in less than 25% of VT). If cannot find RS (only QS, QR, monophasic R, or rSR complexes) this favors VT.
   (b) Onset of R to nadir of S >.10 ms in any pre-cordial lead.
   (c) AV disassociation.
   (d) Fusion beats, capture beats.
   (e) Concordance—all positive or all negative pre-cordial lead deflections.
   (f) Frontal plane QRS axis—usually abnormal.
   (g) If RBBB-like, then look for monophasic R orRSR' in V1 and for R/S <1 in V6. If LBBB-like, then look for wide R (>30 ms), onset of R to nadir of S > 100 ms in V1 or V2, and QR or QS in V6.
8. If still unsure treat for VT.
9. Best treatment is cardioversion.
10. Stabilize rhythm before admission.

Treatment

A. Unstable Patients

Patients with VT or WCT of unknown origin who are hemodynamically unstable with serious signs and symptoms require immediate synchronized DC cardioversion.

Recommendations are to start with 50–100 J and then increase the initial dose by 50 J as needed until sinus rhythm is restored.

B. Stable Patients

Traditionally, patients with stable VT are administered an antiarrhythmic agent for chemical cardioversion. A number of medications are available. The choice for a particular patient is often based on physician preference and experience, findings of preserved or impaired cardiac function, and the underlying cause of the VT.

1. Lidocaine—Lidocaine is a class Ib antiarrhythmic with sodium channel blocking properties. Because it can be administered rapidly with few side effects, some authors consider it the agent of choice for ventricular arrhythmias associated with acute myocardial ischemia or infarction. The recommended intravenous loading dose is 1.0–1.5 mg/kg. If required, a second bolus dose of 0.75–1.5 mg/kg can be administered in 5–10 minutes. If ventricular ectopy persists, an additional bolus dose of 0.5–0.75 mg/kg can be administered every 5–10 minutes to a maximum dose of 3 mg/kg. After rhythm suppression, start a maintenance infusion at 2–4 mg/min. Lidocaine has the lowest incidence of toxicity of all currently used antiarrhythmic medications.

2. Other drugs—Procainamide is an alternative agent to lidocaine for the treatment of stable monomorphic VT. Amiodarone may be preferable to other antiarrhythmic agents for VT in patients with CHF. Although recommended, amiodarone's efficacy may not be fast enough for use on an emergency basis.

Disposition

Hospitalization is recommended for all patients who present with VT.

2. Polymorphic Ventricular Tachycardia (Including Torsades de Pointes)

Clinical Findings

(See Appendix, Figure 35–18) Polymorphic ventricular tachycardia is a form of VT with varying QRS complex morphology. The rhythm is often irregular and hemodynamically unstable, and it can degenerate to VF.

Torsades de pointes is a form of PMVT associated with a prolonged QT interval on the baseline ECG. The rhythm is often described as having a twisting-on-point appearance and can be either paroxysmal or sustained. The heart rate is usually 200–250 beats/min. Hereditary long QT syndromes associated with torsades de pointes include Lange-Nielsen syndrome and Romano-Ward syndrome. Torsades de pointes may also occur as a result of numerous medication interactions. A complete list of medications that have been reported to prolong the QT interval is available at www.qtdrugs.org.

PMVT can also occur in the absence of a prolonged QT interval. In this case, cardiac ischemia or underlying structural heart disease is often the cause.

▶ Treatment and Disposition

Patients with PMVT who are hemodynamically unstable with serious signs and symptoms require immediate cardioversion or defibrillation. Recommendations are to start with 200 J. To prevent recurrence, discontinue all agents that can prolong the QT interval.

Magnesium is the medication of choice for the management of torsades de pointes associated with congenital and acquired forms of long QT syndrome. It may be effective even when serum levels are normal. A 2-g intravenous dose can be administered as a slow push over 5 minutes. Follow the bolus dose by a maintenance infusion of 1–2 g/h. Consider supplemental potassium as an adjunctive therapy to maintain serum potassium levels in the high normal range. Temporary transvenous pacing at rates around 100 beats/min may be useful to prevent recurrences, especially in patients with bradycardia or pauses. Hospitalization is recommended for all patients who present with PMVT.

3. Ventricular Fibrillation

▶ Clinical Findings

(See Appendix, Figure 35–19) Ventricular fibrillation is characterized by an irregular ventricular rhythm with no discernible distinction between the QRS complex, ST segment, and T waves. VF is a common cause of sudden cardiac death and remains a significant contributor to mortality in the first 24 hours after an acute myocardial infarction. In the absence of early bystander cardiopulmonary resuscitation and initiation of advanced cardiac life support, including defibrillation, survival rates are poor.

▶ Treatment and Disposition

Witnessed VF or pulseless VT, is treated with immediate treatment is asynchronous defibrillation followed by CPR for 2 minutes before rhythm check. If VT or pulseless VT persists, repeat defibrillation followed by either epinephrine or vasopressin and continued CPR for 2 minutes. If VT or pulseless VT still persists again repeat defibrillation followed by either amiodarone or lidocaine and CPR for 2 minutes. All patients who have been successfully resuscitated from VF or pulseless VT should be started on a drip of the last antiarrhythmic administered and admitted to the intensive care unit for close observation. If an acute coronary syndrome is suspected as the cause of the arrest, the patient may require cardiac catheterization for evaluation and treatment. Chapter 9 offers a more in-depth discussion of the management of cardiac arrest.

ACC/AHA/ESC 2006 Guidelines for management of patients with ventricular arrhythmias and the prevention of sudden cardiac death—executive summary. Circulation 2006;114:1088–1132 [PMID: 16949478].

Goldberger ZD, Rho RW, Page RL: Approach to the diagnosis and initial management of the stable adult patient with a wide complex tachycardia. Am J Cardiol 2008;101:1456–1466 [PMID: 18471458].

Hollowell H, Mattu A, Perron AD, Holstege C, Brady WJ: Wide-complex tachycardia: beyond the traditional differential diagnosis of ventricular tachycardia vs supraventricular tachycardia with aberrant conduction. Am J Emerg Med 2005;23:876–889 [PMID: 16291445].

Huang DT, Traub D: Recurrent ventricular arrhythmia storms in the age of implantable cardioverter defibrillator therapy: a comprehensive review. Prog Cardiovasc Dis 2008;51:229–236 [PMID: 19026857].

Marrill KA, deSouza IS, Nishijima DK, Stair TO, Setnik GS, Ruskin JN: Amiodarone is poorly effective for the acute termination of ventricular tachycardia. Ann Emerg Med 2006;47:217–224 [PMID: 16492484].

Stahmer SA, Cowan R: Tachydysrhythmias. Emerg Med Clin North Am 2006;24:11-40. [PMID: 16308111]

Vohra J: The Long QT Syndrome. Heart Lung Circ 2007;16: S5–S12 [PMID: 17627884].

▼ BRADYARRHYTHMIAS, CONDUCTION DISTURBANCES, AND ESCAPE RHYTHMS

As in tachycardia management, if a bradycardic patient is hemodynamically unstable, immediate intervention is required regardless of the origin of the underlying arrhythmia (eg, SA block, AV block, and ventricular escape rhythm). Transcutaneous cardiac pacing followed as soon as possible with transvenous pacing is the initial intervention of choice for patients with serious signs and symptoms that occur as a result of a bradyarrhythmia. In stable patients, or in patients with mild symptoms (eg, dizziness, lightheadedness), pharmacologic treatment is often initiated with or without standby pacing. Medical management can be initiated in patients with symptomatic bradycardia as a bridge to cardiac pacing, or may be initiated if emergency cardiac pacing is unavailable.

Primary conduction system disturbances account for 15% of bradyarrhythmias encountered in the emergency department setting. The remaining 85% occur as a result of various secondary causes such as acute coronary ischemia (40%), medications or toxicological causes (20%), metabolic causes (5%), neurological causes (5%), permanent pacemaker failure (2%), and other miscellaneous causes (13%). Symptomatic bradycardia resulting from AV conduction disturbances or sick sinus syndrome is more common in the elderly; the majority of patients present at age 65 years or older.

SINUS BRADYCARDIA

▶ Clinical Findings

(See Appendix, Figure 35–4) Sinus bradycardia occurs when the sinus rate is slower than 60 beats/min. Usually the rate is 45–59 beats/min, but on rare occasion it may be as slow as 35 beats/min. Sinus bradycardia is commonly associated with sinus arrhythmia and is often a normal finding in young, healthy, athletic individuals. Sinus bradycardia is often benign and does not necessarily indicate sinus node dysfunction. Although commonly physiologic, sinus bradycardia may be pathologic when patients experience symptoms of cerebral hypoperfusion or when the heart rate does not increase appropriately with activity or exercise. Certain underlying conditions have been associated with a slowing of the heart rate, including hypothermia, hypothyroidism, and increased intracranial pressure. In addition, a number of different medications, including β-blockers, calcium channel blockers, clonidine, digoxin, and lithium, can cause bradycardia.

▶ Treatment and Disposition

Usually no treatment is required for asymptomatic sinus bradycardia. When serious signs and symptoms are present, medical management, pacemaker placement, and hospital admission are indicated.

SINUS ARREST

Sinus arrest is defined as a failure of sinus node impulse formation. On the ECG, random periods of absent cardiac activity may be noted. Unless escape beats occur, lengthy pauses are noted. When pauses occur, patients may complain of dizziness or lightheadedness or may have syncope. If untreated, pauses longer than 2.5 seconds may progress to asystole.

SINOATRIAL BLOCK

SA block differs from sinus arrest in that SA block is a form of exit block rather than failure of impulse formation. Like sinus arrest, SA block may occur as a result of a number of conditions, including acute myocardial infarction, myocarditis, fibrosis of the SA node, excessive vagal tone, and digoxin toxicity. Analogous to AV block, SA block can be classified into first-, second-, and third-degree heart block.

1. First-degree Sinoatrial Block

First-degree SA block does not produce any ECG changes. The diagnosis can be made only through electrophysiologic testing.

2. Second-degree Sinoatrial Block (Mobitz Type I)

(See Appendix, Figure 35–24) Second-degree Mobitz type I SA block, also known as SA Wenckebach, is characterized

by PP intervals that gradually shorten while the PR interval remains constant. This cycle terminates with a blocked P wave. The length of the pause is shorter than twice the preceding PP cycle.

3. Second-degree Sinoatrial Block (Mobitz Type II)

Second-degree Mobitz type II SA block is characterized by fixed pauses. On the ECG, the PP interval remains constant and is then followed by a blocked P wave. The PP interval, including the blocked P wave, will be twice the length of the normal PP interval.

4. Third-degree Sinoatrial Block

Third-degree SA block may be difficult to distinguish from sinus arrest. Patients with either conduction disturbance present with variable pauses on the ECG until an escape rhythm occurs or sinus rhythm is restored.

5. Sick Sinus Syndrome

▶ Clinical Findings

Sick sinus syndrome is a manifestation of sinus node dysfunction. Patients with the syndrome may present with a wide range of bradyarrhythmias. Numerous arrhythmias are associated with sick sinus syndrome, including marked sinus bradycardia, sinus pause, sinus arrest, and SA block. On occasion, patients may also present with ventricular or atrial tachyarrhythmias.

▶ Treatment and Disposition

Treatment may be indicated when pauses of more than 2–3 seconds occur or if the patient is symptomatic. Administration of atropine or initiation of temporary cardiac pacing may be required. Symptomatic patients will require hospital admission, often for permanent pacemaker placement.

ATRIOVENTRICULAR BLOCK

AV block refers to a group of conduction disturbances within the AV junctional tissue. In general, AV block is characterized by prolonged conduction time or a failure to conduct impulses through the AV node. The conduction disturbance can be partial (first- or second-degree AV block) or complete (third-degree AV block). In general, the hemodynamic effects will depend on the ventricular rate and the presence of underlying heart disease. AV conduction blocks are traditionally classified as first-, second-, or third-degree heart block.

1. First-degree Atrioventricular Block

(See Appendix, Figure 35–25) First-degree AV block is the most common conduction disturbance and is characterized by a PR interval that is prolonged for greater than 0.2 seconds. In general, the PR interval is constant, and each atrial impulse is conducted to the ventricles. First-degree AV block can be a normal variant in young or athletic individuals due to excessive vagal tone. First-degree AV block is also common in elderly patients without underlying heart disease. It may occur in patients with myocarditis, mild digoxin toxicity, and inferior wall myocardial infarction secondary to AV nodal ischemia.

2. Second-degree Atrioventricular Block (Mobitz Type I)

(See Appendix, Figure 35–26) Second-degree Mobitz type I AV block is also known as Wenckebach AV block. This type of block is characterized by a progressive lengthening of the PR interval followed by a nonconducted P wave leading to a dropped QRS complex. Classically, the PP interval remains constant except when sinus arrhythmia is present. The RR interval will have a characteristic cycle throughout the conduction disturbance. The RR interval that includes the blocked P wave is the longest in duration. This is then followed by RR intervals that subsequently become shorter until the next P wave is blocked.

On a rhythm strip, grouped beating is often evident and can further help distinguish second-degree from third-degree AV block. The blocked P waves may occur frequently or periodically, and may or may not occur with regularity. Because Mobitz type I AV block is at the level of the AV node, the QRS complex is normal in configuration unless aberrant ventricular conduction or an underlying BBB exists. In general, Mobitz type I AV block does not usually produce hemodynamically significant symptoms. It can be seen in patients with acute myocardial infarction (usually inferior wall) and does not commonly progress to complete heart block (CHB). If CHB does occur, the escape rhythm pacemaker is usually located in the AV junctional tissue and is often fast enough to maintain an adequate cardiac output.

3. Second-degree Atrioventricular Block (Mobitz Type II)

(See Appendix, Figure 35–28) Second-degree Mobitz type II AV block is characterized by a constant PR interval, either normal or prolonged, that is followed by a nonconducted P wave. In Mobitz type II AV block, the QRS complex is usually wide. This occurs because Mobitz type II AV block represents an infranodal block. At times, every other P wave is blocked. This is described as 2:1 AV conduction. When this occurs, one cannot distinguish between Mobitz type I or type II AV block (see Appendix, Figure 35–27). Mobitz type II AV block is common in patients with acute myocardial infarction (usually anterior wall) and can suddenly progress to CHB resulting in syncope.

4. Third-degree Atrioventricular Block (Complete Heart Block)

▶ Clinical Findings

(See Appendix, Figures 35–29 to 35–31) Third-degree AV block, or CHB, is characterized by independent atrial and ventricular activity. As a result of complete AV block, no atrial impulses are conducted through the AV node. The ventricular rate is determined by the intrinsic escape rhythm, AV junctional escape (usually 45–60 beats/min), or an idioventricular escape rhythm (usually 30–40 beats/min). The atrial rate may be sinus in origin or may be from an ectopic atrial focus. In CHB the atrial rate is typically faster than the ventricular rate. As noted with second-degree AV block, the hemodynamic consequences depend on the ventricular rate and the presence of underlying heart disease. Syncope or CHF commonly accompany acute acquired CHB. Complete AV block is most commonly caused by coronary artery disease or by degeneration of the cardiac conduction system.

▶ Treatment

A. Unstable Patients

Emergency cardiac pacing is indicated for patients with hemodynamically unstable bradycardia, especially for patients who have failed medical therapy, patients with malignant escape rhythms, and patients in bradyasystolic arrest. Transcutaneous cardiac pacing is the initial intervention because of its ease of application, compared to temporary transvenous pacing. In unstable patients, medical management can be initiated, although at times its utility is only temporary.

B. Stable Patients

1. Atropine—Atropine is an anticholinergic medication with parasympatholytic properties leading to enhanced SA node automaticity and AV node conduction. The initial intravenous dose of atropine is 0.5–1.0 mg, which can be repeated every 5 minutes to a total dose of 0.04 mg/kg (3 mg for the average adult). The maximal dose produces complete vagal blockade. Atropine is recommended for, but not limited to, patients with symptomatic bradycardia or relative bradycardia, bradycardia with malignant escape rhythms, and asystole.

Rarely, a paradoxic reduction in heart rate has been observed in patients with advanced AV block after administration of atropine. Therefore, use atropine with caution in patients with infranodal AV block (Mobitz type II, and CHB with wide QRS complexes). Other rarely encountered side effects of atropine administration include worsening of cardiac ischemia in patients with an acute myocardial infarction, or the development of a ventricular tachyarrhythmia. These adverse effects are uncommon, but knowledge of such responses may assist with proper patient selection. Atropine is not effective in the management of the heart transplant patient with symptomatic bradycardia because of surgical denervation of the vagus nerve.

2. Isoproterenol—Isoproterenol is a nonspecific β-adrenergic agonist that causes an increase in heart rate and cardiac contractility. The combined effects lead to increases in cardiac output and systolic blood pressure and decreases in systemic and pulmonary vascular resistance and diastolic blood pressure. As a result, no significant change in mean arterial pressure occurs. Myocardial oxygen demand is increased as a result of the increased heart rate and contractility. In addition, isoproterenol causes smooth muscle relaxation and bronchodilation. Isoproterenol may be used to treat symptomatic bradycardia in heart transplant patients. The initial intravenous dose of isoproterenol is 1 μg/min, titrated slowly until the desired hemodynamic effects are achieved. The maximum infusion rate is 4 μg/min.

3. Dopamine—Dopamine is an endogenous catecholamine with dose-related effects. At doses of 3.0–7.5 μg/kg/min, it has β-agonist properties resulting in increased heart rate and cardiac output. The β-agonist effects are less pronounced than those of isoproterenol. Dopamine is the preferred catecholamine for symptomatic bradycardia refractory to atropine.

4. Aminophylline—Aminophylline, a methylxanthine derivative, is a competitive antagonist of adenosine. Conduction disturbances during an acute myocardial infarction may be partially mediated by the endogenous release of adenosine. Aminophylline can be administered intravenously at a dose of 5–6 mg/kg infused over 5 minutes. A maintenance infusion may be required and can be initiated at 0.5 mg/kg/h.

5. Glucagon—Glucagon stimulates cyclic adenosine monophosphate production. It may be beneficial in the treatment of bradycardia associated with β-blocker or calcium-channel-blocker toxicity. An initial intravenous dose of 0.05–0.15 mg/kg is recommended, although optimal doses have not been determined.

▶ Disposition

Hospitalize all patients who have symptomatic bradycardia. Discontinue medications with AV nodal blocking properties. Although some patients with advanced AV conduction blocks will be asymptomatic, it is recommended that all patients with newly diagnosed second-degree Mobitz type II AV block and CHB be hospitalized.

Often patients with Wenckebach AV block will be asymptomatic. Treatment is usually not necessary unless symptoms occur. In general, no treatment is necessary for patients with first-degree AV block. At times, hospitalization will be necessary to treat the underlying condition such as myocardial ischemia or digoxin toxicity.

▼ IDIOVENTRICULAR RHYTHM

▶ Clinical Findings

Idioventricular rhythm refers to the occurrence of six or more consecutive ventricular escape beats. The rate of an idioventricular escape rhythm is usually 30–40 beats/min. The duration of the QRS complex often exceeds

0.16 seconds. The morphology of the QRS complex is similar to that in premature ventricular contractions (PVCs) but varies depending on the location of the ectopic ventricular focus. Escape rhythms often develop in response to severe bradycardia or an advanced AV block. If the rate is 50–100 beats/min, the rhythm is called accelerated idioventricular rhythm (AIVR). AIVR can also be seen after administration of thrombolytic therapy for acute myocardial infarction and may serve as a marker of reperfusion.

▶ Treatment and Disposition

Treatment may be indicated if the ventricular escape rhythm is unable to maintain adequate cerebral perfusion or if the patient is unstable. If ventricular escape beats occur in response to advanced AV block, it could be dangerous to abolish the escape rhythm. In this case, the escape rhythm may be helping to maintain adequate perfusion. Management is directed at treating the underlying AV block. If AIVR occurs secondary to reperfusion, no treatment is generally needed. Because an idioventricular escape rhythm often occurs as a result of advanced AV block, the majority of patients will require hospitalization.

▼ ATRIOVENTRICULAR JUNCTIONAL RHYTHM

▶ Clinical Findings

AV junctional escape rhythm refers to the occurrence of six or more consecutive junctional escape beats. The ventricular rate is usually 45–60 beats/min. AV junctional rhythm, like AV junctional premature beats, may originate from any location in the AV junctional tissue. Because the origin of the rhythm is the AV junctional tissue, the QRS complex is narrow unless the patient has a preexisting BBB. If the junctional escape rhythm is faster than 60 beats/min, the term AV junctional tachycardia is applied. If this rhythm is present, digoxin toxicity should be ruled out.

▶ Treatment and Disposition

Patients with sinus bradycardia and occasional or intermittent AV junctional escape beats do not generally require intervention. Treatment including hospitalization will depend on the underlying cause of the cardiac arrhythmia.

Hayden GE, Brady WJ, Pollack M, Harrigan RA: Electrocardiographic manifestations: Diagnosis of atrialventricular block in the emergency department. J Emerg Med 2004;26:95–106 [PMID: 14751485].

Hood RE, Shorofsky SR: Management of arrhythmias in the emergency department. Cardiol Clin 2006;24:125–133 [PMID: 16326262].

Sherbino J, Verbeek PR, MacDonald RD, Sawadsky BV, McDonald AC, Morrison LJ: Prehospital transcutaneous cardiac pacing for symptomatic bradycardia or bradyasystolic cardiac arrest:

a systematic review. Resuscitation 2006;70:193–200 [PMID: 16814446].

Ufberg JW, Clark JS: Bradydysrhythmias and atrioventricular conduction blocks. Emerg Med Clin North Am 2006;24:1–9 [PMID: 16308110].

PERMANENT CARDIAC PACEMAKERS AND IMPLANTABLE CARDIOVERTER-DEFIBRILLATORS

It is estimated that more than 100,000 implantable cardioverter-defibrillators (ICDs) and more than 200,000 permanent cardiac pacemakers are implanted in the United States annually. These devices have dramatically reduced death from sudden cardiac death and other arrhythmias. However, they occasionally fail and emergency medicine physicians should be familiar with both normal pacemaker and AICD common malfunctions. It is estimated that permanent pacemakers have a 6% yearly incidence of malfunction and although many of these malfunctions will be identified during routine evaluation, some malfunctions will occur unexpectedly, resulting in an emergency department visit.

► Types of Pacemakers

Pacemakers are either single-chamber (right atrium or right ventricle) dual-chamber (right atrium and right ventricle) or biventricular (right atrium, right ventricle and left ventricle) devices. In single-chamber pacemakers, a single lead paces and senses in the same chamber, most often the right ventricle. In dual-chamber pacemakers, one pacing and sensing lead is in the right atrium and the other is in the right ventricle. The biventricular pacemaker is similar to the dual chamber units except that there is also a left ventricular lead. Biventricular pacing is used with increasing frequency to optimize treatment of CHF with conduction delay or dysynchrony.

Since 1990, almost all pacemaker leads are bipolar. Bipolar leads have two electrodes on the same pacing lead, a distal cathode, and a proximal anode located approximately 1 cm apart near the distal tip of the pacemaker lead. Bipolar leads produce a small electrical field between the two electrodes. This produces a small, sometimes barely noticeable, pacing spike on the ECG. Older pacemaker leads were unipolar in design. The cathode was located at the distal end of the lead and the pulse generator served as the anode. Unipolar leads produce a larger electrical field and give rise to larger pacemaker spikes on the ECG. Unipolar leads are more likely to sense noncardiac electrical events such as pectoralis muscle activity. This can result in inappropriate inhibition of pacemaker activity (myopotential inhibition). The introduction of bipolar leads has virtually eliminated this type of oversensing malfunction.

► Types of ICDs

Since receiving US Food and Drug Administration approval in 1985, ICDs have undergone significant technologic advances. Initially, devices were implanted in the abdominal wall and epicardial patches were sewn in place via a median sternotomy. Newer third-generation devices are smaller, and most are implanted in the subpectoral fascia using a transvenous lead system, similar to permanent pacemaker systems. As compared to earlier models, third-generation devices have more advanced tachycardia detection and termination features with longer battery life (7–8 years). The advanced tachycardia termination features include anti-tachycardia pacing (ATP), low-energy cardioversion, and high-energy defibrillation. Newer ICDs are also capable of rate-responsive dual-chamber back-up pacing.

COMPLICATIONS OF IMPLANTABLE CARDIAC PACEMAKERS AND ICDS

► Venous Access

Although uncommon, the majority of venous access complications occur early after implantation. Venous access complications include bleeding, pneumothorax, hemothorax, and rarely air embolism. Venous thrombosis is another rare complication of pacemaker placement. Patients may present with unilateral upper extremity pain and swelling.

► Pacemaker and ICD Pocket Site

Usually placed in the left subclavicular area, early device pocket site complications include bleeding with hematoma formation, wound dehiscence, or infection. Early pocket site infections are usually caused by *Staphylococcus aureus*. Late complications (greater than 30 days after implantation) can include pacemaker site erosion, keloid formation, pacemaker migration, and infection. Late infections are usually caused by *Staphylococcus epidermidis*. Approximately 6% of patients with permanent pacemakers develop pocket site infections.

► Lead Complications

A number of complications can occur with endocardial pacemaker and ICD leads. Lead dislodgement is uncommon for pacemakers; rates are less than 2% for ventricular leads and less than 5% for atrial leads. ICD lead dislodgement approaches 10%. If lead dislodgement is suspected, obtain posteroanterior and lateral chest radiographs and compare them with prior chest X-ray. Lead fracture or insulation break may also occur. Lead fractures generally occur at three sites: (1) close to the pulse generator, (2) at the venous entry site, and (3) with the heart. Lead fractures may be diagnosed by chest X-ray or by pacemaker interrogation.

Cardiac perforation is another uncommon but potentially serious lead complication. Suspect perforation in the patient with a new paced right bundle branch block (RBBB) pattern on ECG, intercostal muscle or diaphragmatic contractions (hiccups), pericardial effusion, or tamponade. Cardiac perforation may also be identified by a plain chest radiograph demonstrating the tip of the pacemaker lead outside the cardiac silhouette. Echocardiography may be invaluable in diagnosing a pericardial effusion. Most cases (80%) of perforation occur within the first 4 days of pacemaker insertion. Another uncommon lead complication is Twiddler's syndrome. This occurs when a patient wiggles or rotates the pacemaker generator, eventually dislodging the pacemaker leads.

DEVICE MALFUNCTION

▶ General Considerations

The most common pacemaker malfunctions are sensing abnormalities. Sensing malfunctions are further subdivided into undersensing or oversensing. Undersensing occurs when the pacemaker fails to sense intrinsic electrical cardiac activity (P wave or QRS complex). On the ECG, a pacing spike is preceded by an intrinsic P wave or QRS complex. Oversensing or crosstalk—misinterpretation by one lead of the signal generated by the other lead—can cause the pacemaker to inappropriately inhibit a pacing stimulus. On the ECG, this is evident by a pause that is longer than the programmed pacemaker rate.

Other pacemaker malfunctions include failure to pace and failure to capture. Failure to pace is characterized by an absence of an appropriate pacing stimulus. Failure to capture occurs when a pacing stimulus fails to depolarize the myocardium. Physiologic failure to capture may occur if the pacing stimulus occurs during the ventricular refractory period (within 300 ms after a native depolarization). This is not a malfunction, but reprogramming may still be necessary.

Lead complications are common causes of pacemaker malfunction. An increase in the pacing threshold may also cause sensing malfunctions and failure to capture. This can occur as a result of fibrosis at the lead tip, hyperkalemia, hypoxemia, myocardial ischemia, and antiarrhythmic drug toxicity. Battery depletion or component failure may result in failure to pace or undersensing. Electromagnetic interference from electrocautery or magnetic resonance imaging (MRI) can lead to over-sensing. Patients with implantable cardiac pacemakers should not undergo MRI. Variable effects have been documented, including pacemaker motion, function modification, heating of the pacemaker generator, and induction of voltage or current in the pacing leads.

Pacemaker-mediated tachycardia (PMT) is an uncommon complication that can occur with dual-chamber pacemakers. PMT can be triggered by a PVC with ventricular-to-atrial (VA) conduction. Retrograde atrial activity triggers a ventricular paced beat. As the ventricular paced beat undergoes VA conduction, another ventricular paced beat is triggered and the cycle continues. PMT will be evident by sustained pacing at the upper limit of the programmed pacing rate (100–140 beats/min). The ECG will characteristically reveal a wide complex paced tachycardia. PMT is often not life-threatening because the heart rate does not usually result in hemodynamic instability. Runaway pacemaker is another rare cause of a wide QRS complex paced tachycardia. In this case, the malfunctioning pulse generator discharges at a rate above its preset upper limit.

▶ Clinical Findings

Patients may present with a number of symptoms suggestive of pacemaker or ICD malfunction. These include dizziness, lightheadedness, near syncope, syncope, palpitations, shortness of breath, or chest pain. The symptoms most concerning are those associated with cerebral hypoperfusion. Patients may present after blunt chest trauma or external defibrillation leading to pacemaker malfunction. Bradycardia may be an indicator or malfunction because the lower limit of fixed rate pacing is typically 50–60 beats/min. This may occur as a result of oversensing or failure to pace. The upper limit of rate responsive pacemakers is generally 100–140 beats/min. A paced rhythm at this rate may or may not be pacemaker malfunction.

Although uncommon, frequent or recurrent shocks may represent an ICD malfunction. An increased frequency of shocks may be caused by a number of conditions including an increased frequency of ventricular arrhythmias, device inefficacy, or an ICD sensing malfunction. The most common cause of an increased frequency of ICD shocks is an increased frequency of VT or VF. Ventricular arrhythmias can occur as a result of worsening left ventricular dysfunction, myocardial ischemia, or changes in antiarrhythmic therapy. An ICD sensing malfunction may lead to double counting of the T waves or inappropriate recognition of SVT as VT. Lead complications may also cause inappropriate ICD shocks.

Occasionally a patient may present with a sustained ventricular arrhythmia without ICD intervention. Although rare, this may occur as a result of a failure to detect the arrhythmia or exhaustion of therapies. In patients with ICDs, antibradycardia pacing malfunctions will be similar to those experienced by patients with implantable cardiac pacemakers.

Evaluation of the patient suspected of having ICD or pacemaker malfunction includes a 12-lead ICG and rhythm strip. If available, a comparison ECG may be helpful. A chest radiograph should also be obtained. Lab testing, specifically of potassium, magnesium, creatinine, thyroid screening, and antiarrhythmic levels, may be necessary.

A systematic approach to the evaluation of the 12-lead ECG and rhythm strip may help to identify pacemaker malfunction. The ECG should be evaluated to determine the presence or absence of appropriate pacing spikes. A normally functioning pacemaker should be inhibited from firing when the patient's intrinsic rate is faster than the programmed rate. Pacemaker function cannot be evaluated when the intrinsic rate is faster than the programmed rate. When properly inhibited, no pacing spikes are seen on the ECG.

Magnet application may provide information regarding battery depletion or malfunction. When applied correctly over a pacemaker or ICD generator, the magnet triggers a reed switch, which inactivates the sensing function. Pacemakers should revert to an asynchronous pacing mode at a rate (magnet rate) preset by the manufacturer. A magnet rate that is slower than the manufacturer's preset rate suggests battery depletion. If no pacemaker spikes occur after magnet application, lead fracture or another malfunction may be the cause. When applied over an ICD, all antitachycardia functions (ATP and shock therapies) are disabled. Antibradycardia pacing functions are unaffected. Although most pacemakers and ICDs respond immediately when a magnet is applied correctly, there is no industry standard and responses are somewhat manufacturer-dependent. MRI is contraindicated in patients with both implantable pacemakers and ICDs. The strong magnetic field may damage the generator and interfere with normal device functioning.

Major ICD functions include sensing, detection, provision of therapy to terminate VT or VF, and pacing for bradycardia. When a tachycardia is detected two therapies are possible. First, ATP, which commonly consists of burst pacing at a rate 6–10 beats faster than the ventricular rate, is usually attempted. ATP may be felt but is not painful. Second, if ATP does not terminate the tachyarrhythmia, then high-energy shocks (1–40 J) will be delivered between the right ventricle coil electrode and the ICD casing and/or another electrode. These shocks are painful if the patient is conscious.

▶ Treatment and Disposition

Treat venous access complications accordingly. Admit for parenteral antibiotics any patients suspected of having pocket site infections.

For patients presenting with pacemaker malfunction leading to symptomatic bradycardia, institute pharmacologic treatment or emergency pacing measures. If transcutaneous cardiac pacing is initiated, place the anterior pacing pad as far away from the pacemaker generator as possible. In the setting of symptomatic bradycardia, a magnet can also be applied to revert to asynchronous pacing. If a patient requires synchronized DC cardioversion or defibrillation, place the paddles or pads as far from the pulse generator as possible.

In the emergency department, treatment of PMT may be undertaken by a number of different maneuvers. First, a magnet may be applied to terminate the tachycardia. If a magnet is unavailable or unsuccessful, chest wall stimulation using a transcutaneous pacemaker can be attempted. The required stimulus is usually 10–20 mA. This is less than the stimulus generally required for transcutaneous pacing. If unsuccessful, isometric exercises can be tried. Finally, chest

thumps have had success in terminating PMT; no more than two are recommended. Each of the mentioned techniques is designed to affect the sensing function of the pacemaker, inhibit ventricular pacing, and terminate PMT. If these are unsuccessful, cardiology consultation for pacemaker interrogation and reprogramming will be necessary.

Runaway pacemaker is a rarely encountered problem. Pharmacologic intervention or magnet application can be attempted but will most likely be unsuccessful. Definitive treatment may require disconnecting the pacemaker leads or removal of the pulse generator.

Obtain cardiology consultation for patients suspected of having pacemaker malfunction. Unless the pacemaker can be interrogated in the emergency department, the majority of patients with suspected pacemaker malfunction will require hospitalization. For ICD malfunction resulting in frequent inappropriate shocks, temporary device deactivation may be necessary. Similar to cardiac pacemakers, magnet application should trigger a magnetically activated reed switch. This disables all antitachycardia functions (ATP and shock therapies). Antibradycardia pacing functions are unaffected. Although most ICDs are immediately deactivated when a magnet is applied correctly, responses are somewhat manufacturer-dependent. Deactivation is not commonly performed, however, because the most common reason for frequent shocks is an increase in the frequency of VT or VF.

If recurrent ventricular arrhythmias result in frequent ICD shocks, antiarrhythmic administration and sedation may be necessary. If the ventricular arrhythmia is incessant, external cardioversion or defibrillation may be needed. Place the defibrillator pads or paddles as far from ICD generator as possible. Older ICDs with epicardial electrodes have been reported to increase the defibrillation threshold by preventing externally applied current from passing into the myocardium. This may decrease the likelihood of successful defibrillation.

Cesario DA, Turner JW, Dec GW: Biventricular pacing and defibrillator use in chronic heart failure. Cardiol Clin 2007;25:595–603 [PMID: 18063163].

Chan TC, Cardall TY: Electronic pacemakers. Emerg Med Clin North Am 2006;24:179–194 [PMID: 16308119].

Gehi AK, Mehta D, Gomes JA: Evaluation and management of patients after implantable cardioverter-defibrillator shock. JAMA 2006; 296:2839–2847 [PMID: 17179461].

Hood RE, Shorofsky SR: Management of arrhythmias in the emergency department. Cardiol Clin 2006;24:125–133 [PMID: 16326262].

Stevenson WG, Chaitman BR, Ellenbogen KA, Epstein AE, Gross WL, Hayes DL, Strickberger SA, Sweeney MO: Subcommittee on Electrocardiography and Arrhythmias of the American Heart Association Council on Clinical Cardiology; Heart Rhythm Society : Clinical assessment and management of patients with implanted cardioverter-defibrillators presenting to nonelectrophysiologists. Circulation 2004;110:3866–3869 [PMID: 15611390].

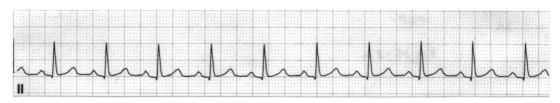

▲ **Figure 35–2.** Normal sinus rhythm at a rate of 90 beats/min.

APPENDIX: COMMONLY ENCOUNTERED CARDIAC ARRHYTHMIAS

▶ Normal Sinus Rhythm

(Figure 35–2) The heart rate is 60–100 beats/min. There is a constant and normal PR interval, and the P wave will be upright in lead II and inverted in lead aVR.

▶ Sinus Tachycardia

(Figure 35–3) The heart rate is faster than 100 beats/min. Usually the rate is 101–160 beats/min. The P wave morphology is the same as in normal sinus rhythm.

▶ Sinus Bradycardia

(Figure 35–4) The heart rate is slower than 60 beats/min. Usually the rate is 45–59 beats/min. Sinus bradycardia is commonly associated with sinus arrhythmia. The P wave morphology is the same as in normal sinus rhythm.

▶ Sinus Arrhythmia

(Figure 35–5) The heart rate is usually 45–100 beats/min. The P wave morphology is the same as in normal sinus rhythm. The PP or RR cycles vary by 0.16 seconds or more. Most commonly, sinus arrhythmia occurs in relation to the respiratory cycle. The sinus rate will gradually increase with inspiration and slow with expiration.

▶ Automatic Atrial Tachycardia

(Figure 35–6) The heart rate is usually 160–250 beats/min but may be as slow as 140 beats/min. The P wave morphology is usually different from that of normal sinus rhythm. The PP and RR cycles are regular in most cases. When the atrial rate is slower than 200 beats/min, 1:1 AV conduction is commonly noted. When the atrial rate is faster than 200 beats/min, the ventricular rate is often half the atrial rate because of the refractoriness of the AV node.

▶ Atrioventricular Nodal Reentrant Tachycardia

(Figures 35–7 to 35–10) The heart rate is usually 180–200 beats/min. The P waves occur concurrent with the QRS complex and are often difficult to visualize on the ECG.

▶ Atrioventricular Reciprocating Tachycardia

(Figure 35–11) The heart rate is usually faster than 200 beats/min. Because activation of the ventricle occurs through normal conduction pathways, the accessory pathway is concealed and the QRS morphology is normal.

▶ Atrial Fibrillation

(Figures 35–12 and 35–13) The atrial rate is disorganized and is 400–650 beats/min. The ventricular rate is irregularly irregular. No P waves are discernible on ECG.

▶ Atrial Flutter

(Figures 35–14) The atrial rate is usually 250–350 beats/min. Characteristic sawtooth flutter waves may be seen on the ECG, particularly in lead II. Variable AV conduction may be noted. Typically, 2:1 AV conduction occurs, resulting in a ventricular rate of approximately 150 beats/min.

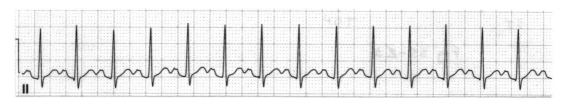

▲ **Figure 35–3.** Sinus tachycardia at a rate of 130 beats/min.

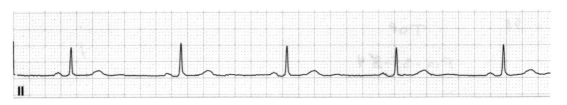

▲ **Figure 35-4.** Sinus bradycardia at a rate of 45 beats/min.

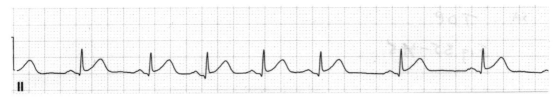

▲ **Figure 35-5.** Sinus arrhythmia. The heart rate varies between 60 and 80 beats/min.

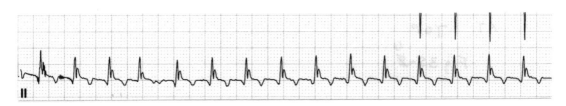

▲ **Figure 35-6.** Automatic atrial tachycardia at a rate of 140 beats/min.

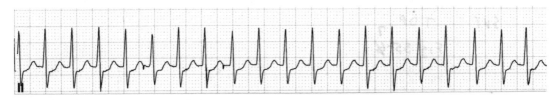

▲ **Figure 35-7.** Atrioventricular nodal reentrant tachycardia at a rate of 175 beats/min. Note the absence of clearly discernible P waves.

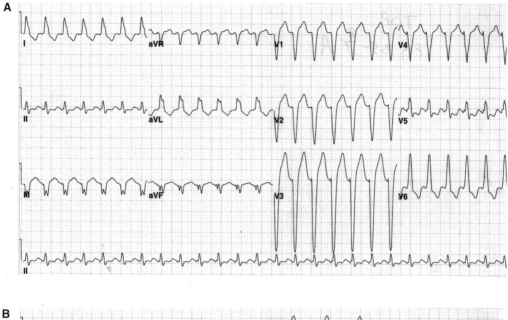

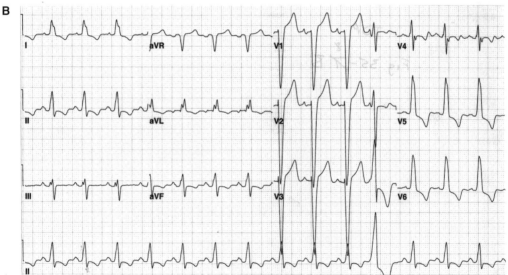

▲ **Figure 35–8.** **A:** AV nodal reentrant tachycardia with a left bundle branch block at a rate of 155 beats/min. **B:** The baseline ECG in the same patient showing sinus rhythm with a LBBB at a rate of 95 beats/min. Note that the 11th beat is a premature ventricular contraction.

▶ Multifocal Atrial Tachycardia

(Figure 35–15) The heart rate is typically 100–130 beats/min. The characteristic ECG finding is at least three different P wave morphologies. Varying PR intervals may also be noted.

▶ Ventricular Tachycardia

(Figures 35–16 and 35–17) The ventricular rate is usually 180–250 beats/min, although rates slower than 160 beats/min may occur. The QRS complex is wide (greater than 0.12 s in duration) and often bizarre in appearance. Fusion beats

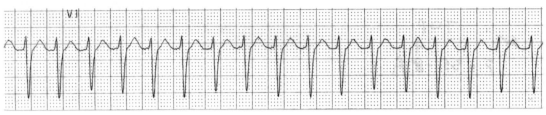

A

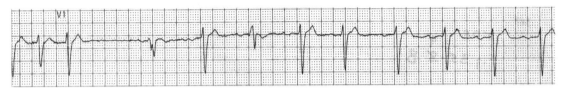

B

▲ **Figure 35–9.** **A:** AV nodal reentrant tachycardia at a rate of 150 beats/min. **B:** Seconds later after the administration of adenosine, the same patient converts to sinus rhythm.

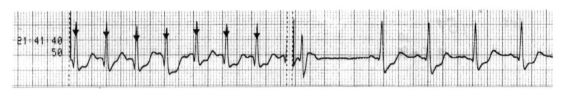

▲ **Figure 35–10.** Paroxysmal supraventricular tachycardia at a rate of 150 beats/min in a patient who is hemodynamically unstable. After the seventh beat, the patient is cardioverted with 50 J to sinus rhythm.

A

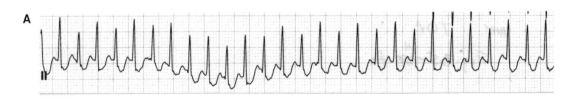

B

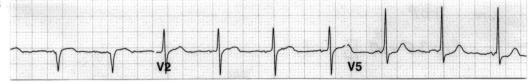

▲ **Figure 35–11.** **A:** AV reciprocating tachycardia at a rate of 250 beats/min. **B:** The same patient after pharmacologic conversion showing sinus rhythm with ventricular preexcitation.

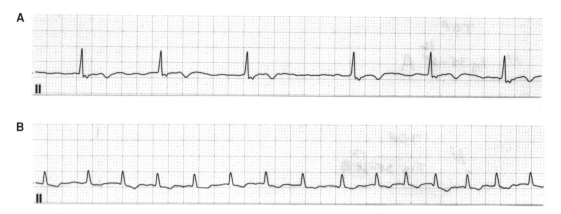

▲ **Figure 35–12.** **A:** Atrial fibrillation with a controlled ventricular response. **B:** Atrial fibrillation at a ventricular rate of 130 beats/min.

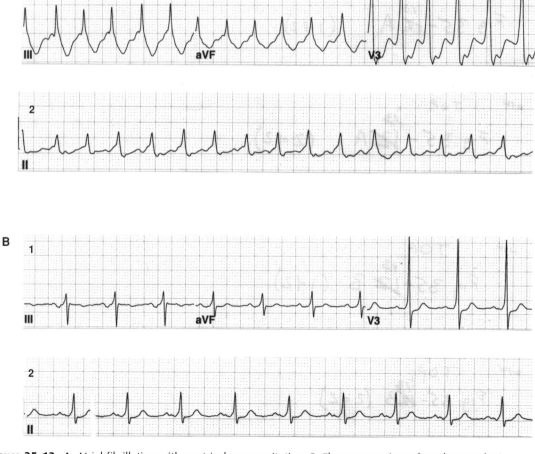

▲ **Figure 35–13.** **A:** Atrial fibrillation with ventricular preexcitation. **B:** The same patient after pharmacologic conversion showing sinus rhythm with ventricular preexcitation.

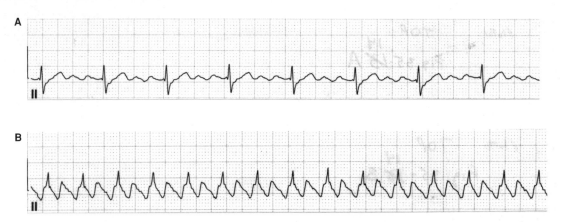

▲ **Figure 35–14. A:** Atrial flutter with 4:1 AV conduction. **B:** Atrial flutter with 2:1 AV conduction. The ventricular rate is 145 beats/min.

or AV dissociation may be noted. If AV dissociation is present, the diagnosis of VT is confirmed.

Polymorphic Ventricular Tachycardia (Torsades de Pointes)

(Figure 35–18) The heart rate is usually 200–250 beats/min. Torsades de pointes is described as having a twisting-on-point appearance.

Ventricular Fibrillation

(Figure 35–19) VF is characterized by an irregularly irregular ventricular rhythm with no discernible distinction between the QRS complex, the ST segment, and T waves.

Premature Atrial Contractions

(Figure 35–20) A premature atrial contraction (PAC) may originate from anywhere in the atria except the sinus node. The P wave morphology is usually different from that of normal sinus rhythm. It is common to see a postectopic pause after a PAC. The QRS complex is narrow unless aberrantly conducted.

Premature Ventricular Contractions

(Figure 35–21) A PVC may originate from anywhere in the ventricles. The QRS complex is 0.12 second or longer in duration and resembles either a LBBB or RBBB. Uniform PVCs originate from the same foci and have the same appearance. Multiform PVCs have different morphology because they originate from different ventricular foci.

Idioventricular Rhythm

(Figure 35–22) The ventricular rate is usually 30–40 beats/min. The morphology of the QRS complexes will be similar to PVCs but will vary depending on the location of the ventricular foci. If the ventricular rate is 50–100 beats/min, the rhythm is called AIVR.

Atrioventricular Junctional Rhythm

(Figure 35–23) The ventricular rate is usually 45–60 beats/min. The QRS complex is narrow unless aberrantly conducted. If the junctional rhythm is faster than 60 beats/min, the term AV junctional tachycardia is applied.

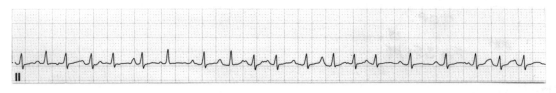

▲ **Figure 35–15.** Multifocal atrial tachycardia at a rate of 145 beats/min. Note the different P wave morphologies.

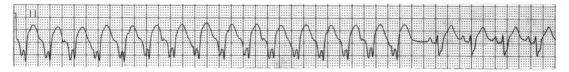

▲ **Figure 35–16.** The rhythm strip shows a run of ventricular tachycardia; the rate is 150 beats/min. After 16 beats the ventricular tachycardia spontaneously converts to sinus tachycardia.

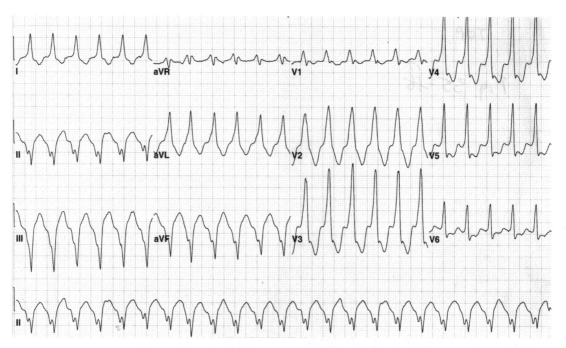

▲ **Figure 35–17.** Ventricular tachycardia at a rate of 145 beats/min.

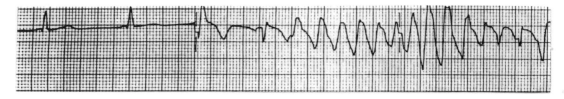

▲ **Figure 35–18.** Polymorphic ventricular tachycardia.

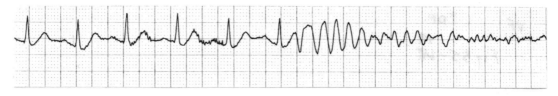

▲ **Figure 35–19.** Ventricular fibrillation. After six beats, sinus rhythm degenerates into ventricular fibrillation.

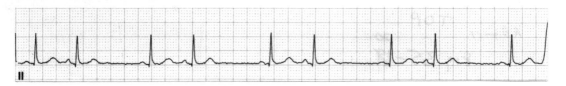

▲ **Figure 35–20.** Sinus rhythm with premature atrial contractions in a bigeminal pattern. The configuration of the P waves of the premature atrial contractions are different from that of normal sinus rhythm.

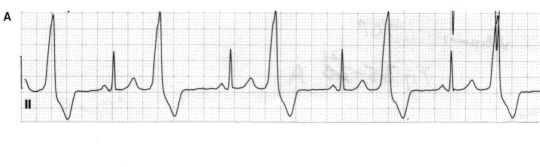

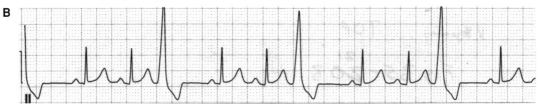

▲ **Figure 35–21.** **A:** Sinus rhythm with frequent premature ventricular complexes in a pattern of bigeminy. **B:** Sinus rhythm with frequent premature ventricular complexes in a pattern of trigeminy.

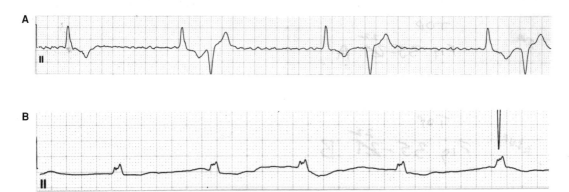

▲ **Figure 35–22.** **A:** Atrial fibrillation with an idioventricular escape rhythm. **B:** Accelerated idioventricular rhythm at a rate of 50 beats/min.

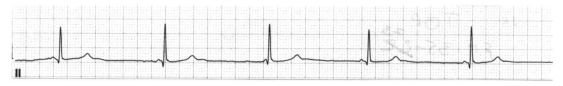

▲ **Figure 35–23.** AV junctional rhythm at a rate of 40 beats/min.

▶ Sinoatrial Block

(Figure 35–24) SA block is characterized by blocked P waves, evident by a long PP interval. The PP intervals before the blocked P wave may gradually shorten (SA Wenckebach), or the PP intervals may be constant (second-degree Mobitz type II SA block).

▶ First-degree Atrioventricular Block

(Figure 35–25) The PR interval is constant but characteristically prolonged greater than 0.2 second.

▶ Second-degree Atrioventricular Block (Mobitz Type I)

(Figure 35–26) There is progressive lengthening of the PR interval followed by a nonconducted P wave leading to a dropped QRS complex. Classically, the PP interval remains constant. The RR interval that includes the blocked P wave is the longest in duration.

▶ Second-degree Atrioventricular Block

(Figure 35–27) When every other P wave is blocked, one cannot distinguish between Mobitz type I or Mobitz type II AV block. This is described as 2:1 AV conduction.

▶ Second-degree Atrioventricular Block (Mobitz Type II)

(Figure 35–28) The PR interval is regular and can be either normal or prolonged. Periodically, a P wave is not conducted, leading to a dropped QRS complex.

▶ Third-degree Atrioventricular Block (Complete Heart Block)

(Figures 35–29 to 35–31) The PP interval (atrial rate) is usually shorter (faster) than the RR interval (ventricular rate). Because no atrial impulses are conducted through the AV node, no relationship exists between the atrial and ventricular activity.

▶ Single-chamber Ventricular Pacing

(Figures 35–32 and 35–33) When the intrinsic heart rate is faster than the programmed pacemaker rate, the pacemaker is inhibited from firing. When the intrinsic rate is slower, the pacemaker is triggered, taking over as the dominant pacemaker of the heart.

▶ Dual-chamber Atrioventricular Pacing

(Figures 35–34 and 35–35) The pacemaker is capable of pacing and sensing the atria and ventricles. Depending on the intrinsic rate, the pacemaker can either be triggered or inhibited.

▶ Failure to Capture

(Figure 35–36) Failure to capture occurs when an appropriate pacemaker discharge fails to depolarize the myocardium. Physiologic failure to capture can occur if the pacing stimulus occurs during the ventricular refractory period.

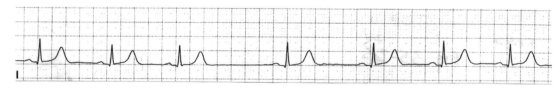

▲ **Figure 35–24.** Sinus rhythm with second-degree Mobitz type I SA block. Note that the PP intervals gradually shorten, whereas the PR intervals remain constant. The cycle terminates with a blocked P wave. The length of the pause is shorter than twice the preceding PP cycle.

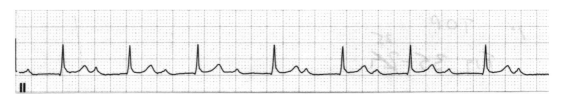

▲ **Figure 35–25.** Sinus rhythm with first-degree AV block. The PR interval is 0.44 s.

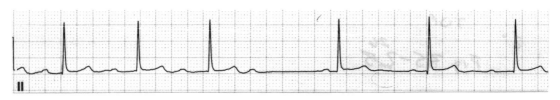

▲ **Figure 35–26.** Sinus bradycardia with second-degree Mobitz type I AV block. Note the progressive lengthening of the PR interval until a QRS complex is dropped.

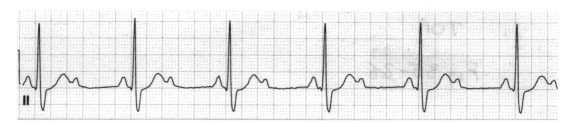

▲ **Figure 35–27.** Sinus rhythm with second-degree AV block.

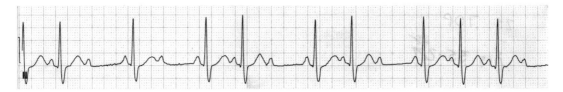

▲ **Figure 35–28.** Sinus rhythm with second-degree Mobitz type II AV block. Note the variable AV conduction.

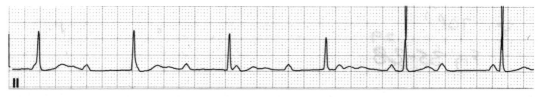

▲ **Figure 35–29.** Third-degree AV block. The atrial rate is 92 beats/min and the ventricular rate is 50 beats/min.

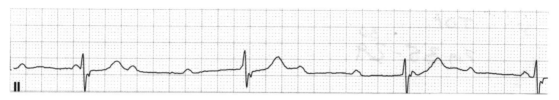

▲ **Figure 35–30.** Third-degree AV block. The atrial rate is 88 beats/min and the ventricular rate is 30 beats/min.

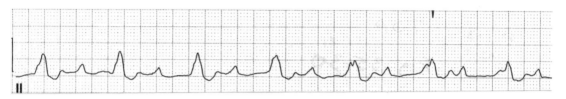

▲ **Figure 35–31.** Third-degree AV block with an accelerated idioventricular escape rhythm with a ventricular rate of 60 beats/min.

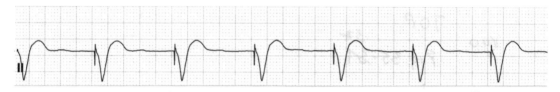

▲ **Figure 35–32.** Asynchronous ventricular pacing. In this case, the intrinsic heart rate is slower than the programmed pacemaker rate. When this occurs, the pacemaker is triggered, taking over as the dominant pacemaker of the heart.

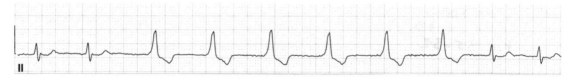

▲ **Figure 35–33.** VVI pacing. Although the pacemaker spikes are difficult to appreciate, beats 3–8 are ventricular paced beats. When the intrinsic heart rate is faster than the programmed rate, the pacemaker is inhibited from firing.

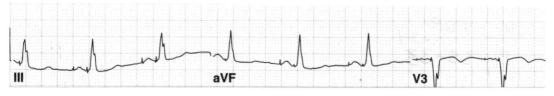

▲ **Figure 35–34.** AV sequential pacing in a dual-chamber pacemaker. In this case, the pacemaker will pace both the atria and ventricles when no intrinsic cardiac activity is sensed.

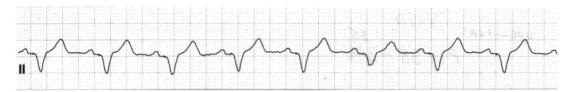

▲ **Figure 35-35.** Dual-chamber pacemaker functioning in the VAT mode. The pacemaker paces the ventricles and senses the atria. If intrinsic atrial depolarizations are sensed, a ventricular pacing spike is triggered. This is evident on the ECG by the presence of atrial tracking.

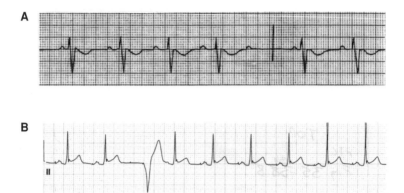

▲ **Figure 35-36. A:** Single-chamber ventricular pacemaker showing failure to capture. The underlying rhythm is second-degree Mobitz type I AV block. A ventricular pacing spike occurs after the fifth atrial complex (P wave). This pacing spike fails to depolarize the ventricular myocardium. **B:** Dual-chamber pacemaker showing failure to capture. Beat 3 shows an atrial pacing spike that fails to depolarize the atrial myocardium. The pacemaker then proceeds to pace the ventricle. Beats 1, 2, and 4-9 show an atrial pacing spike with capture followed by normal AV conduction. (Part A reproduced, with permission, from Garson A: Stepwise approach to the unknown pacemaker ECG. Am Heart J 1990;119:924.)

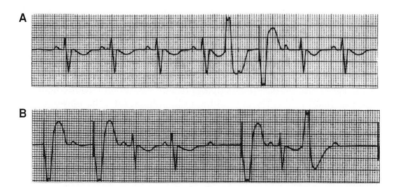

▲ **Figure 35-37. A:** Undersensing. The fifth beat is a premature ventricular contraction (PVC). The next beat is a ventricular paced beat. Note that the paced beat occurs soon after the PVC, indicating a failure to sense the preceding complex. **B:** The first and second beats are paced and the third and fourth beats show normal AV conduction. There is a longer than expected pause between the fourth and fifth beats. This occurs secondary to ventricular oversensing. (Reproduced, with permission, from Garson A: Stepwise approach to the unknown pacemaker ECG. Am Heart J 1990;119:924.)

▶ Failure to Sense (Undersensing)

(Figure 35–37A) Undersensing occurs when the pacemaker fails to detect intrinsic electrical cardiac activity. On the ECG, a P wave or QRS complex is inappropriately followed by a pacing spike.

▶ Oversensing

(Figure 35–37B) Oversensing is the inappropriate inhibition of a pacing stimulus. On the ECG, it is evident by a pause that is longer than the programmed pacemaker rate.

Gastrointestinal Emergencies

Elizabeth Davis, MD
Kimberly J. Powers, MD

Immediate Management of Life-Threatening Problems
Hypotension and Shock
Acute Abdominal Emergencies
Toxic Exposures
Other Emergencies
Further Evaluation of the Patient with Diarrhea and Vomiting
Emergency Evaluation and Management of Infectious Causes of Diarrhea and Vomiting
Viral Gastroenteritis
Bacterial Gastroenteritis
Parasitic Enteritis

Empiric Management and Disposition of Patients with Infectious Gastroenteritis
Inflammatory Bowel Disease
Gastroesophageal Reflux Disease
Esophageal Emergencies
Esophageal Rupture
Esophageal Foreign Body
Acute Gastritis and Peptic Ulcer Disease
Alcoholic Hepatitis
Hemorrhoids

▶ Diarrhea and Vomiting

Diarrhea and vomiting are common reasons for Emergency Department visits. Although the majority of cases are of an infectious, self-limiting nature, the differential diagnosis is broad with the potential for significant morbidity and mortality. Many pathologic processes involve gastrointestinal (GI) symptoms. Included are intracranial pathology (trauma, masses, infections), cardiac disease (myocardial infarction, angina), toxic exposures (digoxin, carbon monoxide, heavy metals), acute abdominal pathology (intestinal obstruction, mesenteric ischemia), and endocrine abnormalities (diabetic ketoacidosis, adrenal insufficiency), among others. In addition, infectious causes of diarrhea and vomiting can cause significant harm, especially in the elderly, in infants, and in immunocompromised individuals (Figure 36–1).

▼ IMMEDIATE MANAGEMENT OF LIFE-THREATENING PROBLEMS

HYPOTENSION AND SHOCK

 ESSENTIALS OF DIAGNOSIS

▶ Signs of decreased perfusion
▶ Hypotension, tachycardia, oliguria, and orthostasis
▶ Cool, pale skin; dry mucous membranes; and altered mentation

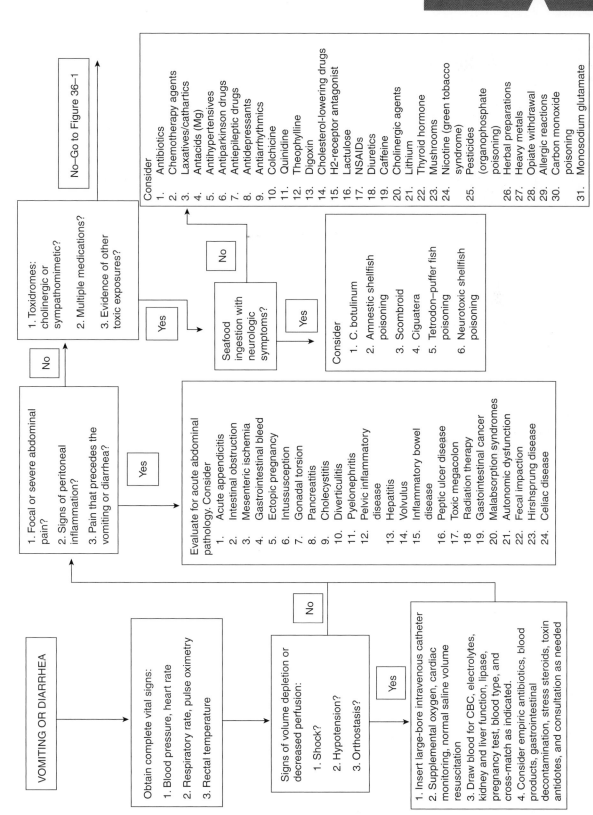

▲ **Figure 36–1.** Approach to the patient with vomiting and diarrhea, part 1. NSAIDs, nonsteroidal anti-inflammatory drugs.

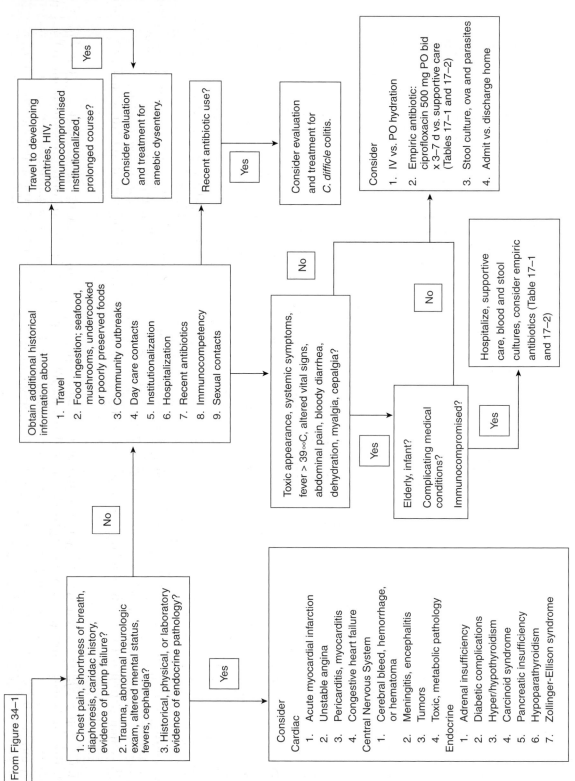

▲ **Figure 36–1.** (Continued) Approach to the patient with vomiting and diarrhea, part 2.

Clinical Findings

Obtain complete vital signs. Look for signs of decreased perfusion (ie, cool, pale skin; altered mentation; decreased urinary output; dry mucous membranes). Hypotension (systolic pressure <90 mm Hg), tachycardia, oliguria, and orthostasis may indicate impending hemodynamic instability. Look for evidence of sepsis, GI bleed, cardiac pump dysfunction, surgical abdominal pathology, toxic exposures, endocrine abnormalities, or anaphylaxis.

Treatment and Disposition

Insert a large-bore intravenous catheter and draw blood for a complete blood count (CBC), electrolytes, renal and liver function, serum lipase, and a pregnancy test, if indicated. Type and crossmatch if significant blood loss is reported or suspected. Start supplemental oxygen, cardiac monitoring, and pulse oximetry together with normal saline volume resuscitation while the underlying cause is sought. If appropriate, initiate empiric antibiotic therapy. Hospitalize the patient for continuous monitoring, supportive treatment, and further investigation if the cause is uncertain. Initiate specific treatment once the cause is determined.

ACUTE ABDOMINAL EMERGENCIES

ESSENTIALS OF DIAGNOSIS

► Focal abdominal pain or signs of peritoneal inflammation (rebound)
► Pain that precedes the vomiting or diarrhea
► Pain out of proportion to the physical examination

Clinical Findings

Patients with acute surgical abdominal pathology may present with diarrhea and vomiting and are at risk of being mislabeled as having gastroenteritis. Inquire about the nature and location of pain and the existence of upper GI symptoms (vomiting) and lower GI symptoms (diarrhea). Determine which symptom began first. Signs and symptoms suggestive of an acute abdominal emergency include focal abdominal pain, an examination consistent with peritoneal inflammation, pain that precedes the vomiting and diarrhea, protracted vomiting with nonspecific abdominal pain, and pain out of proportion to the physical examination. Consider entities such as acute appendicitis, intestinal obstruction, mesenteric ischemia, ectopic pregnancy, GI bleed, intussusception, and gonadal torsion (Table 36–4).

Serial abdominal examinations in the ED may help differentiate early acute abdominal emergencies with vomiting or diarrhea from gastroenteritis. In patients with arteriovascular disease who present with pain out of proportion to the examination, mesenteric ischemia must be ruled out.

Treatment and Disposition

Treatment ultimately depends on the cause of the symptoms. Obtain complete vital signs; gain intravenous access; and draw blood for a CBC, electrolytes, renal and liver function tests, serum lipase, pregnancy test if appropriate, and blood type and crossmatch. An acute abdominal series may demonstrate a small or large bowel obstruction. A computed tomography (CT) scan or ultrasound may help identify the cause of the acute abdomen. If intussusception is suspected, an air contrast or barium enema can be both diagnostic and therapeutic. If the patient's condition is unstable, seek appropriate surgical consultation early.

TOXIC EXPOSURES

ESSENTIALS OF DIAGNOSIS

► Cholinergic or sympathomimetic syndromes
► Ingestion of mushrooms, herbal or plant preparations, or seafood
► Occupational exposures—exposure to heavy metals, pesticides, or carbon monoxide
► Medications—digoxin, salicylates, or others

Clinical Findings

Diarrhea and vomiting are often the presenting symptoms of toxic exposures. The list of toxins is extensive (Figure 36–1). Obtain key historical information including medications, occupational exposures, use of herbal preparations, consumption of mushrooms or plant products, ingestion of seafood, exposures to heavy metals, and a history of allergic reactions. Search for specific toxin-induced syndromes such as cholinergic or sympathomimetic reactions. Consider common toxins such as digoxin, salicylates, and carbon monoxide. If neurologic symptoms exist, consider botulism or shellfish poisoning.

Treatment and Disposition

Begin treatment with the proper decontamination method. Give patients with toxic ingestions activated charcoal and a cathartic. Patients with cutaneous and inhalation exposures should be removed from the source and the contaminant diluted. Initiate supportive care and continuous monitoring. Administer specific antidotes if appropriate.

OTHER EMERGENCIES

ESSENTIALS OF DIAGNOSIS

► Chest pain, shortness of breath, diaphoresis, acute pump failure

► History of cardiac, central nervous system, endocrine disease, or trauma

► Abnormal neurological examination, alteredmentation, fevers, headache

► Laboratory and physical abnormalities

▶ Clinical Findings

Cardiac, central nervous system, or endocrine disorders may include vomiting or diarrhea as presenting symptoms (Figure 36–1). Evidence of a cardiac-related disorder includes chest pain, shortness of breath, diaphoresis, a history of cardiac disease, or evidence of acute pump failure. Indications of central nervous system pathology include a history of trauma, an abnormal neurological examination, fever, headache, and evidence of other toxic or metabolic pathology affecting the central nervous system.

▶ Treatment and Disposition

Patients with a suspected cardiac, central nervous system, or endocrine causes of vomiting or diarrhea should receive aggressive evaluation and management. This may include an ECG, continuous cardiac monitoring, intravenous access, supplemental oxygen, pulse oximetry, and a complete set of labs including clotting studies and cardiac enzymes as indicated. Obtain X-rays, CT scans, and consultations as needed.

▼ FURTHER EVALUATION OF THE PATIENT WITH DIARRHEA AND VOMITING

Once life-threatening conditions have been sought and treatment begun, an attempt should be made to further identify the cause of vomiting and diarrhea. Consider the following historical, physical, and laboratory investigations (Table 36–1).

▶ History

A. Features of the Present Illness

Important features of the present illness include time of onset, the nature of symptoms, and duration of illness. Differentiate acute (less than 2 weeks) from chronic symptoms. Clarify the

patient's use of the term *diarrhea*. Identify associated symptoms. Inquire about fever, abdominal pain, anorexia, diarrhea, constipation, tenesmus, myalgias, vomiting, cephalgia, and neurologic symptoms such as paresthesias, weakness, or cranial nerve palsies. Inquire about the presence of blood or mucus in the stool and about the character of the vomitus (bloody or bilious). Determine the onset and severity of diarrhea and vomiting in relation to other symptoms. Abdominal cramps after copious, watery diarrhea is consistent with gastroenteritis. However, abdominal pain followed by nausea and loose stool could represent appendicitis. The

---

Table 36–1. Evaluation of acute vomiting and Diarrhea.

History
 Present illness: time of onset, duration and nature of symptoms, associated symptoms (fevers, abdominal pain, myalgias, cephalgia, anorexia, neurologic symptoms)
 Travel: international or domestic, backpacking, new water supplies
 Exposures: community outbreaks, daycare exposure, hospitalization, or institutionalization
 Ingestion: mushrooms, plant products, herbal preparations, seafood, 24-hour food history
 Toxins: medications, recreational drugs, recent antibiotic use, exposure to heavy metals, pesticides, carbon monoxide
 Radiation therapy or chemotherapy
 Medical and surgical history: endocrine disorders, HIV, malignancies, gastrointestinal bleeds, abdominal surgeries
 Sexual contacts

Physical examination
 General appearance: patient's overall health, toxic appearance, jaundice or evidence of volume depletion
 Complete set of vital signs: blood pressure, heart rate, respiratory rate, pulse oximetry, rectal temperature
 Abdominal examination: focal tenderness, signs of peritoneal inflammation, pain out of proportion to the examination, distended abdomen
 Rectal examination: fecal impaction, melena, hematochezia, occult blood

Laboratory and diagnostic studies
 Fecal cell count: limited clinical utility because fecal erythrocytes and leukocytes are associated with dysentery and noninfectious processes
 Stool cultures: in patients who appear toxic, patients who are immunocompromised, and those with chronic diarrhea
 Stool for ova and parasites: in patients with chronic diarrhea, those with history of international travel, HIV-infected patients, and daycare exposures
 C. difficile toxin: consider if recent antibiotic use
 Giardia antigen: consider in HIV-infected patients, in patients with history of travel to developing countries, in those with a history of backpacking, and in daycare exposures
 Complete blood count, blood urea nitrogen, creatinine, glucose, lipase, liver function test, and blood cultures: as indicated
 Urinalysis: urinalysis and a urine pregnancy test if indicated
 Radiographic evaluation: consider an acute abdominal series in suspected bowel obstruction; abdominal CT scan or ultrasound as indicated

symptom complex of profuse diarrhea, fever, myalgias, and cephalgia is consistent with dysentery, whereas a symptom complex of sudden severe headache, nausea, vomiting, and loose stool could represent a process such as subarachnoid hemorrhage.

B. Medical and Surgical History

Inquire about the patient's medical and surgical history. Give special attention to immunocompetency. Inquire about a history of HIV, diabetes mellitus, GI bleed, abdominal surgeries, malignancies, and endocrine disease. Ask about recent chemotherapy or radiation therapy.

C. Medications and Antibiotic Use

Inquire about medications including prescription, over-the-counter, herbal preparations, and drugs of abuse. Give particular attention to recent antibiotic or laxative use.

D. Exposure Risk; Similar Illness in Others

Ask about common source exposures such as daycare or community outbreaks. Inquire about a history of hospitalization or institutionalization.

E. Dietary History

Inquire about unusual foods, dairy products, eggs, seafood, or unpasteurized or undercooked food. Ask about the ingestion of mushrooms or other plant products.

F. Travel History

Inquire about recent international travel, especially to developing countries. Forty percent of travelers to endemic regions of Latin America, Asia and Africa acquire traveler's diarrhea. Ask about recent domestic travel or outdoor activities, especially backpacking or exposure to new water sources.

G. Toxin Exposures

Assess the risk of exposure to toxins, including heavy metals, carbon monoxide, salicylates, and digoxin (see Figure 36–1). Ask about occupational history as it relates to toxin exposures. In farm workers, consider pesticides (organophosphate poisoning) and nicotine (green tobacco syndrome). Inquire about a history of allergic reactions.

H. Sexual Exposures

Inquire about sexual contacts. Amebiasis, giardiasis, campylobacteriosis, salmonellosis, and shigellosis can be transmitted by sexual contact. *Chlamydia trachomatis,* herpes simplex, and *Neisseria gonorrhoeae* are also possible causes of lower GI symptoms. HIV-positive and immunocompromised individuals are subject to infections with *Cryptosporidium,* cytomegalovirus, and *Mycobacterium avium intracellulare.*

▶ Physical Examination

Use the physical examination to assess the patient's hydration status, evaluate for sepsis, rule out the acute abdomen, and determine the presence of blood in the stool.

A. General Appearance

Assess the patient's overall health. Look for evidence of volume depletion, a toxic appearance, or jaundice.

B. Fever

Fever is consistent with invasive bacterial or parasitic causes of gastroenteritis (ie, dysentery). Fever could also indicate a process requiring acute surgical intervention. Less commonly, fever may be associated with a viral or noninvasive bacterial gastroenteritis. Food poisoning should not be associated with fever.

C. Blood Pressure and Pulse Rate

Hypotension and tachycardia are typical responses to volume depletion. If the volume status is not apparent, evaluate for orthostasis with the patient supine, sitting, and standing to detect more subtle degrees of volume depletion (systolic pressure drop ≥10 mm Hg and pulse rise ≥15 beats/min). Young, healthy adults may maintain normal vital signs even with significant dehydration. Look for a blunted response in patients who are taking atrioventricular nodal blockers.

D. Abdominal Examination

Significant abdominal pain should prompt the search for causes other than infectious gastroenteritis. If abdominal examination elicits focal tenderness, or if signs of peritoneal inflammation are present, consider acute surgical pathology. However, subjective, diffuse, and crampy abdominal pain or tenderness may occur after extensive vomiting or diarrhea. In addition, several infectious agents, most notably *Yersinia enterocolitica* and *Campylobacter* sp., may mimic appendicitis and cause right lower quadrant pain, anorexia, low-grade fever, and vomiting preceding the onset of diarrhea. Appendicitis must be ruled out in patients with this presentation.

E. Rectal Examination

Perform rectal examination to detect fecal impaction, melena, or hematochezia.

▶ Laboratory and Diagnostic Studies

Laboratory and diagnostic tests are of limited value in the routine evaluation of diarrhea and vomiting. Testing should be carried out, as indicated, in patients with a suspected noninfectious cause of vomiting or diarrhea, in those who are hemodynamically unstable, the very young, the elderly, and immunosuppressed individuals. In addition, testing may be necessary in patients with a prolonged course or in those not responding to conservative management.

A. Fecal Cell Count

Fecal erythrocytes and, to a greater degree, leukocytes have been used as a guide to determine who should receive empiric antibiotics. Both findings are associated with inflammatory diarrhea, of which bacterial dysentery is a common cause. However, there are many noninfectious causes of inflammatory diarrhea, which may also produce fecal red and white cells. These include inflammatory bowel disease (IBD), chemotherapy and radiation therapy, hypersensitivity, and autoimmune disorders. Just as the presence of erythrocytes and leukocytes is not specific for a bacterial process, their absence by stool smear does not rule it out. Furthermore, the cell count has not been shown to be a good indicator of which patients will benefit from empiric antibiotic treatment.

B. Bacterial Culture of Stool

Consider bacterial culture of stool in patients experiencing a prolonged course, in infants, in the elderly, in immunocompromised patients, and in patients who appear toxic. Stool for culture can be collected in the emergency department, and, in the event that the diarrhea persists, results can be used to guide future treatment.

C. Stool for Ova and Parasites

Consider testing for ova and parasites in patients with chronic diarrhea, those with a history of travel to developing countries, patients with HIV infection, and those with exposure to infants in daycare.

D. *Clostridium Difficile* Toxin

Consider testing for *C. difficile* toxin if the patient reports recent antibiotic use or recent hospitalization. Diarrhea may be delayed as long as 12 weeks after antibiotic therapy. Clindamycin, penicillins, and cephalosporins are commonly implicated. The incidence of community-acquired infection without recent antibiotic use is well established. Consider testing in patients with severe diarrhea, abdominal pain, and foul-smelling stool, even in those without recent antibiotic use.

E. *Escherichia coli* O157:H7 Toxin

Test patients with suspected hemolytic-uremic syndrome for *E. coli* O157:H7 toxin through a stool culture looking specifically for O157:H7 or if available by identifying the toxin through rapid immunoassay.

F. *Giardia* Antigen

Consider testing for *Giardia* antigen in HIV-infected patients, in those with a history of travel to developing countries or a history of backpacking, and in those with daycare exposure.

G. CBC, Blood Urea Nitrogen/Creatinine, Glucose, Lipase, and Liver Function Tests

Order other blood tests as indicated, especially if significant dehydration is suspected. Liver function testing is helpful if biliary colic or cholecystitis is suspected as the cause of vomiting. Lipase should be ordered in the patient with a history of pancreatitis, significant alcohol use or epigastric pain.

H. Urinalysis

A urinalysis and a urine pregnancy test should be obtained if indicated.

I. Radiographic Evaluation

Radiographic evaluation is indicated for patients thought to have a surgical abdomen. If abnormal bowel sounds, bilious vomiting, or abdominal distention are present, consider an acute abdominal series. An abdominal CT scan or an ultrasound may be appropriate as indicated.

J. Referral

Referral to a gastroenterologist may be indicated in the evaluation of chronic diarrhea.

▼ EMERGENCY EVALUATION AND MANAGEMENT OF INFECTIOUS CAUSES OF DIARRHEA AND VOMITING

The specific agent responsible for an episode of infectious gastroenteritis is difficult to identify in the acute setting. However, viral agents account for the majority of episodes, up to 70% by some estimates. Of the remaining infectious causes, bacterial agents account for approximately 24% and parasitic agents account for 6%.

VIRAL GASTROENTERITIS

ESSENTIALS OF DIAGNOSIS

► Mild systemic symptoms; generally no fever or abdominal pain

► Fecal erythrocytes and leukocytes are uncommon

► Dehydration may be mild to severe

▶ Clinical Findings

Most viral agents produce a secretory diarrhea. Viral cytotoxins lead to an increased cellular permeability and result in the secretion of water and electrolytes into the intestinal lumen. Unlike invasive dysentery, viral gastroenteritis usually lacks significant systemic symptoms and is not generally associated with fever and abdominal pain. Fecal erythrocytes and leukocytes are uncommon. The most frequently identified agents are Norwalk virus and rotavirus.

▶ Treatment and Disposition

Like other causes of nondysenteric gastroenteritis (Table 36–2), viral gastroenteritis tends to be self-limiting

and to require only supportive care. However, significant dehydration can occur and lead to severe illness, especially in those at the extremes of age or those with other compromising medical conditions. Patients without underlying disease, who are nontoxic, can tolerate oral intake, have normal vital signs, and have a supportive/appropriate social situation at home can usually be discharged. Patients should be given discharge instructions to return if they are unable to tolerate oral intake or have worsening symptoms.

Table 36–2. Differential Diagnostic Features of Common Types of Nondysenteric Gastroenteritis.

Cause	Mode of Transmission	Incubation	Comments	Therapy in Adults
S. aureus	Previously cooked proteinaceous foods (ham, shrimp, cream-filled goods, potato salad, chicken, and egg salads)	1–6 hours	Nausea, severe vomiting, mild diarrhea, and abdominal cramps; fever is rare; the source is an infected food handler; symptoms are caused by preformed enterotoxins	Supportive care; intravenous versus oral rehydration; symptomatic treatment; antibiotics ineffective against preformed enterotoxins
Bacillus cereus	Previously cooked meats, fried rice, vegetables, dried fruit, and powdered milk	1–6 hours	Abrupt onset of nausea and vomiting, mild diarrhea; fever is rare; induced by preformed enterotoxins	Self-limiting; supportive care; oral or intravenous rehydration and symptomatic treatment
Clostridium perfringens	Previously cooked or poorly reheated meats, gravy, and poultry	8–24 hours	Abdominal cramps, nausea, watery diarrhea with minimal vomiting; fever is rare; caused by enterotoxins formed both before and after gastrointestinal colonization	Supportive care; self-limiting illness; intravenous versus oral rehydration and symptomatic treatment
Clostridium botulism	Home-canned fruits and vegetables; commercial fish products	12–36 hours	Very rare; mild gastrointestinal symptoms, followed by weakness, malaise, fatigue, dry mouth, diplopia, dysphagia, and muscle incoordination; progressive cranial nerve palsies and muscle weakness may lead to respiratory failure	Hospitalization, supportive care, and ventilatory support as needed; consider gastrointestinal decontamination and intravenous trivalent antitoxin administration if appropriate
Enterotoxigenic Escherichia coli	Most outbreaks are due to contaminated water	12–72 hours	Accounts for 30–70% of traveler's diarrhea; a major cause of infantile diarrhea in the developing world; adults are usually afebrile; infants may have a fever; causes a cholerae-like illness with profuse watery diarrhea	Usually self-limiting; prevention is through good hygiene; supportive care; if severe, ciprofloxacin, 500 mg orally twice daily for 3–5 days
V. cholerae	Raw or undercooked seafood (oysters, crabs, shrimp); contaminated water or fecal-oral transmission	12–72 hours	Summer and early fall; in North America most cases are along the Gulf Coast of Texas and Louisiana; explosive rice-water diarrhea up to 1 L/h; vomiting, fever, abdominal cramps, dehydration, lactic acidosis, and death if untreated; enterotoxins are formed after bacterial colonization	Fluid resuscitation is the essential treatment; antibiotics may shorten the disease course; ciprofloxacin, 1.0 g orally for 1 dose; alternatively tetracycline or TMP-SMZ
Scombroid poisoning	Contaminated scombroid fish (tuna, bonito, mackerel); dolphin fish (mahi-mahi)	1–2 hours	Numbness and tingling of the mouth; dysphagia; headache; dizziness; diffuse flushing of the face, neck, and upper trunk; may develop palpitations, nausea, vomiting, abdominal pain, and diarrhea; bronchospasm occurs rarely; caused by histamine-like substance released form contaminated fish muscle	Antihistamines: parenteral diphenhydramine, 50 mg; histamine receptor antagonist, cimetidine, or ranitidine; give fluid and bronchodilators as needed

(continued)

Table 36–2. Differential Diagnostic Features of Common Types of Nondysenteric Gastroenteritis. (*Continued*)

Cause	Mode of Transmission	Incubation	Comments	Therapy in Adults
Paralytic shellfish poisoning	Bivalve shellfish (clams, oysters, mussels, scallops)	Up to 1 hour	Nausea, vomiting, diarrhea, abdominal cramps, paresthesias of face and extremities, headache, ataxia, vertigo, cranial nerve palsies, and muscle weakness; in severe ingestions, paralysis	Gastrointestinal decontamination and supportive care; hospitalization for 24-hour observation; may require ventilatory support
Viral gastroenteritis	Fecal-oral, person-to-person transmission; contaminated food or water; daycare; cooler months	12–72 hours	Norwalk and rotavirus are the most common agents; nausea, vomiting, and watery diarrhea; may have mild abdominal cramps and myalgias; usually afebrile; occasionally epidemics occur, especially in infants and small children	Self-limiting; supportive care; oral or intravenous rehydration and symptomatic treatment
Giardia lamblia	Contaminated food or water; fecal-oral, person-to-person transmission	1–4 weeks	Backpackers, travelers, elderly; most common intestinal parasite in the United States; causes bloating, crampy abdominal pain, excessive flatus, and malabsorptive diarrhea; vomiting is rare; a common cause of chronic diarrhea	Metronidazole, 250 mg orally three times daily for 7 days.

TMP-SMZ, trimethoprim–sulfamethoxazole

BACTERIAL GASTROENTERITIS

ESSENTIALS OF DIAGNOSIS

► Cytotoxin-mediated bacterial gastroenteritis is clinically similar to viral gastroenteritis

► Invasive bacterial enteritis produces dysentery with fever, diarrhea, abdominal cramps, and other systemic symptoms

► Fecal erythrocytes and leukocytes are common in invasive disease

► Clinical Findings

Bacterial agents may produce either an inflammatory or a secretory diarrhea. Secretory diarrhea is cytotoxin mediated and may be caused by toxins that are preformed and therefore rapid acting, as with *Staphylococcus aureus* food poisoning, or by toxins formed after bacterial colonization, as with *Vibrio cholerae* (see Table 36–2). Secretory diarrhea that affects the upper small bowel generally produces watery diarrhea. Inflammatory diarrhea is caused by direct bacterial invasion of the intestinal mucosa and often affects the distal small bowel and colon. The result is release into the intestinal lumen of water, electrolytes, blood, proteins, and mucus. The clinical presentation is dysentery and may include fever, abdominal pain, bloody diarrhea, anorexia, myalgia, cephalgia, dehydration, and weight loss. With invasive enteritis, stool smears generally contain both erythrocytes and leukocytes.

► Treatment and Disposition

Among patients with gastroenteritis, those with dysentery tend to experience the greatest morbidity and mortality. Several invasive bacterial agents, most notably *Salmonella* and *Shigella*, may result in bacteremia, sepsis, and death. This is especially of concern in the elderly, infants, and the immunocompromised. However, any bacterial agent can cause significant harm in susceptible patients. Worldwide, *V. cholerae* accounts for a significant number of deaths annually. Treatment depends on the causative agent; however, in the acute setting an empiric strategy is often required (see below). Consider collecting stool for laboratory analysis in the patient with prolonged dysentery to guide future treatment.

PARASITIC ENTERITIS

ESSENTIALS OF DIAGNOSIS

► Acute amebic dysentery may be clinically similar to bacterial dysentery

► Consider parasitic causes in patients with chronic diarrhea, a travel history to developing countries, or a history of institutionalization or immunocompromise

Clinical Findings

Parasitic agents are rarely identified in the ED. Acute amebic dysentery, caused by *Entamoeba histolytica*, may be difficult to distinguish clinically from dysentery of a bacterial cause. Consider parasitic causes in patients with a travel history to developing countries, in institutionalized patients, or in immunocompromised patients. Also consider parasitic causes in those with a prolonged course and in those not responding to conventional treatment. Laboratory analysis of stool may be of benefit for diagnosing suspected parasitic enteritis.

Treatment and Disposition

Treatment is best determined by the results of stool analysis. In the acute setting, empiric treatment may be required (see next section).

EMPIRIC MANAGEMENT AND DISPOSITION OF PATIENTS WITH INFECTIOUS GASTROENTERITIS

Supportive Care

Initial treatment consists of supportive care with special attention to the patient's hydration status. For many patients, this may be the only treatment necessary. Oral rehydration may be used for mild to moderate dehydration. In pediatric patients, oral rehydration can be accomplished by giving 50–100 mL/kg of a glucose–electrolyte solution over 4 hours.

In patients with evidence of more severe dehydration, initiate intravenous fluid resuscitation with normal saline or lactated Ringer's solution. Give pediatric patients a bolus of 20 mL/kg of normal saline and repeat as needed. Because children are particularly susceptible to hypoglycemia after prolonged vomiting and poor oral intake, a rapid bedside glucose determination should be performed in ill-appearing pediatric patients.

Empiric Chemotherapy

Interruption of the fecal–oral pathway should be the initial treatment for infectious gastroenteritis and can be accomplished by adherence to strict hygiene. Viral and noninvasive bacterial gastroenteritis, as well as many cases of bacterial dysentery, tend to be self-limiting and to require only supportive therapy. Initiate empiric antibiotic treatment in patients with a suspected invasive bacterial process and severe diarrhea, systemic symptoms, fever, and abdominal pain or in those who appear toxic. Fecal cell count is of limited utility in deciding whom to treat. Admit patients with this presentation if they are immunocompromised, have complicating medical conditions, are elderly, or are infants. For these patients, base ultimate treatment on culture results. Young, healthy adults may be candidates for outpatient treatment if they meet basic discharge criteria including ability to tolerate oral intake and having normal vital signs.

Because the results of cultures are usually unavailable in the acute setting, treatment must be empiric and guided by knowledge of common causes of dysentery (Table 36–3). Ciprofloxacin, 500 mg orally twice daily for 3–5 days, is the drug of choice. Azithromycin is an option in children and pregnant women. Use empiric treatment with caution in pediatric patients and the elderly because of an association with hemolyticuremic syndrome (HUS). This association has been shown with both ciprofloxacin and TMP-SMZ and is most strongly associated with treatment of enterohemorrhagic *E. coli* 0157:H7. HUS follows a diarrheal illness and is characterized by hemolytic anemia, renal failure, and thrombocytopenia. Most cases are in children and the elderly, but people of any age can be affected. *Salmonella* and *Shigella* have also been implicated. If possible, treatment in these patients should be based on culture results. If *C. difficile* infection is suspected, stool should be tested for C. difficile toxin and treatment initiated with metronidazole.

Because no broad empiric strategy exists for the treatment of parasitic agents, drug therapy is best guided by laboratory analysis. However, if amebic dysentery is of concern, treatment with metronidazole should be considered. A second agent, such as iodoquinol, is needed after initial treatment.

Symptomatic Treatment

A. Antiemetics

Intravenous hydration helps reduce emesis and should be used as initial therapy. Often this is the only therapy needed. For patients with uncontrollable, protracted vomiting, the use of an antiemetic can be considered. However, these agents may cause somnolence and complicate evaluation in a potentially septic population. In addition, side effects are common, especially dystonic reactions with the phenothiazines (prochlorperazine or promethazine). If patients can tolerate some oral intake, a trial of oral antiemetics is reasonable. In children, ondansetron given as a single oral dose may prevent the need for intravenous rehydration. A single oral dose can be followed by repeated small doses of an oral rehydration solution. The following are some available antiemetic options:

- Prochlorperazine (Compazine)—Adults, 5–10 mg intravenously, or 25 mg rectally; children >10 kg, 0.1 mg/kg rectally every 6 hours (use is contraindicated in children <10 kg)

- Ondansetron (Zofran)—Adults, 4–8 mg intravenously or orally every 4–6 hours; children, 0.1 mg/kg

- Promethazine (Phenergan)—Adults, 12.5–25.0 mg intravenously or rectally; children, 0.25–1.0 mg/kg rectally every 4–6 hours; use promethazine with caution in the elderly as it can alter mental status

Table 36–3. Differential Diagnostic Features of Common Types of Dysentery.

Cause	Mode of Transmission	Incubation	Comments	Therapy in Adults
Salmonella sp.	Contaminated food or water (eggs, poultry, milk). Animals or pets (turtles, chicks, lizards). Group gatherings.	8–72 hours	Very common. Fever, abdominal pain, headache, myalgia, diarrhea with little vomiting. Risk of sepsis in the young, elderly, or the compromised (sickle cell disease, diabetes, HIV, intravenous drug abusers, the asplenic). Rare fecal RBCs; common WBCs.	Treat infection in those with severe illness or sepsis, the immunocompromised, or the hospitalized. Ciprofloxacin, 500 mg orally (400 mg intravenously) twice daily for 3–7 days. Alternative: azithromycin or ceftriaxone.
Shigella sp.	Fecal-oral, person-to-person transmission, or contaminated food. Daycare and institutions. Poor sanitation. Highly contagious.	1–3 days	Very common. Children aged 1–5 years, institutionalized patients. Fever, headache, myalgia, diarrhea with little vomiting. Febrile seizures and a toxic appearance may prompt lumbar puncture. Diarrhea may begin during the procedure. Fecal RBCs common; sheets of WBCs.	Treat infection in those with severe dysentery, sepsis, or institutional outbreaks. Ciprofloxacin, 500 mg orally (400 mg intravenously) twice daily for 3–5 days. Alternative: TMP-SMZ or azithromycin.
Campylobacter sp.	Unchlorinated water, contaminated food (unprocessed milk, poultry). Animals or pets. Natural water supplies in the national parks.	1–7 days	Very common. Backpacker's diarrhea, summer months, children and young adults. Fever, headache, abdominal pain, myalgias for several days followed by diarrhea with little vomiting. May mimic appendicitis. Fecal RBCs and WBCs common.	Treat infection in those who are compromised or appear toxic. Ciprofloxacin, 500 mg orally twice daily for 5 days. Alternative: azithromycin.
Yersinia enterocolitica	Contaminated food or water (pork, milk). Fecal-oral, person-to-person transmission. Wild and domestic animals.	1–5 days	Children and young adults. Anorexia, low-grade fever, right lower quadrant abdominal pain, and vomiting may precede diarrhea and mimic appendicitis. Bacteremia is rare. Fecal RBCs and WBCs common.	Treat infection in severely ill patients. Usually self-limiting. Ciprofloxacin, 500 mg orally twice daily for 3–5 days. Alternative: TMP-SMZ.
Vibrio parahaemolyticus	Contaminated food or water. Raw or undercooked shellfish.	8–72 hours	Most common during the summer months and in adults; common in Japan; diarrhea, abdominal cramps, low-grade fever, headache, and nausea with minimal vomiting; bacteremia is rare; fecal RBCs and WBCs common	None proven; usually self-limiting; in vitro sensitivity to fluoroquinolones or doxycycline
Enterohemorrhagic *E. coli* 0157:H7	Contaminated food or water; raw undercooked meats, hamburger; fecal-oral, person-to-person transmission; institutions, daycare	3–8 days	Children and the elderly; fever, abdominal pain, vomiting, grossly bloody diarrhea; may mimic gastrointestinal bleed or mesenteric ischemia; hemolytic uremic syndrome (common cause of renal failure in children) occurs in 5%, 5–20 days postinfection; fecal RBCs and WBCs common	Supportive care; antibiotics are not recommended; may increase the risk of complications (hemolytic uremic syndrome)
Aeromonas hydrophilia	Contaminated water.	1–5 days	More common in the elderly or the compromised; more severe in children; cause of 10–15% of cases of pediatric diarrhea; diarrhea, vomiting, and abdominal cramps with or without fever; chronic infection may mimic inflammatory bowel disease; fecal RBCs and WBCs common	Ciprofloxacin, 500 mg orally twice daily for 3–7 days; alternative: TMP-SMZ or tetracycline

Table 36–3. Differential Diagnostic Features of Common Types of Dysentery. (*Continued*)

Cause	Mode of Transmission	Incubation	Comments	Therapy in Adults
Strongyloides stercoralis	Soils with fecal contamination. Warm climates, poor sanitation, institutions.	Weeks to months	Fever, abdominal pain, vomiting, diarrhea, and sepsis in the immunocompromised; the compromisedmay develop cutaneous, pulmonary, or central nervous system symptoms.	Thiabendazole, 25 mg/kg orally twice daily for 3–5 days.
Clostridium difficile (antibiotic associated)	Recent antibiotic use. Clindamycin, penicillins, and cephalosporins are most commonly implicated.	1–12weeks	More common in adults; more severe in children; fever, abdominal pain, diarrhea, rarely vomiting; may cause significant illness especially in the elderly, the compromised, or the very young; fecal RBCs and WBCs common	Discontinue associated antibiotics; metronidazole, 500 mg orally three times daily for 10–14 days, or vancomycin, 125 mg orally four times daily for 10–14 days.
Entamoeba histolytica (amebic dysentery)	Contaminated food or water. Poor sanitation, institutions. Travel to developing countries.	1–12weeks	Patients with acute amebic dysentery present with abrupt onset of fever, abdominal pain, tenesmus, and bloody diarrhea; vomiting is rare; chronic dysentery causes malaise, weight loss, bloating, and blood-streaked diarrhea; may develop an hepatic abscess; fecal RBCs and WBCs common	Metronidazole, 750 mg orally three times daily for 10 days followed by iodoquinol, 650 mg orally three times daily for 20 days.

RBCs, red blood cells; TMP-SMZ, trimethoprim–sulfamethoxazole; WBCs, white blood cells.

- Metoclopramide (Reglan)—Adults, 5–10 mg intravenously; children, 0.1–0.2 mg/kg intravenously every 6–8 hours

B. Antidiarrheal Agents

Antimotility and antisecretory agents should be used with caution. Of concern is the association of morphine administration with *Salmonella* and *Shigella* bacteremia. An additional association has been suggested between the use of opiates, loperamide, or diphenoxylate with atropine and the precipitation of toxic megacolon in patients with ulcerative colitis or antibiotic-associated colitis. Antimotility and antisecretory agents should generally not be used in febrile patients with dysentery. They can generally be used in patients that do not have fever and have nonbloody diarrhea that is not severe. In the acute setting, benefits often do not outweigh possible risks of using these agents. Commonly used agents and some associated risks are listed below:

- Loperamide (Imodium)—avoid in patients with antibiotic-associated colitis, IBD, or dysentery
- Bismuth subsalicylate suspension (Pepto-Bismol)—avoid in pediatric patients because of concern about Reye syndrome; it may cause salicylate toxicity
- Kaolin-pectin suspension (Kaopectate)—may cause constipation, bloating; avoid if intestinal obstruction is suspected

- Diphenoxylate with atropine (Lomotil)—avoid in pediatrics patients; may precipitate toxic megacolon in patients with IBD; may cause central nervous system depression
- Opiates—avoid in patients with antibiotic-associated colitis, IBD, or dysentery

C. Treatment of Dehydration

A patient with vomiting and diarrhea is at risk for dehydration. The clinician must assess hydration status using vital signs, and examination of mucous membranes and capillary refill. Associated symptoms such as lightheadedness on standing also provide insight into the patient's hydration status. The severely dehydrated patient generally needs intravenous volume replacement with isotonic fluids. For mild or impending dehydration, oral fluid replacement is often adequate. Infants with impending dehydration or even mild to moderate dehydration can usually be successfully rehydrated over 3–4 hours with the administration of frequent, small amounts of an oral rehydration solution.

▶ Disposition

Hospitalization is rarely required for vomiting or diarrhea due to food poisoning or viral gastroenteritis. Even though symptoms may be severe, the vomiting or diarrhea rarely persists long enough to require inpatient parenteral hydration. Patients with dysentery and a toxic appearance, severe dehydration, or persistent vomiting or diarrhea; those with complicating medical conditions; and the very young or elderly may require hospitalization. Patients should meet basic discharge criteria including stable vital signs, benign abdominal exam, and ability to tolerate oral intake before leaving the emergency department. Hospitalization may be required in the following cases:

- extremes of age—newborns and the very elderly tolerate fluid depletion poorly;

- systemic toxemia, as indicated by high fever and rigors;

- possible toxic exposures requiring further evaluation or treatment;

- massive diarrhea or extreme dehydration;

- severe vomiting (preventing oral replenishment) with diarrhea;

- for further evaluation of unexplained causes of vomiting or diarrhea;

- poor home environment where required support cannot be provided.

Dial S, Kezouh A, Dascal A, et al: Patterns of antibiotic use and risk of hospital admission because of *Clostridium difficile* infection. CMAJ. 2008 Oct 7;179(8):767–772 [PMID: 18838451].

Kuijper EJ, van Dissel JT: Spectrum of *Clostridium difficile* infections outside health care facilities. CMAJ. 2008 Oct 7; 179(8):747–748 [PMID:18838443].

Koletzko S, Osterrieder S: Acute infectious diarrhea in children. Dtsch Arztebl Int 2009;106(33):539–547 [PMID: 19738921].

Levine DA: Antiemetics for acute gastroenteritis in children. Curr Opin Pediatr 2009;21(3):294–298 [PMID: 19381093].

Manteuffel J. Use of antiemetics in children with acute gastroenteritis: are they safe and effective? J Emerg Trauma Shock 2009;2(1):3–5 [PMID: 19561947].

Yates J: Traveler's Diarrhea. Am Fam Physician 2005;71(11): 2095–2100 [PMID: 15952437].

INFLAMMATORY BOWEL DISEASE

ESSENTIALS OF DIAGNOSIS

▶ Usually longstanding diarrhea, abdominal pain, malaise, weight loss, and fever are some of the nonspecific signs and symptoms

▶ In general, Crohn's patients have nonbloody diarrhea and ulcerative colitis patients have bloody diarrhea

▶ Patients often have family history of inflammatory bowel disease

▶ Clinical Findings

IBD is the term used to describe the two likely autoimmune disorders, Crohn's disease and ulcerative colitis that cause chronic and often debilitating GI symptoms. Patients with Crohn's disease or ulcerative colitis may have ongoing symptoms for years without a specific diagnosis of the disease. Because symptoms may worsen slowly, patients may delay presenting for evaluation. Crohn's disease can involve any segment of the GI tract from the mouth to the anus and causes a transmural inflammation of the bowel. With transmural involvement, complications such as fistulae, abscesses, small bowel obstruction, or perforation can occur. Perianal disease (fistulae and abscesses) can occur as well in Crohn's disease. Patients with ulcerative colitis have disease limited to the mucosa and submucosa of the colon beginning in the rectum and spreading proximally with no skip areas. Typical symptoms include pain, tenesmus, and rectal bleeding. The typical course for patients with Crohn's disease includes intermittent exacerbations of abdominal pain, vomiting, and severe nonbloody diarrhea and fever followed by relatively symptom-free periods of remission. Many patients with the disease have frequent exacerbations requiring treatment with immunosuppressants. Because Crohn's disease often involves the terminal ileum, patients may have right lower quadrant pain that can be confused with appendicitis if a more careful history of recurrent symptoms is not obtained. Frequent diarrhea and rectal bleeding are common with exacerbations of ulcerative colitis. Diagnosis of IBD is suggested by history but can be more firmly established with endoscopy and histology of biopsies. During exacerbations, patients may present to the ED for evaluation. Especially for Crohn's disease, contrast enhanced CT of the abdomen is the study of choice to determine if complications such as abscess, microperforation, or obstruction have developed. Consider toxic megacolon, a condition in which the bowel dilates and may become ischemic leading to the clinical picture of sepsis, if severe abdominal pain or distention is evident. This condition, which has a mortality of 50%, can occur during severe exacerbations of IBD.

▶ Management and Disposition

When patients with IBD present to the ED during exacerbations, management depends on the degree of dehydration, ability to maintain oral intake, and abdominal examination findings. If available, consultation with a patient's gastroenterologist is usually advisable for an IBD patient in the ED. Typical medical therapy for exacerbations includes bowel rest, intravenous fluids, close monitoring of electrolytes, intravenous antibiotics and steroids, and often will require admission for control of symptoms. If surgical conditions such as obstruction, abscess, fistula, or toxic megacolon are identified, consult a surgeon on an emergency basis.

Loftus EV Jr et al: The epidemiology and natural history of Crohn's disease in population-based patient cohorts from North America: a systematic review. Aliment Pharmacol Ther 2002;16(1):51–60 [PMID: 11856078].

GASTROESOPHAGEAL REFLUX DISEASE

ESSENTIALS OF DIAGNOSIS

▶ Substernal midline burning pain after eating and when recumbent

▶ Postprandial reflux of gastric contents into the posterior pharynx or the mouth

▶ Clinical Findings

Gastroesophageal reflux disease (GERD) is a common disorder causing substernal burning discomfort often radiating toward the neck. Symptoms are usually worse after eating or when reclining and are often improved, if only temporarily, by antacids. The condition develops when high-concentration acidic gastric secretions damage the protective epithelial mucosa and cause esophagitis. Other symptoms of GERD include nausea, sore throat, hoarseness, and wheezing. Occasionally gastric fluids and small amounts of undigested food will reflux into the posterior pharynx, mouth, or upper airway. Because symptoms of acute coronary syndrome may overlap with those of GERD, consider an ECG and rule out myocardial infarction protocol for patients in which it is difficult to accurately differentiate the two conditions.

▶ Management and Disposition

Patients with GERD are usually given recommendations for lifestyle modification such as a list of foods to avoid (eg, caffeine, chocolate, fatty foods, alcohol, and peppermint) which lower the esophageal sphincter pressure. Patients with GERD should be advised to stop smoking for two reasons: (1) smoking decreases salivation that neutralizes acidic secretions in the distal esophagus and (2) smoking lowers the esophageal sphincter pressure. Other foods to avoid include those that lower the gastric pH such as orange juice, red wine, and colas. Medications that can exacerbate reflux symptoms by lowering the esophageal sphincter pressure include calcium channel blockers, β-agonists, anticholinergics, diazepam, estrogen, narcotics, progesterone, and theophylline. One simple modification includes raising the head of the bed at least 6 inches if heartburn or other symptoms such as coughing, wheezing, or laryngospasm are prominent at night. Pharmacologic treatment consists of H2-blockers twice daily for mild symptoms or proton pump inhibitors once daily for moderate to severe disease. Patients should follow up with a primary-care physician for further evaluation. Some patients may benefit from outpatient esophagogastroduodenoscopy, since long-standing GERD is associated with Barrett's esophagitis and esophageal cancer.

Liu JJ, Saltzman JR: Management of gastroesophageal reflux disease. South Med J 2006;99:735–741 [PMID: 16866056] (Review).

▼ ESOPHAGEAL EMERGENCIES

ESOPHAGEAL RUPTURE

ESSENTIALS OF DIAGNOSIS

▶ Classic triad of vomiting, lower chest pain, and subcutaneous emphysema is occasionally present

▶ Hamons sign is a crunch-like sound from movement of mediastinal air

▶ More likely to occur today from instrumentation of the esophagus than spontaneous rupture with vomiting

▶ Hypotension, tachycardia, dyspnea, and fever are ominous signs, and rapid diagnosis and treatment are essential to achieve the best chance at survival

▶ Clinical Findings

Esophageal rupture also known as Boerhaaves syndrome may occur from a variety of causes. Forceful vomiting, instrumentation of the esophagus, or blunt or penetrating trauma to the chest can all cause esophageal rupture. Once gastric and oral secretions leak out of the esophagus into the mediastinum or pleural cavity, an inflammatory and septic process begins. Patients may develop severe tachycardia, hypotension, respiratory distress, or other signs of sepsis associated with mediastinitis. Clinicians must keep a high index of suspicion for this condition because the longer the mediastinal soilage persists, the worse the patient's chances for a successful outcome. The classic triad of vomiting, lower chest pain, and subcutaneous emphysema is unfortunately not common. Hamons sign is a crunch-like sound caused by the presence of air moving within the mediastinum. Esophageal rupture should be considered in patients with vomiting, fever, and chest pain. While rarely normal in Boerhaaves syndrome, chest X-ray may demonstrate pneumomediastinum, pneumoperitoneum, either-sided pleural effusions, or pneumothoraces. For patients with fever or chest pain in setting of chest trauma, recent esophageal instrumentation, or forceful vomiting, an aggressive approach to diagnosis is recommended. Esophageal fluoroscopy using water soluble contrast may be required for diagnosis. If the initial study is negative, a barium esophagram should be performed for complete evaluation. For critically ill patients who are unable to tolerate a fluoroscopic study, a contrast-enhanced CT of the chest may demonstrate extra esophageal air and/or paraesophageal fluid and suffice for diagnosis.

Management and Disposition

Successful management of esophageal rupture depends on timely definitive treatment including decontamination of soilage in the mediastinum and in general primary repair of the esophageal injury. In the ED, management of the patient should focus on rapid stabilization of the ABCs, including intubation if respiratory compromise is developing or already present. Large-bore peripheral or central intravenous access is required for fluid resuscitation. Intra-arterial pressure monitoring is advisable. To prevent further contamination of the mediastinum, patients should be kept NPO and a nasogastric tube placed for gastric decompression. Broad-spectrum intravenous antibiotics should be initiated. Emergency consultation with a cardiothoracic surgeon is necessary as treatment is almost always surgical, however potential management options include esophagectomy, stent placement, surgical repair of the tear, and conservative treatment. Early referral should be initiated if the patient presents to a facility without the surgical or critical care expertise to manage esophageal rupture.

Vallböhmer D et al: Options in the management of esophageal perforation: analysis over a 12-year period. Dis Esophagus. 2010 Apr;23(3):185–190; [Epub ahead of print] [PMID: 19863642].

ESOPHAGEAL FOREIGN BODY

1. Pediatric Esophageal Foreign Body

See also Chapter 50.

Clinical Findings

Children commonly swallow foreign bodies, which are most often coins. Fortunately, most pass from the hypopharynx into the esophagus without causing airway obstruction. (See Chapter 50 regarding management of pediatric airway foreign body obstruction). Because of the size of coins, children may have difficulty spontaneously clearing the foreign body from the esophagus. A radiograph that visualizes the neck, chest, and abdomen is very useful to identify and track the progress of metallic foreign bodies such as a coin (see Figure 50–10). One other metallic foreign body that deserves special mention includes the button battery. Button batteries are small discs about the size of a pill or a piece of candy that can cause significant mucosal irritation and even perforation if left in place.

Management and Disposition

Once a coin or other object passes through the lower esophageal sphincter into the stomach, it is very likely to traverse the entire GI tract without difficulty. Objects that become stationary in the esophagus or those associated with pain, difficulty swallowing, drooling, or difficulty breathing should be removed on an emergency basis. To prevent significant complications, button batteries should be removed on an emergency basis by endoscopy when identified. Once a coin enters the stomach in an asymptomatic patient, outpatient follow-up with a primary-care physician is acceptable. Parents should be instructed to return to the ED if abdominal pain, vomiting, or fever develops.

2. Food Bolus Impaction

Clinical Findings

Adults more commonly become symptomatic with esophageal foreign bodies in the setting of food bolus impaction. When food bolus impaction occurs, it is usually a combination of the nature of the food that was swallowed and presence of pathology in the esophagus. Meat that is partially chewed is a common source of impaction. Esophageal abnormalities that predispose to impaction include benign stricture, Shatzki's ring, or esophageal spasm with esophagitis in the distal esophagus. Patients are usually symptomatic with dysphagia, chest pain, inability to handle oral secretions, and vomiting. A chest X-ray is unlikely to demonstrate the food bolus impaction, but it may demonstrate an air–fluid level in the esophagus. A contrast radiographic study is not recommended as it will complicate endoscopy if the food bolus impaction does not spontaneously clear.

Management and Disposition

Glucagon 1 mg intravenous has been used to relax the lower esophageal sphincter and potentiate clearance of the esophageal impaction. Studies suggest that if the food bolus is meat, glucagon is unlikely to facilitate passage of the bolus but most gastroenterologists still recommend its use. Symptomatic patients require urgent endoscopy to relieve the esophageal obstruction. Endoscopy has a high success rate of removing the obstruction. If obstructive symptoms improve, a trial of fluids is reasonable to determine if the food bolus has moved and the obstruction has resolved. If spontaneous clearance occurs, patients should have outpatient follow-up with possible endoscopy arranged to determine if underlying esophageal pathology contributed to the problem.

Katsinelos P et al: Endoscopic techniques and management of foreign body ingestion and food bolus impaction in the upper gastrointestinal tract: a retrospective analysis of 139 cases. J Clin Gastroenterol 2006;40(9):784–789 [PMID: 17016132].

ACUTE GASTRITIS AND PEPTIC ULCER DISEASE

ESSENTIALS OF DIAGNOSIS

▶ Nausea, vomiting, epigastric abdominal pain, and mild tenderness to palpation

▶ May have coffee ground hematemesis or guaiac positive stool

▶ History of exposure to GI irritants such as NSAIDs or alcohol

▶ Clinical Findings

Patients with acute gastritis often present complaining of epigastric abdominal burning type pain associated with nausea or vomiting. Food may relieve or exacerbate symptoms. Often there is a history of exposure to GI irritants such as NSAIDs, alcohol, and cocaine. Other etiologies include radiation exposure during cancer therapy, infectious causes such as *Helicobacter pylori*, or other bacteria, viruses, fungi, or parasites. The pain associated with peptic ulcer disease is nonradiating, burning, and classically occurs 2–3 hours after a meal. Gastric and duodenal ulcers are associated with *H. pylori* infection and NSAID use. Duodenal ulcers are also are linked to cigarette smoking. Laboratory evaluation should include hepatic function tests, lipase, hemogram (if significant blood loss is a concern), urinalysis, and urine pregnancy test if indicated. If abdominal discomfort is severe, consider an acute abdominal series or CT of the abdomen to exclude perforated viscus. Consider a gallbladder ultrasound if the patient is at risk for gallstones (hypercholesterolemia or positive family history of cholelithiasis) or has right upper quadrant abdominal tenderness or pain. Remember to include acute coronary syndrome in the differential of epigastric abdominal pain in patients with risk factors for the condition such as age over 40, hypertension, diabetes, and positive family history. In such cases consider an ECG and/or rule out myocardial infarction protocol if symptoms are suspicious for anginal equivalent.

▶ Treatment and Disposition

Acute gastritis is a clinical diagnosis that can be definitively confirmed by endoscopy. Endoscopy for acute gastritis is in general a nonemergency diagnostic procedure. Patients diagnosed with acute gastritis who have mild abdominal discomfort, no peritoneal signs, and are tolerating oral fluids may be discharged from the ED. Discharge instructions should include avoidance of irritants that may be contributing to the condition (NSAIDs or alcohol). Pharmacologic treatment can be with over-the-counter antacids, H2-blockers (cimetidine, ranitidine or famotodine), or proton pump inhibitors (omeprazole). Patients should follow-up with a primary-care physician for reevaluation and possible referral for endoscopy. Patients with severe dehydration and/or intractable nausea and vomiting should be admitted to the hospital or to an observation unit for serial abdominal examinations and rehydration. Intravenous omeprazole may provide symptomatic relief.

Patients with suspected gastric or duodenal ulcers should be counseled to eliminate risk factors such as smoking and NSAID use. They should be referred to primary care for *H. pylori* testing and treatment if indicated. Proton pump inhibitors, though more expensive than H2 blockers, have been shown to produce faster healing rates of ulcers. Proton pump inhibitors may also provide more rapid pain relief.

Patients with severe pain, significant confirmed or suspected blood loss from ulcers should be admitted. Patients with confirmed or suspected perforated ulcer should receive emergent surgical consultation and admission.

ALCOHOLIC HEPATITIS

ESSENTIALS OF DIAGNOSIS

▶ History of heavy alcohol consumption

▶ Nausea, malaise, and low-grade fever

▶ Evidence of hepatic dysfunction such as abnormal coagulation studies, hyperbilirubinemia, or moderately elevated AST

▶ Clinical Findings

Alcoholic hepatitis (AH) should be suspected in any patient with a history of heavy alcohol use presenting with nausea, malaise, and low-grade fever. Other presenting symptoms and signs may include jaundice, anorexia, right upper quadrant pain, hepatomegaly, or ascites. Alcoholic hepatitis develops in up to 35% of heavy drinkers and can present on a spectrum from slightly tender hepatomegaly to fulminant hepatic failure. Stigmata of chronic liver disease are often present including palmar erythema, spider angiomata, and gynecomastia. While low-grade fever (usually not higher than 101°F) is often present in AH, infectious etiologies should also be considered. Because abdominal pain is not common with AH, suspect other etiologies such as spontaneous bacterial peritonitis, pancreatitis, or hollow viscus perforation in alcoholic patients with abdominal pain complaints. Right upper quadrant tenderness and hepatomegaly are com-

Table 36–4. The Glasgow Alcoholic Hepatitis Score.

GAHS	Score Given		
	1	2	3
Age	<50	≥50	—
WBC (10⁹/l)	<15	≥15	—
BUN (mmol/l)	<5	≥5	—
PT ratio (INR)	<1.5	1.5–2.0	>2.0
Bilirubin (μmol/l)	<125	125–250	>250

Patients with a combined GAHS ≥9 on day 1 had a survival of 46 and 40% at days 28 and 84, respectively. Those patients with GAHS <9 on day 1 had a survival of 87 and 79% at days 28 and 84. Reproduced with Permission from the BMJ Publishing Group Ltd. *Source:* Forrest EH, Evans CDJ, Stewart S et al. Analysis of factors predictive of mortality in alcoholic hepatitis and derivation and validation of the Glasgow alcoholic hepatitis score. Gut 2005;54:1174–1179.

mon findings related to hepatic inflammation and swelling associated with AH. Common abnormal laboratory studies include elevated PT, elevated unconjugated hyperbilirubinemia, moderately elevated AST, and only mildly elevated ALT with the ratio of AST:ALT typically in a 2:1 pattern.

A long used objective scoring system, the Maddrey Discriminant Function (MDF) score has been employed to determine the severity of an episode of AH. Taking into account the bilirubin and absolute value of the prothrombin time, this system has been criticized as being only moderately sensitive and specific and perhaps missing those patients with a low score but significant mortality.

The Glasgow Alcoholic Hepatitis Score (GAHS) is a new tool to help accurately predict mortality at 28 and 84 days when measured at days 1 and 7 (See Table 36–4). It is a simple system incorporating five variables (age, serum bilirubin, blood urea, prothrombin time, and white blood cell count) and has been shown to be a more accurate predictor of outcome than the MDF score. Additionally, it can help identify those patients who would benefit from corticosteroids.

▶ Treatment and Disposition

While controversial, treatment of AH with corticosteroids (prednisolone 40 mg/d for 4 weeks followed by a taper) is generally recommended for patients with MDF >32 or GAHS ≥9 with spontaneous encephalopathy and no contraindications such as GI bleed, hepatorenal syndrome, sepsis, or viral hepatitis. Patients with severe AH or who are symptomatic should be hospitalized preferably in an ICU setting until the condition stabilizes. Close attention should also be paid to blood glucose levels, coagulation studies, signs and symptoms of Wernicke encephalopathy, and acute alcohol withdrawal. For

patients with coagulopathy and concurrent bleeding, transfusion with fresh frozen plasma should be considered. In general, AH is an inflammatory condition that is likely to resolve slowly if alcohol is avoided. With persistent alcohol intake, patients with AH are likely to develop progressive cirrhosis and hepatic failure. Patients with mild AH who can tolerate fluids and are hemodynamically stable may be candidates for outpatient treatment. These patients should be counseled to undergo treatment for alcoholism, as abstinence from alcohol is the only treatment available to prevent the condition from deteriorating into advanced hepatic failure. Unfortunately, even with total abstinence from alcohol, some patients will continue to have progressive hepatic dysfunction from alcoholic liver disease and often will develop residual cirrhosis.

Forrest EH, Evans CDJ, Stewart S et al: Analysis of factors predictive of mortality in alcoholic hepatitis and derivation and validation of the Glasgow alcoholic hepatitis score. Gut 2005;54:1174–1179 [PMID: 16009691].

Forrest EH, Morris AJ, Stewart S et al: The Glasgow alcoholic hepatitis score identifies patients who may benefit from corticosteroids. Gut 2007;56:1743–1746 [PMID: 17627961].

Haber PS, Warner R, Seth D et al: Pathogenesis and management of alcoholic hepatitis. J Gastroenterol Hepatol 2003;18(12):1332–1344 [PMID: 14675260] (Review).

HEMORRHOIDS

ESSENTIALS OF DIAGNOSIS

▶ Perianal mass associated with itching, bleeding, and/or pain

▶ Bleeding is usually bright red blood

▶ Careful inspection of the perineum and digital rectal examination are necessary for diagnosis as other causes of rectal pain such as perianal abscess or anal fissure are common

▶ Clinical Findings

Careful history and physical examination should be performed in patients with anorectal complaints. Bleeding is the most common presenting symptom associated with hemorrhoids. Usually the bleeding from hemorrhoids is bright red although significant blood loss or associated anemia is rare. Darker bleeding or blood mixed in with stool are not characteristic of hemorrhoidal bleeding and suggest that the source is more proximal. General guidelines recommend that patients with rectal bleeding should undergo a more complete evaluation including anoscopy and sigmoidoscopy as an outpatient. Careful inspection may reveal an anal fissure, which can cause severe anal pain that is classically worst after defecation. Patients with portal hypertension from chronic liver disease develop anal canal varices, which are clinically different from hemorrhoids. Pain from hemorrhoids is generally associated with thrombosis. An important clinical distinction is origin of the hemorrhoid relative to the dentate line. Hemorrhoids that originate above the line are "internal" and those that originate below are "external." Internal hemorrhoids are less common and do not have overlying sensory epithelium, and therefore they are generally nonpainful. Determine the origin (internal vs external), degree of prolapse, and reducibility of hemorrhoidal tissue. Thrombosed external hemorrhoids are common and cause acute pain, a perianal lump, and bleeding when overlying skin becomes eroded from irritation. Thrombosed internal hemorrhoids produce bleeding and mucus production and when prolapsed may be tender. If gangrenous, however, internal hemorrhoids are extremely painful. Although fortunately rare, fever and urinary retention can be ominous signs of severe perineal necrotizing infection associated with infected hemorrhoids.

▶ Treatment and Disposition

Treatment depends on the degree of thrombosis and whether the hemorrhoid is an internal or external hemorrhoid. Most nonthrombosed and nonincarcerated hemorrhoids are treated medically with instructions for sitz baths and good perianal hygiene, stool softeners, high-fiber diet, and pain control. While over-the-counter topical medications and suppositories including steroids are often recommended for symptomatic control of hemorrhoids, there is no evidence that these measures alter the time course of the disease. Acutely painful thrombosed external hemorrhoids are usually bluish to purple in color, are firm, and very tender to touch. Patients with symptomatic thrombosed external hemorrhoids may be excised in the ED using local anesthesia with epinephrine and removal of the overlying skin with an elliptical incision and completely evacuating the clot. Only hemorrhoids that are clearly thrombosed should be excised in the emergency department to avoid significant bleeding. Contraindications to excision of external hemorrhoids in the ED include bleeding disorders, immunocompromised state, or significant hemodynamic instability. After excision, the wound can be packed with gauze or gelfoam, and sitz baths initiated within 24 hours. Consult a general surgeon for incarcerated thrombosed internal hemorrhoids or those associated with excessive bleeding, which should be surgically treated in the operating room. Patients discharged from the ED should have specific instructions to return to the ED for fever, significant bleeding, or severe pain or inability to void as these may be indicative of significant complications such as infection. After excision, patients should also return to the ED or a primary-care physician in 48–72 hours for a wound check.

Mounsey AL, Henry SL: Clinical inquiries. Which treatments work best for hemorrhoids? J Fam Pract 2009;58(9):492–493 [PMID: 19744418].

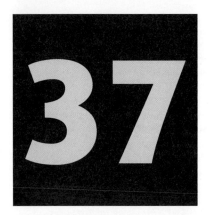

Neurologic Emergencies

C. Keith Stone, MD

IMMEDIATE MANAGEMENT OF LIFE-THREATENING PROBLEMS

STROKE

ISCHEMIC STROKE

▶ General Considerations

Stroke is a cerebrovascular disorder resulting from impairment of cerebral blood supply by occlusion (eg, by thrombi or emboli) or hemorrhage. It is characterized by the abrupt onset of focal neurologic deficits. The clinical manifestation depends on the area of the brain served by the involved blood vessel. Stroke is the most common serious neurologic disorder in adults and occurs most frequently after age 60 years. The mortality rate is 40% within the first month, and 50% of patients who survive will require long-term special care.

Ischemic strokes, comprising thrombotic, embolic, and lacunar occlusions, account for over 80% of all strokes and result in cerebral ischemia or infarction. A variety of disorders of blood, blood vessels, and heart can cause occlusive strokes, but the most common by far are atherosclerotic disease (especially of the carotid and vertebrobasilar arteries) and cardiac abnormalities.

▶ Stabilize Ventilation

A. Establish Airway

Assess adequacy of airway and ventilation in all stroke patients, especially in the presence of depressed level of consciousness, absent gag reflex, respiratory difficulty, or difficulty managing secretions.

B. Consider Intubation

Patients with inadequate ventilation (respiratory acidosis) or difficulty managing secretions will require intubation.

▶ Search for Head Trauma

Stroke patients may sustain head injury due to incoordination or weakness. Conversely, patients with focal neurologic findings due to head trauma may be mistakenly diagnosed as suffering from stroke. If head injury is suspected from the history or clinical findings, immobilize the cervical spine. Refer to Chapter 22 for management.

▶ Treat Cerebral Edema

Deterioration of neurologic status or the presence of brain-stem involvement (depressed sensorium, pupillary or extraocular movement abnormality, decorticate or decerebrate posturing) suggests significant cerebral edema and impending herniation. Mannitol 20% 0.5–1.5 g/kg hourly or 23.4% hypertonic saline solution 0.5–2.0 ml/kg, maintaining the head of the bed at greater than a 30° angle are medical therapies for elevated intracranial pressure associated with cerebral edema from ischemic stroke. However, medical therapy for cerebral edema associated with ischemic stroke does not appear to alter the patient's outcome.

▶ Treat Seizures

(See Chapter 19 for management of seizures.) Consider prophylaxis for seizure. Give intravenous phenytoin, 15–18 mg/kg at a rate not greater than 50 mg/min, or fosphenytoin, 15–20 mg/kg PE (phenytoin equivalents) intravenously.

▶ Treat Hypoglycemia

Occasionally patients with hypoglycemia may have focal neurologic deficits that may mimic a stroke. Confirm the presence of hypoglycemia using a glucometer or reagent strips before giving 50 mL of 50% dextrose solution. Stroke patients with elevated serum glucose may have a worsened outcome.

▶ Obtain Emergency CT Scan

Emergency CT scan of the head should be obtained early. This is the most readily available method for reliably detecting the presence of hemorrhage and focal cerebral edema. MRI, especially diffusion weighted, has enhanced the diagnosis of ischemic stroke.

▶ Further Evaluation of the Patient with Stroke

Accurate diagnosis and identification of the underlying cause of the stroke are important for appropriate evaluation and treatment. Conditions that predispose to strokes should be sought and corrected. A systematic approach to the evaluation of the patient with stroke is detailed below and can be modified depending on the urgency of the patient's condition.

▶ History

A. Determine Time Course of Deficits

The goal is to determine the exact time of onset of symptoms since the current recommended window of opportunity for thrombolytic therapy is 3 hours. Patients who awake with symptoms are considered to have symptom onset at the time they were last "normal" neurologically; when they went to sleep.

B. Identify Risk Factors

Hypertension, diabetes mellitus, TIAs, hyperlipidemia, smoking, family history, and use of oral contraceptives predispose to atherosclerotic disease. Cardiac disorders such as changing cardiac rhythms (especially atrial fibrillation), dyskinetic myocardium, and valvular heart disease are associated with increased risk for embolic strokes (Table 37–1). Bleeding dyscrasias, hypercoagulable states, blood disorders (especially sickle cell disease), and vascular disorders are also associated with a risk for stroke. Carotid artery bruits in patients with TIAs or stroke suggest the possibility of emboli derived from atheromatous plaques.

Table 37-1. Sources of Emboli.

Cardiac
    Changing rhythms, especially atrial fibrillation
    Valvular disease
        Rheumatic heart disease
        Valve prosthesis
        Bacterial and fungal endocarditis
        Myxomatous vegetation
        Congenital heart disease
        Mitral valve prolapse
    Atrial tumor
    Myocardial dysfunction
        Myocardial infarction
        Ventricular aneurysm
Noncardiac
    Foreign body
    Air, nitrogen, or other gases
    Fat
    Tumor
    Atheromatous material
    Thrombus

► Physical Examination

A. General

A thorough examination may reveal the underlying cause for the stroke and direct treatment.

1. Vital signs—Record the body temperature. Hypertension is a risk factor for stroke, and markedly elevated blood pressure may require treatment.

2. Head—Arteriovenous malformations may be detected by auscultation of the head for bruits. Palpate the temporal arteries for tenderness, nodularity, or absence of pulse suggestive of giant cell arthritis. Search for any evidence of trauma.

3. Eyes—Examination of the retina may reveal visible emboli in the retinal vessels.

4. Neck—The carotid arteries should be examined (one at a time) for presence of bruits and reduction of pulsation. Although these findings are not specific for carotid disease, further carotid studies may be warranted to evaluate for possible carotid endarterectomy.

5. Heart—Changing cardiac rhythms and murmurs or valvular disease are associated with increased risk of embolization from the heart.

6. Skin—Ecchymosis and petechiae may suggest blood disorders or vasculitis as causative factors. Presence of recent needle tracks or subungual splinter hemorrhages suggests the possibility of septic emboli derived from infected heart values.

7. Lung sounds—Auscultate for possible aspiration pneumonia or pulmonary edema.

B. Neurologic Examination

A rapid neurologic examination should be performed in the emergency department and should focus on (1) localizing the anatomic site of deficit as an aid in determining the specific stroke syndrome and (2) assessing the degree of neurologic impairment, from which improvement or worsening can be assessed.

1. Level of alertness—Reduced mental alertness can be a sign of extensive injury from hemorrhage, brain-stem infarction or herniation, or metabolic changes.

2. Cognitive—Assess response to commands and fluency of speech. Aphasia and apraxia are associated with involvement of the cerebral cortex and anterior (carotid) circulation; lacunar infarction or disturbance of posterior (vertebrobasilar) circulation is unlikely.

3. Cranial nerves—Visual field abnormalities exclude lacunar infarction. Abnormal pupillary reflexes and ocular palsies are brain-stem findings and are associated with disturbance of posterior circulation or impending brain herniation.

4. Motor—Hemiparesis can be associated with disturbance of the anterior or posterior circulation. Generally, in anterior circulation strokes, the face, hand, and arm are affected more than the leg. In lacunar infarction and posterior circulation strokes, this pattern is less common. Hemiparesis involving one side of the face and the other side of the body is due to disturbance of posterior circulation.

5. Sensory—Hemisensory deficits without associated motor involvement are usually due to lacunar infarcts. Astereognosis (inability to identify objects by touch) and agraphesthesia (inability to recognize figures traced on the skin) are cortical sensory deficits and are due to disturbance of anterior circulation.

6. Cerebellar—Hemiataxia suggests involvement of the cerebellum or the brain stem, or lacunar infarction deep in white matter.

C. Perform NIH Stroke Scale

The NIH stroke scale (Table 37–2) is a 13-item scoring system integrating neurologic examination components, language, and levels of consciousness that indicate the severity of neurologic dysfunction. The maximum score is 42, signifying devastating stroke, and 0 is normal. Score of 1–4 is considered minor stroke, 5–15 moderate stroke, 15–20 moderately severe stroke, and >20 a severe stroke.

► Clinical Findings

The neurologic deficits may evolve over minutes to hours and are typical for a specific vascular distribution. Motor

Table 37–2. NIH Stroke Scale Summary.

1a. Level of consciousness	0 = Alert 1 = Drowsy 2 = Stuporous 3 = Comatose
1b. LOC questions: Ask the month and the patient's age	0 = Answers both questions correctly 1 = Answers one question correctly 2 = Answers neither question correctly
1c. LOC commands: Close your eyes and make a fist	0 = Performs both tasks correctly 1 = Performs one task correctly 2 = Performs neither task correctly
2. Best gaze	0 = Normal 1 = Partial gaze palsy 2 = Forced deviation
3. Visual fields	0 = No visual loss 1 = Partial hemianopia 2 = Complete hemianopia 3 = Bilateral hemianopia
4. Facial paresis	0 = Normal symmetrical movements 1 = Minor paralysis 2 = Partial paralysis 3 = Complete paralysis
5–8. Best motor (repeat for each arm and leg)	0 = No drift 1 = Drift 2 = Some effort against gravity 3 = No effort against gravity 4 = No movement
9. Limb ataxia	0 = Absent 1 = Present in one limb 2 = Present in two limbs
10. Sensory (pinprick)	0 = Normal 1 = Partial loss 2 = Dense loss
11. Best language	0 = No aphasia 1 = Mild-to-moderate aphasia 2 = Severe aphasia 3 = Mute
12. Dysarthria	0 = Normal 1 = Mild-to-moderate dysarthria 2 = Severe dysarthria
13. Neglect/inattention	0 = No abnormality 1 = Partial neglect 2 = Complete neglect
Total score	0–42

and sensory pathways are impaired. Headache and vomiting are rare. The diagnosis is made on the basis of the clinical findings and exclusion of hemorrhage by CT scan. MRI and repeat CT scan at 48–72 hours will often confirm the diagnosis when the initial study is normal.

▶ Laboratory Tests

A. Blood Tests

The following blood tests should be obtained in most patients with focal neurologic deficits:

- Complete blood count and platelet count (to detect blood dyscrasias), and prothrombin time and partial thromboplastin time for coagulation disorders.

- Glucose level, because both hyperglycemia and hypoglycemia may cause focal neurologic findings that can mimic stroke.

- Erythrocyte sedimentation rate to detect vasculitis or arteritis.

- Toxicologic screen if drug use is suspected.

B. Electrocardiogram

An electrocardiogram may reveal new arrhythmias or conversion to a normal rhythm, both of which are associated with increased risk for emboli. Presence of myocardial infarction or persistent changes suggestive of a ventricular aneurysm also increases the risk for stroke.

C. CT

These studies are essential for localizing the lesion; distinguishing hemorrhagic from ischemic stroke; and identifying other intracranial disease, such as tumor or abscess, which can be confused with strokes. A noncontrast CT scan should be obtained in any suspected stroke patient.

▶ Treatment

A. Intravenous Thrombolysis

Thrombolytic therapy for acute ischemic stroke may be considered. The American Heart Association in conjunction with American Stroke Association and others have published guidelines for its use. Management of acute ischemic stroke is handled on a case-by-case basis. Intravenous tissue plasminogen activator (t-PA) can be used if the following criteria are met.

- Ischemic stroke in patient with a measurable deficit, the deficit must not be resolving spontaneously and the nuerological signs should not be minor and isolated.

- Caution should be used with major deficits (NIHSS >22).

- Patient has symptoms consistent with subarachnoid hemorrhage.

- The time of onset of the stroke is clearly defined, and treatment is started within 3 hours after the onset of symptoms.

- A noncontrast CT without evidence of (1)hemorrhage and (2) a multilobar infarction (hypodensity of >1/3 of cerebral hemisphere).

- No history of head trauma or previous stroke in the previous 3 months.

- No myocardial infarction in the previous 3 months.

- No gastrointestinal or urinary tract hemorrhage in the previous 21 days.

- No major surgery in the previous 14 days.

- No arterial punctures in a noncompressible site in the previous 7 days.

- No previous history of intracranial hemorrhage.

- Systolic blood pressure is less than 185 mm Hg and diastolic blood pressure is less than 110 mm Hg.

- No evidence on examination of trauma or active bleeding.

- Patient is not taking oral anticoagulants or an INR of ≤1.7 if taking or anticoagulants.

- Platelet count >100,000/mm³.

- If the patient has received heparin within the previous 48 hours the PTT must be in the normal range.

- Blood glucose must be ≥50 mg/dL.

- Seizure with post ictal residual neurologic deficits (Todds Paralysis) or seizure with onset of stroke.

- Full discussion with the patient and or family members to understand the potential risks and benefits of t-PA treatment.

  Dosage and Administration of t-PA:

- Give 0.9 mg/kg body weight of intravenous t-PA up to a maximum of 90 mg.

- Give 10% of the dose as a bolus and then administer the rest of the dose as a continuous infusion over 1 hour.

- Do not give anticoagulants or antiplatelet drugs for 24 hours after treatment.

Acute stroke patients that receive t-PA should be admitted to an intensive care setting.

B. Intra-Arterial Thrombolysis

Patients with a major stroke due to occlusions of the middle cerebral artery that present within 6 hours or less and are not candidates for intravenous t-PA may be considered for intra-arterial thrombolysis. This procedure should only be done in an experienced stroke center by qualified interventionalists with immediate access to angiography.

C. Disposition

All patients with an acute ischemic stroke should be hospitalized in a location based on their clinical condition. Patients that receive t-PA should be admitted to an intensive care unit.

HEMORRHAGIC STROKE

1. Subarachnoid Hemorrhage

ESSENTIALS OF DIAGNOSIS

- ▶ Sudden onset of severe headache
- ▶ Nausea and vomiting
- ▶ Photophobia, visual changes
- ▶ Loss of consciousness

▶ General Considerations

Subarachnoid hemorrhage (SAH) occurs secondary to bleeding in the subarachnoid space. It is a medical emergency. Approximately 80% are due to saccular or berry aneurysms. The rest may be due to trauma or arteriovenous malformation. Risk factors include family history of SAH, autosomal dominant polycystic kidney disease, connective tissue diseases, hypertension, smoking, and heavy alcohol use.

▶ Clinical Findings

Patients usually complain of "the worst headache of my life" or "thunderclap" headache. Commonly associated symptoms include nausea and vomiting, neck stiffness, and photophobia. Patients who present with stupor or coma are at high risk for mortality.

A high index of suspicion must be raised in patients presenting with early warning signs of a sentinel leak. They are frequently misdiagnosed and early diagnosis can be lifesaving. Grading of subarachnoid bleeds is based on the patient's condition on presentation. The World Federation of Neurological Surgeons grading scale is as follows:

Grade	Glasgow Coma Score
I	15
II	14 or 13 without motor deficit
III	14 or 13 with motor deficit
IV	12-7 with or without deficit
V	6-3 12-7 with or without deficit

A CT scan should be performed as the first diagnostic study (Figure 37–1). CT scan is up to 98% accurate within the first 12 hours. Lumbar puncture should be performed if the CT scan does not demonstrate blood but the suspicion for SAH remains high. Spinal fluid demonstrating xanthochromia is diagnostic. However, it takes 12 hours after the bleeding for the spinal fluid to become xanthochromic and

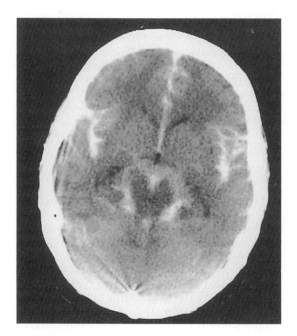

▲ **Figure 37–1.** A noncontrast head CT demonstrating diffuse subarachnoid blood.

it will remain xanthochromic for approximately 2 weeks. Blood in the CSF may be due to SAH or a traumatic lumbar puncture. The reliability of decreasing erythrocyte count to identify a traumatic lumbar puncture is questionable. If the diagnosis is still in doubt angiography may be indicated.

Angiography is the gold standard for detecting aneurysms but the newer imaging modalities of MR angiography (MRA) and CT angiography (CTA) are improving. CTA is easier to perform in critically ill patients compared to MRA. CTA has a sensitivity between 77 and 100%.

▶ Complications and Treatment

A. Aneurysmal Rebleeding

Aneurysmal rebleeding may be secondary to uncontrolled hypertension or aneurysmal clot fibrinolysis. Surgical clipping or endovascular coiling is strongly recommended to reduce the rate of rebleeding.

B. Seizure

Because seizures increase the risk of rebleeding after an SAH, prophylactic use of an anticonvulsant, for example, intravenous fosphenytoin or phenytoin, 15–20 mg/kg, is recommended.

C. Hypovolemia and Hyponatremia

Hypovolemia and hyponatremia can occur secondary to the syndrome of inappropriate secretion of antidiuretic hormone. Treatment involves intravenous hydration with isotonic crystalloid. A central intravenous monitor is desirable.

D. Hydrocephalus

1 Acute obstructive hydrocephalus—This form of hydrocephalus occurs in about 20% of patients after SAH. Ventriculostomy is recommended, although it may increase the risk of rebleeding or infection.

2. Chronic communicating hydrocephalus—This form of hydrocephalus is a frequent occurrence after SAH. A temporary or permanent cerebrospinal fluid diversion is recommended in symptomatic patients.

E. Vasospasm

Vasospasm, or delayed cerebral ischemia, remains a frequent complication with high morbidity and mortality rates. Nimodipine, 60 mg orally every 4 hours, is strongly recommended.

F. Hypertension

The acute management of elevated blood pressure in SAH is controversial. There is no evidence that lowering blood pressure decreases rebleeding or the rate of cerebral infarction. Antihypertensive therapy should be reserved for severe blood pressure elevations and should be controlled balancing the risk of hypertension related rebleeding and maintenance of cerebral perfusion pressure.

G. Neurosurgical Consultation

Surgical clipping or endovascular coiling, depending upon the resources available, should be performed to reduce the rate of rebleeding.

2. Intracerebral Hemorrhage

 ESSENTIALS OF DIAGNOSIS

▶ No specific signs or symptoms reliably distinguish between intracerebral hemorrhage and ischemic stroke

▶ Symptoms vary depending on affected area and extent of bleeding

▶ Patients are more likely to exhibit signs of increased intracranial pressure; seizures more common

▶ Headache often severe and sudden

▶ Nausea and vomiting, hypertension, altered sensorium

▶ General Considerations

Intracerebral hemorrhage is twice as common as SAH and even more likely to result in a major disability or death. Bleeding occurs primarily in the brain parenchyma, although blood may appear in the cerebrospinal fluid. Symptoms are due to mass effect of the hematoma with displacement and compression of adjacent brain tissue. The most common cause is advancing age and damage of intracerebral arterioles by long-standing systemic hypertension. Other causes include anticoagulation, alcohol abuse, thrombolytic therapy, bleeding diathesis, neoplasms, cerebral amyloid angiopathy, infections, and arteriovenous malformations.

▶ Clinical Findings

Clinical findings depend on the site of the hemorrhage but occur abruptly and progress within minutes to a few hours. Headache and vomiting are frequent symptoms. Focal neurologic deficits are prominent, since most bleeding sites about the basal ganglia, thalamus, and internal capsule. Abrupt onset of coma and prominent brainstem findings (pinpoint pupils, absent extraocular movements) are characteristic of pontine hemorrhage. A CT scan is diagnostic and is the imaging study of choice (Figure 37–2). MRI, MRA, and CTA are useful in detecting structural abnormalities such as malformations and aneurysms.

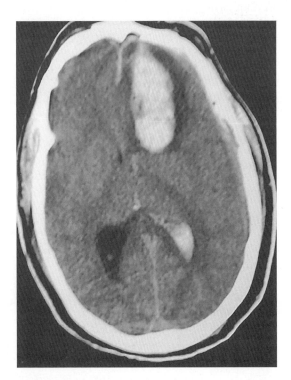

▲ **Figure 37–2.** A noncontrast head CT demonstrating a large frontal intercerebral hemorrhage.

Ataxia and cerebellar abnormalities, with absent or mild hemiparesis, are characteristic of cerebellar hemorrhage. It is particularly important to diagnose hypertensive intracerebellar hemorrhage rapidly, because fatal brain-stem compression may occur rapidly. Emergency surgical decompression of intracerebellar hemorrhage can be lifesaving. Because the clinical differentiation from acute vestibular dysfunction may be difficult, patients with sudden onset of disequilibrium and vomiting require a CT scan of the brain to exclude cerebellar hemorrhage.

▶ Treatment

As with all other emergencies, initial management of a patient with intracerebral hemorrhage is directed toward airway, breathing, and circulation. A directed history and physical examination are essential to assess for underlying clues and deficits. If the patient exhibits need for airway protection, tracheal intubation should be performed.

A. Blood Pressure Management

Blood pressure management is based on a theoretical rationale: lower the blood pressure and decrease the risk of ongoing bleeding from ruptured small arterioles. The converse theory therefore holds that aggressive treatment of blood pressure may decrease cerebral perfusion pressure and worsen brain injury. If the patient's systolic blood pressure is >200 mm Hg or MAP is >150 mm Hg, institute aggressive blood pressure reduction with continuous IV medications such as labetalol 20 mg bolus followed by 2 mg/min infusion nitroprusside 0.1–10 micrograms/kg/min or nicardipine 5–15 mg/h. If systolic blood pressure is >180 mm Hg or MAP is >130 mm Hg and there is evidence of elevated intracranial pressure (ICP), along with monitoring of ICP, blood pressure should be reduced with intermittent or continuous medications to keep the cerebral prefusion pressure between 60 and 80 mm Hg. If systolic blood pressure is >180 mm Hg or MAP is >130 mm Hg and there is no clinical evidence of ICP elevation, a more modest decrease in MAP to 110 mm Hg is appropriate using intermittent or continuous medications.

B. Intracranial Pressure

Treatment of suspected elevation of ICP should be treated in the ED with simple measures such as elevation of the head of the bed, analgesia and sedation.

C. Surgical Treatment

Neurosurgical consultation should be obtained. The decision about whether and when to operate remains controversial. Patients with a cerebellar bleed of >3 cm who are demonstrating neurologic deterioration, have brainstem compression or hyrocephalus from ventricular obstruction, should undergo surgical decompression.

Table 37-3. Conditions Associated with Acute Confusion or Delirium That May Cause Rapid Cerebral Damage.

Hypoglycemia
Wernicke encephalopathy
Hypotension and shock
Respiratory failure (hypercapnia or hypoxemia)
Hyperthermia or hypothermia
Meningitis or encephalitis
Stroke
Mass lesions (including intracranial bleeding)
Poisoning (methanol, ethylene glycol, carbon monoxide)

D. Disposition

All patients with an intracerebral hemorrhage should be monitored and treated in an intensive care unit.

ACUTE CONFUSIONAL STATE

Delirium and acute confusional states are among the most difficult problems confronting the emergency physician. The patient's mental status can be assessed quickly using a classification scheme. Such schemes classify patients according to whether or not they are alert, their ability to attend, and their memory capability, allowing the physician to differentiate among coma, delirium, and dementia.

Confused patients are often uncooperative or combative, making evaluation difficult. Signs and symptoms may be manifestations of a life-threatening underlying condition demanding prompt diagnosis and treatment to prevent irreversible brain damage (Table 37-3). Although evaluation may be difficult, every patient with an acutely altered state of consciousness must be examined and a history taken so that the cause can be established, if possible, in the emergency department. If the diagnosis cannot be established with certainty, the patient should be hospitalized.

▶ Immediate Measures

A. Maintain Airway

Clear secretions as needed. Begin oxygen, if necessary, 5–10 L/min, by mask or nasal cannula. Restrain the patient only if necessary.

B. Gain Intravenous Access

Insert a large-bore (≥18-gauge) intravenous catheter. Administer the following intravenously: (1) thiamine, 100 mg by slow bolus injection; (2) 50% dextrose in water, 50 mL over 3–5 minutes, if the patient is hypoglycemic by bedside finger stick glucose testing; and (3) naloxone 0.4–2 mg by bolus injection. *Caution*: Administration of glucose may worsen brain injury by increasing lactate in ischemic areas. Do not give glucose to patients during

the acute phases of stroke or after cardiac arrest if serum glucose is normal.

C. Treat Shock

Hypotension and shock with associated peripheral hypoperfusion may be associated with delirium or confusion. Treat shock with immediate intravenous administration of crystalloid solutions unless the patient is in cardiogenic shock, and follow with more specific measures (Chapter 11).

D. Correct Respiratory Failure

Hypoxemia or hypercapnia that develops abruptly may be associated with delirium. Assess ventilatory status by means of arterial blood gases, and correct hypoxemia or hypercapnia by administration of oxygen, assisted ventilation, or both, as needed.

E. Treat Hyperthermia or Hypothermia

Markedly elevated body temperatures (40.6°C [105°F]) may be associated with delirium or acute confusional states. Hypothermia is likely to produce confusion at body temperatures below 32.2°C (90°F) and unconsciousness at temperatures below 26.6°C (80°F). Treat by lowering or raising core temperature, as needed (Chapter 46).

F. Treat Severe Hypertension

Severe hypertension (when associated with papilledema and encephalopathy) is a medical emergency requiring rapid reduction of mean arterial pressure toward 110 mm Hg (Chapter 35). The diagnosis of hypertensive encephalopathy must be firmly established before antihypertensive therapy is started, however, because reduction of blood pressure when cerebral ischemia is present can severely exacerbate ischemic brain injury.

▶ Initial Evaluation

1. Obtain complete vital signs, including temperature.

2. Assess for shock (peripheral hypoperfusion).

3. Measure oxygen saturation and consider blood gas analysis if appropriate.

4. Does the delirium lighten after administration of intravenous glucose, thiamine, and naloxone? If so, consider the following possibilities:

   • Hypoglycemia (diagnosis is confirmed by finding of low serum glucose)

   • Wernicke encephalopathy (look for associated alcoholism, malnutrition, ataxia, ophthalmoplegia, and peripheral neuropathy)

   • Opiate overdose (diagnosis is confirmed by positive response to naloxone and toxicology screen)

▶ Further Evaluation

A. Examination and Diagnostic Tests

1. History—Obtain a brief history from the patient, family, friends, neighbors, ambulance attendants, or bystanders. Ask in particular about prior episodes of confusion or delirium, duration and other features of the present episode, drug usage, and previous illness.

2. Physical and neurologic examination—Perform a general physical examination, and look especially for signs of trauma, meningeal irritation, and cardiac disease. Signs of meningeal irritation (meningismus: stiff neck, positive Kernig and Brudzinski signs) are almost invariably present in meningitis or SAH except in very young or very old patients. The most helpful diagnostic maneuver is passive flexion of the patient's neck, which elicits reflex knee flexion (usually unilateral) if meningeal irritation is present (positive Brudzinski sign). Perform lumbar puncture immediately in patients with meningismus in the absence of signs of increased intracranial pressure (papilledema, focal neurologic findings) for evaluation of cerebrospinal fluid. In patients with fever and focal neurologic findings, a brain abscess must be considered along with meningitis and encephalitis. A lumbar puncture is contraindicated until a CT scan has eliminated the possibility of a mass lesion. To avoid delay of needed treatment for possible meningitis while awaiting the results of the CT scan, obtain blood cultures and begin antibiotics immediately (Chapter 42).

Complete a basic neurologic examination, including tests of orientation and memory. Although focal signs may be found in metabolic brain disease (notably the fluctuating hemiparesis that may occur with hypoglycemia and hepatic encephalopathy), such asymmetric findings should be assumed to reflect a structural brain lesion until proved otherwise and a CT scan obtained for evaluation.

3. Laboratory studies—Send blood to the laboratory for CBC; serum electrolyte, glucose, calcium, and magnesium determinations; renal and liver function tests; carboxyhemoglobin level; and toxicology studies. Obtain urine for urinalysis and toxicology studies.

4. Electrocardiogram—Obtain an electrocardiogram in order to seek any abnormalities that might suggest a cardiac cause of the confusional state (eg, myocardial infarction, cardiac arrhythmias, prolonged intervals). T-wave changes, however, are nonspecific and may be seen with acute intracranial events.

5. Special studies—CT scan is indicated in most patients with an acute change in mental status. Other special studies may be indicated based on the results of history and physical examination (eg, lumbar puncture for cerebrospinal fluid in the patient with confusion and fever or signs of meningeal irritation).

6. Gastric decontamination—Administer an activated charcoal slurry (50–100 mg of activated charcoal admixed with water or sorbitol) and consider gastric lavage if ingestion or overdose of a toxin is a diagnostic possibility.

B. Trauma

If there is evidence of trauma—even if the head itself appears uninjured—consider the possibility of traumatic brain damage (eg, subdural or epidural hematomas). CT scan may be indicated (Chapter 22).

C. Other Causes of Delirium or Confusion

Once life-threatening conditions have been ruled out, a more specific diagnosis can be attempted. Main causes are shown in Table 37–4. Delirium or confusion occurring in patients with AIDS is discussed in Chapter 42.

▶ Treatment and Disposition

Almost all patients presenting with an acute confusion will require hospitalization.

Adams HP Jr, del Zoppo G, Alberts MJ et al: Guidelines for the early management of adults with ischemic stroke: a guideline from the American Heart Association/American Stroke Association Stroke Council, Clinical Cardiology Council, Cardiovascular Radiology and Intervention Council, and the Atherosclerotic Peripheral Vascular Disease and Quality of Care Outcomes in Research. Stroke 2007;38:1655–1711 [PMID: 17431204].

Benderson JB, Connolly ES, Batjer RG et al: Guidelines for the management of aneurismal subarachnoid: a ststement for healthcare professionals from a special writing group of the Stroke council, American Heart Association. Stroke 2009;40:994–1025 [PMID: 19164800].

Broderick J, Connolly S, Feldman E et al: Guidelines from the American Heart Association/American Stroke Council, High Blood Pressure Research Council, and the Quality of Care and Outcomes in Research Interdisciplinary Working Group. Stroke 2007;38:2001–2023 [PMID: 17478736].

Diedler S, Sykora M, Juttler E, Steiner T, Hacke W: Intensive care management of acute stroke: general management. Int J Stroke 2009;4:365–378 [PMID: 1976512].

Dringer MN: Management of aneurismal subarachnoid hemorrhage. Crit Care Med 2009;37:432–440 [PMID: 19114880].

Fulgham JR, Ingall TJ, Stead LG, Cloft HJ, Wijdicks EF, Flemming KD: Management of acute ischemic stroke. Mayo Clin Proc 2004;79:1459–1469 [PMID: 15544028].

Manno EM: Subarachnoid hemorrhage. Neurol Clin 2004;22:347–366 [PMID: 15062516].

Provenzale JM, Hacein-Bey L: CT evaluation of subarachnoid hemorrhage: apractial review for the radiologist interpreting emergency room studies. Emerg Radiol 2009;16:441–451 [PMID: 19543757].

Seder DB, Mayer SA: Critical care management of subarachnoid hemorrhage and ischemic stroke. Clin Cheat Med 2009;30:103–122 [PMID: 19186283].

Washburn LA: Altered mental status: Cause determines treatment. JAPPA 2005;18:16–22 [PMID: 15742778].

Table 37–4. Differential Diagnosis of Conditions Causing Delirium or Confusion.

Etiologic Category	Clinical Findings
Central nervous system mass lesion (subdural hematoma, cerebral infarction, brain tumor)	Somnolence; neurologic examination shows focal or asymmetric abnormality. Posterior nondominant parietal lobe strokes present with an agitated delirium, without hemiparesis.
Meningitis or meningoencephalitis Infectious, carcinomatous, or chemical meningitis secondary to subarachnoid hemorrhage	Headache, fever, meningeal signs, cerebrospinal fluid pleocytosis
Seizure disorders Confusional states following seizures (postictal states) Psychomotor status epilepticus	History or evidence of seizures, especially seen in seizure patients with superimposed metabolic abnormality, encephalitis, or diffuse cerebral damage, in whom postictal state may be prolonged
Amnestic states	Findings confined to recent memory loss
Fluent aphasias	Sudden onset; patient alert; mild right hemiparesis (may be absent). Excessive speech with frequent word substitutions and nonsense phrases
Psychiatric disease (thought disorders and hysteria)	Paranoia prominent; auditory hallucinations common; disorientation as to person, which is greater than that as to place, which is greater than that as to time. Recent memory preserved
Head trauma (acute posttraumatic delirium, post-concussion syndrome) Metabolic encephalopathy; drug intoxication or withdrawal	Recent history or evidence of head trauma Fluctuations in mental status (lucid intervals); asterixis; myoclonus; tremor; visual hallucinations; disorientation as to time, which is greater than that as to place, which is greater than that as to person; nystagmus

▼ EMERGENCY MANAGEMENT OF SPECIFIC CENTRAL NEUROLOGIC DISORDERS

LACUNAR STROKE

ESSENTIALS OF DIAGNOSIS

- ▶ Most frequent in basal ganglia and internal capsule
- ▶ Five classical lacunar syndromes
  Pure motor stroke/hemiparesis
  - ▶ Most common syndrome
  - ▶ Usually affects face, arm, leg equally
  - ▶ Transient sensory symptoms (but not signs) may be present
  Ataxic hemiparesis
  - ▶ Second most common syndrome
  - ▶ Weakness and clumsiness on one side of body; legs affected more commonly than arms
  Dysarthria/clumsy hand
  - ▶ Facial weakness
  - ▶ Severe dysarthria
  - ▶ Slight weakness and clumsy hand

Pure sensory stroke (Thalamus)
- ▶ Persistent numbness or tingling on one side of the body (face, arm, leg, trunk)
- ▶ Unpleasant sensation
Mixed sensorimotor stroke
- ▶ Hemiparesis or hemiplegia noted
- ▶ Ipsilateral sensory impairment

▶ Clinical Findings

Lacunar stroke results from occlusion of the small penetrating arteries of the brain by lipohyalinotic deposits, which are a product of long-standing hypertension. The areas of infarction are generally small, and multiple old infarct sites may also be identified on CT scan. The clinical findings are distinct and may range from pure motor or pure sensory deficits to incoordination and clumsiness of the hand or ataxia of the arm or leg. CT scan is often normal or may show small areas of reduced attenuation in the affected areas, usually in the internal capsule, basal ganglia, or upper brain stem.

▶ Treatment and Disposition

Treatment is supportive and consists mainly of blood pressure control. The prognosis is generally good. Patients should usually be hospitalized for observation.

ARTERIAL DISSECTION

ESSENTIALS OF DIAGNOSIS

► Nonspecific presenting signs and symptoms, neurologic deficits

► Headache, facial pain, neck swelling, pulsatile tinnitus

► More common in young adults

► May follow traumatic event or simple manipulation of the neck, or may be spontaneous

► Horner syndrome/bruit

► Clinical Findings

An acute progressive syndrome of carotid or vertebral artery ischemia almost invariably associated with anterior or posterior neck pain suggests carotid or vertebral artery dissection, respectively. A history of recent neck trauma is frequent and may be relatively trivial, such as chiropractic manipulation. However, dissection may occur spontaneously. The patient will complain of pain, transient monocular visual loss. They may also present with Horner's Syndrome. Emergent CT scan of the head is usually indicated to evaluate for ischemic complications. MR or CT angiography has displaced conventional catheter angiography as the imaging study of choice to diagnose arterial dissection.

► Treatment and Disposition

Current opinion favors anticoagulation acutely and for several months thereafter to reduce the potential for distal embolization of platelet aggregates formed on the damaged vessel wall. Surgical or endovascular treatment is usually not primarily indicated and should be considered in patients whom medical management has failed to prevent further ischemic signs or those who have contraindications to anticoagulation.

TRANSIENT ISCHEMIC ATTACKS (TIA)

ESSENTIALS OF DIAGNOSIS

► Rapid onset of neurologic symptoms lasting typically less than 60 minutes and rarely up to 24 hours

► Clinical Findings

The definition of a TIA has changed from focal neurologic deficits that persist less than 24 hours to a focal neurological event lasting less than one hour with a normal neuroimaging study. Most stroke nuerologist accept the new definition but the general nuerologist and the wider medical community continue to prefer the classic definition. Most TIA symptoms last less than one hour and they typically resolve within 30 minutes. Studies using the 24 hour definition demonstrate that between 8.6 and 11.5% of patients will have a stroke within seven days of a TIA, The 90-day stroke risk ranges from 10.5 to 17.3% in patients who have had a TIA. One study showed that 50% of the strokes occurred within 2 days of the TIA. A TIA should therefore be promptly evaluated to institute therapy to decrease the risk of stroke. Clinical findings depend on the area of the brain affected. Transient monocular blindness due to embolus in the retinal artery (amaurosis fugax) usually signifies ipsilateral carotid artery disease, but unlike hemispheric TIA, amaurosis fugax is associated with less risk for subsequent carotid stroke.

► Treatment

Treatment is directed at identifying and correcting the underlying cause (eg, treat hypertension, evaluate for carotid endarterectomy). Antiplatelet agents are typically the treatment of choice for prevention of future strokes in patients who have experienced a TIA of presumed atherosclerotic origin. The selection of a specific agent is typically based on interpretation of the results of randomized trials that have tested these agents in populations of patients who have had a recent TIA or stroke. Anticoagulation and surgical intervention may be appropriate in selected patients.

A. Aspirin

Aspirin is the most economical and frequently chosen (except in intolerant patients) antiplatelet regimen in patients with TIA. Aspirin can be used in doses of 75–1300 mg/d for the prevention of stroke.

B. Ticlopidine

Ticlopidine prevents platelet aggregation induced by adenosine diphosphate. Its use has been approved in the United States for prevention of stroke in patients with TIA or minor stroke. Typically used in patients who are intolerant to aspirin or who have had an ischemic event despite taking aspirin, its usefulness is limited by its side effects. The recommended dosage is 250 mg two times a day.

C. Clopidogrel

Clopidogrel works by inhibiting platelet aggregation by adenosine diphosphate. It offers another alternative to patients intolerant to aspirin or to those who have had an ischemic event despite taking aspirin. It has a good safety profile. The recommended dosage is 75 mg/d.

D. Anticoagulation

Oral anticoagulation with warfarin continues to be the therapy of choice for stroke prevention in atrial fibrillation and is preferred for those with prosthetic valves. In patients in whom oral anticoagulation is contraindicated, aspirin is recommended. Current recommendations suggest a target range INR of 2.0–3.0 for most indications for oral anticoagulation.

E. Surgical Interventions

1. Carotid endarterectomy—This intervention is used to remove atherosclerotic plaque from a carotid artery when the vessel is blocked. It has proved beneficial in preventing future strokes in certain patients with minor strokes or TIAs. The procedure is indicated when the vessel has a 70–99% blockage. When the vessel is 50–69% blocked, carotid endarterectomy is recommended; and when the vessel is less than 50% stenosed, there is no benefit from the procedure and medical management is recommended.

2. Carotid angioplasty and stent placement—This method has had a high degree of technical success, and low complication rates have been reported. This technology is not yet widely available.

▶ Disposition

Most patients with TIAs should be hospitalized. Patients who have had recent thorough evaluation for TIAs or who are not candidates for surgical or interventional therapy may be referred to their primary care physician for outpatient follow-up.

SPINAL CORD COMPRESSION

ESSENTIALS OF DIAGNOSIS

▶ Acute or rapidly progressing neurologic deficit
▶ May be from trauma, cancer, infection, spinal stenosis, or disc herniation

Spinal cord compression is most commonly caused by metastatic cancers representing 85–95% of spinal cord compression cases. Other causes include spinal epidural abcess, epidural hematomas and central disc herniation. Patients present with back pain and neurologic impairment referred to the spinal level of the lesion. Rapid assessment and diagnosis is the key since emergency surgery or radiation therapy may be needed to prevent permanent paraplegia or quadriplegia.

A. Locate Level of Lesion

Acute spinal cord compression is associated with weakness and sensory loss caudad to the level of involvement. Cord-mediated functions cephalad to this level and cranial nerve (CN) examination will be normal.

1. Cervical level—Both upper and lower extremity weaknesses are present, but CN function is normal. Respiratory insufficiency is especially likely with high cervical cord lesions.

2. Thoracic level—Lower extremity weakness is present, but the upper extremities and CNs are spared. Because spinal cord compression involves sensory and motor pathways, a sensory level should be carefully sought by eliciting reactions to pinprick or a cold object placed against the skin.

3. Lower spinal cord, or cauda equina, involvement—Signs and symptoms include bladder or bowel incontinence, sensory loss in sacral (saddle) distribution, and lower extremity weakness.

4. Vertebral body involvement—If spinal cord compression is due to a process that also involves the vertebral bodies (eg, metastatic tumor, epidural abscess), focal tenderness during vertebral percussion will be noted. Radiologic evidence of bony erosion or collapse of the vertebral column at the spinal cord level responsible for the abnormal neurologic findings virtually establishes the diagnosis.

B. Perform Emergency Imaging

Patients with suspected spinal cord compression due to any cause require emergency imaging preferably with MRI, if available. Unfortunately, CT scans are of limited value. Emergent neurosurgical or orthopedic consultation is indicated for documented spinal cord compression. If metastatic cancer is responsible, additional consultation with radiation oncologist is warranted.

METASTATIC TUMORS CAUSING SPINAL COMPRESSION

ESSENTIALS OF DIAGNOSIS

▶ Slowly progressive
▶ Stuttering neurologic deficit

▶ Clinical Findings

The most common primary malignant neoplasms producing epidural metastases and spinal cord compression are breast cancer (20%), lung cancer (10%), Hodgkin disease (10%), and prostate cancer (7%).

A. Symptoms and Signs

Local vertebral column pain at the level of the spinal cord lesion is the presenting symptom in the vast majority of patients. This symptom usually precedes neurologic deterioration by weeks to months, but occasionally it may be present for only a few hours.

Onset of radicular radiation of the pain (involvement of the territory of a nerve root) heralds progression. Radiation of the pain may be bilateral, especially when the thoracic spine is involved. This is followed by signs and symptoms of myelopathy to include extremity weakness, paresthesias, sensory impairment, and bladder and bowel dysfunction. Sensory and motor impairment soon ascends to a spinal cord level just below the site of the lesion.

B. Imaging

X-rays of the spine may reveal bony destruction by the tumor at the involved vertebral level. However, in a cancer patient with new onset back pain, or worsening back pain, an MRI of the spine is indicated. If the patient has neurologic deficits, emergency MRI is indicated. Pain without signs or symptoms of myelopathy should have an MRI within 24 hours.

▶ Treatment and Disposition

Patients with this diagnosis should be given corticosteroids immediately to reduce peritumoral edema (eg, dexamethasone, 10–40 mg intravenously, followed by 4 mg every 6 hours intravenously or orally). Obtain emergency neurosurgical consultation if spinal cord compression is demonstrated on MRI and the patient has neurologic symptoms. Hospitalization is required for decompression by laminectomy or local radiotherapy.

TRANSVERSE MYELITIS

ESSENTIALS OF DIAGNOSIS

▶ Rapid onset of motor and sensory loss
▶ Sphincter disturbances

▶ General Considerations

Transverse myelitis is a poorly defined entity that is usually idiopathic but may be a manifestation of a known systemic disease (multiple sclerosis or systemic lupus erythematosus).

▶ Clinical Findings

A. Symptoms and Signs

The presenting symptoms are equally divided between motor weakness, sensory loss or paresthesia, and back and radicular pain. Symptoms and signs of transverse (bilateral)

cord involvement may progress to a maximum level within hours. Vertebral tenderness to percussion is noted in about half of cases.

B. Imaging

An MRI or myelogram is required to exclude a compressive lesion; myelography will almost always demonstrate free flow of contrast material.

▶ Treatment and Disposition

Treatment is supportive care only. Partial to full recovery may occur over a period of weeks to months. Hospitalization is recommended for diagnosis and supportive care. Steroid treatment is frequently used, but its benefit is uncertain. Plasma exchange may be of benefit.

SPINAL EPIDURAL ABSCESS

ESSENTIALS OF DIAGNOSIS

▶ Fever, localized back pain; radiating pain (along nerve root); sensory disturbances
▶ Tenderness to percussion or palpation
▶ Reflexes may be hypoactive, absent, brisk, or spastic

Spinal epidural abscess is one-eighth as common as transverse myelitis, but it may be associated with remarkably similar signs and symptoms.

▶ Clinical Findings

The most common predisposing conditions include local staphylococcal infections of the skin and surgical wounds (including intravenous sites), bacteremia, vertebral osteomyelitis, spondylodiscitis, and intravenous drug abuse.

A. Symptoms and Signs

Patients are usually febrile and appear acutely ill on presentation. Focal pain and localized tenderness over the abscess are nearly consistent findings. Classically, symptoms progress over a few days from local vertebral column pain to radiating radicular pain. Cord compression with weakness and sensory loss below the level of the lesion follows.

B. Imaging

Plain X-rays of the spine reveal osteomyelitic lesions in about some cases, especially in patients with symptoms of long duration (weeks). MRI is the imaging modality of choice for suspected spinal abscess

C. Laboratory Findings

Lumbar puncture should not be done as part of the diagnostic workup. Meningitis may result if the needle is advanced through the abscess, allowing pus to enter the subarachnoid space. Almost all patients will have an elevated ESR and CRP. Blood cultures should be obtained and may provide the causative organism in 60% of the cases.

▶ Treatment and Disposition

Hospitalization is required for emergency surgical decompression by laminectomy, abscess drainage, and intravenous antimicrobial therapy. Selected patients without significant weakness can be managed with antibiotics alone.

Bluman EM, Palumbo MA, Lucas PR: Spinal epidural abscess in adults. J Am Acad Orthop Surg 2004;12:155–163 [PMID: 15161168].

Costello F: Carotid artery dissection and vertebrobasilar insufficiency. Int Prhthalmol clin 2009;49:1–14 [PMID: 19584618].

Flemming KD, Brown RD, Jr, Petty GW, Huston J, 3rd, Kallmes DF, Piepgras DG: Evaluation and management of transient ischemic attack and minor cerebral infarction. Mayo Clin Proc 2004;79:1071–1086 [PMID: 15301338].

Kaplin AI, Krishnan C, Deshpande DM, Pardo CA, Kerr DA: Diagnosis and management of acute myelopathies. Neurologist 2005;11:2–18 [PMID: 15631640].

Lewandowski CA, Rao CP, Silver B: Transient ischemic attack: definitions and clinical presentations. Ann emerg Med 2008; 52:S7–S16 [PMID: 18655918].

Nguyen-Huynh MN, Johnston SC: Transient ischemic attack: a neurologic emergency. Curr Neurol Neurosci Rep 2005;5(1): 13–20 [PMID: 15676103].

Ruckdeschel JC: Early detection and treatment of spinal cord compression. Oncology 2005;19:81–86 [PMID: 15743153].

Winters ME, Kluetz P, Zilberstein J: Back pain emergencies. Med Clin North Am 2006;90:505–523 [PMID: 16473102].

EMERGENCY MANAGEMENT OF PERIPHERAL NEUROPATHIES

MONONEUROPATHIES

BELL'S PALSY

ESSENTIALS OF DIAGNOSIS

- ▶ Cranial nerve VII paralysis
- ▶ Abrupt, isolated, unilateral, peripheral facial paralysis
- ▶ Diagnosis of exclusion; unknown cause
- ▶ Entire face is involved on affected side (unlike in cortical stroke, where upper third of face is spared)

▶ General Considerations

Bell's palsy is a common condition of unknown cause (although some authorities suggest a link with herpes simplex infection). Although manifestations of the disorder are dramatic, recovery usually begins within 1 month, and complete resolution of symptoms occurs in 70–85% of patients. All patients with initial subtotal facial paralysis will make a cosmetically complete functional recovery.

▶ Clinical Findings

Diagnostic features include the following:

- Development of symptoms in over less than 24–48 hours
- Unilateral involvement of the facial nerve
- No signs of other nervous system involvement
- Postauricular pain (not required for diagnosis)

▶ Differential Diagnosis

The major differential diagnostic possibilities—and those of most concern to patients—are stroke and tumor. Tumors in the region of the facial nerve rarely cause sudden onset of symptoms and usually produce abnormalities of other facial nerves, resulting in nystagmus, decreased hearing, and ataxia. Facial numbness may suggest involvement of the trigeminal nerve, but patients with Bell's palsy often describe pure facial weakness in sensory terms (eg, "My face is numb.").

Stroke with facial weakness is associated with weakness of the ipsilateral arm and probably the ipsilateral leg also (most easily detectable in the extensors of the arm and the flexors of the leg). Stroke produces an upper motor neuron lesion, thereby sparing the muscles of the forehead. Bell's palsy, however, involves the facial nerve itself and produces unilateral weakness of all facial muscles (those of the forehead, those responsible for eye closure, and those around the mouth). Other facial nerve functions may be involved, such as unilateral decrease of lacrimation and taste and increase in apparent intensity of sounds (eg, when talking on the telephone).

▶ Laboratory Tests and Other Examinations

When the diagnosis is clear on clinical grounds, no further evaluation or radiographic studies (CT scans or MRI) are indicated.

▶ Treatment and Disposition

Although Bell's palsy is cosmetically disfiguring during the acute phase, the more serious concern is the risk for eye injury owing to inability to close the eyelid completely. Artificial tears should be instilled frequently during waking hours, and the lid should be taped closed (under careful instruction) when the patient is asleep to prevent corneal abrasions and ulcers. Corticosteroids may affect the ultimate recovery of motor function such as prednisone, 40–60 mg/d orally for 10 days, decrease the postauricular pain often associated with acute Bell's palsy. Acyclovir, 400 mg five times daily for 10 days with steroids, may possibly provide a faster recovery. All patients should be referred to a neurologist, otolaryngologist, or primary care physician within a few days, regardless of whether corticosteroids have been given. Hospitalization is not required.

COMPRESSIVE MONONEUROPATHIES

▶ General Considerations

Compressive mononeuropathies usually occur because of prolonged compression of a superficial peripheral nerve producing injury. This may result from repeated stress to connective tissues, sleep in an unusual position or from prolonged fixed position of a limb due to drug intoxication or general anesthesia.

▶ Carpal Tunnel Syndrome

Median nerve neuropathy at the wrist is the most common upper extremity neuropathy. It is found more often in females and is typically bilateral with more prominent symptoms in the dominant hand. Patients complain of pain in the hand and wrist with paresthesias in the in the medial thumb, index, middle and lateral fouth fingers. Exam findings may include decreased sensation to light touch, a positive Tinel's sign and production of paresthesias in the median nerve distribution with wrist flexion (Phalen's maneuver).

Treatment consists of conservative treatment, removing causative maneuvers, a wrist splint in the neutral position and nonsteroidal anti-inflammatory medications. Refer all to primary care or a hand specialist is indicated for further evaluation with nerve conductive studies and more aggressive treatment with local corticosteroid injections or surgery if conservative treatment fails or symptoms progress.

▶ Radial Nerve Palsy

Paralysis of the radial nerve produces complete but isolated wrist and finger drop (inability to extend the wrist or fingers) with numbness over the lateral dorsum of the hand. Such injuries occur from compression of the nerve against the humerus in patients sedated with alcohol or other drugs (Saturday night palsy) or during sleep with a partner (bridegroom's palsy). If the radial nerve is compressed in the axilla, as occurs in crutch palsy, the triceps muscle is affected as well, resulting in the additional finding of weakness of extension at the elbow.

Complete recovery over weeks to months is the rule. Immediate treatment measures include cockup splint to the wrist with fingers extended. Refer the patient to a primary care physician, hand specialist, or neurologist.

▶ Ulnar Palsy

Acute injury of the ulnar nerve occurs at the elbow following fracture or dislocation. Delayed ulnar nerve palsies result from repeated trauma, such as resting of upper body weight on the elbows. Wasting and weakness of the hands ultimately produce a claw posture (hyperextension at the metacarpophalangeal joint and flexion at the interphalangeal joints that are maximal in the fourth and fifth digits). Sensory loss occurs in the ulnar border of the dorsal and palmar aspects of the hand below the wrist, extending to involve the fourth and fifth fingers. Injury to the ulnar nerve in the palm (eg, cycle-racing palsy) spares the sensory fibers.

Initial management consists of padding of the elbow and referral to a primary care physician, hand specialist, or neurologist.

▶ Peroneal Nerve Palsy

Nerve compression occurs at the head of the fibula as a result of acute trauma (eg, fibular fracture, or sleeping or sitting with the legs crossed). The resulting footdrop produces a high-stepping gait in the involved limb, with inability to dorsiflex or evert the foot on examination. Some sensory loss may be found over the dorsum of the foot and the lateral aspects of the calf.

Lesions at the root of L5 (eg, disk disease) also produce footdrop but involve other muscles innervated by L5 as well (eg, foot invertors and knee flexors).

Immediate management in the emergency department or upon referral to an orthopedist, primary care physician, neurologist, or physical medicine specialist consists of splinting the foot at a right angle (cock-up splint) to normalize the gait.

POLYNEUROPATHIES

GUILLAIN-BARRÉ SYNDROME

ESSENTIALS OF DIAGNOSIS

- ▶ Acute ascending progressive neuropathy starting in lower extremities; weakness is symmetric
- ▶ Paresthesias, hyporeflexia
- ▶ Muscle weakness may lead to respiratory failure
- ▶ Labile autonomic dysfunction (labile vital signs)
- ▶ History of gastrointestinal or respiratory infection approximately 1–3 weeks prior to onset of weakness

▶ General Considerations

Guillain-Barré syndrome is a common disease of uncertain cause involving the peripheral nerves and occurring in both sexes and all age groups. In two thirds of cases, a mild upper respiratory infection or gastroenteritis precedes the onset of the neurologic disease by 1–3 weeks. Well-documented cases have also been recorded following surgery, other viral infections, immunization (eg, influenza vaccine), and acute glomerulonephritis or as an acute seroconversion reaction to HIV infection. Marked hypophosphatemia can produce a nearly identical syndrome.

▶ Clinical Findings

A. Symptoms and Signs

Symmetric motor weakness is the major symptom. It may be either proximal or distal at onset and usually begins in the lower extremities. The weakness classically progresses in an ascending manner, involving first the lower and then the upper extremities and finally the cranial nerves (CN) within 1–3 days of symptom onset. The weakness does not ascend in all cases, however.

Subjective and objective sensory disturbances (numbness or paresthesias) of brief duration are common initially and may be the presenting complaint. These dysesthesias most commonly occur in a distal (stocking-glove) distribution. Muscle pain or tenderness is also an early symptom in about half of cases.

Absence of the deep tendon reflexes (or, rarely, only distal areflexia with definite hyporeflexia of biceps and knee jerks) almost always occurs by the time of presentation to a physician. *Note*: This loss of reflexes is the most important clue to diagnosis and is found even in muscles that cannot yet be shown to be weak by objective testing.

CN involvement is common; involvement of every nerve except CNs I and II (olfactory and optic) has been described. The nerve most commonly affected is CN VII (facial); facial weakness (usually bilateral) occurs in half of the cases. CN palsies may be the most prominent feature of the illness, as in the Guillain-Barré variant of ophthalmoplegia, ataxia, and areflexia.

Peripheral autonomic nervous system involvement also occurs and may be manifested by hypertension, tachycardia, facial flushing, postural hypotension, and electrocardiographic changes. Respiratory musculature weakness requiring assisted ventilation occurs in 25% of cases.

B. Laboratory Findings

Increased spinal fluid pressure is seen only in severe cases. The cerebrospinal fluid cell count is normal initially in most patients; less than 10% of patients have more than 10 leukocytes per microliter. The classic elevation in cerebrospinal fluid protein to levels as high as 100–400 mg/dL in the absence of significant pleocytosis (so-called albuminocytologic dissociation) may not be seen until several days after the onset of symptoms. These cerebrospinal fluid findings support the diagnosis of Guillain-Barré syndrome, but they are not specific and may be seen occasionally in any acute

or chronic polyneuritis. Nerve conduction studies can aid in the diagnosis.

▶ Treatment and Disposition

Endotracheal intubation and ventilatory support should be considered in the emergency department for patients in respiratory failure. High-dose immunoglobulin IVIg and plasmapheresis are equally effective treatments. Corticosteroids are ineffective and may prolong the disease in elderly patients. All patients should be hospitalized.

ARSENICAL NEUROPATHY

See also Chapter 47.

ESSENTIALS OF DIAGNOSIS

▶ Painful peripheral neuropathy

▶ Acute poisoning: vomiting and severe diarrhea leading to dehydration and shock

▶ Chronic poisoning: classical dermatitis, peripheral neuropathy, and chronic renal and hepatic damage

▶ General Considerations

The neuropathy of arsenic poisoning is a rapidly progressive sensorimotor polyneuropathy that in many ways mimics Guillain-Barré syndrome. It manifests weeks after exposure. Common sources of arsenic include rat and ant poison and the copper acetoarsenite contained in insecticides (eg, Paris green). Fowler's solution, once used for psoriasis, also contains arsenic. Patients with chronic symptoms may represent attempted murder.

▶ Clinical Findings

A. Symptoms and Signs

Abdominal pain, nausea and vomiting, and diarrhea occur minutes to hours following ingestion. A rapidly progressive polyneuropathy ensues 7–14 days later. Symmetric ascending paresthesias, initially distal, begin in the lower extremities and progress to overt sensory loss. Diffuse muscle aches and tenderness are common, as is a burning pain on the soles of the feet that is markedly aggravated by touching the skin. Deep tendon reflexes are depressed early and in the same distribution as the sensory loss.

Symmetric motor impairment follows as the neuropathy progresses over days to a few weeks and is typically more severe distally and in the lower extremities and can lead to flaccid paralysis. The CNs, rectal sphincter, and respiratory muscles are unaffected.

Cutaneous stigmata of arsenical poisoning include increased skin pigmentation and marked exfoliation (especially of the hands and feet). Mees's lines (transverse white, nonpalpable lines on the nails) are especially suggestive of arsenic poisoning but do not appear until 40–60 days after ingestion because of the slow rate of nail growth.

B. Laboratory Findings

The diagnosis is established by documenting elevated concentrations of arsenic in urine with more than 50 μg/L in a single sample or more than 100 μg/L in a 24-hour urine collection. Hair protected from external contamination, most commonly pubic hair (upper limits of normal: 0.1–0.5 mg/kg) can be used as well.

C. Imaging

If continued ingestion of arsenic is suspected, abdominal X-ray may be helpful, since arsenic is radiopaque.

▶ Treatment

(See also Chapter 47) Symptomatic patients should be given a chelating agent to facilitate excretion of arsenic. Treatment must be started within 24 hours after ingestion to influence the course of the neuropathy. Give dimercaprol, 3–4 mg/kg/dose intramuscularly every 4 hours for 48 hours, then 3 mg/kg every 12 hours for a total of 10 days. Follow urine arsenic levels, because hair and nail levels do not reflect acute changes.

▶ Disposition

If arsenic poisoning is diagnosed or suspected, hospitalization is indicated for evaluation and treatment.

TICK PARALYSIS

ESSENTIALS OF DIAGNOSIS

▶ Acute ascending paralysis a few days after tick attachment

▶ Constitutional symptoms are absent

▶ Rapid reversal of clinical and physiologic deficits post tick removal

▶ General Considerations

Tick paralysis is a rapidly ascending motor paralysis caused by an injected neurotoxin from the female *Dermacentor andersoni* (wood tick) and *Dermacentor variabilis* (dog tick). Symptoms begin after the ticks have been attached to the patient for 5–7 days.

▶ Clinical Findings

A. Symptoms and Signs

Most cases occur in children. Neurologic symptoms begin with ataxia and lower extremity weakness, the latter progressing over 24–48 hours to involve the upper extremities and CNs. Reflexes are diminished or absent early. Respiratory depression occurs and may be fatal. Distal extremity paresthesias are common, but objective sensory loss is rare.

B. Laboratory Findings

Cerebrospinal fluid and peripheral blood examinations are normal.

▶ Treatment

The tick may be attached to any portion of the body but is most commonly hidden in long hair about the head and neck. Removal of the entire tick is followed by symptomatic improvement within hours. Complete resolution of symptoms occurs within a few days to a week.

▶ Disposition

Patients in the acute phase must be hospitalized for supportive management.

DISEASES OF THE NEUROMUSCULAR JUNCTION

BOTULISM

ESSENTIALS OF DIAGNOSIS

▶ Progressive, symmetric, descending weakness, first in muscles innervated by cranial nerves, then neck, arms, and legs

▶ Dry mouth, diplopia, dysarthria, generalized weakness

▶ General Considerations

Clostridium botulinum toxin attacks the neuromuscular junction by impairing the release of acetylcholine at all peripheral synapses. Paralysis occurs mainly following the ingestion of foods contaminated with the toxin and only rarely from infected wounds. In infants, cases result from colonization of the gastrointestinal tract by *C. botulinum* (originating, in some cases, from ingested honey). Although commercially canned foods have caused epidemics, most cases have been due to improperly home-canned vegetables, fruits, meat, and fish. Ingestion of even a few drops of contaminated food

Table 37–5. Symptoms and Signs of Botulism in Approximate Order of Frequency.

Symptoms	Signs
Nausea and vomiting	Extraocular muscle weakness
Generalized weakness	Ptosis
Blurred vision	Bilaterally dilated and unreactive pupils
Diplopia	Dry mucous membranes
Dysphagia	Limb weakness
Dyspnea	Respiratory impairment
Dry mouth	Postural hypotension
Dizziness (especially postural)	
Constipation	
Abdominal fullness	

may cause botulism. The distribution of the toxin in the contaminated vehicle may not be uniform. Fruits or vegetables contaminated with type A or B toxin will taste spoiled; other foods may not.

▶ **Clinical Findings**

A. Symptoms and Signs

Symptoms usually begin 12–48 hours following toxin ingestion and may progress over hours to days (Table 37–5). The shorter the interval between ingestion and the appearance of symptoms, the more severe the disease. The nervous system is involved in descending fashion, beginning with the muscles innervated by the CNs. This contrasts with Guillain-Barré syndrome, in which there is usually ascending involvement.

Nausea and vomiting are the initial symptoms in one-third of the cases (prominent with type E toxin). Blurring of vision (due to paralysis of muscles of accommodation) is the most common initial neurologic symptom. Diplopia, dysphagia, and dysphonia come on in sequence as lower bulbar muscles become involved. Weakness of respiratory and extremity muscles follows as the paralysis descends. Ptosis, extraocular muscle paralysis, and pupillary dilatation and fixation follow, and then weakness of jaw and palate function. Some deep tendon reflex activity remains until muscle paralysis is complete.

Dryness of mucous membranes and orthostatic hypotension have been prominent features in some patients. There are no sensory abnormalities.

Infant botulism is characterized by poor feeding, poor muscle tone, episodes of aspiration, and constipation.

B. Laboratory Findings

Examination of cerebrospinal fluid and peripheral blood smears is not helpful unless a superimposed condition develops (eg, aspiration pneumonia). Specimens of blood or contaminated food should be saved for laboratory assay for botulinum toxins (available through local public health departments). Blood samples should consist of 30 mL of clotted, nonheparinized blood, which need not be centrifuged or separated but must be collected before the antitoxin is started. In infants, save a sample of stool for culture for *C. botulinum* (consult the local public health department for details).

▶ **Treatment**

A. Antitoxin

Trivalent equine antitoxin (type A, B, and E) should be given as soon as possible after diagnosis. Skin testing should be performed before administration of antitoxin because of the risk of anaphylaxis. The current recommended dose of licensed botulinum antitoxin is a single 10 mL vial (per patient), diluted 1:10 in a 0.9% saline solution and given in a slow intravenous infusion. The local health department should be notified immediately. With rapid diagnosis and adequate supportive care, the mortality rate has dropped to less than 10%. Recovery of neurologic function occurs over weeks to months; complete recovery is common.

B. Antibiotics

The treatment of wound botulism is debridement and penicillin, 300,000 units/kg/d intravenously, in addition to other measures described above. Clindamycin, 30 mg/kg/d intravenously, or chloramphenicol, 50 mg/kg/d intravenously, may be used in penicillin-allergic patients. Aminoglycosides may worsen neuromuscular blockade and should be avoided.

C. Additional Measures

Careful monitoring of vital capacity, maximum inspiratory force, and arterial blood gases is mandatory, because respiratory insufficiency may develop rapidly. Cathartics and enemas must be given early to remove any toxin remaining in the bowel. Emesis or gastric lavage is indicated if the contaminated food was ingested less than 6–8 hours before arrival at the emergency department.

▶ **Disposition**

The patient must be hospitalized for observation and treatment.

ORGANOPHOSPHATE POISONING

See also Chapter 47.

General Considerations

Organophosphates exert their toxic effect by inhibiting acetylcholinesterase, producing stimulation and then inhibition at the myoneural junction by the uncatabolized acetylcholine. Poisoning is most commonly due to insecticides (eg, parathion, malathion) and occurs during spraying or dusting of crops. Organophosphates can be absorbed through lungs, skin, gastrointestinal tract, and mucous membranes.

Clinical Findings

Rapidity of onset and severity of symptoms vary with the dose and route of administration; symptoms of poisoning may occur within 5 minutes to 12 hours after exposure.

A. Symptoms and Signs

Initial symptoms are fatigue, headache, dizziness, nausea and vomiting, and increased salivary and sweat production. Weakness of skeletal and bulbar muscles with marked fasciculations follows, and finally loss of consciousness occurs.

Lacrimation is common, and pupils are pinpoint and may be unreactive to light. Muscle fasciculations and complete motor paralysis may be present.

B. Laboratory Findings

Hyperglycemia with prominent glycosuria may occur. Polymorphonuclear leukocytosis is common. Laboratory demonstration of depressed plasma and erythrocyte cholinesterase activity confirms the clinical diagnosis.

Treatment

A. Decontamination

Maintain airway and respiratory function, and remove residual organophosphate by washing the skin and removing exposed clothing. Ingested organophosphates should be removed by lavage and catharsis. Induction of emesis is usually contraindicated because of the early onset of drowsiness and risk of aspiration. In this case, protect the airway and perform gastric lavage.

B. Specific Measures

Atropine, a specific antidote, is the treatment of choice; however, it does not reverse paralytic symptoms. Large doses may be required. Start with 0.5 mg/kg up to 2–4 mg IV, followed by repeated doses of 2–4 mg every 5–10 minutes until signs of atropinization occur: flushing, mydriasis, drying of secretions, and tachycardia. The use of up to 50 mg in 24 hours is not unusual.

Pralidoxime (Protopam, 2-Pam) releases organophosphates from acetylcholinesterase and should be given to all patients with significant poisoning. It should not be used for carbamate poisoning, because carbamates are not irreversibly bound to acetylcholinesterase. The dose is 20–40 mg/kg up to 1 g in saline intravenously over 20–30 minutes. The dose may be repeated in 1–2 hours. Adequate renal function is a prerequisite for use of pralidoxime, because it is excreted in the urine.

Benzodiazepines may be used for seizure control.

Disposition

All patients except for the very mildly ill with stable or improving symptoms require hospitalization. The earlier treatment is instituted, the lower the mortality rate.

MYASTHENIA GRAVIS

Clinical Findings

Musculature innervated by the CNs is commonly the earliest and most severely involved in myasthenia gravis, as manifested by ptosis and by impaired eye movements, facial expressions, chewing, swallowing, and speaking. Pupillary responsiveness is preserved. There is increasing weakness on repetitive muscle use ("fatigability"). Sensory abnormalities are absent.

The diagnosis in previously untreated myasthenia gravis is confirmed by objective and unequivocal improvement following anticholinesterase drugs, for example, edrophonium (Tensilon) or the longer-acting neostigmine (Prostigmin). Stable patients with myasthenia gravis will be taking one of the drug regimens listed in Table 37–6.

The acute occurrence of respiratory insufficiency or the inability to handle oropharyngeal secretions in a previously

Table 37–6. Drug Therapy of Stable Myasthenia Gravis.

Drug	Preparation	Dose	Duration of Action (h)
Pyridostigmine (mestinon)	60-mg tablets	1-4 tablets orally every 3-6 h	3-5
Pyridostigmine (mestinon)	180-mg sustained release capsules	1-3 capsules orally at bedtime	6-12
Neostigmine bromide (prostigmin)	15-mg tablets	1-4 tablets orally every 36 h	2-4
Neostigmine methylsulfate (prostigmin, others)	Solution for injection; 1:1000, 1:2000, 1:4000	1 mg (2 mL of 1:2000) intramuscularly or subcutaneously	2-4

stable myasthenic patient constitutes a myasthenic crisis. Crises may be precipitated by intercurrent infection or surgery or may have no obvious cause. The subjective complaint of dyspnea in such patients demands immediate and careful evaluation.

▶ Treatment

Immediately evaluate the need for respiratory assistance and endotracheal intubation, as described above. Temporizing with drug therapy may have disastrous consequences, because the patient may worsen within minutes. Discontinue anticholinesterase therapy in the intubated patient. Treat precipitating causes if present (eg, infection), but avoid aminoglycoside antibiotics because they may worsen myasthenia gravis. Plasmapheresis may temporarily reduce symptoms or help the patient to recover from the crisis. Intravenous immunoglobulin appears to have a role in acute treatment intervention when other modalities have failed.

▶ Disposition

All patients in myasthenic crisis require immediate hospitalization. Stable patients without any respiratory symptoms (not in crisis) may receive medical treatment and be referred for outpatient care. Patients newly diagnosed as having myasthenia gravis may be hospitalized for evaluation and treatment or started on a medical regimen (Table 37–6) and referred.

Cherington M: Botulism: update and review. Semin Neurol 2004;24:155–163 [PMID: 15257512].

Gilden DH: Clinical practice. Bell's Palsy. N Engl J Med 2004;351:1323–1331 [PMID: 15385659] (A comprehensive review of management of Bell's palsy).

Goonetilleke A, Harris JB: Clostridial neurotoxins. J Neurol Neurosurg Psychiatry 2004;75(Suppl 3):iii35–iii39 [PMID: 15316043].

Juel VC: Myasthenia gravis: management of myasthenic crisis and perioperative care. Semin Neurol 2004;24:75–81 [PMID: 15229794].

Kuwabara S: Guillain-Barre syndrome: epidemiology, pathophysiology and management. Drugs 2004;64:597–610 [PMID: 15018590].

Li Z, Turner RP: Pediatric tick paralysis: discussion of two cases and literature review. Pediatr Neurol 2004;31:304–307 [PMID: 15464647].

Newswanger DL, Warren CR: Guillain-Barré syndrome. Am Fam Physician 2004;69:2405–2410 [PMID: 15168961].

Rusyniak DE, Nanagas KA: Organophosphate poisoning. Semin Neurol 2004;24:197–204 [PMID: 15257517].

Scherer K, Bedlack RS, Simel DL: Does this patient have myasthenia gravis? JAMA 2005;293(15):1906–1914 [PMID: 15840866].

Shapiro BE, Preston DC: Entrapment and compressive neuropathies. Med clin North Am 2009; 93:285–315 [PMID: 19272510].

Vahidnia A, van der Voet GB, de Wolff FA: Arsenic neurotoxicity-a review. Hum Exp Toxicol 2007;26:823–832 [PMID: 18025055].

Vedanarayanan V, Sorey WH, Subramony SH: Tick paralysis. Semin Neurol 2004;24:181–184 [PMID: 15257515].

EMERGENCY MANAGEMENT OF MYOPATHIES

PRIMARY ACUTE MYOPATHIES

PERIODIC PARALYSIS

 ESSENTIALS OF DIAGNOSIS

▶ Usually presents after puberty, but may occur from early childhood up to age 30 years, rare after age 50 years

▶ Severe symmetric complete weakness

▶ Symptoms can last up to 1 week

▶ Exacerbated by strenuous exercise, high carbohydrate or sodium meals, cold temperatures

▶ Potassium may be decreased but is not necessarily below normal

▶ Increased urinary sodium, potassium, chloride

▶ Decreased serum phosphorous

Table 37–7. Disorders of Serum Potassium Causing Acute Muscle Weakness.

Hyperkalemia
   Potassium administration, orally or intravenously
   Renal insufficiency
   Potassium-retaining drug therapy: triamterene or spironolactone
   Acute tissue necrosis secondary to trauma or chemotherapy
   Addison disease
   Myoglobinuria
   Rhabdomyolysis
   Hypoaldosteronism
Hypokalemia
   Gastrointestinal potassium wastage
      Chronic vomiting or nasogastric suction
      Chronic diarrhea or laxative abuse
      Villous adenoma
      Draining gastrointestinal fistulas or ureteroileostomy
   Renal potassium wastage
      Drugs (diuretics, amphotericin B)
      Hyperaldosteronism
      Cushing disease or corticosteroid therapy
      Renal tubular acidosis
      Licorice (glycyrrhizic acid) intoxication

▶ General Considerations

Periodic paralysis is a rare disease characterized by episodes of profound weakness that may occur at intervals ranging from several times weekly to once in a lifetime. The episodes of paralysis are associated with blood potassium levels. There are three forms: hypokalemic, normokalemic, and hyperkalemic periodic paralysis. The first episode is usually during the teenage years and the disease is more common in males. Males also have more frequent attacks than females. The primary form of the disease is genetic, with secondary causes such as potassium loss from GI or renal disease or chronic hyperkalemia from renal or endocrine disease (Table 37–7). The normokalemic from of the disease does exist but is extremely rare.

▶ Clinical Findings

A. Symptoms and Signs

An attack of weakness usually lasts 2–24 hours. The weakness is painless and generalized, often beginning in the lower extremities and becoming more severe proximally. Paralysis of cranial and respiratory musculature is rare, and for this reason fatal episodes are uncommon. Extremity musculature is hypotonic during attacks. Reflexes are reduced in proportion to the muscle weakness. Sensory examination is normal. In all types, attacks are precipitated by rest after exercise. In the hypokalemic form a meal rich in carbohydrates is also a typical trigger. Hyperkalemic attacks are often associated with fasting and cold exposure.

The episodes typically occur more frequently in the hyperkalemic form but are milder then hypokelmic periodic paralysis.

B. Laboratory Findings

In primary hypokalemic periodic paralysis the potassium level is reduced from the patient's usual level. In patients with markedly reduced potassium, the disorder should be considered secondary and causes for loss of potassium, usually renal or gastrointestinal, should be sought. Serum phosphorus may also be decreased and should be measured. Thyroid function testing should be done to rule out thyrotoxic periodic paralysis. In hyperkalemic or hypokalemic periodic paralysis, the serum potassium levels are abnormal only during attacks making the differentiation between primary and secondary disease relatively easy.

▶ Treatment

Hypokalemic periodic paralysis is treated with potassium. Potassium may be given 1 mEq/kg orally at hourly intervals or as intravenous potassium chloride, with the rate of administration not exceeding 20 mEq/h. Clinical improvement usually occurs within 3–4 hours. The frequency and severity of attacks can be reduced with acetazolamide, 250 mg orally two or three times a day.

Hyperkalemic periodic paralysis attacks are mild and rarely result in the need for emergent treatment. If treatment is required glucose should be given and calcium and loop dirutics considered.

▶ Disposition

Patients having acute attacks can usually receive treatment in the emergency department and be sent home.

Fontaine B: Periodic Paralysis. Adv Genet 2008;63:3–23 [PMID: 19185183].

RHABDOMYOLYSIS

ESSENTIALS OF DIAGNOSIS

▶ Myalgias and muscle weakness

▶ Dark urine

▶ Tenderness, decreased muscle strength, swelling, bruising, and soft extremities (vs compartment syndrome) may be present

▶ Many causes, including trauma, toxic exposure, heat injury, strenuous exertion, infection, inflammatory disorders, and metabolic and endocrine disorders

Table 37–8. Common Causes of Rhabdomyolysis.

Muscle compression and necrosis secondary to prolonged coma (alcoholism, drug overdose, stroke)
Vigorous exercise, especially with poor conditioning and high environmental temperature
Status epilepticus
Delirium tremens
Chronic potassium depletion
Influenza or other acute viral infections

▶ General Considerations

Rhabdomyolysis is a syndrome where muscle injury leads to calcium release into the intracellular space triggering a cascade resulting in muscle protein destruction and release of potassium, phosphate, myoglobin, creatinine phosphokinase (CPK), and urate into the blood stream. Some of the many causes of rhabdomyolysis are summarized in Table 37–8. Weakness is the primary presenting complaint. Common life-threatening complications include acute renal failure and hyperkalemia.

▶ Clinical Findings

A. Symptoms and Signs

Pain and swelling of the involved muscles and weakness of the limbs occur, especially in proximal distribution. Reflexes are depressed in proportion to muscle weakness. Sensory examination is normal. Half of patients with rhabdomyolysis will have vague symptoms or be asymptomatic. Gross evidence of frank injury to muscle is frequently lacking.

B. Laboratory Findings

Serum CK will rise 2–12 hours post muscle injury and peak in 1–3 days. Typically, an elevation of CPK that is five times the upper limit of normal, is the definition used to make the diagnosis of rhabdomyolysis. However, there is no correlation between CPK levels and disease severity or complications. The urine may be red-tinged and turns dark brown on standing. Myoglobinuria may be suggested by a heme-positive (dipstick) test in erythrocyte-free urine and confirmed by specific chemical testing. Serum potassium should be measured since hyperkalemia is a life threatening complication of the disease.

▶ Treatment

Treatment consists of hydration to ensure high urine volumes and prevent precipitation of myoglobin in renal tubules to prevent renal failure or lessen its severity. A recommended regimen is normal saline at a rate of 1.5 L/h. Maintain urine output at 2 mL/kg. Diuretics should not be employed as they may worsen renal outcome especially if there is preexisting hypovolemia. There is no evidence to support their use.

Sodium bicarbonate to alkalinize the urine and prevent breakdown of myoglobin into the nephrotxic metabolites is often used. However, it has not been shown to be superior to saline alone. Bicarbonate use may also lead to worsening of initial hypocalcemia and deposition of calcium phosphate in various tissues. Monitor urine output closely. Do not treat an initial hypocalcemia unless the patient is symptomatic or having ECG changes related to their hyperkalemia. Hypercalcemia is a common development in the recovery phase of rhabdomyolysis. Some patients may require hemodialysis secondary to development of acute renal failure.

▶ Disposition

Hospitalization is mandatory. It may be necessary to admit elderly patients and those with preexisting renal dysfunction to the ICU for closer monitoring. Serum potassium levels should be followed closely. Generally, the prognosis of this disorder is good even with profound muscle necrosis and renal failure.

Bagley WH, Yang H, Shah KH: Rhabdomyolysis. Intern Emerg Med 2007;2:210–218 [PMID: 17909702].

▼ EMERGENCY MANAGEMENT OF METABOLIC ENCEPHALOPATHIES

DRUG-RELATED ENCEPHALOPATHIES

1. Alcohol Withdrawal

▶ General Considerations

Several well-recognized syndromes are associated with acute withdrawal from alcohol. Complications of alcohol withdrawal include alcohol withdrawal seizures and delirium tremens. Seizures usually occur 48 hours after ingestion ceases while classic delirium tremens syndrome typically appears after 3–4 days of abstinence (range: 24 hours to 7 days).

▶ Clinical Findings

A. Delirium Tremens

Note: Delirium tremens is an uncommon but life-threatening illness that requires prompt recognition and treatment for the best outcome. Symptoms and signs include the following:

- Profoundly delirious state associated with tremulousness and agitation.

- Excessive motor activity (most notable as a tremor that affects the face, tongue, and extremities but that may also involve speech) and purposeless activity such as picking at the bedclothes.

- Hallucinations, classically visual rather than auditory, are a prominent feature, especially if patients are specifically asked, "What do you see? What's over there? Is there anything frightening you?" These patients may be quite suggestible and may be persuaded to light an imaginary cigarette or identify the color of a nonexistent piece of string.

- Autonomic nervous system hyperactivity: tachycardia, dilated pupils, fever, and hyperhidrosis.

- Loss of orientation as to time and place. Such patients are often oblivious to the most obvious features of the surrounding environment.

B. Withdrawal Seizures

Withdrawal seizures, a syndrome distinct from delirium tremens, may result from abrupt decrease or cessation of alcohol consumption. About 90% of such convulsions occur 6–48 hours after abstinence. Seizures may occur with the patient still consuming alcohol if there is a rapid drop in blood alcohol levels. Since alcoholics are high risk for fall, head trauma must be considered and CT imaging done to rule out any intracranial process as the cause of the seizure.

Because delirium tremens requires a longer period of abstinence than do withdrawal seizures, pure withdrawal seizures (ie, those occurring only during periods of withdrawal) always occur before delirium tremens. Therefore, any seizures occurring after delirium tremens must be assumed to be due to some cause other than alcohol withdrawal, and further evaluation is required.

▶ Treatment

A. Delirium Tremens

Note temperature, pulse, and blood pressure, and record results twice hourly to monitor for hyperpyrexia and hypotension. Consider lumbar puncture to rule out meningitis if fever or meningismus is present.

1. Fluids—Fluid requirements on the first day of treatment may be as if profound dehydrationis present. Intravenous fluid should contain glucose to prevent hypoglycemia.

2. Thiamine—Thiamine, 100 mg/d, prevents Wernicke encephalopathy.

3. Benzodiazepines—Benzodiazepines are the primary form of treatment. They may also prevent patients with impending delirium tremens from developing a full-blown case.

A. **INITIAL DOSE**—A suggested regimen is diazepam 10 mg intravenously given over at least 2 minutes, followed by 5 mg intravenously every 5 minutes until the patient is calm. The total dose required to calm a patient may be as high as 200 mg. Lorazepam has a longer duration of action and is an alternative. Drug-induced hypotension and respiratory depression during administration of benzodiazepines for delirium tremens are uncommon if adequate hydration is maintained and overzealous treatment avoided. After delirium tremens has been controlled, the patient may sleep without interruption for up to 36 hours but can nonetheless be easily aroused.

B. **MAINTENANCE DOSES**—Administer diazepam, 5–10 mg, intravenously or orally as needed. Avoid intramuscular administration, because absorption by this route is erratic. Sedation is achieved within a few minutes following intravenous injection.

4. Phenothiazines—Phenothiazines have been used and may promptly control hallucinatory symptoms; however, these drugs are not recommended, because they may cause hypotension or precipitate seizures.

5. β-Blockers—The concomitant administration of β-blocking drugs helps decreases the associated autonomic hyperactivity but there is no evidence that their use is of any benefit in the treatment of delirium tremens.

B. Withdrawal Seizures

Pure withdrawal seizures are self-limited and usually do not require anticonvulsant therapy. Observation is necessary, because about 60% of patients will have more than one seizure, 95% of which will occur within 12 hours after the initial seizure and 80% within 6 hours. Benzodiazepines are the first line treatment and may lower the incidence of the second seizure. Lorazepam or diazepam is appropriate. Patients with withdrawal seizures, unless previously investigated, should receive outpatient follow-up. Most should be investigated at least once for structural causes. Hospitalization is rarely required.

2. Drug Intoxication

▶ Centrally Acting Anticholinergic Drugs

Intoxication with a wide variety of anticholinergic medications that penetrate the central nervous system may produce agitated and confusional states. Table 37–9 lists representative prescription and over-the-counter medications.

Delirium, psychosis, anxiety, hallucinations, breathlessness, hyperactivity, disorientation, seizures, and coma are typically associated with signs of peripheral cholinergic blockade: tachycardia, mydriasis, hyperpyrexia, urinary retention, decreased bowel motility, decreased sweating, and decreased bronchial, pharyngeal, and salivary secretions. The patient is hot, dry, red, and mad (delirious). Treatment

Table 37–9. Drugs That May Cause a Central Anticholinergic Syndrome.[a]

Anticholinergics
   Atropine (eg, belladonna, donnatal)
   Scopolamine (also found in Jimsonweed [*Datura* sp.])
Tricyclic antidepressants
   Amitriptyline (elavil, many others)
   Doxepin (adapin, sinequan, others)
   Imipramine (tofranil, many others)
Phenothiazines
   Chlorpromazine (thorazine, many others)
   Trifluoperazine (stelazine, many others)
   Thioridazine (mellaril, many others)
Antihistamines
   Chlorpheniramine (omade, teldrin, many others)
   Diphenhydramine (benadryl, many others)
   Promethazine (phenergan, many others)
Ophthalmic preparations
   Atropine, 1% ophthalmic solution
   Cyclopentolate (AK-pentolate, cyclogyl, others)
   Tropicamide (mydriacyl, others)
Antispasmodics
   Methantheline (banthine)
   Propantheline (Probanthine, others)
Antiparkinsonism agents
   Benztropine (cogentin, many others)
   Biperide (akineton)
   Trihexyphenidyl (artane, others)
Over-the-counter drugs (hypnotics, analgesics)
   Sominex (diphenhydramine)
   Sleep-Eze (diphenhydramine)
   Contac (chlorpheniramine)
   Dristan (chlorpheniramine)

[a]Only selected representatives from each group are listed.

is discussed in Chapter 47. Hospitalization is required for supportive care.

Stimulants and Hallucinogenic Drugs

Some commonly abused drugs, for example, cocaine, amphetamine, LSD (lysergic acid diethylamide), jimsonweed, and PCP (phencyclidine), can cause an agitated confusional state. Cocaine and methamphetamine are currently the most frequent culprits and can produce agitation, anxiety, depression, psychosis, paranoia, suicidal ideation, or any combination of these conditions. Symptoms are independent of the route of drug administration. Treatment is discussed in Chapter 47. Short-term psychiatric admission often is required.

Al-Sanouri I, Dikin M, Soubani AO: Critical care aspects of alcohol abuse. South Med J 2005;98:372–381 [PMID: 15813165].

McKeon A, Frye MA, Delanty N: The alcohol withdrawl syndrome. J Neurosurg Psychiatry 2008;79:854–862 [PMID: 17986499].

Table 37–10. Precipitating Causes of Hepatic Encephalopathy.

Constipation
GI bleeding
Renal failure
Dehydration
Infection
Surgery
Drug exposure
Electrolyte abnormalities
Hypoxia
Dietary protein overload

HEPATIC ENCEPHALOPATHY

 ESSENTIALS OF DIAGNOSIS

► Acute or chronic alteration of mental status

► History of cirrhosis, hepatic failure, congenital abnormality of portal circulation

► Elevation in ammonia level

► Episodes are usually related to a precipitating cause

► Commonly a recurrent problem

General Considerations

Hepatic encephalopathy is a life threatening, potentially reversible metabolic encephalopathy. Cirrhosis is present in the majority of patients and they will usually have a history of liver failure or portal hypertension. Precipitating causes are detailed in Table 37–10.

Clinical Findings

A. Symptoms and Signs

Patients may present with a wide range of alterations in mental status. A clinical grading scale can be applied to describe the severity of symptoms (Table 37–11). Physical examination may also reveal classic signs of chronic liver disease to include hepatomegaly, jaundice, scleral icterus, ascites, asterixis, gynecomastia, and spider angiomas.

B. Laboratory Findings

An elevated ammonia level may lead to the diagnosis of hepatic encephalopathy in a patient presenting with altered mental status. Although the level does not correlate directly with severity of symptoms, it may serve as an assay for

Table 37–11. Clinical Grading of Hepatic Encephalopathy.

Grade 0: Subtle mental status changes noted on testing of memory, concentration, cognition, and coordination
Grade 1: Mood disorder, sleep cycle derangement, inattention, difficulty with intellectual tasks
Grade 2: Lethargy, confusion, ataxia, slurred speech, asterixis, inappropriate behavior
Grade 3: Significant confusion, somnolence, delirium, incomprehensible speech, amnesia, hyperreflexia
Grade 4: Stupor, coma

monitoring the effect of short- and long-term therapy. Laboratory investigation of other causes of altered mental status should be considered.

▶ **Treatment**

Emergency department therapy is primarily directed at supportive care and reversal of any underlying conditions. Lactulose, oral or rectal, is generally administered to decrease ammonia levels. Oral neomycin, vancomycin or metronidazole is sometimes given acutely in an attempt to decrease ammonia production by eliminating intestinal flora, especially in patients intolerant of, or refractory to, lactulose therapy. However, there is little evidence to support their use.

▶ **Disposition**

Patients considered grade 1–4 should be admitted. Patients may require ICU admission if they are in advanced stages or are suffering from any other life-threatening sequel of liver disease or alcoholism. Patients with mild symptoms who are known to have chronic or intermittent hepatic encephalopathy may be discharged if they respond to therapy and have reliable social support and close follow-up.

Eroglu Y, Byrne WJ: Hepatic encephalopathy. Emerg Med Clin North Am 2009; 27:401–414 [PMID: 19646644].

WERNICKE ENCEPHALOPATHY (ACUTE THIAMINE DEFICIENCY)

 ESSENTIALS OF DIAGNOSIS

▶ Present with ophthalmoplegia, ataxia, and confusion
▶ Wernicke encephalopathy is a medical emergency and should be treated promptly with thiamine

▶ **Clinical Findings**

Wernicke encephalopathy is a medical emergency characterized by ophthalmoplegia, ataxia and mental status changes resulting from thiamine deficiency. However up to 19% of patients will demonstrate none of the classic triad of symptoms. Most cases are associated with alcoholism, malnutrition, or both. Failure to initiate prompt thiamine therapy in a patient with any of these features may result either in death or in permanent neuropathy or loss of cognitive function.

A. Ocular Abnormalities

Occular symptoms occur in roughly 29% of patients. Nystagmus (horizontal alone or horizontal and vertical) may occur. Isolated vertical nystagmus is rare. Bilateral lateral rectus muscle (sixth CN) palsies and conjugate gaze palsies may be present. Other types of ophthalmoplegia may occur. The response to irrigation of the external ear canal with ice water (caloric test) is invariably abnormal and reveals unilateral or bilateral absence of ocular movement.

B. Ataxia

Ataxia is similar to that associated with alcoholic cerebellar degeneration and occurs in approximately. Truncal ataxia is most common, with a wide-based, unsteady gait as the major finding. Limb ataxia is less common than ataxia of gait and affects the lower extremities much more than the upper extremities.

MENTAL STATUS CHANGES

Mental status changes occur in about 82% of patients with frank delirium occurring in about 20% of cases. Blatant apathy, manifested as inattention, drowsiness, and decreased spontaneous speech, is present in most cases. In the recovery phase, Korsakoff's psychosis may become more prominent, with marked impairment of recent memory and inability to retain new information. Confabulation is common.

▶ **Treatment**
A. Vitamins

Give thiamine, 100 mg intravenously, immediately upon the suspicion of the diagnosis of Wernicke encephalopathy. Patients should be hospitalized and thiamine continued in doses of 50 mg/d intravenously until adequate diet and bowel function are reestablished. Other water-soluble vitamins (B complex and C) should be given, because multiple deficiencies are common in these patients. The need for folate or vitamin B_{12} should be assessed based on the CBC (presence of hypersegmented polymorphonuclear leukocytes, and macrocytosis). Deficiencies of fat-soluble vitamins (A, D, and E) are rare.

Magnesium deficiency is common in alcohol withdrawal states, and magnesium should be replaced based on blood levels (Chapter 44).

B. Outcome

With thiamine therapy, oculomotor abnormalities may begin to improve within minutes to hours, and complete recovery will occur within 1–4 weeks, except for persistent lateral gaze nystagmus. Global confusional state, ataxia, peripheral neuropathies, and Korsakoff's psychosis in particular clear much less quickly, and permanent disability is common.

▶ Disposition

All patients with thiamine deficiency syndromes should be hospitalized for supportive care and continued administration of thiamine.

Sechi G, Serra A: Wernicke's encephalopathy; new clinical settings and recent advances in diagnosis and management. Lancet Neurol 2007;6:442–455 [PMID: 17434099].

REYE'S SYNDROME

ESSENTIALS OF DIAGNOSIS

- ▶ Acute noninflammatory encephalopathy
- ▶ Hepatic dysfunction, with fatty degeneration
- ▶ Recent viral illness with exposure to salicylates
- ▶ Patient is younger than 18 years

▶ General Considerations

Reye's syndrome, an encephalopathy associated with fatty degeneration of the liver, is a rare but severe cause of delirium progressing to coma in infants and children with a mortality rate of 21%. The degree of central nervous system impairment does not correlate well with the degree of hepatic dysfunction. The disease is extremely rare in individuals older than 20 years. Seasonal occurrence from November to April with a peak incidence in February has been noted. There may be a history of a preceding viral illness. Epidemiologic evidence has firmly linked Reye's syndrome with chickenpox and influenza virus infections. Other viruses, including parainfluenza, adenovirus, coxsackie and herpes simplex, have also been implicated. An association between Reye's syndrome and the use of salicylates during an antecedent illness has been demonstrated.

The number of cases has dropped dramatically since the 1980s. Several authors have noted a correlation between the decrease in reported cases to almost zero and the discovery of many new metabolic disorders that have a common pathophysiology. New diagnostic techniques to identify these inborn errors of metabolism have revealed that many cases of Reye's syndrome mimicked these disorders. It is now recommended that any infant or child suspected of having Reye's syndrome undergo extensive testing to rule out the treatable inborn metabolic disorders.

▶ Clinical Findings

Illness begins with protracted vomiting and delirium, which progresses to coma within 2 days. Seizures are common but are usually self-limited. Decerebrate posturing is common, but focal neurologic signs are rare once coma is established. Sustained hyperventilation and hepatomegaly are usually noted.

▶ Laboratory Findings

Cerebrospinal fluid examination reveals normal protein and cell count. Blood glucose is frequently reduced because of hepatic failure and may be reflected in low levels of cerebrospinal fluid glucose. Serum transaminase and blood ammonia levels are characteristically elevated. Prothrombin time is prolonged. Serum bilirubin is normal, so that icterus makes the diagnosis of Reye's syndrome doubtful.

▶ Treatment and Disposition

Hospitalization is required for control of intracranial pressure and supportive care. Early placement of an intracranial pressure monitor and measures to lower intracranial pressure may be helpful. There is no specific treatment.

Pugliese A, Beltramo T, Torre D: Reye's and Reye's-like syndromes. Cell Biochem funct 2008;26:741–746 [PMID: 18711704].

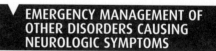

EMERGENCY MANAGEMENT OF OTHER DISORDERS CAUSING NEUROLOGIC SYMPTOMS

AMNESTIC SYNDROMES

ESSENTIALS OF DIAGNOSIS

- ▶ Recall must be specifically tested for the identification of memory loss
- ▶ Amnestic syndromes are identified by their onset, duration, and specific type of memory loss

1. Amnestic Episodes

▶ Clinical Findings

Memory loss is difficult to assess without specifically testing recall. Amnestic patients may present with only memory loss and no alteration of consciousness, basic cognition, or other physical examination findings. Recent memory is usually affected without significant alteration in distant memory. Some patients may appear obviously confused while other will attempt to deny their symptoms. The history and type of memory loss are critical in establishing the correct diagnosis. Cerebrospinal fluid examination, CT or MRI scan, along with other basic labs may be helpful. When combined with an accurate clinical history and associated findings these studies will help establish the cause in most cases.

▶ Treatment and Disposition

In addition to any necessary supportive care, administration of thiamine, 100 mg intravenously, may be appropriate because Korsakoff's syndrome is a diagnostic possibility. All patients with new onset of memory loss should be hospitalized for evaluation.

2. Transient Global Amnesia

▶ Clinical Findings

Transient global amnesia is a sudden onset of severe anterograde amnesia usually lasting several hours. There is a higher incidence in patients older than 50 years. Men are affected more frequently than women. Attacks predominate in the early morning. Previously the disorder was thought to be associated with migraines, seizure activity, or transient ischemic attack but the pathophysiology remains unclear.

Patients remain alert and are able to communicate. In addition, they have no loss of personal identity. They demonstrate a profound amnesia to recent events and are unable to form new memory. They repeatedly ask the same questions regarding their current condition. They do not become agitated and they maintain intellectual functioning. Physical exam and neurologic exam will be normal. During the episode, retrograde amnesia is present and may vary from days to months or even years. Recovery usually occurs within 2 hours and almost always within 12 hours. Anterograde amnesia for the entire episode is usually total and permanent.

▶ Treatment and Disposition

No specific treatment is available. Hospitalization may be indicated if the diagnosis is in question or if there is a lack of social support required for a safe discharge with close follow-up.

Shekhar R: Transient global amnesia-a review. Int J Clin Pract 2008;62:939–942 [PMID: 18248369].

CONFUSION ASSOCIATED WITH PSYCHIATRIC DISEASE

 ESSENTIALS OF DIAGNOSIS

▶ All forms of organic causes must be evaluated and ruled out prior to considering the possibility of psychiatric disease

▶ Patients tend to be fully oriented to place and time, and disorientation tends to be to person

▶ Short-term memory is preserved, and hallucinations are typically auditory in nature

▶ General Considerations

Differentiation between organic and psychiatric causes of confusion (psychosis or hysteria) may be difficult. Careful evaluation is required to ensure the correct diagnosis. Differentiating features of organic and psychiatric for confusion are summarized in Table 37–12.

1. Psychotic Confusional States

▶ Clinical Findings

The presentation of patients with psychotic confusional states differs from that of patients with confusional states due to organic causes. Psychotic patients may be fully oriented or, if disoriented, exhibit disorientation as to person that is at least as great as or greater than their disorientation to time and place. In organic brain disease, by contrast, disorientation as to time and place is invariably greater than to person.

Psychotic patients usually retain recent memory and are able to perform simple calculations and other cognitive tasks adequately. In contrast, these functions are rarely preserved in organic confusional states. Auditory hallucinations are the mainstay with psychotic states, as opposed to the visual hallucinations seen in organic confusional states.

▶ Treatment and Disposition

Obtain psychiatric consultation. Hospitalization in a secure ward is required for patients with acute psychosis or abrupt worsening of chronic psychosis. Parenteral antipsychotics may be required for the acutely psychotic patient who is at risk for harming themselves or others.

2. Hysteria

▶ Clinical Findings

Hysteria is a diagnosis of exclusion and should be made only after all other possibilities have been ruled out. The

Table 37–12. Differentiating Features of Organic and Psychiatric Disorders of Mentation.

Features	Organic	Psychiatric (Hysteria or Psychosis)
Age	Any; older more susceptible	Younger; puberty to mid 30s
Premorbid personality	Any	Previous functional illness common
Onset	Often acute	Usually gradual and insidious
Weakness, fatigue	Rare	Common
Level of awareness	Fluctuates between confusion and lucidity	Usually consistent
Hallucinations	Common; predominantly visual, tactile, and olfactory	Common; predominantly auditory
Orientation	Impaired: disorientation as to time is greater than that as to place, which in turn is greater than that as to person	Impaired: disorientation to person is greater than that as to place, which is greater than that as to time; may be unimpaired, however
Memory	Usually affected; recent memory more affected than remote memory	Total amnesia, including self-identity; or memory may be completely unimpaired
Other evidence of organic central nervous system disease	Present	Usually absent
Electroencephalogram	Frequently abnormal, usually slow	Usually normal
Asterixis and multifocal myoclonus	Diagnostic if present	Never seen

differential features listed in Table 37–12 are helpful, but few guidelines are absolute. It is useful to remember that amnesia is probably the most common hysterical disturbance of mental function. Hysterical amnesia usually includes the inability both to form new memories and especially to recall any past experience with certainty. For example, such patients often deny knowledge of their own name, a finding that in an awake and alert person is essentially restricted to the hysterical personality. The disparity between alleged mental incapacity and the ability to function in the immediate surroundings is often quite striking.

The most helpful differentiating features on physical examination are asterixis and myoclonus, which, when present, point to a metabolic cause of the symptoms. Asterixis and myoclonus do not occur as features of psychiatric or hysterical illness.

An electroencephalogram is often helpful in diagnosis, because it is nearly always normal in psychiatric disease and is frequently abnormal (usually slowed) in organic or metabolic disease. The presence of very fast b-wave activity on the tracing may be seen with sedative–hypnotic drug intoxication and provides a helpful clue to proper diagnosis.

▶ **Treatment and Disposition**

Refer the patient for psychiatric consultation. Anxiolytics may be helpful. Hospitalization may be required if a protected home environment is not available.

CONFUSIONAL STATES OF UNCERTAIN CAUSE

Even after all the above diagnoses have been considered, for many patients in confusional states, no clear diagnosis can be established in the emergency department. These patients, especially the elderly, are often found to have subclinical mild metabolic or drug-induced abnormalities or infection, and correction of the underlying disorder may restore patients to their customary normal state. Hyperthyroidism or hypothyroidism must be considered, especially in elderly patients.

Hospitalization is indicated for further evaluation of all patients with confusional states of uncertain cause.

Attard A, Ranjith G, Taylor D: Delerium and its treatment: CNS Drugs 2008;22:631–644 [PMID: 18601302].

Saxena S, Lawley D: Delerium in the elderly: a clinical review. Postgrad Med J 2009;85:405–413 [PMID: 19633006].

Obstetric and Gynecological Emergencies and Rape

Ryan Tucker, MD
Melissa Platt, MD

IMMEDIATE MANAGEMENT OF LIFE-THREATENING PROBLEMS

ABNORMAL VAGINAL BLEEDING

See Table 38–1. Patients with active vaginal bleeding are at risk of exsanguination and require immediate evaluation and treatment.

▶ Emergency Evaluation and Treatment

A. Assess for Hemodynamic Instability

Examine the patient for hypotension or tachycardia due to depletion of intravascular volume.

1. Hypotension—If blood pressure and pulse are normal in the supine position, measure them in the sitting position. If they are still normal, measure them in the standing position to detect more subtle volume depletion. Supine or postural hypotension can indicate life-threatening hemorrhage.

2. Tachycardia—Tachycardia while the patient is resting or when she assumes the upright posture also may indicate vascular depletion.

3. Poor Peripheral Perfusion—Cool, mottled skin and delayed capillary refill may indicate significant volume loss.

B. Treat Shock, if Present

(See Chapter 11) Briefly, the procedure is as follows:

1. Insert at least 2 large-bore (≥16-gauge) intravenous catheters. A central venous catheter may be preferable if peripheral venous access is not readily obtainable. Intraosseus access is an acceptable alternative (Chapter 8).

2. Determine the amount of blood loss and draw blood for (a) typing and crossmatching (reserve four units

Table 38–1. Causes of Abnormal Vaginal Bleeding.

Premenarcheal vaginal bleeding
  Menarche
  Tumor (vaginal, uterine)
  Genital trauma
  Foreign body
  Precocious puberty
  Hematuria
  Miscellaneous
Reproductive age bleeding
  Variations in normal cycle
    Hypermenorrhea (excessive bleeding at time of period)
    Polymenorrhea (menstrual periods < 21 days apart)
  Metrorrhagia (including ectopic)
    Abortion
    Pregnancy (including ectopic)
    Endocrine abnormality (idiopathic, estrogens, thyroid)
    Salpingitis
    Cervictis
    Coagulopathy (factor VIII deficiency)
    Malignant neoplasm or polyps (cervical, vaginal, uterine)
    Ovarian cyst
    Myoma of uterus
    Trophoblastic tumor
  Miscellaneous (mittelschmerz)
Postmenopausal bleeding
  Carcinoma (cervical, uterine)
  Estrogen excess
  Atrophic vaginitis
  Cervical polyps
  Trauma
  Miscellaneous

of fresh-frozen plasma and two to four units of packed red cells), (b) platelet count, prothrombin time, and partial thromboplastin time to uncover any bleeding abnormality, (c) complete blood count (CBC), (d) renal function tests and measurement of serum electrolytes, and (e) blood gas measurements and pH (useful in assessing adequacy of ventilation and perfusion).

3. Insert a Foley catheter.

4. If the patient is of child-bearing age, obtain a serum or urinary pregnancy test.

5. Begin rapid infusion of crystalloid solution (Ringer's solution or normal saline), the rate depending on vital signs (eg, 200–1000 mL/h), to restore intravascular volume and maintain blood pressure until compatible blood becomes available for transfusion.

6. Infuse crossmatched blood as soon as possible. If the patient is unstable and crossmatched blood is unavailable, transfuse O-negative blood. Give two or more units depending on vital signs.

C. Determine the Cause of Bleeding

1. Pelvic ultrasonography—In the evaluation of a pregnant patient with vaginal bleeding, ultrasound can be used to rapidly identify fluid in the pelvis or abdomen (presumed to be blood in the setting of shock), which is highly suggestive of ruptured ectopic pregnancy. In the setting of symptomatic vaginal hemorrhage in the first trimester of pregnancy, ultrasound may show retained intrauterine products of conception, indicative of an incomplete spontaneous abortion. For the nonpregnant patient, an ultrasound showing significant pelvic or intraabdominal fluid may be representative of a hemorrhagic ruptured ovarian cyst, which occasionally requires surgical intervention.

D. Treatment

The measures described here should not be used in third-trimester pregnancy.

1. Compression of the uterus—Insert one hand in the vagina, elevate the uterus, and compress it against the abdominal wall and the opposite hand. Alternately, tamponade may be attempted by inserting a foley catheter into the uterine cavity and inflating the balloon until bleeding subsides.

2. Medical Therapy—Conjugated Estrogen therapy 25 mg q 4 hrs IV may be used alone, or in combination with direct compression until bleeding is controlled.

E. Treat for Trauma

If trauma has occurred, determine the extent of injury, and apply pressure to the bleeding site.

F. Obtain Consultation

Obtain urgent gynecologic or surgical consultation for possible emergency dilation and curettage, laparoscopy, or laparotomy in any hemodynamically unstable patient

▶ Disposition

Patients with vaginal bleeding resulting in abnormal hemodynamics or significant anemia should be hospitalized.

PELVIC PAIN WITH OR WITHOUT BLEEDING

See Table 38–2.

▶ Clinical Findings

A. History

Obtain information about the following points:

- Possible pregnancy (recent amenorrhea or abnormal period, intercourse without contraception, morning sickness, or tenderness of breasts of recent onset)

- History of trauma, including rape or nontherapeutic abortion

Table 38-2. Differential Diagnosis of Pelvic Pain.

	History and Symptoms				Signs					Laboratory Findings	
	Relationship to Menstrual Period	Quality of Pain	Prior Salpingitis	Type of Vaginal Discharge	Fever	Cervix	Uterus	Adnexal Mass	Adnexal Tenderness	Urine Immunologic Pregnancy Test	Leukocytosis
Salpingitis	Accompanying or just after period	Constant and severe	+	Scant to purulent	+	Tender with motion	Tender	None	Usually bilateral	Indicated	++
Salpingitis plus tubo-ovarian abscess								+			Also, elevated erythrocyte sedimentation rate
Incomplete abortion	Period of amenorrhea with recent spotting or frank blood	Cramping and suprapubic	±	Heavy blood clots	-	Dilated	Enlarged, tender	None	None	±	±
Septic abortion				Thick and bloody; foulsmelling	+	Dilated, tender	Enlarged, tender	±	Bilateral	±	++
Ectopic pregnancy	Amenorrhea with recent spotting	Intermittent; variable severity	±	Scant but rarely none	±	Slightly tender	Normal to slightly enlarged	+	Unilateral	±	±
Ruptured ovarian cyst	Precedes period	Sudden and severe	-	None	±	Normal	Normal	±	Unilateral	Indicated	±
Mittelschmerz	Midcycle	Sudden	-	Spotting	-	Normal	Normal	None	Unilateral	-	-
Torsion of ovarian tumor	None	Intermittent; radiates to thigh	-	None	±	Slightly tender	Slightly tender	None	Unilateral	±	-
Endometritis with or without IUD	Variable	Cramping	±	Scant or none	+	Variable	Slightly tender	+if tubal abscess	Variable	±	±
Dysmenorrhea	Accompanies period	Cramping	±	Normal menses	-	Normal	Variable tenderness	Negative	Seldom	-	-
Appendicitis	None	Periumbilical; cramping; progressing to constant right lower quadrant	-	None	±	Normal	Normal	None	Unilateral	±	±

- History of salpingitis
- History of ectopic pregnancy
- Duration of symptoms and relation to menses
- Type of pain (cramping or constant)
- Type and amount of vaginal bleeding or discharge
- Use of intrauterine device (IUD)

B. Symptoms and Signs

Fever is often the first sign of infection, and pelvic warmth (from local inflammation) may be noted on bimanual examination. Pelvic organs are tender and engorged.

C. Laboratory Tests and Special Examinations

1. Blood tests—The white cell count, differential, and erythrocyte sedimentation rate may reflect inflammation or infection but are nonspecific tests.

2. Pregnancy test—A pregnancy test is important if pain or bleeding is present (Table 38–3). Qualitative tests of blood

Table 38–3. Clinical Manifestations of Common Pelvic Disorders.

Clinical Findings	Possible Causes
Bleeding	Trauma Postpartum hemorrhage Dysfunctional uterine bleeding Carcinoma
Pain	Salpingitis and tubo-ovarian abscess Ruptured ovarian cyst Torsion of tube and ovary Mittelschmerz Abdominal disorders (appendicitis, etc.)
Pain and bleeding	Dysmenorrhea Endometriosis Endometritis
Pregnancy and bleeding	Placenta previa Ectopic pregnancy Spontaneous abortion Abruptio placentae
Pregnancy and pain	Ectopic pregnancy Degenerating fibroid (leiomyoma) Normal labor
Pregnancy with pain and bleeding	Labor with placenta previa Abruptio placentae Septic abortion Puerperal sepsis Ectopic pregnancy

or urine are sensitive and may provide positive test results within 7 days of conception. They are also relatively inexpensive, easy to do, and can be performed in 5–10 minutes. Quantitative blood tests are more sensitive and may assist in the evaluation of gestational age.

3. Cultures—Obtain cervical swab cultures for gonococci and *Chlamydia trachomatis* if infection is a possible diagnosis.

4. Ultrasound—Ultrasound may show an ectopic pregnancy, intrauterine pregnancy, inflamed fallopian tubes, ovarian cysts, or pelvic abscesses (Figures 38–1 and 38–2).

5. Laparoscopy—Laparoscopy may be helpful when the diagnosis is uncertain.

▶ Treatment and Disposition

If the diagnosis is uncertain but either ectopic pregnancy or septic abortion is a possibility, consultation with a gynecologist for hospitalization or daily follow-up on an outpatient basis is mandatory.

▼ EMERGENCY MANAGEMENT OF GYNECOLOGIC DISORDERS

ECTOPIC PREGNANCY

ESSENTIALS OF DIAGNOSIS

- ▶ Unilateral pelvic pain in early pregnancy
- ▶ Vaginal bleeding present or absent
- ▶ Risk factor assessment
- ▶ Unilateral adnexal tenderness or mass
- ▶ Uterine size less than dates
- ▶ Quantitative human chorionic gonadotropin (hCG) and pelvic ultrasound

▶ General Considerations

Ectopic pregnancy is the leading cause of pregnancy-related death in the first trimester. Patients with ectopic pregnancy are often encountered in the emergency department, and the disorder may be difficult to identify given the varied presentations that occur. Because ectopic pregnancy can be life threatening, it should be suspected in any patient presenting with amenorrhea, vaginal bleeding, and lower abdominal pain. For some women, the initial presenting symptom of an ectopic pregnancy is syncope. The most common presenting

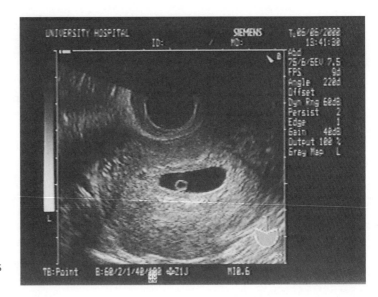

▲ **Figure 38–1.** Bedside endovaginal ultrasound of an intrauterine pregnancy. An intrauterine gestational sac with a yolk sac is clearly visualized.

complaint is vaginal bleeding, often scant at first, with cramping lower abdominal pain.

The incidence of ectopic pregnancy is increased in women using an IUD and in those with a history of pelvic infection (eg, salpingitis), tubal surgery, infertility treatments, or previous tubal pregnancies. About 98% of ectopic pregnancies are tubal.

The clinical presentation of ectopic pregnancy is variable, ranging from the asymptomatic patient to the patient with hemorrhagic shock. Rupture of the fallopian tube followed by free intraperitoneal bleeding from tubal vessels is the principal cause of illness and death.

With improved resolution of ultrasound and rapidly available quantitative hCG assays, the diagnosis of ectopic pregnancy can be made more accurately and earlier than in the past (Figure 38–3).

▶ **Clinical Findings**

A. Symptoms and Signs

Patients have a history of the following: (1) missed or abnormal menses or vaginal bleeding—however, 30% of patients with ectopic pregnancy have no vaginal bleeding; (2) pelvic pain, which may be unilateral, following amenorrhea; and

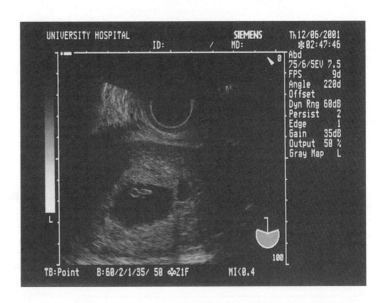

▲ **Figure 38–2.** Bedside endovaginal ultrasound of an intrauterine pregnancy. An intrauterine gestational sac containing both a yolk sac and fetal pole is noted.

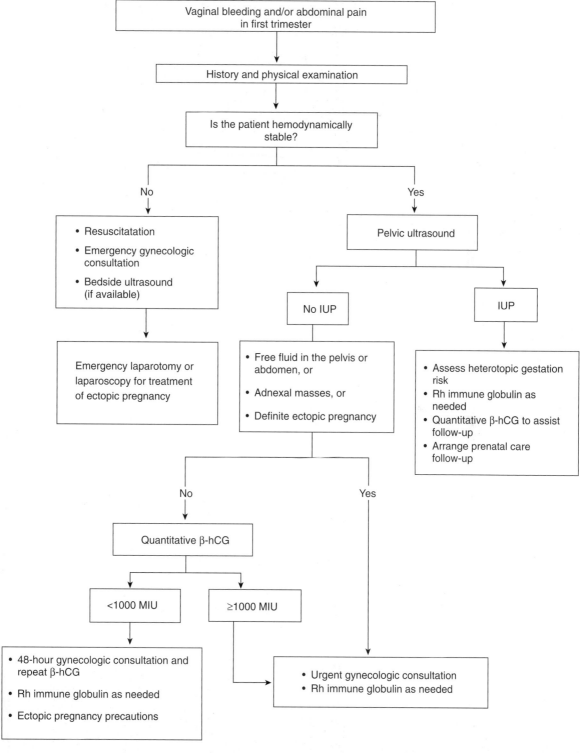

▲ **Figure 38–3.** Diagnostic algorithm for the patient with possible ectopic pregnancy. IUP, intrauterine pregnancy.

(3) possible intermittent pain; rupture of the fallopian tube may bring temporary relief of pain.

Symptoms of early pregnancy (eg, breast tenderness and nausea) may be present. Unilateral abdominal or pelvic pain may be present. Referred shoulder pain, syncope, or lightheadedness may also occur. Peritoneal pain may develop after tubal rupture with bleeding into the peritoneum.

In the early stages of ectopic pregnancy, the results of pelvic examination may be normal. Initially, symptoms may be completely nonspecific, because the tubal pregnancy producing them may be in the early stages of development. In advanced cases, a tender adnexal mass, enlarged uterus, or blood in the peritoneal cavity (eg, doughy cul-de-sac) may occur.

Obtain complete vital signs, including supine, sitting, and standing pulse and blood pressure measurements to look for supine or orthostatic hypotension.

B. Laboratory Tests and Special Examinations

1. Pregnancy test—The qualitative urine and serum pregnancy test may be positive at levels as low as 10 mIU/mL. Check with the laboratory. The most specific and sensitive test is the serum quantitative hCG. It may detect levels as low as 5 mIU/mL depending on laboratory assay. Quantitative hCG values are invaluable in the interpretation of pelvic ultrasound in this setting. In a normal intrauterine first-trimester pregnancy, the hCG level should double about every 1.5 days.

2. Ultrasound—Endovaginal and transabdominal sonography have become key diagnostic tools in the differentiation of normal (see Figures 38–1 and 38–2) from abnormal early pregnancy (Figure 38–4). Occasionally, a mass can be seen in the adnexa or cul-de-sac, or products of conception can be visualized outside the uterine cavity, and ectopic pregnancy can be readily diagnosed (see Figure 38–4).

Ultrasound is often useful in excluding an ectopic pregnancy by ruling in an intrauterine pregnancy. If the patient reports a history of infertility treatments, avoid making premature conclusions because the possibility of a heterotopic pregnancy (ie, simultaneous intrauterine and ectopic) has been reported to be as low as 1 in 4000. With an hCG of 6000–6500 mIU/mL, an intrauterine pregnancy can be visualized transabdominally 94% of the time. Likewise, a yolk sac can be identified at the discriminatory hCG values of 1000–1500 mIU/mL utilizing endovaginal sonography. With endovaginal scanning, a small intrauterine collection of blood, or pseudosac, may be seen associated with an ectopic pregnancy. In very early pregnancy, at levels below the discriminatory values, the uterus may appear empty. Fluid in Morison's pouch on transabdominal scanning strongly suggests ruptured ectopic pregnancy, usually requiring operative intervention (Figure 38–5).

3. Laparoscopy or laparotomy—Laparoscopy or laparotomy may be necessary to make a definitive diagnosis of ectopic pregnancy.

▶ **Treatment and Disposition**

Treatment of possible ectopic pregnancy is determined by the patient's risk factors for ectopic pregnancy (ie, infertility treatments, history of tubal ligation, or pelvic inflammatory disease), hemodynamic stability, and physical examination findings. Sonography is important in the evaluation of pregnant patients with either abdominal pain or vaginal bleeding (see Figure 38–3). Quantitative hCG results may help in the interpretation of ultrasound findings. In addition, Rh-negative mothers should receive Rho(D) immune globulin.

A. High Probability of Ectopic Pregnancy

Obtain emergency pelvic sonography if hemodynamic stability allows. If the quantitative hCG value is greater than 1500–2000 mIU/mL in a patient with an empty uterine cavity on endovaginal ultrasound, ectopic pregnancy should be strongly suspected. An adnexal mass or extrauterine products of conception may or may not be readily identified. A large amount of pelvic or intraperitoneal fluid is highly suggestive of ectopic pregnancy (Figures 38–4C and 38–5). If ultrasound is unavailable for evaluation of a patient with a positive pregnancy test, physical findings worrisome for ectopic pregnancy include adnexal tenderness or an adnexal mass. However, do not be misled by a lack of peritoneal signs during your examination.

Prevent or correct hemorrhagic shock by inserting 2 large-bore (≥16-gauge) intravenous catheters and infusing crystalloid solution for volume replacement. Type and cross-match for 2–4 units of packed red blood cells. Insert a Foley catheter, and send urine for analysis.

Obtain emergency obstetric consultation, and prepare the patient for surgery. Obtain CBC, serum electrolyte, blood urea nitrogen, creatinine, coagulation profile, and other studies as required.

B. Ectopic Pregnancy Equivocal

Vaginal bleeding, pelvic pain, and tenderness without explanation may be present in a patient with a positive pregnancy test.

Insert an intravenous catheter, and send blood for CBC and crossmatching. Obtain pelvic sonogram. A transvaginal sonogram may not show definite evidence of an ectopic pregnancy, but worrisome signs include fluid in the cul-de-sac or an empty uterus with a quantitative hCG at or above the discriminatory zone. Urgent gynecologic consultation is recommended in these situations.

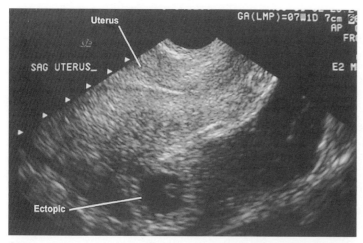

A

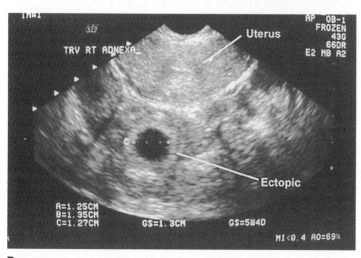

B

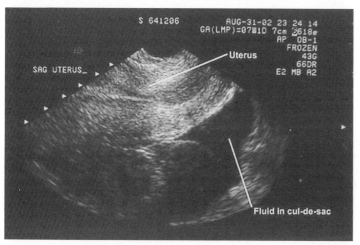

C

▲ **Figure 38–4.** Endovaginal ultrasound clearly demonstrating an ectopic pregnancy. **A:** Longitudinal view of the uterus with a well-defined endometrial stripe and no intrauterine gestational sac. A gestational sac is noted posterior to the uterus. **B:** Transverse view of the uterus and right adnexa also demonstrating an extrauterine gestational sac. **C:** Longitudinal view demonstrating free fluid in the cul-de-sac.

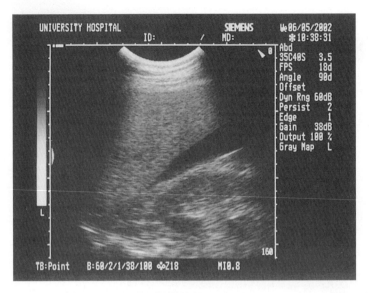

▲ **Figure 38–5.** Bedside transabdominal ultrasound of free fluid in Morison's pouch (hepatorenal space) secondary to a ruptured ectopic pregnancy.

C. Low Probability of Ectopic Pregnancy

Vaginal bleeding or pelvic pain is present. The results of physical examination and laboratory studies are normal. Some authors have developed clinical criteria for prediction of ectopic pregnancy. Suggested low-risk clinical criteria (ectopic pregnancy risk <1%) for patients with pain or bleeding include absence of signs of peritoneal irritation on palpation, no cervical, adnexal, or uterine tenderness, and no abdominal or pelvic pain other than in the midline.

Send blood for quantitative hCG. If a pelvic sonogram demonstrates an intrauterine pregnancy, and the patient is at low risk for a heterotopic pregnancy (ie, no fertility medications or procedures), discharge the patient with 24–48 hours follow-up. Other patients who can be managed as outpatients with close gynecologic follow-up include those with quantitative hCG below the discriminatory zone (1000 mIU/mL) with an empty uterus and no abnormalities on endovaginal ultrasound suggestive of ectopic pregnancy. Patients with an isolated quantitative hCG below 1000 are not necessarily low risk because nearly one-third of patients with ectopic pregnancies have a quantitative hCG level below 1000 mIU/mL. A decision based only on a single hCG value below the discriminatory values lacks specificity and needs to be carefully evaluated.

Discharge the patient from the emergency department to outpatient care with a definitive follow-up appointment for reevaluation within 1–2 days. Give the patient *written* instructions explaining that ectopic pregnancy is a possible diagnosis and she must be alert to the following symptoms, which would require that she return to the hospital immediately: (1) increased vaginal bleeding, (2) increased pelvic or abdominal pain, or (3) syncope.

SPONTANEOUS ABORTION

ESSENTIALS OF DIAGNOSIS

- ▶ Vaginal bleeding in early pregnancy
- ▶ Pelvic and back pain common
- ▶ Variable pelvic examination findings
- ▶ Quantitative hCG and pelvic ultrasound
- ▶ Exclude ectopic pregnancy

▶ General Considerations

At least 20% of all pregnancies terminate in abortion, usually because of serious defects in the ovum. Half of abortions occur before the 8th week of gestation and another quarter before the 16th week. Many of these early spontaneous abortions go unnoticed as a delayed menstrual period. Nevertheless, early spontaneous abortions are also a common cause of visits to the emergency department.

Fetal demise and failed expulsion of the products of conception from the uterus, with a closed cervix, is termed missed abortion. If this state persists for longer than 4–6 weeks, the patient is at increased risk for infection and disseminated intravascular coagulation. Table 36–4 describes the various types of spontaneous abortion.

Table 38–4. Classification of Spontaneous Abortion.

Type	Symptoms and Signs
Threatened abortion	Mild, transient uterine cramps with minimal transient vaginal bleeding. The cervix is long and closed. Uterine size is compatible with the presumed length of pregnancy.[a] Symptoms of pregnancy continue, and the conceptus remains viable
Inevitable abortion	Persistent uterine cramps and moderate vaginal bleeding. The cervical os is open (ie, a 0.5-cm [3/16-in] diameter sponge stick passes easily). Passage of some or all of the products of conception is inevitable or is about to occur; ie, fetal or placental tissue is found in the vagina or protrudes through the cervical os, or the patient gives a history of passage of tissue. Symptoms and signs of pregnancy disappear.
Incomplete abortion	Uterine cramps and vaginal bleeding are persistent and excessive. Symptoms of pregnancy may disappear. Products of conception are noted in the vagina, or the patient gives a history of passage of tissue.
Complete abortion	Uterine cramps markedly diminish or stop. Vaginal bleeding ceases. The entire conceptus is expelled. Symptoms of pregnancy disappear.
Missed abortion	The products of conception are retained. Symptoms and signs of pregnancy abate, and results of pregnancy tests change to negative. Brownish vaginal discharge (rarely, frank bleeding) occurs. Uterine cramps are rare. Examination shows a small and irregularly softened uterus. Ultrasonography fails to demonstrate a live fetus; ie, fetal heart motion is absent.

[a]Uterine size in centimeters measured from the top of the symphysis pubica to the top of the uterine fundus is a useful approximation of gestational age in weeks from 15–16 weeks through 32–33 weeks. A normal 20-week gestational age uterine size should be at the level of the umbilicus.

▶ Clinical Findings

A. Symptoms and Signs

Almost all patients have a history suggesting possible pregnancy:

- Sexual intercourse
- Period of amenorrhea or abnormal menses
- Nausea and vomiting; breast tenderness
- Uterine cramps and vaginal bleeding
- Passage of fetal or placental tissue (incomplete or complete abortion)

Caution: Pelvic examination should be performed on all patients with suspected abortion and on all pregnant patients with vaginal bleeding who have reached less than 20 weeks' gestation. Extreme care, however, must be exercised in examining patients in the second trimester; instruments should not be introduced into the cervical os. Beyond 20 weeks' gestation, pelvic examination should be done by an obstetrician because of the increasing risk of placenta previa.

B. Laboratory Tests and Special Examinations

In the first trimester of pregnancy, an hCG level that does not double in 48 hours suggests fetal demise or an abnormal pregnancy. Real-time ultrasonography, using abdominal or vaginal probes, can be diagnostic, for example, demonstrating a fetus without heartbeat or movement. Pathologic examination of tissue expelled by the uterus confirms passage of the products of conception.

▶ Treatment and Disposition

Blood typing and antibody screening are required in all patients with abortion of any type. If patients are Rh-negative, give $Rh_o(D)$ immune globulin (RhoGAM 300 mcg IM, many others), within 72 hours after any event in which fetal–maternal transfusion may occur, including abortion.

A. Threatened Abortion

Advise the patient to rest. Do not use hormones, douches, or tampons. The patient should not engage in coitus. Ultrasound may reveal a gestational sac or evidence of fetal cardiac activity. Discharge instructions must include follow-up instructions and indications for return to the emergency department, including passage of fetal tissue, severe vaginal bleeding greater than one pad per hour, significant abdominal or pelvic pain, or fever. The patient should also be given adequate analgesia.

B. Incomplete or Inevitable Abortion

Hospitalize the patient if hypovolemia or anemia is present or if the pregnancy is past the first trimester. Treat hypovolemia if present. An obstetrical or gynecological consult should be obtained to perform possible suction curettage or dilation and curettage.

C. Complete Abortion

The patient may be discharged to home care if vital signs and hematocrit are stable and if vaginal bleeding is clearly decreasing. Pain must also be clearly decreasing and the cervical os closed. A physician must differentiate a complete abortion from an incomplete abortion. Several clues can help the physician determine that a complete abortion has occurred:

- A reliable history.
- Ultrasound revealing a clean uterine stripe.
- The products of conception are brought to the physician and confirmed by pathology. If pathology is not readily available, a physician can differentiate between blood clots and products of conception by rubbing the specimen between a wet gauze pad. Unlike blood clots, true products of conception will not dissolve.

D. Missed Abortion (Retained Conceptus)

Obtain CBC, differential, and coagulation panel (platelet count, prothrombin time, and partial thromboplastin time). Obtain disseminated intravascular coagulation screening tests if abnormal values are found. Hospitalize the patient, and prepare to perform dilation and curettage if evidence indicates infection or disseminated intravascular coagulation or if the products of conception have been retained more than 4 weeks.

Outpatient management of early missed abortion is possible if the patient has close follow-up.

SEPTIC ABORTION

ESSENTIALS OF DIAGNOSIS

- ▶ History of gynecologic procedure or abortion
- ▶ Pelvic pain
- ▶ Systemic signs of infection
- ▶ Tender uterus
- ▶ Profuse, malodorous vaginal discharge

▶ General Considerations

Septic abortion is a rare complication after some obstetric–gynecologic procedures. Septic abortion may also arise as a result of nonsterile nontherapeutic abortion. The usual cause of sepsis is incomplete evacuation of the products of conception. Infection is usually due to mixed aerobic and anaerobic bacteria (bacteroides, *Prevotella*, group B streptococci, Enterobacteriaceae, and *C. trachomatis*) and is rapidly progressive, extending quickly through the myometrium and involving the adnexa and pelvic peritoneum. Septic pelvic thrombophlebitis with or without septic pulmonary embolization is an uncommon but devastating complication.

▶ Clinical Findings

A. Symptoms and Signs

Symptoms and signs are consistent with a history of recent pregnancy and induced abortion followed by pelvic pain and symptoms of infection. Nonjudgmental questioning in a private setting by a physician may be necessary to elicit a history of nontherapeutic abortion; in some cases, such a history is never obtained. Clinical findings include signs of infection (eg, fever and leukocytosis); diffuse pelvic tenderness; and profuse, foul vaginal discharge in most cases. Frank septic shock may be present.

B. Imaging

Ultrasound or other imaging techniques (computed tomography [CT], magnetic resonance imaging) may show retained intrauterine material, uterine emphysema, or intraperitoneal air from uterine perforation.

▶ Treatment and Disposition

Evacuation of the uterine contents and administration of broad-spectrum antibiotics are the mainstay of treatment.

Note: Although antibiotic therapy alone is effective in the earliest stage of infection, many patients require emergency hysterectomy. Death may occur despite the best treatment.

A. Immediate Measures

Hospitalize the patient at once, and start general measures for septic shock (Chapters 11 and 42). Obtain emergency surgical obstetric–gynecologic consultation.

B. Laboratory Tests

Obtain samples of blood and uterine discharge for culture. Draw blood for CBC, hepatic and renal panels, serum electrolyte determination, prothrombin time, partial thromboplastin time, platelet count, and disseminated intravascular coagulation screening tests if initial findings are abnormal.

C. Antibiotics

After taking specimens for culture of aerobic and anaerobic organisms, give antibiotics (eg, doxycycline, 100 mg IV every 12 hours, and one of the following: cefoxitin 2.0 g every 6–8 hours IV, piperacillin/tazobactam 4.5 g IV every 8 hours, ampicillin/sulbactam 3 g IV daily, or ertapenem 1 g IV daily. An alternate regimen consists of clindamycin 900 mg IV every 8 hours, plus ceftriaxone 1 g IV daily.

CARCINOMA AND OTHER TUMORS

Although gynecologic cancers seldom present as emergency situations, the emergency physician should be aware of the various presenting symptoms and risk factors associated with gynecologic cancers. Vulvar cancers are rarely sudden in onset and usually occur in women over age 50 years. They are more common in women with a history of cervical dysplasia or cancer.

Persistent unremitting vaginal pruritus is the single most common symptom of vulvar cancer and should never be dismissed as a frivolous complaint in the post-menopausal patient. Vaginal cancers are rare. Bleeding is typically the presenting complaint. The patient is usually of 50 years or older, but even teenagers have developed clear cell carcinoma (eg, girls whose mothers were given diethylstilbestrol during pregnancy). Patients with ovarian cancer may have abdominal distention from ascites, intestinal obstruction, or rarely, acute abdominal pain. Furthermore, ovarian carcinoma increases the risk for ovarian torsion.

Patients with gestational trophoblastic disease may present with heavy vaginal bleeding and symptoms similar to those of early miscarriage, but the following symptoms and signs suggest trophoblastic disease: (1) heavy vaginal bleeding with or without passage of tissue, or grape clusters of tissue aborted from the cervical os; (2) uterine size inappropriately large for dates; (3) profound anemia; (4) history of molar pregnancy; (5) first-trimester hypertension or preeclampsia; or (6) hCG remarkably elevated over the expected values. The diagnosis can be confirmed by ultrasound examination.

Any patient presenting with neurologic signs and with a recent history of molar pregnancy or trophoblastic disease may have cerebral metastasis. Central nervous system metastasis of trophoblastic disease represents a true oncologic emergency, because cerebral metastasis has the potential for cure as long as rapid growth or hemorrhage does not occur.

Patients with trophoblastic disease should be hospitalized for gynecologic consultation.

For any carcinoma, if the bleeding is severe, it is imperative to try to control the bleeding (ie, vaginal packing), volume resuscitate, and obtain emergency surgical and obstetrical consultation.

A. Carcinoma of the Cervix

Vaginal bleeding is the most common symptom in cervical cancer. Patients may be in their late 20s to (most commonly) early 40s. Patients often complain of persistent watery discharge. Speculum examination reveals a necrotic friable lesion on the cervix.

Uncontrollable bleeding from the cervix may be treated with applications of ferric subsulfate solution or vaginal packing. Manipulation should be kept to a minimum. Biopsy of the lesion at its margin with normal tissue usually confirms the diagnosis, but this procedure should not be performed in an emergency department.

B. Carcinoma of the Endometrium

Postmenopausal bleeding is the most common symptom of endometrial carcinoma. Risk factors associated with endometrial carcinoma include ingestion of exogenous estrogens, obesity, infertility, polycystic ovarian syndrome, and age over 50 years.

The physician should not try to stop postmenopausal bleeding with administration of hormones (eg, estrogens or progesterone) without confirming the diagnosis beforehand. Consultation with a gynecologist should be obtained prior to discharge for further input.

GENITAL TRAUMA

Genital trauma in women almost always occurs as a result of sexual activity, either forced (rape) or voluntary. Penile thrusts rarely produce trauma unless it is the first sexual experience.

▶ Clinical Findings

The most common presenting complaints are vaginal bleeding and pain or dyspareunia. Examination usually reveals bleeding from a tear in the genital mucosa or skin. Bleeding is rarely brisk enough to produce signs of hypovolemia, but if these are present, replace volume losses, and provide supportive care (Chapter 11). In prepubertal patients, general anesthesia may be required for adequate examination.

▶ Treatment and Disposition

Determine whether rape has occurred, and proceed accordingly. Provide sedation or analgesia if necessary.

Treat hypovolemia if present. Control vaginal bleeding temporarily with a vaginal pack, or direct firm pressure if the bleeding is from the external genitalia. A urethrogram may be needed if urethral trauma is suspected.

Hospitalize the patient if bleeding cannot be easily and definitively controlled, and obtain gynecologic consultation. Small lesions at the introitus may be repaired in the emergency department under local anesthesia. However, small and seemingly minor vaginal tears may communicate with either the rectum or the peritoneum; consequently, such repairs are best performed by a gynecologist in an operating room with adequate anesthesia and good exposure.

RUPTURED OVARIAN CYST

ESSENTIALS OF DIAGNOSIS

- ▶ Sudden, moderate to severe unilateral pelvic pain
- ▶ Possible history of initial nausea, diaphoresis, near-syncope
- ▶ Lack of systemic signs of infection
- ▶ Negative pregnancy test
- ▶ Unilateral adnexal tenderness without mass
- ▶ Pelvic ultrasound excludes significant hemorrhage

▶ Clinical Findings

Ruptured ovarian cyst is associated with sudden, moderately severe pelvic or lower abdominal pain. The patient is afebrile, and leukocytosis is variable. Tenderness is found over the affected ovary, and there are no masses. A pregnancy test should be obtained because ectopic pregnancy is a possible diagnosis. Ultrasonography may show the presence of an ovarian cyst or free pelvic fluid and is useful to detect ectopic pregnancy.

▶ Treatment and Disposition

The physician should provide adequate analgesics, including narcotics if needed. The patient should be observed and may require hospitalization if the diagnosis is uncertain or if relief is required for severe pain not relieved by narcotics. Surgery is rarely required unless there is a significant hemoperitoneum from the rupture of a hemorrhagic corpus luteum cyst with hemodynamic instability.

OVARIAN TORSION

ESSENTIALS OF DIAGNOSIS

- ▶ Extremes of age
- ▶ Single or recurrent moderate unilateral pelvic pain
- ▶ Negative pregnancy test
- ▶ Pelvic mass
- ▶ Pelvic ultrasound

▶ Clinical Findings

Torsion of ovary is associated with a history of attacks of severe unilateral pain in the lower abdomen. There is a bimodal age distribution which includes the adolescent and postmenopausal women older than 50. The symptoms may be gradual, or occur suddenly if there is accompanying intraovarian bleeding. Physical examination can be unreliable, therefore imaging studies, usually ultrasonography, is needed. Doppler studies can detect decreased or absent blood flow to the torsed ovary. If other intra-abdominal pathology is suspected, computed tomography may be the better imaging modality.

▶ Treatment and Disposition

Hospitalize the patient, and obtain urgent gynecologic consultation. Laparoscopy is frequently required. Laparotomy is indicated if the diagnosis is confirmed or if the patient's condition deteriorates.

ENDOMETRIOSIS

ESSENTIALS OF DIAGNOSIS

- ▶ Recurrent pelvic, flank, or abdominal pain with menses
- ▶ Negative pregnancy test

▶ Clinical Findings

The patient with endometriosis gives a history of attacks of crampy lower abdominal pain associated with menstruation. Symptoms may be gradual, or sudden if bleeding is present. Acquired dysmenorrhea is most commonly due to endometriosis. Other symptoms include painful defecation and dyspareunia.

▶ Treatment and Disposition

Refer the patient for further gynecologic evaluation. Definitive diagnosis usually requires laparoscopy. Provide oral analgesia as needed.

DYSMENORRHEA

ESSENTIALS OF DIAGNOSIS

- ▶ Painful menstruation
- ▶ Negative pregnancy test
- ▶ Exclude pelvic infection

▶ Clinical Findings

Many women experience painful menstruation (dysmenorrhea). The pain is cramping in nature, may be debilitating, and is usually relieved by menses. The pain occurs because of elaboration of excessive quantities of prostaglandins by the endometrium with subsequent increased uterine tone. It is not psychological in origin.

Idiopathic dysmenorrhea usually begins at menarche and is probably more common than the acquired form. Acquired dysmenorrhea, occurring in the late teens and early 20s, may suggest endometriosis and is common in chronic pelvic inflammatory disease.

▶ Treatment and Disposition

Both types of dysmenorrhea may be seen by the emergency physician and may be treated by prostaglandin inhibitors (eg, ibuprofen, 400 mg orally every 6 hours; naproxen, 250–500 mg twice daily; or controlled release, 750–1000 mg every day). Local application of heat to the lower abdomen may be helpful.

MITTELSCHMERZ

Midcycle pain (mittelschmerz) is common in women with regular menstrual periods who are not taking birth control pills. These patients may commonly have mid-cycle spotting caused by an estrogen surge. There is no fever and no other abnormal bleeding such as that resulting from trauma to the cervix (eg, coitus and douching). Pain usually occurs over several cycles. There is no history of intermittent lower abdominal pain. Examination at the time of mittelschmerz may reveal some lower quadrant tenderness with or without rebound. Bimanual examination may show localized tenderness. A palpable ovary may be present, but a history of regular menses, lack of fever, and negative pregnancy tests confirm the diagnosis.

Mild analgesics and reassurance are usually adequate for these patients.

UTERINE PROLAPSE

ESSENTIALS OF DIAGNOSIS

- ▶ Prior vaginal deliveries
- ▶ History of pelvic heaviness, low back pain
- ▶ Patient may present with urinary retention
- ▶ Firm, muscular mass in or protruding from vagina

▶ Clinical Findings

Uterine prolapse typically occurs because of muscular defects in the pelvic floor arising from childbirth. Prolapse is characterized by variable symptoms of pelvic heaviness or a dragging sensation and lower back pain. Urinary retention of sudden onset may be a presenting complaint. Examination reveals a firm, muscular mass in the vagina or protruding from the vagina (procidentia) and having the shape and size of the uterus and cervix. Cystocele, rectocele, and enterocele are commonly associated with procidentia.

▶ Treatment and Disposition

Uterine prolapse associated with delivery requires immediate obstetric–gynecologic consultation, as significant hemorrhage and hemodynamic instability may occur. Reversion of the uterus should be attempted by manual pressure, directing the fundus back through the introitus. Tocolytics may be used to relax the uterus if needed. After repositioning, oxytocin is given to facilitate uterine contraction and prevent further prolapse. Patients with acute urinary retention or procidentia should have urgent gynecologic consultation. Patients with mild prolapse should be referred within 5–7 days for gynecologic evaluation and possible surgery.

SALPINGITIS AND TUBO-OVARIAN ABSCESS

See Chapter 42.

▶ Rape (Men and Women)

Proper care of the reported rape victim requires concern for the social and emotional consequences of the event as well as for the medical sequelae. The best care fulfills the requirements of the law while providing proper support and reassurance to the patient. Every state has its own laws and regulations concerning rape; however, some general principles apply. The physician's responsibilities include the following:

- recognizing and managing life-threatening trauma (eg, hemorrhagic shock);
- obtaining informed written consent for physical examination, collection of evidence, photographic documentation, and treatment;
- shielding the rape victim from other patients, bystanders, and visitors;
- accurately diagnosing and treating all physical injuries, both genital and nongenital;
- recording a detailed and explicit history of the event in the patient's own words;
- carefully collecting specimens for evidence, with accurate documentation and protection of the chain of evidence;
- providing psychological support and follow-up;
- offering prophylaxis against pregnancy and sexually transmitted disease;

- the physician should avoid judgmental or conclusive language;
- being willing to testify in court;
- ensuring that discharge from the emergency department is to a safe place;
- encouraging a physical examination even if the patient declines forensic examination.
- Unless required to do so by statute, the emergency physician does not have a legal obligation to notify the police when providing treatment to a victim of the rape. Notifying the police is appropriate when the patient has consented (preferably in writing) to such notification. The physician may wish to refer the patient to a counseling organization that aids rape victims.
- The responsibilities described above may be fulfilled by having a multidisciplinary team who follows an established protocol.

1. Management of the Rape Victim (Man or Woman)

▶ Evaluation

A. Initial Steps

If required by law or with the patient's consent, inform the police (see below). Obtain written informed consent for examination.

B. History

Obtain and record the history in the patient's own words. Obtain answers to other specific questions including the specific time in which the reported rape occurred (if they have not already been answered). A detailed account of the events leading up to the assault, however, is not helpful and should not be documented. Record the victim's general appearance and demeanor, and note whether clothing is torn or stained.

C. Evidence

Collect and label relevant evidence following your state and local protocol, use a rape kit if available and protect the chain of evidence. Your examination should be complete and thorough but guided by the history of the assault to include all pertinent evidence. Most evidence includes but is not necessarily limited to

1. scrapings under the fingernails;
2. pubic hair;
3. collecting any other loose hairs or dried blood;
4. dried slides of vaginal contents as well as vaginal secretions;
5. specimens from oral cavity or rectum if penetration has occurred;
6. photograph all external lesions, but only with the patient's written consent.

D. Physical Examination

Thoroughly examine the patient for other signs of bodily trauma or bleeding; record the results of the examination; and photograph all lesions (the last only with the patient's written consent). Examine the mouth and the rectum for injuries. Proctoscopy may be advisable if penetration has occurred and if foreign objects were used, because peritoneal perforation may occur from rectal trauma.

E. Pelvic Examination

Look carefully for signs of trauma to the external genitalia. Note and record whether the hymen is intact and whether any hymenal tags are fresh (indicating trauma) or healed.

Using a warm, water-moistened speculum, carefully examine the vagina for lacerations. Topical application of toluidine blue may enhance identification of genital skin tears. Colposcopy enhances the identification of traumatic injury. Rarely, peritoneal perforation may occur. If examination must be delayed for a short while, some methods to enhance future collection include insertion of tampon (send tampon with evidence) and do not have the patient urinate, douche, or defecate.

F. Laboratory Tests

Obtain blood for chemistry studies (if indicated), a serologic test for syphilis, and blood typing (to compare the alleged assailant's type with that of the victim). Blood sampling may also be used for hepatitis B and C and human immunodeficiency virus (HIV) serologic testing. Rapid HIV testing in the perpetrator should also be sought if advisable. To exclude pregnancy, a urine pregnancy test is indicated.

▶ Treatment

The physician should be empathic and concerned, never skeptical or judgmental.

A. Prevent Sexually Transmitted Disease

Treatment for gonorrhea, *C. trachomatis*, and syphilis (Chapter 40) should be offered. Only about 3% of rapes result in gonorrhea and only about 0.1% result in syphilis. Follow-up cultures for *Neisseria gonorrhoeae* are essential. Perform follow-up serologic tests for syphilis 1 and 3 months after the rape.

B. Prevent Infectious Diseases

Offer the hepatitis B vaccine as well as follow-up in 3–4 weeks for repeat hepatitis vaccination and testing. HIV is also of concern. Offer postexposure prophylactic medications based on risk factors with a follow-up for repeat HIV testing.

C. Prevent Pregnancy

Treatment for the prevention of pregnancy should be offered. Only about 1% of rapes result in pregnancy; the chances are much less if the victim is using an effective method of contraception. Levonorgestrel 0.75 mg, two tablets taken 12 hours apart, or Levonorgestrel 1.5 mg taken as a single dose, is approved for emergency contraception. Accepted alternate regimens include ethinyl estradiol, 200 μg, and norgestrel, 2 mg, orally over 12 hours in two divided doses (eg, norgestrel [Ovral], two tablets orally, repeating in 12 hours) to prevent implantation if it is certain that the patient is not already pregnant. Advise the patient that nausea and vomiting may occur. Give an antiemetic 40 minutes prior to the oral contraceptives.

Caution: Existing pregnancy is an absolute contraindication to the use of oral contraceptives. Warn the patient that this regimen may not be effective, and explain that a return visit within 1–2 weeks is essential for another pregnancy test.

D. Report the Incident

If required by law or if the patient consents, report the incident to the proper authorities before the patient leaves the emergency department because the police will want to question her. If the reported victim is a child, the incident should be reported to the appropriate child welfare authorities (Chapter 50).

E. Start Rape Counseling Immediately

Preferably, counseling should be directed by experienced personnel who are part of an established rape counseling program.

F. Arrange Follow-up

A definite appointment (time, place, and physician or clinic) should be made.

INTRAUTERINE DEVICES

▶ Problems with IUDs

A. "Lost" IUD

In the emergency department, the most common problem relating to these devices is the "lost" IUD. Check to see if the IUD is still properly placed by looking for the removal string protruding from the cervix (most women soon learn to feel for it with a finger). If no string can be found, the IUD may be located by uterine sonography or abdominal X-ray (for metallic IUDs). The IUD may be in an extrauterine position, in which case it should be removed surgically by laparoscopy or laparotomy.

B. Emergency Removal of IUD

1. Infection—The principal indication for removal of an IUD in the emergency department is infection (salpingi-tis, endometritis, pyosalpinx, or pelvic peritonitis). The incidence of endometritis, salpingitis, and tubal abscess is increased in women using IUDs. Any of these conditions requires removal of the IUD so that infection can be completely cleared. If possible, the patient should be started on appropriate antibiotics before the device is removed (see Salpingitis section in Chapter 40).

2. Bleeding and pain—Persistent vaginal bleeding or pelvic pain usually requires removal of an IUD but not often on an emergency basis. Referral to the physician who inserted the device is preferable.

If referral is impractical, grasp the string of the IUD with a Kelly clamp or other long grasping forceps and pull with gentle but increasing force until the IUD emerges from the uterus. Do not jerk the string, because it may detach from the device and make removal more difficult. If the string is not easily seen after manipulation with a speculum, use a special IUD remover to locate and grasp the string.

C. Serious but Rare Problems

1. Perforation of the uterus—Perforation of the uterus is a probable diagnosis in patients with IUDs who have symptoms of endometritis, salpingitis, or peritonitis. Physical examination, an abdominal X-ray, and sonography show that the IUD is embedded in the uterine wall or free in the peritoneum. Emergency hospitalization is required.

2. Pregnancy with IUD in place—If pregnancy is confirmed by a positive pregnancy test, and an IUD is still in place, seek emergency obstetric consultation. Ectopic pregnancy is a distinct possibility in the pregnant patient with an IUD still in place.

POSTCOITAL EMERGENCY CONTRACEPTION

Postcoital emergency contraception, also known as the morning-after pill, can be given to prevent implantation. The US Food and Drug Administration has approved plan B (levonorgestrel 0.75 mg) within 72 hours of intercourse and repeated again 12 hours later. Several prescriptive equivalents are available. Nausea and emesis frequently occur, and an antiemetic should be prescribed. Although the morning-after pill is reported to be 98% effective, a pregnancy test should be performed if menstruation does not occur within 21 days of treatment.

DISORDERS OF THE VULVA AND VAGINA

Vaginal and vulvar cancers and other lesions are discussed earlier in this chapter. Vaginitis, gonorrhea, genital herpes virus infection, and genital abscesses are discussed in Chapter 42.

WARNING ABOUT DISCONTINUING CONTRACEPTION

Treatment of gynecologic problems in the emergency department may require discontinuing the patient's current form of contraception. The emergency physician advising this course of action must warn the patient of the possibility of pregnancy and offer appropriate contraceptive advice. Discontinuation of oral contraceptives or IUD use because of treatment in the emergency department should not result in an unwanted pregnancy.

EMERGENCY MANAGEMENT OF OBSTETRIC DISORDERS

PREGNANCY

▶ Clinical Findings

The physician should have a high index of suspicion for the diagnosis of pregnancy even with the patient's denial, history of contraception, or recent menses. Initial presentation of pregnancy may be at the exact time as a presenting pregnancy complication.

A. Early Symptoms and Signs

Amenorrhea, nausea and vomiting, syncopal attacks, breast tenderness or tingling, and urinary symptoms (especially frequency) are early symptoms of pregnancy. Early signs of pregnancy include cervical cyanosis and softening, vaginal cyanosis, softening and enlargement of the uterus, and breast enlargement and tenderness.

B. Laboratory Tests

Urinary tests for pregnancy may occasionally be negative early in the pregnancy. False-positive results are rare at any time, unless trophoblastic tumors are present.

Ectopic pregnancies and spontaneous abortions may rarely cause false-negative results on urine immunologic pregnancy tests.

▶ Differential Diagnosis of Pregnancy

The differential diagnosis of pregnancy includes disorders producing secondary amenorrhea (endocrinopathies, emotional stress, drugs, malnutrition, and menopause) and those producing abdominal or uterine enlargement (obesity, tumors, pseudopregnancy [pseudocyesis]).

DISCOMFORTS OF PREGNANCY

Pregnant women are subject to many discomforts, any of which may cause a visit to the emergency department. Common discomforts include vomiting, backache, syncopal attacks, urinary symptoms (with and without demonstrable urinary tract infection), heartburn, constipation, hemorrhoids, varicose veins, leg swelling, and cramps.

If drug therapy of these complaints is contemplated, only drugs generally recognized as safe in pregnancy should be used, and the patient should be informed of potential benefits and risks. Rarely, pregnant women may have severe abdominal pain localized to one or another quadrant. Patients with round ligament pain may present in this manner. The pain tends to be fairly constant, not cramping. Temperature and white blood cell count are usually normal. Treatment consists of oral analgesics and bed rest.

Nausea and vomiting are common in the first trimester and usually occur in the morning. Symptomatic treatment of nausea and vomiting is preferred, for example, eating soda crackers immediately on arising in the morning, or consuming small, frequent, low-fat meals.

HYPEREMESIS GRAVIDARUM

▶ Clinical Findings

Hyperemesis gravidarum presents with persistent vomiting and dehydration, elevated specific gravity of urine, ketonuria, and hemoconcentration. Patients may require hospitalization for parenteral hydration and nutrition. Other causes of vomiting, such as infection, diabetes mellitus, or abdominal disorders must be excluded.

A. Symptoms and Signs

Patients who are known to be pregnant or have symptoms and signs of pregnancy (see above) complain of persistent vomiting, often with postural dizziness, presyncope, weight loss, or other signs of dehydration. Hyperemesis gravidarum usually resolves early in the second trimester. Physical examination reveals signs of dehydration: hypotension or postural hypotension, tachycardia, dry mucous membranes, and collapsed neck veins. Patients are rarely in severe shock.

B. Laboratory Tests

The test for pregnancy usually is positive, although rarely urinary tests may be negative early in pregnancy. Blood tests may show hemoconcentration, elevated blood urea nitrogen or creatinine, hypokalemia, or metabolic alkalosis. The urine usually appears concentrated with high specific gravity and ketonuria. Initial liver function tests may be mildly elevated.

▶ Treatment

A. Initial Steps

Insert an 18-gauge intravenous catheter (a larger bore is rarely needed). Draw blood for CBC, electrolytes, and renal/liver function. Infuse crystalloid solution containing glucose (eg, 0.9% saline with 5% dextrose) to correct hypovolemia. Consider thiamine replacement prior to glucose containing solutions, as Wernicke's Encephalopathy is a rare but serious complication. The amount and rate of administration depend on the severity of dehydration. Replace potassium as needed.

B. Antiemetics

If emesis persists, administer an antiemetic. Ondansetron (Class B safety in pregnancy) 4–8 mg IV every 8 hours or promethazine (Class C safety in pregnancy)12.5–25 mg IV every 6 hours can be used. While controlled, randomized studies of these medications are limited, they are both generally accepted as safe in pregnancy. Alternately, vitamin B_6 10–25 mg orally three times daily has been shown to reduce nausea in pregnancy.

Medications should be avoided during the first 10 weeks of pregnancy because of fetal organogenesis, but a risk-to-benefit ratio must be weighed on a case-by-case basis. The patient should be made aware of such risks before being given antiemetics.

▶ Disposition

Hospitalize patients who have persistent vomiting or ketonuria. Patients whose emesis is controlled and whose ketonuria resolves may be discharged with follow-up in 1–2 days. Antiemetic tablets or suppositories may be prescribed for the patient to use only as needed.

THIRD-TRIMESTER BLEEDING

▶ General Considerations

The most common causes of third-trimester bleeding are abruptio placentae, placenta previa, lower genital tract bleeding, or systemic coagulopathy. The least severe cause, lower genital tract bleeding, should be diagnosed only after the more severe conditions have been excluded systematically.

Third-trimester bleeding must be treated as a grave emergency threatening the life of both the mother and the fetus. Digital pelvic examination should be deferred until the relationship of the cervical os and placenta can visualized on ultrasound.

▶ Clinical Findings

A. Placental disorders

1. Abruptio placentae—Premature separation of the placenta from the endometrium, with hemorrhage into the subplacental space (between the uterus and the placenta). In most cases, patients present with vaginal bleeding. Pelvic pain may or not be present depending on the level of uterine irritability. Risk factors include advanced maternal age, multiparity, smoking, hypertension, external abdominal trauma, cocaine use, and prior history of abruption. Signs and symptoms include uterine tenderness, vaginal bleeding, and back or abdominal pain. Tocometry may demonstrate increased uterine contractility and signs of fetal distress. Ultrasound may miss early abruption. Larger placental abruptions are associated with disseminated intravascular coagulation, fetal demise, and/or maternal exsanguination.

2. Placenta previa—A placenta implanted in the lower uterine wall usually causes painless bleeding in small volumes that occurs regularly over a short period of observation. Such seemingly small blood loss may produce a false sense of security, because sudden massive hemorrhage can occur at any time. Risk factors for placenta previa include increased age, increased parity, multiple gestations, and previous cesarean sections or abortions. Abdominal or transvaginal ultrasound is safe and is imaging modality of choice.

B. Systemic Coagulopathies

Coagulation disorders are uncommon as the sole cause of third-trimester bleeding. Diagnosis is confirmed by routine coagulation studies.

▶ Treatment

A. Initial Steps

Obtain emergency obstetric consultation. Evaluate the patient for hypovolemia (as shown by supine or postural hypotension), and if present, correct it with intravenous infusion of crystalloid solution or whole blood.

B. Laboratory Tests

Insert a large-bore (≥16-gauge) intravenous catheter. Draw blood for CBC, coagulation studies (prothrombin time, partial thromboplastin time, fibrinogen, and platelet count), and measurement of blood urea nitrogen and serum creatinine. Type and crossmatch for four units of blood.

Monitor fetal heart tones and toxicology especially looking for the presence of cocaine. Obtain urine for urinalysis, and monitor urine output with an indwelling urinary catheter.

C. Other Considerations

Ultrasound should be used to determine the placental location, but this should not delay delivery if the fetus is in distress.

The pregnant patient should never be maintained for any length of time in the supine, recumbent position (see Trauma in Pregnancy section).

▶ Disposition

Hospitalize the patient immediately, and move her to a delivery unit as soon as possible. Fetal bradycardia increases the urgency of the need for cesarean section.

PREGNANCY INDUCED HYPERTENSION (PREECLAMPSIA–ECLAMPSIA)

▶ Clinical Findings

Pregnancy induced hypertension describes a condition that covers a spectrum of symptoms and a continuum of severity. Gestational hypertension is defined by a blood pressure measurement of 140/90 or higher. Preeclampsia is characterized by pregnancy-induced hypertension and proteinuria. Eclampsia manifests as seizures in a patient with signs of preeclampsia. Blood pressure measurements should be checked and urinalysis performed in every pregnant patient that presents to the emergency department to detect early signs of preeclampsia–eclampsia.

A. Symptoms and Signs

Symptoms and signs are variable and may include headache, various visual symptoms, and vertigo. Nausea and vomiting, hyperreflexia, and abdominal pain may occur. Especially alarming is pain in the upper right quadrant and epigastrium (so-called hepatic pain), which is due to compression of the swelling liver by its capsule. Nervousness, irritability, and even frank seizures may occur.

Hypertension or rising blood pressure relative to the patient's normal blood pressure is a significant sign. Note that blood pressure may not be sufficiently elevated to be considered abnormal because of the physiologic decline in blood pressure usually associated with pregnancy.

Peripheral edema is usually present. Spasm of retinal arterioles and hemorrhage may occur. Hepatomegaly or hepatic tenderness (or both) may be present.

B. Laboratory Findings

Critical laboratory findings supporting the diagnosis of preeclampsia–eclampsia are decreased urine output, elevated blood urea nitrogen and serum creatinine levels, decreased creatine clearance, proteinuria, and evidence of disseminated intravascular coagulation.

▶ Treatment and Disposition

Patients with suspected preeclampsia–eclampsia should be emergently evaluated by an obstetrician.

A. Gestational Hypertension

Gestational hypertension is defined as a blood pressure measurement above 140/90. There should be no proteinuria, and liver function and coagulation panels should be normal. Physical examination should demonstrate normal deep tendon reflexes and mental status. The patient with gestational hypertension may be appropriate for discharge with short term follow up after consultation with an obstetrician.

B. Mild Preeclampsia

Mild preeclampsia is characterized by diastolic blood pressure under 105 mm Hg, trace to proteinuria >300/24 hrs, good urinary output, and absence of other symptoms. Obstetric consultation should be obtained, and if not admitted, instructions for patient bedrest should be given at discharge with and short term follow-up arranged.

C. Severe Preeclampsia

Severe preeclampsia is characterized by proteinuria, diastolic blood pressure greater than 110 mm Hg, headaches, vision changes, anuria, or severe edema. Signs of end organ damage

are often present. HELLP Syndrome is a severe form of preeclampsia in which laboratory findings of *H*emolysis, *E*levated *L*iver enzymes, and *L*ow *P*latelets. The patient is said to have eclampsia when the above finds are present with seizures.

Hospitalization is indicated for patients with signs of moderate to severe preeclampsia. Treat hypertension with intravenous hydralazine (Alazine, Apresoline), 5–10 mg intravenously followed by 5–10 mg intravenously every 20–30 minutes as needed for blood pressure control. Labetolol can be used as an alternative. Do not reduce blood pressure to "normal" levels (120/80 mm Hg), because end organ hypoperfusion may result. Magnesium sulfate is indicated for seizure prophylaxis., given 4–6 g given over 30 minutes as an intravenous loading dose, followed by 2 g/h. Continued seizure activity raises the possibility of intracranial pathology such as a cerebral hemorrhage, and a CT scan of the head may be in order.

When neurologic and cardiovascular status is stable, transfer the patient to a hospital equipped to manage high-risk obstetric patients.

TRAUMA IN PREGNANCY

Trauma due to gunshot wounds, assault, or automobile accident may cause abruptio placentae, ruptured fetal membranes, or direct fetal trauma.

A. Normal Physiologic Changes

An awareness of the normal physiologic changes in pregnancy is important in evaluating and providing treatment to the mother and fetus:

- Systolic and diastolic blood pressure decreases approximately 10 mm Hg by the middle of the second trimester.
- Resting heart rate increases by 10–15 beats.
- Uterine blood flow increases to 17% of the cardiac output.
- Hematocrit decreases to a range of 30–36%.
- Tidal volume increases by 30–40%.
- Residual volume and functional residual capacity decrease.
- Leukocytosis is common by the second trimester.
- Pco_2 decreases to approximately 35 mm Hg (mild respiratory alkalosis).

B. Injuries

1. Blunt abdominal trauma—Motor vehicle accidents account for most trauma. Be aware of abruptio placentae or uterine rupture.

2. Penetrating abdominal injuries—During pregnancy, the physical response to intraperitoneal irritation may be decreased. Also, a cephalad and lateral displacement of maternal intraabdominal viscera occurs.

C. Laboratory Findings

Rh blood typing is indicated. The Kleihauer–Betke test detects fetal blood cells in the maternal circulation and placental disruption; it may help identify fetal hypovolemia before obvious fetal distress occurs.

▶ Treatment

A. Blunt Abdominal Trauma

Beyond 24 weeks' gestation the patient should be placed in the left lateral decubitus position unless potential spinal injury is a concern. Maintain spinal immobilization on a long, rigid spine board tilted slightly to the left when necessary. Ensure that ventilation and resuscitative measures are adequate. Anticipate rapid oxygen desaturation and aggressively treat any acidosis. A complete physical examination including a bimanual examination for evaluation of the cervical os should be completed. Maternal vital signs, vaginal bleeding, and any abdominal tenderness should be the focus of examination.

For a pregnancy greater than 20 weeks' gestation, use a standard fetal monitor to monitor fetal heart tones and contractions. A sonograph should be used for confirmation of gestation age. Fetal distress may precede maternal hemodynamic instability as an indicator of inadequately resuscitated shock. The need for aggressive resuscitation measures cannot be overemphasized because blood loss is easily underestimated. Early notification of surgical and obstetrical consultants is important. Radiologic studies should proceed as indicated.

Because of the possibility of a fetal–maternal transfusion with even minor blunt trauma, Rh negative patients should receive RhoGAM™ to prevent a serious isoimmunization reaction which could severely complicate the current or future pregnancies.

B. Penetrating Trauma

Most gunshot wounds to the abdomen should be explored surgically. In a pregnant patient, unstable vital signs with any penetrating abdominal wound is an indication for a laparotomy. However, not all penetrating trauma requires surgery. For instance, stab wounds to the lower abdomen are less likely to cause visceral injuries than upper abdominal wounds and may not need exploratory laparotomy. Although generally considered contraindicated in pregnancy, diagnostic peritoneal lavage (Chapter 8) may help diagnose hemoperitoneum and the need for surgery.

The decision to perform surgery with or without delivery should be made in conjunction with a surgeon and an obstetrician. Several factors are used to make an interventional decision, including gestational age, penetration of amniotic cavity, and fetal injury. This needs to be a multidisciplinary approach to include obstetrics and surgery.

▶ Perimortem Cesarean Delivery

A. Indications

A fetus has been reported to survive up to 30 minutes after maternal cardiac arrest, but the greatest likelihood for fetal survival is if delivery occurs within 4–5 minutes after maternal cardiac arrest. Another indication for a perimortem cesarean section is to improve the possibility of returning spontaneous maternal circulation as part of her ongoing resuscitation.

B. Technique

1. Cardiopulmonary resuscitation should continue throughout the procedure.

2. Make an abdominal incision approximately 4–5 cm below the xiphoid to 2–3 cm above the pubis.

3. Separate the rectus muscles bluntly in the midline and enter the peritoneum with a midline incision usually below the umbilicus.

4. Make a vertical incision from the top of the uterine fundus to above the opaque insertion of the bladder.

5. Remove the fetus.

6. Remove the placenta.

7. Close the uterus in one or two layers using large sutures.

LABOR AND DELIVERY

In many hospitals, patients in active labor are seen initially in the emergency department. A calm and orderly approach to evaluation of these patients—as well as established policies for transfer of responsibility from emergency department staff to obstetric staff—is essential for proper management.

▶ Evaluation

A. History

If records from prenatal visits are not available, ask the patient about recent or intercurrent illness and risk factors such as diabetes mellitus, valvular heart disease, or previous cesarean section delivery. Ask whether the membranes have ruptured. Determine parity and multiparity gestation. Estimate the due date and gestational age of the fetus.

B. Physical Examination

Record complete maternal vital signs. Perform brief physical examination of the mother. Determine frequency and intensity of uterine contractions.

Check for vaginal discharge by speculum examination (blood or meconium). The presence of amniotic fluid may be detected by an alkaline reaction (yellow turning to blue) with Nitrazine paper.

Determine fetal position. Determine the fetal heart rate during and between uterine contractions.

Perform vaginal examination. *Note*: Do not perform digital examination if vaginal bleeding is present. Determine the presenting part and the degree of dilation and effacement of the cervix by speculum.

▶ Clinical Findings

Progressive labor is characterized by uterine contractions occurring every 3 minutes and dilation of the cervical os. Abnormal signs requiring emergency obstetric consultation include fetal bradycardia (<100 beats/min during or after uterine contractions, vaginal bleeding (on history or examination), transverse, breech, or cord presentations, and maternal illness (eg, eclampsia, coma, major trauma).

▶ Treatment

A. Premature Birth

Infants under 36 weeks' gestational age are likely to require neonatal intensive care. If there is no such nursery in the facility where the mother has sought treatment, consider transferring her to another facility unless she is in active labor and delivery is imminent or likely during transport (ie, baby is crowning or very low station). See Chapter 5 for further discussion.

Give crystalloid solution, 1000 mL over 3–4 hours, and monitor cardiovascular status carefully. In consultation with an obstetrician, decisions can be made about the use of tocolysis, administration of maternal betamethasone for fetal lung maturity, and prophylaxis against group B streptococci by administration of penicillin G.

B. Emergency Department Delivery

If delivery is imminent, give nothing (or sips of clear fluids only) by mouth. Maintain or reinstate adequate hydration with intravenous fluids. Give analgesia if there are no contraindications. Obtain a baby warmer, a precipitous delivery kit, and try to have a labor and delivery nurse present.

1. Delivery—Analgesia may be given as needed to the mother with an uncomplicated term pregnancy. Delivery may be accomplished in either the lithotomy or the Sims position. Prepare a clean field (wash the vulva and perineum). Prevent sudden uncontrolled delivery of the fetal head.

Suction the infant's nasal passages and airway with a suction bulb (or DeLee suction trap, if available) after the head is delivered but before the body is delivered. If thick meconium staining of the amniotic fluid is present, you may use direct laryngoscopy and subglottic suctioning techniques. The physician may need to intubate the infant immediately, before spontaneous respirations occur, and apply suction to the trachea.

Cut the umbilical cord after ligating it about 2–3 in (5.0–7.5 cm) from the infant's abdomen.

Within 20–30 minutes, deliver the placenta with gentle traction on the cord if it comes out easily. Massage the fundus to help obtain hemostasis and uterine tone. If the patient is not bleeding vigorously, the placenta may be left in place while the patient is sent to the delivery room for further measures (eg, suture of lacerations). Delivery of an incomplete placenta is an obstetrical emergency.

2. Postpartum measures—Dry and examine the infant, and resuscitate if necessary. *Keep the baby warm.*

Monitor the mother's blood pressure every 5 minutes for 15 minutes and then every 15 minutes for 1 hour. Uncontrolled bleeding from vaginal lacerations may be packed to await definite repair from an obstetrician. A sample of the infant's clotted cord blood should be sent for ABO and Rh typing and a serologic test for syphilis.

▶ Disposition

A. Premature Birth

Hospitalize the newborn infant and mother for evaluation and supportive care.

POSTPARTUM HEMORRHAGE

ESSENTIALS OF DIAGNOSIS

- ▶ History of recent delivery
- ▶ Painless, sudden, brisk vaginal bleeding

▶ Clinical Findings

Rarely, a patient returns to the hospital a few days after delivery with brisk vaginal bleeding that may or may not be associated with hemorrhagic shock. The usual causes of postpartum hemorrhage are uterine atony, retention of products of conception, or uterine rupture following cesarean section. Other possible causes are subinvolution of the placental site, vaginal tears, or bleeding from an episiotomy. Signs of postpartum hemorrhage may include an enlarged uterus suggestive of atony, a vaginal mass suggestive of an inverted uterus, or uterine bleeding with good uterine tone and a normal size suggestive of retained products of conception.

▶ Treatment and Disposition

A. Initial Steps

Treat hemorrhagic shock, if present (Chapter 11). If bleeding is brisk, insert the fingers of one hand into the vagina, and compress the uterus against the abdominal wall.

B. Laboratory Tests

Draw blood for CBC, coagulation studies (prothrombin time, partial thromboplastin time, and platelet count), blood urea nitrogen, and serum creatinine. Type and crossmatch for 4 units of blood.

C. Consultation

Obtain emergency obstetric–gynecologic consultation.

D. Medications

Oxytocin, 10–40 units in 1 L normal saline for intravenous infusion at 20–40 milliunits per minute, may be used for uterine atony. After an obstetrical consult is obtained, methylergonovine (Methergine) by mouth may be recommended prior to discharge.

E. Definitive Treatment

The definitive treatment is dilation and curettage, which should be performed by an obstetrician, because post-partum surgery may result in uterine perforation.

 Disposition

If the cause of bleeding is definitively treated and the patient is otherwise stable, she can be discharged with close follow-up in 2–3 days. All other patients should be hospitalized and obstetric consultation obtained as needed.

PUERPERAL SEPSIS AND ENDOMETRITIS

 ESSENTIALS OF DIAGNOSIS

► History of recent delivery
► Systemic signs of infection
► Abdominal pain, vaginal discharge
► Peritoneal signs
► Boggy, tender uterus and purulent lochia

 Clinical Findings

Symptoms of puerperal sepsis in the early postpartum period are fever, peritoneal pain, and vaginal discharge. Examination reveals abdominal tenderness, exquisite uterine tenderness, and purulent lochia with leukocytes and bacteria on Gram stain.

 Treatment and Disposition

If signs of sepsis are present, obtain obstetric–gynecologic consultation, and hospitalize the patient immediately.

Patients with minimal symptoms may be managed as outpatients. Obtain samples of blood and discharge for diagnostic culture and sensitivity testing. Start antibiotics in accordance with the following recommendations as follows.

A. Severely Ill Patients

Give cefoxitin 2 g every 6–8 hours intravenously, ticarcillin–clavulanate 3.1 g every 6 hours intravenously, imipenem–cilastatin 500 mg intravenously every 6 hours, or meropenem 1 g intravenous every 8 hours.

PUERPERAL MASTITIS

 ESSENTIALS OF DIAGNOSIS

► Postpartum breast infection
► Increased localized breast pain
► Variable systemic signs of infection
► Localized tenderness, redness, induration, or warmth

 Clinical Findings

Postpartum infection of the breast is almost always due to infection with *Staphylococcus aureus*. Pain, induration, redness, and warmth in the affected breast characterizes mastitis. Fever, chills, malaise, and axillary adenopathy may be present.

The diagnosis of puerperal mastitis is based on systemic signs of infection, pain, and tenderness of the involved breast. Abscess formation may occur, and blood cultures are occasionally positive.

 Treatment and Disposition
A. Mild Cases (Afebrile)

Apply warm compresses to the affected breast. The patient may continue to breast feed. The patient should be given dicloxacillin, 500 mg by mouth four times a day, or cephalexin, 500 mg by mouth four times a day. Consider trimethoprim-sulfamethoxazole double strength two tablets twice daily, or clindamycin 300 mg four times daily in patients with risk factors for community-acquired methicillin-resistant staphylococcus aureus (MRSA). Close follow-up with the obstetrician is recommended, and consultation with a lactation expert may be in order. Analgesia may be indicated.

B. Severe Cases (Suspected Abscess)

Hospitalize the patient, and obtain surgical consultation. Give nafcillin 2 g every 4 hours intravenously. Penicillin-allergic patients may be given clindamycin, 450 mg intravenously every 8 hours, or erythromycin, 0.5 g intravenously every 6 hours.

Achanna S et al: Puerperal uterine inversion : A report of four cases. J Obstet Gynaecol Res 2006;32(3):341–345 [PMID: 16764627].

Emergency Medicine ultrasound guidelines. Ann Emerg Med 2009;53:550–570 [PMID: 19303521]. ACEP Policy Statement (revision of 2001 Guidelines).

Benjamins LJ. Practice Guideline: evaluation and management of abnormal vaginal bleeding in adolescents. J Pediatr Health Care 2009;23(3):189–193 [PMID: 19401253].

Brown HL. Trauma in pregnancy. Obstet Gynecol 2009;114(1): 147–160 [PMID: 19546773].

Brown MA et al: Screening sonography in pregnant patients with blunt abdominal trauma. J Ultrasound Med 2005;24(2): 175–181 [PMID: 15661948].

Condous G, Kirk E, Lu C et al: Diagnostic accuracy of varying discriminatory zones for the prediction of ectopic pregnancy in women with a pregnancy of unknown location. Ultrasound Obstet Gynecol 2005;26:770 [PMID: 16308901].

Goodwin TM. Hyperemesis gravidarum. Obstet Gynecol Clin North Am 2008;35(3):401–417, viii [PMID: 18760227].

Graeber B et al: Lase postpartum eclampsis as an obstetric complication seen in ED. Am J Emerg Med 2005;23(20):168–170 [PMID: 15765338].

Griebel CP et al: Management of spontaneous abortion. Am Fam Physician 2005;72(7):1243–1250 [PMID: 16225027].

Hansen LB, Saseen JJ, Teal SB. Levonorgestrel-only dosing strategies for emergency contraception. Pharmacotherapy 2007; 27:278 [PMID: 17253917].

Kirk E, Condous G, Bourne T. The non-surgical management of ectopic pregnancy. Ultrasound Obstet Gynecol 2006;27:91 [16374758].

Leeman L, Fontaine P. Hypertensive disorders of pregnancy. Am Fam Physician 2008;78(1):93–100 [PMID: 18649616].

Luce H, Schrager S, Gilchrist V. Sexual assault of women. Am Fam Physician 2010;81(4):489–495 [20148503].

Mirza FG, Devine PC, Gaddipati S. Trauma in pregnancy: a systemic approach. Am J Perinatol. 2010;27(7):579–586. Epub 2010 Mar 2. Review. [PMID: 20198552].

Oyelese et al: Postpartum hemorrhage. Obstet Gynecol Clin North Am 2007;34(3):421–441 [17921008].

Sakornbut E, Leeman L, Fontaine P. Late pregnancy bleeding. Am Fam Physician 200715;75(8):1199–1206 [PMID: 17477103].

Sexually transmitted diseases treatment guidelines 2006. Centers for Disease Control and Prevention. MMWR Recomm Rep 2006;55(11).

Sibai BM. Diagnosis, prevention, and management of eclampsia. Obstet Gynecol 2005;105:402 [PMID: 15684172].

Snell BJ. Assessment and Management of Bleeding in the first trimester of pregnancy. Midwifery Womens Health 2009;54(6):483–491 [19879521].

Thorp JM. Utilization of anti-RhD in the emergency department after blunt trauma. Obstet Gynecol Surv 2008;63(2):112–115 [PMID: 18199384].

van Mello NM, Mol F, Adriaanse AH et al: The METEX study: methotrexate versus expectant management in women with ectopic pregnancy: a randomised controlled trial. BMC Womens Health 2008;8:10 [PMID: 18565217].

Vandermeer FQ, Wong-You-Cheong JJ. Imaging of acute pelvic pain. Clin Obstet Gynecol 2009;52(1):2–20 [PMID: 19179858].

Genitourinary Emergencies

Joseph Heidenreich, MD[1]

IMMEDIATE MANAGEMENT OF SERIOUS AND LIFE-THREATENING CONDITIONS

OLIGURIA OR ANURIA

▶ General Considerations

It is helpful to categorize the mechanism as prerenal (eg, resulting from decreased or abnormal renal perfusion), renal (eg, resulting from intrinsic renal disease), or postrenal (eg, disease of the urinary collecting system distal to the renal parenchyma). Prerenal and postrenal causes are often suggested by the history and physical examination. Additionally, it is be helpful to determine the presence and extent of acute kidney injury (AKI) that frequently accompanies oliguria and anuria.

A. Prerenal Causes

Prerenal causes include hypovolemia, sepsis, and heart failure.

B. Renal Causes

Renal causes include tubular, glomerular, vascular, or interstitial disease.

C. Postrenal Causes

1. Supravesical obstruction—Supravesical obstruction rarely causes oliguria or anuria, because bilateral disease is required to reduce decreased urine flow. There are two types of supravesical obstruction: (1) ureteral obstruction (usually tumor) and (2) ureteropelvic or ureterovesical obstruction.

2. Intravesical or infravesical obstruction—Intravesical or infravesical obstruction is more common than supravesical obstruction and may be from many causes (Table 39–1).

▶ Clinical Findings

A. History

1. Obstruction—Differentiate between reduced urine output (with normal or nearly normal voiding patterns) and oliguria associated with difficult in voiding, feeling of incomplete voiding, and diminished urinary stream. The latter findings suggest obstruction.

2 Associated medical conditions—Ask about coexisting cardiac, pulmonary, renal, or other underlying disease that might contribute to renal or prerenal oliguria.

3. Drugs—The patient's medications might cause problems with urination or be nephrotoxic. Anticholinergics and sympathomimetics are most often the culprits of urinary retention.

---

[1]This chapter is a revision of the chapter by Charles F. McCuskey, MD, from the 6th edition.

Table 39-1. Diagnostic Clues to the Cause of Bladder Outlet Obstruction.

Cause	Frequency of Occurrence	Results of History and Physical Examination	Laboratory Tests and Other Studies
Prostatic hypertrophy	Common	Gradually increasing difficulty in voiding, often with abrupt worsening. Enlarged prostate on rectal examination is common	Urethral catheterization may be difficult.
Urethral strictures or valves	Uncommon	Often previous attacks of urethritis or urethral trauma. Onset may be gradual or abrupt	Urethral catheterization often difficult. Urethrogram or urethroscopy is diagnostic
Bladder stones or tumor	Uncommon	Hematuria is common. Obstruction may be intermittent	Urethral catheter is passed without difficulty. Cystogram or cystoscopy is diagnostic
Neuropathic bladder	Very common	Onset may be gradual and painless or abrupt and painful. Look for associated neurologic abnormalities (sacral dermatomal hypesthesia, poor rectal sphincter tone, neuralgic pain)	Urethral catheter passed without difficulty. Cystometrogram is diagnostic
Traumatic urethral injury	Uncommon	Male; history of trauma, prostatic dislocation, urethral bleeding	*Do not pass catheter.* Retrograde urethrogram and percutaneous cystogram are diagnostic

B. Physical Examination

1. Vital signs—Obtain a complete set of vital signs. Correct volume depletion, if present (Chapter 11).

2. General examination—Focus on signs of cardiac, pulmonary, renal, or hepatic disease that might contribute to oliguria of a prerenal or renal origin. Look for signs of volume depletion, such as dry mucous membranes or poor skin turgor.

3. Abdominal examination—Palpate the lower abdomen to determine whether a suprapubic mass, consistent with a distended bladder, is present. A distended bladder is manifested as a firm (but not hard) mass that is adjacent to the symphysis pubica and is dull to percussion.

4. GU examination—Examine the prostate for masses, prostatic hypertrophy, prostatic tenderness, or prostatic dislocation (associated with trauma).

C. Detection of Bladder Outlet Obstruction

Bladder outlet obstruction (complete or partial) is strongly suggested by a palpable bladder in a patient who is unable to void or who has a weak urinary stream or a feeling of incomplete voiding. Severe lower abdominal pain is more likely to be present with acute obstruction and rapid bladder distention than gradually progressive obstruction.

The diagnosis may be confirmed by calculating postvoid residual using either catheter drainage, ultrasonography, or CT scanning immediately after the patient's attempt to completely empty their bladder. Diagnostic features of some of the common causes of bladder outlet obstruction are set forth in Table 39–1.

D. Acute Kidney Injury

Oliguria and anuria are frequently accompanied by AKI. A standardized definition as well as objective grading system for AKI has been developed to help predict outcomes and aid in treatment (Table 39–2). It is important to note that laboratory markers of AKI such as serum creatinine usually lag behind oliguria or anuria.

Table 39-2. Acute Kidney Injury Network Staging Criteria for Acute Kidney Injury.

AKIN Stage	Serum Creatinine	Urine Output
1	Increased by 1.5–2 times baseline or by ≥0.3 mg/dL	<0.5 mL/kg/hr for 6 hrs
2	Increased between 2 and 3 times baseline	<0.5 mL/kg/hr for 24 hrs
3	Increased by >3 times baseline or to ≥4mg/dL with an acute rise of ≥0.5 mg/dL	<0.3 mL/kg/hr for 24 hrs

▶ Treatment

A. Serious Underlying Disease

If the patient appears to be acutely ill, in shock, septic, in decompensated heart failure or has other serious coexisting conditions that might cause prerenal oliguria, these disorders must be evaluated and treated before those of the urinary tract.

B. Distended Bladder (Presumed Bladder Outlet Obstruction)

1. Gain intravenous access—Draw blood for complete blood count (CBC), electrolyte determination, and blood urea nitrogen and serum creatinine measurements.

2. Drain the bladder

A. URETHRAL CATHETER—Try to pass an indwelling urethral (Foley) catheter. If this maneuver is successful, drain the bladder, record the volume of urine obtained, and send a specimen for urinalysis and culture. Monitor the patient for postobstructive diuresis. Gradual bladder draining is not a proven method of decreasing bladder atony or mucosal hemorrhage. If bladder outlet obstruction is relieved by passage of a Foley catheter and is apparently due to a transient cause (eg, drugs), the catheter may be removed and the patient observed for ability to void after the effects of any drugs are presumed to have dissipated. In patients with fixed bladder outlet obstruction (eg, benign prostatic hypertrophy), leave the catheter in place, and obtain urologic consultation within 1 week. If a standard Foley catheter cannot be passed secondary to prostatic hypertrophy, reattempt passage using a coudé catheter (which has a curved tip that usually allows passage beyond the enlarged prostate). Inability to pass the catheter beyond the proximal urethra is suggestive for urethral stricture.

B. SUPRAPUBIC CATHETER—If the coudé catheter is unsuccessful and a urologist is not available, insert a suprapubic catheter for temporary drainage (Chapter 7). A large (16-gauge) needle-clad catheter (eg, Intracath) will provide satisfactory emergency bladder drainage.

3. Treat cystitis and prostatitis, if present—See Dysuria section, below.

4. Hospitalize patients as needed—Hospitalize patients who have systemic symptoms (fever, rigors, intractable emesis) and those who need additional diagnosis and treatment (eg, for management of postobstructive diuresis, azotemia, sepsis, or electrolyte abnormalities).

C. Bladder Not Palpable; Patient Able to Void

If the patient can void on command but continues to have subjective or objective evidence of a weak urinary stream or if the patient experiences a feeling of incomplete voiding, partial bladder outlet obstruction is likely.

Draw blood for CBC, electrolyte, blood urea nitrogen, and serum creatinine measurements. Send a urine specimen for urinalysis and culture. Treat cystitis or prostatitis, if present. If blood chemistry results and urinalysis are normal, refer the patient to a urologist. The presence of azotemia or electrolyte abnormalities indicates severe or long-standing obstructive uropathy, and the patient likely requires hospitalization.

D. Bladder Not Palpable; Patient Unable to Void

Consider the following in the differential diagnosis (1) intrinsic renal disease, (2) occult prerenal disease (unlikely, because most causes would be obvious on brief physical examination), (3) occult bladder outlet obstruction, or (4) supravesical obstructive uropathy (rare).

Draw blood for CBC; serum glucose, electrolyte, calcium, and phosphorus; and tests of renal and hepatic function. Obtain chest and abdominal X-rays to help evaluate the size of the kidneys and bladder. Ultrasonography is the best noninvasive test for evaluating kidney and bladder size.

Ensure adequate hydration. In an adult without obvious volume overload (eg, pulmonary or peripheral edema), give 1–2 L of fluid orally or intravenously, and observe the patient for 1–2 hours. In an individual with normal kidneys, this amount should produce a brisk flow of urine.

If anuria persists despite adequate hydration and if the bladder is not distended, the cause of the anuria is likely to be proximal to the bladder (prerenal, renal, or, rarely, bilateral ureteral obstruction). Bladder catheterization, with strict adherence to sterile technique, should be performed to confirm the lack of urine output. Hospitalize the patient for further evaluation.

▶ Disposition

Hospitalization is required for patients with persistent unexplained anuria or severe oliguria (<500 mL/d), those with systemic symptoms, and those with markedly abnormal electrolytes or renal function.

Patients with partial bladder outlet obstruction (ie, weak urinary stream, with or without palpable bladder) should be referred to a urologist if renal function is normal or nearly normal. Asymptomatic patients with an indwelling urethral catheter should be reexamined or referred to a urologist within 1 week.

SCROTAL PAIN

See Table 39–3.

ESSENTIALS OF DIAGNOSIS

▶ Trauma is a common cause

▶ Infection accounts for orchitis and epididymitis

▶ Flank pain, hematuria, and scrotal pain usually indicates urolithiasis

▶ Incarcerated hernias cause scrotal pain

▶ Testicular torsion requires urgent diagnosis to salvage the testicle. A torsed testis may be high riding or horizontally lying; ultrasound will show diminished blood flow to the torsed testis

▶ Clinical Findings

A. Trauma

(See also Chapter 26) Trauma commonly causes testicular or scrotal pain. Careful questioning may be required to elicit the circumstances under which the trauma occurred.

B. Viral Orchitis

Mumps virus and the enteroviruses may cause acute unilateral or bilateral orchitis. In orchitis due to mumps virus, associated parotitis is usually present.

C. Urolithiasis

Rarely, patients with urolithiasis present with pain localized mainly in the scrotum; however, in most cases, back or flank pain has preceded the scrotal pain, or a history of nephrolithiasis is present. In such cases, the testicle and epididymis are normal to palpation. Hematuria is an important diagnostic clue.

D. Incarcerated Hernia

Inguinal hernias incarcerated in the scrotum may cause scrotal pain that may be confused with testicular pain. Bowel sounds are heard in the scrotum early in incarceration; if the hernia strangulates, bowel sounds are no longer audible. Intestinal hernia into the scrotum is almost always associated with clinical findings of intestinal obstruction (Chapter 15). Ultrasonography is diagnostic.

E. Testicular Torsion, Epididymitis, and Torsion of the Testicular Appendages

(See Table 39–3) Torsion of a testicular appendage, epididymitis, and testicular torsion are the three most common causes of acute scrotal pain and account for approximately 85–90% of cases. Because of the urgency to diagnose and treat testicular torsion within 6 hours to prevent loss of the testis, testicular torsion must be promptly ruled out in all patients with scrotal pain. It may be difficult to distinguish from epididymitis or torsion of testicular appendages as edema and inflammation progress to involve the entire scrotal sac and contents.

1. Testicular torsion—Testicular torsion tends to occur in young men and is rare in men older than 30 years; however, it can and does occur at all ages and a smaller peak also occurs in the first year of life. There is often a history of episodes of similar scrotal pain representing torsion with spontaneous repositioning of the testicle. The pain is abrupt in onset, severe, unilateral, and often associated with nausea and vomiting. Tenderness is initially noted only in the testicle; however, with persistent torsion and the resulting testicular hypoxia, pain and tenderness spread to involve contiguous intrascrotal structures.

Examination early in the illness shows an elevated testicle that is apt to have a horizontal lie (Bell clapper deformity). The epididymis may be felt in an abnormal position (eg, anteriorly) in the early stages. Later, the entire scrotal contents become swollen and tender, making the examination extremely difficult and less informative because the epididymis becomes indistinguishable from the testis on palpation.

2. Epididymitis—Epididymitis tends to occur in sexually active men older than 20 years and is the most common misdiagnosis for testicular torsion. There may be a history of urinary tract infection or urethritis. Pain begins gradually and is less severe than in testicular torsion. The Prehn's sign is present if the pain is reduced when the scrotum is elevated. This finding is not specific to epididymitis nor is it a reliable discriminating clinical sign. Physical examination reveals a tender epididymis, often unilateral and often with erythema and edema of the scrotal skin. Early on, the testicle may be normal or minimally tender. However, as edema worsens, the epididymis becomes indistinguishable from the testicle on palpation, and a reactive hydrocele may develop, making it difficult to differentiate epididymitis from testicular torsion. Urinalysis frequently shows pyuria and possibly bacteriuria if a concomitant urethritis or urinary tract infection is present. Doppler ultrasound shows increased blood flow to the affected testis, in contrast to the decreased blood flow seen in testicular torsion.

3. Torsion of testicular or epididymal appendages—Of the four appendages, the appendix testis, located on the anterosuperior pole of the testis, is the most frequently (92%) torsed appendage followed by the appendix epididymis (7%), located on the head of the epididymis. Pain is usually sudden in onset and can be severe, with nausea and vomiting. Physical examination occasionally (21%) reveals a small, tender, firm nodule ("blue dot" sign), representing the infarcted appendage in the anterosuperior pole of the

Table 39–3. Diagnostic Clues to the Cause of Acute Scrotal Pain.

	History	Physical Examination	Urinalysis Results	Other Laboratory Studies	Treatment and Disposition
Trauma	History of injury	Scrotal hematoma	Variable; may have hematuria	Sonogram	Obtain urologic consultation (Chapter 24)
Urolithiasis	Antecedent flank or back pain; occasionally abdominal pain	Testicle minimally tender or nontender	Hematuria	Stones on excretory urogram	Obtain urologic consultation
Viral (eg, mumps) orchitis	Gradual onset, coexisting mumps parotitis common	Tender testicles (unilateral or bilateral); epididymis rarely involved	Normal	Viral cultures (throat, stool) if available; characteristic fourfold rise in serum antibody titer.	Elevate and immobilize testicle (eg, athletic supporter), give analgesics, and discharge for follow-up care.
Incarcerated hernia	Gradual onset; crampy pain	Fluid rushes heard in scrotum (early); abdominal tenderness consistent with intestinal obstruction	Normal	Characteristically abnormal results on ultrasound studies; abdominal X-ray results often abnormal (intestinal obstruction)	Obtain general surgical consultation; hospitalize
Epididymitis	Gradual onset; history of urethritis or urinary tract infection common; older men (>age 25 yrs)	Tender epididymis (often unilateral) with normal testicle early in course; pain relieved by elevating scrotum.	Leukocytes; bacteriuria in some cases (coexisting urinary tract infection)	Normal results on Doppler and ultrasound studies; nuclide scan shows uptake in epididymis	1. Prescribe bed rest and elevation of scrotum, with analgesics as needed. 2. Treat underlying urethritis or urinary tract infection with antimicrobials (Chapter 40) 3. Discharge all patients for follow-up care.
Testicular torsion	Abrupt onset (minutes to hours); history of testicular pain in some; boys and young men (< age 25 yrs)	Tender testicle, often elevated and horizontally displaced; normal epididymis (if palpable)	Normal	Characteristically abnormal results on Doppler examination and radionudidescan	Obtain emergency urologic consultation; hospitalize for surgery. Attempt manual detorsion (see text)
Torsion of testicular appendage	Abrupt onset	Firm nodule with point tenderness on upper anterior pole of testis; testicle normal	Normal	Transillumination may reveal affected appendage as "blue dot," normal results on Doppler ultrasound and radionuclide studies.	1. Prescribed bed rest and elevation, with analgesics as needed 2. Surgery is often needed to relieve pain 3. Obtain urologic follow-up care

testis. The scrotal skin and testicle are usually normal and minimally tender. In advanced cases, marked edema and appearance of a reactive hydrocele may obscure the diagnosis of testicular torsion.

4. Specialized diagnostic tests for differentiating torsion from epididymitis—

These tests should not delay emergency urologic consultation and surgical treatment of patients with high probability of testicular torsion (ie, patients younger than 18 years with acute unilateral testicular pain and no signs or recent history of urinary tract infection).

A. COLOR-FLOW DOPPLER ULTRASONOGRAPHY—Color-flow Doppler ultrasonography is the diagnostic study of choice in most institutions. It is widely available and has a sensitivity of 86–100% and a specificity of 100% as compared with a sensitivity of 80–100% and a specificity of 86–100% for radionucleotide imaging. The most frequent sonographic finding is absent or diminished blood flow to the affected testis, compared with the unaffected side. If the diagnosis is still unclear, then a nuclear study should be pursued. Ultrasound is more advantageous than nuclear scanning for elucidating other scrotal pathology including varicoceles, hydroceles, hernias, and masses.

B. RADIONUCLIDE SCAN—In epididymitis, scanning of the scrotum after intravenous injection of technetium-99m sodium pertechnetate reveals increased scrotal uptake on the affected side, whereas torsion shows decreased uptake.

▶ Treatment and Disposition

(See Table 39–3) If testicular torsion is present, obtain urgent urologic consultation, and prepare the patient for immediate surgery. Manual detorsion should be attempted if the urologist is not immediately available but definitive treatment should not be delayed. Detorsion of the testicle (either manual or surgical) must be accomplished within 6 hours to prevent testicular infarction. Torsion causes the patient's left testicle to rotate counterclockwise and the right to rotate clockwise (Figure 39–1); the affected testicle should be twisted in the opposite direction when detorsion is attempted. Because the testis affected by torsion is usually rotated a minimum of 360° (one turn), the physician should initially attempt to untwist the testicle by counter rotating it one turn. The testis will usually return to normal position on its own after this maneuver, even if it was originally twisted more than one complete revolution.

Regardless of the result of manual detorsion, emergency surgery is indicated to perform detorsion—if necessary—and to secure the testicle. Without surgery, torsion may occur again at any time.

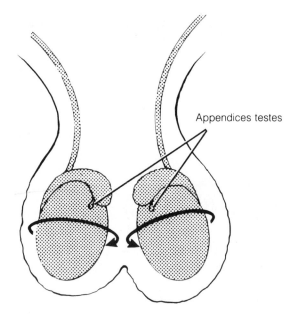

▲ **Figure 39–1.** Torsion of the testicle. View of the testicles, epididymides, testicular appendages, and scrotum, showing direction of rotation of the testicles during torsion (as seen by the physician standing at the foot of the patient's bed and looking down at the patient). Manual detorsion should rotate the testicles in the opposite direction.

In patients with suspected epididymitis or orchitis, urologic consultation should be sought if the diagnosis is in doubt. If epididymitis is present, see Chapter 42 for treatment. Torsion of the testicular appendage (after testicular torsion is excluded) is managed with bed rest, scrotal elevation, analgesics, and follow-up care within 1–2 days. Surgical excision is often needed for adequate pain control.

PAINLESS SCROTAL MASS LESIONS

See Table 39–4.

ESSENTIALS OF DIAGNOSIS

► Malignancy is often painless

► A tense hydrocele or a firm spermatocele must be differentiated from a tumor. Ultrasound is the diagnostic study of choice

► Sudden onset of a varicocele in an older male may be a late sign of a renal tumor

Table 39–4. Diagnostic Clues to the Cause of Common Painless Scrotal Masses.

	History and Physical Examination	Other Diagnostic Studies
Varicocele	Usually asymptomatic mass; some patients have mild pain. Mass is separate from testis; feels like "bag of worms," especially in upright position. Size increased by Valsalva maneuver. Right-sided varicocele should raise suspicion for inferior vena cava and intra-abdominal pathology. Sudden left-sided varicocele should raise suspicion for left renal vein obstruction	Not usually required, physical examination is diagnostic. Ultrasonography also helpful in diagnosis of enigmatic cases
Hydrocele	Gradually enlarging painless cystic mass that transilluminates. *Note:* Hydrocele may complicate tumor	Aspiration yields clear fluid. Ultrasonography helpful in diagnosis
Spermatocele	Asymptomatic mass separate from and superior to the testicle	Aspiration reveals white cloudy fluid with immotile sperm. Ultrasonography also helpful in diagnosis
Testicular tumor	Patient often a young adult. Asymptomatic enlargement of testis, rarely painful. Examination shows firm, nontender mass that does not transilluminate. Gynecomastia, virilization, or feminization rarely occur	Ultrasonography helpful in confirming mass lesion. Surgical exploration required for exact diagnosis of all testicular mass lesions

▶ General Considerations

Conditions causing painless (relatively painless) scrotal swelling are not true emergencies, although testicular tumors are life-threatening and require urgent evaluation (within a few days). Table 39–4 sets forth helpful diagnostic features of conditions associated with painless scrotal swelling. Patients with newly diagnosed testicular enlargement or mass lesions should be referred to a urologist.

DYSURIA

ESSENTIALS OF DIAGNOSIS

▶ Painful urination that represents acute inflammation of the urethra, bladder, or prostate

▶ Frequency and urgency may also be present

▶ Workup should be guided by other associated symptoms, ie, hematuria or discharge

▶ Urinalysis or sexually transmitted disease testing usually confirms the diagnosis

▶ General Considerations

Common causes of dysuria and their associated clinical findings are given in Table 39–5. Urethral diverticula, urolithiasis, endocervical gonorrhea, balanitis, and urethral warts are uncommon causes of dysuria.

▶ Clinical Findings

A. Dysuria in Males

1. Urethritis—In males, urethritis is a much more common cause of dysuria than is urinary tract infection. Attempt to express urethral discharge by milking the urethra, and send the material for culture and smear. If no discharge can be obtained, sample the anterior 2–3 cm (¾–1³/₁₆ in) of the urethra with a calcium alginate, Dacron, or cotton swab, or wire loop and send the swab for PCR or culture for *Neisseria gonorrhoeae* and *Chlamydia trachomatis. Do not use a wood-handled cotton swab, because wood is toxic to the* Chlamydia *organism.* The presence of more than 5 leukocytes per × 400 field indicates urethritis; the presence of intracellular diplococci (gram-negative if a Gram stain was done)—especially without other bacteria—indicates gonococcal urethritis. See Chapter 42 for treatment of gonorrhea and nongonococcal urethritis.

Dysuria without evidence of urethral or urinary tract inflammation (<5 white blood cells per × 100 field, negative culture) is rare in men and may represent low-grade infection. Treatment for urethritis is usually indicated.

2. Prostatitis—If no evidence of urethritis is found, obtain a midstream clean-voided urine specimen. Polymorphonuclear neutrophils in the urine in the absence of urethritis are diagnostic of urinary tract inflammation. Prostatitis (either alone or associated with urinary tract infection) may be excluded by rectal examination. For further information on treatment, see Chapter 42.

3. Urinary tract infection—Leukocytes, usually with bacteria, are found on microscopic examination of a midstream urine specimen. Urine dip reagent strips that test for the presence of leukocyte esterase and nitrite are equivalent

Table 39–5. Diagnostic Clues to Common Causes of Dysuria.

Condition	Sex More Commonly Affected	History and Physical Examination	Diagnostic Studies
Urethritis	Men	Dysuria, usually severe. Clear or purulent urethral discharge	Leukocytes in urethral discharge or on urethral swab. Tests for gonococcal or chlamydial infection are often positive
Prostatitis	Men only	Pelvic pain and dysuria. Fever common. Tender, boggy prostate on examination	Prostatic massage produces leukocytes and bacteria in urethral discharge or urine ("3-glass test")
Urethral stricture	Men	Dysuria, may have split or reduced urinary stream	Urethroscopy or urethrogram
Urethral caruncle	Women (usually postmenopausal)	Mild dysuria; examination may show lesion	Urethroscopy
Dysuria-frequency syndrome	Women only	Dysuria and urgency. May have urethral discharge	Pyuria; leukocytes in urethral discharge or on urethral swab
Vaginitis	Women only	External dysuria, vaginal discharge dyspareunia	Vaginal smear or culture shows Candida, *Gardnerella vaginalis*, or *Trichomonas vaginalis*
Genital herpes	Women	History of herpes (if recurrent); vesicles and ulcers on external genitalia	Positive results on tests for herpes simplex
Urinary tract infection	Mainly women	Dysuria, urgency, frequency; cloudy or foul-smelling urine. May have fever, flank, or suprapubic tenderness	Pyuria and bacteriuria, urine culture shows more than 10^3 bacteria/mL (often >10^5/mL)
Urethral trauma	Either (mainly children)	History or evidence of genital manipulation or trauma	Hematuria occasionally
Psychogenic	Either	No logical pattern to symptoms. Examination normal	Normal results on urinalysis. No leukocytes on urethral swab. Tests for gonococcal and chlamydial infection negative

to the urine sediment analysis at detecting pyuria when both are positive. They are increasingly being used as a screening tool and often eliminate the need for microscopic examination. Culture usually shows bacteria of a single species (usually >10^5 colony-forming units per milliliter but occasionally only 10^2–10^4, especially with certain organisms [eg, *Candida* species or enterococci]). *Note:* Urinary tract infection is unusual in men younger than 60 years unless associated urinary tract abnormalities are present or the patient engages in anal intercourse.

4. Local causes—Inspect the penis and urethral meatus for balanitis and intrameatal pathologic structures (warts, herpetic ulcers) that are commonly associated with dysuria. Urethral strictures often cause dysuria, and patients may describe a split or intermittent urinary stream.

B. Dysuria in Females

1. Collection of urine—Obtain an uncontaminated urine specimen for microscopic analysis. Contamination of the specimen is usually indicated by the presence of squamous (vaginal) epithelial cells visible microscopically (eg, ≥5 cells per × 100 field); if these are seen, discard the specimen and

obtain another uncontaminated specimen. Proper collection techniques for adults are as follows:

A. MIDSTREAM CLEAN-VOIDED URINE—This method of collection is satisfactory in most cases but requires a cooperative patient and some coordination.

B. CATHETERIZATION—A small, straight (9 F) catheter should be used for quick "in and out" catheterization, because it is more comfortable than the 14–19 F Foley-type catheter. Contamination may occur.

C. SUPRAPUBIC ASPIRATION—(See Chapter 7) Suprapubic aspiration is useful in special situations (eg, for infants) and is associated with a very low contamination rate.

2. Clinical differentiation of causes of dysuria in women—

A. DYSURIA-FREQUENCY SYNDROME (URETHRAL SYNDROME) AND URINARY TRACT INFECTION—These conditions are characterized by dysuria without vaginal symptoms (eg, discharge) and by pyuria (<5 white cells per × 400 field). If bacteria are seen in the urinary sediment, urinary tract infection is a more likely diagnosis than urethral syndrome. Occasionally women with dysuria-frequency syndrome may have no pyuria.

B. Local causes—If results on urinalysis are normal, if vaginal symptoms associated with dysuria are present, or if pain is felt outside the urinary tract (external dysuria), perform a pelvic examination to look for vaginitis, genital herpes, or a urethral caruncle. Urethral caruncle is found in postmenopausal woman and is a small, nontender red lesion resembling a strawberry on the dorsal aspect of the urethral meatus. In addition, it is helpful to culture endocervical mucus for gonococci, because gonococcal infection in women may be associated with dysuria.

C. Dysuria Associated with Hematuria in Either Sex

The presence of large numbers of erythrocytes in the urine in either sex should suggest hemorrhagic cystitis, concomitant urolithiasis, or urethral manipulation (see Hematuria section, below).

▶ Treatment and Disposition

Treat the various causes of dysuria as follows:

A. Urinary Tract Infections

For treatment of cystitis, pyelonephritis, and urethral syndrome, see Chapter 42.

B. Gonorrhea

See Chapter 42.

C. Vaginitis

See Chapter 42.

D. Prostatitis

See Chapter 42.

E. Other Conditions

Patients with other conditions (eg, urethral stricture or diverticulum) should be referred to a urologist or gynecologist for evaluation.

ATRAUMATIC HEMATURIA

ESSENTIALS OF DIAGNOSIS

▶ Hematuria is often an early sign of genitourinary cancer

▶ Hematuria with associated flank or groin pain is suggestive of urolithiasis

▶ Dysuria and frequency may accompany hematuria of an infectious cause

▶ General Considerations

Common causes of hematuria (microscopic defined as >3 red blood cells per high-power field) and their associated clinical findings are set forth in Table 39–6. See Chapter 26 for management of hematuria associated with trauma or genitourinary manipulation. In all cases of atraumatic hematuria, nonglomerular diseases including infection account for 25% of cases, stones account for 20% of cases, cancer accounts for 12% of cases, and 10% of cases have an unknown cause.

Renal vein thrombosis, renal arterial embolization, drug-induced (cyclophosphamide, penicillins) interstitial cystitis, glomerular diseases, abdominal aortic aneurysm, and malignancy are less common causes of hematuria. In the elderly, painless gross hematuria is malignancy until proven otherwise.

▶ Clinical Findings

A. History

Hematuria associated with abdominal or flank pain and tenderness suggests urolithiasis or, less commonly, renovascular disease. Diagnostic clues may come from timing of the hematuria. Initial, terminal, or total stream hematuria suggests bleeding from the following respective areas: anterior urethral, posterior urethra to trigone, or bladder sources or beyond.

Hematuria associated with dysuria and urinary urgency and frequency suggests hemorrhagic cystitis (drug-induced, infectious, or idiopathic). Systemic conditions associated with hematuria include thrombotic thrombocytopenic purpura, Henoch-Schönlein purpura, sickling hemoglobinopathies, excessive anticoagulation therapy, or coagulopathies.

Bleeding from other perineal areas, especially menstrual flow, may be mistaken for hematuria.

B. Physical Examination

Examine the external genitalia for local causes of hematuria (eg, intraurethral trauma). Examine the abdomen, back, and pelvis for tenderness and evidence of trauma.

In males, perform a rectal examination for evaluation of the prostate after a urine specimen has been obtained, because prostatic manipulation can induce pyuria.

C. Laboratory Examination

1. Urinalysis—Perform urinalysis to confirm the diagnosis of hematuria. Carefully performed microscopic examination of a freshly voided midstream urine specimen is essential to the evaluation of hematuria; look especially for erythrocyte casts, which suggest glomerulonephritis. In men, fractionate urinalysis (initial, midstream, and terminal specimens) is also helpful in localizing the source of hematuria.

2. Other laboratory tests—Further laboratory testing (except possibly urine culture) is not usually needed for bacterial

Table 39–6. Diagnostic Clues to Common Causes of Hematuria.

	History and Physical Findings	Diagnostic Studies
Trauma	History or evidence of local genital, abdominal (renal), or pelvic trauma or recent genitourinary instrumentation	See Chapter 24
Tumor	Often long-standing painless hematuria	Intravenous pyelogram reveals upper urinary tract tumors; cystogram or cystoscopy shows bladder tumor
Urolithiasis	Intermittent hematuria usually associated with pain. Bladder stones may be painless but may be associated with intermittent urinary obstruction	Intravenous pyelogram reveals ureteral stone, obstruction, or postobstructive hydroureter; cystoscopy or cystography shows bladder stones
Infection	Dysuria common	Pyuria often present. Urine culture shows bacteria (usually $\geq 10^5$ colonies/ml)
Glomerulonephritis	May follow streptococcal infection; often associated with autoimmune diseases (eg, systemic lupus erythematosus). Gradual onset. Hypertension common	Urinalysis shows leukocytes, red cell casts, and frequently proteinuria; blood urea nitrogen and serum creatinine elevated
Prostatitis	Dysuria often present. Abnormal (large or tender) prostate	Pyuria often present
Urethral stricture, foreign body, or manipulation	Often painful. Local abnormality may be obvious on examination	Urethroscopy reveals stricture or foreign body
Sickle cell or sickle cell trait	Intermittent hematuria that may be painless (trait) or painful (disease)	Urinalysis shows red blood cells and isosthenuria. Hemoglobin electrophoresis abnormal
Bleeding diathesis	Painless hematuria. History of coagulation defect. Evidence of bleeding elsewhere (eg, purpura). Anticoagulant use	Coagulation tests show thrombocytopenia, prolonged prothrombin time, etc. (Chapter 39)

hemorrhagic cystitis. Patients with urolithiasis may require baseline serum electrolyte determinations and renal function tests. Patients in whom a bleeding disorder is suspected or the cause of hematuria is unknown should have the following laboratory examinations: CBC with differential; prothrombin time, partial thromboplastin time, and international normalization ratio; serum electrolytes; and renal function.

D. Special Studies

A CT scan may be necessary for the evaluation of urolithiasis, trauma, tumors, and other causes. Compared with ultrasound, CT scanning is a better diagnostic study for evaluation of intra-abdominal pathology and tumors, especially those that are less than 3 cm in size. In pregnant females, ultrasound is the test of choice for evaluating hematuria.

Cystoscopy is essential for evaluation of bladder or urethral hematuria due to tumors and other causes. It may also be helpful for localizing hematuria of the upper genitourinary tract to one side or the other. The need for cytoscopy should be determined by the consulting urologist.

Other studies such as radionuclide scans or angiograms may be needed in special situations, but urologic consultation should be obtained before these studies are requested.

▶ Treatment and Disposition

Treat the various causes of hematuria as follows:

A. Trauma

See Chapter 26.

B. Urinary Tract Infection

See Chapter 42.

C. Suspected Tumor

Refer the patient to a urologist for evaluation. Consider hospitalization in order to expedite diagnostic procedures.

D. Urolithiasis

See below.

E. Glomerulonephritis

Hospitalize the patient, and obtain consultation with a nephrologist.

F. Prostatitis

See Chapter 42.

G. Urethral Strictures and Foreign Bodies

Refer the patient to a urologist.

H. Unknown Cause

Patients with hematuria of an unknown cause need urgent urologic consultation.

Dogra V, Bhatt S: Acute painful scrotum. Radiol Clin North Am 2004;42:349–363 [PMID: 15136021].

Edwards TJ, Dickinson AJ, Natale S et al: A prospective analysis of the diagnostic yield resulting from the attendance of 4020 patients at a protocol-driven haematuria clinic. BJU Int 2006;97:301 [PMID: 17407528].

Gatti JM, Murphy JP: Current management of the acute scrotum. Semin Pediatr Surg 2007;16:58–63 [PMID: 17210484].

Hicks D, Li CY: Management of macroscopic haematuria in the emergency department. Emerg Med J 2007;24:385–390 [PMID: 17513531].

Kellum JA: Acute kidney injury. Crit Care Med 2008;36:S141–145 [PMID: 18382185].

Khalil P, Murty P, Palevsky PM: The patient with acute kidney injury. Prim Care 2008;35:239–264 [PMID: 18486715].

Lamm WW, Yap TL, Jacobsen AS et al: Colour Doppler ultrasonography replacing surgical exploration for acute scrotum: Myth or reality? Pediatr Radiol 2005;35:597–600 [PMID: 15761770].

Ludwig M: Diagnosis and therapy of acute prostatitis, epididymitis and orchitis. Andrologia 2008;40(2):76–80 [PMID: 18336454].

Malhotra SM, Kennedy WA: Urinary tract infections in children: treatment. Urol Clin North Am 2004;31:527–534 [PMID: 15313062].

Mori R, Lakhanpaul M, Verrier-Jones K: Diagnosis and management of urinary tract infection in children: summary of NICE guidance. BMJ 2007;335:395–397 [PMID: 17717369].

Nicolle LE: Uncomplicated urinary tract infection in adults including uncomplicated pyelonephritis. Urol Clin North Am 2008;35:1–12 [PMID: 18061019].

O'Regan KN, O'Connor OJ, McLoughlin P et al: The role of imaging in the investigation of painless hematuria in adults. Semin Ultrasound CT MR 2009;30:258–270 [PMID: 19711639].

Ringdahl E, Teague L. Testicular torsion. Am Fam Physician 2006;74:1739–1743 [PMID: 19378875].

Sahsi RS, Carpenter CR: Evidence-based emergency medicine/rational clinical examination abstract. Does this child have a urinary tract infection? Ann Emerg Med 2009;53:680–684 [PMID: 19380042].

Selius BA, Subedi R: Urinary retention in adults: diagnosis and initial management. Am Fam Physician 2008;77:643–650 [PMID: 18350762].

Trojian TH, Lishnak TS, Heiman D: Epididymitis and orchitis: an overview. Am Fam Physician 2009;79:583–587 [PMID: 19378875].

Vilke GM, Ufberg JW, Harrigan RA, Chan TC: Evaluation and treatment of acute urinary retention. J Emerg Med 2008;35:193–198 [PMID: 18280090].

▼ **EMERGENCY TREATMENT OF SPECIFIC DISORDERS**

UROLITHIASIS (RENAL COLIC)

 ESSENTIALS OF DIAGNOSIS

- ▶ Patients usually present with sudden onset of unilateral flank pain that may radiate to the ipsilateral lower quadrant, groin, scrotum, or labia
- ▶ Hematuria is present in approximately 90% of cases
- ▶ Spiral CT scan is the diagnostic study of choice but KUB, intravenous pyelogram, and ultrasound may also be used

▶ General Considerations

Patients with stones in the urinary tract commonly present to the emergency department. Stones usually form in the renal pelvis, and symptoms occur with passage of the stone into the ureter, as the result of infection, or both. The incidence of stones is highest among whites with a peak incidence between ages 20 and 50 years, and the male to female ratio is 3:1. Bladder stones are less common, and patients may present with hematuria or intermittent urinary obstruction.

▶ Clinical Findings

A. Symptoms and Signs

The initial symptom is usually acute, unilateral flank pain (stones near kidney) that rapidly becomes excruciating, radiating to the ipsilateral lower quadrant and often referred to the ipsilateral groin, testicle, or labia (stones near ureterovesical junction). The pain may cause vasovagal syncope; occasionally patients are asymptomatic except for hematuria. Eliciting a history of pain that shifts anteriorly and inferiorly from the flank as the stone moves distally in the urinary tract may be helpful in differentiating renal colic from other types of abdominal pain.

Some patients note gross hematuria. Nausea and vomiting are frequent. If complicating infection is present, signs and symptoms of pyelonephritis also may be present. Inquire about a history of similar attacks or a pre-disposing condition (eg, previous documented urolithiasis, gout, hypercalcemia).

Vital signs are usually normal in the absence of infection, although bradycardia from vagal hypertonicity or tachycardia from pain may be seen. Some degree of ileus is usually present. Tenderness over the affected kidney (costovertebral angle tenderness) and ureter can be elicited.

B. Laboratory Findings

Obtain a urinalysis. Hematuria (gross or microscopic) is present in approximately 90% of cases. Occasionally a patient presents with pain and no hematuria. A urine or serum human chorionic gonadotropin level should be obtained in all females of child-bearing age. Urine culture should be sent if an infected stone is suspected by bacteriuria and fever. Blood urea nitrogen and serum creatinine levels are usually normal. Although they will not change the emergency department management, calcium, magnesium, phosphorus, and uric acid levels may be helpful to the urologist in assessing for metabolic causes of stone formation.

C. Imaging

Imaging studies should be performed during the first episode of suspected renal colic or if the diagnosis is uncertain. Patients with recurrent stones with typical historical and physical examination consistent with urolithiasis may be managed symptomatically without any diagnostic studies unless obstruction or infection is of concern.

1. Unenhanced helical (spiral) CT—(see Figure 39–2) Helical CT scan is widely used and currently the study of choice for the diagnosis of renal colic. Not only is it accurate, but it is less time consuming, no contrast is required, and additional intra-abdominal information may be obtained. It has a sensitivity of 98%, a specificity of 97%, and positive and negative predictive values of 100 and 97%, respectively. It does not provide information regarding the functional status of the kidney. Even without contrast an aortic aneurysm may be seen; therefore, the helical CT scan is the preferred imaging choice for an elderly patient.

2. Ultrasound—Renal ultrasound may be useful to detect stones or hydronephrosis but is not as sensitive (64%) as helical CT or intravenous pyelogram, particularly for detection of small stones. It may be of value in patients with a history of hypersensitivity to intravenous contrast and with radiolucent stones. Pregnant women and pediatric patients should be evaluated with ultrasound as the first screening modality.

3. Intravenous pyelogram—An intravenous pyelogram has a 90% sensitivity for detecting urolithiasis or the related obstruction as well as for assessing functional status and visualization of the entire urinary tract. *Caution*: This method is relatively contraindicated in the following settings: (1) patients with creatinine above 1.4 mg/dL, (2) elderly patients with proteinuria and elevated creatinine, and (3) patients with documented allergy to contrast media unless they are premedicated with antihistamines and steroids.

4. KUB—KUB, a study of the kidneys, urethras, and bladder, is less than 70% sensitive but may be useful because 90% of calculi are radiopaque. When the stone is visualized on KUB, its progress can usually be followed on subsequent KUBs.

▶ Treatment

About 90% of renal stones are passed spontaneously. The likelihood of renal stone passage decreases with increasing stone size. Stones larger than 6 mm will pass without intervention in only 10% of patients. Basic treatment is as follows:

A. Provide Analgesia

Begin analgesics as soon as the diagnosis has been established with reasonable certainty. Opioids and antiemetics

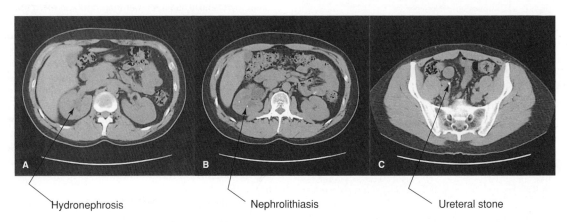

▲ **Figure 39–2.** Unenhanced helical CT scan demonstrating (A) right-sided hydronephrosis (B) right nephrolithiasis, and (C) stone in right ureter.

are mainstays of therapy. Ketorolac is as equipotent as mild narcotic analgesics. Ketorolac provides analgesia, and given its antiprostaglandin effects, it can decrease the inflammatory response, promote relaxation of the ureteral spasm, and alleviate capsular distention. Most comparison studies show little difference between opiates and NSAIDs with a trend toward fewer complications with the NSAIDs. For patients who are not hospitalized, an antiemetic, an anti-inflammatory agent, and a narcotic may be required for control of pain and emesis.

B. Ensure Adequate Hydration

Although authorities usually recommend drinking 2–3 L of fluid per day, this is probably of more value in preventing the formation of more stones than in facilitating passage of an existing stone.

C. Medical Expulsive therapy

The use of medication to expidite passage of the stone should be considered. Corticosteroids, calcium channel blockers and alpha-blockers, such as terazosin, and the alpha-1 selective blocker tamsulosin, can promote relaxation of ureteral musculature to aid in the passage of stones.

D. Strain Urine

Patients with their first episode of urolithiasis or those who pass stones of unknown composition should strain their urine through a urine strainer or a coffee filter and submit the stone for chemical analysis.

▶ Prevention

Specific preventive therapy can be recommended after the composition of the stone has been determined by chemical analysis.

▶ Disposition

Patients with any of the following conditions require hospitalization:

- Intractable pain
- Intractable emesis
- Coexisting pyelonephritis
- Documented or suspected renal dysfunction (elevated blood urea nitrogen or serum creatinine levels, bilateral ureteral stones, oliguria or anuria, hydronephrosis)

Patients who do not require hospitalization should be referred to a urologist within 24–48 hours for further evaluation and treatment.

DISEASES OF THE MALE GENITOURINARY SYSTEM

1. Torsion of the Testicle

ESSENTIALS OF DIAGNOSIS

- ▶ Rare in males older than 30 years but occurs at all ages
- ▶ The testicle may be high riding with "bell clapper" deformity
- ▶ Detorsion must occur within 6 hours for testicular salvage
- ▶ Attempt manual detorsion
- ▶ Color-flow Doppler ultrasound demonstrates diminished blood flow to affected testis

▶ Clinical Findings

Testicular torsion has a bimodal incidence with peaks occurring in neonates and pubescent males; however, it can occur in all age groups. Torsion of the testicular or epididymal appendages can also present as acute unilateral scrotal pain. Of the four appendages, the appendix testis becomes torsed the most often (99%) and usually requires only supportive care.

The history for testicular torsion is most often a sudden onset of moderate to severe, unilateral scrotal pain. Patients may recount similar episodes that resolved spontaneously in the past. On physical examination, the testis can be high-riding with a transverse rather than vertical lie, slightly larger than the unaffected testis, and diffusely tender and erythematous. An absent cremasteric reflex on the affected side is the most sensitive physical finding. Nausea, vomiting, and abdominal pain may occur as a result of the ischemia.

Epididymitis, orchitis, neoplasms, peritonitis, hernia, abdominal aortic aneurysm, Fournier gangrene, and other scrotal diseases need to be considered in the differential diagnosis (see Table 39–3). Urinalysis is usually normal. Color-flow Doppler ultrasonography or radionucleotide scanning may confirm the diagnosis.

Epididymitis and orchitis may be confused with torsion of the testicle; helpful differentiating features are discussed in the section on scrotal pain and in Table 39–3. The diagnosis may be confirmed by Doppler ultrasound examination or radionuclide scanning.

▶ Treatment and Disposition

A. Provide Analgesia

Parenteral narcotic analgesics usually are required.

B. Prepare for Surgery

Give nothing orally, obtain blood for CBC and renal function tests, and begin an intravenous infusion.

C. Obtain Immediate Urologic Surgical Consultation

If a delay in urologic consultation is anticipated, attempt manual detorsion as discussed earlier in this chapter. Testicular salvage approaches 100% if detorsion (manual or surgical) is performed within 6 hours.

2. Epididymitis

See Chapter 42.

3. Orchitis

Orchitis is commonly associated with epididymitis. It usually has an infectious cause, for example, from viral, bacterial, or mycobacterial agents. Viral orchitis is most often due to mumps. The orchitis commonly presents 5 days after the parotitis. Mumps orchitis may result in atrophy. If the diagnosis is in doubt or specific treatment appears warranted, obtain urologic consultation. Symptomatic relief may be achieved with recumbency and analgesics.

4. Priapism

▶ Clinical Findings

Priapism is a persistent involuntary, painful erection, unrelated to sexual stimulation and unrelieved by ejaculation. About 25% of cases are associated with leukemia, metastatic carcinoma, or sickling hemoglobinopathies. If the medical history is unclear, consider a CBC and sickling test. Alcohol, marijuana, cocaine, and now MDMA (Ecstasy) are among some of the recreational drugs known to induce priapism, but many prescription drugs are culprits as well. Regardless of treatment, there is a high incidence of corporal fibrosis and erectile dysfunction.

▶ Treatment

Management is mainly to provide analgesia and hydration and to abort the erection to prevent permanent damage. Several modalities can be attempted, but success is often limited. Ice packs have limited success. Hydration, oxygenation, and sometimes exchange transfusion is necessary for sickle cell patients. Terbutaline, either subcutaneous or oral, has had some favorable results. Corporal aspiration and irrigation with a phenylephrine solution can be used and is more effective than systemic sympathomimetic therapy but should be done in conjunction with urologic consultation.

▶ Disposition

Hospitalize all patients with persistent priapism or those with serious underlying disease (sickling hemoglobinopathy, leukemia). Obtain urgent urologic consultation.

5. Fournier Gangrene

ESSENTIALS OF DIAGNOSIS

- ▶ Necrotizing fasciitis of the perineum
- ▶ Fever, pain, edema, and erythema of the scrotum are typically present
- ▶ Chiefly affects diabetic males

Fournier gangrene is a necrotizing fasciitis of the perineum that primarily affects diabetic males aged 20–50 years. Patients typically present with fever, pain, edema, and erythema of the scrotum or penis. The most common causes are infection and trauma. Aerobes or anaerobes may be the causative infectious agents. A CT scan often shows the infection to have spread beyond what is clinically apparent on the skin. Treatment includes antibiotic therapy, wide surgical incision, and drainage. Mortality is approximately 60–70%.

6. Phimosis and Paraphimosis

ESSENTIALS OF DIAGNOSIS

- ▶ Chronic balanoposthitis, due to a bacterial or fungal infection, is a risk factor for phimosis (inability to retract the foreskin)
- ▶ Physiologic phimosis is normal in the first few years of life
- ▶ Paraphimosis (retracted, constricted foreskin proximal to the glans) may cause necrosis to the glans and urethra if not treated

Phimosis is a fibrous constriction of the foreskin preventing retraction; it is often associated with balanitis and may cause urinary retention. Phimosis or paraphimosis rarely results from chronic balanoposthitis, which is categorized as either irritant or infectious. Balanoposthitis is inflammation of the glans penis and the prepuce. Treatment for acute irritant balanoposthitis is sitz baths, cleansing with the foreskin retracted, and 0.5% hydrocortisone cream. Candidal infections are the most common infectious cause and are treated with good hygiene and topical antifungal cream. Phimosis without balanitis may be an indication for elective circumcision, but it is not an emergency. Surgical correction should not be attempted in the emergency department.

Paraphimosis occurs when the retracted foreskin develops a fixed constriction proximal to the glans. The penis distal to the constricting foreskin may become swollen and painful, or even gangrenous, and urinary retention may result. Attempt manual reduction: Squeeze the glans firmly for 5–10 minutes to reduce its size. Then move the prepuce distally while the glans is pushed proximally. Additionally ice, sugar and multiple punctures to the glans with a small bore needle have each been described and reported to be successful. If manual reduction is unsuccessful, a dorsal slit of the foreskin is necessary (Figures 39–3 and 39–4). Refer the patient to a urologist for elective circumcision to reduce risk of recurrence. In addition, a complication of the Plastibell device for pediatric circumcision occurs if the ring inadvertently slips behind the glans, creating a paraphimosis and causing penile ischemia. The ring should be removed immediately.

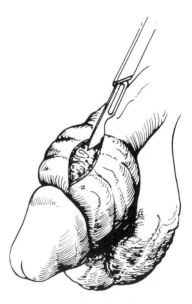

▲ **Figure 39–3.** Method of performing a dorsal slit of the foreskin for balanitis and paraphimosis. An incision made through the tight band of skin as shown will relieve the paraphimosis.

Burnett AL, Bivalacqua TJ: Priapism: current principles and practice. Urol Clin North Am 2007;34:631–642 [PMID: 17983902].

Gatti JM, Patrick Murphy J: Current management of the acute scrotum. Semin Pediatr Surg 2007;16:58–63 [PMID: 17210484].

Holgate A, Pollock T: Nonsteroidal anti-inflammatory drugs (NSAIDs) versus opioids for acute renal colic. Chochrane Database Syst Rev 2005;2:CD004137 [PMID: 15846699].

Kobayashi S: Fournier's gangrene. Am J Surg 2008;195:257–258 [PMID: 18083136].

Lin EP, Bhatt S, Rubens DJ et al: Testicular torsion: twists and turns. Semin Ultrasound CT MR 2007;28:317–328 [PMID: 17874655].

Mackway-Jones K, Teece S: Best evidence topic reports. Ice, pins, or sugar to reduce paraphimosis. Emerg Med J 2004;21:77–78 [PMID: 14734388].

McGregor TB, Pike JG, Leonard MP: Pathologic and physiologic phimosis: approach to the phimotic foreskin. Can Fam Physician 2007;53:445–448 [PMID: 17872680].

Ringdahl E, Teague L: Testicular torsion. Am Fam Physician 2006;74:1739–1743 [PMID: 19378875].

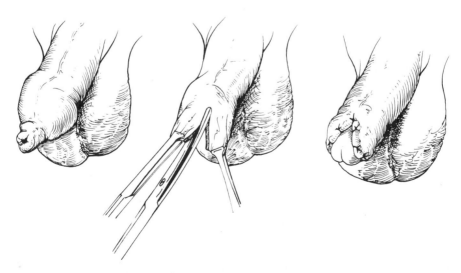

▲ **Figure 39–4.** Method of performing a dorsal slit of the foreskin for phimosis.

Rucker CM, Menias CO, Bhalla S: Mimics of renal colic: alternative diagnoses at unenhanced helical CT. Radiographics 2004;24:S11–S28 [PMID: 15486235].

Teichman JM: Clinical Practice. Acute renal colic from ureteral calculus. N Engl J Med 2004;350:684–693 [PMID: 14960744].

Thwaini A, Khan A, Malik A et al: Mammen K. Fournier's gangrene and its emergency management. Postgrad Med J 2006;82:516–519 [PMID: 16891442].

Vilke GM, Harrigan RA, Ufberg JW et al: Emergency evaluation and treatment of priapism. J Emerg Med 2004;26:325–329 [PMID: 15028333].

Vascular Emergencies

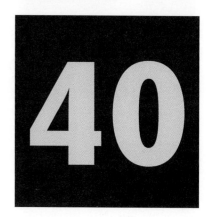

David A. Fritz, MD, FACEP

Most vascular emergencies are due to either disruption of the blood vessel wall with bleeding (eg, from penetrating trauma) or to occlusion of the blood vessel lumen (eg, by an embolus or thrombus). The major consequences of these events are blood loss or acute distal ischemia. If vascular injury is untreated, hypotension or tissue necrosis may occur.

VASCULAR EMERGENCIES DUE TO TRAUMA

IMMEDIATE MANAGEMENT OF LIFE-THREATENING VASCULAR INJURIES

▶ Maintain Airway and Treat Associated Injuries

Treat associated life-threatening head, thoracic, and abdominal injuries (Chapters 12, 22, 24, and 25).

▶ Stop Hemorrhage

1. Stop active bleeding from arterial or venous hemorrhage by gentle manual compression.

2. Avoid clamping the bleeding vessel because this will cause further injury.

3. Avoid the use of tourniquets.

4. Do not remove embedded objects because they may be preventing further bleeding.

▶ Treat or Prevent Shock

(See also Chapter 11) Insert two or more large-bore (≥16-gauge) intravenous catheters. Two intravenous access sites are preferable if the patient is already in shock or is bleeding profusely.

While intravenous catheters are being inserted, draw blood for complete blood count (CBC), serum electrolytes, glucose and creatinine measurements, prothrombin time (PT), partial thromboplastin time (PTT), and typing and crossmatching (reserve 6–8 units of packed red blood cells or whole blood).

Begin intravenous infusion of crystalloid solutions (eg, normal saline or lactated Ringer's) to support blood pressure. Up to 2–3 L of crystalloid solution may be given before blood products are administered. Replace blood. The number of units administered depends on the severity of existing blood loss and on anticipated loss from projected surgery. Use fresh whole blood whenever possible.

▶ Prevent Further Vascular and Nerve Injury

All fractures and joint dislocations associated with abnormal pulses should be carefully reduced and splinted to reduce further neurovascular damage. Control hemorrhage by pressure; avoid clamping vessels to stop hemorrhage. Consider adjunctive studies for further evaluation as appropriate (eg, computed tomography [CT] scan, angiography).

▶ Minimize Ischemia

Keep ischemic limbs horizontal. Do not use tourniquets.

▶ Relieve Pain

Provide adequate analgesia; if necessary, give narcotic analgesics.

▶ Obtain Surgical Consultation

All documented or suspected vascular injuries should be examined promptly by a general or vascular surgeon before the patient is transferred from the emergency department.

▶ Hospitalize Patients as Required

Hospitalize all patients with arterial or major venous injuries.

▶ General Considerations

Acute vascular injury may result in either hemorrhage or tissue ischemia.

A. Arterial Injury

1. Hemorrhage—Obvious external hemorrhage is present in many patients. Occult bleeding into soft tissue, the retroperitoneum, the pelvis, or body cavities may also occur.

2. Ischemia—Ischemia from arterial injury must be recognized and treated promptly, because increased tissue pressure and swelling from ischemia further compromise arterial perfusion, and prolonged ischemia results in irreversible tissue damage.

B. Venous Injury

1. Hemorrhage—Obvious or occult bleeding usually occurs following venous injury. It is rarely life-threatening except in the case of injuries to central veins (eg, vena cava) or their immediate branches (eg, femoral vein).

2. Ischemia—Tissue ischemia from venous trauma alone is rare, although venous obstruction and resultant tissue congestion may worsen preexisting tissue ischemia resulting from arterial injury.

C. Causes of Vascular Injury

1. Penetrating trauma—Penetrating trauma is the most common cause of peripheral vascular injury and ranges in severity from innocuous simple puncture wounds to extensive wounds caused by high-velocity missiles. Penetrating injuries to the central vessels may lead to massive hemorrhage and death.

2. Blunt trauma—Blunt trauma may also cause vascular injury. Contusions or crushing injuries of an artery may cause either transmural disruption with hemorrhage, or partial disruption of the artery and elevation of the intima from an intramural hematoma (ie, dissection). Thrombosis of a segment of artery may also occur. Blunt trauma with dislocation of a joint may result in disruption of the arteries crossing that joint line, leading to ischemia distal to the site of injury (eg, disruption of the popliteal artery with posterior dislocation of the knee). Blunt trauma may also contribute indirectly to vascular occlusion by creating large hematomas near a blood vessel. Hematoma formation may lead to arterial spasm, distortion, or compartment syndromes, all of which may interfere with arterial flow.

3. Chemicals—Chemical injury to blood vessels is increasing in frequency. It is generally iatrogenic or associated with parenteral drug abuse. Intra-arterial injection of drugs that are chemically irritating to tissues (eg, barbiturates) causes occlusion of small peripheral vessels. If occlusion is severe, all or part of the limb may be lost. Extravasation of an intravenously administered chemical may also cause associated arterial spasm or tissue necrosis. Barbiturates, phenytoin, vasopressors, and chemotherapeutic agents (eg, doxorubicin) are notable examples. High doses of certain intravenously administered vasopressors (eg, dopamine) can cause intense peripheral vasoconstriction with ultimate digital ischemic necrosis.

D. Sequel

Late sequelae associated with major vascular injuries include the development of false aneurysms and arteriovenous fistulas.

1. False aneurysms—False aneurysms do not contain all three layers of the vessel wall (intima, media, and adventitia). They result from walled-off disruptions of vessel walls. They enlarge over time, may compress adjacent veins or nerves, and may rupture without warning.

2. Fistulas—Fistulas may occur after adjacent arteries and veins are injured simultaneously, usually as a result of stab wounds or missile injury. The fistula may enlarge over time and cause increased cardiac output if a large left-to-right shunting of blood is present. If the fistula involves the blood supply to an extremity, dilated veins may be observed in that extremity. Turbulent blood flow through the fistula results in an obvious thrill or bruit. Fistulas may also compress adjacent nerves or impede collateral circulation, or they may rupture, causing a severe hemorrhage.

▶ Principles of Diagnosis

A. Physical Examination

If there is a wound in the vicinity of a major blood vessel, assume that vascular injury has occurred. The findings listed below may not appear for hours to days following a significant vascular injury, and absence of these findings does not rule out the possibility of vascular injury.

1. Signs—Clinical manifestations of vascular injury include an expanding or pulsating hematoma, to-and-fro or continuous murmurs of arteriovenous fistulas, a false aneurysm, loss of pulses, progressive swelling of the injured part, unexplained ischemia or dysfunction, and unilateral cool or pale extremities.

2. Pulses—Perform a complete vascular examination unless treatment of other life-threatening injuries precludes it.

A. PALPATION—Palpate all peripheral pulses: carotid, axillary, brachial, radial, femoral, popliteal, dorsalis pedis, and posterior tibial.

B. DOPPLER ULTRASOUND EXAMINATION—The presence of blood flow in a peripheral vessel can be detected using a standard pocket Doppler apparatus. Any assessment of the normality of this flow requires concomitant pressure measurements or waveform analysis.

3. Murmurs and bruits—Auscultate over injured areas to detect bruits or murmurs.

4. Neurologic function—Assess neurologic function. Paresthesia may be an early sign of developing vascular problems (eg, compartment syndrome).

B. Diagnostic Imaging

Arteriography and CT scan with contrast or CTA are the imaging modalities to evaluate vascular injury. In addition, ultrasonography may be useful in specific circumstances (discussed below).

Caution: Diagnostic imaging should not be performed in a patient whose condition is unstable and who needs emergency laparotomy or thoracotomy. The procedure should be delayed until after resuscitation and treatment of the life-threatening emergency, either in the emergency department or in the operating room.

EMERGENCY MANAGEMENT OF SPECIFIC VASCULAR INJURIES

NECK INJURIES

See also Chapter 23.

ESSENTIALS OF DIAGNOSIS

- ▶ History of blunt or penetrating trauma
- ▶ Consider concomitant injury to nonvascular structures
- ▶ CT scan and/or arteriography confirms diagnosis

▶ General Considerations

Vascular injury to the neck is most often due to penetrating injuries; however, blunt trauma to the cervical vessels can result in intimal disruption, dissection, and thrombosis. Concomitant injury to nonvascular structures of the neck (eg, trachea, esophagus, and spinal cord) may also occur. The cervical spine must be protected until injury is excluded.

▶ Penetrating Trauma

In penetrating trauma to the neck, two immediate concerns are massive hemorrhage and airway compromise secondary to a rapidly expanding hematoma.

A. Emergency Treatment

Control hemorrhage, preferably with direct pressure, along with ongoing fluid resuscitation; neither of these measures should delay transport to the operating room for definitive repair. If a rapidly expanding hematoma is suspected, tracheal intubation via direct laryngoscopy or intubating bronchoscope should be conducted before compression of the trachea makes this procedure more difficult or impossible. Transtracheal jet insufflation and cricothyrotomy are methods of last resort; in this setting, emergency tracheostomy in the operating room is preferable.

B. Further Treatment

Further management is a function of the patient's hemodynamic stability and the location of the wound. All actively bleeding, hemodynamically unstable patients are taken immediately to the operating room for surgical exploration. For stable patients with wounds that penetrate the platysma muscle, management is a function of the zone of the neck affected (Figure 40–1). Wounds should never be probed beyond the level of the platysma muscle in the emergency department.

1. Zone I injuries—These wounds are frequently associated with injury to the great vessels and require imaging with CT or angiography to exclude major arterial injury.

2. Zone II injuries—These injuries may be further evaluated by surgical exploration or imaging of the vessels and nonvascular structures with CT or angiography at the discretion of the attending surgeon.

3. Zone III injuries—Because the relationship of the blood vessels to the base of the skull makes surgical exploration and distal control of hemorrhage difficult, preoperative imaging with CT or angiography should be conducted to define the injury and help plan the surgical approach.

▶ Blunt Trauma

Blunt trauma to the carotid artery can result in intimal disruption, dissection, and thrombosis leading to acute cerebral ischemia manifest as a gross hemispheric neurologic deficit not explained by intracranial trauma. Conduct emergent imaging of the neck arteries with CTA or conventional angiography.

▶ Diagnostic Imaging

The use of multiplanar CT scanning with arterial enhanced imaging allow the neck vessels to be evaluated for injuries to include complete or partial transection, arteriovenous fistula, pseudoaneurysms or thrombosis. In addition, conventional arteriography may be required in addition to CT in zone I and III injuries.

▶ Disposition

Asymptomatic patients with mild neck injuries due to blunt trauma or penetrating injuries that do not cross the platysma muscle may be discharged from the emergency department. Hospitalize all other patients with neck injuries, and consult with a general or vascular surgeon.

CHEST INJURIES

See also Chapter 24.

ESSENTIALS OF DIAGNOSIS

▶ Significant mechanism of thoracic trauma

▶ Tearing retrosternal or interscapular pain, dysphagia, hoarseness, or dyspnea

▶ In blunt trauma, less than half of patients will have visible signs of chest wall injury

▶ CT scan or TEE confirms diagnosis

▶ General Considerations

Vascular injury to the chest occurs secondary to both penetrating and blunt trauma. If bleeding is not contained within fascial planes, these injuries can lead to exsanguination and death, often before the patient arrives in the emergency department. A high degree of suspicion for this type of injury must be maintained in any patient with a significant mechanism of thoracic trauma. CT with contrast has become the diagnostic study of choice in evaluating vascular injury in a hemodynamically stable patient with chest trauma.

▶ Thoracic Aortic Injury

Penetrating and blunt trauma may cause thoracic aortic injury (TAI). Though penetrating TAI may be caused by any variety of objects or weapons, blunt TAI involves large,

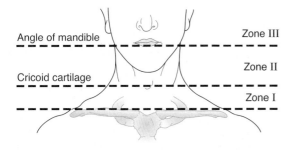

▲ **Figure 40–1.** Zones of vascular injury in the neck.

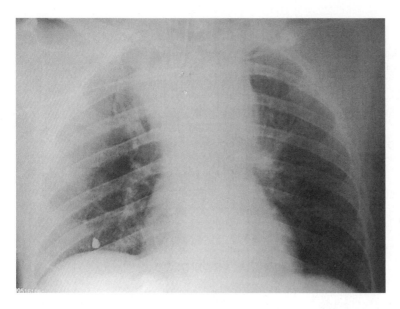

▲ **Figure 40–2.** Chest X-ray from a patient with a traumatic aortic injury demonstrating a wide mediastinum, blurring of the aortic arch, left apical cap, and deviation of the nasogastric tube.

violent deceleration forces (eg, falls, motor vehicle collisions including occupant ejection or auto-pedestrian). The greatest risk of TAI in a motor vehicle collision exists when the impact occurs on the same side of the vehicle as the occupant, when there is greater than 15 in of intrusion into the passenger compartment, and when the overall change in velocity experienced by the vehicle and its occupants is greater than 20 miles/h. A significant mechanism of injury should heighten suspicion of blunt TAI, because less than half of these patients will have visible signs of chest wall injury.

► Clinical Findings

A. Symptoms and Signs

Patients may complain of tearing retrosternal or interscapular pain. Less frequently, dysphagia, hoarseness, stridor, or shortness of breath is present. The physical examination often reveals no external evidence of chest wall injury. Classically, a difference in upper-extremity pulses and a harsh systolic murmur across the precordium and in the interscapular area are noted. Signs and symptoms of shock may be present.

B. Imaging

The chest X-ray is frequently the first imaging study obtained (Figure 40–2); the classic chest X-ray findings associated with TAI are listed in Table 40–1. However, 7% of patients with TAI can have a normal chest X-ray and further imaging studies may be warranted, based on clinical suspicion and mechanism of injury. In the past,

aortography had been the study of choice in evaluating TAIs. However, CT scan has emerged as the study of choice after initial chest X-ray. It is more readily available than aortography and less invasive, and prospective clinical trials have shown spiral CT scan to be 100% sensitive and 99.7% specific in diagnosing TAI following blunt trauma. In centers where transesophageal echocardiography (TEE) is readily available, it is a highly sensitive (98%) and specific (100%) modality for diagnosing TAI. TEE can be done at the bedside, requires no contrast dye, and evaluates real-time cardiac function.

► Treatment and Disposition

Patients with TAI will require emergency consultation with a vascular or thoracic surgeon. In the emergency department, it is important to maintain intravascular volume with crystalloid solutions and blood products. Systolic blood pressure should be lowered to less than 120 mm Hg. Exsanguinating hemorrhage may require emergency thoracotomy for the control of bleeding.

Table 40–1. X-ray Findings Associated with Traumatic Rupture of the Thoracic Aorta.

Left apical "cop" (fluid in the apical pleural space)
Widened mediastinum
Deviation of trachea to the right
Depression of left mainstem bronchus
Obscuration of the aortic arch
Hemothorax

PULMONARY VASCULAR INJURIES

ESSENTIALS OF DIAGNOSIS

▶ Usually due to penetrating thoracic or abdominal injury
▶ Rapidly expanding hemothorax on chest X-ray

▶ Clinical Findings: General Considerations

Most patients present with penetrating chest or abdominal trauma and rapidly expanding hemothorax, visible on chest X-ray. Rarely, blunt chest trauma is associated with pulmonary vascular injury.

▶ Treatment and Disposition

Most patients can be managed with a 36–42 F chest tube that uses suction and allows the lung to reexpand and tamponade the bleeding vessel. Continued massive bleeding requires prompt surgery. Consider the use of autotransfusion. Prompt consultation with a general, vascular, or thoracic surgeon is required, because exsanguination can occur rapidly. Hospitalization is indicated for all patients.

ABDOMINAL INJURIES

See also Chapter 25.

ESSENTIALS OF DIAGNOSIS

▶ History of abdominal trauma
▶ Signs and symptoms of shock that fail to respond to resuscitation efforts

▶ Clinical Findings

Patients with injuries to major vessels within the abdominal cavity present mainly with hemorrhagic shock that fails to respond to resuscitative efforts. In hemodynamically stable patients, CT with contrast is used to evaluate intrabdominal vascular and solid organ injury.

▶ Treatment and Disposition

Immediate operation is the only effective treatment for abdominal vascular injuries. Support blood pressure with infusion of intravenous fluids (colloid or crystalloid solutions) until surgery can be performed. Packed red blood cells or whole blood should be used as soon as available.

INJURIES TO THE EXTREMITIES

ESSENTIALS OF DIAGNOSIS

▶ History of blunt or penetrating trauma
▶ Presence of a pulse does not rule out vessel injury
▶ Use CT or arteriography to evaluate

▶ Clinical Findings

A. Penetrating Trauma

Vascular injuries are present in 25–35% of patients with penetrating trauma to the extremities. Occasionally vascular trauma is present without the usual physical findings, and the presence of a pulse does not rule out injury to the vessel. Imaging should be considered whenever the weapon's trajectory has passed close to major blood vessels.

B. Blunt Trauma

Vascular injury may also occur after blunt trauma, especially if fractures and joint dislocations are present. Even if the pulse is restored with splinting and traction, an arteriogram is necessary to rule out significant injury to the intima.

C. Posterior Dislocation of the Knee

Posterior dislocation of the knee is associated with popliteal artery injury in half of cases, and arteriography is therefore mandatory.

▶ Treatment

Stabilize the patient, and stop hemorrhage as outlined above. Splint fractures. Do not clamp vessels or use a tourniquet.

▶ Imaging and Disposition

All patients with suspected vascular injury should undego diagnostic imaging. CT angiography (CTA) in now the primary limaging modality for evaluating extremity arterial injuries in both blunt and penetratig extremity injuries. Obtain general or vascular surgical consultation for all penetrating extremity injuries.

MAJOR VENOUS TRAUMA

ESSENTIALS OF DIAGNOSIS

▶ History of trauma

▶ Injuries to major venous structures manifested by progressive hemorrhagic shock (not ischemia)

▶ Venography may aid diagnosis

▶ General Considerations

Trauma to peripheral veins without associated arterial injury usually does not require operative correction; however, disruption of the central large veins (vena cava or its immediate branches, subclavian or iliac veins)—especially where they are not enclosed by dense fascia or muscles—requires prompt operation.

▶ Clinical Findings

Venous injury is usually manifested by hemorrhage, not ischemia. Patients with bleeding from the central veins present with progressive hemorrhagic shock (Chapter 9). Superior vena cava and subclavian vein hemorrhage is usually associated with hemothorax visible on chest X-ray.

In contrast, hemorrhage from the inferior vena cava and iliac vein is more difficult to detect. The only common finding is progressive hemorrhagic shock, and many of these injuries are not suspected before they are discovered at surgery.because most patients are too unstable to allow detailed radiologic evaluation.

▶ Treatment and Disposition

Surgical correction in the operating room is indicated.

Arthurs ZM, Sohn VY, Starnes BW: Vascular trauma: endovascular management and techniques. Surg Clin North Am 2007;87:1179–1192 [PMID: 17936481].

Cook CC, Gleason TG: Great vessel and cardiac trauma. Surg Clin North Am 2009; 89:797–820 [PMID: 19782838].

Foster BR, Anderson SW, Soto JA: CT angiography of extremity trauma. Tech Vasc Interv Radiol 2006;9:156–166 [PMID: 17709080].

Isenhour JL, Marx J: Advances in abdominal trauma. Emerg Med Clin North Am 2007;25:713–733 [PMID: 17826214].

Rathlev NK, Medzon R, Bracken ME: Evaluation and management of neck trauma. Emerg Med Clin North Am 2007;25:679–694 [PMID: 17826212].

Stallmeyer MJ, Morales RE, Flanders AE: Imaging of traumatic neurovascular injury. Radiol Clin North Am 2006;44:13–39 [PMID: 16297680].

Steenburg SD, Ravenel JG, Ikonomidis JS, Schönholz C, Reeves S: Acute traumatic aortic injury: imaging evaluation and management. Radiology 2008;248:748–762 [PMID: 18710974].

Tisherman SA, Bokhari F, Collier B, Cumming J, Ebert J, Holevar M, Kurek S, Leon S, Rhee P: Clinical practice guideline: penetrating zone II neck trauma. J Trauma 2008; 64:1392–1405 [PMID: 18469667].

▼ VASCULAR EMERGENCIES NOT DUE TO TRAUMA

ACUTE ISCHEMIA

ACUTE PERIPHERAL ISCHEMIA DUE TO MAJOR ARTERIAL OCCLUSION

ESSENTIALS OF DIAGNOSIS

▶ History of arrhythmia, myocardial infarction, valvular disease, or atherosclerosis may be presen

▶ Pain, paresthesias, and coolness of affectedextremity

▶ Pale, mottled, cyanotic limb with decreased or absent pulses

▶ Angiography confirms diagnosis

▶ Clinical Findings

Acute arterial occlusion may be caused by an embolus, thrombosis, or trauma to an artery. Occlusion leads to distal ischemia, which if not corrected can progress to irreversible tissue damage and necrosis.

A. Embolic Occlusion

Embolic occlusion is caused by the dislodgment of an intravascular thrombus that travels distally and occludes a smaller artery. The majority of thrombi originate in the heart, but they may come from anywhere within the vascular system. A history of arrhythmia, myocardial infarction, or valvular heart disease suggests an embolic cause for acute peripheral ischemia.

1. Cardiac emboli—Cardiac emboli generally originate in the left atrium in patients with atrial fibrillation or mitral valve disease and in the left ventricle in patients with recent myocardial infarction or ventricular aneurysm.

2. Vascular emboli—Vascular emboli originate on irregular luminal surfaces of atherosclerotic vessels (eg, ulcerative plaques or aneurysms). These emboli may contain cholesterol in the clot.

3. Tumor emboli—Tumor emboli are rare, the most common sources are atrial myxomas.

B. Thrombotic Occlusion

Thrombosis of an atherosclerotic artery resulting in acute ischemia is uncommon but may occur secondary to plaque disruption and resultant clot formation. A history of peripheral vascular disease, claudication, progressive rest pain, or nonhealing wounds of the distal extremities is suggestive of occlusion secondary to thrombosis, because these patients often lack sufficient collateral flow that can minimize ischemia.

C. Consequences of Occlusion

Acute occlusion of a previously patent major artery results in ischemia of the nerves, muscles, and skin distal to the occluded site. The severity of symptoms is a function of the adequacy of flow through collateral vascular channels. Within a few hours after persistent and severe occlusion, irreversible anesthesia, paralysis, and tissue infarction occur. During this time, the developing thrombus progressively occludes the distal vessels, reducing the likelihood of restoration of blood flow to distal parts. For these reasons, early recognition and appropriate treatment, before irreversible damage occurs, are critical.

▶ Clinical Findings

A. Symptoms and Signs

Patients typically present with extremity pain but may also complain of paresthesias and even paralysis of the affected limb. Physical examination may reveal a pale, mottled, cool, or cyanotic limb. Pulses will be reduced or absent, and there may be tenderness to palpation of affected muscle groups.

B. Imaging Studies

Angiography of the affected limb confirms the diagnosis and is useful for planning surgical intervention. In addition, other imaging modalities such as CTA, MRA, and arterial duplex ultrasonography may be useful.

▶ Treatment

Obtain an immediate general or vascular surgery consultation. Insert a large-bore (≥16-gauge) intravenous catheter. Obtain baseline laboratory studies, including CBC, PT, PTT, and blood chemistries. Also send a blood sample for typing and crossmatching. Begin intravenous heparin at full anticoagulation dosage as soon as possible.

Definitive treatment involves clot lysis through the use of localized intravascular thrombolytics, endovascular or open surgical treatment to avoid lim loss.

▶ Disposition

All patients with acute arterial insufficiency should be hospitalized for management.

ACUTE PERIPHERAL ISCHEMIA DUE TO SMALL-VESSEL OCCLUSION ("BLUE TOE SYNDROME")

ESSENTIALS OF DIAGNOSIS

▶ Abrupt onset of small painful area on affected digit
▶ Affected area is tender, cool, and cyanotic
▶ Asymmetric distribution
▶ Livedo reticularis may be present

▶ General Considerations

Acute occlusion of a digital artery by microemboli results in ischemia of the affected digit. The most common sources of these microemboli are proximal atherosclerotic plaques or aneurysms. Debris consisting of cholesterol, calcium, and platelet aggregates breaks off from these areas, travels distally through the vasculature, and lodges in the small digital arteries. Other sources of microemboli are clots on prosthetic heart valves and septic emboli from infected heart valves.

▶ Clinical Findings

The diagnosis is based on clinical findings. Patients typically report the abrupt onset of a small painful area on the affected digit that is tender, cool, and cyanotic. If multiple areas are affected, the distribution of lesions is asymmetric. Pulses in the affected extremity are intact. A fine, lace-like rash (livedo reticularis) may be noted. If the patient presents late, gangrene may be present.

▶ Treatment

Treatment is directed at identifying and treating the proximal source of the emboli because recurrence is likely if the source is not removed. Consult a vascular surgeon.

▶ Disposition

Hospitalize the patient for evaluation and treatment of the source of the microemboli.

ACUTE PERIPHERAL ISCHEMIA DUE TO VENOUS OCCLUSION

ESSENTIALS OF DIAGNOSIS

- ▶ Massive acute swelling of affected leg
- ▶ Leg has doughy consistency
- ▶ Cyanosis and gangrene may occur
- ▶ Color-flow Doppler ultrasound or contrast venography confirms diagnosis

▶ General Considerations

Phlegmasia cerulea dolens (venous gangrene) is a severe form of iliofemoral thrombosis characterized by massive venous occlusion. Rapidly progressive venous hypertension results in diffuse limb swelling to the level of the groin. Distal ischemia occurs secondary to increased venous and tissue pressure. Cyanosis develops and gangrene can occur.

▶ Clinical Findings

Massive acute swelling of the entire leg and cutaneous cyanosis occur early. Distal pulses are diminished or absent. The leg has a doughy consistency, and bullae may be present. Gangrene is a late finding. The diagnosis is confirmed by color-flow Doppler ultrasound or contrast venography.

▶ Treatment

Obtain immediate general or vascular surgery consultation. Begin intravenous heparin at full anticoagulant dosage. The first step in definitive treatment is catheter-directed intrathrombus thrombolysis. If this approach fails, or if the use of thrombolytics is contraindicated, the treatment is thrombectomy.

▶ Disposition

Hospitalize all patients for definitive management.

ACUTE VISCERAL (INTESTINAL) ISCHEMIA

ESSENTIALS OF DIAGNOSIS

- ▶ Severe, poorly localized abdominal pain
- ▶ May have history of intestinal angina
- ▶ Pain out of proportion to physical examination findings
- ▶ Gross or occult intestinal bleeding
- ▶ Mesenteric arteriography or CT confirms diagnosis

▶ General Considerations

Significant arterial insufficiency can cause ischemia that results in necrosis of the bowel mucosa. This may progress to full-thickness involvement in 6–48 hours. The extent of necrosis depends on the vessel involved, the adequacy of collateral perfusion, and the degree of hypoperfusion. Untreated severe intestinal ischemia results in intestinal gangrene, diffuse peritonitis, cardiovascular collapse, and death.

▶ Causes

A. Acute Mesenteric Vascular Occlusion

Acute mesenteric vascular occlusion is the cause of acute visceral ischemia in two-thirds of patients. Occlusion may be due to an embolus from a cardiac mural thrombus or to arterial thrombosis that is the end result of atherosclerotic stenosis of the involved vessel. Some patients give a history of intestinal angina (pain after eating, often relieved by vomiting). Rarely, arterial thrombosis is due to a dissecting aneurysm (aortic or mesenteric artery), connective tissue disease (eg, polyarteritis), or other conditions.

Venous thrombosis occurs occasionally and is associated with portal hypertension, abdominal sepsis, hypercoagulable state, trauma, or use of oral contraceptives.

B. Nonocclusive Arteriolar Intestinal Ischemia

Nonocclusive arteriolar intestinal ischemia is the cause of acute visceral ischemia in one-third of patients and can occur with cardiac arrhythmia, sepsis, or any prolonged hypotensive state. Splanchnic vasoconstriction causes ischemia secondary to a low-flow state.

▶ Clinical Findings

Obscure abdominal pain and intestinal bleeding in elderly patients should suggest the diagnosis of intestinal ischemia.

A. Symptoms and Signs

Severe, poorly localized diffuse abdominal pain is invariable in intestinal ischemia. Classically the pain is out of proportion to that expected based on physical examination findings. See Chapter 15 for differential diagnosis of disorders causing acute abdominal pain. With major acute occlusion, the onset of pain is sudden. With nonocclusive ischemia, pain may develop more insidiously.

Usually, few abdominal findings occur early in the disease; later, abdominal distention and tenderness generally occur. Gross or occult intestinal bleeding may be present. Systemic toxicity may precede abdominal findings. Shock and generalized peritonitis occur late.

B. Laboratory and Other Findings

1. Laboratory tests—Laboratory tests show leukocytosis, metabolic acidosis, and elevated serum lactate.

2. X-ray findings—Upright plain films show ileus, absence of intestinal gas, or diffuse distention with an air–fluid level. Ischemia and intestinal necrosis are late findings. Abdominal plain films are abnormal in only 20% of cases. A barium enema (not recommended if vascular disease is strongly suspected) may show "thumbprinting" of the colonic mucosa.

3. Mesenteric arteriography—When performed early in the course of the disease, mesenteric arteriography is the definitive diagnostic procedure, because it demonstrates major vascular occlusion, if present. If it is done later, it merely delays necessary surgery and permits development of more extensive bowel necrosis and peritonitis. The catheter inserted in the superior mesenteric artery may be used to infuse vasodilating agents when the cause of disease is non-occlusive arteriolar intestinal ischemia and after the primary occlusive lesion is corrected.

4. CT Scan—CT scan is useful in evaluating acute visceral (intestinal) ischemia. In addition, it is useful to help exclude other causes of abdominal pain. CT angiography has a sensitivity ranging from 71 to 96% and a specificity ranging from 92 to 94%. CT angiography is noninvasive as well as being readily available compared to standard angiography and can be considered first line imaging modality.

▶ Treatment

Treat hypotension and shock with infusion of intravenous crystalloid solutions and blood, if bleeding is present. Notify a vascular or general surgeon immediately to prepare for surgery. Prompt operation is required to resect necrotic bowel. In some cases, the embolus can be removed or the arterial obstruction bypassed.

Vasodilator drugs may be used as an adjunct to management of the vascular disease in selected cases of nonocclusive ischemia; however, operation is usually required to resect necrotic bowel. Begin parenteral administration of broad-spectrum antimicrobials.

▶ Disposition

All patients with suspected or proved acute visceral ischemia should be hospitalized.

Lyden SP, Joseph D: The clinical presentation of peripheral arterial disease and guidance for early recognition. Cleve Clin J Med 2006;73:S15–S21 [PMID: 17385387].

Menke J: Diagnostic accuracy of multidetector CT in acute mesenteric ischemia: systematic review and meta-analysis. Radiology 2010;256:93–101 [PMID: 20574087].

Shamoun F, Sural N, Abela G: Peripheral artery disease: therapeutic advances. Expert Rev Cardiovasc Ther 2008;6:539–553 [PMID:18402543].

Sontheimer DL: Peripheral vascular disease: diagnosis and treatment. Am Fam Physician 2006;73:1971–1976 [PMID: 16770929].

Wyers MC: Acute mesenteric ischemia: diagnostic approach and surgical treatment. Semin Vasc Surg 2010;23:9–20 [PMID: 20298945].

ARTERIAL ANEURYSMS

RUPTURED ABDOMINAL AORTIC ANEURYSM

ESSENTIALS OF DIAGNOSIS

▶ Sudden onset of abdominal or flank pain, pulsatile abdominal mass, and hypotension

▶ Bedside ultrasound or CT scan with contrast confirms diagnosis

▶ General Considerations

An artery is described as aneurysmal once it reaches more than twice its normal diameter. The exact mechanism behind the formation of an abdominal aortic aneurysm (AAA) is unknown and is likely multifactorial. The belief that aneurysms are due to atherosclerosis alone has undergone serious challenge in the past several years. Risk factors include a family history of AAA, male gender, age more than 70 years, long-term smoking, and systemic hypertension. Ninety-five percent of AAA's are infrarenal with a small amount extending proximally to involve the renal and splachnic vessels. This condition is fairly common, affecting 2–5% of the population over age 60 years. The primary complication of AAA is spontaneous rupture, which carries a high mortality rate of 80%. The chance of rupture increases exponentially as the diameter of the aneurysm increases (Table 40–2).

Table 40–2. Annual Risk of Rupture of an Abdominal Aortic Aneurysm as a Function of the Size of the Aneurysm.

Aneurysm Diameter	Annual Risk of Rupture
Less than 4 cm	Rare
4–5 cm	1–3% per year
5–6 cm	5–10% per year
Greater than 7 cm	Greater than 20% per year

If the aneurysm ruptures into the peritoneal space, exsanguination and death occur rapidly, usually prior to arrival in the emergency department. When rupture occurs into the retroperitoneal space, a tamponade effect may temporarily control hemorrhage and allow time for diagnosis and treatment.

▶ Clinical Findings

A. Symptoms and Signs

The classic symptoms of AAA rupture include sudden-onset abdominal or flank pain, pulsatile abdominal mass, and hypotension. However, because this triad is seen in only 50% of patients presenting with AAA rupture, a high level of suspicion must be maintained. The most common misdiagnosis given to patients with AAA is symptomatic nephrolithiasis. Consider the diagnosis of AAA in patients with hypotension and shock of uncertain cause and in patients presenting with myocardial ischemia or infarction. Additionally, patients who have undergone previous aortic bypass grafting can present with gastrointestinal bleeding caused by erosion of the graft into the duodenum and subsequent rupture.

B. Laboratory Findings

The hematocrit may be normal or low.

C. Electrocardiogram

The electrocardiogram (ECG) may show signs of myocardial ischemia.

D. Imaging

Bedside ultrasound is rapidly becoming the standard of care in the diagnosis of symptomatic AAA with reported sensitivities of 100%. Images of the aorta can be obtained by the emergency physician concurrently with the initial history and physical examinations and facilitate the early mobilization of surgeons and additional staff. Ultrasound is particularly useful in the hemodynamically unstable patient who presents with abdominal pain, allowing for rapid diagnosis without transfer to a distant radiology suite.

In the clinically stable patient, CT scanning allows for more detailed imaging and helps exclude other etiologies of abdominal pain. Abdominal X-ray may reveal the presence of an AAA due to calcification of the wall of the aneurysm (70% of AAAs). Aortography is used to investigate the vascular anatomy in the workup for elective (nonemergency) AAA repair.

▶ Treatment

Act quickly. Even if the patient appears hemodynamically stable at the time of initial evaluation, the contained rupture may progress rapidly to exsanguinating hemorrhage at any time.

Treat hypotension and shock (see Chapter 9 for more detail):

1. Begin oxygen, 4 L/min, by nasal cannula or mask.

2. Insert two large-bore (≥16-gauge) peripheral intravenous catheters.

3. Obtain blood for CBC, electrolytes, and renal function tests; type and crossmatch for 10 units of packed red blood cells or whole blood. It is also imperative to replace other blood components such as platelets and FFP with massive transfusions. Measure the hematocrit immediately and at frequent intervals thereafter. Remember that the delay in equilibration of blood volume may keep the hematocrit falsely elevated for 12–18 hours.

4. Give 1–3 L of crystalloid solution intravenously to restore adequate blood pressure, and follow with crossmatched blood. If the initial hematocrit is below 20%, either "universal donor" blood or type-specific blood may be necessary.

5. Insert a urinary catheter, send urine for analysis, and monitor urine output.

Request urgent consultation with a general or vascular surgeon, since emergency surgery is the only definitive treatment.

▶ Disposition

Hospitalize all patients with suspected or documented ruptured AAA.

VISCERAL AND HYPOGASTRIC ARTERY ANEURYSMS

ESSENTIALS OF DIAGNOSIS

▶ Abrupt onset of diffuse abdominal pain

▶ Signs and symptoms of shock may be present

▶ CT scan with contrast or visceral angiography confirms diagnosis

▶ General Considerations

Congenital aneurysm occurs in younger patients, whereas atherosclerotic aneurysm occurs more commonly in older patients. The splenic artery is the most commonly involved vessel. Bleeding may be confined to the lesser sac of the peritoneal cavity for the first 24–48 hours. However, free rupture into the general peritoneal cavity invariably causes exsanguination. Rupture is most common during pregnancy. Hypogastric artery aneurysms may rupture into the retroperitoneum or erode into contiguous organs, in which case gastrointestinal bleeding or hematuria occurs.

Clinical Findings

There is abrupt onset of diffuse abdominal pain. Hypotension occurs secondary to blood loss. The hematocrit is low if the bleeding is more than a few hours old. CT scan with contrast is an excellent tool for diagnosis in the hemodynamically stable patient. Peritoneal lavage may reveal gross blood. A plain film of the abdomen may show an aneurysm if it has calcified.

The only definitive diagnostic procedure is selective visceral angiography, which should be performed in the hemodynamically stable patient in whom an aneurysm is not present on a plain film.

Treatment

Start resuscitative measures, including insertion of a large-bore (≥16-gauge) intravenous catheter, nasogastric tube, Foley catheter, and the like (see Ruptured Abdominal Aortic Aneurysm section above and Chapter 9). Draw blood for CBC, and type and crossmatch for 8 units of packed red blood cells or whole blood.

Notify a vascular surgeon at once, because early operation is imperative.

Disposition

Immediately hospitalize all patients with suspected or documented visceral and hypogastric artery aneurysms.

THORACIC AORTIC ANEURYSM (AORTIC DISSECTION)

Introduction

ESSENTIALS OF DIAGNOSIS

▶ Abrupt chest or abdominal pain, often radiating to the back, pulse differential, murmur of aortic regurgitation

▶ Chest CT with contrast or TEE are imaging studies of choice

General Considerations

Aortic dissection, a rare but deadly disease, is often misdiagnosed at first presentation. Sir William Osler, perhaps the most astute diagnostician of his day, suggested that no other disease could cause as much humility in a clinician. In one study of hospitalized patients with aortic dissection, the correct diagnosis was delayed over 24 hours in 31–53% of patients. An initial misdiagnosis rate of 85% in patients ultimately diagnosed with aortic dissection has been described.

Left untreated or misdiagnosed, aortic dissection is associated with a mortality rate of almost 1% per hour initially, 40–50% in the first 48 hours, and 90% at 1 year. Modern treatment has reduced the in-hospital mortality rate to 10–27% and the 10-year survival rate is now approximately 55%.

The annual incidence of aortic dissection is from 5 to 30 cases per million; incidence varies depending on risk factors of the population studied. Since this disease is often fatal prior to arrival at the hospital, the incidence may be underestimated.

Pathophysiology

Aortic dissection occurs when the intima (the innermost layer of the aorta) tears and allows blood to dissect between the intima and adventitia (the outermost layer of the aorta). Cystic medial necrosis, a weakening of the media (the central layer of the aorta) and hypertension contribute to this process although the exact mechanism is not known. The dissection may propagate either proximally or distally and a second tear often occurs, creating a false lumen through which blood flows freely. Approximately 90% of all dissections occur in the right lateral wall of the proximal ascending aorta, where shear forces are the highest. The next most common site of dissection is just distal to the origin of the left subclavian artery.

Risk factors for aortic dissection include hypertension, trauma, pregnancy, Marfan syndrome, Ehlers-Danlos syndrome, Turner syndrome, cocaine abuse, coarctation of the aorta, bicuspid aortic valve, previous aortic valve replacement, and intra-aortic catheterization.

Classification

The more commonly used Stanford Classification divides aortic dissections into type A dissections, which involve the ascending aorta, and type B dissections, which do not involve the same. The DeBakey system describes three categories (Table 40–3). Stanford type A and DeBakey types I and II usually require surgery, while Stanford type B and DeBakey III may be treated medically. Type A dissections managed medically have been demonstrated to have double the mortality (58% vs 26%) of surgically corrected cases. Type B dissections demonstrated a mortality of only 11% with medical management versus 31% of the surgically repaired patients. Beyond open surgical revision, endovascular repair has become an optimal alternative in selected patients with aortic dissection. Recent studies evaluating endovascular repair with medical management in acute Type B dissections have

Table 40–3. Aortic Dissection Classification Systems.

DeBakey system	
Type I	Involves both the ascending and descending thoracic aorta
Type II	Involves only the ascending thoracic aorta
Type III	Involves only the descending thoracic aorta
Type IIIb	Involves the descending thoracic and abdominal aorta
Stanford system	
Type A	Involves the ascending aorta
Type B	All others

concluded medical management remains the gold standard in uncomplicated, asymptomatic Type B dissections.

History

The classic description of symptoms of aortic dissection is the abrupt onset of a tearing chest pain radiating to the back. The International Registry of Acute Aortic Dissection (IRAD) found that these classic symptoms are insensitive and nonspecific. Chest pain, for example, was found in only 72.7% of patients while back pain was found in only 53.2%. Only half of patients described the pain as "tearing or ripping," and abdominal pain was the chief complaint in a third of the patients. The majority (84.8%) of patients described an abrupt onset of pain (when pain was present), and 9.4% of patients in the registry presented with syncope.

Physical Findings

Classic findings in aortic dissection include aortic regurgitation murmur and pulse deficit; however, these were present in only 31.6 and 15.1%, respectively, of patients in the IRAD study. Forty-nine percent of patients were hypertensive while 34.6% were normotensive, and 8.4% presented with a systolic blood pressure below 80 mm Hg. Neurological deficits were noted in 4.7% of IRAD patients, while congestive heart failure was described in 6.6%.

Physical findings are caused by ischemia due to the occlusion of thoracoabdominal aortic branch vessels, systolic failure due to severe aortic regurgitation, cardiac tamponade, or aortic rupture. Ascending dissections may cause cardiac tamponade and hemopericardium. Severe aortic regurgitation is the second most common cause of death after aortic rupture. Rupture of the aorta leads to sudden cardiovascular collapse and death.

Bruits may be auscultated in the carotid, subclavian, or femoral arteries. Painless bilateral lower extremity ischemia has been reported and bowel infarction may be the predominant presentation. Reports of aortic dissections rupturing into the esophagus or bowel and causing gastrointestinal hemorrhage are exceptionally rare.

Neurologic involvement occurs in 4.7–30% of aortic dissections and usually manifests as stroke, although a history of antecedent chest pain is usually elicited. Spinal cord ischemia may cause para- or quadriplegia or anterior spinal cord syndrome, or mimic transverse myelitis. Peripheral nerve involvement occurs rarely, leading to Horner's syndrome, hoarseness, or limb paresthesias.

Diagnosis

Aortic dissection is a life-threatening, time-dependent diagnosis. Patients may quickly become hemodynamically unstable. Clinical suspicion is paramount—if the diagnosis is not considered and pursued aggressively, valuable time will be lost. First line tests are unreliable; a widened mediastinum is present in 61.6%, abnormal aortic contour in 49.6%, and pleural effusion in 19.2% of initial chest radiographs. ECGs are normal 31.3% of the time, with 41.4% revealing nonspecific ST segment or T-wave changes. A critical misdiagnosis can occur in the 18.3% of patients who present with definite ischemic changes on ECG; anticoagulation or thrombolysis can be fatal in patients mistakenly believed to have ischemic coronary syndromes.

The classic gold-standard test for the diagnosis of aortic dissection was aortography. Because it is invasive, time-consuming, and usually requires transport of a potentially unstable patient to a distant angiogram suite, this modality is becoming less favored. MRI, TEE, and CT scanning are all sensitive for the diagnosis. Because of the difficulty in obtaining an MRI or TEE on an emergency basis, CT has become the test of choice for the initial diagnosis of aortic dissection with a sensitivity of 83–94% and specificity of 87–100%.

Difficulties with CT scanning include need for contrast dye administration and limited evaluation of branch vessel involvement and degree of aortic regurgitation.

Transthoracic echocardiography is an insensitive tool for the diagnosis of aortic dissection and is not considered a conclusive test. TEE, on the other hand, is exceptionally sensitive (98%) and specific (96%) for proximal dissections in the hands of an experienced echocardiographer. It can be performed at the bedside and requires no contrast administration. Distal segments of the abdominal aorta cannot be visualized by TEE.

Treatment

Goals of treatment are fourfold:

- Prevent extension of dissection.
- Control pain.

- Involve cardiothoracic or vascular surgeons early.
- Proper disposition of patient.

The primary goal in the normotensive or hypertensive patient is to reduce the shear forces caused by the rapid increase in arterial pressure (dP/dT). This is best achieved by both pulse rate and blood pressure reduction. Typically an esmolol infusion is begun, titrated to reduce pulse rate to 60 beats/min, followed by a nitroprusside infusion titrated to reduce the mean arterial pressure to 60–70 mm Hg. The β-blocker infusion is started first to blunt the reflex tachycardia often associated with nitroprusside infusions. Blood pressure should not be lowered to a level where end-organ perfusion is compromised. If these infusions are not immediately available, intravenous labetalol may be administered, 10–40 mg every 5 minutes until pressure and rate goals are achieved.

Pain control is achieved with intravenous opiates. Fentanyl is often used, 50–100 μg intravenously, due to its short half-life and few hemodynamic side effects.

The hemodynamically unstable patient should receive two large-bore peripheral intravenously; maintain ABCs and consult cardiothoracic or vascular surgeons on an emergency basis to discuss optimal management. The critically ill patient with persuasive indications of aortic dissection may best be managed with immediate surgery without further imaging.

All patients with acute aortic dissection must be admitted into the hospital, mostly to the intensive care unit setting where intravenous infusions and close monitoring may be administered. Surgical consultation is indicated for all dissections regardless of location and initial treatment choices.

POPLITEAL AND FEMORAL PERIPHERAL ANEURYSMS

ESSENTIALS OF DIAGNOSIS

▶ Symptoms are due to thrombus, embolization, or pressure from an expanding aneurysm

▶ Pulsatile mass on physical examination (if not thrombosed)

▶ Ultrasound confirms diagnosis

▶ Arteriography defines distal arterial circulation

▶ General Considerations

Occlusion or distal embolization of the friable lining of peripheral aneurysms results in symptoms of distal ischemia. Unlike AAA or visceral aneurysm, rupture is rare. The most common locations of peripheral aneurysms are the popliteal artery and, secondarily, the femoral artery. Popliteal aneurysms are often bilateral and associated with AAAs.

Acute occlusion can result in severe distal ischemia. Distal embolization can also result in severe distal ischemia; however, it is often associated with episodes of moderate ischemia that decrease as collateral circulation improves.

▶ Clinical Findings

A. Symptoms and Signs

Symptoms are due to thrombosis, embolization, pressure from an expanding aneurysm, or (rarely) rupture. There may be an arterial mass in the popliteal fossa or the groin. The aneurysm is pulsatile unless it is thrombosed. Signs of acute arterial occlusion often coexist.

Popliteal aneurysms can cause symptoms (eg, signs of venous obstruction, weakness, and sensory defects) when they compress the popliteal vein or tibial nerve. Rupture of the aneurysm is rare.

B. Imaging

1. Plain X-ray—A rim of calcification may be apparent in the wall of the aneurysm.

2. Arteriography—Arteriography may not demonstrate the aneurysm if it is thrombosed, but this procedure is generally advised to define the status of the arterial circulation distal to the aneurysm.

3. Ultrasonography—Ultrasonography is helpful in identifying the presence of an aneurysm.

▶ Treatment

Notify a vascular surgeon, because immediate operation is required when severe distal ischemia has occurred secondary either to acute thrombosis or to distal embolization. Elective operation is recommended for any aneurysm producing compression of adjacent structures as well as for most documented popliteal aneurysms, because the rate of complication is high if these are left untreated.

▶ Disposition

All symptomatic patients should be hospitalized immediately.

Bergqvist D: Aneurysms---from traumatology to screening. Ups J Med Sci 2010;115:81–87 [PMID: 20370596].

Karthikesalingam A, Holt PJ, Hinchliffe RJ, Thompson MM, Loftus IM: The diagnosis and management of aortic dissection. Vasc Endovascular Surg 2010;44:165–169 [PMID: 20308170].

Moon MR: Approach to the Treatment of Aortic Dissection. Surg Clin N Am 2009;89: 869–893 [PMID: 19782842].

Moore CL, Holliday RS, Hwang JQ, Osborne MR.: Screening for abdominal aortic aneurysm in asymptomatic at-risk patients using emergency ultrasound. Am J Emerg Med 2008; 26:883–887 [PMID: 18926345].

Shanley CJ, Weinberger JB: Acute Abdominal Vascular Emergencies. Med Clin N Am 2008; 92:627–647 [PMID: 18387379].

R J Hinchliffe, Halawa M, Holt PJ, Morgan R, Loftus I, Thompson MM: Aortic dissection and its endovascular management. J Cardiovasc Surg 2008; 49:449–460 [PMID: 18665107].

Adams JD, Garcia LM, Kern JA.: Endovascular repair of the thoracic aorta. Surg Clin N Am 2009;89:895–912 [PMID: 19782843].

VENOUS DISEASE

LOWER-EXTREMITY DEEP VENOUS THROMBOSIS

 ESSENTIALS OF DIAGNOSIS

► Unilateral swelling, warmth, and redness of affected limb

► Physical examination is unreliable in diagnosing deep venous thrombosis (DVT)

► Contrast venography or ultrasound confirms diagnosis

▶ General Considerations

DVT results in 600,000 hospitalizations each year in the United States. If untreated, DVT commonly results in pulmonary embolism, thus making it a significant source of morbidity and mortality.

As described by Virchow in 1856, venous thrombosis is predisposed by stasis of blood flow, hypercoagulopathy, and vascular endothelial injury. Specific conditions associated with development of DVT are shown in Table 40–4.

▶ Clinical Findings

A. Symptoms and Signs

Patients with symptomatic DVT typically complain of unilateral lower-extremity pain and swelling that begins gradually and progresses over days. The described sense of fullness may worsen with standing or walking. Physical examination is of little help in diagnosing DVT and should not be used to exclude diagnosis. Possible findings include unilateral lower-extremity edema, warmth, or erythema. There may be tenderness along the course of the affected vessel, and rarely the clot will be palpable. The time-honored Homans sign (pain in posterior calf with passive dorsiflexion of the foot)

Table 40–4. Factors Predisposing to Deep Venous Thrombosis.

Stasis of blood flow
Recent travel
Bedrest
Immobilization (casting)
Sedentary lifestyle
Hypercoagulopathy
Malignancy
Smoking[a]
Exogenous estrogen[a]
Intrinsic coagulopathies
Factor V Leyden
Protein C deficiency
Protein S deficiency
Antithrombin III deficiency
Homocysteinemia
Trauma
Surgery, particularly orthopedic surgery hip or lower extremity

[a]Causes secondary protein S deficiency.

has been shown to be unreliable in diagnosing DVT. Because the DVT results in a systemic inflammatory response, the patient may be febrile. Adjunctive testing is required because physical examination is unreliable in diagnosing DVT.

B. Imaging and Laboratory Findings

1. Contrast venography—Although contrast venography remains the gold standard for diagnosing DVT, it has been largely replaced by ultrasonography in most institutions. The advantages of contrast venography include a sensitivity and specificity of nearly 100% and the ability to detect DVTs of the calf, iliac vessels, and inferior vena cava that can be missed by ultra-sound. Its primary disadvantages include its invasive nature, use of contrast material, and availability. Additionally, 5–15% of studies performed are technically inadequate.

2. Ultrasonography—Ultrasonography is the most accurate noninvasive study for diagnosing lower-extremity DVT, with a sensitivity of 93–100% and a specificity of 97–100% in detecting proximal DVTs. The limitations of ultrasonography are its ability to detect pelvic and calf DVTs (20% of which will extend into the popliteal vein and thigh). The sensitivity for detecting distal (calf) DVT is only 70%.

3. D-Dimer assay—D-dimer is formed when fibrin is degraded by plasmin. The testing for the presence of D-dimer is by latex agglutination (least sensitive), whole blood agglutination (bedside, qualitative), and enzyme-linked immunoassay (ELISA) (most accurate). When combined with ultrasound, the whole blood agglutination and ELISA have an almost 100% negative predictive value.

▶ Treatment

For DVT of proximal veins of the thigh, put the patient on bed rest and elevate the limb. Start anticoagulation with intravenous heparin, subcutaneous low-molecular-weight heparin (enoxaparin or dalteparin) or fondaparinux (a factor X_a inhibitor). Alternatively, catheter-directed thrombolytic therapy with streptokinase or urokinase is effective in treating acute DVT less than 7 days old and may prevent postphlebitic complications. Obtain consultation with a vascular surgeon in cases of massive iliofemoral thrombosis. Surgery may be required for certain patients.

Management of calf DVT and the need for hospitalization are controversial. Isolated calf thrombi do not commonly produce pulmonary emboli, although they may propagate into proximal vessels. Traditional treatment has been low-dose heparin (eg, 5000 units subcutaneously twice a day), although some authors advocate serial noninvasive studies (eg, ultrasound) and treatment only if propagation occurs.

▶ Disposition

All patients with proximal DVT should be hospitalized. Because of the association between DVT and malignancy, patients with a new diagnosis of DVT should be referred to a primary-care provider for further evaluation.

SUPERFICIAL THROMBOPHLEBITIS

ESSENTIALS OF DIAGNOSIS

- ▶ Pain, tenderness, induration, and erythema along course of affected vein
- ▶ Affected extremity shows only slight to no edema (no other signs of impaired venous return)

▶ General Considerations

Superficial venous thrombosis of the upper extremity is usually iatrogenic, occurring secondary to intravenous catheterization. Lower-extremity superficial venous thromboses may be associated with varicose veins, bacterial infection of surrounding tissues, trauma, or thromboangiitis obliterans. Trauma may play a part in the development of thrombi or may cause recurrences.

▶ Clinical Findings

Pain, tenderness, induration, and erythema are noted along the course of the involved vein, which may feel like a cord.

The extremity shows only slight or no swelling, and there are no other signs of impaired venous return.

Septic thrombophlebitis usually occurs following intravenous injections (especially among intravenous drug abusers) and at venous catheter sites. It should be suspected in the presence of the above symptoms or fluctuance along a superficial vein. Fever and rigors may be present. The diagnosis is confirmed if pus can be aspirated from the vein.

▶ Treatment

A. Cases with No Complications

For uncomplicated superficial venous thrombosis, only symptomatic treatment is required. Neither bed rest nor anticoagulation is indicated. An elastic bandage at and above the level of thrombosis helps to speed remission. Elevation of the leg when the patient is sitting and nonsteroidal anti-inflammatory drugs are also helpful.

B. Cases with Complications

Obtain general or vascular surgical consultation for all complications. If clinical examination suggests that the thrombosis is approaching the saphenofemoral junction, ligation and division of the saphenous vein are indicated, because pulmonary embolization can result from deep venous involvement.

If septic thrombophlebitis occurs, parenteral antimicrobials are required and the involved segment of vein must be excised or ligated and drained to prevent persistent bacteremia.

▶ Disposition

Patients with mild, localized superficial thrombosis may be discharged. Patients with more serious disease, including suspected or documented septic thrombophlebitis, should be hospitalized.

UPPER-EXTREMITY VENOUS THROMBOSIS

ESSENTIALS OF DIAGNOSIS

- ▶ Pain and swelling of affected limb
- ▶ Occurs in 3% of patients with a central venous catheter
- ▶ Examination reveals nonpitting edema, normal skin color, and intact distal pulses
- ▶ Contrast venography or ultrasonography confirms diagnosis

General Considerations

Upper-extremity DVT (UEDVT) is much less common (4% of all DVT cases) than lower-extremity DVT but remains an important cause of morbidity because of its association with pulmonary embolism and postphlebitic sequelae (persistent upper-extremity pain and swelling). Nearly 15–33% of cases of UEDVT will be complicated by pulmonary embolism. Mortality from UEDVT is approximately 1% overall, but one study was able to demonstrate that one third of UEDVT patients died within 3 months of a confirmed diagnosis.

The most common risk factor for UEDVT is central venous catheter placement, with clinically significant thrombus formation in 3% of patients with a central line. The second most common category of UEDVT is spontaneous (effort related) thrombosis. Risk factors include repetitive activities involving hyperabduction of the shoulder and aberrant anatomy of the costoclavicular space. Other causes include intravenous drug use, thoracic tumors, and radiation. The most commonly affected site of thrombosis is the axillary–subclavian venous system.

Clinical Findings

A. Symptoms and Signs

Patients typically present with pain and swelling of the affected limb. The risk factors discussed above may be present. Physical examination may reveal nonpitting edema of the affected side forearm (occasionally the whole arm), normal skin color, and intact distal pulses. Venous cords may be palpable.

B. Imaging

As with lower-extremity DVT, contrast venography remains the gold standard for diagnosis of UEDVT. However, it is slowly being replaced by ultrasonography, which has been shown to have a high degree of sensitivity and specificity for diagnosing UEDVT. Compression ultrasonography has been shown to have a sensitivity of 96% and a specificity of 94% for UEDVT found along the axillary and subclavian veins. As one moves more centrally in the exam towards the bony structures of the chest, the sensitivity and specificity decrease significantly.

Treatment

Initial treatment involves immobilization, elevation, and the application of heat to the affected limb. This is followed by systemic anticoagulation with intravenous heparin, subcutaneous low-molecular-weight heparin (enoxaparin or dalteparin) or fondaparinux (a factor X_a inhibitor). Other options include catheter-directed thrombolysis and surgical thrombectomy. Frequently surgery is required to correct underlying anatomic defects to prevent recurrence. Consult a vascular surgeon.

Disposition

Hospitalize all patients for definitive management.

RUPTURED VENOUS VARICOSITIES (VARICOSE VEINS)

ESSENTIALS OF DIAGNOSIS

▶ Bleeding from varicose veins, usually due to minor trauma

General Considerations

Rupture is an uncommon complication of varicose veins. The skin overlying varices can become thin, and erosion can occur spontaneously or with minor trauma.

Clinical Findings

Bleeding from varicose veins is present and may be brisk.

Treatment

Gentle digital pressure over the bleeding site and elevation of the leg control the initial bleeding. Suture ligature of the ruptured vein may be necessary to definitively stop the bleeding. When the initial bleeding has been controlled, the leg should be wrapped in an elastic bandage or Unna's paste boot. Consult a vascular or general surgeon about elective stripping of varicose veins.

Disposition

Brief hospitalization may be advisable.

PULMONARY EMBOLISM

Pulmonary embolism is an occasional complication of venous thrombosis. It is discussed in Chapter 33.

ARTERIOVENOUS FISTULA

ESSENTIALS OF DIAGNOSIS

▶ Abnormal connection between arteries and veins
▶ Constant systolic and diastolic (to-and-fro) murmur and palpable thrill at site
▶ Arteriography confirms diagnosis

General Considerations

Arteriovenous fistulas are abnormal connections between arteries and veins. They may be congenital or acquired. Congenital lesions tend to have more diffuse connections and may involve an extremity. Acquired arteriovenous fistulas—other than those constructed to gain access for dialysis—generally occur secondary to trauma and result from erosion of the artery into a contiguous vein. Other causes include malignancy, infection, and arterial aneurysm. The physiologic effect depends on the size of the communication.

Clinical Findings

A constant systolic and diastolic (to-and-fro) murmur is heard, and a thrill is palpable over most arteriovenous fistulas. Cardiac output may be high if significant left-to-right shunting of blood exists. Patients with congenital arteriovenous fistulas may show increased muscle mass, increased bone length, clubbing, and cyanosis of the involved limb. Polycythemia may also be present.

Complications

Complications include cosmetic deformity due to limb disproportion, congestive heart failure, severe arterial insufficiency, expanding false aneurysm, and hemorrhage. Arteriography delineates the precise outlines of the lesion and may be used for therapeutic embolization.

Treatment and Disposition

Patients with pain, expanding mass, heart failure, or obvious high cardiac output require hospitalization. Others may be discharged from the emergency department and referred to a vascular surgeon or general surgeon.

Davies MG: Deep venous thrombosis: prevention and treatment. Methodist Debakey Cardiovasc J 2009;5:25–31 [PMID: 20143592].

Lee JT, Kalani MA: Treating superficial venous thrombophlebitis. J Natl Compr Canc Netw 2008;6:760–765 [PMID: 18926088].

Naz R et al: Diagnostic yield of color Doppler ultrasonography in deep vein thrombosis. J Coll Physicians Surg Pak 2005;15:276 [PMID: 15907237].

Malhotra S et al: Upper extremity deep vein thrombosis. J Assoc Physicians India 2004;52:237 [PMID: 15636316].

Scarvelis D, Wells PS: Diagnosis and treatment of deep-vein thrombosis. CMAJ 2006;175:1087–1092 [PMID: 17060659].

Tan M, van Rooden CJ, Westerbeek RE, Huisman MV: Diagnostic management of clinically suspected acute deep vein thrombosis. Br J Haematol 2009;146:347–360 [PMID: 19466972].

OTHER VASCULAR SYNDROMES

THORACIC OUTLET SYNDROME

 ESSENTIALS OF DIAGNOSIS

► Signs and symptoms caused by compression of the neural, arterial, or venous structures at the thoracic outlet

► Hand or arm fatigue with use, especially with abduction of the arm

► Elevated arm stress test may elicit symptoms

General Considerations

Thoracic outlet syndrome comprises a variety of disorders caused by abnormal compression of the neural, arterial, or venous structures at the superior aperture of the thorax (thoracic outlet); the most common is compression of nerve structures against the first rib. Symptoms of dysfunction of branches of the brachial plexus are far more common than symptoms secondary to compression of the axillary–subclavian artery or vein, accounting for approximately 95% of cases. Compression of the eighth cervical and first thoracic nerve roots (C8 and T1) is most common. The second most common pattern is involvement of the three uppermost nerve roots of the brachial plexus, the fifth through seventh cervical nerve roots (C5–C7). Thoracic outlet syndrome is rarely an emergency.

Clinical Findings

A. Symptoms

The diagnosis is typically made on clinical grounds with patients complaining of hand or arm fatigue with use, especially with activities involving abduction of the arm. More subtly, patients may note wasting of the muscles of the hand.

If symptoms are due to nerve compression, patients may complain of positional paresthesias in the distribution of one or more trunks of the brachial plexus. Compression of C8–T1 nerve roots results in paresthesias in the ulnar nerve distribution, whereas symptoms referable to C5–C7 compression may involve the ear, neck, upper thorax, or lateral aspect of the shoulder. Raynaud symptoms, secondary to compression of sympathetic nerve fibers may also be reported.

Symptoms of venous compression and thrombosis include pain and swelling of the affected limb. Patients with arterial thoracic outlet syndrome with resultant subclavian–axillary artery stenosis or aneurysm formation may present with symptoms of acute arterial occlusion or embolization.

B. Signs

Physical examination should include the elevated arm stress test (EAST) in an attempt to provoke symptoms. In this test, the patient externally rotates and abducts both arms to 90° with elbows flexed 90° and shoulders braced posteriorly. The patient then opens and closes both hands for a 3-minute period. Patients with thoracic outlet syndrome will complain of the rapid onset of fatigue and heaviness of the arms and are often unable to complete the entire test. Paresthesias may also be reproduced.

In neurologic thoracic outlet syndrome, wasting of the lateral thenar muscles of the hand, weakness of the intrinsic muscles of the hand, and patchy sensory deficits in the distribution of the involved nerve roots may be seen. Reproducible paresthesias during the EAST may be elicited.

Findings in arterial thoracic outlet syndrome include a blood pressure differential in the upper extremities, a bruit with auscultation over the subclavian or axillary artery, and radial pulse deficit on the affected side during the EAST. Findings of acute arterial occlusion or embolization may be found. Thoracic outlet syndrome secondary to venous occlusion or thrombosis may be associated with swelling of the affected extremity and normal pulses.

C. Imaging

1. X-rays—Plain film radiographs of the cervical spine or chest may reveal skeletal abnormalities predisposing to thoracic outlet syndrome (cervical rib, first rib, or clavicle deformity).

2. Angiography—Angiography may be indicated for evaluation of acute arterial occlusion or embolization.

3. Ultrasonography—Ultrasonography may be indicated for evaluation of arterial aneurysms or venous thrombosis.

4. Venography—Venography may be indicated for evaluation of venous thrombosis.

▶ Treatment and Disposition

Patients with neurologic thoracic outlet syndrome can be discharged with a referral to a neurologist or thoracic surgeon. Patients with evidence of a venous or arterial abnormality and stable symptoms should be referred to a vascular or thoracic surgeon. If venous thrombosis or arterial occlusion or embolization is present, the patient should be hospitalized with immediate surgical consultation.

COMPLICATIONS OF PERCUTANEOUS TRANSLUMINAL ANGIOPLASTY AND RETROGRADE ANGIOGRAPHY

 ESSENTIALS OF DIAGNOSIS

► History of recent percutaneous procedure
► May see complications at puncture site or signs and symptoms due to thrombosis or embolization

Increasing number of patients are undergoing percutaneous transluminal angioplasty (balloon dilatation of the arteries) and angiography via the femoral artery. These patients are observed for the development of immediate complications but usually discharged from the hospital within 24–48 hours and may subsequently present to the emergency department with complications (Table 40–5).

Hospitalize the patient and obtain prompt vascular or cardiothoracic surgical consultation, because many of these complications require surgical treatment.

INTRA-ARTERIAL INJECTION OF DRUGS

 ESSENTIALS OF DIAGNOSIS

► History of parenteral drug injection
► Severe burning pain distal to injection site

Table 40–5. Complications of Percutaneous Transluminal Angioplasty.

Puncture site complications
  Bleeding: massive, expanding, or pulsatile hematoma
  False aneurysm: pulsatile mass at puncture site
  Femoral artery occlusion: loss of pulse at or proximal to puncture site, due to thrombosis at catheter site or arterial injury (eg, luminal flap)
  Infection: superficial or deep, with or without arterial involvement
Dilatation site complications
  Thrombosis of dilated vessel (most commonly coronary, iliac, femoral, or renal artery)
Complications distal to insertion site
  Embolization (usually occurs before patient leaves the hospital)

General Considerations

Inadvertent or intentional intra-arterial injection of drugs can cause intense vasospasm followed by arterial occlusion, with distal gangrene as a possible result. This is commonly known as a "hand trip" by intravenous drug abusers. Vasospasm may occur while the drug is being given, or the reaction may be delayed. Unfortunately, many patients with delayed reactions fail to seek medical attention until ischemia is advanced.

Clinical Findings

There is a history of therapeutic or illicit drug injection by the parenteral route. Severe burning pain in distal arterial distribution is followed by intense vasospasm. If the vasospasm has been prolonged, gangrene of the fingers or entire hand may occur even though the arterial vasoconstriction subsequently resolves.

Treatment and Disposition

Hospitalize the patient, and obtain vascular surgical consultation. If the needle is still in place, irrigate distally with heparinized saline. Start systemic anticoagulation with heparin. Systemic vasodilating agents may be necessary to treat the intense vasospasm. Intra-arterial injection of vasodilators (eg, reserpine) is not usually beneficial. If sympathetic nerve block is indicated because of persistent severe peripheral ischemia, consult an anesthesiologist or vascular surgeon.

Huang JJH, Zager EL: Thoracic outlet syndrome. Neurosurgery 2004;55:897–902 [PMID: 15458598].

Koknel Talu G: Thoracic outlet syndrome. Agri 2005;17:5–9 [PMID: 15977087].

Hematologic Emergencies

MK Strecker-McGraw, MD

Mark Andrew Wilson, MD

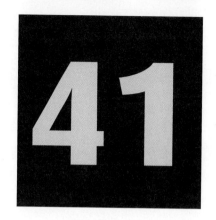

41

▼ HEMOSTATIC DISORDERS: GENERAL CONSIDERATIONS

Most bleeding seen in the emergency department is due to trauma, the result of local wounds, lacerations, or other structural lesions that occur in patients with normal hemostasis. Conversely, bleeding from multiple sites, bleeding from untraumatized sites, delayed bleeding several hours after trauma, and bleeding into deep tissues or joints suggest the possibility of a bleeding disorder. Historical data for the presence of a congenital bleeding disorder include the presence or absence of unusual or abnormal bleeding in the patient and other family members and the possible occurrence of excessive bleeding after dental extractions, surgical procedures, or trauma. Many patients with abnormal bleeding have an acquired disorder, commonly due to liver disease or drug use (particularly ethanol, aspirin, nonsteroidal anti-inflammatory drugs [NSAIDs], warfarin, and antibiotics).

The site of bleeding may provide an indication of the hemostatic abnormality. Mucocutaneous bleeding, including petechiae, ecchymoses, epistaxis, or gastrointestinal,

Table 41–1. Standard Tests of Hemostasis.

Test	Normal Value	Comments
Platelet count	150,000–400,000 platelets/mL	Traumatic bleeding not a serious concern unless platelet count <50,000/μL, and spontaneous bleeding unlikely unless platelet count <10,000/μL.
Prothrombin time and international normalized ratio (INR)	11–13 s, depending on reagent; INR 1.0	Tests extrinsic and common pathways: factors VII, X, V, prothrombin, and fibrinogen.
Activated partial thromboplastin time	22–34 s, depending on reagent	Tests intrinsic and common pathways: factors XII, XI, IX, VIII, V, prothrombin, and fibrinogen.
Fibrinogen level	150–450 mg/dL	Fibrinogen is cleaved by thrombin into fibrin monomer, which then polymerizes into cross-linked fibrin clot.
Fibrin degradation products by latex agglutination	<2.5 mg/L, depending on assay methodology	Breakdown products of fibrinogen and fibrin monomer.
D-dimer by enzyme-linked immunoassay	<500 μg/L, depending on assay methodology	Breakdown products of cross-linked fibrin.

genitourinary, or heavy menstrual bleeding, is characteristic of qualitative or quantitative platelet disorders. Purpura is often associated with thrombocytopenia and commonly indicates a systemic illness. Bleeding into joints and potential spaces, such as between fascial planes and into the retroperitoneum, as well as delayed bleeding, is most commonly associated with coagulation factor deficiencies. Patients who demonstrate both mucocutaneous bleeding and bleeding in deep spaces may have disorders such as disseminated intravascular coagulation (DIC), in which both platelet abnormalities and coagulation factor abnormalities are present. Basic hemostatic tests and clinical evaluation are generally adequate for diagnosis (Table 41–1). Additional hemostatic studies are ordered as indicated (Table 41–2).

▼ HEMOSTATIC DISORDERS: PLATELET DISORDERS

DISORDERS OF DECREASED PLATELET PRODUCTION

Neonatal infections, such as cytomegalovirus (CMV) or rubella, may cause isolated thrombocytopenia. Many medications impair platelet production and produce thrombocytopenia (Table 41–3). Chronic alcohol use is a common cause of thrombocytopenia and will generally resolve if the patient abstains from drinking for longer than 7 days. If multiple cell lines are affected, the differential diagnosis includes aplastic anemia, marrow infiltration from lymphoma or leukemia, or myelofibrosis. Usually, the history and physical examination

Table 41–2. Specialized Tests of Hemostasis.

Test	Normal Value	Comments
Bleeding time	2.5–10 min	Tests interaction between platelets and subendothelium.
Thrombin clotting time	10–12 s	Tests conversion of fibrinogen to fibrin monomer.
Mixing test	Variable	1:1 mixing of abnormal plasma with normal plasma will correct any single coagulation factor deficiency and normalize PT or PTT. If mixing does not normalize the PT or PTT, a coagulation inhibitor is present.
Specific factor assays	60–130% (0.6–1.3 units/mL)	Used to identify specific factor deficiencies.
Inhibitor screens	Variable	Used to detect inhibitors to coagulation factors (e.g., lupus-anticoagulant).

PT, prothrombin time; PTT, partial thromboplastin time.

Table 41–3. Drugs That Impair Platelet Production or Function.

Impair Platelet Production (Thrombocytopenia)[a]	Impair Platelet Function (Prolonged Bleeding Time)
Heparin 4+	Aspirin
Gold salts 4+	Nonsteroidal anti-inflammatory drugs
Sulfa-containing antibiotics 4+	Antiplatelet agents: ticlopidine and
Quinine and quinidine 4+	clopidogrel
Ethanol (chronic use) 4+	Penicillins and cephalosporins
Aspirin 3+	Calcium channel blockers
Indomethacin 3+	Propranolol
Valproic acid 3+	Nitroglycerin
Heroin 3+	Antihistamines
Thiazides 2+	Phenothiazines
Furosemide 2+	Tricyclic antidepressants
Procainamide 2+	
Digoxin 2+	
Cimetidine and ranitidine 2+	
Phenytoin 1+	
Penicillins/cephalosporins 1+	

[a]The numerals following each drug indicate relative incidence based on case reports.

determines the most likely source of thrombocytopenia; however, bone marrow biopsy is sometimes needed.

IMMUNE THROMBOCYTOPENIA

Antibody-mediated platelet destruction can be related to medications, infections, or autoimmune diseases. Two of the more common antibody-mediated thrombocytopenic disorders are idiopathic thrombocytopenic purpura (ITP) and drug-induced immune thrombocytopenia.

1. Idiopathic Thrombocytopenic Purpura

▶ General Considerations

Idiopathic thrombocytopenic purpura is an acquired autoimmune disease characterized by thrombocytopenia, the presence of purpura or petechiae, normal bone marrow, and no other identifiable cause for the thrombocytopenia. Platelet destruction is mediated by the production of autoantibodies that attach to circulating platelets, and the antibody-coated platelets are removed by the reticuloendothelial system. The bone marrow usually responds by increasing platelet production, but sometimes the same antibodies that bind to the platelets also bind to the megakaryocytes, limiting the bone marrow response. Despite the presence of antibodies, the circulating platelets function properly, and many people with ITP may not have significant bleeding despite low platelet counts.

ITP occurs in all age groups and may have an acute or chronic course. Acute ITP is more common among younger children, affects males and females equally, and typically resolves within 6 months. Chronic ITP lasts more than 3 months, is more common in adults, and rarely remits spontaneously. Additionally, patients with chronic ITP are more likely to exhibit an underlying disease or autoimmune disorder, such as HIV infection, systemic lupus, Graves' disease, Hashimoto's thyroiditis, or antiphospholipid antibody syndrome.

▶ Clinical Findings

The most common symptom of ITP is petechiae; mild bleeding may also be seen at mucosal surfaces, including epistaxis, gingival bleeding, and menorrhagia in women of childbearing age. The physical examination is otherwise normal. The presence of lymphadenopathy, hepatosplenomegaly, anemia, or hyperbilirubinemia should suggest an alternative diagnosis, such as leukemia, lymphoma, systemic lupus erythematosus, infectious mononucleosis, or hemolytic anemia. The complete blood count (CBC) should be normal in all cell lines except for the platelets. In some patients with bleeding, a mild anemia may be present. The peripheral blood smear should show large, well-granulated platelets that are few in number. The diagnosis of ITP is based primarily on the history, physical examination, CBC, and peripheral smear.

▶ Treatment

Minimize bleeding risks in patients with ITP, for example, by avoiding the use of antiplatelet medications (eg, aspirin and NSAIDs), avoiding unnecessary invasive procedures, maintaining good blood pressure control, treating exacerbating comorbid conditions (eg, liver disease, renal disease), and addressing fall risks. Treatment of ITP depends on severity, comorbid conditions, and presence of bleeding.

Asymptomatic patients, who are otherwise healthy, with platelet counts greater than 50,000/μL require no treatment. Treatment is indicated for (1) nonbleeding patients with platelet counts less than 20,000/μL and (2) patients with bleeding or significant risk factors for bleeding and platelet counts less than 50,000/μL.

Initial therapy in adults is prednisone started at 60–100 mg/d (children, 1–2 mg/d) and tapered after the platelet count reaches normal (usually requires 4–8 weeks). For patients who do not respond to steroids, the main alternative therapy is splenectomy. For life-threatening bleeding, the current recommendation is high-dose steroid therapy (methylprednisolone 1–2 g/d intravenously for 2–3 days) with or without intravenous immunoglobulin. Additional research is being conducted using several days (4–8 days) of high dose dexamethasone (40 mg/d) in cycles separated by up to 28 days for up to 6 cycles with promising results. However, more study of this approach is needed before it can be recommended. Transfuse platelets as needed following the first dose of methylprednisolone or immunoglobulin; holding the platelet transfusion until the first dose of either is completed results in a better response. Conjugated estrogen, 25 mg intravenously one time, can be given for severe uterine bleeding.

► Disposition

Hospitalization is required for ITP-related bleeding. It is generally not required for asymptomatic patients with platelet counts greater than 20,000/μL. At counts below 20,000/μL, hospitalization may not be required if patients are asymptomatic or have only mild purpura. Hospitalization is prudent when arranging patient follow-up is difficult, when compliance is in doubt, or when significant additional bleeding risk factors are present.

2. Drug-Induced Immune-Mediated Thrombocytopenia

Heparin is the drug most commonly associated with drug-induced immune-mediated thrombocytopenia. Platelet counts typically fall after the 5th day of therapy, even in heparin-naive patients, to usually to below 100,000/μL. Less than 10% of patients develop profound thrombocytopenia with counts less than 20,000/μL. Paradoxically, the complications from heparin-induced thrombocytopenia are usually thromboembolic (deep venous thrombosis, pulmonary embolism, stroke), the conditions heparin is used to treat. Immediate cessation of heparin therapy is indicated when the platelet count falls to below 100,000/μL or more than 50% from baseline. Substitute alternative agents (eg, danaparoid, hirudin, argatroban) for heparin. Although platelet transfusion in heparin-induced thrombocytopenia is typically considered contraindicated, recent data and clinical practice guidelines suggest that in patients with significant bleeding platelet transfusion may be both efficacious and safely performed. Avoid future exposure to either unfractionated heparin or the low-molecular-weight heparins.

The platelet glycoprotein IIb/IIIa receptor antagonists are associated with a 3–7% incidence of modest thrombocytopenia (platelet counts of 50,000–100,000/μL), typically occurring within the first 24 hours of treatment. Severe thrombocytopenia (below 20,000/μL) occurs in less than 1% of patients. Petechiae, wound hematomas, mucosal bleeding, and hematuria are the most common hemorrhage complications. Platelet counts return to normal within 2–3 days after drug discontinuation.

Other drugs rarely cause immune-mediated thrombocytopenia; the sulfonamide, penicillin, and cephalosporin antibiotics have been most commonly reported. In this circumstance, thrombocytopenia typically develops 7–10 days after start of the medications, platelet counts typically fall to below 20,000/μL, and the most common symptoms are petechiae and oral mucosal hemorrhagic blisters.

THROMBOTIC THROMBOCYTOPENIC PURPURA AND HEMOLYTIC UREMIC SYNDROME

Thrombotic thrombocytopenic purpura (TTP) and hemolytic uremic syndrome (HUS) involve platelet aggregation in the microvascular circulation via the mediation of von Willebrand factor (vWF). This leads to consumption thrombocytopenia and microangiopathic hemolytic anemia (MAHA) or schistocyte-forming hemolysis as red blood cells (RBCs) are fragmented during travel through these occluded arterioles and capillaries. TTP and HUS are clinical syndromes with characteristic features, but overlap between the syndromes makes differentiation sometimes difficult. TTP is traditionally more common in adults, whereas HUS is more common in children. TTP typically induces more prominent neurologic deficits with deposition of platelet aggregates in a broader, systemic distribution; HUS more specifically impairs the renal system. In general, adults presenting with clinical and laboratory evidence of MAHA accompanied by thrombocytopenia should receive treatment for TTP once other diagnoses have been excluded (eg, sepsis, metastatic cancer, systemic vasculitis, preeclampsia–eclampsia, Evans syndrome, heparin-induced thrombocytopenia with thrombosis, and malignant hypertension). Untreated TTP has an 80–90% mortality rate.

Pallor, jaundice or scleral icterus, fatigue, and dyspnea on exertion are common because of the hemolytic anemia. With significant thrombocytopenia, purpura or mucosal bleeding may be evident. Focal neurologic deficits (often vacillating), aphasia, seizure, coma, visual disturbance, chest pain, cardiac conduction disorders, abdominal pain, oliguria, and hypertension indicate end-organ involvement.

1. Thrombotic Thrombocytopenic Purpura

► Clinical Findings

A. Symptoms and Signs

TTP classically comprises the following pentad of symptoms and signs: (1) thrombocytopenia, (2) MAHA, (3) fever, (4) renal impairment, and (5) neurologic impairment. It is uncommon for all five features to occur in any one patient, but if they are, severe end-organ ischemia or damage has likely taken place. In comatose patients with extensive brain abnormalities on MRI, resolution of imaging abnormalities and near-full neurologic recovery is possible. As a result, aggressive interventions should still be pursued. Thrombocytopenia and MAHA are the most common features, and fever is the least frequent finding.

A common feature of acquired TTP is the development of autoantibodies to a vWF-cleaving metalloprotease termed ADAMTS-13. Pregnancy is the most common precipitating event for TTP. Preeclampsia has some features similar to TTP, but TTP usually presents earlier during pregnancy, around 23–24 weeks. Delivery does not affect the course of TTP. Other triggers of TTP include infection (particularly HIV), vaccination, and autoimmune disorders such as systemic lupus erythematosus. Several drugs have been associated with TTP, including quinidine, cyclosporine, tacrolimus, and the antiplatelet agents ticlopidine and clopidogrel. A particularly refractory form of TTP has been seen in post-bone marrow transplant patients after treatment with the cancer chemotherapeutic agents mitomycin and gemcitabine.

B. Laboratory Findings

TTP is still a clinical diagnosis, but characteristic laboratory findings include severe anemia, thrombocytopenia, schistocytes or helmet cells on peripheral smear, decreased haptoglobin, elevated reticulocyte count, and elevated unconjugated (indirect) bilirubin from intravascular hemolysis. Additional study suggests that an under recognized cause of morbidity and mortality among patients with TTP is acute myocardial infarction. An LDH elevated above 1000 U/L and an initial troponin I greater than 0.2 ng/mL (troponin T is also used) are excellent predictors of poor outcome. The direct Coombs' test (DAT) is characteristically negative, because the hemolysis seen in TTP does not involve anti-RBC autoantibodies. Because TTP thrombi do not involve fibrin, TTP is distinguished from DIC based on normal coagulation studies.

▶ Treatment

Acquired TTP is treated with daily plasma exchange consisting of (1) plasmapheresis to remove large vWF multimers and autoantibodies and (2) plasma infusion to give the patient back one calculated daily volume of fresh frozen plasma (FFP) or cryoprecipitate-poor plasma (cryosupernatant). The advent of plasma exchange has decreased TTP mortality rates from 90% to 10–20%, and remains the mainstay of treatment. When TTP is suspected, plasma exchange should be initiated without delay for a final definitive diagnosis. If plasmapheresis cannot be performed immediately, initial FFP infusion should be started but infusion should never replace exchange. Plasma exchange is performed daily until several days after remission is achieved. Remission usually occurs within 1 week but may require up to 4 weeks. Remission is defined by normalization of the platelet count and lactate dehydrogenase (LDH) combined with clinical resolution of tissue ischemia and thrombosis. Corticosteroids (usually prednisone, 1–2 mg/kg/d) may be helpful in the presence of a high-autoantibody titer and if plasma exchange does not provide the desired response.

Supportive measures may be needed to address systemic complications associated with TTP, including RBC transfusion for anemia, anticonvulsants for seizures, antihypertensives for hypertension, and hemodialysis for severe renal insufficiency. The general recommendation regarding platelet transfusion is to avoid it unless life-threatening bleeding or intracranial hemorrhage is present since thrombosis may worsen acutely, leading to rapid renal failure and potentially death. While this remains a standard recommendation, recent evidence suggests the warning may be overstated. Aspirin can worsen hemorrhagic complications in the setting of severe thrombocytopenia and also should be avoided. Heparin is not beneficial in TTP. Relapse rates after appropriate treatment may be as high as 30%, and maintenance therapies have not been shown to prevent relapse.

2. Hemolytic Uremic Syndrome
▶ Clinical Findings

HUS is a disease primarily of early childhood, with a peak incidence between ages 6 months and 4 years. The adult form of HUS may be very difficult to distinguish from TTP. The overall mortality rate is 5–15% with the prognosis being worse in older children and adults. HUS is characterized by acute renal failure, MAHA, and thrombocytopenia. HUS often follows a viral or bacterial illness.

Although several infectious agents have been implicated, *Escherichia coli* serotype O157:H7 is a well-recognized factor. Between 20% and 40% of patients with *E. coli* O157:H7 infection have bloody diarrhea, and 15% of children and 5% of adults go on to develop HUS. Onset of HUS is typically 2–14 days after diarrhea develops. Other organisms implicated in HUS include *Shigella, Yersinia, Campylobacter, Salmonella, Streptococcus pneumoniae,* varicella, echovirus, and coxsackievirus A and B.

In HUS the microthrombi are confined mostly to the kidneys, whereas in TTP they occur throughout the microcirculation. Laboratory studies reflect the presence of MAHA, and thrombocytopenia may be present but generally not to the degree seen in TTP. The serum creatinine may be markedly elevated, and urine contains protein and RBCs (although the urine can be normal). Increasingly TTP and HUS are considered to be similar diseases within a spectrum, with some experts simply using the term TTP-HUS syndrome. The sometimes blurred lines between the many varied disease presentations are beyond the scope of this text and likely impossible to fully define within the patient stay in the emergency department. In general, the presence of a preceding diarrheal illness and the predominant laboratory finding of renal failure with minimal to no neurologic changes makes the HUS diagnosis and treatment algorithm more appropriate.

▶ Treatment

Patients with mild HUS with less than 24 hours of urinary symptoms require only fluid and electrolyte correction and supportive care. Steroid therapy may be beneficial. In the setting of more severe disease, plasma exchange or infusion have been performed with equivocal results. Patients whose disease resembles TTP may respond to plasma exchange, but the overall low mortality of HUS makes routine use of plasma exchange questionable.

Hemodialysis may be required in the setting of acute renal failure, especially in adults because acute renal failure tends to be more severe. A shorter duration of dialysis therapy is associated with increased likelihood of recovery from HUS. Do not treat infection with *E. coli* O157:H7 with antimotility drugs because these agents appear to increase the risk of developing HUS. Antibiotic treatment of *E. coli* O157:H7 dysentery is controversial, but meta-analysis has found no evidence that antibiotic treatment increases or decreases the risk of developing HUS.

QUALITATIVE PLATELET ABNORMALITIES

Several disease processes can cause acquired qualitative or functional platelet abnormalities (Table 41–4). In the myeloproliferative diseases, despite frequently elevated platelet counts, the platelets are often dysfunctional and patients can develop mucosal hemorrhages or clinically significant bleeding. To control acute bleeding, consider transfusion to raise the level of normal platelets to 50,000/μL. In macroglobulinemia and related disorders, the elevated serum proteins interfere with platelet function, and patients with clinically significant bleeding may require plasmapheresis to reduce the protein level and correct hemostatic function.

Many commonly used drugs can influence platelet function (see Table 41–3). Of these, the most commonly used are aspirin, the NSAIDs, and clopidogrel. Aspirin inhibits platelet function by acetylating and irreversibly inactivating platelet cyclooxygenase, which inhibits platelet aggregation. This antithrombotic effect can be seen in doses as small as 30 mg, occurs within 1 hour after ingestion, and continues for the lifespan of the platelets. Because the NSAIDs reversibly inhibit platelet cyclooxygenase, the impairment of platelet aggregation lasts only as long as the active drug is present in the circulation, usually less than 24 hours. An exception is the drug piroxicam, which has a 2-day half-life.

Ticlopidine and clopidogrel are related substances that inhibit platelet function by impairing fibrinogen binding to glycoprotein IIb/IIIa receptors and by inhibiting platelet binding. Platelet inhibition occurs within 24–48 hours after ingestion and continues for approximately 4–10 days after discontinuation of therapy.

Table 41–4. Conditions Associated with Functional Platelet Disorders.

Renal failure
Liver disease
Myeloproliferative disorders: polycythemia vera, chronic myelogenous leukemia
Paraproteinemias: multiple myeloma, Waldenström macroglobulinemia
Antiplatelet antibodies: autoimmune disorders such as systemic lupus
von Willebrand's syndrome

Burrus TM, Wijdicks EF, Rabinstein AA: Brain lesions are most often reversible in acute thrombotic thrombocytopenic purpura. Neurology 2009 Jul 7;73:66–70 [PMID: 19564586].

Bussel J: Treatment of immune thrombocytopenic purpura in adults. Semin Hematol 2006;43:S3–S10 [PMID: 16815346].

Cines DB, Blanchette VS: Immune thrombocytopenic purpura. N Engl J Med 2002;346:995–1008 [PMID: 11919310].

Forzley BR, Sontrop JM, Macnab JJ, Chen S, Clark WF: Treating TTP/HUS with plasma exchange: a single centre's 25-year experience. Br J Haematol 2008;143:100–106 [PMID: 18691172].

George JN: Clinical practice. Thrombotic thrombocytopenic purpura. N Engl J Med 2006;354:1927–1935 [PMID: 16672704].

Greinacher A, Kohlmann T, Strobel U, Sheppard JA, Warkentin TE: The temporal profile of the anti-PF4/heparin immune response. Blood 2009;113:4970–4976 [PMID: 19109231].

Hawkins BM, Abu-Fadel M, Vesely SK, George JN: Clinical cardiac involvement in thrombotic thrombocytopenic purpura: a systematic review. Transfusion 2008;48:382–392 [PMID: 18028268].

Hopkins CK, Goldfinger D: Platelet transfusions in heparin-induced thrombocytopenia: a report of four cases and review of the literature. Transfusion 2008;48:2128–2132 [PMID: 18657085].

Hughes C, McEwan JR, Longair I, Hughes S, Cohen H, Machin S, Scully M: Cardiac involvement in acute thrombotic thrombocytopenic purpura: association with troponin T and IgG antibodies to ADAMTS 13. J Thromb Haemost 2009;7:529–536 [PMID: 19175494].

Kennedy AS, Lewis QF, Scott JG, Kremer Hovinga JA, Lämmle B, Terrell DR, Vesely SK, George JN: Cognitive deficits after recovery from thrombotic thrombocytopenic purpura. Transfusion 2009;49:1092–1101 [PMID: 19222817].

Lowe EJ, Werner EJ: Thrombotic thrombocytopenic purpura and hemolytic uremic syndrome in children and adolescents. Semin Thromb Hemost 2005;31:717–730 [PMID: 16388423].

Mazzucconi MG, Fazi P, Bernasconi S, et al: Therapy with high-dose dexamethasone (HD-DXM) in previously untreated patients affected by idiopathic thrombocytopenic purpura. A GIMEMA experience. Blood 2006;109:1401–1407 [PMID: 17077333].

McCrae KR, Bussel JB, Mannucci PM, Remuzzi G, Cines DB: Platelets: An update on diagnosis and management of thrombocytopenic disorders. Hematology Am Soc Hematol Educ Program 2001:282–1305 [PMID: 11722989].

Michael M, Elliott EJ, Ridley GF, Hodson EM, Craig JC: Interventions for haemolytic uraemic syndrome and thrombotic thrombocytopenic purpura. Cochrane Database Syst Rev 2009:CD003595 [PMID: 19160220].

Moake JL: Thrombotic microangiopathies. N Engl J Med 2002;347:589–600 [PMID: 12192020].

Patschan D, Witzke O, Dührsen U, Erbel R, Philipp T, Herget-Rosenthal S: Acute myocardial infarction in thrombotic microangiopathies—clinical characteristics, risk factors and outcome. Nephrol Dial Transplant 2006;21:1549–1554 [PMID: 16574680].

Swisher KK, Terrell DR, Vesely SK, Kremer Hovinga JA, Lämmle B, George JN: Clinical outcomes after platelet transfusions in patients with thrombotic thrombocytopenic purpura. Transfusion 2009;49:873–887 [PMID: 19210323].

Terrell DR, Williams LA, Vesely SK, Lämmle B, Hovinga JA, George JN: The incidence of thrombotic thrombocytopenic purpura-hemolytic uremic syndrome: all patients, idiopathic patients, and patients with severe ADAMTS-13 deficiency. J Thromb Haemost 2005;3:1432–1436 [PMID: 15978100].

Warkentin TE, Greinacher A, Koster A, Lincoff AM; American College of Chest Physicians: Treatment and prevention of heparin-induced thrombocytopenia: American College of Chest Physicians Evidence-Based Clinical Practice Guidelines (8th Edition). Chest 2008;133:340S [PMID: 18574270].

▼ HEMOSTATIC DISORDERS: COAGULATION FACTOR DISORDERS

HEMOPHILIA

▶ General Considerations

Hemophilia is a disorder of coagulation caused primarily by a deficiency or defect in one of two circulating plasma proteins. Hemophilia A, or classic hemophilia, is caused by a deficiency of factor VIII and is the most common cause of hemophilia in the United States, affecting 1 in 10,000 males. Hemophilia B, or Christmas disease, is caused by a deficiency of factor IX. This form of hemophilia is less common, affecting approximately 1 in 30,000 males.

Hemophilia A and B are clinically indistinguishable from each other, and specific factor testing is required for diagnosis. Both hemophilia A and B are X-linked recessive disorders; therefore, hemophilia is a disease of men, and women are asymptomatic carriers.

▶ Clinical Findings

A. Symptoms and Signs

Bleeding manifestations in patients with all forms of hemophilia (Table 41–5) are directly attributable to the decreased plasma levels of either factor VIII or IX. Individuals with factor levels below 1% of normal are classified as having severe disease, and these people will experience severe spontaneous bleeding episodes and difficult-to-control bleeding related to traumatic events. Patients with factor levels of 1–5% of normal are classified as having moderate disease; although they may bleed spontaneously, more commonly their bleeding is related to a traumatic event. Patients with factor levels of 5–50% of normal are classified as having mild disease and usually bleed only after trauma.

As a result of exposure to blood products, many hemophiliacs have chronic viral hepatitis or are infected with HIV. Fortunately, as a result of newer viral inactivation procedures and recombinant technology, few seroconversions have resulted from the use of currently available factor replacement products.

An interesting clinical feature is the apparent protective effect of hemophilia and for carriers of hemophilia for coronary heart disease (CHD) for which studies have shown up to an 80% reduction in coronary disease related mortality.

B. Laboratory Findings

Routine coagulation studies (prothrombin time [PT] or activated partial thromboplastin time [aPTT]) require only 30% of normal factor VIII or IX level to be normal; therefore, patients with mild disease may have normal values. Coagulation studies are unlikely to yield new information in the known hemophiliac and are not routinely indicated when the patient presents with mild to moderate bleeding episodes.

▶ Treatment

A general principle in managing major or life-threatening bleeding in a hemophilic patient is early and complete factor replacement, before or at the same time as other resuscitative and diagnostic maneuvers. Spontaneous or traumatic bleeding into the neck, tongue, retropharynx, or pharynx has a high potential for airway compromise. Any patient with hemophilia who complains of a new headache, localizing neurologic symptoms, or a blunt head injury requires immediate factor replacement therapy followed by urgent CT

Table 41–5. Common Bleeding Locations in Hemophilia Patients.

Location	Comments
Joint (hemarthrosis)	Common, can lead to joint destruction and chronic arthropathy.
Soft tissue (hematomas)	Can occur in any location, dangerous in the neck (asphyxia), limb (compartment syndrome), and retroperitoneum (hemorrhagic shock).
Mucosa	Epistaxis, bleeding after dental extractions, and gastrointestinal bleeding.
Central nervous system	Can occur with minimal trauma, common cause of death.
Kidney (hematuria)	Common, rarely serious.

scanning of the head. Hemophilic patients with complaints of back, thigh, groin, or abdominal pain may have bleeding into the retroperitoneum. At times the initial manifestations of bleeding can be subtle. Simple injuries such as ankle and wrist sprains may at first appear benign but can be complicated by bleeding. Compartment syndromes result from muscle bleeds within the fascial compartments of the extremities, both spontaneously and after minimal trauma to an extremity.

One of the most common manifestations of hemophilia is hemarthrosis. Clinical evidence of an acute problem with the joint may or may not present, but these patients can reliably report when bleeding is occurring. Prompt treatment of hemarthroses can prevent or reduce the long-term sequelae of hemophilic arthropathy. Recent research has investigated using regular factor infusions versus episodic infusions at the time of injury for comparison of joint damage seen on MRI years following initiation and has shown that episodic infusions are inferior. The cost and communicable disease risk of infusions, however, is probably to blame for this practice

not being the standard in most institutions. Many patients and their families have a sophisticated understanding of the disease. These patients will know to seek treatment at the first sign of a problem, and as stated earlier, little outward evidence of pathology may be present initially. Despite minimal findings, take seriously the concerns of these patients. Additionally, many known hemophiliacs will have in their medical records a detailed treatment plan for how to manage acute bleeding episodes. Consult these records when they are available.

Do not place central lines, including femoral lines and external jugular lines, in patients with hemophilia without giving factor replacement therapy. Similar rules apply to arterial blood gases or lumbar puncture. Patients with hemophilia should never receive intramuscular injections unless factor replacement is given and maintained for several days. Do not give compounds that contain aspirin for pain relief.

Two different factor replacement types are available: recombinant or plasma derived (Table 41–6). The highest

Table 41–6. Available Products for Hemophilia Treatment.

Hemophilia Type	Available Products	Comments
Hemophilia A	Human-plasma-derived factor VIII products: Koate-HP Humate-P Alphanate	All have a low risk of HIV and hepatitis transmission.
	Human-plasma-derived factor VIII with immunoaffinity purification: Hemofil M Monoclate-P	Both products have reduced amounts of von Willebrand factor. Monoclate-P is highly purified source of factor VIII.
	Recombinant factor VIII products: Recombinate Gelixate Bioclate Kogenate	Low to no risk of hepatitis or HIV.
	Porcine factor VIII products: Antihemophilic factor Hyate C	No evidence of porcine viral transmission to humans.
Hemophilia B	Factor IX complex products: Koyne-80 factor IX complex Proplex T factor IX complex Profilnine SD Bebulin VH	Proplex T: HIV seroconversion has occurred. Other products have low risk of HIV and hepatitis transmission.
	Activated factor IX complex products: Autoplex T Feiba VH	Low risk of HIV and hepatitis transmission.
	Purified factor IX products: AlphaNine SD Mononine	Low risk of HIV and hepatitis.
	Recombinant factor IX: BeneFix	No known risk of viral transmission.

Table 41–7. Initial Factor Replacement Guidelines.

Site	Minimum Initial Factor Level (%)	Hemophilia A Initial Dose (U/kg)	Hemophilia B Initial Dose (U/kg)	Details
Deep muscle	40–50	20–40	40–60	Monitor total blood loss, watch for compartment syndrome. Duration of replacement: 1–3 d.
Joint	30–50	20–40	30–40	Orthopedic consult for splinting, physical therapy, and follow-up. Duration of replacement: 1–3 d.
Epistaxis	80–100	40–50	80–100	Local measures should be used. Replacement is given until bleeding resolves.
Oral mucosa	50	25	50	Local measures and antifibrinolytic therapy will decrease need for additional factor replacement. Duration of replacement: 1–2 d.
Gastrointestinal bleeding	100	40–50	80–100	Consultation with gastroenterologist is appropriate to identify a lesion. Duration of replacement: 7–10 d.
Central nervous system	100	50	100	Early neurosurgical consultation. Lumbar puncture requires factor replacement.

level of purity comes from the recombinant factors, but these products cost 2–3 times more than plasma-derived products, and they are not available everywhere. Another concern with the plasma-derived factors is that some of the preparations may contain other coagulation factors, some partially activated. Prolonged use of the less pure concentrates may increase the risk of DIC or, in some cases, cause paradoxical clotting. Safety, cost, and availability must be considered when choosing the product to use in replacement therapy, but because the recombinant forms are perceived to be safer, approximately 60% of patients with severe hemophilia in the United States receive these preparations.

The dosing regimen used in the hemophilic patient is based on the clotting factor's volume of distribution, the factor's half-life, and the hemostatic level of factor required to control the bleeding (Table 41–7). Clotting factor is dosed in units (U) of activity; 1 unit of factor represents the amount of factor present in 1 mL of normal plasma. For hemophilia A, 1 unit of factor VIII per kilogram of body weight raises the plasma level by approximately 0.02 U/mL (2%) with a half-life of approximately 8–12 hours. For hemophilia B, 1 unit of factor IX per kilogram of body weight will raise the plasma level by approximately 0.01 U/mL (1%) with a half-life of approximately 16 hours.

Bleeding from the mouth is common in hemophiliacs, particularly children. If an oral bleed is present, identify the area, clean it of inadequate clot, and place a dry topical thrombin on the bleeding site. In addition to factor replacement, antifibrinolytic agents such as ε-aminocaproic acid (EACA) and tranexamic acid are useful to prevent bleeding when the clot falls off. For superficial mucosal injuries, it

may be possible to manage the bleeding with antifibrinolytic therapy alone. The dose of EACA is 75–100 mg/kg for children (6 g for adults) every 6 hours, given orally or intravenously. Topical hemostatic agents used to help control oral or nasal bleeding include microfibrillar collagen hemostats, thrombin, and absorbable gelatin sponges.

Patients with mild hemophilia A (factor levels of 5% or greater) who have mild bleeding may not always require factor replacement. Rather, these patients may be given desmopressin, which causes endothelial storage sites to release vWF that is capable of carrying additional amounts of factor VIII in the plasma. This medication is well tolerated, and patients can administer it at home by subcutaneous injection or intranasal spray. The dose of intravenous desmopressin is 0.3 μg/kg (maximum dose, 20 μg) over 30 minutes. The concentrated intranasal form of desmopressin is an antidiuretic agent, and fluid restriction may be needed during use. For children older than 5 years, a single spray in a single nostril (150 μg total dose) is adequate. For adolescents and adults, a single spray in each nostril is used (300 μg total dose). This dose of intranasal desmopressin increases the factor VIII level by 2–3 times. This treatment can be repeated in 8–12 hours, but the patient's stores of factor VIII will be depleted, and subsequent effect will be less.

In response to the clotting factors used to treat bleeding episodes, some people will develop inhibitors, or antibodies against the replacement factor. Inhibitors tend to occur most commonly in patients with severe hemophilia because of frequent factor replacement. These inhibitors not only interfere with the effectiveness of factor replacement therapy but also cause anaphylaxis to factor administration in patients with hemophilia B. Inhibitors occur in 10–25% of those with hemophilia A and in 1–3% of those with hemophilia B. The use of factor replacement in hemophilic patients with inhibitors is guided by the concentration of inhibitor (measured in Bethesda Inhibitor Assay [BIA] units) and by the type of response the patient has to factor concentrates. Bleeding episodes are more difficult to treat in these patients, but options do exist. Given the complexity of these patients, consultation or transfer to a center with hematology is recommended.

▶ Disposition

Many patients with hemophilic bleeding episodes can receive factor replacement in the emergency department or clinic and then be discharged home with follow-up in 12–24 hours. Hemophilic patients with bleeding episodes that require hospital admission include (1) those with bleeding involving the central nervous system, neck, pharynx, retropharynx, or retroperitoneum, (2) those with potential compartment syndrome, (3) those for whom treatment requires more than three doses (relative indication), (4) those unable to use, or lacking access to, factor replacement, or (5) those in whom pain cannot be controlled with oral analgesics.

von WILLEBRAND DISEASE

▶ General Considerations

von Willebrand disease is the most common congenital bleeding disorder; it is present in 1–2% of the population. This disease is a group of disorders caused by abnormalities of vWF. The disease is heterogeneously inherited and expressed, and although multiple subtypes exist, these can be classified into three major groups (Table 41–8). Type I is the most common and is a partial quantitative disease, type II is a qualitative (abnormal function) disease, and type III is a severe and almost complete deficiency of vWF (this type is a rare autosomal recessive form). vWF is a glycoprotein that, as opposed to most other coagulation factors, is synthesized, stored, and then secreted by the vascular endothelial cells. It is a cofactor for platelet adhesion and the carrier protein for factor VIII.

Table 41–8. Classification of von Willebrand Disease.

Type	Occurrence in Patients with von Willebrand Disease	von Willebrand Factor (vWF) Defect
I	70–80% of patients	All multimeric forms are present, but their quantity is diminished.
II	10–15% of patients	vWF is abnormal, missing some of the multimers.
III	<10%	Essentially no vWF is present.

▶ Clinical Findings

A. Symptoms and Signs

Bleeding symptoms are common in people with von Willebrand disease, particularly in children and adolescents. Symptoms include recurrent epistaxis, gingival bleeding, unusual bruising, gastrointestinal bleeding, and menorrhagia in young women. Hemarthrosis is not typical unless severe disease is present. In mild cases of von Willebrand disease, patients may be unaware of the disease until they undergo a surgical procedure or experience a traumatic event. Von Willebrand disease is relatively common, and its presence influences the treatment of other medical problems, because patients with this disease should not take medications with known antiplatelet effects, including aspirin, NSAIDs, antiplatelet agents, heparin, and some antibiotics.

B. Laboratory Findings

Common abnormalities on hemostatic testing include a prolonged bleeding time, low or normal vWF antigen, and low vWF activity. The PT is usually normal, but this can be variable, as can the factor VIII level. This variability sometimes makes von Willebrand disease difficult to differentiate from mild hemophilia A. The patient's blood type affects the vWF level; blood type O has as much as a 30% reduction in vWF levels compared to the other blood types.

▶ Treatment

Desmopressin has become a mainstay of therapy for many patients with type I von Willebrand disease and may work in conjunction with other plasma products that contain vWF for types II and III. In responsive individuals, desmopressin causes a transient two- to fourfold increase in vWF. It also seems to have an effect on the endothelium that promotes hemostasis. The dose is 0.3 μg/kg (maximum dose, 20 μg) administered subcutaneously or intravenously every 12 hours for a total of 3–4 doses; after 4 doses, tachyphylaxis develops. Desmopressin can also be used as an intranasal spray. For children older than 5 years, a single spray in a single nostril is adequate (150 μg total dose). For adolescents and adults, administer a single spray in each nostril (300 μg total dose).

Plasma derivatives that contain vWF are used for patients with type I disease that does not or no longer responds to desmopressin and for patients with type II or III disease. To be effective the chosen product must have vWF in the high-molecular-weight form. Cryoprecipitate meets this objective (contains factor VIII and vWF), but the potential for viral transmission is a concern. If cryoprecipitate is used, 10 bags every 12–24 hours will usually control bleeding. Humate-P is an intermediate-purity factor VIII concentrate that has significant amounts of vWF and can be used to treat bleeding episodes. Platelet transfusions may benefit patients with certain types of von Willebrand disease (especially type III) that do not respond to vWF-containing concentrates of cryoprecipitate.

Local measures to control bleeding in von Willebrand disease include (1) intranasal application of porcine strips (eg, Surgicel), porcine strips sprinkled with microfibrillar collagen (eg, Avitene), or cauterization for epistaxis, (2) birth control pills to help raise vWF levels and limit the degree of menstrual bleeding, and (3) EACA for dental injury or planned intraoral procedures.

LIVER DISEASE

▶ Clinical Findings

Acute and chronic diseases of the liver can be associated with many hemostatic abnormalities. Hepatocytes synthesize all of the coagulation factors and related regulatory proteins, with the exception of factor VIII. Malabsorption of vitamin K can occur with processes that interfere with the absorption of fat-soluble vitamins, including impaired bile acid metabolism (ie, primary biliary cirrhosis), intrahepatic or extrahepatic cholestasis, and treatment with bile acid binders.

Thrombocytopenia in severe liver disease is most often due to portal hypertension, which leads to congestive hypersplenism and splenic sequestration. Patients with significant liver disease have increased fibrinolysis due to decreased synthesis of α_2-plasmin inhibitor. In some patients with liver disease, abnormal fibrinogen molecules are synthesized, which, when cleaved to fibrin monomers, do not polymerize correctly.

Patients with mild to moderate hepatic dysfunction frequently have subclinical hemostatic abnormalities. Patients with severe liver disease may have life-threatening bleeding. Laboratory studies should include a PT, aPTT, and platelet count. Also consider obtaining fibrinogen levels and measurement of fibrin degradation products (FDP) or d-dimer. In general, prolongation of the PT and a plasma fibrinogen level of less than 100 mg/dL is a poor prognostic sign in patients with liver disease.

▶ Treatment and Disposition

Patients who have liver disease and laboratory abnormalities without clinically significant bleeding usually require only close observation. If clinically significant bleeding is present or an invasive procedure or surgery is pending, the coagulopathic state will need to be treated. Transfuse packed RBCs to maintain an adequate hemoglobin level and to maintain hemodynamic stability. Give oral or intravenous vitamin K to all patients. FFP can be used to replace coagulation factors temporarily, but the volume needed to completely replenish the coagulation factors may limit the amount given.

Cryoprecipitate may be used to replace fibrinogen in patients with fibrinogen levels less than 100 mg/dL. Platelet transfusions may be appropriate if platelet counts are low. Desmopressin (either 0.3 μg/kg subcutaneously or intravenously [maximum dose, 20 μg] or 300 μg intranasal spray) shortens the prolonged bleeding time in some patients with liver disease. Although controlled trials are lacking, there are few side effects.

RENAL DISEASE

Patients with end stage renal disease typically develop complications due to two opposing hemostatic processes: bleeding and clotting. Platelet dysfunction is the main factor responsible for hemorrhagic disorders, although platelet counts are frequently normal. Platelet dysfunction occurs as a result of intrinsic platelet abnormalities such as impaired platelet adhesiveness and abnormal platelet–endothelial interaction. Anemia and complications from hemodialysis are major contributors to bleeding in advanced kidney disease.

Dialysis partially improves platelet function and may reduce bleeding likely due to the reduction of dialyzable toxins. Platelet function is optimized when the hematocrit is maintained at approximately 30% because anemia contributes to bleeding. Desmopressin administration intravenously or intranasally may improve the bleeding time in end stage kidney disease and can also be used prior to procedures that carry a risk of bleeding. Conjugated estrogen, 25 mg intravenously, also improves both bleeding time and clinical bleeding in more than 80% of uremic patients. Cryoprecipitate carries the risk of viral transmission, and platelet transfusions are relatively ineffective because the infused platelets quickly acquire the uremic defect.

WARFARIN AND VITAMIN K DEFICIENCY

▶ General Considerations

The vitamin K-dependent coagulation factors produced in the liver are prothrombin factor II, VII, IX, and X, as well as the anticoagulant proteins C and S. Nutritional deficiency of vitamin K is rare in adults. However, patients with liver disease can have vitamin K deficiency due to a combination of poor nutrition and malabsorption. Additionally, deficiency of the vitamin K-dependent factors can occur in patients receiving antibiotics, particularly the third-generation cephalosporins that contain the N-methylthiotetrazole side chain (ie, moxalactam, cefamandole, cefotaxime, cefoperazone).

Warfarin, the major oral anticoagulant used in the United States, inhibits the production of the vitamin K-dependent coagulation factors. The half-life of warfarin is approximately 36 hours with normal hepatic function. The standard starting dosage is usually 5 mg/d with subsequent dose adjustment guided by the international normalized ratio (INR). Observable anticoagulation effect is expected in 2–7 days. The goal INR is 2.0–3.0 for all indications except in patients with prosthetic mechanical valves and with antiphospholipid antibody syndrome; these patients require a higher INR of 2.5–3.5. Maintenance dosage can be influenced by different variables, including the patient's vitamin K stores, malnutrition, liver function, concurrent medical disorders, and numerous drug interactions.

► Clinical Findings

The major adverse effects associated with warfarin treatment include warfarin embryopathy, warfarin-induced skin necrosis, and bleeding. Warfarin interferes with a vitamin K-dependent protein used to build the bone matrix, resulting in fetal bone abnormalities. This toxicity occurs with warfarin exposure during the 6th–12th weeks of gestation, but warfarin should be avoided during the entire pregnancy. Warfarin-induced skin necrosis is an uncommon complication occurring during the 1st week after initiating therapy. Some patients who develop this complication have a hereditary heterozygous protein C deficiency or protein S deficiency.

► Treatment

Treatment of warfarin complications includes discontinuation of warfarin, heparinization if anticoagulation is required, vitamin K administration, and screening for protein C and protein S deficiencies. The fear of creating a hypercoagulable state in persons with undiagnosed protein C deficiency is unfounded, but persons with a known hypercoagulable state should receive anticoagulation therapy with heparin before starting warfarin.

Bleeding is the most common complication of warfarin treatment; the risk of bleeding is related directly to the degree of anticoagulation. Additionally, individual risk factors for bleeding include age greater than 65 years, hypertension, anemia, prior cerebrovascular disease, gastrointestinal lesions, and renal disease. Medications that increase warfarin activity and antiplatelet medications can also increase bleeding risks. Management of bleeding depends on the type of bleeding and the INR value (Table 41–9).

The anticoagulated state can be reduced by withholding warfarin, administering oral or intravenous vitamin K, or substitution of clotting factors such as (but not exclusive) FFP (widely used) or prothrombin complex concentrates (PCCs), which are increasingly being recommended and used.

Subcutaneous administration of vitamin K has an unpredictable and delayed response, whereas oral vitamin K is convenient to administer, is effective, and produces less resistance to subsequent warfarin use. Additionally, hypersensitivity reactions and anaphylaxis are uncommon with the oral administration of vitamin K. Intravenous administration of vitamin K results in the rapid reversal of hypercoagulation but is associated with anaphylaxis or hypersensitivity reactions, including flushing, diaphoresis, hypotension, dyspnea, and chest pain. Doses of vitamin K above 10 mg are associated with overcorrection of hypercoagulation and warfarin resistance for up to 1 week upon reinstitution of anticoagulation. In general, restrict the intravenous use of vitamin K to patients with life-threatening bleeding or to those with an INR greater than 20.

Two additional hemostatic agents are available for rapid correction of life-threatening bleeding. Recombinant factor VIIa (FVIIa) and PCC. FVIIa is a potent procoagulant agent that can generate thrombin even in the absence of tissue factor. It is a recombinant agent, it will not transmit viruses, and it will rapidly correct FVII deficiency. However, PCCs are now recommended for anticoagulation reversal in patients with life-threatening bleeding and an increased INR. Compared with FFP, PCCs provide quicker correction of the INR and improved bleeding control. Compared to FVIIa, PCCs correct not only the FVII deficiency but all of the warfarin-induced coagulation deficiencies, resulting in a true physiologic correction to normal.

Table 41–9. Warfarin Reversal Guidelines.

International Normalized Ratio (INR) Value	Bleeding	Recommendations
Any elevation	Major to life-threatening	Withhold warfarin. Replace coagulation factors with FFP or factor complex concentrates. Vitamin K, 5-10 mg IV (dose dependent on INR). Consider Prothrombin Complex Concentrate administration Consider Factor VIIa administration
Any elevation	Mild to moderate	Withhold warfarin. Vitamin K, 2-4 mg PO (dose dependent on INR).
<5	None	Withhold warfarin until INR therapeutic and then restart at same or lower dose.
5-9	None	Withhold warfarin until INR therapeutic and then restart at same or lower dose. Vitamin K, 1-2 mg PO.
>9	None	Withhold warfarin until INR therapeutic and then restart at same or lower dose. Vitamin K, 2-4 mg PO.

DISSEMINATED INTRAVASCULAR COAGULATION

General Considerations

Disseminated intravascular coagulation is characterized by both widespread activation of the coagulation system (resulting in fibrin formation and consumption of hemostatic factors) and activation of the fibrinolytic system (resulting in the breakdown of fibrin clots, consumption of coagulation factors, and bleeding). DIC is associated with a variety of disorders such as infection (usually bacterial and occasionally viral), malignancy (adenocarcinoma, acute leukemia, lymphoma), trauma (burns, fat embolism), liver disease, and environmental disorders (hyperthermia, envenomation). DIC may be acute and life-threatening or chronic and compensated.

Clinical Findings

A. Symptoms and Signs

Clinical features of DIC vary with the underlying precipitating medical illness. The clinical complications of DIC are bleeding, thrombosis, purpura fulminans, and multiple organ failure. Although hemorrhage and thrombosis may occur simultaneously, in an individual patient, one manifestation usually predominates and the most common one is bleeding. Bleeding can range from petechiae and ecchymoses to bleeding from the gastrointestinal tract, genitourinary tract, surgical wounds, mucocutaneous sites, and venipuncture sites. Intravascular coagulation and fibrin deposition can cause multiple organ failure. Clinical signs include mental status changes, focal ischemia or gangrene, oliguria, renal cortical necrosis, and adult respiratory distress syndrome. Purpura fulminans results when widespread arterial and venous thromboses occur and is most commonly seen with significant bacteremia. In chronic DIC, the pathophysiology of disease is essentially the same, but the destruction of coagulation factors and platelets is balanced by hepatic and bone marrow production.

B. Laboratory Findings

The typical laboratory results in acute DIC include prolonged PT, low platelet count, and low fibrinogen level. The most commonly observed abnormality is thrombocytopenia. Fibrinogen levels may remain normal because fibrinogen is an acute-phase reactant. FDP and D-dimer may help differentiate DIC from other causes of prolonged coagulation times and low platelets; the D-dimer may be more specific than FDP in diagnosing DIC. Additional laboratory findings include increased LDH, decreased haptoglobin levels, and a peripheral smear with schistocytes. Patients with chronic DIC will have minor abnormalities on the screening assays, reflecting the limited consumption of coagulation factors that are being replaced by hepatic synthesis.

Treatment

Treatment of acute DIC rests on supportive measures and specific and vigorous management of the underlying illness. Circulatory stabilization requires fluid, RBCs, and sometimes inotropic agents. Secondary treatment involves replacement therapy with platelets, fibrinogen, and coagulation factors. Many patients with DIC require no specific therapy if evidence of bleeding or thrombosis is lacking and laboratory study results are not deteriorating. Replacement therapy should be given only to the patients with bleeding or an impending invasive procedure and should use specific replacement products: fibrinogen repletion with cryoprecipitate to raise the plasma fibrinogen level to 100–150 mg/dL, platelet concentrates to raise platelet count above 50,000/μL, and FFP to replace coagulation factors. Patients with DIC also should be given vitamin K and folate.

Heparin administration usually has a limited role in the treatment of acute DIC. It is usually considered in patients with documented DIC in whom thromboembolic complications predominate the clinical picture. Consider heparin for patients with chronic DIC and thrombosis.

Brown DL: Congenital bleeding disorders. Curr Probl Pediatr Adolesc Health Care 2005;35:38–62 [PMID: 15692557].

Cox Gill J: Diagnosis and treatment of von Willebrand disease. Hematol Oncol Clin North Am 2004;18:1277–1299 [PMID: 15511616].

Crowther MA, Warkentin TE: Managing bleeding in anticoagulated patients with a focus on novel therapeutic agents. Haemost 2009;7:107–110 [PMID: 19630780].

Darby SC, Kan SW, Spooner RJ, Giangrande PL, Hill FG, Hay CR, Lee CA, Ludlam CA, Williams M: Mortality rates, life expectancy, and causes of death in people with hemophilia A or B in the United Kingdom who were not infected with HIV. Blood 2007;110:815–825 [PMID: 17446349].

Foley, CJ, Nichols L, Jeong K, Moore CG, Ragni MV: Coronary atherosclerosis and cardiovascular mortality in hemophilia. J Thromb Haemost 2010;8:208–811 [PMID: 19874455].

Franchini M: Pathophysiology, diagnosis and treatment of disseminated intravascular coagulation: An update. Clin Lab 2005;51:633–639 [PMID: 16329621].

Gando S: Microvascular thrombosis and multiple organ dysfunction. Crit Care Med 2010;38: S35–S42 [PMID: 20083912].

James AH: Von Willebrand disease. Obstet Gynecol Surv 2006;61:136–145. [PMID: 16433937].

Kaw D, Malhotra D: Platelet dysfunction and end stage renal disease. Semi Dial 2006;19:317–322 [PMID: 16893410].

Kitchens CS: Thrombocytopenia and thrombosis in disseminated intravascular coagulation. Hematology Am Soc Hematol Educ Program 2009;240–246 [PMID: 20008204].

Lankiewicz MW, Hays J, Friedman KD, Tinkoff G, Blatt PM: Urgent reversal of warfarin with prothrombin complex concentrate. J Thromb Haemost 2006;4:967–970 [PMID: 16689743].

Lee JW: Von Willebrand disease, hemophilia A and B, and other factor deficiencies. Int Anesthesiol Clin 2004;42:59–76 [PMID: 15205640].

Levi M; Disseminated intravascular coagulation. Crit Care Med 2007;35:2191–2195 [PMID: 17855836].

Levy JH, Tanaka KA, Dietrich W: Perioperative hemostatic management of patients treated with vitamin k antagonists. Anesthesiology 2008;109:918–926 [PMID: 18946305].

Manco-Johnson MJ, Abshire TC, Shapiro AD, et al: Prophylaxis versus episodic treatment to prevent joint disease in boys with severe hemophilia, N Engl J Med 2007;357:535–544 [PMID: 17687129].

Rodeghiero F, Castaman G: Treatment of von Willebrand disease. Semin Hematol 2005;42:29–35 [PMID: 15662613].

Wiedermann CJ, Stockner I: Warfarin induced bleeding complications—clinical presentation and therapeutic options. Thromb Res 2008;122:S13–S18 [PMID: 18549907].

Recombinant human activated protein C may be considered in treating patients with severe sepsis and DIC. If a patient is at high risk of bleeding, activated protein C should not be used.

Table 41–10. Normal Red Blood Cell (RBC) Values for Adults.[a]

Measure	Male	Female
RBC count (million/μL)	4.5-6.0	4.0-5.5
Hemoglobin (g/dL)	14-17	12-15
Hematocrit (%)	42-52	36-48
Mean corpuscular volume (fL)	78-100	78-102
Mean cellular hemoglobin (pg/cell)	25-35	25-35
Mean corpuscular hemoglobin concentration (g/dL)	32-36	32-36
Red cell distribution width (%)	11.5-14.5	11.5-14.5
Reticulocyte count (%)	0.5-2.5	0.5-2.5

[a]Normal values may vary depending upon the equipment used, patient's age, and altitude.

ANEMIA

Anemia is a common problem, affecting an estimated one-third of the world's population. Worldwide, the most common causes of anemia include iron deficiency, thalassemia, hemoglobinopathies, and folate deficiencies. Within the United States, the most common causes are iron deficiency, thalassemia, and anemia of chronic disease. Not only is anemia common in the general population, but also the prevalence of anemia increases with age. Given the ubiquity of this entity, some patients who present to the emergency department with anemia will be symptomatic, whereas anemia will be an incidental finding in other patients.

Anemia is defined as a reduced concentration of RBCs. Erythropoiesis ensures that the number of RBCs present is adequate to meet the body's demand for oxygen and that RBC destruction equals production with an average lifespan of 120 days for circulating erythrocytes. Any process or condition that impairs the production, increases the rate of destruction, or increases the loss of erythrocytes will result in anemia if the body cannot produce enough new RBCs to keep up with the loss.

Quantification of the RBC concentration is reflected in the RBC count per microliter, hemoglobin concentration, or hematocrit. Normal RBC values for adults vary slightly between males and females (Table 41–10). Anemia has been categorized into three types on the basis of RBC values (Table 41–11).

Regardless of the cause of anemia, many of the clinical manifestations are the same. The severity of symptoms and signs related to anemia depends on several factors: the rate of development of anemia, the extent of anemia present, the patient's age, the patient's general physical condition, and other existing comorbid illnesses. Patients with chronic and slowly developing anemia may have almost no complaints even with hemoglobin levels as low as 5–6 g/dL. More typically, most people will begin to be symptomatic with hemoglobin levels at about 7 g/dL. Patients with chronic anemia may complain of weakness, fatigue, lethargy, dyspnea with minimal exertion, palpitations, and orthostatic symptoms. Physical examination findings in patients with significant chronic anemia may include orthostatic hypotension; tachycardia; skin, nail bed, and mucosal pallor; systolic ejection murmur; bounding pulse; or widened pulse pressure.

Patients who develop anemia in a rapid fashion frequently have more pronounced symptoms. Additionally, these patients may have hypotension, resting and exertional dyspnea, palpitations, diaphoresis, anxiety, severe weakness that may progress to lethargy, and altered mental status. Loss of more than 40% of blood volume leads to severe symptoms that are due more to intravascular volume depletion than to anemia.

The diagnosis of anemia is established by the finding of a decreased RBC count, hemoglobin, or hematocrit on the routine CBC. A specific cause of anemia need not be established in the emergency department; however, appropriate workup should be initiated to help expedite a diagnosis, and initial studies should be started before the transfusion of packed RBCs. The basic evaluation of a patient newly diagnosed with anemia includes the following: RBC indices (provided with the CBC), reticulocyte count, and peripheral blood smear. The mean cellular volume (MCV) is the most useful guide to the possible cause of an anemia. The reticulocyte count reflects activity in the bone marrow. The red cell distribution width (RDW) measures the size variability of the RBC population, and in early nutritional-deficiency anemias (iron, vitamin B_{12}, or folate) the RDW may be increased before the MCV becomes abnormal. As part of the general evaluation, the two

Table 41–11. Classification of Anemias.

Type	Mean Corpuscular Volume (fL)	Mean Corpuscular Hemoglobin Concentration (g/dL)	Cause	Other Hematologic Findings
Microcytic	<80	<32	Iron deficiency	Low reticulocytes, low serum ferritin and iron, high total iron-binding capacity
	<80	Variable, but usually <32	Thalassemias	Elevated reticulocytes, target cells, normal or elevated serum ferritin and iron
	<80	<32	Chronic lead poisoning	Basophilic red blood cell stippling
	<80	Variable, but usually <32	Sideroblastic anemia	Elevated serum iron; ring sideroblasts in bone marrow
Normocytic	80–100	32–36	Acute blood loss	Elevated platelets
	80–100	32–36	Hemolytic anemia	Elevated reticulocytes, low haptoglobin, elevated LDH, and indirect bilirubin
	80–100	32–36	Chronic disease	Low reticulocytes; low serum iron and total iron-binding capacity
Macrocytic	>101 (usually >130)	>36	Vitamin B_{12} or folate deficiency	Macroelliptocytes, hypersegmented neutrophils
	>101–120	>36	Liver disease	Decreased platelets

most common sources of blood loss should be investigated: gastrointestinal (eg, checking the stool for occult blood) and uterine bleeding (eg, history of hypermenorrhea).

IRON-DEFICIENCY ANEMIA

Iron-deficiency anemia occurs when body iron content is insufficient for erythropoiesis; it manifests as a microcytic, hypochromic anemia. Iron deficiency is seen with either inadequate iron intake (usually in undeveloped countries with little meat in the diet) or from a combination of iron loss (hemorrhage) and inadequate intake (in developed countries). Heme iron (as found in meat) is absorbed more efficiently than is nonheme iron (found in vegetables) and accounts for the higher incidence of iron deficiency in vegetarians. Total body iron content varies with age and gender at 35–60 mg/kg of body weight. Each gram of hemoglobin contains 3.47 mg of iron. The recommended daily intake of iron is about 7 mg in a man, 12–16 mg in a menstruating woman, and 5–7 mg in a postmenopausal woman.

▶ Clinical Findings

A. Symptoms and Signs

The symptoms of iron-deficiency anemia (fatigue and weakness) are primarily those seen with any chronic anemia. Occasionally, patients may describe a desire to chew ice or cold food (termed pagophagia) or leg cramps on climbing stairs. Gastrointestinal epithelial (angular stomatitis, glossitis, esophageal webs, and gastric atrophy) and nail (koilonychia) abnormalities have been described in iron deficiency, although their frequency varies and these findings are uncommon in the United States.

B. Laboratory Findings

Patients with iron-deficiency anemia have both microcytic (low MCV) and hypochromic (low MCHC) erythrocytes. The platelet count is often elevated. Examination of the peripheral smear is useful to exclude thalassemia; target cells are not seen in iron-deficiency anemia. Combined iron deficiency and folate deficiency produces variation in red cell size, some macrocytic and others microcytic, such that the measured MCV can be within the normal range, although the RDW should be significantly increased. Iron-deficiency anemia produces a low serum ferritin, low serum iron, and elevated total iron-binding capacity.

The most accurate initial diagnostic test for iron-deficiency anemia is the serum ferritin measurement. Serum ferritin values greater than 100 ng/mL (100 μg/L) indicate adequate iron stores and low likelihood of iron-deficiency anemia. Serum ferritin levels of 25 ng/mL (25 μg/L) have a very high probability of being iron deficient. The use of serum iron, total iron-binding capacity, and transferrin saturation are recommended as follow-up tests in patients with an intermediate ferritin level as a strategy to reduce the need for bone marrow biopsy.

The gold standard is the absence of stainable iron on bone marrow aspirate and establishes the diagnosis without other tests. Possible blood loss should be investigated in a patient with iron-deficiency anemia and often requires testing for occult blood loss from either the gastrointestinal tract (stool for occult blood) or the kidneys (hemoglobinuria or hemosiderinuria).

▶ Treatment

The first line of therapy for iron-deficiency anemia is oral iron therapy using ferrous sulfate, 325 mg (children, 1–2 mg/kg), with each meal 3 times daily. A response with increased reticulocytes is seen within 3–4 days and peaks in 7–10 days, with the hemoglobin level increasing about 1 g/dL per week. Once normal hemoglobin levels are achieved, oral iron therapy should continue to replenish total body iron stores.

Transfusion should be considered for patients of any age who are symptomatic with complaints of fatigue or dyspnea on exertion. Cardiac patients with a hemoglobin level less than 10 g/dL should also be considered for transfusion therapy.

Parenteral iron therapy is reserved for the rare patient who cannot absorb oral iron, but parenteral preparations are expensive and associated with adverse effects, including fatal anaphylactic reactions. Red cell transfusion is used for the patient with ongoing blood loss or acute symptoms of inadequate oxygen delivery to the brain or heart.

ACUTE HEMOLYTIC ANEMIA

The immune-mediated hemolytic anemias traditionally have been divided into three categories: autoimmune, alloimmune, and drug related.

AUTOIMMUNE HEMOLYTIC ANEMIA

▶ General Considerations

Individuals with autoimmune hemolytic anemia (AIHA) make antibodies against their own RBCs or against the body's higher-incidence antigens. The overall incidence of AIHA is approximately 1–3 cases per 100,000 population per year. The incidence of AIHA in infants and children is less, approximately 0.2 cases per 100,000 population per year in those younger than 20 years. AIHA in children is commonly associated with viral or respiratory infections; is mediated by immunoglobulin G (IgG); and causes acute, fulminant hemolysis. Pregnant women have a 5 times greater risk of developing autoantibodies, but significant RBC destruction is not common.

Diagnosis of AIHA requires evidence of an autoantibody against RBCs in the form of (1) detection of the autoantibody on the patient's red cells (positive DAT) and (2) identification of an autoantibody. To make the diagnosis of AIHA, serologic evidence of autoantibodies should be correlated with clinical and other routine laboratory evidence of hemolytic anemia, including decreased hemoglobin, decreased haptoglobin,

Table 41–12. Causes of Secondary Autoimmune Hemolytic Anemia.

Lymphoproliferative disease: chronic lymphocytic leukemia, lymphoma, Hodgkin disease, Waldenström macroglobulinemia, multiple myeloma.
Autoimmune disease: systemic lupus, rheumatoid arthritis, polyarteritis nodosa, pernicious anemia, autoimmune thyroid disease, scleroderma, ulcerative colitis, Crohn's disease
Infection: infectious mononucleosis, cytomegalovirus infection, viral hepatitis, malaria, pediatric viral respiratory illness
Immunodeficiency syndrome: HIV, X-linked agammaglobulinemia, common variable immunodeficiency, IgA deficiency, Wiskott-Aldrich syndrome, dysglobulinemia
Nonlymphoid tumors: ovarian carcinoma and dermoid cysts, teratomas, Kaposi sarcoma, thymoma

elevated reticulocyte count, elevated unconjugated (indirect) bilirubin, elevated LDH, or hemoglobinuria.

AIHA can be divided into primary and secondary varieties. Primary AIHA refers to cases without an underlying cause (idiopathic), and secondary AIHA refers to cases seen with an underlying disorder (Table 41–12). Primary AIHA is more common in women, with peak incidence during the 4th and 5th decades. The hemolytic process in AIHA can take place within the vascular space or in the liver or spleen. AIHA is also categorized according to autoantibody type: warm type, cold type, and mixed type.

A. Warm-Type AIHA

▶ Clinical findings

Warm-type AIHA comprises 70% of AIHA cases and is usually mediated by an IgG antibody directed against surface antigens of the RhD-erythrocyte system. Autoantibodies of the warm type react most strongly near 37°C. These autoantibodies are usually pan-reactive and produce hemolysis both in the patient's RBCs and in transfused RBCs. Warm-type autoantibody-mediated hemolysis is predominantly extravascular, occurring in the spleen. Warm-type AIHA carries a 2:1 female preference but has no racial predilection. About half of warm-type AIHA cases can be labeled as primary or idiopathic. Secondary cases are most often associated with lymphoproliferative disorders (in about half) or a systemic autoimmune disease. Viral-induced or HIV-associated warm-type AIHA is often mild and self-limited.

▶ Treatment

Warm-type AIHA is initially treated with oral prednisone, 1–1.5 mg/kg/d for 1–3 weeks. Improvement is usually noted within 1 week, and 70–80% of patients are improved within 3 weeks. Once the patient's hemoglobin level stabilizes, the steroids can be tapered. Complete remission is achieved in 15–20% of new-onset cases of warm-type AIHA, but half of patients will need low-dose prednisone for several months.

Between 10% and 20% of steroid-treated patients will fail to respond adequately or will require unacceptably high doses to maintain the desired response. In such patients the AIHA is treated with either splenectomy or cytotoxic drugs. Splenectomy removes both the main site of extravascular hemolysis and a major site of general autoantibody production. Splenectomy produces a 65–70% response rate and has the potential for long-term remission or a complete cure.

Cytotoxic drugs produce a 40–60% response rate and have been used for patients who have not responded to steroids or splenectomy. Severe hemolysis in cases of warm-type AIHA may be treated with plasmapheresis as a transient stabilizing measure while waiting for steroids or cytotoxic agents to take effect. Intravenous immunoglobulin has been used in children with mixed results and should only be considered in the most refractory cases. Danazol, an attenuated androgen with fewer side effects than glucocorticoids, can produce remission in occasional patients.

For patients with life-threatening anemia, RBC transfusion of the least incompatible units may be carried out slowly with close monitoring. Transfusion may precipitate further production of autoantibodies as well as introduce a source for the production of allogeneic antibodies.

2. Cold-Type AIHA: General Considerations

Cold-type AIHA autoantibodies are usually immunoglobulin M (IgM) and are most strongly hemolytic at 0–4°C. The presence of cold-type autoantibodies leads to clumping or agglutination of RBCs on peripheral smear at cooler temperatures. Hemolysis occurs in both the extravascular and intravascular spaces, and Kupffer cells in the liver are responsible for most of the extravascular RBC destruction. The two common cold-type AIHA disorders are cold agglutinin syndrome (CAS) and paroxysmal cold hemoglobinuria (PCH). Fifty percent of secondary cold-type AIHA cases are associated with lymphoproliferative disorders.

3. Cold-Type AIHA: Cold Agglutinin Syndrome

Cold agglutinin syndrome (CAS) accounts for up to one-third of all AIHA cases and is typically IgM mediated and directed against the I/i blood group antigens. Primary CAS is seen in older adults, particularly females, with a peak incidence at age 70 years. The hemolysis associated with the primary and chronic secondary forms of CAS tends to be mild and stable with hemoglobin levels of 9–12 g/dL. Secondary CAS can also occur as an acute attack, such as that seen in patients who have preceding infectious illnesses, including from *Mycoplasma pneumoniae*, Epstein–Barr virus (EBV), adenovirus, CMV, influenza, varicella zoster virus

(VZV), HIV, *E. coli*, *Listeria monocytogenes*, and *Treponema pallidum*.

▶ Clinical findings

Symptom onset corresponds with the peak antibody response to infection, usually 2–3 weeks after the onset of illness. The triggered cold-type AIHA resolves approximately 2–3 weeks later. Chronic cold-type AIHA associated with lymphoproliferative diseases, such as chronic lymphocytic leukemia, lymphomas, and Waldenström macroglobulinemia, produces high autoantibody levels with the potential for significant hemolysis. Cold weather exacerbates CAS with more episodes of acute hemolysis seen during winter. Patients are apt to develop acrocyanosis because the peripheral circulation is typically cooler than the central circulation. Raynaud phenomenon, vascular occlusion, and tissue necrosis may complicate CAS. Clumping of cold agglutinins will elevate the MCV and decrease the RBC count. Peripheral smear findings include the spherocytosis caused by RBC membrane destruction as well as anisocytosis, poikilocytosis, polychromasia, and agglutination. As with other forms of hemolytic anemia, patients will have elevated LDH and unconjugated bilirubin with moderate disease, and decreased haptoglobin, hemoglobinemia, and hemoglobinuria with severe, intravascular hemolysis.

▶ Treatment

In primary and chronic CAS with mild anemia, treatment is symptomatic and involves simply keeping extremities, noses, and ears warm in cold weather. Patients with CAS should take daily folate supplements. Treatment for severe hemolysis has been successful with immunosuppressive or cytotoxic agents. As in warm-type AIHA, plasmapheresis may prove helpful as a temporizing measure by removing autoantibodies. Unlike warm-type AIHA, CAS rarely responds to steroids, although such treatment may be considered in atypical cases. Splenic macrophages play a lesser role in IgM-mediated cold-antibody disease; thus splenectomy is not as helpful for cold-antibody-mediated extravascular hemolysis. Transfusions should be limited because they may worsen ongoing hemolysis. Transfusion carries the risk of producing alloantibodies to transfused RBCs. RBC transfusion can be performed for patients at risk for significant cardiac or cerebrovascular ischemia, but transfused blood should be kept at 37°C using a blood warmer.

4. Cold-Type AIHA: Paroxysmal Cold Hemoglobinuria

Paroxysmal cold hemoglobinuria (PCH) is caused by a biphasic IgG autoantibody called the Donath–Landsteiner antibody. The PCH autoantibody is directed against the P antigen system found on most RBCs. Despite the name, hemolysis may occur at both cold and normal temperatures.

▶ Clinical Findings

Symptoms include high fever, chills, headache, abdominal cramps, nausea and vomiting, diarrhea, and leg and back pain that develops with cold exposure. Cold urticaria, extremity paresthesias, and Raynaud phenomenon may also develop. Primary PCH and PCH secondary to congenital or late-stage syphilis are characterized by chronic disease with cold-induced relapses. Secondary PCH caused by other infectious agents is most common in children and is one of the more common causes of childhood hemolytic anemia. Postinfection PCH is usually associated with measles, mumps, EBV, CMV, VZV, adenovirus, influenza A, *M. pneumoniae, Haemophilus influenzae,* and *E. coli.* Most cases of postinfectious PCH are self-limited, but severe cases may take weeks to resolve. With severe hemolysis, hemoglobinuria is common and methemoglobinuria may be seen. Acute renal failure may develop as a complication of PCH.

▶ Treatment

Keep patients with PCH warm. Consider steroids in children with severe hemolytic anemia but because infection-related PCH tends to be self-limited, the benefit is uncertain. PCH secondary to syphilis responds to effective antibiotic treatment. Splenectomy is not helpful, and plasmapheresis should be used only as a temporizing measure in life-threatening cases. RBC transfusion using a blood warmer should be limited to patients with severe hemolysis because most donor units are P antigen positive and may stimulate further production of PCH autoantibodies.

5. Mixed-Type AIHA

Mixed-type AIHA occurs as primary or secondary disease (usually lymphoproliferative or autoimmune diseases). The course of illness is usually chronic with severe exacerbations. Like warm-type AIHA, mixed-type AIHA is steroid responsive, can be treated with splenectomy, and responds to cytotoxic therapy. Because relapses are not triggered by cold exposure, acrocyanosis and the Raynaud phenomenon are not characteristically seen. As with any secondary AIHA, treatment of the underlying disorder will reduce hemolytic activity.

ALLOIMMUNE HEMOLYTIC ANEMIA

Alloimmune hemolytic anemia requires exposure to allogeneic RBCs with subsequent formation of alloantibodies that react specifically with the allogeneic RBCs that triggered their production. These antibodies do not react against a patient's own RBCs. A well-known example of alloimmune hemolytic anemia is when the RhD-negative maternal immune system develops IgG alloantibodies on exposure to RhD-positive fetal RBCs. The maternal alloantibodies can then cross the placenta to inflict fetal RBC destruction in a condition termed hemolytic disease of the newborn. Anemia can range

from mild to potentially fatal producing intrauterine fetal death. By still uncertain mechanisms, administration of anti-D IgG with any fetomaternal hemorrhage event and soon after delivery will suppress maternal alloantibody formation and prevent hemolytic disease of the newborn. Treatment of established disease employs intrauterine and intravascular fetal transfusion and may include plasma exchange or intravenous immunoglobulin therapy.

Most adults who develop alloimmune hemolytic anemia have a history of RBC transfusion, which sensitizes patients to allogeneic RBC antigens. A subsequent transfusion can result in immediate alloantibody production, resulting in the fever, chest and flank pain, tachypnea, tachycardia, hypotension, hemoglobinuria, and oliguria seen in the hemolytic transfusion reaction. In patients with high alloantibody titers, the hemolytic reaction can be immediate. Patients with lower alloantibody levels develop delayed hemolysis occurring 3–7 days posttransfusion.

DRUG-RELATED AIHA

Drug-related AIHA can be divided into three types: autoimmune, drug adsorption, and neoantigen. Steroids can be used in cases of drug-related severe hemolysis. RBC transfusion will aggravate hemolysis if the recipient's serum contains antibodies against antigens found on the transfused RBCs.

▶ Autoimmune Drug-Related AIHA

Autoimmune drug-related AIHA results when the offending drug triggers formation of autoantibodies that bind with RBC self-antigens, leading to a hemolytic process serologically indistinct from that seen in warm-type AIHA. The diagnosis is proved when the hemolytic process abates on withdrawal of the offending drug. Drugs implicated include α-methyldopa, levodopa, mefenamic acid, procainamide, diclofenac, quinidine, phenacetin, and the second- and third-generation cephalosporins (particularly cefotetan and ceftriaxone). Up to 71 drugs have been associated with development of a positive DAT (direct antiglobulin test); however, significant hemolysis is seen only occasionally. An extended drug exposure is usually required for autoantibodies to form. A positive DAT does not indicate that hemolysis will occur or that a drug must be discontinued. Within days of stopping the offending drug, hemolysis usually stops, although it may take months to see full resolution of the process.

▶ Drug Adsorption–Type AIHA

Drug adsorption–type AIHA requires that the drug incite the formation of antidrug antibodies and that the drug bind to the RBCs with significant affinity. Antibodies formed against the drug will react against the drug bound to the RBC surface, producing hemolysis. This type of hemolysis has also been called drug requiring because the absence of the offending drug eliminates the hemolytic reaction completely.

Neoantigen-Type Drug-Related AIHA

Neoantigen-type drug-related AIHA involves weak binding of the offending drug to normal RBCs. The body's immune system, seeing the formed immune complexes as foreign, will generate an immune response that then produces hemolytic disease. The classic causative agent is penicillin, and isolated cases of diphtheria–tetanus–pertussis vaccination in children have been associated with hemolysis possibly via this neoantigen mechanism.

SICKLE CELL ANEMIA

General Considerations

Sickle cell anemia is caused by the substitution of the amino acid valine for glutamine at position 6 in the β-globin chain, producing an abnormal hemoglobin tetramer termed hemoglobin S (HbS). As a result of this mutation, deoxygenated HbS polymerizes, deforming the RBC and producing the characteristic sickled appearance. The distorted cell results in premature RBC destruction and also increases the viscosity of blood, leading to obstruction within the microvasculature. The overall effect is chronic ongoing hemolysis and episodic periods of vascular occlusion resulting in tissue ischemia affecting most organ systems.

This defect is inherited as an autosomal recessive trait, and disease is seen in patients who are homozygous for the sickle gene (*HbSS*). People with sickle cell trait (*HbAS*; heterozygous with one gene for normal β-globin chain and one gene for a β-globin chain with the sickle mutation) have a normal lifespan and are usually asymptomatic except in rare cases of severe physiologic stress when they may have an acute pain crisis, splenic infarction, or cerebrovascular complications. Approximately 8% of the African-American population carries sickle cell trait (heterozygous for the sickle cell gene), and approximately 0.15–0.2% of African-American newborns have sickle cell disease (homozygous for the sickle gene). A lesser percentage of individuals of Middle Eastern, eastern Mediterranean, and Indian descent may have the *HbS* gene.

Clinical Findings

A. Symptoms and Signs

Patients with sickle cell disease typically present to the emergency department because of complications (Table 41–13). Acute painful (vaso-occlusive) sickle cell crisis is a common problem, and the average patient with sickle cell disease has 1–4 severe attacks per year. The initiating event may not be identifiable, but stressors such as infection, cold, dehydration, and altitude have been implicated. As a result of intravascular sickling and small vessel occlusion, infarction of bone, viscera, and soft tissue occurs. Infarction manifests as diffuse bone, muscle, and joint pain and, in some cases, symptoms related to a specific affected organ. Initial

Table 41–13. Emergencies in Sickle Cell Disease.

Type	Specific Emergencies
Vaso-occlusive crises	Musculoskeletal pain (typical painful crisis) Dactylitis (hand-foot syndrome) Acute chest pain syndrome Stroke Priapism
Hematologic crises	Splenic sequestration Aplastic crisis Hemolytic crisis
Infections	Pneumonia Meningitis Sepsis Osteomyelitis Urinary tract infections

management includes aggressive pain management and hydration, an assessment of the cause of the current crisis, and a search for additional complications.

B. Laboratory Findings

Generally, a CBC and reticulocyte count help assess the degree of anemia and ensure that the marrow is still producing red cells. If the reticulocyte count is not available, the presence of polychromasia in the peripheral blood smear can indicate continued red cell production. Patients with sickle cell disease sometimes have a low-grade fever and an elevated white blood cell (WBC) count. This combination can make it difficult to determine whether an infection is present during a crisis. Consider infection if the WBC count has a left shift and is elevated above 20,000/μL. Because of the chronic hemolysis, mild elevations in bilirubin and serum LDH are common.

Treatment

Supplemental oxygen is commonly used for painful crises, but unless the patient is systemically hypoxemic, it has not proved to be of routine benefit. Treatment of acute pain requires opioids, and patients with severe pain should receive parenteral agents. A potent opioid, such as morphine or diamorphine, is recommended, whereas meperidine, with the potential for neurotoxicity from the metabolite normeperidine, is not recommended. Some patients may be tolerant because of prior opioid treatment, and large doses may be required. Regular doses of analgesics for a few hours to several days are typically required. Patient-controlled analgesia can be used in selected patients. NSAIDs can be used for their additive effect in pain management of sickle cell crisis. Because patients with sickle cell disease and a painful crisis have an absolute or relative hypovolemia due to their disease (deficient renal concentrating ability) or crisis (anorexia, vomiting, fever), aggressive oral or intravenous rehydration is commonly carried out. Induced hyponatremia and purified poloxamer 188 shorten the duration and severity of an acute crisis, but the effect is small, and no approach to shortening the duration and severity of a painful sickle cell crisis has proved reliable, safe, and appropriate for routine use. A common and recommended practice is to develop an individualized assessment and treatment protocol for specific patients who frequently present to the emergency department with painful crises. Sickle cell pain is complex and varied, and often requires extraordinary doses of narcotics. Nonpharmacologic treatments (distraction, massage, TENS units) may be helpful, and nonanalgesic adjuvants such as antihistamines, TCAs, and anticonvulsants may be more effective than narcotics at relieving chronic and neuropathic components of sickle cell pain.

The goal of treating sickle cell disease is to prevent complications. Specific treatments such as penicillin prophylaxis, pain medications, and blood transfusions can be instituted in the emergency department. Hydroxyurea has now been shown to be successful in reducing the number and recurrences of pain crisis and acute chest syndrome, but is useful only in compliant patients as it requires daily dosing, and is outside the scope of the emergency department.

▶ Sickle Cell Complications

A. Bone Pain

Bone pain is common during a sickle cell crisis and may include the back and the extremities. Usually, the pain is diffuse, and no physical findings are present. However, redness, warmth, or swelling suggests infection (cellulitis or osteomyelitis). The complaint of localized pain to the hip with difficulty ambulating suggests the possibility of aseptic necrosis of the femoral head, and approximately 30% of those with sickle cell disease develop hip pathology by age 30 years. Bone infarctions may cause symptoms similar to osteomyelitis. Plain radiographs may show evidence of aseptic necrosis or osteomyelitis, whereas bone infarcts are not usually visible on radiographs. Joint effusions are occasionally seen as a complication of sickle cell crisis, but arthrocentesis is often necessary to determine if the joint is infected.

B. Dactylitis

In young children an early manifestation of sickle cell disease is dactylitis (hand-foot syndrome). The syndrome is thought to be due to infarction of the red marrow with associated periosteal inflammation. It manifests as fever and painful swelling of the hands, feet, or both, and some redness and warmth may be present. As the child grows, the hematopoietic tissue in the metacarpal and phalangeal marrow is replaced by fatty tissue, making this entity less likely.

C. Chest Syndrome

The acute chest syndrome is used to describe a sickle cell crisis with pulmonary symptoms and a new pulmonary infiltrate found on radiograph. The patient might have pleuritic chest pain, shortness of breath, fever, nonproductive cough, and tachypnea. The exact cause of the chest syndrome is unclear, but infection, infarction (ribs or lung), and pulmonary fat embolism (from ischemic marrow fat necrosis) have all been implicated. Although a chest radiograph is not routinely required in all patients with painful sickle cell crisis, it is indicated in those with pulmonary symptoms or signs of fever. The onset of acute chest syndrome may be associated with a fall in hemoglobin level from the normal baseline. Pulmonary infiltrates may be present in one lobe or be diffuse and bilateral, and pleural effusions may be present. Severe cases may progress rapidly to respiratory failure. Treatment involves close monitoring of fluid status, oxygen, and pain control. Broad-spectrum antibiotics to cover *S. pneumoniae* and *M. pneumoniae* are recommended. In severe cases, simple transfusion or exchange transfusion can be done. Acute chest syndrome is currently the leading cause of death from sickle cell disease in the United States.

D. Abdominal Pain

Generalized and constant abdominal pain is a common complaint during an acute sickle cell crisis, and it may be difficult to distinguish between infarction of the abdominal and retroperitoneal organs associated with a sickle cell crisis and a focal abdominal problem such as cholecystitis or appendicitis. Frequently, the patient can determine that the pain is similar to or different from prior episodes. Patients with a typical vaso-occlusive episode should not have evidence of peritonitis (rebound). Hepatic infarction may cause the acute onset of jaundice and abdominal pain and can be difficult to distinguish from hepatitis or cholecystitis. Biliary disease is common because pigment-related cholelithiasis is seen in 30–70% of patients with sickle cell disease. Severe right upper quadrant pain and marked elevations of bilirubin may be due to intrahepatic cholestasis.

E. Genitourinary System

Vaso-occlusive events involving the kidneys are common but often asymptomatic. Infarction in the renal medulla may cause flank pain, renal colic-type pain, and costovertebral angle tenderness, mimicking pyelonephritis. Papillary necrosis may result in either gross or microscopic hematuria, but red cell casts are uncommon. Renal imaging studies are generally necessary for correct diagnosis. Priapism occurs in up to 30% of males with sickle cell disease. Initial treatment is fluid hydration, pain control, and transfusion. Urinary tract infections are more common in patients with sickle cell disease, and urinalysis is recommended.

F. Splenic Infarction

The spleen is particularly susceptible to the effects of sickled cells. During childhood, microinfarctions result in a nonfunctional spleen (in 14% of patients by age 6 months and 94% by age 5 years). Immunizations, prophylactic penicillin therapy, and parental education are critical to minimize the risk of infection and prompt early evaluation of fever in these patients. As sickle cell patients age, their risk of overwhelming sepsis decreases, but they remain predisposed to infection.

G. Splenic Sequestration

Splenic sequestration is more common in children than in adults, and it is a potential cause of death that can be averted with treatment. This syndrome is manifested by sudden enlargement of the spleen with an acute fall in the hemoglobin level due to sequestration of the blood volume within the spleen. Symptoms include tachycardia, hypotension, pallor, lethargy, and abdominal fullness. Left upper quadrant pain may or may not be present. The spleen is usually enlarged and firm. Platelets may also be sequestered, resulting in moderate thrombocytopenia. Therapy includes volume resuscitation, which may mobilize some of the red cells trapped within the spleen. Transfusion or exchange transfusion may be necessary; rarely, splenectomy is necessary. Unfortunately, recurrence of this syndrome is common.

H. Hemolytic Anemia

Patients with sickle cell disease have a chronic hemolytic process with a baseline hemoglobin level usually between 6 and 9 g/dL; the reticulocyte count is 5–15%. With infections the hemolytic process may worsen and hemoglobin may drop from previous baseline. Typically, reticulocytosis will increase in response to the increased red cell destruction but may not be enough to compensate for the increased hemolysis. Acutely, the patient may notice symptoms of worsening fatigue, shortness of breath, dyspnea on exertion, and scleral icterus. The hemolysis is rarely severe enough to require transfusion.

I. Aplastic Crisis

Aplastic crisis results when the production of red cells declines significantly, producing a rapid decrease in the hemoglobin level with reticulocytopenia. The most common cause of aplastic crisis appears to be infection, specifically from parvovirus. Folate deficiency and bone marrow necrosis also may play a role. Aplastic crisis is more common in pediatric patients than in adults. The hemoglobin level will be unusually low, and few or no reticulocytes will be present (reticulocyte count typically <0.5%). The WBC and platelet levels are usually normal. Generally, this syndrome is self-limiting, and the marrow will begin producing red cells

spontaneously within a week. Transfusion may be required in the interim.

J. Neurologic Complications

Complications of sickle cell disease include stroke and subarachnoid hemorrhage. The cause of strokes in most patients is cerebral infarction due to occlusion or narrowing of large cerebral vessels. Approximately 10% of patients with sickle cell disease experience a stroke before age 20 years. Acute treatment is simple or partial exchange transfusion on an emergency basis. Unfortunately, children who suffer a stroke are at 70–90% risk for recurrence. Chronic transfusion therapy is indicated to prevent recurrent stoke after the initial event. Cerebral aneurysms are also more common in sickle cell patients, perhaps due to local vessel occlusion or ischemia.

K. Infections

Patients with sickle cell disease are functionally asplenic after early childhood, making them susceptible to infections from encapsulated organisms, such as *H. influenzae* and *S. pneumoniae*. Other common infections associated with sickle cell disease include pneumonia caused by these organisms as well as *M. pneumoniae*, meningitis, and osteomyelitis due to *Salmonella typhimurium, Staphylococcus aureus,* and *E. coli.* Although low-grade fever sometimes occurs during an acute crisis, unexplained fevers of 38°C (101°F) or higher require evaluation for bacterial infection and consideration for early treatment with broad-spectrum antibiotics.

L. Cardiac Complications

Cardiomegaly is common and correlates with the degree of chronic anemia. Additionally, cardiac dysfunction may occur from microinfarcts and hemosiderin deposition from hemolysis and blood transfusion. Because of the chronic anemia, enhanced cardiac contractility is present to maintain adequate systemic oxygen delivery producing a widely radiating systolic ejection murmur.

M. Dermatologic Complications

Chronic, poorly healing leg ulcers around the malleoli are common in older patients with sickle cell disease. Minor injury, impaired microcirculation due to repeated sickling episodes and microinfarcts, and infections all contribute to the development and persistence of these ulcers.

▶ Disposition

Most sickle cell pain crises last 2–3 days. Patients with adequate clinical response and no indications for hospital admission can be discharged with oral pain medications and referred for follow-up with their primary care physician in the next 24–48 hours. The following are guidelines for hospital admission for sickle cell patients: (1) pulmonary or neurologic complications, (2) significant bacterial infection, (3) splenic sequestration or aplastic crisis, or (4) pain that remains poorly controlled or patients are unable to maintain adequate hydration.

THALASSEMIAS

The thalassemias are a diverse group of disorders characterized by defective synthesis of globin chains, resulting in the inability to produce normal adult hemoglobin. With β-thalassemias, unpaired α_4 tetramers accumulate in the cell membrane of RBCs, causing intravascular hemolysis. With α-thalassemias, b_4 tetramers accumulate, but are less severe due to HbH being more soluble and stable, resulting in less precipitate. The hallmark of these disorders is a microcytic, hypochromic, hemolytic anemia. These disorders are most common in individuals of Mediterranean, Middle Eastern, African, or Southeast Asian descent. Thalassemia red cells contain decreased hemoglobin, which accounts for the hypochromia and target cell formation. Individuals with either α- or β-thalassemia can be minimally to severely affected due to the specific genotype and whether the mutation produces complete or partial reduction in globin chains.

α-THALASSEMIA CARRIER AND TRAIT

α-Thalassemia carriers have normal RBC size, shape, and number and have no clinical consequences from this inherited gene. Those with α-thalassemia trait are detected by the findings of microcytic RBCs and a normal hemoglobin level.

HEMOGLOBIN H DISEASE

Hemoglobin H disease is a disorder in which one out of four α-globin chain genes is functional. Patients with hemoglobin H disease usually present in the neonatal period with a severe hypochromic anemia. Later in life the clinical picture includes a hypochromic, microcytic anemia with jaundice and hepatosplenomegaly. These patients may not require regular transfusions, but a transfusion may be necessary in conditions of increased oxidative stress (which may cause precipitation of the unstable hemoglobin H resulting in hemolysis) or infection. Most of these patients will know their diagnosis, and the emergency physician needs to provide only supportive care and blood transfusion when necessary. Medications that may precipitate hemolysis should be avoided in this population (Table 41–14).

β-THALASSEMIA MINOR (β-THALASSEMIA TRAIT)

Patients with β-thalassemia minor are heterozygous for the β-globin mutation and have only mild microcytic anemia. Splenomegaly may be present. These patients may exhibit microcytosis, hypochromia, and basophilic stippling on blood smear. An elevated hemoglobin A_2 level, typically 4–6%, confirms the diagnosis. These patients will generally not have clin-

Table 41–14. Drugs That Produce Oxidative Stress on Red Blood Cells and May Induce Hemolysis.

Class	Drug
Sulfonamides	Sulfacetamide Sulfamethoxazole Sulfanilamide Sulfapyridine
Antimalarials	Primaquine Chloroquine Pamaquine Pentaquine
Urinary agents	Nitrofurantoin Nalidixic acid Phenazopyridine
Miscellaneous antibiotics	Ciprofloxacin niridazole Norfloxacin Chloramphenicol
Mothballs	Naphthalene
Miscellaneous	Vitamin K analogs Methylene blue Acetanilid Doxorubicin Isobutyl nitrite Phenylhydrazine

ical manifestations, and this form of thalassemia may come to the clinician's attention only during routine blood work.

β-THALASSEMIA MAJOR (COOLEY ANEMIA)

In patients with β-thalassemia major, both β-globin genes are defective and production of β-globin chains is severely impaired. β-Thalassemia major is characterized by a severe anemia that begins within the first year of life after the conversion from fetal hemoglobin synthesis to adult hemoglobin synthesis. These children develop hepatosplenomegaly, jaundice, expansion of the erythroid marrow (causing bone changes and osteoporosis), and increased susceptibility to infection. The anemia is severe and requires regular and lifelong blood transfusions. These transfusions and enhanced iron absorption eventually cause iron overload, which, if untreated, results in hemochromatosis with cardiac, hepatic, and endocrine dysfunction. The RBCs of these children show a low MCV with microcytic and hypochromic cells. Variation in size and shape of the RBCs will be notable (increased RDW) as will the presence of nucleated cells. Consider this diagnosis in any child with a severe microcytic anemia and the appropriate ethnic background. For those with a known diagnosis, who present to the emergency department with significant symptoms related to anemia or hemolysis, consider transfusion and search for precipitating events.

GLUCOSE-6-PHOSPHATE DEHYDROGENASE DEFICIENCY

Glucose-6-phosphate dehydrogenase deficiency is the most common enzyme deficiency world wide. Glucose-6-phosphate dehydrogenase (G6PD) is an enzyme responsible for preventing oxidative damage to intraerythrocytic hemoglobin. Over 300 variant mutations are described for G6PD; the highest prevalence is in individuals of African, Asian, or Mediterranean descent. Because the gene for G6PD is carried on the X chromosome, males are affected when they are hemizygous. Females must carry two defective genes to be severely affected, but because expression of this gene is variable, women with one dysfunctional gene may show some symptoms. The severity of G6PD disease is related to the magnitude of enzyme deficiency; patients with severe deficiencies have less than 10% of normal enzyme activity, and patients with moderate deficiencies have 10–60% of normal activity. G6PD deficiency is seen in approximately 10–15% of black males in the United States.

Oxidization of the hemoglobin sulfhydryl groups causes hemoglobin to precipitate within the cell; it is recognized by the presence of Heinz bodies on the peripheral blood smear. The affected RBC is removed from the circulation by the spleen. Oxidant damage also occurs at the RBC membrane, producing both extravascular and intravascular hemolysis.

A history of neonatal jaundice 1–4 days after birth is common. Patients with severe variants may have a severe chronic hemolytic anemia. In the more common variants of G6PD deficiency, the patient is usually asymptomatic except for acute hemolytic crises that occur due to bacterial and viral infections, exposure to oxidant drugs (most commonly sulfonamides, antimalarials, and nitrofurantoin), metabolic acidosis (such as diabetic ketoacidosis), renal failure, and, in some patients, ingestion of fava beans (see Table 41–14). These episodes are usually self-limited and well tolerated because only the older RBCs will hemolyze. The incidence of pigmented gallstones and splenomegaly is increased in patients with G6PD deficiency. Treatment for this disease is supportive and preventative.

HEREDITARY SPHEROCYTOSIS

Hereditary spherocytosis is a common hereditary disorder that is characterized by anemia, jaundice, and splenomegaly. It is a result of an erythrocyte membrane defect and is the most prevalent hereditary hemolytic anemia among people of northern European descent. The disease is typically inherited in an autosomal dominant pattern, although a less common autosomal recessive variant exists; in up to 20% of patients the disease is the result of an apparent spontaneous mutation. The abnormal shape of the RBC results from molecular abnormalities in the cytoskeleton of the cell membrane, resulting in red cells with a microspherocytic shape, which is not pliable enough to pass through the spleen, leading to an increased rate of destruction and a compensatory increase in RBC production. The clinical spectrum of hereditary spherocytosis includes (1) mild disease, occurring in 20–30% of cases, with an autosomal dominant inheritance, (2) moderate disease, occurring in 60–75% of cases, with primarily autosomal dominant inheritance, and (3) severe disease, in about 5% of cases, occurring with autosomal recessive inheritance.

Neonatal jaundice during the 1st week of life occurs in 30–50% of hereditary spherocytosis patients. After the neonatal period, the symptoms and signs depend on the severity of ongoing hemolysis. Patients with mild disease usually have a normal hemoglobin level and little or no splenomegaly but are susceptible to hemolytic or aplastic episodes triggered by infection. Patients with moderate disease have mild to moderate anemia, modest splenomegaly, periodic episodes of hemolysis with jaundice, and an increased incidence of pigmented gallstones. The rare patient with severe hereditary spherocytosis has chronic jaundice, an enlarged spleen, and significant hemolytic anemia requiring episodic blood transfusions. Folate therapy is only indicated for patients with severe hemolysis.

The peripheral blood smear shows spherocytes with a normal to low MCV and increased MCHC (>36%). The diagnosis of hereditary spherocytosis is established by the osmotic fragility test. In severe cases, splenectomy will generally reverse the anemia except in the unusual cases of autosomal recessive variants. After splenectomy, spherocytes are still present.

Ballas SK: Pain management of sickle cell disease. Hematol Oncol Clin N Am 2005;19:785–802 [PMID: 16214644].

Buchanan G, Vickinsky E, Krishnamurti L, Shenoy S: Severe sickle cell disease-pathophysiology and therapy. Biol Blood Marow Transplant 2010;16:S64–S67 [PMID: 19819341].

Cappellini MD, Fiorelli G: Glucose-6-phosphate dehydrogenase deficiency. Lancet 2008;371:64–74 [PMID: 18177777].

Chui DH: Alpha-thalassemia: Hb H disease and Hb Barts hydrops fetalis. Ann NY Acad Sci 2005;1054:25–32 [PMID: 16339648].

Cook JD: Diagnosis and management of iron-deficiency anaemia. Best Pract Res Clin Haematol 2005;18:319–332 [PMID: 15737893].

Coyer SM: Anemia: Diagnosis and management. J Pediatr Health Care 2005;19:380–385 [PMID: 16286225].

Creary M, Williamson D, Kulkarni R: Sickle cell disease: current activities, public health implications and future directions. Report from CDC: J Women's Health 2007;16:575–582 [PMID: 17627395].

Cunningham MJ: Update on thalassemia: clinical care and complications. Hematol Oncol Clin N Am 2010;24:215–227 [PMID: 20113904].

Field JJ, Knight-Perry JE, DeBaun MR: Acute pain in children and adults with sickle cell disease: management in the absence of evidence-based guidelines. Curr Opin Hematol 2009;16:173–178 [PMID: 19295432].

Frank JE: Diagnosis and management of G6PD deficiency. Am Fam Physician 2005;72:1277–1282 [PMID: 16225031].

Garratty G: Immune hemolytic anemia-a primer. Semin Hematol 2005;42:119–121 [PMID: 16041660].

Garratty G: Drug-induced immune hemolytic anemia. Clin Adv Hematol Oncol 2010;8:98–101 [PMID: 20386530].

Hick JL, Nelson SC, Hick K, Nwaneri MO: Emergency management of sickle cell disease complications: Review and practice guidelines. Minn Med 2006;89:42–44, 47 [PMID: 16700347].

Inati A, Chabtini L, Mounayar M, Taher A: Current understanding in the management of sickle cell disease. Hemoglobin 2009;33:S107–S115 [PMID: 20001613].

Kato GJ, Gladwin MT, Steinberg MH: Deconstructing sickle cell disease: reappraisal of the role of hemolysis in the development of clinical subphenotypes. Blood Rev 2007;21:37–47 [PMID: 17084951].

Killip S, Bennett JM, Chambers MD: Iron deficiency anemia. Am Fam Physician 2007;75:671–678 [PMID: 17375513].

King KE, Ness PM: Treatment of autoimmune hemolytic anemia. Semin Hematol 2005;42:131–136 [PMID: 16041662].

Muncie HL, Campbell JS: Alpha and beta thalassemia. Am Fam Physician 2009;80:339–344, 371 [PMID: 19678601].

Perrotta S, Gallagher PG, Mohandas N: Hereditary spherocytosis. Lancet 2008;372, 1411–1426 [PMID: 18940465].

Raphel RI: Pathophysiology and treatment of sickle cell disease. Clin Adv Hematol Oncol 2005;3:492–505 [PMID: 16167028].

Rund D, Rachmilewitz E: Beta-thalassemia. N Engl J Med 2005;353:1135–1146 [PMID: 16162884].

Schrier SL, Angelucci E: New Strategies in the treatment of the thalassemias. Annu Rev Med 2005;56:157–171 [PMID: 15660507].

▼ POLYCYTHEMIA

The term *polycythemia* means increased cellular components in peripheral blood—RBCs, WBCs, and platelets—but in common practice is used to describe increased red cells or erythrocytosis. Polycythemia can be primary, due to malignant transformation of a hematopoietic stem cell (called polycythemia vera), or can be secondary to an event outside the bone marrow driving erythropoiesis. It is characterized by an increased red cell mass. In relative or false polycythemia, the red cell mass is normal, but decreased plasma volume results in elevated hemoglobin and hematocrit values.

PRIMARY POLYCYTHEMIA (POLYCYTHEMIA VERA)

Polycythemia vera is an unregulated neoplastic proliferation of red cells, usually accompanied by increased WBC and platelet production. Peak age of onset is 50–70 years, although it can occur in young adults.

▶ Clinical Findings

A. Symptoms and Signs

Onset is gradual, and symptoms are usually due to hyperviscosity and impaired circulation in the brain (headache, dizziness), eyes (impaired vision), heart (chest pain), or peripheral circulation (claudication). Increased production of basophils and mast cells can lead to pruritus after a hot shower from the associated histamine release. Hemorrhagic or thrombotic complications are rare. Physical findings include hypertension (common), plethora or ruddy complexion, splenomegaly (in about 75% of cases), and hepatomegaly (in about 30% of cases).

B. Laboratory Findings

Determination of red cell mass with a radionuclide technique will show an elevated value (>36 mL/kg in males or >32 mL/kg in females) but is unnecessary when the hemoglobin value is above 20 g/dL or hematocrit is above 60% in males or above 56% in females, as these values are always associated with an elevated red cell mass. The WBC and platelet counts are commonly elevated.

▶ Treatment and Disposition

Standard treatment is periodic phlebotomy to remove excess red cells, reduce blood viscosity, and improve microcirculation and low dose aspirin. Patients with altered mentation should have emergency phlebotomy of 500 mL of blood. Hydroxyurea is the mainstay of treatment, although this is outside the scope of treatment in the emergency department.

SECONDARY POLYCYTHEMIA

Secondary polycythemia is produced by erythropoietin stimulation of bone marrow red cell production. Systemic hypoxia (eg, from chronic obstructive pulmonary disease, right-to-left cardiac shunts) or local renal hypoxia (eg, atherosclerotic renal vascular disease) can lead to stimulation of erythropoietin production by the kidney. Because of widespread tobacco abuse, chronic obstructive pulmonary disease is the most common cause of secondary polycythemia. Less common causes include chronic carbon monoxide exposure, erythropoietin secreting renal tumors, use of androgenic steroids, and familial hemoglobinopathies associated with high oxygen affinity.

▶ Clinical Findings

Polycythemia should be suspected when the hematocrit is greater than 52% in males or 47% in females. Confirmation of red cell mass and plasma volume requires measurement via radionuclide techniques. Systemic hypoxia (arterial oxygen saturation <92%) or chronic carbon monoxide exposure (carboxyhemoglobin levels >8%) should be considered. Blood viscosity increases and impairs microcirculation with hematocrit values above 60–65%.

▶ Treatment and Disposition

Symptomatic patients should undergo phlebotomy to reduce blood viscosity and improve microcirculation. Phlebotomy on an emergency basis may be necessary in the emergency department for acute symptoms. Long-term management of secondary polycythemia depends on the primary disorder.

Cao M, Olsen RJ, Zu Y: Polycythemia vera: New clinicopathologic perspectives. Arch Pathol Lab Med 2006;130:1126–1132 [PMID: 16879013].

Finazzi G, Barbui T: Evidence and expertise in the management of polycythemia vera and essential thrombocythemia. Leukemia 2008;22:1494–1502 [PMID: 18596737].

McMullin MF: The classification and diagnosis of erythrocytosis. Int J Lab Hem 2008;30:447–459 [PMID: 18823397].

Silver RT: Treatment of polycythemia vera. Semin Thromb Hemost 2006;32:437–442 [PMID: 16810620].

Tefferi A: Polycythemia vera: a comprehensive review and clinical recommendations. Mayo Clin Proc 2003;78:174–194 [PMID: 12583529].

Zhan H, Spivak JL: The diagnosis and management of polycythemia vera, essential thrombocythemia and primary myelofibrosis in the JAK2 V617F era. Clin Adv Hematol Oncol 2009;7:334–342 [PMID: 19521323].

▼ WHITE CELL DISORDERS

NEUTROPENIA

▶ General Considerations

Neutropenia is defined as a decrease in circulating neutrophils as detected by measuring the absolute neutrophil count (ANC) in the peripheral blood. The ANC is determined by multiplying the total WBC count by the percentage of segmented neutrophils and bands from the WBC differential. The ANC is normally greater than 1500 cells/μL in individuals of European descent and greater than 1000 cells/μL in African-Americans. Neutropenia produces an increased susceptibility to bacterial infections inversely related to the ANC. Severe neutropenia is defined as an ANC less than 500 cells/μL.

▶ Clinical Findings

Neutropenia can be congenital, associated with inherited immune defects and phenotypic abnormalities. A form of congenital neutropenia is chronic benign neutropenia, either familial with an autosomal dominant inheritance pattern or nonfamilial. Patients with chronic benign neutropenia do not have significantly increased susceptibility to bacterial infections. Acquired neutropenia can be due to drugs, toxins, nutritional deficiencies, autoimmune disorders, or diseases that impair bone marrow granulocyte cell production. The list of drugs that can produce neutropenia is extensive, but the most common agents are the cytotoxic chemotherapeutic agents used to treat malignancies.

Neutropenia should be suspected when a cancer patient receiving chemotherapy presents with fever or when an otherwise healthy patient presents with an infection that has not responded as expected to antibiotic treatment. Patients with febrile neutropenia typically have a temperature greater than or equal to 100.4°F and an ANC of <500–1000 cells/mL. The evaluation of the febrile neutropenic patient requires a careful evaluation for clinically occult infection. Because of the neutropenia, the patient may not be able to generate pus in a local site or wound, an infiltrate on chest radiograph, or pyuria in response to infection. Carefully examine the skin, mouth, sinuses, and rectal area for evidence of local infection. Obtain blood cultures, urine culture, and a chest radiograph. When present, culture other body secretions such as diarrhea, wound exudate, or sputum.

▶ Treatment and Disposition

The decision to initiate empiric antibiotic therapy is based on the patient's clinical condition and on the estimated risk of serious bacterial infection as judged by the cause, severity, and expected duration of neutropenia. The severely ill cancer patient with severe neutropenia (ANC < 500 cells/μL) due to recent chemotherapy clearly requires broad-spectrum empiric antibiotic therapy and hospital admission. Conversely, a mildly ill cancer patient with no obvious source of bacterial infection, with mild neutropenia (ANC of 1000–1500 cells/μL), and who has not received recent chemotherapy can likely be discharged home with symptomatic therapy and close follow-up. If indicated, initiate empiric antibiotics in the emergency department after obtaining appropriate cultures. Multiple antibiotic regimens are used, typically a broad-spectrum agent such as a third-generation cephalosporin (ceftazidime), or a fluoroquinolone (levofloxacin), or a carbapenem (imipenem and cilastatin) with or without a specific antistaphylococcal agent such as vancomycin.

LEUKOCYTOSIS

Elevated WBC counts may represent an appropriate response to infection or may constitute an autonomous proliferation of cells due to a primary hematologic disorder. Elevated WBC count is not a problem by itself except in the unusual case of leukemia associated with hyperleukocytosis, when WBC counts exceed 100,000–300,000 cells/μL, causing increased blood viscosity and circulatory compromise. This can lead to central nervous system impairment and respiratory insufficiency; urgent treatment with leukocytapheresis is indicated. As a temporizing measure, intravenous hydration and exchange transfusion can be performed.

ACUTE LEUKEMIA

▶ General Considerations

Acute leukemia is a malignancy of hematopoietic stem cells in which the leukemic cell population replaces and suppresses normal bone marrow cells, resulting in bone marrow failure with anemia, functional or absolute neutropenia, and thrombocytopenia. The usual causes of illness and death are infectious or hemorrhagic. These rapidly progressive disorders are uniformly fatal without treatment. Fortunately, effective treatment is now available for most patients with acute leukemia, and depending on cell type, 20–40% of adult patients and 50–70% of pediatric patients with acute leukemia survive longer than 5 years. Acute leukemias have historically been classified according to neoplastic cell morphology (acute lymphocytic leukemia [ALL] and acute myelocytic leukemia [AML]), but immunologic analysis has found a wide diversity in neoplastic cell origin.

▶ Clinical Findings

Patients with acute leukemia typically develop symptoms over a few weeks and present with fatigue (due to anemia), fever (due to neutropenia), or bleeding problems (due to thrombocytopenia or DIC). Leukemic organ infiltration accounts for symptoms such as bone pain (ALL), swollen gums (AML), and abdominal pain due to splenomegaly (ALL and AML)

The diagnosis of acute leukemia is suspected when the WBC count is elevated and the peripheral blood smear shows a large number of immature white cells (blast cells), along with anemia and thrombocytopenia. Uncommonly, blast cells may be absent from the peripheral blood (termed *aleukemic leukemia*), and the hemoglobin value and platelet count may be normal. Definitive diagnosis of acute leukemia is based on bone marrow examination showing more than 30% immature blast cells. Differentiation between the types of acute leukemia is made using morphologic, histochemical, and immunochemical staining.

▶ Disposition

Hospitalize patients with suspected acute leukemia. Evaluate fever, if present, and initiation of empiric antibiotic treatment in the neutropenic patient is prudent. Patients with hyperleukocytosis (>300,000 cells/μL) may develop symptoms of impaired microcirculation and require emergency treatment.

CHRONIC LEUKEMIA

Chronic leukemias are indolent diseases, typically found in older adults and producing nonspecific systemic symptoms (malaise, fatigue, weight loss, low-grade fever) and signs of leukemic organ infiltration (splenomegaly, lymphadenopathy). Chronic leukemias have historically been classified according to neoplastic cell morphology (chronic lymphocytic leukemia [CLL] and chronic myelocytic leukemia [CML]), but immunologic analysis has found a wide diversity in neoplastic cell origin.

1. Chronic Lymphocytic Leukemia

Chronic lymphocytic leukemia is the most common leukemia seen in the adult population of Western countries. Most cases of CLL are seen in patients older than 55 years, and the majority of cases have a slow progression lasting up to 10 years before they enter a final terminal stage. These patients commonly experience repeated infections such as

pneumonia, herpes simplex, and herpes zoster because the lymphocytes are functionally incompetent. Patients often have fatigue, lymphadenopathy, mucosal surface bleeding, or hepatosplenomegaly. Diagnosis is suggested by a peripheral blood smear with absolute B-lymphocyte count exceeding 5000 cells/μL. Peripheral blood smear typically shows numerous mature lymphocytes with a dense nucleus and a narrow cytoplasmic border. Bone marrow biopsy and genetic testing are not required to diagnose CLL. Patients with an initial diagnosis of CLL and without any of the complications can be followed up by a hematologist. Patients with any of the above-mentioned complications (bleeding, fever, symptoms of hyperviscosity, bone marrow failure) may need hospitalization and consultation with a hematologist.

2. Chronic Myelocytic Leukemia

Chronic myelocytic leukemia is a clonal disorder of hematopoietic stem cells most commonly due to a reciprocal translocation between the long arms of chromosomes 22 and 9, resulting in a shortened chromosome 22, termed the Philadelphia chromosome.

Patients typically present with fatigue, malaise, and weight loss. Often, findings of leukocytosis and splenomegaly with or without hepatomegaly are found incidentally on routine examination. The CBC often shows a moderate leukocytosis of 20,000–60,000 cells/μL, a mild anemia, and variable platelet counts. The peripheral blood smear shows a predominance of myeloid progenitor cells (myeloblasts, myelocytes, metamyelocytes) and nucleated RBCs.

Most patients are clinically stable and responsive to therapy for 3–5 years, then develop an acute blastic crisis (generally myeloid but occasionally lymphoid) that is refractory to treatment, and progress to death. A small subset of CML patients bypass the initial chronic phase and enter a rapidly progressive leukemic phase wherein they have profound leukocytosis and thrombocytopenia as evidenced by bleeding, petechiae, and ecchymoses. A serious complication is the hyperviscosity syndrome in which WBC counts exceed 300,000 cells/μL or the leukocrit is greater than 10%. This is evidenced by neurologic and ophthalmologic manifestations and respiratory failure.

Exchange transfusion can be a useful temporizing measure in the acute setting with severe stupor or seizure, but urgent leukocytopheresis is the most effective treatment. Typical initial treatment by hematology is with imatinib (tyrosine kinase inhibitor).

INFECTIOUS MONONUCLEOSIS
▶ General Considerations

Infectious mononucleosis is a primary infection with EBV characterized by fever, pharyngitis, adenopathy, and greater than 10% atypical lymphocytes in the peripheral smear. Only a minority of primary EBV infections come to medical attention; population studies indicate that as many as 90% of young adults have serologic evidence of prior EBV infection, but only a minority of individuals describe a prior episode of infectious mononucleosis, supporting the concept that most primary EBV infections are mild or asymptomatic. After the primary infection, the EBV is carried for a lifetime.

▶ Clinical Findings

A. Symptoms and Signs

The incubation period of infectious mononucleosis is 1–2 months. Initial symptoms are fatigue, malaise, and sore throat. Fever is usually low grade and chills are uncommon. The pharyngitis of infectious mononucleosis may be exudative or nonexudative, and tonsillar enlargement is common. The lymphadenopathy is usually bilateral and most common in the posterior cervical nodes, although other lymph nodes may be affected, and generalized lymphadenopathy is possible. Splenic tenderness is common early in the disease, whereas splenomegaly is a later finding. A variety of other symptoms or signs are well described in infectious mononucleosis: (1) an early, faint, evanescent generalized maculopapular rash, (2) early bilateral periorbital edema, (3) hepatitis with liver tenderness and jaundice, (4) uvular edema, and (5) neurologic disorders such as Bell's palsy, optic neuritis, other cranial nerve mononeuropathies, aseptic meningitis, encephalitis, Guillain–Barré syndrome, and transverse myelitis.

B. Laboratory Findings

Common laboratory findings of infectious mononucleosis include (1) leukocytosis (usually 12,000–20,000 cells/μL), (2) lymphocytosis (usually >60% on the white cell differential), (3) atypical lymphocytosis (>10% and frequently >30%), (4) mild elevations in serum transaminases, and (5) elevated erythrocyte sedimentation rate. EBV infection induces the production of host antibodies that form the basis for serologic diagnosis of infectious mononucleosis. The most commonly used antibody test is the Monospot, which detects an IgM antibody to the viral capsid antigen (historically named heterophile antibody). The Monospot is considered to have approximately 85% sensitivity and almost 100% specificity. However, the sensitivity of this test is lower early in the clinical disease (up to 6 weeks is required for maximal sensitivity) and in children younger than 2 years, who are frequently Monospot negative. False-positive Monospot tests have been seen in patients with CMV, rubella, systemic lupus erythematosus, rheumatoid arthritis, HIV, and herpes simplex infections. Specific antibody testing is available for additional characterization but not useful in the emergency department.

▶ Differential Diagnosis

The differential diagnosis of infectious mononucleosis includes (1) streptococcal pharyngitis (complicated by the observation that up to 30% of infectious mononucleosis patients have

detectable group A streptococci in the oropharynx), (2) primary CMV infection (the closest clinical mimic of infectious mononucleosis), (3) acute toxoplasmosis (usually with unilateral lymphadenopathy), and (4) viral hepatitis.

▶ Treatment

There is no effective antiviral therapy for infectious mononucleosis. Steroid treatment is controversial with a recent Cochran Review revealing unsufficient evidence to support steroid use. Antibiotic treatment of coexistent group A streptococci is controversial. Some clinicians recommend withholding antibiotic treatment because a positive throat culture or streptococcal antigen test represents colonization rather than infection, and antibiotic treatment may induce a rash that, although due to the infectious mononucleosis and not the drug, may be judged as a drug allergy and may complicate future antibiotic therapy. Patients should be instructed to refrain from strenuous physical activity and especially sports for 3 weeks.

MULTIPLE MYELOMA

▶ Clinical Findings

A. Symptoms and Signs

Multiple myeloma is a disease of malignant plasma cell proliferation and excessive secretion of monoclonal paraproteins. Multiple myeloma usually presents during the sixth to seventh decades of life. The most common initial symptoms are bone pain (in up to 70% of patients; involving the lumbar region) sometimes with pathologic fractures; constipation, nausea, confusion, and somnolence from hypercalcemia; fatigue from anemia; infection with impaired immunity; bleeding from thrombocytopenia or hyperviscosity; and paresthesias from peripheral neuropathies. Complications of multiple myeloma include renal impairment, amyloidosis from paraproteinemia, hypercalcemia, and spinal cord compression from extradural compression. Physical examination findings include bony tenderness, soft tissue plasmacytoma masses, pallor from anemia, ecchymoses or petechiae, epistaxis, or findings of spinal cord compression (lower extremity weakness or dysesthesias with incontinence of bowel or bladder with associated decreased rectal tone or saddle anesthesia).

B. Laboratory Findings

The diagnosis is suspected when the serum globulin protein level is elevated and is confirmed with serum protein immunoelectrophoresis demonstrating a monoclonal spike. Evaluate the patient's hematologic (CBC), hemostatic (PT, PTT), renal (blood urea nitrogen and creatinine), and metabolic (electrolytes, calcium, uric acid) status. Quantification of urinary protein excretion (Bence Jones proteinuria; ie, lambda light chains) is sometimes useful for diagnosis and for determining response to therapy. A skeletal series looking for sites of lytic lesions (commonly in the skull and long bones) can be helpful to identify potential pathologic fracture sites and to differentiate multiple myeloma from Waldenström macroglobulinemia (which does not typically have lytic bone lesions). Bone marrow examination typically finds sheets or clumps of plasma cells replacing normal marrow contents.

▶ Treatment and Disposition

Many patients with multiple myeloma are asymptomatic, and specific treatment can be delayed until the patient shows signs of disease progression without affecting efficacy of treatment. Treatment is usually with melphalan and prednisone. In occasional patients, multiple myeloma is treated with irradiation and high-dose chemotherapy followed by hematopoietic stem cell transplant. Adjunctive therapy may include bisphosphonates to prevent hypercalcemia and pathologic fractures, erythropoietin to treat anemia, and radiation to lytic lesions to prevent pathologic fractures. Complications of hypercalcemia, hyperviscosity, pathologic fracture, or spinal cord compression may require hospitalization for specific therapy.

WALDENSTRÖM MACROGLOBULINEMIA

▶ General Considerations

Waldenström macroglobulinemia is a rare malignancy of B lymphocytes characterized by excessive production of monoclonal IgM. Symptoms and signs are due to the elevated serum viscosity and infiltration of organs (bone marrow, spleen, liver, lymph nodes) from the neoplastic lymphocytes. The disease most commonly occurs in the elderly with median age of onset around 60 years.

▶ Clinical Findings

The onset is typically gradual, and common symptoms are weakness, anorexia, and weight loss. Additional symptoms due to hyperviscosity include mental status changes, Raynaud phenomenon, peripheral neuropathy, and visual changes. Ocular signs of hyperviscosity include papilledema, enlarged retinal veins, and retinal hemorrhage. Hepatosplenomegaly and lymphadenopathy are common. Purpura can occur due to thrombocytopenia, and functional platelet impairment from the IgM paraproteinemia. The laboratory diagnosis of Waldenström macroglobulinemia is supported by (1) an IgM level above 3 g/dL and (2) hematologic abnormalities of anemia and thrombocytopenia and occasionally leukopenia. The malignant nature is identified with high-resolution serum protein immunoelectrophoresis or bone marrow biopsy with immunochemical staining.

▶ Treatment and Disposition

Consider hyperviscosity for any Waldenström macroglobulinemia patient who presents with mental status or visual changes. Plasma exchange is indicated for the acute management of patients with symptoms of hyperviscosity because 80% of the IGM protein is intravascular. Chemotherapy with alkylating agents (chlorambucil, melphalan, or cyclophosphamide) is used to reduce production of the IgM paraprotein and control symptoms of neoplastic organ infiltration. Prednisone is used to control autoimmune symptoms such as digital ischemia from cryoglobulinemia or immune hemolysis from agglutination. Other chemotherapeutic agents are sometimes used, but no combination is superior or changes median survival. Stable, asymptomatic patients typically do not receive treatment.

Abbott BL: Chronic lymphocytic leukemia: recent advances in diagnosis and treatment. Oncologist 2006;11:21–30 [PMID: 16401710].

Barzi A, Sekkeres MA: Myelodysplastic syndromes: a practical approach to diagnosis and treatment. Cleve Clin J Med 2010;77:37–44 [PMID: 20048028].

Courtney DM, Aldeen AZ, et al: Cancer-associated neutropenic fever: clinical outcome and economic costs of emergency department care. Oncologist 2007;12:1019–1026 [PMID: 17766662].

Dickens KP, Nye AM, Gilchrist V, Rickett K, Neher JO: Should you use steroids to treat infectious mononucleosis? J Fam Pract 2009;57:754–755 [PMID: 19006627].

Dimopoulos MA, Anagnostopoulos A: Waldenstrom's macroglobulinemia. Best Pract Res Clin Haematol 2005;18:747–765 [PMID: 16026748].

Fausel C: Targeted chronic myeloid leukemia therapy: seeking a cure. Am J Health Syst Pharm 2007;64:S9–S15 [PMID: 18056932].

Goldman JM: Initial treatment for patients with CML. Hematology Am Soc Hematol Educ Program 2009:453–460 [PMID: 20008231].

Gulley ML, Tang W: Laboratory assays for Epstein-Barr virus related disease. J Mol Diagn 2008;10:279–292 [PMID: 18556771].

Halfdanarson TR, Hogan WJ, Moynihan TJ: Oncologic emergencies: diagnosis and treatment. Mayo Clinic Proc 2006;81:835–848 [PMID: 16770986].

Heerema-McKenney A, Arber DA: Acute myeloid leukemia: Hematol Oncol Clin N Am 2009;23:633–654 [PMID: 19577164].

Higdon ML, Higdon JA: Treatment of oncologic emergencies. Am Fam Physician 2006;74:1873–1880 [PMID: 17168344].

Jabbour E, Estey E, Kantarjian HM: Adult acute myeloid leukemia. Mayo Clin Proc 2006;81:247–260 [PMID: 16471082].

Kaufman M, Rubin J, Rai K: Diagnosis and treating chronic lymphocytic leukemia in 2009. Oncology 2009;23:1030–1037 [PMID: 20017285].

Klein E, Kis LL, Klein G: Epstein-Barr virus infection in humans: from harmless to life endangering virus-lymphocyte intractions. Oncogene 2007;26:1297–1305 [PMID: 17322915].

Macsween KF, Higgins CD, McAulay KA, Williams H, Harrison N, Swerdlow AJ, Crawford DH: Infectious mononucleosis in university students in the United Kingdom: evaluation of the clinical features and consequences of the disease. Clin Infect Dis 2010;50:699–706 [PMID: 20121570].

Meckler G, Lindemulder S: Fever and neutropenis in pediatric patients with cancer. Emerg Med Clin N Am 2009;27:525–544 [PMID: 19646652].

Moon JM, Chun BJ: Predicting the complicated neutropenic fever in the emergency department. Emerg Med J 2009;26:802–806 [PMID: 19850806].

Neparidze N, Dhodapkar M: Waldenstrom's macroglobulinemia: recent advances in biology and therapy. Clin Adv Hematol Oncol 2009;7:677–681, 687–690 [PMID: 20040909].

Pui C, Evans WE: Treatment of acute lymphoblastic leukemia. N Engl J Med 2006;354:166–178 [PMID: 16407512].

Quintas-Cardama A, Cortes J: Chronic myeloid leukemia: Diagnosis and treatment. Mayo Clin Proc 2006;81:973–988 [PMID: 16835977].

Raab MS, Breitkreutz I, Richardson PG, Anderson KC: Multiple myeloma. Lancet 2009;374:324:39 [PMID: 19541364].

Rajkumar SV, et al: Multiple myeloma: Diagnosis and treatment. Mayo Clin Proc 2005;80:10 [PMID: 16212152].

Ravandi F, Kebriaei P: Philadelphia chromosome-positive acute lymphoblastic leukemia. Hematol Oncol Clin N Am 2009;23:1043–1063 [PMID: 19825452].

Ribera JM, Oriol A: Acute lymphoblastic leukemia in adolescents and young adults. Hematol Oncol Clin N Am 2009;23:1033–1042 [PMID: 19825451].

Schwartz RN, Vozniak M: Current and emerging treatments for multiple myeloma. J Manag Care Pharm 2008;14:12–19 [PMID: 18774881].

Sweetenham JW: Treatment of lymphoblastic lymphoma in adults. Oncology 2009:23:1015–1020 [PMID: 20017283].

Te Poele EM, Tissing WJE, Kamps WA, de Bont ESJM: Risk assessment in fever and neutropenia in children with cancer: What did we learn? Crit Rev Oncol Hematol 2009;72:45–55 [PMID: 19195908].

Vijay A, Gertz MA: Waldenstom macroglobulinemia. Blood 2007;109:5096–5103. [PMID: 17303694].

Yee KW, O'Brien SM: Chronic lymphocytic leukemia: diagnosis and treatment. Mayo Clin Proc 2006;81:1105–1129 [PMID: 16901035].

▼ TRANSFUSION THERAPY

Transfusion in the emergency department is primarily used for acute blood loss and circulatory shock. As medical care is moved to outpatient settings and emergency departments become more crowded, emergency physicians may be responsible for transfusion therapies once relegated to inpatient settings. An understanding of the available blood products, their indications, and potential complications is important.

PACKED RED BLOOD CELLS

Total blood volume is estimated to be 2.5 L/m^2, 75 mL/kg, or approximately 5 L in a 70-kg person. Fresh whole blood transfusion would be ideal to replace acute blood loss; however, during the storage of whole blood, platelets and other factors become inactive. In addition, the storage life of whole blood is less than that of individual components. Therefore, by necessity and convenience, whole blood is fractionated to its components for storage and transfusion.

Packed red blood cells (PRBCs) are prepared by the centrifugation of whole blood to remove about 80% of the plasma. Each unit of PRBCs has a hematocrit of 65–80% and a volume of approximately 250–350 mL (Table 41–15).

Table 41–15. Characteristics of Blood Products and Doses.

Component	Shelf-Life	Volume/Unit (mL)	Approximate Content/Unit[a]	Typical Dose	Typical Dosage Effect
Packed red blood cells	21–42 d	250–350	Red cells, 65–80%; plasma, 20–35%	2 units or 15 mL/kg	Raises hemoglobin concentration about 2g/dL.
Platelets (random-donor platelet concentrate)	5 d	50–60	Platelets, 7.5×10^{10}	6 units or 5 mL/kg	Raises platelet count about 50,000/μL
Platelets (apheresis-collected single-donor platelet concentrate)	5 d	250–300	Platelets, 3.6×10^{11}	1 unit	Raises platelet count about 50,000/μL.
Fresh frozen plasma	1 yr frozen and 24 h thawed	200–250	Each coagulation factor, 200–250 units; and fibrinogen, 400–500 mg	4 units or 15 mL/kg	Raises most coagulation factor levels about 20%.
Cryoprecipitate	1 yr frozen	20–50	Factor VIII, 80 units; fibrinogen, 225 mg; von Willebrand factor, variable amounts	10 units or 1 unit/5 kg	Raises fibrinogen about 75 mg/dL.

[a]Blood-derived components often contain white blood cells, red blood cells, platelets, and plasma unless they have been specially prepared.

Transfusion of 1 unit of PRBCs into a typical adult will increase the hematocrit by 3% or the hemoglobin by 1 g/dL.

The primary reason for emergency transfusion of PRBCs is acute blood loss or profound anemia with impaired oxygen delivery. According to various animal and human studies, lactic acid production increases, oxygen extraction ratio exceeds 50%, and the mortality rate starts to increase in otherwise stable patients with hemoglobin levels of 3.5–4.0 g/dL. In an animal model of coronary stenosis, adverse cardiac effects are seen with hemoglobin levels of 6.0 g/dL. However, there are reports of Jehovah's Witnesses, who generally refuse blood products, tolerating surgery with hemoglobin levels below 6.0 g/dL as long as intravascular volume is maintained. Patients with chronic anemia have developed compensation mechanisms so that chronic anemia is likely better tolerated than acute anemia. At least one recent study supports this hypothesis where patients undergoing cardiac surgery had no statistically significant risk of adverse outcome when the intraoperative hemoglobin nadir dropped below 7 g/dL. However, in the same study those patients whose hemoglobin nadir was less than 50% of the pre-operative level, a clear increase in adverse events was observed. This adds to the argument that guidelines should perhaps be focused more on the relative and not the absolute hemoglobin level as the trigger for transfusion. Common practice currently is based on consensus panels that have recommended transfusion for hemoglobin level less than 7 g/dL, whereas patients with hemoglobin levels greater than 10 g/dL rarely will benefit from transfusion. Some patients with cardiac or vascular disease may benefit from transfusion when hemoglobin levels are 7–10 g/dL. Transfusion thresholds for children may be higher and depend on the cause of their anemia.

Depending on the urgency of transfusion, most patients can be typed (ABO and RhD blood group type) and crossmatched against the blood intended for transfusion. The blood type can be determined in about 15 minutes, whereas typing and crossmatching takes approximately an hour. In critically ill patients, type O RhD-negative blood (universal donor) may be transfused. Type O RhD-positive blood may also be used if type O RhD-negative blood is not available, but it is not the blood of choice for women of childbearing potential. If an RhD-negative patient is transfused with 1 unit of RhD-positive PRBCs, approximately 80% will develop anti-D antibodies. Because the effect of 1 unit of PRBCs is small and clinically inconsequential, it is standard practice to transfuse a minimum of 2 units.

PRBCs may be further treated to meet specific uses, for example, leukocyte-reduced PRBCs, irradiated PRBCs, washed PRBCs, and frozen PRBCs. Leukocyte-reduced PRBCs have had 70–85% of the leukocytes removed. The advantages of leukocyte-reduced PRBCs are (1) to prevent or avoid nonhemolytic febrile reactions due to antibodies to WBC and platelets, if the patient has been exposed to previous transfusions or pregnancies, (2) to prevent sensitization in patients who may be eligible for bone marrow transplantation, and (3) to minimize the risk of virus transmission such as HIV and CMV. The leukocytes can be reduced by filtration or other methods before storage of the PRBCs or during transfusion. Irradiation of PRBCs eliminates the capacity of T cells to proliferate, therefore preventing the donor's T cells from reacting to the recipient's cells and causing graft-versus-host disease. Consider using irradiated cells in transplant patients, neonates, and immunocompromised patients.

Washed PRBCs are indicated in patients who have a hypersensitivity to plasma, such as IgA deficiency. For rare blood types, PRBCs may be frozen and saved for up to 10 years for later use. This process is more expensive than normal storage, and once thawed the blood must be washed and transfused within 24 hours.

One unit of PRBCs, about 250–350 mL in volume, is generally transfused over 1–2 hours. However, blood may be transfused more rapidly in patients with hemodynamic instability. During standard transfusions the initial rate is slower over the first 30 minutes, so that if there is incompatibility, the transfusion may be stopped.

PLATELETS

Platelet transfusions may be used either prophylactically to prevent bleeding or therapeutically when patients with thrombocytopenia are actively bleeding. Platelets are collected from whole blood donation or, more commonly, from single donors using apheresis techniques. One random-donor platelet concentrate prepared from 500 mL of donated whole blood contains an average of 7.5×10^{10} platelets (see Table 41–15). One apheresis-collected single-donor platelet concentrate generally contains $3–6 \times 10^{11}$ platelets, depending on local collection practice. Platelets should be given according to ABO compatibility, if available. A dose of one random-donor platelet concentrate per 10 kg (approximately 6–8 random-donor platelet concentrates for an adult) or one apheresis-collected single-donor platelet concentrate in an adult will increase the platelet count by about $50,000/\mu L$. Response to platelet transfusions is variable; therefore, platelet levels should be checked at 1 hour and 24 hours posttransfusion. Failure of platelets to rise appropriately may be due to increased consumption of platelets from an underlying process, destruction due to platelet antibodies, or sequestration due to hypersplenism. Transfused platelets should survive 3–5 days, unless a consumptive process is present.

The cause of thrombocytopenia is important in the decision to transfuse platelets. With ITP, an antiplatelet antibody-mediated consumptive process, the platelets are larger, younger, and more functional; therefore, prophylactic transfusion is rarely indicated despite very low platelet counts. However, with platelet hypoplasia, platelet function is impaired, making the risk of bleeding greater. Patients with comorbid diseases such as infection, fever, medications, and central nervous system involvement may be more likely to bleed or may be at higher risk if they bleed; therefore, the threshold for platelet transfusion is higher.

The dose of platelets should reflect the indication. In general, spontaneous bleeding is possible, and prophylactic transfusion is indicated with platelet counts less than 10,000/μL. Platelet counts of greater than 50,000/μL rarely cause significant bleeding. Indications for platelet transfusion include the following:

- Platelet count 10,000 μL in asymptomatic patients.
- Platelet count 15,000 μL and coagulation disorder or minor bleeding.
- Platelet count 20,000 μL and major bleeding.
- Platelet count 50,000 μL and invasive procedure (thoracentesis, paracentesis, LP) or general surgery required, or during massive transfusion (1–2 blood volumes).
- Platelet count 100,000 μL and neurologic or cardiac surgery required.

Like PRBCs, platelets can be leukocyte reduced or washed. Patients who have had repeated transfusions may become alloimmunized and refractory to platelet transfusion, noted by the lack of expected rise of platelet count after transfusion. Such patients need HLA-matched or crossmatched platelets. Other disorders may affect the efficacy of platelet transfusion including duration of platelet storage, sepsis, antibiotics, graft-versus-host disease, DIC, and splenomegaly.

Relative contraindications to platelet transfusion are consumptive processes such as TTP, hemolytic uremic syndrome, or heparin-induced thrombocytopenia, in which transfusion may worsen thrombosis and thereby renal failure and neurologic manifestations. Although as previously mentioned this warning may be overstated, in these diseases, platelet transfusion should be performed in consultation with a hematologist unless life-threatening hemorrhage is present.

FRESH FROZEN PLASMA

Fresh frozen plasma is plasma obtained after the separation of whole blood from RBCs and platelets, and then frozen within 6 hours. Each unit of FFP is 200–250 mL and contains about 1 unit of each coagulation factor and 2 mg of fibrinogen per milliliter (see Table 41–15). FFP is appropriate for rapid replacement of multiple coagulation deficiencies such as those occurring during liver failure, warfarin overdose, DIC, and massive transfusion in bleeding patients. Administration of FFP prophylactically to nonbleeding patients is not indicated, and prophylaxis is not always needed for some procedures in patients with a coagulopathy. For example, patients undergoing paracentesis and thoracentesis are not at increased risk of bleeding until the INR is greater than 2 times control. During massive transfusion with replacement of an entire blood volume, coagulation factor levels are about one-third of normal, and although PT and PTT may

be abnormal, clinical coagulopathy does not always occur. Indications for FFP transfusion include the following:

- Rapid reversal of warfarin therapy
- Bleeding and multiple coagulation defects as evidenced by prolonged PT, INR, and aPTT greater than 1.5 control (eg, liver disease, DIC)
- Correction of coagulation defects for which no specific factor is available (specific factor replacement is safer and better but may not always be available)
- Transfusion of more than one total blood volume with evidence of active bleeding and prolonged PT or PTT

Other possible indications for FFP in consultation with an appropriate specialist include TTP, antithrombin III deficiency, and hereditary angioedema (FFP contains C1 esterase and may reverse this potentially life-threatening condition when C1 esterase inhibitor concentrates are not immediately available).

Because the efficacy of transfused coagulation factors varies, the increase in specific coagulation factors seen after FFP infusion also varies. In general, 1 unit of FFP will increase most coagulation factors by 3–5% in a 70-kg adult. The common adult dose of 7–8 mL/kg (or 2 units of FFP in a 70-kg individual) will increase coagulation factors by only 10%, a clinically inconsequential benefit in most circumstances. For clinically relevant correction of coagulation factor deficiencies, a dose of 15 mL/kg (or 4 units in a 70-kg adult) is required (see Table 41–15). As indicated by the name, FFP is stored frozen, and there may be a delay while it is thawed. FFP should be ABO compatible. After transfusion, reevaluate bleeding and coagulation studies. If consumption is present, repeated FFP transfusion should be guided by the PT, INR, and aPTT response.

CRYOPRECIPITATE

Cryoprecipitate is the cold-insoluble protein fraction of FFP. Each unit of cryoprecipitate is about 20–50 mL and contains about 225 mg of fibrinogen, 80 units of factor VIII, and variable amounts of vWF (see Table 41–15). It also contains some factor XIII and fibronectin. With the development of recombinant factor VIII products for use in hemophilia, the primary role of cryoprecipitate is now replacement of fibrinogen or vWF. Bleeding patients with fibrinogen levels below 100 mg/dL due to severe liver disease, DIC, and dilutional coagulopathy may benefit from cryoprecipitate. The dose of cryoprecipitate is 1 unit/5 kg (or 10 units in an adult), which will raise fibrinogen by about 75 mg/dL.

OTHER PLASMA-DERIVED PRODUCTS

▶ Immunoglobulin for Intravenous Administration

Immunoglobulin for intravenous administration is a pooled IgG product that has been virally attenuated. Labeled indications for its use are ITP, pediatric HIV infection, and primary humoral immunodeficiency; it is also indicated for several new and off-label treatments such as for Kawasaki disease and autoimmune disorders. Dose and administration vary by the indication. Adverse reactions include anaphylaxis, especially in IgA deficiency (rare), febrile reactions, headache, and renal failure. Some patients develop transient positive serology to hepatitis C and CMV.

▶ Albumin

Albumin is a virally inactivated purified plasma protein that usually accounts for 50% of circulating protein and 75% of plasma oncotic pressure. Albumin transfusion in patients with decreased oncotic pressures may transiently increase oncotic pressure; however, the albumin rapidly distributes to extravascular spaces. Therefore, because of its cost and the lack of proved efficacy over crystalloid, there is no advantage of using albumin.

▶ Antithrombin III

Antithrombin III is a serum coagulation inhibitory protein. Deficiency can be acquired or congenital and is usually associated with difficult-to-treat thrombosis. Antithrombin III replacement is indicated in antithrombin III deficiency-related thrombosis and for thrombosis prophylaxis. This product should be considered in antithrombin III-deficient patients when difficulty is encountered in achieving adequate heparinization or when recurrent thrombosis is observed despite adequate anticoagulation. It is also reasonable to give concentrate to antithrombin III-deficient subjects before major surgeries or in obstetric situations where the risks of bleeding from anticoagulation are unacceptable. Currently, antithrombin III therapy is under investigation in sepsis, DIC, and other thrombotic diseases. The dose depends on the indication. An infusion of 50 units (1 unit is the amount in 1 mL of pooled plasma) of antithrombin III concentrate per kilogram will usually raise the plasma antithrombin III level to about 120% of normal in a congenitally deficient individual. Monitor plasma antithrombin III levels to ensure that they remain above 80%. Subsequent administration of antithrombin III at 60% of the initial dose at 24-hour intervals is recommended to maintain antithrombin III levels in the normal range.

MASSIVE TRANSFUSION

Massive transfusion is defined as the replacement of one blood volume or about 10 units of PRBCs within a 24-hour period. Patients receiving less than one blood volume rarely need hemostatic factor (ie, FFP, platelets) replacement. In patients receiving two blood volumes or more than 20 units of PRBCs, transfusion of coagulation factors and platelets may be empirically helpful. For patients who receive 1–2 times total blood volume, hemostatic factor replacement should be guided by considerations noted above: (1) If the

platelet count is less than 50,000/μL, platelet transfusion is warranted; (2) if the INR is greater than 1.5, FFP may be given; and (3) if fibrinogen levels are below 100 mg/dL, it may be replaced with cryoprecipitate. In massive transfusion, hypothermia is a risk, and blood and crystalloid as well as the patient should be warmed. Hypocalcemia from the preservative citrate-chelating calcium is rare but should be considered in massive transfusion if symptoms or signs of hypocalcemia are present.

▶ Massive Transfusion in the Trauma Patient

Recent data suggest that improved outcomes can be achieved in trauma patients when massive transfusion protocols approach a 1:1:1 ratio of PRBCs to platelets to FFP. Although still somewhat controversial practice, one study compared giving high (1:1.4) and low (1:8) ratios of FFP to PRBCs to trauma patients. In the high-ratio group the survival was 81% compared to 35% in these combat trauma patients. In the same study, just increasing to an intermediate ratio (1:2.5) almost doubled the survival rate to 66%. Other studies looking at similar high transfusion ratios of platelets as well as FFP have shown similar promising results.

COMPLICATIONS OF TRANSFUSION THERAPY

Up to 20% of all transfusions may lead to some type of adverse reaction. Although most of these reactions are minor, some are life threatening (Table 41–16). In critically ill patients, transfusion reactions may be difficult to identify; therefore, attention should be paid to unexpected changes in patient status during a transfusion.

▶ Infectious Complications of Blood Transfusion

Improved blood donor screening, serologic testing, safer handling of blood products, and viral inactivation of many blood products have reduced the risk of infection from blood transfusion (Table 41–17). Most cases of viral transmission are thought to occur during the window period between infection and antibody production in the donor. This window is reduced but not eliminated by the use of antigen testing. The prevalence of CMV-positive antibodies in the general population is 50–80%. Therefore, blood is not routinely tested for CMV unless the recipient is seronegative and is (1) pregnant, (2) a potential or present transplant candidate, (3) immunocompromised, or (4) a premature infant. Use of leukocyte-reduced blood components further decreases the risk of CMV transmission to susceptible populations because most of the virus resides in the leukocytes. Bacterial sepsis resulting from RBC transfusion is most commonly due to *Yersinia enterocolitica*, which is able to grow easily in refrigerated blood. The risk of bacterial sepsis is highest with random-donor platelet concentrates.

Table 41–16. Acute Transfusion Reactions.

Reaction Type	Symptoms and Signs	Management	Evaluation
Acute intravascular hemolytic reaction	Fever, chills, low back pain, dyspnea, tachycardia, shock	Immediately stop transfusion. Intravenous hydration to maintain diuresis.	Retype and crossmatch. Direct and indirect Coombs' tests. Serum haptoglobin, free hemoglobin, and indirect bilirubin. Urine hemoglobin.
Acute extravascular hemolytic reaction	Low grade fever, but may be asymptomatic	Stop transfusion. Rarely causes hemodynamic instability.	Retype and crossmatch. Direct and indirect Coombs' tests. Serum haptoglobin, free hemoglobin, and indirect bilirubin. Urine hemoglobin.
Febrile transfusion reaction	Fever, chills	Stop transfusion. Treat fever with acetaminophen.	Evaluate for intravascular hemolysis reaction and infection.
Allergic reaction	Mild: urticaria, pruritus. Severe: dyspnea, wheezing, hypotension, tachycardia, and shock	Stop infusion. Treat urticaria and pruritus with antihistamines; bronchospasm with inhaled β-adrenergic agonists; and shock with intravenous fluids and epinephrine.	For mild symptoms that resolve with antihistamines: no further evaluation. For severe symptoms: evaluate for intravascular hemolysis.

▶ Acute Hemolytic Transfusion Reactions

Hemolytic transfusion reactions occur when the recipient's antibodies recognize and induce hemolysis in the donor's RBCs. The reaction is usually acute when antibodies already exist in sufficient levels but can be delayed when an amnestic response occurs to a transfused RBC antigen to which the recipient is already sensitized. Acute transfusion reactions are most commonly caused by ABO incompatibility and are usually the result of technical errors made during the collection of blood, during pretransfusion testing, or in patient identification. The majority of transfusion-related fatalities are due to acute hemolytic reactions.

Table 41–17. Risk of Infection from Transfusion of Blood Products.

Cause	Estimated Frequency[a]
HIV-1	1:1,000,000 (200,000–2,000,000)
HIV-2	Unknown
HTLV-I/II	1:500,000 (250,000–2,000,000)
Hepatitis B	1:40,000 (30,000–250,000)
Hepatitis C	1:40,000 (30,000–150,000)
Parvovirus B19	1:10,000
Bacterial contamination	1:12,000 random-donor platelet concentrates 1:500,000 packed red blood cells

[a]One infection per number of units transfused (95% confidence interval where available).

The risk of acute hemolytic transfusion reaction due to incompatible blood is 1–4 per million units transfused; the fatality rate is approximately 50%. With acute hemolytic reaction, most of the transfused cells are destroyed, which may result in activation of the coagulation system with DIC and release of anaphylotoxins and other vasoactive amines. Evidence of this type of reaction includes back pain, pain at the site of the transfusion, headache, alteration of vital signs (fever, hypotension, dyspnea, tachycardia), chills, bronchospasm, pulmonary edema, bleeding due to developing coagulopathy, and evidence of new or worsening renal failure. Recognition of transfusion reactions in critically ill patients who may already be hypotensive and tachycardiac is difficult and requires a high degree of suspicion. Ongoing transfusion should be stopped immediately on first indication of potential problems. While laboratory confirmation is being performed, treat the sequelae of hemolysis supportively. Check renal function (serum creatinine, urinalysis), electrolytes, and coagulation status (PT, INR, aPTT). Maintain renal blood flow and urine output with fluids, mannitol, and furosemide as needed. Treat shock with volume and vasopressors to support blood pressure. Treat coagulopathy with FFP. Send the remaining donor blood, along with a posttransfusion blood specimen from the recipient, to the blood bank for analysis. Diagnosis is made by evidence of hemolysis (hemoglobinuria or hemoglobinemia) and by blood incompatibility. The blood bank will be able to test the blood, review records, confirm blood types, and should be able to determine if the patient's syndrome is from a transfusion reaction.

Since the risk of morbidity and mortality is proportional to the amount of blood received, in nonemergent transfusions, a low initial rate of infusion for the first 30 minutes allows for the identification of a transfusion reaction while minimizing the volume of blood transfused.

Extravascular Hemolytic Reactions

Extravascular hemolytic reactions occur in about 1 per 1000 PRBC units transfused. Hemolysis most commonly occurs in the spleen and occasionally in liver and bone marrow. This type of reaction is less serious than acute hemolytic transfusion reactions and is rarely fatal. It may be confirmed by a positive DAT, elevated unconjugated bilirubin, and poor response to transfusion. Treatment is supportive.

Febrile Transfusion Reactions

Febrile transfusion reactions are characterized by the onset of fever during or within a few hours of a blood transfusion. It is more common in multiparous women or multiply-transfused patients. The clinical presentation can range from a mild elevation in temperature to fever with rigors, headache, myalgias, tachycardia, dyspnea, or chest pain. Initially it may be difficult to differentiate a febrile reaction from the more serious hemolytic transfusion reaction or sepsis. Febrile transfusion reactions result from a combination of recipient antibody against donor leukocytes and the release of cytokines produced during storage. For non-leukocyte-reduced platelets, the risk of fever during transfusion is about 20%, and with leukocyte reduction, the incidence of febrile reactions is about 2%. For the first-time febrile reaction, or in any severe reaction, the transfusion should be stopped and the product returned to the blood bank. Laboratory investigation similar to that done for possible hemolytic transfusion reaction should be done and blood cultures should be obtained. Febrile transfusion reactions are usually self-limited and respond to antipyretics. Premedication with diphenhydramine has been recommended and indeed is common practice in some centers; however, recent data failed to show any benefit from this practice. For patients with recurrent febrile reactions, the use of leukocyte-reduced blood products and pretreatment with antipyretics may be helpful.

Allergic Transfusion Reactions

Allergic transfusion reactions are associated with onset of urticaria and pruritus during the transfusion and occur in approximately 1% of transfusions. Fortunately, only a small percentage of patients will have more severe reactions such as bronchospasm, wheezing, and anaphylaxis. These reactions are caused by an immune response to plasma proteins. Conservative therapy with an antihistamine usually controls the symptoms. The transfusion does not typically have to be stopped. For more severe symptoms the transfusion may need to be stopped and more aggressive management initiated. In patients with IgA deficiency, more severe anaphylactoid reactions can occur in response to exposure to the IgA in donor products. Washing the plasma from the cells minimizes this type of reaction.

Alderson P, Bunn F, Lefebvre C, Li WP, Li L, Roberts I, Schierhout G: Human albumin solution for resuscitation and volume expansion in critically ill patients. Cochrane Database Syst Rev 2002:CD001208 [PMID: 11869596].

Borgman MA, Spinella PC, Perkins JG, Grathwohl KW, Repine T, Beekley AC, Sebesta J, Jenkins D, Wade CE, Holcomb JB: The ratio of blood products transfused affects mortality in patients receiving massive transfusions at a combat support hospital. J Trauma 2007;63:805–813 [PMID: 18090009].

Carson JL, Hill S, Carless P, Hébert P, Henry D: Transfusion triggers: A systematic review of the literature. Transfus Med Rev 2002;16:187–199 [PMID: 12075558].

Cotton BA, Au BK, Nunez TC, Gunter OL, Robertson AM, Young PP: Predefined massive transfusion protocols are associated with a reduction in organ failure and postinjury complications. J Trauma 2009;66:41–48 [PMID: 19131804].

Gilstad CW: Anaphylactic transfusion reactions. Curr Opin Hematol 2003;10:419–423 [PMID: 14564171].

Goodnough LT, Brecher ME, Kanter MH, AuBuchon JP: Transfusion medicine. First of two parts—blood transfusion. N Engl J Med 1999;340:438–447 [PMID: 9971869].

Goodnough LT, Brecher ME, Kanter MH, AuBuchon JP: Transfusion medicine. Second of two parts—blood conservation. N Engl J Med 1999;340:525–533 [PMID: 10021474].

Holcomb JB, Wade CE, Michalek JE, Chisholm GB, Zarzabal LA, Schreiber MA, Gonzalez EA, Pomper GJ, Perkins JG, Spinella PC, Williams KL, Park MS: Increased plasma and platelet to red blood cell ratios improves outcome in 466 massively transfused civilian trauma patients. Ann Surg 2008;248:447–458 [PMID: 18791365].

Karkouti K, Wijeysundera DN, Yau TM, McCluskey SA, van Rensburg A, Beattie WS: The influence of baseline hemoglobin concentration on tolerance of anemia in cardiac surgery. Transfusion 2008;48:666–672 [PMID: 18194382].

Janatpour K, Holland PV: Noninfectious serious hazards of transfusion. Curr Hematol Rep 2002;1:149–155 [PMID: 12901137].

Kennedy LD, Case LD, Hurd DD, Cruz JM, Pomper GJ: A prospective, randomized, double-blind controlled trial of acetaminophen and diphenhydramine pretransfusion medication versus placebo for the prevention of transfusion reactions. Transfusion 2008;48:2285–2291 [PMID: 18673350].

Kleinman SH, Kamel HT, Harpool DR, Vanderpool SK, Custer B, Wiltbank TB, Nguyen KA, Tomasulo PA: Two-year experience with aerobic culturing of apheresis and whole blood-derived platelets. Transfusion 2006;46:1787–1794 [PMID: 17002636].

Kopko PM, Holland PV: Mechanisms for severe transfusion reactions. Transfus Clin Biol 2001;8:278–281 [PMID: 11499977].

Pekdemir M, Ersel M, Aksay E, Yanturali S, Akturk A, Kiyan S: Effective treatment of hereditary angioedema with fresh frozen plasma in an emergency department. J Emerg Med 2007;33:137–139 [PMID: 17692764].

Rebulla P: Platelet transfusion trigger in difficult patients. Transfus Clin Biol 2001;8:249–254 [PMID: 11499971].

Repine TB, Perkins JG, Kauvar DS, Blackborne L: The use of fresh whole blood in massive transfusion. J Trauma 2006;60:S59–S69 [PMID: 16763483].

Tobian AA, King KE, Ness PM: Transfusion premedications: a growing practice not based on evidence. Transfusion 2007;47:1089–1096 [PMID: 17524101].

Infectious Disease Emergencies

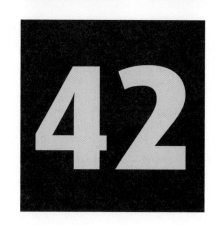

Jon Jaffe, MD
Taylor Ratcliff, MD

IMMEDIATE MANAGEMENT OF LIFE-THREATENING PROBLEMS

SEPTIC SHOCK

ESSENTIALS OF DIAGNOSIS

► Hyperthermia or hypothermia

► Tachycardia

► Tachypnea

► Leukocytosis or leukopenia

► Clinical evidence of infection

Sepsis is a state of systemic inflammation triggered by infection, affecting virtually every organ system. Although the mortality rate from sepsis has been falling, its incidence is increasing and septic shock now accounts for 10% of admissions to ICUs. Septic shock peaks in the sixth decade of life, and factors that can predispose to it include immunodeficiency, cancer, malnutrition, and genetics. Early recognition of sepsis is essential to providing effective care.

The systemic inflammatory response syndrome (SIRS) is characterized by a complicated interplay of multiple inflammatory mediators and may result from trauma, infection, burns, or diseases such as pancreatitis. It is defined as two or more alterations in the following physiologic parameters:

- Body temperature >38°C or <36°C

- Heart rate >90 beats per minute

- Respiratory rate >20, $Paco_2$ <32 mm Hg, or need for mechanical ventilation

- White blood count (WBC) >12,000/mm³ or <4000/mm³, or >10% bands

Sepsis is defined as SIRS with a documented infection, with the identification of microorganisms from a normally sterile fluid or visual inspection of a focus of infection. Severe sepsis consists of sepsis with evidence of end-organ hypoperfusion or dysfunction (eg, prolonged capillary refill, ARDS, mental status changes, or elevated lactate). Septic shock is severe sepsis with persistent hypotension despite adequate fluid resuscitation, with refractory septic shock defined as septic shock requiring high doses of vasopressors.

▶ Immediate Measures

A. Maintain Airway and Ventilation

Provide supplemental oxygen in order to maintain pulse oximetry >92%. Patients with profound mental status changes or hypoxia unresponsive to noninvasive ventilation may require intubation. Early on, arterial blood gas samples may show a respiratory alkalosis, with a metabolic acidosis becoming more prominent as the disease state progresses.

B. Establish Adequacy of Circulation

Adequate intravenous access should be obtained early on; consideration should be given to placing a central venous line that will allow monitoring of central venous pressure (CVP) as well as central venous oxygen saturation and allow the rapid infusion of crystalloid. Central venous lines also allow for the prolonged infusion of vasopressors if necessary; norepinephrine and dopamine are first-line agents. Routine use of low-dose ("renal protective") dopamine is not recommended. An arterial line should be considered for all patients receiving vasopressors.

Traditional clinical measures of perfusion (urine output, capillary refill, tachycardia) may miss hypoperfusion in a significant number of patients. In patients with an elevated lactate >4 or systolic pressure <90, early goal-directed therapy (EGDT) should be considered and aggressive resuscitation with crystalloid should be initiated until a CVP of 8–12 is reached.

C. Early Goal-Directed Therapy (EGDT)

EGDT reduces mortality in patients with sepsis. Although not completely clear, treatment should be initiated aggressively in a 6-hour window for optimal results. Patients who meet the SIRS criteria mentioned above and have a suspected infectious etiology along with either a SBP <90 or a lactate >4 mmol/L are candidates for EGDT. Patients should initially be given crystalloid infusion until a CVP of 8–12 is reached. Vasoactive agents are then added to maintain a mean arterial pressure (MAP) greater than 65 mm Hg using either norepinephrine or dopamine. There may be some benefit from addition of low-dose vasopressin in refractory shock. Once the desired MAP is reached, check a mixed venous or central venous oxygen saturation. Those with <70% saturation should be transfused with PRBCs to maintain a hematocrit of at least 30%. Patients with a mixed venous O_2 saturation <70% despite an adequate hematocrit should be given inotropic support with dobutamine starting at 2.5 $\mu g/kg/min$ and titrating to a maximum dose up to 20 $\mu g/kg$ to improve cardiac output.

D. Antibiotic Therapy

In accordance with current guidelines, appropriate antibiotics should be given within the first hour after sepsis is recognized. Remember to obtain needed cultures such as blood, urine, and fluid cultures prior to initiation of therapy, but do not delay treatment for such purposes. Recent literature has suggested that β-lactam monotherapy or later generation cephalosporins such as cefepime are effective and demonstrate equal efficacy compared to β-lactam and aminoglycoside dual therapy without the added nephrotoxicity. Local resistance patterns in the hospital and community as well as the patient's particular risk for resistant organisms should be considered in antibiotic selection. Gram-positive organisms are now more common as a source for sepsis than gram-negative organisms. Sepsis due to fungal organisms, although carrying a high mortality rate, is rare; routine antifungal coverage is not recommended unless the clinical picture dictates.

E. Source Control

When possible, the infectious etiology should be identified and removed surgically. A thorough examination for the source of infection is warranted, particularly in debilitated patients in whom complaints that would prompt evaluation of perineal infection or perirectal abscesses may be absent.

F. Adjunctive Therapies

Glycemic control is still encouraged with most sources recommending "moderate" control keeping glucose levels below 150 mg/dL but not in the normal range Corticosteroid therapy has been well researched with most recommendations indicating a "low-dose" steroid approach with no more than 200–300 mg of hydrocortisone per day. This has a higher grade of evidence in patients who fail to respond to a cosyntropin test or have fluid and vasopressor refractory hypotension. Continuation of this low dose and gradual tapering is encouraged. Efficacy regarding recombinant human activated protein C (RhAPC) is still debated but current guidelines continue to recommend RhAPC for patients with an APACHE II score >25 who are at high risk for mortality. Contraindications continue to include recent surgery or other risks for increased bleeding. The presence of disseminated intravascular coagulation (DIC) should not influence the decision to give RhAPC.

▶ Laboratory Findings

A. Cultures

Obtain cultures of blood, urine, and sputum if indicated on all patients with severe sepsis. Other sources such as wound, CSF, peritoneal fluid, intravenous catheter sites, and joint fluid may be sent for Gram stain and culture if clinically indicated.

B. Other Laboratory Studies

A CBC may show an increased or, more ominously, decreased WBC with evidence of left shift. Thrombocytopenia should prompt evaluation for DIC, with evaluation of fibrinogen and fibrin split products as well as partial thromboplastin (PT) and partial thromboplastin time (PTT). Elevated blood urea nitrogen (BUN) and creatinine may result from renal hypoperfusion, and elevated liver function tests (LFTs) may result from hepatic hypoperfusion. Blood glucose may be increased or decreased, and electrolyte abnormalities are common.

C. Radiologic Studies

Chest X-ray as well as focused imaging of other potential sources of infection should be pursued as needed.

▶ Pediatric Considerations

Vasopressors should only be initiated after adequate fluid resuscitation. Bolus of 20 mL/kg crystalloid should be given initially, with most patients responding after 40–60 mL/kg although larger amounts may be required. Dopamine is the first choice of support for pediatric patients with refractory hypotension despite fluid resuscitation. Patients with low cardiac output and high peripheral resistance may benefit from short-acting vasodilators such as nitroprusside. Infants are at higher risk for hypoglycemia and warrant more frequent monitoring. Blood pressure is not a reliable end point of resuscitation in children as they are able to maintain pressure by peripheral vasoconstriction and increased heart rate to a much greater degree than adults. Hypotension often heralds cardiovascular collapse.

▶ Disposition

All patients with severe sepsis or septic shock require hospitalization in an ICU.

Alejandria MM, Lansang MAD, Dans LF, Mantaring III JB: Intravenous immunoglobulin for treating sepsis and septic shock. Cochrane Database of Sys Rev 2002;CD001090 [PMID: 11869591].

Annane D, Bellissant E, Bollaert PE, Briegel J, Keh D, Kupfer Y: Corticosteroids for treating severe sepsis and septic shock. Cochrane Database Sys Rev 2004;CD002243 [PMID: 14973984].

Badaró R, Molinar F, Seas C, Stamboulian D, Mendonça J, et al: A multicenter comparative study of cefepime versus broad-spectrum antibacterial therapy in moderate and severe bacterial infections. Braz J Infect Dis 2002;6:206–218 [PMID: 12495602].

Dellinger RP, Levy MM, Carlet JM, et al: Surviving Sepsis Campaign: International guidelines for management of severe sepsis and septic shock: 2008. Intensive Care Med 2008;34:17–60 [PMID: 18058085].

Lindenauer PK, Rothberg MB, Nathanson BH, Pekow PS, Steingrub JS: Activated protein C and hospital mortality in septic shock: A propensity-matched analysis. Crit Care Med 2010;38:1101–1107 [PMID: 20154607].

Martí-Carvajal AJ, Salanti G, Cardona-Zorrilla AF: Human recombinant activated protein C for severe sepsis. Cochrane Database Sys Rev 2008;CD004388 [PMID: 18254048].

Paul M, Grozinsky S, Soares-Weiser K, Leibovici L: Beta lactam antibiotic monotherapy versus beta lactam-aminoglycoside antibiotic combination therapy for sepsis. Cochrane Database Sys Rev 2006;CD003344 [PMID: 16437452].

Sinert R, Bright L: Evidence-based emergency medicine/systematic review abstract. Empiric antibiotic therapy for sepsis patients: Monotherapy with beta-lactam or beta-lactam plus an aminoglycoside? Ann Emerg Med 2008;52:557–560 [PMID: 18294731].

IDENTIFICATION AND EVALUATION OF THE IMMUNOCOMPROMISED PATIENT WITH SUSPECTED INFECTION

▶ Classification of Immune Dysfunction

Those who have acquired their immunodeficiencies at birth or later in life through disease or medical treatment provide the emergency physician with a challenge to both recognize the specific problem and treat it appropriately. Excluding a defect in the skin, our primary host defense, we encounter problems associated with diseases of cell mediated and humoral immunity. In addition, there are infections associated with granulocytes in both function and quantity.

1. Neutropenia—Neutrophils ordinarily make up the majority of circulating WBCs. An absolute neutrophil count below 1000 is clinically significant. Most of these patients have undergone chemotherapy or irradiation. However, acquired neutropenia can come from an untoward response to a drug. The presence of fever >38.5°C, with neutropenia, suggests a related infection. For the evaluation of the source of infection, empiric therapy with admission to the hospital is indicated. Infections with pyogenic organisms such a *Staphylococcus aureus* and *Pseudomonas aeruginosa* are common. People with short-term neutropenia have a better prognosis than those chronically affected.

2. Cellular immune dysfunction—Problems with cell-mediated immunity involve the relationships between tissue macrophages, effector T cells, and cytotoxic T cells. Persons with AIDS, immunosuppression with antirejection drugs or antineoplastic drugs, as well as those with congenital T cell problems suffer from this. What is unique is that they are plagued by infections that are caused by intracellular pathogens. Mycobacteria, cytomegalovirus (CMV), and herpes simplex are a few examples.

3. Humoral immune dysfunction—It refers to decrease in antibody production or function as well as cytokine production, including pathogen and toxin neutralization, complement activation, and opsonin promotion of phagocytosis. From skin infection and vaginitis to frank sepsis, defects in humoral immunity result in a variety of conditions.

▶ Clinical Findings

A. Symptoms and Signs

Fever is the most reliable sign of infection in immunocompromised patients and must never be ascribed to an underlying disease until infection has been excluded. In patients with neutropenia with skin and soft tissue infections, there may be lack of abscess formation with persistent redness and pain being the only symptom. A careful evaluation of the lungs, mucous membranes, and the skin may give clues. Because of the relatively low pathogenicity of some of the offending organisms, even infections of the meninges may be subtle.

B. Laboratory and X-Ray Findings

The CBC is useful in evaluating the immunocompromised patient. With it, the absolute neutrophil count may be estimated by multiplying the percent of observed neutrophils by the total. The usual evaluations of the chest and urine as well as cultures of blood and other fluids will be helpful. Evaluation of the spinal fluid may involve testing for *Cryptococcus* or CMV, and also staining for AFB.

▶ Treatment

A. Antibiotics

In febrile patients with granulocyte counts under 1000, antibiotic therapy should be started immediately after material for routine culture has been obtained. Frequently, when the low count has been suspected, the neutropenic patient will have been started on antibiotics by their physician. Antibiotic adsorbing cultures should be used in this case. Circumstances that strengthen the directive for urgent empiric therapy include (1) a rapidly falling granulocyte count, (2) a very low granulocyte count (<500 further increases the risk of infection; <100 is frequently associated with fulminant infection), and (3) other clinical findings suggesting infection.

Current therapy for neutropenic fever varies depending on the illness severity and the "risk classification" of the patient based on disease process and overall health. Current literature identifies successful oral therapy for low risk, otherwise nonseptic, neutropenic patients. Combinations of fluoroquinolones and extended spectrum penicillins have been supported such as ciprofloxacin and amoxicillin/clavulanate.

For high risk or apparently toxic patients, hospital admission and monotherapy are often appropriate. Numerous recent articles support monotherapy, especially with late generation cephalosporins such as ceftazidime and cefepime. Other plausible monotherapy agents include ciprofloxacin and piperacillin–tazobactam. Classical dual therapy combines one of the above with an aminoglycoside such as gentamycin. Patients with risk factors for methicillin-resistant *Staph. aureus* (MRSA) colonization such as indwelling catheters, skin structure infections, or unknown origin sepsis may have vancomycin added to the regimen until cultures identify an organism.

B. Isolation

Neutropenic patients should be hospitalized in private rooms, and strict hand-washing precautions observed. Protective isolation as usually practiced (ie, masks and gowns) does not appear to be effective. Most infections neutropenic patients are derived from their own flora as opposed to infections from other persons and health care providers. This may explain why standard contact isolation procedures are usually minimally effective in preventing infections. Patients should be prescribed a diet free of fresh fruits and vegetables, which are often heavily contaminated with gram-negative bacilli.

3. Disposition

All immunocompromised patients with new findings of fever or other signs of infection should be hospitalized.

Bow EJ, Rotstein C, Noskin GA et al: A randomized, open-label, multicenter comparative study of the efficacy and safety of piperacillin-tazobactam and cefepime for the empirical treatment of febrile neutropenic episodes in patients with hematologic malignancies. Clin Infect Dis 2006;43:447–459 [PMID: 16838234].

Glasmacher A, von Lilienfeld-Toal M, Schulte S, et al: An evidence-based evaluation of important aspects of empirical antibiotic therapy in febrile neutropenic patients. Clin Microbiol Infect 2005;11:17–23 [PMID: 16138815].

Perrone J, et al: Emergency department evaluation of patients with fever and chemotherapy-induced neutropenia. J Emerg Med 2004;27:115 [PMID: 15261351].

Vidal L, Paul M, Bendor I, et al: Oral versus intravenous antibiotic treatment for febrile neutropenia in cancer patients: A systematic review and meta-analysis of randomized trials. J Antimicrob Chemother 2004; 54:29–37 [PMID: 15201227].

▼ EMERGENCY MANAGEMENT OF SPECIFIC DISORDERS

MENINGITIS AND MENINGOENCEPHALITIS

ESSENTIALS OF DIAGNOSIS

- ▶ Fever
- ▶ Nuchal rigidity
- ▶ Mental status change
- ▶ Photophobia
- ▶ Headache
- ▶ CSF findings

▶ General Considerations

Meningitis is defined as inflammation of the meninges; it is the major infectious syndrome affecting the CNS. When meningitis is accompanied by parenchymal involvement, it is referred to as meningoencephalitis. The epidemiology of meningitis has changed drastically since *Haemophilus influenzae* immunizations became available. The incidence of meningitis caused by this agent has decreased by 94%. The average age of meningitis cases peaks in a bimodal fashion. Infants and young adults around the age of 18 are at highest risk in terms of incidence and disease burden. The current mortality according to the Centers for Disease Control (CDC) is 10–14% but with 11–19% of survivors

have some permanent neurologic sequelae. Survival depends on prompt recognition and early treatment.

▶ Clinical Findings

A. Symptoms and Signs

Patients with meningitis present with fever, headache, nuchal rigidity, and mental dysfunction. Seizures and cranial nerve deficits are also common. Infants with meningitis may present with only vomiting, lethargy, irritability, and poor feeding. Elderly patients may present with only low-grade fever and delirium. The headache associated with meningitis is continuous and throbbing and, although generalized, is usually most prominent over the occiput. The pain is increased by jugular vein compression or any other maneuver that increases intracranial pressure (eg, coughing, sneezing, and straining at stool). Neck stiffness and other signs of meningeal irritation must be sought with care because they may not be obvious early and may disappear during coma. Patients with meningitis may be divided into two groups on the basis of the presentation of the disorder.

1. Acute presentation (septic meningitis)—Symptoms and signs have been present for less than 24 hours and are rapidly progressive. The causative organisms are usually pyogenic bacteria, and the mortality rate is approximately 50%.

2. Subacute presentation—Symptoms and signs have been present for 1–7 days. Meningitis is due to bacteria, viruses, or fungi, and the death rate due to bacterial infection is much lower than in patients with acute presentation of disease. Aseptic meningitis is typically caused by viruses (enteroviruses, herpes simplex virus [HSV], or Epstein–Barr virus). Suggestive features such as respiratory tract syndrome and hand–foot–mouth syndrome strengthen the diagnosis. Chronic meningitis is defined as meningitis present for more than 4 weeks; the major infectious causes are tuberculous meningitis and cryptococci.

B. Laboratory Findings

Perform lumbar puncture immediately in the absence of papilledema and focal neurologic findings. For contraindications to lumbar puncture, see Table 42–1. Interpretation of

Table 42–1. Contraindications to Lumbar Puncture.

Impending or established septic shock
Glasgow Coma Scale score of less than 13 or deteriorating score
Other signs of raised intracranial pressure (marked instability of blood pressure or heart rate)
Focal neurologic signs
Confident diagnosis of meningococcal infection
Infection at the planned lumbar puncture site
Bleeding disorder
Immune compromised patient with known decrease in CD4 count w/o therapy

Table 42–2. Cerebrospinal Fluid Findings in Meningitis.

Measure	Normal	Bacterial Meningitis	Viral Meningitis	Fungal Meningitis	Tuberculous Meningitis	Abscess
WBC/mL	0–5	>1000	<1000	100–500	100–500	10–1000
PMNs (%)	0–15	>80	<50	<50	<50	<50
Lymphocytes (%)	>50	<50	>50	>80	Increased monocytes	Variable
Glucose	45–65	<40	45–65	30–45	30–45	45–60
CSF–blood glucose ratio	0.6	<0.4	0.6	<0.4	<0.4	0.6
Protein	20–45	>150	50–100	100–500	100–500	>50
Pressure	6–20	>25–30	Variable	>20	>20	Variable

PMN, polymorphonuclear leukocytes; WBC, white blood cells.

CSF findings is shown in Table 42–2. Draw blood for serum glucose measurement and for culture. Gram staining of CSF will allow presumptive identification of the causative agent. Even if no organisms are seen on Gram-stained smears of CSF, bacterial meningitis is a likely diagnosis and warrants empiric antimicrobial therapy if total CSF leukocytes number more than 1000, if polymorphonuclears (PMNs) make up at least 85% of the white cells in CSF, or if the CSF glucose is less than 50% of the serum glucose level in a simultaneously drawn blood sample. The differential diagnosis in patients in whom PMNs are less than 85% of the CSF white count must include several possible causes of acute lymphocytic meningitis (Table 42–3). Prior treatment with antibiotics could result in sterile cultures of CSF.

▶ Treatment

A. Antimicrobial Therapy

1. Acute presentation—When bacterial meningitis is suspected, begin administration of appropriate empiric antibiotics immediately (Table 42–4). Give the first dose as soon as

Table 42–3. Some Causes of Acute Lymphocytic Meningitis.

Early or partially treated bacterial meningitis
Viral meningitis and meningoencephalitis (including HIV)
Tuberculous or fungal meningitis
Syphilis
Parameningeal infection (e.g., brain abscess)
CNS collagen vascular disease
CNS tumor, leukemia, lymphoma, or carcinomatosis
Intracranial injury (e.g., subdural hematoma)
Subarachnoid hemorrhage

samples of CSF and blood have been collected for tests; the goal is to begin intravenous administration of antimicrobials within 30 minutes after a patient with acute presentation of meningitis has sought treatment. If lumbar puncture must be delayed for computed tomography (CT) scan, obtain two blood samples for culture and begin appropriate antimicrobials. Perform lumbar puncture after mass lesion has been excluded and obtain CSF for microscopic examination as soon as possible. For pathogen-specific antibiotic therapy for bacterial meningitis, see Table 42–5.

2. Subacute presentation—Treatment is based on results of Gram staining of CSF and other tests. If meningitis is likely but Gram staining is negative, begin empiric treatment based on the patient's clinical characteristics pending the results of CSF studies.

3. Suspected brain abscess—In patients thought to have a brain abscess, begin intravenous therapy with a combination of penicillin and metronidazole or a third-generation cephalosporin. Obtain an emergency CT scan.

B. Corticosteroids

Studies have failed to clearly define the utility of corticosteroids in the patient with bacterial meningitis. However, evidence does suggest a potential benefit and no prominent negative effects. Therefore, use is recommended, especially with *S. pneumoniae* meningitis in adults and in children older than 2 months. Dexamethasone 10 mg should be administered to adults preferably prior to, or along with antibiotics. Utilization after antibiotic administration has been found not to be helpful.

C. Supportive Care

General supportive care measures should be started in the emergency department. Protect the patient's airway, and provide padded rails or restraints for agitated or delirious

Table 42–4. Recommended Empiric Antimicrobial Therapy for Bacterial Meningitis Based on Age.

Age	Major Pathogens	Antibiotic Regimen	Alternative Regimens	Comment
Less than 3 months	Group B streptococci, *Listeria monocytogenes*, *Escherichia coli*, *Strep. pneumoniae*	Ampicillin plus ceftriaxone (or cefotaxime)	Chloramphenicol plus gentamicin	CSF levels are not reliable in low-birth-weight infants and should be monitored
3 months– 18 years	*Neisseria meningitidis*, *S. pneumoniae*, *Haemophilus influenzae*	Ceftriaxone (or cefotaxime)	Meropenem or Chloramphenicol	Add vancomycin in areas with greater than 2% incidence of highly drug resistant *S. pneumoniae*
18-50 years	*S. pneumoniae*, *N. meningitides*, *H. influenzae*	Ceftriaxone (or cefotaxime)	Meropenem or chloramphenical	Add vancomycin in areas with greater than 2% incidence of highly drug resistant *S. pneumoniae*
50 years and older	*S. pneumoniae*, *L. monocytogenes*, gram-negative bacilli	Ampicillin plus ceftraxone (or cefotaxime)	Ampicillin plus fluoroquinolone (ciprofloxacin, levofloxacin)	Add vancomycin in areas with greater than 2% incidence of highly drug resistant *S. pneumoniae*; for patients who have major penicillin allergy, TMP-SMZ can substitute for ampicillin to treat *L. monocytogenes* infection

patients. If seizures occur, begin anticonvulsant therapy. Avoid overhydration, which may worsen cerebral edema.

▶ Disposition

Immediate hospitalization is warranted for all patients, except those with aseptic (viral) meningitis who appear well and can be observed at home.

Assiri AM, Alasmari FA, Zimmerman VA, Baddour LM, Erwin PJ, Tleyjeh IM: Corticosteroid administration and outcome of adolescents and adults with acute bacterial meningitis: A meta-analysis. Mayo Clin Proc. 2009;84:403–409. [PMID: 19411436]

Chaudhuri A, Martinez-Martin P, Kennedy PG, Andrew Seaton R, Portegies P, Bojar M, Steiner I; EFNS Task Force: EFNS guideline on the management of community-acquired bacterial meningitis: Report of an EFNS Task Force on acute bacterial meningitis in older children and adults. Eur J Neurol 2008;15:649–659 [PMID: 18582342].

Daley AJ: Meningococcal disease. Aust Fam Phys 2003;32:597 [PMID: 12973866].

van de Beek, de Gans J, Tunkel AR, Wijdicks EF: Community-acquired bacterial meningitis in adults. N Engl J Med 2006 Jan;354:44–53 [PMID: 16394301].

van de Beek D, de Gans J, McIntyre P, Prasad K: Corticosteroids for acute bacterial meningitis. Cochrane Database of Sys Rev 2007;CD004405 [PMID: 17253505].

Tunkel AR, Hartman BJ, Kaplan SL, et al: Practice guidelines for the management of bacterial meningitis. Clin Infect Dis 2004;39:1267–1284 [PMID: 15494903].

Table 42–5. Pathogen-Specific Therapy for Patients Who Have Bacterial Meningitis.

Organism	Preferred Regimen	Alternative Choices	Duration (days)
Group B streptococci	Penicillin G (or ampicillin)	Vancomycin	14-21
Haemophilus influenzae	Ceftriaxone (or cefotaxime)	Chloramphenicol	7-10
Listeria monocytogenes	Ampicillin plus gentamicin	TMP-SMZ	14-21
Neisseria meningitidis	Penicillin G (or ampicillin)	Ceftriaxone (or cefotaxime); chloramphenicol	7-10
Strep. pneumoniae (MIC <0.1)	Ceftriaxone (or cefotaxime)	Penicillin; meropenem	10-14 (MIC <0.1)
S. pneumoniae (MIC <0.1)	Vancomycin plus ceftriaxone (or cefotaxime)	Substitute rifampin for vancomycin; use vancomycin monotherapy if patient is highly allergic to cephalosporins	10-14

MIC, minimum inhibitory concentration.

PNEUMONIA

1. Pneumonia in Neonates (Aged <2 Weeks)

 ESSENTIALS OF DIAGNOSIS

► Grunting, tachypnea
► Focal lung exam
► Radiographic findings

▶ Clinical Findings

A. Symptoms and Signs

The early neonatal period, birth to 2 weeks, is dominated by group B *Streptococcus*, *Listeria*, and gram-negative *Escherichia coli* and *Klebsiella pneumoniae*. These are acquired at birth. These infants will have poor feeding, paradoxical irritability, grunting, and tachypnea. Cough may only be an infrequent feature. Sepsis or meningitis may accompany the pneumonia.

B. Laboratory and X-Ray Findings

A total sepsis workup is clearly indicated for these infants. Laboratory findings will vary, but the diagnosis will be confirmed with the chest X-ray.

▶ Treatment and Disposition

Appropriate antibiotic therapy is outlined in Table 42–6. All neonates should be hospitalized.

2. Pneumonia in Infants and Children (Aged 2 Months to 5 Years)

▶ Clinical Findings

A. Symptom and Signs

In infants over 2 months of age, more classic signs and symptoms of pneumonia are present but tachypnea predominates. Cough, grunting, rales, and wheezing may be seen and fever is variable.

B. Laboratory and X-Ray Findings

As viruses predominate this age group, an elevation of the WBC above 15,000/mm³ is suggestive but not diagnostic for bacterial infection. Arterial blood gas analysis may be obtained to assess the adequacy of ventilation. Electrolyte levels and BUN are useful in assessing the degree of dehydration, the most frequent complication seen in this age group. Obtaining sputum is difficult without direct tracheal aspiration, or pneumocentesis. Blood cultures though frequently obtained are rarely positive as *H. influenzae* and *S. pneumoniae* have become rarer. Indirect identification of respiratory

Table 42–6. Empiric Antibiotic Treatment of Pneumonia in the Pediatric Population.

Age Group	Cause	Primary Treatment	Alternative Treatment
Neonates	Group B streptococcus *Listeria* sp. Coliforms *S. aureus* *P. aeruginosa*	Ampicillin *or* Nafcillin *plus* Gentamicin	Vancomycin *plus* Cefotaxime
1–3 months	*Chlamydia* sp. *S. pneumoniae*	Erythromycin *or* Amoxicillin	Cefuroxime
3 months to 5 years	*S. pneumoniae* *Mycoplasma* spp. *Chlamydia* spp.	Amoxicillin (+/–) Macrolide	Cefuroxime *or* Ceftriaxone
5 years to 18 years	*Mycoplasma* spp. *S. pneumoniae*	Macrolide	Amoxicillin-clavulanate *or* Cefuroxime *plus* Macrolide

syncytial virus (RSV) and influenza have been very helpful in confirming the etiology of the pneumonia.

▶ Treatment and Disposition

Appropriate antibiotic therapy should be guided by age and is outlined in Table 42–6. Severely ill infants (ie, with respiratory distress, hyperthermia, or Po₂ <70) should be hospitalized.

3. Pneumonia in Older Children (Aged 5–18 Years)

▶ Clinical Findings

A. Symptoms and Signs

Infection with *Mycoplasma pneumoniae* begins to predominate. Cough rales and wheezing may be seen. Bullous myringitis helps confirm the etiology and thus tailor appropriate treatment. Fever is very common with pneumonia in this age group, while cough may be present, abdominal pain may be the child's chief complaint.

B. Laboratory and X-Ray Findings

In pneumonia due to *M. pneumoniae*, the white cell count is usually normal or slightly elevated, and chest X-ray reveals scattered segmental infiltrates, atelectasis, interstitial disease, or, less frequently, lobar consolidation.

In pneumonia due to bacteria other than *M. pneumoniae*, the white cell count usually exceeds 15,000. Chest X-ray abnormalities include patchy infiltrates, increased bronchovascular markings, lobar consolidation, cavitary infiltrates, and pleural effusions or empyema. Gram-stained smears of sputum may allow for a presumptive diagnosis if numerous PMNs, few epithelial cells, and a predominant microorganism are found. Pleural fluid should be examined if present.

▶ Treatment and Disposition

Appropriate antibiotic therapy is outlined in Table 42–6. Hospitalization is indicated for patients with pneumonia who require oxygen or have intractable vomiting. In addition, patients with preexisting pulmonary disease and all patients with bilateral bacterial pneumonia should be hospitalized.

4. Pneumonia in Adults

▶ General Considerations

Complete CDC data from 2006 indicates pneumonia and respiratory infection to be the 8th leading cause of death in the United States. Over 1.2 million patients were admitted with pneumonia with an average of 5.1 days hospital stay. This contributes to a multibillion dollar cost related to pneumonia care. *S. pneumoniae* remains the most common cause of community-acquired pneumonia (CAP) in the adult population, with atypical organisms such as *M. pneumoniae* and *Chlamydiapneumoniae* common in young adults. Patients with structural lung disease, the elderly, nursing home residents, alcoholics, those with recent antibiotic exposure, and those who are immunosuppressed (>10 mg/d of prednisone) or have recently been hospitalized are more likely to be infected with resistant *S. pneumoniae* or gram-negative organisms. Influenza, varicella, and RSV (particularly in nursing home residents) are common viral causes of CAP.

▶ Clinical Findings

A. Symptoms and Signs

Atypical or viral pneumonias may develop insidiously with focal respiratory complaints preceded by a 3- to 5-day history of malaise, fever, myalgias, and sore throat. Auscultation of the lungs typically reveals diffuse findings such as wheezing or fine rales, which may be slightly more prominent in the lung bases. Bacterial pneumonias are characterized by an abrupt onset of fever, chills, cough often productive of purulent or blood-tinged sputum, and pleuritic chest pain. Physical examination reveals a focal area of rales and possible consolidation. *Legionella* pneumonia presents as a severe form of lobar pneumonia and is classically associated with diarrhea. The diagnosis of pneumonia in nursing-home residents requires a high index of suspicion as they often have nonspecific presentations, often in the absence of cough, fever, and dyspnea. Aspiration pneumonia is more common in the elderly, those with poor dentition, and alcoholics, and is characterized by very foul-smelling sputum.

B. Laboratory and X-Ray Findings

A chest X-ray should be obtained to confirm the diagnosis of pneumonia, help guide initial treatment, and exclude other etiologies. Chest X-ray findings with the associated organisms are outlined in Table 42–7. A right lower lobe or right upper lobe infiltrate in the setting of aspiration may represent aspiration pneumonitis rather than pneumonia if other clinical indicators of infection are absent. CT may be helpful in differentiating between lung abscess and empyema when the chest X-ray is equivocal. An oxygen saturation should be obtained on all patients with an arterial blood gas reserved for severely ill patients. Gram staining and culture of the

Table 42–7. Chest X-Ray Findings in Pneumonia.

Finding	Description	Associated Organisms
Lobar consolidation	Nonsegmental, homogenous consolidation involving one lobe; may have air bronchograms	*S. pneumoniae* *K. pneumoniae* *L. pneumophila*
Bronchopneumonia	Peribronchial thickening, poorly defined air space opacities ("patchy" consolidation)	*S. aureus* *H. influenzae*, most gram-negative rods, fungi
Interstitial pneumonia	Edema and infiltrate in alveolar septa, surrounding small airway/vessels	Viruses *M. pneumoniae* *P. carinii*
Abscess	Air-fluid level, often with adjacent parenchymal consolidation	Anaerobes *S. aureus* *P. aeruginosa*
Effusion	Assumes shape of pleural space; if air-fluid level present, longer on lateral view	Any; more common in severe pneumonia ~10% *S. pneumoniae*; almost 50% of *L. pneumophila* and *H. influenzae*
Pneumatocele	Thin-walled, gas-filled spaces within parenchyma	Present in up to 50% *S. aureus* pneumonias in children

sputum is the most valuable study for patients in whom it is important to determine an etiology (critically ill, those at risk for resistant organisms). Urinary antigen testing for *Legionella pneumophila* and *S. pneumoniae* is more sensitive at detecting infection with these organisms than are blood cultures but provides no data on antibiotic sensitivity. In patients younger than 50 years with no significant comorbidities, who are not hypoxic, and who do not have any of the abnormal physical examination findings, no further laboratory testing may be needed. Leukocytosis is a common but nonspecific finding, while leukopenia in the setting of clinical infection is often ominous. Elderly patients commonly show prerenal azotemia, and hyponatremia with elevated LFTs are associated with *Legionella* pneumonia.

▶ Treatment

Initial treatment is empiric and based on the presumed causative organism for the patient's clinical presentation. Hospitalized patients should be divided into one of three categories: CAP, health care associated pneumonia (HCAP) early or with no risk factors for multidrug resistant pathogens (MDR), and HCAP late or with risk factors for MDR (Table 42–8).

Recommended empiric antibiotic regimens for both CAP and HCAP are listed in Table 42–9. Current literature reviews have failed to demonstrate any statistically significant research demonstrating higher therapeutic success with any one outpatient regimen for CAP. Prompt recognition and treatment with a variety of agents as initial therapy seem appropriate. Although coinfection with atypical organisms

Table 42–8. Pneumonia Classification.

Community-acquired pneumonia (CAP)—No recent contact with health care system or hospital admissions in past

Health care associated pneumonia, early/low-risk (HCAP)—Includes patients within 5 days of hospital admission to non-ICU setting, not intubated. Otherwise not meeting multi drug resistant (MDR) pathogen risk below.

Health care associated pneumonia, late/MDR risk (HCAP)—Includes patients with the following risk factors:
- Antimicrobial therapy in preceding 90 days
- Current hospitalization of 5 days or more
- High frequency of antibiotic resistance in the community or in the specific hospital unit
- Hospitalization for 2 days or more in the preceding 90 days
- Residence in a nursing home or extended care facility
- Home infusion therapy (including antibiotics) or home wound care
- Chronic dialysis within 30 days
- Family member with multidrug-resistant pathogen
- Immunosuppressive disease and/or therapy

Table 42–9. Empiric Antibiotic Treatment of Pneumonia in Adults.

Age Group	First-Line Treatments	Alternative Treatment
CAP (not hospitalized)	Azithromycin 500 mg PO × 1 then 250 mg/d × 4 d Clarithromycin 500 mg PO b.i.d. × 10 d Erythromcyin 500 mg PO q.i.d. × 10 d Doxycycline 100 mg PO b.i.d. × 10 d	Amoxicillin-clavulanate 875 mg PO b.i.d. × 10 d Levofloxacin 750 mg PO q.d. × 10 d Moxifloxacin 400 mg PO q.d. × 10 d Cefuroxime 500 mg PO b.i.d. × 10 d
CAP (hospitalized medical bed)	Respiratory fluoroquinolone[a]	Macrolide *plus* β-lactam
CAP (hospitalized ICU bed)	Beta-lactamt[b] *plus* Respiratory fluoroquinolone[a]	Respiratory fluoroquinolone[a] *plus* Clindamycin
HCAP (not admitted)	Respiratory fluoroquinolone[a]	Amoxicillin-clavulanate *plus* Macrolide
HCAP Early/Low-Risk MDR	Ceftriaxone or Respiratory fluoroquinolone[a]	Ampicillin/sulbactam
HCAP Late/MDR Risk	Cefepime or ceftazidime *plus* Ciprofloxacin or levofloxacin *plus* Linezolid or vancomycin	Imipenem/meropenem *or* Piperacillin-tazobactam *plus* Cipro or levofloxacin
Aspiration	Clindamycin	Amoxicillin-clavulanate, imipenem, meropenem

[a]Moxifloxacin, levofloxacin, gemifloxacin
[b]Cefotaxime, ceftriaxone, or ampicillin–sulbactam

is common, it is not clear whether adding atypical coverage is beneficial in younger patients. Initial enteral treatment recommendations include macrolides as a common first-line choice with amoxicillin/clavulanate and doxycycline cited as appropriate other choices. Respiratory fluoroquinolones are commonly second-line therapy for failed treatment or high-risk patients and should probably be reserved for this use.

Hospitalized patients should be treated with a β-lactam agent and macrolide or a fluoroquinolone as monotherapy, with consideration given to resistant organisms and appropriate gram-negative coverage, particularly for ICU patients. Administration of antibiotics rapidly following presentation and diagnosis is critical. Although classically the standard goal for administration of parenteral antibiotics has been 4 hours, data has shown that time periods up to 6 hours may still be acceptable. Clearly earlier administration is preferable and decreases mortality, even if the diagnosis remains unclear and the initial antibiotic regimen may not be optimal.

▶ Disposition

The use of validated scoring systems such as the Pneumonia PORT Severity Index has been demonstrated to determine effectively that patients may be safely treated on an outpatient basis (see Table 42–10). Classes I, II, and III (≤ 90 points) patients are at sufficiently low risk for death that they can be considered for outpatient treatment or an abbreviated course of inpatient care. Class IV and V patients should be hospitalized.

American Thoracic Society; Infectious Diseases Society of America: Guidelines for the management of adults with hospital-acquired, ventilator-associated, and healthcare-associated pneumonia. Am J Respir Crit Care Med 2005;171:388–416 [PMID: 15699079].

Bjerre LM, Verheij TJM, Kochen MM: Antibiotics for community acquired pneumonia in adult outpatients. Cochrane Database Sys Rev 2009;CD002109 [PMID: 19821292].

Centers for Disease Control: Fast stats pneumonia. Atlanta, GA, 2010. www.cdc.gov/nchs/fastats/pneumonia.htm (last accessed August 17, 2010).

Cincinnati Children's Hospital Medical Center. Evidence based care guideline for community acquired pneumonia in children 60 days through 17 years of age. Cincinnati, OH, 2006. www.guideline.gov/summary/summary.aspx?doc_id=9690 (last accessed August 17, 2010).

Lutfiyya MN, Henley E, Chang LF, Reyburn SW: Diagnosis and treatment of community-acquired pneumonia. Am Fam Physician 2006;73:442–450 [PMID: 16477891].

Mandell LA, Wunderink RG, Anzueto A, et al: Infectious Diseases Society of America/American Thoracic Society consensus guidelines on the management of community-acquired pneumonia in adults. Clin Infect Dis 2007;44:S27–S72 [PMID: 17278083].

Zhanel GG, DeCorby M, Laing N, et al: Antimicrobial-resistant pathogens in intensive care units in Canada: results of the Canadian National Intensive Care Unit (CAN-ICU) study, 2005-2006. Antimicrob Agents Chemother 2008;52:1430–1437 [PMID: 18285482].

Table 42–10. Pneumonia PORT Severity Index.[a]

Characteristic	Points Assigned
Age	
Men	Age
Women	Age−10
Nursing Home Resident	+10
Coexisting Illnesses	
Neoplastic disease	+30
Liver disease	+20
CHF	+10
Cerebrovascular disease	+10
Renal disease	+10
Physical Examination Findings	
Altered mental status	+20
Respiratory rate ≥30/min	+20
SBP <90 mm Hg	+20
Temperature <35 or > 40	+15
Pulse ≥125/min	+10
Laboratory/X-Ray Findings	
Arterial pH <7.35	+30
BUN >30 mg/dL	+20
Sodium <130 mmol/L	+20
Glucose ≥250 mg/dL	+10
Hematocrit <30%	+10
Pao_2 <60 mm Hg	+10
Pleural effusion	+10
Risk Group (# of points)	Mortality
I (pts not calculated)	0–0.4%
II (≤70)	0.4–0.7%
III (71–90)	0–2.8%
IV (91–130)	8.2–9.3%
V (>130)	27–31.1%

[a]Patients less than 50, without active neoplastic disease, liver disease, CHF, cerebrovascular disease, or renal disease, and who have normal or only mildly deranged vital signs and normal mental status are placed into Risk Group I.

BRONCHIOLITIS

ESSENTIALS OF DIAGNOSIS

▶ Wheezing

▶ Cough

▶ Low-grade fever

▶ Tachypnea

▶ General Considerations

Bronchiolitis is an acute inflammation of the bronchioles, most commonly resulting from a viral infection. It typically affects children from birth to age 2 years and occurs mostly during the winter months (November to March). RSV is the cause in 60–90% of cases; the remaining cases are caused by parainfluenza, adenovirus, rhinovirus, and influenza and human Bocavirus.

▶ Clinical Findings

A. Symptoms and Signs

The child with bronchiolitis typically has a 4-day history of clear profuse rhinorrhea and congestion, usually accompanied by low-grade fever followed by the development of a cough, tachypnea, and wheezing. Signs of respiratory distress including cyanosis and accessory muscle use may be evident, and inspiratory wheezing and crackles are typically heard on auscultation of the patient's lungs. Apnea can occur, and approximately 2–7% of children ill enough to require hospitalization develop respiratory failure, and require intubation.

B. Laboratory and X-Ray Findings

A nasopharyngeal aspirate can be sent for rapid identification of RSV and influenza and have become the standard for diagnosis. A positive test does not preclude the diagnosis of asthma that is also an inflammatory process. A chest X-ray is recommended for all patients who do not already have chronic respiratory problems and may show findings characteristic of bronchiolitis: hyperinflation, atelectasis, peribronchial thickening, and diffuse interstitial infiltrates.

▶ Treatment

Oxygen rapidly relieves hypoxemia and is the most important therapeutic agent for bronchiolitis. A trial of bronchodilators is indicated. Studies evaluating the use of glucocorticoids show no improvement in outcome, provided that asthma can be excluded. Ribavirin is a synthetic nucleoside analogue that has virostatic activity against RSV and is recommended for use in patients with a history of congenital heart disease or chronic lung disease, preterm infants, infants younger than 6 weeks, and infants ventilated for RSV infection.

▶ Disposition

Criteria suggestive of severe disease include the following: ill or toxic appearing, oxygen saturation less than 95%, gestational age less than 34 weeks, respiratory rate greater than 70 breaths/min, atelectasis on X-ray, and age less than 3 months. The infant's oxygen saturation while feeding is the single best objective measure of severe disease.

Allander T, Jartti T, Gupta S, Niesters HG, Lehtinen P, Osterback R, Vuorinen T, Waris M, Bjerkner A, Tiveljung-Lindell A, van den Hoogen BG, Hyypiä T, Ruuskanen O: Bocavirus and acute wheezing in children. Clin Infect Dis 2007;44:904–910 [PMID: 17342639].

Rafei K, Lichenstein R: Airway infectious disease emergencies. Pediatr Clin North Am 2006;53:215–242 [PMID: 16574523].

SEPTIC ARTHRITIS

ESSENTIALS OF DIAGNOSIS

▶ Fever
▶ Painful joint
▶ Joint effusions
▶ Arthrocentesis findings

▶ General Considerations

Left untreated, septic arthritis rapidly destroys articular cartilage, causing permanent joint damage. Delay between the onset of symptoms and treatment is the major determining factor for prognosis. Joint infection may occur by hematogenous route, direct inoculation, or spread of contiguous infections. Hematogenous infection in children was the most common route, but HIB immunization has decreased this significantly. The peak incidence occurs in children under age 3 years, and boys are affected twice as often as girls. However, with the increasing frequency of prosthetic joints, a new group has emerged that may be the most problematic.

Septic arthritis typically affects only one or a few asymmetrically distributed joints. Because joint infection superimposed on rheumatoid arthritis sometimes occurs, any joint that develops inflammation out of proportion to that in other affected joints should be aspirated to rule out the possibility of infection in patients with rheumatoid arthritis. There are about 20,000 cases of septic arthritis in the United States annually with gonococcus being the leading cause and *Staph. aureus* in second place. People with existing joint damage from rheumatoid arthritis and surgery are at risk. Other groups at high risk include intravenous drug abusers and patients on hemodialysis. Aspiration of the affected joint in the emergency department is often necessary to differentiate septic arthritis from other causes of synovitis, such as gout or pseudogout.

▶ Clinical Findings

A. Symptoms and Signs

Patients with septic arthritis usually have acute or subacute onset of pain, erythema, swelling, and limitation of motion in the affected joints. The patients most likely will show signs of systemic infection with fever chills and an ill appearance. The arthritis more commonly affects the large joints, especially the knee. In infants or neonates, failure to feed or pseudoparalysis of the extremity may be present.

B. Laboratory Findings

Definitive diagnosis is established by demonstration of the infecting organism in synovial tissue or joint fluid. Blood

Table 42–11. Treatment of Septic Arthritis.

Age Group	Cause	Primary Treatment	Alternative Treatment
Infant (<3 months)	*S. aureus* Enterobacteriaceae Group B streptococci, *N. gonorrhoeae*	Antistaphylococcal penicillin + third-generation cephalosporin	Antistaphylococcal penicillin + aminoglycoside
Children (3 months–14 years)	*Staph. aureus* *Streptococcus pyogenes* *Strep. pneumoniae* *Haemophilus influenzae*	Antistaphylococcal penicillin + third-generation cephalosporin	Vancomycin + third-generation cephalosporin
Adults (acute monoarticular; sexually active)	*N. gonorrhoeae*	Ceftriaxone or cefotaxime or ceftizoxime	Nafcillin if gram-positive organisms are found
Adults (acute monoarticular; not sexually active)	*Staph. aureus* Streptococci gram-negative bacilli	Antistaphylococcal penicillin + third-generation cephalosporin	Antistaphylococcal penicillin + ciprofloxacin
Adult (polyarticular)	*N. gonorrhoeae*	Ceftriaxone	

cultures may be positive even though cultures of joint fluid are negative and should be obtained for all patients thought to have septic arthritis.

1. Joint fluid analysis—Joint fluid typically shows high leukocyte counts, usually over 50,000, although the count may not be strikingly elevated in early disease. Synovial fluid should be considered inflammatory and possibly infectious if the count is above 7500. The higher the white cell count in joint fluid, the greater the likelihood of bacterial or fungal arthritis. The glucose content of synovial fluid is usually lower than normal but occasionally may be normal. If no antimicrobial therapy has been given, smears and cultures often reveal the causative organism. A synovial fluid lactic acid test may be useful in excluding septic arthritis; the test has a negative predictive value of 97%. Results of other laboratory tests are variable, and plain X-rays of affected joints are usually negative early in the disease.

2. Gonococcal arthritis—In gonococcal arthritis, Gram-stained smears and cultures of joint fluid are negative in 50–75% of cases, although in 86% of patients, cultures of exudates from the cervix, urethra, pharynx, or rectum demonstrate gonococci. Because the gonococcus is a fastidious organism, demonstration of its growth in cultures depends on prompt processing of specimens by the laboratory. Because special handling is also required, all specimens submitted should bear the instruction "Rule out gonorrhea." Prompt response to antimicrobial therapy helps confirm the diagnosis of gonococcal arthritis.

▶ **Treatment**

1. Aspiration

Aspirate affected joints. Aspiration is necessary except for infections in inaccessible joints. Open drainage is almost never required in gonococcal arthritis.

2. Antibiotics

High doses of intravenous antibiotics should be given (Table 42–11). Intra-articular instillation of antibiotics is unnecessary because high antibiotic levels are attained in synovial fluid when drugs are given intravenously. If no organisms are seen on Gram-stained smears of synovial fluid, but other findings suggest septic arthritis, empiric antibiotic therapy based on the type of patient and clinical findings should be started depending on the results of culture and sensitivity.

▶ **Disposition**

Hospitalize all patients with suspected or documented septic arthritis.

OSTEOMYELITIS

 ESSENTIALS OF DIAGNOSIS

▶ Pain, fever
▶ Increased erythrocyte sedimentation rate
▶ Biopsy findings

▶ **General Considerations**

Osteomyelitis is an infection of bone that affects all age groups. The infecting organisms are bacteria, mycobacteria, or fungi. For purposes of discussion, osteomyelitis can be classified according to the pathogenic mechanism: (1) hematogenous osteomyelitis and (2) osteomyelitis secondary to contiguous focus of infection. Hematogenous osteomyelitis is common in children, although its incidence is increasing in older age groups. Hematogenous osteomyelitis in adults usually involves the vertebral bodies. Spread of disease from a contiguous focus of infection is the most common pathogenic mechanism in adults. In both children and adults, the most commonly involved bones are the long bones, especially those of the lower extremities; this is particularly true in children. Orthopedic procedures or traumatic wounds predispose to osteomyelitis of the extremities. Sometimes a third classification of osteomyelitis from peripheral vascular disease is included, but this is likely a predisposing condition to contiguous spread.

▶ Clinical Findings

1. Symptoms and Signs

1. Hematogenous osteomyelitis—The abrupt onset of high fever, systemic toxicity, and physical findings of local suppuration surrounding the involved bone (local pain, swelling, and tenderness) are typical. The disease may be more indolent, particularly in patients with vertebral osteomyelitis. Patients with vertebral osteomyelitis may have low-grade or intermittent fever or back pain that may be either severe or only nagging and may not cause extreme discomfort or immobility until late in the disease. Focal tenderness over the dorsal spines of the involved vertebral bodies may be the only physical finding.

2. Osteomyelitis secondary to contiguous infection—The most common predisposing factor is postoperative infection, such as that following open reduction in fractures. Extension of soft tissue infections to bone from infected fingers and toes, infected teeth, or infected sinuses also occurs. Most patients are over age 50 years and may present with fever, swelling, and erythema in the initial episode. During recurrences, sinus formation and drainage are the major presenting signs.

3. Osteomyelitis associated with vascular insufficiency—Patients with osteomyelitis associated with vascular insufficiency invariably have diabetes mellitus or severe peripheral vascular disease. The toes and small bones of the feet are usually affected. Local signs and symptoms such as pain, swelling, redness, or frank cellulitis with deep ulcers in the soft tissue are prominent. Pain is often absent because of diabetic neuropathy.

B. Laboratory Findings

Routine laboratory tests are of limited value in the diagnosis of osteomyelitis. The leukocyte count is often elevated in acute disease but may be normal in more chronic infection. The erythrocyte sedimentation rate and C-reactive protein are elevated in most patients. Radiographic procedures are the primary diagnostic tool, although plain X-rays may not show signs of disease until 10–14 days after symptom onset. The earliest visible X-ray changes are adjacent soft tissue swelling and periosteal reaction. Lytic lesions and areas of sclerosis may then develop. If osteomyelitis is suspected and plain X-rays fail to reveal signs of disease, MRI or bone scan should be performed. The diagnosis is confirmed by culture and histologic examination of bone. Bacteriologic findings vary, and cultures should be obtained from bone (via needle aspiration or surgical biopsy) or blood (results are positive in 50% of cases in patients with acute hematogenous osteomyelitis).

▶ Treatment

The most important therapeutic measures are systemic antibiotics and surgery to drain abscesses or for debridement of necrotic tissue. The selection of an antibiotic depends on identification of the causative organism. If the disease is uncomplicated (ie, involves a long bone in a patient without underlying medical problems), if the patient is a child, or if the patient is critically ill, then antistaphylococcal therapy should be initiated because *Staph. aureus* is the most common infective organism.

Surgery in acute osteomyelitis should be limited to biopsy for diagnosis, drainage of suppurative areas, and debridement of necrotic bone. Surgical drainage is also indicated if neurologic abnormalities are present or develop in patients with vertebral or cranial osteomyelitis or if infection spreads to the hip joint in a child.

▶ Disposition

Patients with acute osteomyelitis should be hospitalized for intravenous antimicrobial therapy.

Calhoun JH, Manring MM. Adult osteomyelitis. Infect Dis Clin North Am 2005;19:765–786 [PMID: 16297731].

Gutierrez K: Bone and joint infections in children. Pediatr Clin North Am 2005;52:779–794 [PMID: 15925662].

Smith JE, Chalupa P, Shabaz Hasan M: Infectious arthritis: Clinical features, laboratory findings and treatment. Clin Microbiol Infect 2006;12:309–314 [PMID: 16524406].

PHARYNGITIS

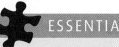

ESSENTIALS OF DIAGNOSIS

▶ Sore throat
▶ Fever
▶ Erythematous pharynx
▶ Odynophagia

Table 42–12. Bacterial Etiologies of Acute Pharyngitis.

Streptococci
  Group A
  Group C and G
Mixed anaerobes
N. gonorrheae
Corynebacterium diphtheriae
Arcanobacterium haemolyticum
Yersinia enterocolitica
Yersinia pestis
Francisella tularensis
Mycoplasma pneumoniae
Chlamydia psittaci
Chlamydia pneumoniae
Fusobacterium necrophorum

▶ General Considerations

Acute pharyngitis is a common presenting complaint, particularly in the winter months, and is caused by a multitude of organisms (see Table 42–12). The vast majority of cases are caused by viruses, although 15–30% of children and 5–10% of adults will have pharyngitis caused by group A β-hemolytic streptococci (GABHS), the single most common etiology. Judicious antibiotic use is warranted to prevent over treatment; over 70% of adults receive antibiotic treatment despite the low prevalence of GABHS in this age group.

▶ Clinical Findings

A. Symptoms and Signs

1. Group A streptococcal infection—GABHS most commonly occurs between the ages of 5 and 15 years and is prevalent in late winter and early spring. Onset is typically sudden and may include fever, sore throat, anterior cervical lymphadenopathy, a "beefy red" uvula and pharynx, and tonsillar exudates. Children more commonly present with headache, vomiting, and abdominal pain with a nontender abdomen. A scarlatiniform rash and palatal petechiae may also be present. The absence of cough, coryza, and diarrhea support the diagnosis of GABHS. Several organizations have published guidelines regarding the use of rapid-antigen testing, but questions remain over whether these guidelines are sufficiently specific.

2. Infectious mononucleosis—Clinical findings in infectious mononucleosis may be identical to those in GABHS, although the onset and course are usually more indolent. Generalized lymphadenopathy, particularly posterior cervical, and hepatosplenomegaly are common and resolve over 3–6 weeks. Laboratory testing for specific antibodies to Epstein–Barr virus, heterophile antibody, and a CBC to document atypical lymphocytosis support the diagnosis.

3. Diphtheria—Diphtheria is rare but should be considered in patient for whom immunization status is uncertain in the face of a membranous or exudative pharyngitis. A "bull neck" appearance due to prominent anterior and posterior cervical lymphadenopathy, tachycardia out of proportion to fever, and a grayish-brown pseudomembrane that may extend down the pharynx to include the tracheobronchial tree are classic findings.

4. Vincent angina—Vincent angina is a polymicrobial infection, typically limited to the gingiva, and characterized by foul breath, cervical lymphadenopathy, and fever. In immunocompromised individuals, it may extend to include a necrotic gray pseudomembrane on the pharynx.

5. Lemierre's Syndrome—Lemierre's Syndrome is a rare complication of the anaerobic bacteria *Fusobacterium necrophorum*. Its hallmark is a thrombosis of the ipsilateral jugular vein and is associated with dissemination of abcesses in the throat, chest and mediastinum.

B. Laboratory Findings

Definitive diagnosis of group A streptococcal pharyngitis can be made by results on culture of exudates from the throat. Rapid streptococcal antigen tests are highly specific but not as sensitive as culture. The American Heart Association has revised its recommendation for throat cultures before antibiotic therapy. Throat cultures are considered "valuable" for children and adolescents and "not as essential" for adults. They are indicated primarily to avoid the unnecessary use of antibiotics for the 70–80% of adult patients with pharyngitis due to virus.

An elevated white cell count (>12,000) suggests bacterial pharyngitis. Obtain a heterophil agglutination test or mononucleosis spot test for patients thought to have infectious mononucleosis. A CBC with differential may also reveal a lymphocytosis with atypical lymphocytes.

▶ Treatment

Treatment of GABHS appears to reduce the duration of symptoms by approximately 1 day when begun in the middle of the illness as is common. Suppurative complications are reduced by antibiotic treatment as in acute rheumatic fever, and there is a trend toward reduction in post-streptococcal glomerulonephritis. Patients with symptoms suggestive of GABHS pharyngitis who have close contact with a documented infection (eg, parents of school-age children) or in high-prevalence areas should be treated without laboratory confirmation, but rapid antigen testing with or without confirmatory culture is warranted in most others.

Cephalosporins are twice as likely to result in clinical and bacteriological cure as oral penicillin. Many antibiotic regimens have been shown to be effective, including oral or intramuscularly penicillin, amoxicillin, cephalosporins, and macrolides. Dexamethasone is beneficial in acute pharyngitis but multiple doses may be required in infectious mononucleosis.

Disposition

Patients with uncomplicated pharyngitis may be discharged home with appropriate supportive therapy and antibiotics, if indicated. Hospitalization with appropriate consultation is indicated for diphtheria, Vincent angina, Lemierre's Syndrome, and epiglottis. Patients with infectious mononucleosis should follow up with their primary-care physician before returning to sports because of the risk of splenic rupture.

Casey JR, Pichichero ME: Meta-analysis of cephalosporins versus penicillin for treatment of group A streptococcal tonsillopharyngitis in adults. Clin Infect Dis 2004;38:1526–1534 [PMID: 15156437].

Gerber MA: Diagnosis and treatment of pharyngitis in children. Pediatr Clin North Am 2005;52:729–747 [PMID: 15925660].

Lai C, Vummidi DR: Lemierre's Syndrome. N Engl J Med 2004 Apr 15;350(16):e14 [PMID: 15084710].

Smith A, Lamagni TL, Oliver I, Efstratiou A, George RC, Stuart JM: Invasive group A streptococcal disease: Should close contacts routinely receive antibiotic prophylaxis? Lancet Infect Dis 2005;5:494–500 [PMID: 16048718].

URINARY TRACT INFECTIONS

ACUTE LOWER URINARY TRACT INFECTION (UNCOMPLICATED CYSTITIS)

ESSENTIALS OF DIAGNOSIS

▶ Dysuria

▶ Frequency and urgency

▶ Suprapubic pain

▶ Hematuria

▶ Pyuria

General Considerations

Uncomplicated bacterial cystitis is defined as a urinary tract infection confined to the bladder. It affects women more commonly than men and tends to recur even in the absence of anatomic abnormalities. Many patients with apparent lower urinary tract infection also have asymptomatic involvement of the upper urinary tract (absence of fever, chills, or flank pain). Children present with cystitis without the complaint of dysuria much more commonly than do adults. Conditions such as vesicoureteral reflux may predispose children to infections, and an aggressive workup to evaluate for these possibilities is required. Prior to age 1 year, the

incidence is nearly equal in males and females, but after age 1 year, females are 30 times more likely to develop a urinary tract infection until age 50 years, when men begin developing an increased incidence of these infections.

Most cystitis is caused by bacterial infection, usually *E. coli* (80%) and other enteric gram-negative bacilli such as *Proteus mirabilis*, *K. pneumoniae*, and *P. aeruginosa*. Gram-positive bacteria such as *Streptococcus faecalis*, *Streptococcus epidermis*, and *Streptococcus viridans* are less common causes. Adenovirus is a common cause of hemorrhagic cystitis in children (typically males) and occasionally young adults.

Clinical Findings

A. Symptoms and Signs

A history of urinary tract infections is frequently elicited. Dysuria and urinary frequency and urgency are the most common symptoms in adults, although they may be absent in children. Patients may report that their urine is cloudy, smelly, or dark.

Suprapubic discomfort and tenderness are common. Patients are usually afebrile or have a low-grade fever. The presence of high fever (>38.3°C [101°F]) or rigors is inconsistent with a diagnosis of uncomplicated cystitis and suggests pyelonephritis. Nausea and vomiting, though uncommon in adults, are not unusual in children with uncomplicated cystitis.

Neonates may present with poor feeding, vomiting, jaundice, or irritability and may not always have fever. Young children may present with new bed-wetting or loss of bladder training.

B. Laboratory Findings

1. Urinalysis—Accurate diagnosis of urinary tract infection depends on obtaining a urine specimen uncontaminated by perineal secretions. The presence of squamous epithelial cells or of mixed flora on Gram-stained smears suggests contamination, and the specimen should be discarded and a better one obtained. Urine should be examined while it is fresh (within 1 hour) or should be refrigerated if delay is expected. Urine should be obtained by catheter or clean-catch specimens only because bagged specimens are usually contaminated.

A. CHEMISTRY—Mild degrees of proteinuria and hematuria are common on dipstick tests of urine. If the infection is caused by a urea-splitting bacterium (eg, *P. mirabilis*), urinary pH may be abnormally high (eg, 6–8). The leukocyte esterase and nitrite dipstick tests are a reliable indicators of infection, made even more likely with the positive presence of both. Chemical tests for the presence of bacteria in urine (eg, nitrate reduction) are not sensitive and specific enough to be generally recommended.

B. SEDIMENT—Many leukocytes and often some erythrocytes are present. Clumps of leukocytes must be differentiated

Table 42–13. Empiric Antibiotic Therapy for Urinary Tract Infection.

Type of Infection	First-Line Therapy	Alternative Regimens	Comments
Uncomplicated cystitis (including mild pyelonephritis)	Fluoroquinolone, Bactrim DS, nitrofurantoin.	Amoxicillin-clavulanate, third-generation cephalosporin	
Urinary tract infection with pyelonephritis (inpatient therapy)	Intravenous fluoroquinolone, ampicillin + gentamicin, third-generation cephalosporin, or antipseudomonal penicillin	Ticarcillin-clavulanate, ampicillin-sulbactam, or piperacillin-tazobactam	
Complicated urinary tract infection (obstruction, reflux, indwelling catheter)	Ampicillin + gentamicin, piperacillintazobactam Ticarcillin-clavulanate, imipenem, or meropenem	Intravenous fluoroquinolone	Rule out obstruction

from WBC casts, which signify upper urinary tract involvement. In most cases, numerous bacteria are visible.

c. GRAM-STAINED SMEARS—Microscopic examination of Gram-stained specimens of urinary sediment from centrifuged urine usually shows bacteria of a single morphologic type. If uncentrifuged urine is examined, and an average of one bacterium is found per oil-immersion field, there is about an 80% probability that there are 10^5 organisms per milliliter of urine (strongly indicative of infection).

2. Urine culture—In women of child-bearing age with a history of recurrent cystitis (two to three times per year) who are otherwise healthy, treatment may be started on the basis of urinalysis results alone, and urine culture may be postponed until 1 week after treatment (test-of-cure culture) or may be omitted in patients who respond well to treatment. In all other patients, quantitative urine cultures should be obtained. Growth of at least 10^5 organisms of a single species per milliliter of urine indicates a high probability of active urinary tract infection.

A urine culture should be ordered for all febrile infants under age 2 years, for children with a history of urinary tract infection, for children who are taking suppressive antibiotic therapy, and for children in whom antibiotic therapy is started regardless of urinalysis results. Smaller numbers (10^2–10^4/mL) of bacteria (especially of a single species) are significant and indicate the need for therapy (see the Dysuria–Frequency Syndrome section below).

▶ **Treatment**

A. Antimicrobials

Nonpregnant women of child-bearing age who have a history of and findings compatible with uncomplicated cystitis may be given a short course (3 days) of therapy. Single-dose therapy has fallen into disfavor because of the frequency of relapse and because it requires that the patient be seen 2–4 days later for a test-of-cure urine culture. All other patients should receive multidose therapy for at least 7–10 days. Because men

often harbor occult infection in the prostate or kidney, some authorities recommend that treatment be extended for at least 3 weeks in an effort to prevent relapse of infection.

Current AAP guidelines recommend treatment for children for 7–14 days with coverage by antibiotics until radiologic studies are completed and urologic referral conducted.

For uncomplicated cystitis, no clear consensus exists on a leading antimicrobial agent for treatment (Table 42–13) Expert data suggests that treatment with trimethoprim/sulfamethoxazole (TMP-SMZ), a fluoroquinolone, nitrofurantoin, or amoxicillin/clavulanate are all effective choices and acceptable treatment. Some authorities suggest that early generation cephalosporins and simple penicillins are less effective than the above. However, as resistance patterns change and specifically E. coli becomes more resistant to fluoroquinolones, one should periodically become familiar with resistance rates in your area to guide TMP-SMZ and ciprofloxacin, because of their good penetration into the prostate and high level of activity against uropathogens, are recommended for men with urinary tract infection who have normal serum creatinine levels.

B. Adjunctive Measures

Phenazopyridine (Pyridium, many others), 200 mg orally three times a day, may help relieve severe dysuria. The drug should be taken for only 2–3 days. Warn patients that their urine will turn orange.

C. Follow-Up

In uncomplicated cystitis, follow-up urine cultures are optional in patients who respond to therapy. Patients given single-dose or 3-day therapy and whose symptoms recur should have urine culture and be given a 10-day course of therapy.

▶ **Disposition**

Infants, children, and men with diagnosed urinary tract infection should receive treatment and be referred to a urologist. Hospitalization is indicated for children younger than age

3 months and for children with dehydration, toxicity, vomiting, or failure of outpatient regimen. Urologic referral is also recommended for women with frequent recurrences of cystitis (monthly) and probably also for those who have had three or more infections in 1 year, although the latter recommendation is controversial. Hospitalization is not indicated for patients with uncomplicated cystitis.

UPPER URINARY TRACT INFECTION (PYELONEPHRITIS)

▶ General Considerations

Acute pyelonephritis is a bacterial infection of the kidney. It is invariably an ascending infection from the bladder. It is usually caused by the same organisms that cause cystitis (ie, *E. coli*, *P. mirabilis*). In elderly men, pyelonephritis may be caused by *Strep. faecalis*. In patients who have received prior antimicrobial therapy (eg, during recent hospitalization, because of chronic indwelling Foley catheter) and in nursing home patients, the infecting organisms may be resistant to commonly used antimicrobials. Because of the changes in anatomy, pregnant women are prone to pyelonephritis. Moreover, pyelonephritis in pregnancy is associated with an increased risk of premature delivery. Thus, pregnant patients with urinary tract infection should always receive multidose antimicrobial therapy.

Chronic pyelonephritis is more indolent. About 20% of people with end-stage renal disease have chronic pyelonephritis causing scaring and decreased function. Patients with multiple urinary tract infections need to be followed up closely to prevent this. Emphysematous pyelonephritis is acute pyelonephritis associated with gas in the collecting system; it typically occurs in patients with diabetes. This disease has a 75% mortality rate and is treated with emergency nephrectomy if required.

▶ Clinical Findings

A. Symptoms and Signs

Pyelonephritis is characterized by symptoms of cystitis (dysuria, urgency, and frequency) accompanied by flank pain and tenderness. Fever, rigors, and, in patients with complicating bacteremia or endotoxemia, systemic signs of sepsis (eg, hypotension, delirium) may be present. In young children, fever is the predominant symptom; only 32% of boys and 40% of girls display dysuria as a symptom, and flank pain is an even less common symptom. In pyelonephritis occurring as a complication of nephrolithiasis, severe flank pain radiating to the groin may be the most prominent symptom.

In patients with sickle cell disease, diabetes, or nephropathy caused by analgesic abuse, necrosis of the renal papillae with sloughing into the ureters occurs as a complication of renal infection, and the patient may present with symptoms of ureteral obstruction that mimic nephrolithiasis.

B. Laboratory Findings

1. Urine—The findings on urinalysis, microscopic examination, and culture are the same as in cystitis (see above), except that leukocyte casts (granular casts) occur only with pyelonephritis. Gross hematuria and pain suggest pyelonephritis-complicating urolithiasis. For all patients with suspected pyelonephritis, send urine for culture and susceptibility testing.

2. Other laboratory studies—Serum electrolyte, BUN, and creatinine measurements should be obtained because azotemia may be present. The white cell count is usually elevated. A normal or low white cell count with a shift to the left in a patient with suspected pyelonephritis is often a sign of sepsis, indicating the need for hospitalization.

C. X-Ray and Other Findings

Some authorities suggest that excretory urography be performed in all nonpregnant women with pyelonephritis after the infection has cleared. In patients with pyelonephritis in whom urinary obstruction is suspected, radiologic and other examinations should be performed as soon as possible. Ultrasonography is a safe and sensitive means of assessing hydronephrosis and may reveal intrarenal and perinephric abscesses. Remember that in pregnancy, some degree of ureteral dilatation (usually greater in the right ureter than the left) is normal.

▶ Treatment

A. Antimicrobials

See Table 42–13.

Patients with anatomic abnormalities of the urinary tract or concomitant prostatitis may require up to 6 weeks of therapy. In patients with suspected bacteremia or suspected infection due to antibiotic-resistant organisms, an aminoglycoside should be added.

B. General Measures

If vomiting or dehydration is present, begin intravenous fluid replacement with crystalloid solutions. Provide analgesia for flank pain if needed. Give antipyretics for high fever regularly (rather than as needed) until the patient is afebrile.

▶ Disposition

Patients who meet the criteria listed below or who have any of the following conditions should be hospitalized:

- Inability to maintain oral hydration or take medications
- Concern about compliance or follow-up
- Diagnostic uncertainty
- Severe illness with high fevers, severe pain, and marked debility

- Comorbid illness (eg, diabetes, renal failure, immunosuppression)
- Failure of outpatient therapy

Patients who are not hospitalized should have a follow-up appointment within 1–2 days to assess their response to therapy.

Some patients with pyelonephritis, especially young women, may not be sick enough for hospitalization but do not appear well enough to go home. For these patients, a 12–24-hour period of intravenous antimicrobial therapy, intravenous hydration, and observation in the emergency department may be indicated. If rapid resolution of signs and symptoms occurs, the patient may be discharged with a prescription for oral antimicrobials and a follow-up appointment in 1–2 days.

DYSURIA–FREQUENCY SYNDROME

▶ General Considerations

The dysuria–frequency syndrome (urethral syndrome) occurs by definition only in women, usually young women. These patients have symptoms of lower urinary tract infection but have urine cultures that are sterile or contain fewer than 10^5 organisms per milliliter of urine. Patients with dysuria–frequency syndrome may be divided into two groups: those with accompanying pyuria (> 10 leukocytes per high power field) and those without. In women with pyuria, symptoms are usually due either to a low-grade bacterial cystitis (bacteriuria with <100,000 organisms per milliliter of urine) or to chlamydial urethritis with or without accompanying chlamydial cervicitis. *Neisseria gonorrhoeae* also causes urethritis. HSV causes urethritis during primary infection and, on occasion, during recurrent infection. In some patients with pyuria and in most patients who lack pyuria, no causative agent can be identified.

▶ Clinical Findings

A. Symptoms and Signs

The principal symptoms are those of cystitis: dysuria, urgency, and frequency. The dysuria is "internal" dysuria as opposed to the "external" dysuria occurring in vaginitis or genital HSV infection and results from urine coming into contact with denuded skin. Findings on physical examination are normal except that there may be urethral inflammation or mucopurulent cervical discharge and cervical edema in patients whose symptoms are due to gonococcal or chlamydial infection. Pelvic examination is important to diagnose vaginitis, which may also cause dysuria.

B. Laboratory Findings

The urine may be normal or may contain PMNs with few or no bacteria. Swabs of urethral discharge should be obtained for smear and culture for *N. gonorrhoeae* in patients with a history of gonorrhea, in those with multiple sexual partners, and in those whose recent sexual partner has had urethritis. Urine culture shows scant growth or no growth of organisms. A cervical swab for *Chlamydia* antigen (fluorescent or ELISA slide test) is indicated in sexually active women with cervicitis accompanying this syndrome because this organism causes concurrent cervicitis and urethritis.

▶ Treatment

Antimicrobial therapy is usually reserved for patients with pyuria. Tetracyclines and erythromycin are the most effective drugs for suspected chlamydial infection; other bacterial pathogens may be resistant to these drugs. Optimal treatment of chlamydial infection requires 7 days of therapy. Short-course, for example, 3-day therapy, may be tried initially in patients with low-grade bacteriuria. None of the single-dose regimens provides reliable empiric therapy for both chlamydial and bacterial infection.

▶ Disposition

Because of the difficulties of empiric therapy in the urethral syndrome, a follow-up visit to a primary-care physician should be arranged. If ordinary bacterial cultures of urine are sterile in patients with pyuria, the patient's sexual partners should be screened for urethritis and *Chlamydia* infection.

American College of Obstetricians and Gynecologists. ACOG Practice Bulletin No. 91: Treatment of urinary tract infections in nonpregnant women. Obstet Gynecol 2008;111:785–794 [PMID: 18310389].

Grabe M, Bishop MC, Bjerklund-Johansen TE, et al: Guidelines on the management of urinary and male genital tract infections. European Association of Urology (EAU), 2008 Mar. pp. 1–116.

Hodson EM, Willis NS, Craig JC: Antibiotics for acute pyelonephritis in children. Cochrane Database of Sys Rev 2007;CD003772 [PMID: 17943796].

DISEASES OF THE FEMALE GENITOURINARY TRACT

See also the Sexually Transmitted Diseases section later in this chapter.

PELVIC INFLAMMATORY DISEASE

ESSENTIALS OF DIAGNOSIS

- ▶ Lower abdominal pain
- ▶ Vaginal discharge
- ▶ Fever
- ▶ Cervical motion tenderness
- ▶ Bilateral lower adnexal tenderness

General Considerations

Infection of the uterine tubes may be acute or chronic and unilateral or bilateral. It may lead to pyosalpinx or tubo-ovarian abscess. Pelvic peritonitis is frequently present. Causative agents include *Chlamydia trachomatis*, *N. gonorrhoeae*, anaerobic bacteria (which include *Bacteroides* and gram-positive cocci), facultative gram-negative bacilli (such as *E.coli*), *Mycoplasma hominis*, and rarely *Actinomyces israelii*. Because it is often impossible to differentiate among these agents in individual patients, treatment regimens that are active against the broadest possible range of these pathogens should be used. Risk factors for pelvic inflammatory disease (PID) include young age, multiple sexual partners, intrauterine device insertion, vaginal douching, tobacco smoking, chlamydial or gonococcal infection, and bacterial vaginosis.

Clinical Findings

A. Symptoms and Signs

Patients are usually young (<age 30 years) and sexually active. Symptoms include fever (sometimes with rigors), severe pelvic pain that may be either continuous or crampy (pelvic pain is usually bilateral and is the most common presenting symptom), dyspareunia, menstrual disturbances, vaginal discharge, and gastrointestinal disturbances (anorexia, nausea and vomiting, constipation). Patients usually are menstruating or just finished their periods (risk of ascending infection is increased secondary to the loss of the cervical mucus plug during menses).

Physical examination in acute cases discloses marked tenderness on manipulation of the cervix and palpation of the adnexa. There is a unilateral tender adnexal mass if tubo-ovarian abscess or pyosalpinx is present. The clinical spectrum in PID includes a gradual progression from subclinical endometritis to salpingitis to pyosalpinx to tubo-ovarian abscess to pelvic peritonitis to perihepatitis. A ruptured tubo-ovarian abscess carries with it a mortality rate of 7% and may require emergency surgery. Table 42–14 presents the physical examination criteria.

Table 42-14. Criteria for Diagnosis of Pelvic Inflammatory Disease.

Minimum Criteria
Lower abdominal tenderness
Adnexal tenderness
Cervical motion tenderness
Additional Criteria
Oral temperature > 101°F
Abnormal cervical or vaginal discharge
Elevated erythrocyte sedimentation rate
Elevated C-reactive protein
Laboratory documentation of cervical infection with *N. gonorrhoeae* or *C. trachomatis*
Elaborate Criteria
Histopathologic evidence of endometritis on endometrial biopsy
Transvaginal sonography or other imaging techniques showing thickened, fluid-filled tubes with or without free pelvic fluid or tubo-ovarian complex
Laparoscopic abnormalities consistent with pelvic inflammatory disease

B. Laboratory Tests and Special Examinations

There is usually leukocytosis or an elevated erythrocyte sedimentation rate or C-reactive protein. Obtain a serum pregnancy test. Purulent fluid should be cultured for aerobic and anaerobic pathogens, specifically for *N. gonorrhoeae* and *Chlamydia*. Ultrasonography may be helpful in detecting or assessing the size of tubo-ovarian abscess.

Treatment

A. Antibiotic Therapy

Table 42–15 presents treatment options. No single agent is active against the entire spectrum of pathogens. Several antibiotic combinations provide a broad spectrum of activity against the major pathogens, but none have been adequately

Table 42-15. Antimicrobial Therapy for Pelvic Inflammatory Disease.

Outpatient Treatment	Inpatient Treatment
Ceftriaxone intramuscularly + doxycycline PO	Cefoxitin intravenously + doxycycline intravenously
Ceftriaxone intramuscularly + ofloxacin PO and clindamycin PO or metronidazole PO	Cefotetan intravenously + doxycycline intravenously
Cefoxitin intramuscularly + probenecid PO + doxycycline PO	Clindamycin intravenously + gentamicin intravenously + doxycycline intravenously
Cefoxitin intramuscularly + probenecid PO + ofloxacin PO and clindamycin PO or metroidazole PO	Unasyn + doxycycline

evaluated. Treatment with penicillin, ampicillin, amoxicillin, or a cephalosporin alone is not recommended.

B. Reevaluation

Patients who are not hospitalized should be reevaluated in 2–4 days and hospitalized if their condition has not improved markedly.

C. Adjunctive Measures

Relieve pain. Narcotics are frequently required. If present, an intrauterine device should be removed as soon as adequate antibiotic levels are achieved in the blood. Surgery should be delayed at least 2–3 days, until the effect of antibiotic therapy can be assessed, even if pyosalpinx or tubo-ovarian abscess is present. Pelvic abscesses often regress with antibiotic therapy alone or may drain externally via the vagina or rectum. Repeated ultrasound examinations help to determine the patient's progress.

▶ Disposition

There is an increasing trend toward the outpatient management of PID. Indications for admission include uncertain diagnosis, pelvic abscess, pregnancy, adolescence, severe illness, failure of outpatient management, inability to arrange follow-up, and HIV-positive status.

VAGINITIS

ESSENTIALS OF DIAGNOSIS

▶ Abnormal vaginal discharge

▶ Pruritus, irritation, odor

▶ Inflamed cervix

▶ General Considerations

Vaginitis is a common and annoying disorder that in the absence of other symptoms or signs rarely indicates serious disease. Common pathogens include *Candida albicans*, *Trichomonas vaginalis*, *Gardnerella vaginalis* with anaerobic bacteria (bacterial vaginosis), and gonococci (in prepubertal girls). Other common causes are estrogen deficiency (atrophic vaginitis) and vaginal foreign body. Systemic antibiotics (especially tetracyclines), oral contraceptives, diabetes mellitus, primary genital HSV infection, and pregnancy predispose to the development of candidiasis. Less common causes include allergy, cervicitis, polyps, tumors, vaginal ulcer, shigellosis, irradiation for cancer, and certain bubble bath preparations.

▶ Clinical Findings

A. Symptoms and Signs

Vaginal discharge and pruritus are the chief symptoms. Vaginal discharge with varying degrees of inflammation of the vaginal wall (minimal in atrophic vaginitis) is usually found. Search for foreign bodies in the vagina, particularly in young girls, and examine for associated disorders (eg, salpingitis).

B. Laboratory Findings

1. Examination of smears—

A. GRAM STAIN—Look for *Candida* and *Gardnerella vaginitis* (small gram-negative rods usually adherent to epithelial cells; "clue cells"). Methylene blue stain also demonstrates clue cells. Vaginitis due to *Candida* or *Trichomonas* is usually associated with a PMN exudate, whereas inflammatory cells are absent in bacterial vaginosis caused by *G. vaginalis*. In prepubertal girls with gonococcal vulvovaginitis, Gram stain of smears usually shows typical gram-negative intracellular diplococci, but cultures should be performed to confirm the diagnosis.

B. SALINE WET MOUNT—Look for motile trichomonads. *Candida* and clue cells of *G. vaginalis* may also be seen.

C. POTASSIUM HYDROXIDE WET MOUNT—Addition of a few drops of potassium hydroxide to a sample of vaginal secretions releases a typical amine odor (fishy) in cases of bacterial vaginosis due to *G. vaginalis*. Microscopic examination reveals *Candida* in cases of *Candida* vaginitis, but Gram staining is more sensitive and specific.

2. Urinalysis—Obtain a clean-catch urine specimen for analysis and culture if dysuria is present.

3. Other tests—Obtain fasting blood glucose measurement in cases of recurrent candidiasis, to rule out diabetes mellitus.

▶ Treatment

A. General Measures

Advise patients to avoid intercourse for a few days after treatment. Partners also should receive treatment, as described below.

B. Specific Measures

1. *C. albicans* vaginitis—

A. IMIDAZOLE REGIMENS—Virtually all azole intravaginal regimens are effective for candidal vaginitis. (1) Miconazole nitrate (vaginal suppositories, 200 mg) or clotrimazole (vaginal suppositories, 200 mg), intravaginally at bedtime for 3 days, or (2) butoconazole (2% cream, 5 g), intravaginally at bedtime for 3 days, or (3) terconazole, 80 mg suppository or 0.4% cream, intravaginally at bedtime for 3 days. (2) Fluconazole 150mg PO single dose.

B. REINFECTION—The male partner should wear a condom, or both partners should abstain from intercourse for 2–3 days. Balanitis due to *Candida* occurs almost exclusively in uncircumcised men. Occasionally the patient's gastrointestinal tract is a reservoir for *Candida*, in which case oral nonabsorbable antifungal preparations (eg, nystatin) are necessary.

2. *T. vaginalis* vaginitis—Give the patient and her sexual partner metronidazole, 2 g orally in a single dose (eight 250-mg tablets). This regimen is curative in about 95% of cases. An alternative regimen involves metronidazole, 500 mg orally three times daily for 7 days. Resistance of *T. vaginalis* to metronidazole has been observed but is rare. Timidazole 2 g and azithromycin 1 g orally can also be used. If treatment fails, the patient should receive the same treatment regimen again.

3. Bacterial vaginosis—Several species of vaginal bacteria (including *G. vaginalis*) interact to produce this syndrome. Some evidence supports the efficacy of intravaginal lactobacillus treatment in low-risk patients. Metronidazole, 500 mg orally two times daily for 7 days, is an effective treatment. Warn the patient about side effects. Clindamycin, 300 mg orally twice daily for 7 days, may be used in pregnant patients. Treatment of pregnant women with BV continues to be debated but current ACOG guidelines do not support routine treatment of normal, low-risk pregnancies. In pregnancy, treatment should be confined to oral therapy only. Treatment of male sexual partners does not reduce the risk of recurrence of bacterial vaginosis in the index case.

4. Atrophic vaginitis—Prescribe estrogen suppositories or creams. Diethylstilbestrol, one 0.5-mg vaginal suppository every 3 days for 3 weeks, followed by 1 week without treatment, may be tried.

5. Gonococcal vaginitis—See the Gonorrhea section below.

Disposition

Patients should have a follow-up appointment with a gynecologist or primary-care physician in 7–10 days so that the results of treatment can be assessed and follow-up cultures obtained.

GENITAL ABSCESSES

ESSENTIALS OF DIAGNOSIS

► Labial pain, swelling
► Fluctuant lesion

General Considerations

Vulvar abscesses may rise in a sebaceous gland or Bartholin gland (Bartholin cyst). Skene glands, adjacent to the urethra, may also be the site of abscess formation. *N. gonorrhoeae* is responsible for some vulvar abscesses; the remainder are caused by a variety of bacteria, often in mixed culture.

Clinical Findings

The patient complains of tender swelling of the labia majora that is confirmed by examination. Gram stain and culture of pus from the abscess help to identify the causative organism. Endocervical culture for *N. gonorrhoeae* should be performed, if possible.

Treatment

A. Nonfluctuant Lesions

If lesions are not fluctuant, incision and drainage are not indicated. If gonorrhea is suspected, give ceftriaxone, 250 mg intramuscularly. In addition, give a broad-spectrum antibiotic such as amoxicillin–clavulanate, 500 mg three times daily. Prescribe sitz baths and application of warm compresses. Ask the patient to return in 1–2 days for reevaluation of the need for incision and drainage.

B. Fluctuant Lesions

When drainage is performed, pack the abscess or place a Word catheter. Administer antimicrobials as described above. Have the patient return in 2–3 days.

Disposition

Gynecologic follow-up is mandatory because surgery may be necessary. Occasionally marsupialization may be performed at the time of diagnosis of acute bartholinitis.

MUCOPURULENT CERVICITIS

ESSENTIALS OF DIAGNOSIS

► Vaginal discharge
► Pruritus
► Cervical exudate

General Considerations

The presence of mucopurulent endocervical exudates strongly suggests cervicitis due to chlamydial or gonococcal infection.

▶ Clinical Findings

A. Symptoms and Signs

Vaginal discharge and pruritus may be present. Mucopurulent endocervical exudate may be observed.

B. Laboratory Findings

1. PCR test—The current gold standard and mainstay of both chlamydial and gonococcal diagnosis is PCR obtained from endocervical and vaginal swabs. This test is both highly sensitive and specific when appropriate samples are obtained. In most cases results will require 48 hours to obtain, and thus empiric treatment usually takes place if clinically indicated.

2. Swab test—Mucopurulent secretion from the endocervix may appear yellow or green when viewed on a white cotton-tipped swab. Cervicitis is present if bleeding occurs when the first swab culture for gonococci is taken or if erythema or edema is present within a zone of cervical ectopy.

3. Slide test—Fluorescent antibody or ELISA slide test should be used to diagnose *Chlamydia*.

4. Gram stain—Gram-stained smears of endocervical secretions show greater than 10 PMNs per microscopic oil-immersion field. The presence of gram-negative, diplococci suggests infection with *N. gonorrhoeae*, but this is not diagnostic. Culture is necessary to confirm infection with *N. gonorrhoeae*.

▶ Treatment

Empiric treatment with ceftriaxone 250 mg intramuscularly or cefixime 400 mg PO or *plus* azithromycin 1 g PO or doxycycline 100 mg PO b.i.d. for 7 days.

DISEASES OF THE MALE GENITOURINARY TRACT

ACUTE BACTERIAL PROSTATITIS

ESSENTIALS OF DIAGNOSIS

- ▶ Fever
- ▶ Low back pain
- ▶ Dysuria
- ▶ Urgency
- ▶ Prostatic tenderness

▶ Clinical Findings

A. Symptoms and Signs

Patients with acute bacterial prostatitis often have chills, fever, low back and perineal pain or pressure, malaise, dysuria, urgency, and difficulty voiding or decreased urinary stream. Recurring attacks of acute prostatitis are common. Urethral discharge may be present if prostatitis is secondary to urethritis (uncommon). The prostate is tender and enlarged. Prostatic abscess should be suspected when localized prostatic tenderness, swelling, or fluctuance is present. Prostatic massage is contraindicated in severe, acute prostatitis because it may induce bacteremia. A simple rectal examination may be performed, however. Prostatitis is the most common urologic diagnosis in men over age 50 years; as many as 50% of men are affected in their lifetime. Consider *N. gonorrhea* and *C. trachomatis* in males younger than 35 years with prostatitis.

B. Laboratory Findings

When acute bacterial prostatitis is suspected based on the patient's symptoms and physical examination, presumptive diagnosis may be made based on the results of urinalysis and urine Gram stain and culture. The bacterial pathogen found in the urine will usually be the same as that infecting the prostate. The presence of bacteria should be confirmed by culture and susceptibility testing. Leukocytosis is common. Azotemia suggests obstructive uropathy. Obtain blood cultures for all patients who have high fever or rigors.

▶ Treatment

A. Antimicrobials

Fluoroquinolones are the first-line agents of choice for outpatient therapy. For patients under age 35 years, give ofloxacin 400 mg PO X1 then 300 mg PO b.i.d. for a 28-day course. An alternative regimen is ceftriaxone 250 mg intramuscularly followed by doxycycline 100 mg PO b.i.d. for 10–14 days. For those over age 35, give ciprofloxacin 500 mg PO b.i.d. for 28 days. An alternative is TMP-SMZ one double strength tablet b.i.d. for 28 days.

Enterococcal prostatitis may require inpatient treatment with intravenous ampicillin and gentamicin. Other inpatient regimens include TMP-SMZ intravenously in two divided doses or an aminoglycoside. Although there is no US consensus on treatment, European consensus statements advocate late generation cephalosporins plus gentamycin for inpatient parenteral treatment. Other regimens include stand-alone aminoglycoside and TMP-SMZ regimens. The addition of ampicillin may be warranted if enterococcal species are suspected.

B. Adjunctive Measures

Analgesics (often including a narcotic) should be provided. Hot sitz baths may provide relief. Bed rest is usually helpful. α-1-Blockers may be useful to decrease pain and recurrence rates.

▶ Disposition

Patients with acute bacterial prostatitis causing systemic symptoms (high fever, rigors) or with suspected prostatic abscess should be hospitalized for treatment with parenteral antibiotics and consultation with a urologist.

Patients who are not hospitalized should return for follow-up in 3–4 days to ensure that recovery is progressing and again 7–10 days after stopping antimicrobial therapy for a test-of-cure culture of expressed prostatic secretions or of urine. Refer the patient to a urologist or to a source of regular medical care.

ACUTE EPIDIDYMITIS

ESSENTIALS OF DIAGNOSIS

- ▶ Testicular pain
- ▶ Epididymal tenderness

1. General Conditions

Epididymitis usually results from retrograde spread of urethral or urinary tract infection into the epididymis. Epididymitis is therefore usually caused by the same pathogens causing urethritis (eg, gonococci, *Chlamydia*) or urinary tract infection (eg, *E. coli*). The former pathogens are found more commonly in men younger than 35 years, and *E. coli* is seen more often in men over age 35 years.

▶ Clinical Findings

A. Symptoms and Signs

Pain and tenderness of the epididymis is present on one or both sides. Epididymitis must be differentiated from testicular torsion and from torsion of the testicular appendage. Ultrasound with Doppler flow will demonstrate an increased flow in epididymitis and a decreased or absence of flow in testicular torsion. In orchitis the testicle is diffusely and tensely swollen, warm, firm, and tender.

Urethritis or urinary tract infection usually coexists with epididymitis, and evidence of these conditions must be sought with appropriate laboratory tests. At a minimum, Gram or methylene blue stain of urethral exudates (or swab of material in the anterior urethra if no exudates can be obtained) and a clean-voided midstream urine specimen should be obtained for analysis.

▶ Treatment

A. Antimicrobials

1. Epididymitis with urinary tract infection—Give TMP-SMZ for 10 days. This regimen may be added onto that below if clinical concern exists for sexually transmitted infection (STI).

2. Epididymitis in sexually active heterosexual men younger than age 35 years—Regardless of whether *N. gonorrhoeae* is demonstrated, the (CDC) recommends treatment for gonorrhea and *Chlamydia*. Administer ceftriaxone 250 mg intramuscularly followed by doxycycline 100mg or tetracycline for 10 days. Levofloxacin 500mg daily for 10 days is an alternative.

3. Epididymitis in sexually active heterosexual men older than age 35 years—Empiric therapy with ciprofloxacin 500 mg PO b.i.d. 10 days or levofloxacin 500 mg daily for 10 days is recommended. TMP-SMZ double strength for 14 days is an alternative. Again, if any concern for STI exists, treat concurrently with ceftriaxone and doxycycline.

B. Adjunctive Measures

Prescribe analgesics as needed. Hot sitz baths may be helpful. Bed rest and scrotal elevation for 1–2 days will provide symptomatic relief. If the patient must be ambulatory, an athletic supporter may be helpful.

▶ Disposition

Refer the patient to a urologist or primary-care physician within a few days. Hospitalization is indicated for orchitis that does not respond within 48 hours to oral therapy and adjunctive measures.

SEXUALLY TRANSMITTED DISEASES

The management of all sexually transmitted diseases should include counseling regarding safe sex practices and the performance of HIV antibody test in consenting patients.

GONORRHEA

N. gonorrhoeae causes primary genitourinary tract infections, localized infections, and the disseminated arthritis–dermatitis syndrome. Approximately 600,000 new cases are diagnosed each year.

▶ Clinical Findings

A. Symptoms and Signs

In men, gonococcal urethritis is characterized by acute onset of dysuria, sometimes with hematuria, and a copious creamy urethral discharge. Less profuse urethral discharge requiring milking of the penile urethra may also occur. Local extension of infection may produce inflammation of preputial glands, epididymitis, seminal vasculitis, and prostatitis.

In women, gonococcal cervicitis may be asymptomatic or patients may present with vaginal discharge or symptoms of accompanying urethritis (eg, dysuria, frequency). Occasionally a Bartholin gland abscess is the initial complaint. Patients with gonococcal salpingitis complain of lower abdominal pain (unilateral or bilateral), vaginal discharge, and metromenorrhagia. Pain on cervical motion and adnexal tenderness are usual; nausea and vomiting and marked abdominal tenderness or rebound suggest pelvic peritonitis.

Rectal infection with *N. gonorrhoeae* is usually asymptomatic, although patients occasionally present with proctitis (rectal pain, discharge, tenesmus, and constipation). Pharyngeal infection is almost always asymptomatic.

Patients with gonococcal conjunctivitis present with marked conjunctival erythema and purulent discharge, often unilateral. In adults, it usually follows contact between contaminated fingers and the eye.

B. Laboratory Findings

In men, obtain a Gram-stained smear of urethral discharge, examine it microscopically, and obtain culture and antimicrobial susceptibility testing. The presence of leukocytes (usually PMNs) and intracellular gram-negative diplococci on the smear is more than 99% specific for gonorrhea. A smear showing only PMNs with no gram-negative diplococci is a predictor of a negative gonococcal culture in over 90% of patients, although culture for gonorrhea is generally recommended. These patients should receive treatment for nongonococcal urethritis. Culture of the pharynx and rectum is necessary if there is a history of oral or receptive rectal intercourse because negative results on Gram-stained smears from these areas do not rule out gonorrhea.

In women, findings on Gram-stained smears of cervical secretions may suggest gonorrhea (PMNs with intracellular gram-negative diplococci), but culture should be performed to confirm the diagnosis. Culture of rectal secretions is recommended in all women because sometimes it is the only site yielding positive cultures.

Culture of pharyngeal secretions is necessary in patients with a history of oral sexual intercourse. Express the exudates in purulent conjunctivitis, and examine a Gram-stained smear. Gram-negative diplococci confirm a diagnosis of gonococcal conjunctivitis. Send a sample of the exudates for culture.

Culture on Thayer–Martin media remains the gold standard for diagnosis. The Gonorrhea PCR test is 97–99% sensitive, with specificity of 99%. A serologic test for syphilis (eg, VDRL) should be ordered for all patients.

▶ Treatment

Because there has been worldwide spread of strains of *N. gonorrhoeae* that are resistant to penicillin, amoxicillin, tetracycline, and fluoroquinolones, these agents are no longer recommended for empiric treatment of gonococcal infections.

Use ceftriaxone, 125 mg intramuscularly. Alternative treatment includes cefotaxime 500 mg intramuscularly. In the β-lactam allergic patient, fluoroquinolone therapy can be used but sensitivity of the patient's strain to quinolones must be evaluated and test of cure obtained, or azithromycin 2 g single dose can be considered. Because of the high frequency of coexisting chlamydial infection (up to 45%), a tetracycline, doxycycline, or azithromycin regimen should follow the treatment of gonococcal infections.

Patients with gonococcal conjunctivitis may be hospitalized and should receive ophthalmologic consultation. Therapy consists of ceftriaxone, 1 g intramuscularly or intravenously once daily for at least 5 days, combined with immediate and at least hourly irrigation of the eye with saline or buffered ophthalmic solutions. Simultaneous ophthalmic infection with *C. trachomatis* can also occur. Careful ophthalmic follow-up is necessary to prevent ocular complications.

▶ Disposition

Hospitalization is not required for patients with localized gonococcal infection, except for gonococcal conjunctivitis. Sexual partners with gonorrhea must be notified and receive treatment. Cases of gonorrhea must be reported to the local public health department.

NONGONOCOCCAL URETHRITIS (NONSPECIFIC URETHRITIS)

Nongonococcal urethritis, or nonspecific urethritis, is due to infection with *C. trachomatis* in over half the cases. Genital *Mycoplasmas* (*Ureaplasma*), HSV, and *Trichomonas* are occasional causes.

▶ Clinical Findings

A. Symptoms and Signs

Most male patients have urethral discharge and dysuria. Symptoms are often insidious in onset, with urethral discharge that is scanty, mucoid, watery, and most prominent in the morning. Women may be asymptomatic or may complain of dysuria or frequency. Infection may involve the cervix as well and extend to the oviducts, producing low-grade fever.

B. Laboratory Findings

Urethral discharge should be stained with Gram stain and examined microscopically. The presence of more than four leukocytes per high-power field confirms the diagnosis of urethritis. If no organisms morphologically consistent with gonococci are found, then presumptive diagnosis of nongonococcal urethritis can be made. A Gram-stained smear with findings diagnostic of gonorrhea does not exclude nongonococcal urethritis because dual infection with *Chlamydia* and the gonococcus is common, particularly in a heterosexual population. The specimen should be sent for culture but because of difficulties in culturing this organism, culture is 80% sensitive. PCR testing is the most sensitive (93–99%), with specificity of 99–100%. A serologic test for syphilis should also be considered.

► Treatment

First-line agents recommended by the CDC include single-dose azithromycin or a 7-day course of doxycycline or levofloxacin 500 mg PO for 7 days. If nongonococcal urethritis is suspected (negative or equivocal findings on Gram-stained smear with culture results pending) or documented (culture negative for nongonococcal urethritis), sexual partners should also receive treatment.

► Disposition

Patients with nongonococcal urethritis can receive treatment on an outpatient basis.

GENITAL HERPES SIMPLEX VIRUS INFECTION

ESSENTIALS OF DIAGNOSIS

▶ Fever, adenopathy

▶ Vesicles on an erythematous base

▶ Pain

► General Considerations

HSV is a major cause of recurrent genital lesions. The initial (primary) infection is the most severe, although it is sometimes asymptomatic. After the primary lesion has healed, the virus remains latent in the paraspinous ganglia, where it periodically causes reactivation of infection. Genital infection is usually caused by HSV type 2, and about 99% of patients with recurrent disease will be infected by type 2 virus. Spread of infection is almost exclusively by sexual intercourse.

► Clinical Findings

A. Symptoms and Signs

1. First clinical episode of genital HSV—The first clinical attack of HSV is usually the most severe. Patients may present with fever, malaise, myalgias, and arthralgias. Aseptic meningitis occurs in 10–20% of cases, particularly in women. Associated symptoms may include dysuria, dyspareunia, and urinary retention. Successive crops of grouped vesicles on an erythematous base denude, form ulcers, and heal by secondary intention, usually in 2–3 weeks but sometimes not until after 6 weeks. Genital edema is common. Local pain and

regional adenopathy are usually marked. In men, the glans and penile shaft are involved. In women, the vulva, vagina, and cervix are the usual sites of involvement. Male or female patients with herpetic proctitis present with fever, tenesmus, constipation, and rectal pain.

2. Recurrent HSV episodes—Recurrent infection is common and may be triggered by a variety of stimuli (eg, friction, menstruation, sexual intercourse, pregnancy, or stress). Recurrent attacks are frequently heralded by a prodrome consisting of local itching, pain, or aching in the buttocks or leg. Initially, a papule develops that rapidly vesiculates, breaks down into an ulcer, and then heals, usually within 7–10 days. The virus may be recovered as long as lesions are moist. Patients should avoid direct skin-to-skin contact until the area is completely dried and healed.

The presence of HSV may be confirmed by the Tzanck test (about 60% sensitivity and 80% specificity) or virus culture. Virus culture is recommended in most cases.

► Treatment

Antipyretics and analgesics may help to relieve systemic symptoms. Antiviral regimens (Table 42–16) accelerate resolution of the signs and symptoms of herpetic eruptions but do not affect the subsequent risk, frequency, or severity of recurrences after the drug is discontinued. Immunocompromised patients (especially AIDS patients) with extensive, ulcerative, or progressive mucocutaneous herpes should receive oral therapy. Continuous therapy is necessary in some patients.

Hospitalization for intravenous therapy may be warranted if the patient is unable to take medications orally or if the lesions are extensive. Antibiotics are not necessary unless Gram-stained smears suggest bacterial superinfection. Women with primary genital herpes frequently have associated *Candida* vaginitis, which should be treated as described above. The patient should bathe the exposed affected areas with warm tap water, or apply warm compresses every

Table 42–16. Outpatient Treatment of Genital Herpes Infections.

Type of Therapy	Agent and Dosing
Primary outbreak	Acyclovir 200 mg PO five times a day for 10 days Valacyclovir 1000 mg PO b.i.d. for 7–10 days Famciclovir, 250 mg PO t.i.d. for 7–10 days
Recurrent	Acyclovir 200 mg PO five times a day for 5 days Valacyclovir, 500 mg PO b.i.d. for 3 days Famciclovir 125 mg PO b.i.d. for 5 days
Suppression	Acyclovir, 400 mg PO b.i.d. Valacyclovir 1000 mg PO q.d. Famciclovir 250 mg PO b.i.d.

4 hours. Because lesions shed infectious virus, patients should avoid manipulating lesions with their bare hands and should wash their hands after exposure (autoinoculation of the eye or other sites may occur). Any other contact with the lesions (eg, sexual) should be avoided until they have healed.

▶ Disposition

Hospitalization is occasionally indicated for patients with primary HSV infection because of severe pain, systemic symptoms, and other complications (urinary retention, obstipation, aseptic meningitis, dehydration). Hospitalization is also required for patients with extensive, large, or rapidly progressive lesions.

Patients with genital HSV infection are often frightened and confused about the nature and transmission of the disease and may suffer both physically and psychologically. Counseling should be initiated and provided in the emergency department, if possible, and patients should be referred to a gynecologist or primary-care provider who is experienced in treating HSV infection and can explain the disease, answer any questions, and provide information on various methods of treatment so that the patient can make an informed evaluation of the associated efficacy, risks, and side effects. Obtain obstetric consultation for pregnant patients with HSV infection.

SYPHILIS

ESSENTIALS OF DIAGNOSIS

- ▶ Chancre (painless)
- ▶ Rash
- ▶ Positive VDRL, RPR, FTA-ABS

▶ General Considerations

Disease following infection due to *Treponema pallidum* may be divided into primary, secondary, latent, and tertiary stages. Infection with *T. pallidum* has been identified as an important risk factor for HIV infection. An HIV antibody test should be obtained for all consenting patients with syphilis.

▶ Clinical Findings

A. Symptoms and Signs

1. Primary stage—A chancre develops at the site of entry of the spirochete between 10 days and 6 weeks after exposure. The ulcer, located on the genitals or occasionally on extragenital sites (finger, mouth), is nontender and has a depressed center and rolled, pearly edges. Associated inguinal adenopathy, if present, is usually firm, hard, and nontender.

2. Secondary stage—Secondary disease develops about 4 weeks after the appearance of the chancre. Clinical manifestations reflect the presence of spirochetes in the bloodstream. Most common is a rash that ranges from macular to maculopapular to plaques (condyloma lata). The rash is generally distributed over the thorax, abdomen, and extremities; it may involve the palms and soles; and it is nonpruritic. Associated findings may include low-grade fever, generalized lymphadenopathy, hepatitis, meningitis, alopecia, and weight loss.

3. Latent stage—A positive serologic test is the only sign, and this stage may last from 1 to 2 months up to more than 20 years.

4. Tertiary stage—This stage is characterized by destructive lesions of the aorta, CNS, skeletal structures, and skin.

B. Laboratory Findings

The diagnosis of infectious syphilis is confirmed by serologic testing or by positive results on microscopic darkfield examination of scrapings from the chancre or lesions of secondary disease. Obtain blood for serologic testing (eg, VDRL or RPR); if results are positive, perform a treponemal antibody test (eg, FTA-ABS or MHA-TP).

▶ Treatment

A. Infectious Syphilis

1. Benzathine penicillin G—The treatment of choice is benzathine penicillin G (2.4 million units intramuscularly). Patients who claim to be allergic to penicillin should be tested (ie, skin testing) and desensitized, if necessary.

2. Doxycycline—An alternative regimen for penicillin-allergic patients is doxycycline, 100 mg orally twice daily, or tetracycline, 500 mg four times daily for 14 days.

3. Erythromycin—Patients who cannot take penicillin, doxycycline, or tetracycline and who are reliable and can be followed closely can take erythromycin, 500 mg orally four times daily for 14 days.

B. Jarisch–Herxheimer Reaction

Aspirin or acetaminophen may be prescribed for the Jarisch–Herxheimer reaction that commonly occurs within a few hours after treatment of secondary syphilis has been started. The reaction is characterized by malaise, fever, faintness, and intensification of the rash. Patients with secondary syphilis who are released from the emergency department following penicillin therapy should be warned about the symptoms of the reaction and should be told that it is not due to penicillin allergy.

C. Syphilis in HIV-Infected Patients

A lumbar puncture should be performed in HIV-infected patients with early syphilis because of increased risk of treatment failure and CNS relapse. If the CSF cell count is normal and the VDRL test nonreactive, give one to three doses of benzathine penicillin G therapy. Serum VDRL testing must be repeated at monthly intervals for at least 3 months. Tetracyclines are probably inadequate therapy for HIV-infected patients with syphilis. Ceftriaxone, 250 mg intramuscularly once daily for 10 days, can be tried.

▶ Disposition

Patients may receive treatment on an outpatient basis. Cases of syphilis must be reported to the local public health department. Sexual partners of patients should be notified and receive treatment. Arrangements must be made for follow-up serologic testing.

CHANCROID

ESSENTIALS OF DIAGNOSIS

- ▶ Erythematous pustule
- ▶ Adenopathy
- ▶ Pain
- ▶ Gram stain or culture

▶ General Considerations

Chancroid is an ulcerating genital infection caused by *Haemophilus ducreyi*. It is common in tropical and subtropical regions and is believed to be underdiagnosed in the United States.

▶ Clinical Findings

Chancroid is manifested by the appearance of a small pustule that rapidly ulcerates with an irregular and purulent exudative base that is painful. It is associated with tender inguinal lymphadenopathy in 50% of cases.

Definitive diagnosis requires growth on culture media, and the diagnosis should be considered for any patient who has painful genital ulceration and for whom darkfield fluoroscopy and HSV testing are negative.

▶ Treatment

Recommended treatments include azithromycin orally or ceftriaxone intramuscularly; ciprofloxacin and erythromycin are alternatives.

TRICHOMONIASIS

▶ Clinical Findings

A. Symptoms and Signs

Most men with *T. vaginalis* infections develop nongonococcal urethritis, but women typically develop malodorous yellow–green frothy discharge, dysuria, dyspareunia, vulvar irritation, and pruritus.

B. Laboratory Findings

Motile parasites are seen on a wet-mount smear.

▶ Treatment

Single-dose metronidazole or metronidazole therapy for 7 days is the only treatment option. No effective alternatives are available. While some intravaginal dosing regimens have been identified, therapy in pregnant women should be confined to the PO route.

Centers for Disease Control: Update to CDC's sexually transmitted diseases treatment guidelines, 2006: Fluoroquinolones no longer recommended for treatment of gonococcal infections. MMWR Morb Mortal Wkly Rep 2007;56:332–336 [PMID: 17431378].

Centers for Disease Control and Prevention, Workowski KA, Berman SM: Sexually transmitted diseases treatment guidelines, 2006. MMWR Recomm Rep 2006;55:1–94 [PMID: 16888612].

Nurbhai M, Grimshaw J, Watson M, Bond C, Mollison J, Ludbrook A: Oral versus intra-vaginal imidazole and triazole anti-fungal treatment of uncomplicated vulvovaginal candidiasis (thrush). Cochrane Database of Sys Rev 2007;CD002845 [PMID: 17943774].

Nygren P, Fu R, Freeman M: Evidence on the benefits and harms of screening and treating pregnant women who are asymptomatic for bacterial vaginosis: An update review for the U.S. Preventive Services Task Force. Ann Intern Med 2008;148: 220–233 [PMID: 18252684].

Oduyebo OO, Anorlu RI, Ogunsola FT: The effects of antimicrobial therapy on bacterial vaginosis in non-pregnant women. Cochrane Database Sys Rev 2009;CD006055 [PMID: 19588379].

Clinical Effectiveness Group, British Association for Sexual Health and HIV (BASHH): United Kingdom national guideline on the management of prostatitis. www.guideline.gov/content.aspx?id=14278. London, United Kingdom, 2008 (last accessed August 17, 2010).

SKIN AND SOFT TISSUE INFECTIONS

SUPERFICIAL SOFT TISSUE INFECTIONS

▶ General Considerations

Initial evaluation of soft tissue infections should focus on three factors: (1) what is the probable organism; (2) what is the depth of infection; and (3) is the infection life- or limb-threatening? Most infections are caused by gram-positive organisms, particularly *Staphylococcus pyogenes* and *Staph. aureus*. Although most infections are benign, complicating factors such as comorbid conditions (diabetes, HIV), high-risk areas (face, hands, perineum), or signs of deep-tissue involvement should prompt more aggressive interventions, including possible surgical consultation in the case of deep-tissue involvement.

Clinical Findings

A. Symptoms and Signs

1. Impetigo—Impetigo is a superficial infection most commonly seen in children and may manifest in bullous and nonbullous forms. Nonbullous impetigo begins as vesicles that rupture and form a golden-yellow, "honey-crusted" purulent discharge. Bullous impetigo results from toxin formation and begins as a small vesicle that rapidly enlarges to a bulla. Lesions are painless and systemic symptoms are rare.

2. Ecthyma—Ecthyma is a slightly deeper form of impetigo with resultant scarring and ulceration.

3. Staphylococcal scalded skin syndrome (SSSS)—SSSS is a toxin-mediated disease resulting in widespread bulla formation and exfoliation, often in the extremities. Children are affected more commonly than adults.

4. Erysipelas—Erysipelas is an acute inflammation of the superficial layers of skin particularly involving cutaneous lymphatics. It most often occurs on the face and results in fiery red, edematous lesion that is raised and clearly demarcated from the surrounding tissue. Lymphangitis and lymphadenopathy are common, as are systemic symptoms such as fever and chills. Approximately 10% of cases will progress to involve deeper soft tissue layers.

5 Cellulitis—Cellulitis is an infection of the lower dermis and subcutaneous tissue that is characterized by an ill-defined erythema, swelling, warmth, and pain. Systemic symptoms are common in more severe cases. Diabetes and peripheral vascular disease places the patient at higher risk for infection with gram-negative organisms and anaerobes.

B. Laboratory Findings

Laboratory studies are of little utility in uncomplicated cases. Blood cultures are rarely positive but should be obtained in rapidly progressive or otherwise severe infection. Gram stain and culture of material from the leading edge of the lesion or vesicles may be helpful in rare cases.

Treatment

A. Impetigo and Ecthyma

Topical treatment with warm soaks to remove crusting and mupirocin is effective for most cases. Oral anti-staphylococcal agents should be considered in bullous impetigo.

B. Staphylococcal scalded skin syndrome

Oral antistaphylococcal agents and a meticulous search for the initiating infection with appropriate treatment are necessary. Cool saline compresses and local wound care as needed should be applied to desquamated areas. Corticosteroids are not beneficial.

C. Erysipelas

Penicillin remains the first-line treatment of uncomplicated erysipelas. In the presence of lymphedema or chronic venous insufficiency, a first-generation cephalosporin, clindamycin, or macrolide may be used.

D. Cellulitis

Mild cases may be treated with oral agents such as a first-generation cephalosporin, dicloxacillin or clindamycin. More severe infection thought to be due to streptococci or staphylococci in patients who are not critically ill may be treated with intravenous first-generation cephalosporin, nafcillin. Addition of an aminoglycoside should be considered when gram-negative bacteria are suspected. Immobilization and elevation of the affected extremity are helpful.

Disposition

Patients with early, mild disease may be discharged home on oral antibiotics. Nontoxic patients with cellulitis that has progressed over 12–24 hours may be given parental therapy and discharged with follow-up within 24 hours. Failure to respond to outpatient therapy, cellulitis of the face or hand, and complicating factors such as diabetes, venous/lymphatic insufficiency, or systemic toxicity may require inpatient treatment.

COMMUNITY-ACQUIRED MRSA

General Considerations

A growing number of skin and soft tissue infections are caused by a strain of MRSA that appears to be clinically and epidemiologically distinct from that traditionally associated with nosocomial infection. Unlike health care associated MRSA, CAMRSA is commonly resistant only to β-lactams. CAMRSA isolates often produce a Panton-Valentine leukocidin toxin, which is associated with soft tissue infections and a severe necrotizing pneumonia. Populations at higher risk for CA-MRSA infection include children (particularly in day-care centers), soldiers, prisoners, intravenous drug users, homeless persons, and men who have sex with men. The apparent common demographic feature seems to center around increased population density.

Clinical Findings

Recurrent furunculosis and cutaneous abscesses are the most common presentation of CA-MRSA infection, with dermonecrotic lesions occasionally present. Recurrent furunculosis and transmission to close contacts such as family members or sports teammates are also suggestive of CAMRSA. CA-MRSA pneumonia, although rare, may occur following influenza.

▶ Treatment

Surgical drainage of any abscesses should be performed. For those in whom outpatient treatment is appropriate, TMP-SMZ, doxycycline, minocycline, and clindamycin are all appropriate agents. However, treatment failure may result from inducible clindamycin resistance. If infection with β-hemolytic streptococci is considered likely, cephalexin may be added. Hospitalized patients may be treated with vancomycin or linezolid.

DEEP SOFT TISSUE INFECTIONS

Deep soft tissue infections, characterized by involvement of subcutaneous tissues with possible extension to the muscles and fascial planes, are uncommon and often difficult to diagnose. Various classification systems have been used to help delineate various microbiologic or anatomic features of the infection; however, the utility of these systems in the emergency department is limited. Instead, a uniform approach to all patients with necrotizing soft tissue infections (NSTIs) may help minimize misdiagnosis and ensure timely treatment.

▶ General Considerations

NSTIs are usually associated with introduction of pathogenic organisms through minor trauma, insect bites, or surgical incision. "Skin popping" by intravenous drug users is a significant risk factor. Spontaneous infections are most likely to occur in the perineum (Fournier gangrene). Most infections are polymicrobial and GABHS are frequently present, rarely as the only organism isolated. Rapidly progressive surgical infections in the first 24 hours postoperatively frequently harbor Clostridium species as well. Chronic illnesses such as diabetes, renal insufficiency, and alcoholism are commonly present, although up to 30% of cases occur in otherwise healthy individuals.

▶ Clinical Findings

A. Symptoms and Signs

NSTIs may occur anywhere on the body, with the perineum and extremities most frequently involved. Early physical findings may be minimal and include cellulitis or a small ulcer with erythema, warmth, and edema in overlying skin, skin anesthesia, and pain out of proportion to examination findings. Later findings include tense edema with bronze discoloration of the skin progressing to hemorrhagic bullae and a seropurulent ("dishwater pus"), foul-smelling exudate. Crepitus is common with clostridial infections but may

be absent in GABHS infections. As the disease progresses, patients may become septic with tachycardia, hyperthermia, and hypotension, with 10% of patients with massive GABHS meeting the criteria for streptococcal toxic shock syndrome (STSS). Key early findings include tachycardia and fever out of proportion to the apparent extent of the skin lesion and tenderness that extends well beyond the lesion.

B. Laboratory Findings

Common laboratory abnormalities include leukocytosis, hyponatremia, azotemia, and hypocalcemia. Radiographic imaging may confirm the presence of subcutaneous emphysema on plain films, but this finding is absent 50% of the time and a negative result does not rule out the diagnosis. CT scanning may show asymmetric thickening or stranding of fascial planes and is more useful for suspected perineal NSTIs. Needle aspiration with gram staining may also be useful in equivocal cases.

▶ Treatment

Aggressive resuscitation with fluids and broad-spectrum antibiotic coverage should be initiated early when a NSTI is suspected. Triple coverage with a penicillin, clindamycin or metronidazole, and an aminoglycoside is appropriate pending the results of cultures. Prompt surgical debridement is imperative and appropriate surgical consultation should be obtained as soon as possible.

▶ Disposition

All patients with NSTIs should be admitted for surgical exploration and debridement, followed by hospitalization in an intensive care setting.

Adam HJ, Allen VG, Currie A, McGeer AJ, Simor AE, Richardson SE, Louie L, Willey B, Rutledge T, Lee J, Goldman RD, Somers A, Ellis P, Sarabia A, Rizos J, Borgundvaag B, Katz KC; EMERGENT Working Group: Community-associated methicillin-resistant *Staphylococcus aureus*: Prevalence in skin and soft tissue infections at emergency departments in the Greater Toronto Area and associated risk factors. CJEM 2009; Sep;11(5):439–446 [PMID: 19788788].

Centers for Disease Control and Prevention: MRSA Infections. Atlanta, GA, August 9, 2010. http://www.cdc.gov/mrsa/index.html (last accessed August 19, 2010).

Loeb MB, Main C, Eady A, Walkers-Dilks C: Antimicrobial drugs for treating methicillin-resistant *Staphylococcus aureus* colonization. Cochrane Database of Sys Rev 2003;CD003340 [PMID: 14583969].

Stevens DL, Bisno AL, Chambers HF, et al: Practice guidelines for the diagnosis and management of skin and soft-tissue infections. Clin Infect Dis 2005 Nov 15;41(10):1373–1406 [PMID: 16231249].

Vinh DC, Embil JM: Rapidly progressive soft tissue infections. Lancet Infect Dis 2005;5:501–513 [PMID: 16048719].

MANAGEMENT OF INFECTIONS CAUSED BY SPECIFIC ORGANISMS

ACUTE MENINGOCOCCEMIA

ESSENTIALS OF DIAGNOSIS

▶ Fever

▶ Petechial rash

▶ Hypotension

▶ Shock

▶ Clinical Findings

A. Symptoms and Signs

Invasive meningococcal disease is often associated with a recent or current upper respiratory infection and is most common in infants, with a second peak around 18 years of age. Meningococcemia may present as meningitis, sepsis, pneumonia, epiglottitis, conjunctivitis, pericarditis, or arthritis, although meningitis and sepsis are the most common and rapid progression is typical. Overcrowding, smoking, and complement deficiencies are risk factors for invasive disease. Mucosal petechiae may appear first, followed by skin petechiae that may become confluent as microvascular thrombosis progresses. However, petechiae may be absent in up to 20% of children with meningococcemia. Peripheral circulatory failure is common in meningococcal sepsis, and ventricular dysfunction with elevated CVP is also seen in severe disease. Waterhouse-Friderichsen syndrome results from adrenal hemorrhage with resultant corticosteroid deficiency and causes circulatory collapse.

B. Laboratory Findings

Routine laboratory studies should be obtained, including blood cultures and CSF studies, if septic shock or coagulopathy does not preclude lumbar puncture. Evaluation for DIC (PT, INR, PTT, fibrinogen, and fibrin degradation products) should also be performed. CSF antigen detection is no more sensitive than microscopy and culture. PCR is the gold standard of diagnosis and does not require that the meningococci be alive at the time material is collected. Although it is preferable to obtain material for culture prior to the administration of antibiotics, antibiotics should not be unduly delayed.

▶ Treatment

Empiric treatment with ceftriaxone or cefotaxime should be instituted as soon as possible when the diagnosis is seriously entertained, along with EGDT for severe sepsis or septic shock as indicated. Steroids are indicated for the treatment of adrenal insufficiency, and dexamethasone should be given in meningococcal meningitis. Chemoprophylaxis of close contacts of those with invasive disease (including health-care workers directly involved in their care) may be accomplished with rifampin, ciprofloxacin, or ceftriaxone.

▶ Disposition

All patients with invasive meningococcal disease should be hospitalized, preferably in an intensive care setting.

Milonovich LM: Meningococcemia: Epidemiology, pathophysiology, and management. J Pediatr Health Care 2007;21:75–80. [PMID: 17321906].

ROCKY MOUNTAIN SPOTTED FEVER

ESSENTIALS OF DIAGNOSIS

▶ Fever

▶ Headache

▶ Petechial rash (palms or soles)

▶ General Considerations

Rocky mountain spotted fever (RMSF) is an acute febrile tick-borne illness caused by *Rickettsia rickettsii*. Although it has been reported in most states in the United States, it is most common in the southern Atlantic and south central states and in Oklahoma. Most cases occur in warm months, when ticks are most active. Eighty percent of patients have a history of tick bite.

▶ Clinical Findings

A. Symptoms and Signs

The classic triad of fever, headache, and rash associated with a recent tick bite is absent in most patients who develop RMSF, and 30–40% will have no history of tick bite. Virtually all adults and older children will have a headache initially, accompanied by myalgias and malaise. Children will often have gastrointestinal complaints, including nausea, vomiting, and abdominal pain. The rash of RMSF typically begins as a maculopapular exanthem on the ankles or wrists and progressing toward the body that then evolves into a petechial rash. Neuropsychiatric symptoms indicate a more severe course and worse prognosis.

B. Laboratory Findings

Thrombocytopenia is typical, and hyponatremia with elevated transaminases may also be seen. Elevated serum creatinine is associated with increased mortality. IFA testing for IgG and IgM can confirm the diagnosis but is not readily available, and early treatment may result in negative testing.

▶ Treatment

Treatment must begin on clinical grounds and is most effective when begun in the first 3–5 days of illness. Doxycycline is the treatment of choice for both adults and children. In the past, chloramphenicol was recommended for younger children, although studies have demonstrated that brief courses of tetracyclines do not result in perceptible staining of teeth in younger children and both the AAP and CDC recommend doxycycline for children younger than age 9.

▶ Disposition

Patients with neurologic symptoms, vomiting, elevated creatinine, or unstable vital signs should be admitted.

Dantas-Torres F: Rocky Mountain spotted fever. Lancet Infect Dis 2007;7:724–732. [PMID: 17961858]

INFECTIVE ENDOCARDITIS

ESSENTIALS OF DIAGNOSIS

- ▶ Fever, chills
- ▶ New or changing murmur
- ▶ Cutaneous lesions

▶ General Consideration

Infective endocarditis denotes infection of the endothelial surface of the heart, most often the cardiac valves. The disease may either be acute or subacute and may affect normal valves, previously damaged cardiac valves, or prosthetic valves. It is usually caused by bacteria, but fungi are also common pathogens in intravenous drug abusers with acute endocarditis. Seeding of bacterial emboli or deposition of immune complexes in the skin may cause characteristic skin lesions that can alert the physician to the correct diagnosis before progressive damage to the heart leads to circulatory collapse. Common pathogenic organisms include *Strep. viridans*, *Streptococcus bovis*, and the HACEK group of gram-negative organisms (*Haemophilus*, *Actinobacillus*, *Cardiobacterium*, *Eikenella*, and *Kingella*). *Staph. aureus* is particularly virulent, and infection is associated with a high mortality rate. *S. epidermis* and coagulase-negative staphylococci

are the leading causes of infective endocarditis in patients with prosthetic valves.

▶ Clinical Findings

A. Symptoms and Signs

Patients usually present with fever and malaise. In subacute endocarditis, there may be a history of anorexia, night sweats, and weight loss. Patients may also present in cardiac failure, with a stroke due to cerebral embolism, or with a cold extremity due to arterial emboli. Patients with infective endocarditis of the tricuspid valve (usually seen in intravenous drug abusers) commonly present with acute, often bilateral, embolic pneumonia. Examination of the heart often reveals a murmur, although heart murmurs are commonly absent in right-sided endocarditis.

Characteristic (but not specific) cutaneous and mucosal lesions in bacterial endocarditis include conjunctival and palatal petechiae, subungual (splinter) hemorrhages, Osler nodes, and Janeway lesions. Osler nodes are tender erythematous nodules with opaque centers that appear on the pulp of the fingertips and toes. Janeway lesions are nontender, red or maroon macules or nodules that develop on the palms and soles. Careful ophthalmologic examination may also reveal Roth spots (pale oval areas surrounded by hemorrhage) near the optic disk.

The Duke criteria were developed to aid in the diagnosis of endocarditis. The diagnosis requires two major criteria, or one major and three minor criteria, or five minor criteria (Table 42–17).

Table 42–17. Duke Criteria for Diagnosis of Infective Endocarditis.

Major Criteria
Positive blood cultures
    Typical microorganisms for endocarditis on two separate blood cultures
    Persistently positive blood cultures
Evidence of endocardial involvement: positive echocardiogram (oscillating intracardiac mass on valve or supporting structures; in the path of regurgitant jets; or on implanted material, abscess, or new partial dehiscence of a prosthetic valve)
New valvular regurgitation (increase or change in preexisting murmur not sufficient)
Minor Criteria
Fever >38°C
Predisposing heart conditions or intravenous drug abuse. Vascular phenomenon: major arterial emboli, septic pulmonary infarcts, mycotic aneurysms, intracranial hemorrhage, conjunctival hemorrhages, Janeway lesions
Immunologic phenomena: glomerulonephritis, Osler nodes, Roth spots, rheumatoid factor
Microbiological evidence: positive blood culture but not meeting major criteria
Echocardiogram: consistent with endocarditis but not meeting major criterion

B. Laboratory Findings

Laboratory findings are variable and nonspecific for infective endocarditis. A normochromic normocytic anemia may be present, especially for patients with subacute disease. The white cell count may be elevated, especially in acute disease. The erythrocyte sedimentation rate is usually elevated. Microscopic hematuria is present in 30–50% of patients. Immune complex glomerulonephritis with renal failure may occur. Transthoracic echocardiography is 98% specific for endocarditis, but sensitivity may be less than 60%. Transesophageal echocardiography is close to 100% sensitive for examination of native valves and 84–94% sensitive for prosthetic valves.

Definitive diagnosis depends on isolating the causative organisms in blood cultures; however, 5–20% of patients with clinical endocarditis have persistently negative blood cultures (termed culture-negative endocarditis). Gram-stained smears of aspirates from skin lesions (usually Janeway lesions) occasionally permit rapid diagnosis. In patients with embolic pneumonia, Gram-stained smears of sputum may demonstrate the causative agent (usually *Staph. aureus*); however, in intravenous drug abusers, possible concurrent infection with other organisms (streptococci, gram-negative bacilli) must be treated pending blood culture results.

Treatment

In patients who are not acutely ill and in whom symptoms and signs of cardiac failure or major emboli are absent, antibiotic therapy may be withheld pending blood culture results. In all other patients, empiric antibiotic therapy should be initiated after samples of blood, urine, and (when present) sputum and aspirates from skin lesions have been obtained for culture.

A. Abnormal Cardiac Valve or Congenital Heart Disease

Usual pathogens in patients with abnormal cardiac valves or congenital heart disease are *Strep. viridans* and group D streptococci. Aqueous penicillin G intravenously is an acceptable empiric regimen. Vancomycin intravenously may be substituted for penicillin.

B. Prosthetic Cardiac Valves

Many pathogens cause prosthetic cardiac valve endocarditis. Infection occurring less than 6 months postoperatively may be caused by *Staph. aureus*, *S. epidermidis*, gram-negative aerobic bacilli, diphtheroids, or fungi. Infection occurring more than 6 months after prosthetic valve insertion is usually caused by *Strep. viridans*, aerobic gram-negative bacilli, enterococci, or staphylococci. Because growth of some of these organisms requires multiple blood cultures using special techniques, it is best to avoid early empiric therapy whenever possible. In a patient who requires immediate surgery because of hemodynamic decompensation, empiric therapy may be started with vancomycin and gentamycin.

C. Parenteral Drug Abuse

The usual pathogens in intravenous drug abusers are *Staph. aureus*, *Pseudomonas* sp., and streptococci, including group D streptococci. Empiric treatment should include vancomycin and gentamicin with substitution for vancomycin with penicillin and nafcillin, oxacillin, or methicillin in patients with compromised renal function.

Disposition

Patients with suspected bacterial endocarditis should be hospitalized. Obtain cardiothoracic surgical consultation for patients with infected prosthetic heart valves, new onset of cardiac failure, or emboli in major vessels because emergency valve replacement is often necessary.

Lester SJ, Wilansky S: Endocarditis and associated complications. Crit Care Med 2007;35:S384–S391 [PMID: 17667463].

McDonald JR: Acute infective endocarditis. Infect Dis Clin North Am 2009;23:643–664 [PMID:19665088].

DISSEMINATED GONOCOCCEMIA

ESSENTIALS OF DIAGNOSIS

► Fever
► Skin lesions
► Septic arthritis
► Positive culture results

General Considerations

As bacteremia occurs in 3% of patients, it is not surprising that it is the leading cause of septic arthritis in adults. It should be recognized easily in the adolescent with arthritis or dermatitis.

Clinical Findings

A. Symptoms and Signs

Frequently, there is two distinct phases with disseminated gonorrhea. Initially there is bacteremia associated with fever arthralgias and dermatitis. This is followed by a frank septic arthritis. The skin lesions usually develop on the extremities. Lesions vary and range from petechiae and erythematous, palpable purpura to vesiculopustules with an erythematous halo, and they often have necrotic centers. About one-fourth of patients have tenosynovitis, usually affecting the wrist or ankle. Acute septic arthritis, affecting one or more large joints, may follow disseminated gonococcemia or may occur in its absence.

B. Laboratory Findings

The white cell count may be elevated. Blood cultures are often positive in disseminated gonococcemia. Although Gram stains and culture of skin lesions are generally negative, cultures of all sites are negative in as many as 50% of patients, and a presumptive diagnosis is based instead on the prompt response to ceftriaxone therapy.

▶ Treatment

A. Antimicrobial Therapy

Give ceftriaxone (1 g intravenously or intramuscularly every 24 hours).

▶ Disposition

Most patients with septic arthritis should be hospitalized, but outpatient treatment with daily visits for joint aspiration is an acceptable alternative for reliable patients. Many patients with only dermatitis or tenosynovitis may receive outpatient treatment with close follow-up.

> Rice PA: Gonococcal arthritis (disseminated gonococcal infection). Infect Dis Clin North Am 2005;19:853 [PMID: 16297736].

TOXIC SHOCK SYNDROME

ESSENTIALS OF DIAGNOSIS

- ▶ Erythroderma
- ▶ Hypotension
- ▶ Multisystem organ dysfunction

▶ General Considerations

Toxic shock syndrome results from absorption of toxin from localized *Staph. aureus* colonization or infection. In the past, most cases occurred in young women who had vaginal colonization with *Staph. aureus* that produce toxic shock syndrome toxin-1 (TSST-1); however, nonmenstrual-related cases currently outnumber menstrual-related cases. Most of the nonmenstrual cases occur in the postoperative setting. The toxin functions as a superantigen that allows the antigen to bind directly to the MHC-II (major histocompatibility complex) receptor in a nonspecific fashion. This may result in activation of 5–30% of the total T-cell population, leading to massive cytokine production. The mortality rate in STSS is five times higher than in toxic shock syndrome.

▶ Clinical Findings

Menstrual-related toxic shock syndrome usually starts abruptly during menses. It occurs most commonly in women using tampons or contraceptive sponges. In nonmenstrual cases associated with postoperative infection, signs of localized infection in the wound may be absent.

A. Symptoms and Signs

There is a short prodrome consisting of various combinations of the following symptoms and signs: fever, myalgias, vomiting, diarrhea, and pharyngitis. Patients then develop shock (SBP <80 mm Hg) with fever (>39°C) and signs of multiple organ dysfunction. At the time of presentation to the emergency department or within 24 hours of admission to the hospital, a diffuse, blanching, macular erythema appears, accompanied by signs of mucous membrane inflammation (pharyngitis, conjunctivitis, vaginitis, and strawberry tongue). The rash fades in about 3 days, but desquamation of the hands and feet occurs in all patients 5–12 days after the rash disappears. Patients typically prefer to remain motionless in bed because of intense myalgias. Confusion and agitation occur in about half of patients. Pedal edema is common.

B. Laboratory Findings

Laboratory findings reflect dysfunction of several organ systems. There may be leukocytosis and thrombocytopenia, elevated BUN and creatinine levels, hyperbilirubinemia, elevated hepatic enzymes, or sterile pyuria. The prothrombin, INR, and PTTs may be elevated, with or without thrombocytopenia. Other laboratory abnormalities include acidosis, elevated creatine kinase levels (indicating rhabdomyolysis), hypocalcemia, decreased serum albumin and total protein due to capillary leakage, and elevated liver enzyme levels. Cultures of material from the vagina or cervix are usually positive for *Staph. aureus*. Blood cultures are negative in 85% of patients with toxic shock syndrome and in 50% of patients with STSS.

▶ Treatment and Disposition

Remove the vaginal tampon or nasal or wound packing if present. Begin volume replacement with saline or colloid solutions and with vasopressors, if necessary. Admit the patient to an ICU, and monitor hemodynamic status. Start treatment with a first-generation cephalosporin, penicillinase-resistant synthetic penicillin, or vancomycin intravenously.

GROUP A STREPTOCOCCAL INFECTIONS ASSOCIATED WITH A TOXIC SHOCK–LIKE SYNDROME

An infection with group A streptococci that is remarkable for severity of local tissue destruction, life-threatening systemic toxicity, and toxic-shock-like syndrome has been described in adults. Clinical isolates frequently produce pyrogenic exotoxin A. The portal of entry may be the skin or the mucous membranes, or infection may occur subsequent to a surgical procedure, but many patients do not have obvious evidence of a portal of entry.

▶ Clinical Findings

A. Symptoms and Signs

Pain is the most common initial symptom and is frequently severe and abrupt in onset. The pain usually involves the extremity but may be intra-abdominal. Before symptom onset, some patients complain of an influenza-like syndrome characterized by fever, chills, myalgia, vomiting, and diarrhea. Patients often have oral temperatures above 37°C, may have confusion that rapidly deteriorates into coma, or may be combative. Shock is apparent at the time of presentation or within hours with evidence of hypotension, renal dysfunction, and respiratory failure. Most patients present with soft tissue infection, such as cellulitis or necrotizing fasciitis. Deeper infections may be present, including osteomyelitis, myometritis, peritonitis, suppurative phlebitis, or endophthalmitis. The mortality rate is approximately 30%.

B. Laboratory Findings

Laboratory findings reflect dysfunction of several organ systems. There may be leukocytosis and thrombocytopenia. The hematocrit is initially normal but may drop within 48–72 hours. Serum creatinine and creatine kinase levels are elevated, but calcium and albumin levels are low. Microscopic hematuria is often present and correlates with the presence of renal impairment. Group A streptococci are cultured from the blood, body fluid, or tissues of all patients who have not received antibiotic therapy.

▶ Treatment and Disposition

Intensive fluid replacement, central venous or pulmonary capillary wedge pressure monitoring, and timely surgical debridement are essential. Start antibiotic therapy with intravenous penicillin or a cephalosporin. Admit patients to the ICU.

Murry RJ: Recognition and management of Staphylococcus aureus toxin-mediated disease. Intern Med J 2005;35:S106 [PMID: 16271055].

LYME BORRELIOSIS

Lyme borreliosis (Lyme disease, Lyme arthritis) is a chronic disease caused by the spirochete *Borrelia burgdorferi*. Transmission is by several tick vectors (*Ixodes, Amblyomma, Rhipicephalus*) and occurs throughout the United States. The highest prevalence is found in the Northeast and Midwest. In stage 1, a rash is present, sometimes accompanied by fever. Timely treatment at this stage may prevent disease progression.

▶ Clinical Findings

A. Symptoms and Signs

Between 3 and 32 days following the tick bite, which the patient may not notice, a gradually expanding area of redness with clearing (erythema migrans) occurs at the bite site. The involved skin is warm but not particularly tender to touch. About half of affected patients will develop smaller lesions of similar morphology at areas remote from the bite site over ensuing days to weeks.

In stage-1 disease (erythema migrans), often there are fever, chills, malaise, and regional lymphadenopathy. In stage 2 (days to weeks after infection), symptoms related to the multisystemic nature of Lyme borreliosis often appear, such as meningitis, hepatitis, sore throat, dry cough, heart block and other cardiac abnormalities, musculoskeletal pain, and neuropathy. Fatigue and lethargy are prominent and may persist for months after the skin lesions have disappeared.

A persistent illness (stage 3) may linger for months to years and usually involves the musculoskeletal system (chronic arthritis), neurologic system (both central and peripheral), and skin (acrodermatitis chronica atrophicans). Stage-3 illness responds more slowly to treatment, and treatment at this stage has higher failure rates compared to stages 1 and 2.

B. Laboratory Findings

Laboratory testing is currently not reliable or standardized. Diagnosis depends on recognition of the pathognomonic rash. Serodiagnosis by either indirect immunofluorescence or ELISA may be negative in early infection. Nonspecific laboratory abnormalities include an elevated erythrocyte sedimentation rate, mild anemia, and transient elevations in SGOT (AST), SGPT (ALT), and lactate dehydrogenase enzyme levels.

▶ Treatment and Disposition

The treatment of choice for early Lyme borreliosis is tetracycline for at least 10 days, or for 20 or 30 days if symptoms persist or recur. For children under age 12 years, give amoxicillin or penicillin V. In pediatric patients with penicillin allergy, give erythromycin for 15–30 days. For more serious disease (eg, Lyme carditis or meningitis), use intravenous therapy with ceftriaxone or penicillin G for 14–21 days.

Marques AR: Lyme disease: A review. Curr Allergy Asthma Rep 2010;10:13–20 [PMID: 20425509].

Table 42–18. Common HIV Emergencies.

Findings	Common Causes	Helpful Diagnostic Tests
Pulmonary Cough, dyspnea, pulmonary infiltrates	*P. carinii, Mycobacterium tuberculosis, Pneumococci Haemophilus influenzae*	Arterial blood gas measurements, chest X-ray Giemsa, acid-fast, and gram-staining of sputum; culture bronchoscopy with lavage with biopsy
Neurologic Seizures; focal neurologic deficit; encephalopathy, hydrocephalus	*Toxoplasma gondii,* crytococcal or tuberculous meningitis, cerebral lymphoma, encephalitis (HIV, herpes virus)	CT scan, MRI lumbar puncture (after CT scan), brain biopsy
Systemic Fever, rigors, night sweats	Neutropenia with sepsis crytococcal infection, disseminated mycobacterial infection (several species), sinusitis *P. carinii,* cytomegalovirus *Salmonella* sp.	Complete blood count, blood cultures (viruses, bacterial, fungi, mycobacteria), lumbar puncture and CSF examination, chest X-ray
Gastrointestinal Diarrhea, dehydration	*Cryptosporidium* sp., *Shigella* sp., *Salmonella* sp., *Campylobacter jejuni, Entamoeba histolytica*	Culture of stool and microscopic examination for parasites
Hematologic Bleeding, purpura	Thrombocytopenia, intestinal or pulmonary Kaposi sarcoma (rare)	CBC and platelet count, endoscopy

▼ AIDS AND HIV INFECTION

See Table 42–18.

▶ General Considerations

AIDS is the end stage of chronic infection by HIV, a lymphotrophic retrovirus. Transmission occurs by sexual contact, perinatally, and by contact with infected blood. The virus causes slow destruction of the helper T-cell subset and in most affected individuals leads to fatal immunosuppression.

AIDS patients can present in extremis, with shock, ARDS, or multiple organ failure secondary to overwhelming infection. Acute adrenal failure can occur secondary to CMV and tuberculosis affecting the adrenals. AIDS and HIV can complicate virtually any organ system, and a detailed history and physical examination are necessary.

▶ Clinical Findings

Assess mental status carefully because mental status changes may be early signs of CNS infection or neuropsychiatric problems such as HIV dementia. Examine the eyes carefully for retinal lesions such as yellowish exudates and large hemorrhages seen in CMV or toxoplasma retinitis. The presence of nuchal rigidity may not be a presenting symptom of meningitis in an HIV-positive patient but should be assessed. Examine the mouth for evidence of oral candida (thrush) or leukoplakia, herpes, and Kaposi sarcoma. Pulmonary examination could reveal tachypnea or unequal breath sounds. A cardiac examination is essential in evaluating for murmurs that could be secondary to an infectious endocarditis (especially in intravenous drug abusers). Examine genitalia for lesions such as the chancre of syphilis. An anorectal examination can reveal fissures or fistulas, perianal abscesses, or prostatitis. A careful neurologic examination can disclose a CNS lesion that could be either infectious or neoplastic in origin.

▶ Organ-System-Specific Presentations

A. Pulmonary

The most common presenting complaint for an HIV-positive patient is pulmonary in origin. *Pneumocystis carinii* pneumonia (PCP) is the most common identifiable cause of death in AIDS patients and remains common (70% of HIV-positive patients will get it, and 70% of those will get reinfected). PCP is typically associated with fever and nonproductive cough, in contrast to bacterial pneumonia, in which the cough tends to be productive. Other causes of pulmonary pathology include tuberculosis, CMV, *Cryptococcus, Histoplasma,* and neoplasms (Kaposi sarcoma, lymphoma).

B. Neurologic

Ninety percent of patients with AIDS and 10–20% of HIV-positive patients will present with neurologic symptoms at some point (eg, seizure, mental status change, and headache). It is crucial not only to rule out infectious causes (*Cryptococcus,* bacterial meningitis, *Histoplasma,* CMV, progressive multifocal leukoencephalopathy, HSV, neurosyphillis, tuberculosis) but also to consider HIV encephalopathy (also known as AIDS dementia or subacute encephalitis; occurring in up to 15% of AIDS patients), lymphoma, cerebrovascular accident, and metabolic encephalopathy.

C. Gastrointestinal

Fifty percent of HIV-positive patients will have a gastrointestinal complication, presenting with complaints such as odynophagia, abdominal pain, bleeding, or diarrhea. Common infections include *Shigella, Salmonella, E. coli, Campylobacter, Cryptosporidium, Isospora,* CMV, or *Mycobacterium avium* complex (MAV). Bacterial infection is typically fulminant. If bacterial infection is suspected, give a fluoroquinolone empirically. Hepatitis is commonly seen secondary to high rates of coinfection with hepatitis B and C but can also be due to CMV, *Cryptosporidium,* or MAV. Proctocolitis is common in HIV-positive patients, and unless a careful examination is carried out, this diagnosis is easily overlooked (common causative organisms include *Campylobacter, Shigella, Salmonella,* gonococcus, and *Chlamydia*).

D. Systemic

Acute HIV infection causes an acute flulike illness in 50–90% of patients. Patients may present with fever, weight loss, adenopathy, or fatigue. MAV causes disseminated disease in up to 50% of AIDS patients (with fever, weight loss, and diarrhea). Fever is a common symptom and, in the absence of organ-specific clues, needs to be evaluated carefully. It may be due to HIV infection itself or another infectious cause. Patients with PCP may present with fever in the absence of respiratory symptoms. Cryptococcal meningitis can begin as fever without headache. Also consider *Mycobacterium* tuberculosis, MAV, endocarditis (especially if the patient is an intravenous drug abuser), and fever associated with neoplasm (lymphoma).

E. Ophthalmologic

The most common ocular finding is retinal microvasculopathy ("cotton wool spots"). CMV retinitis is common, and patients with this disorder present with visual loss, blindness, photophobia, scotomata, and floaters. On examination, CMV retinitis appears as fluffy white perivascular lesions with hemorrhage. HSV ophthalmicus is a worrisome complication; patients present with conjunctivitis, episcleritis, iritis, and keratitis.

F. Renal

HIV-positive patients not only commonly display prerenal azotemia secondary to volume depletion but also must deal with the consequences of drug nephrotoxicity, HIV nephropathy (focal segmental glomerulosclerosis), and renal tubular acidosis (hyperchloremic metabolic acidosis nonanion-gap acidosis), which are common in HIV infection and AIDS.

G. Skin

Patients can display a multitude of symptomology related to the skin. Infections are common (eg, *Staphylococcus, Pseudomonas,* HSV, herpes zoster, syphilis, intertriginous *Candida*), as are xerosis or pruritus associated with HIV infection.

H. Drug Reactions

Complications of the antiviral medications are common and are summarized in Table 42–19.

Table 42–19. Side Effects of HIV Antiviral Therapy.

Drug	Side Effects
Abacavir	Nausea, vomiting, fever, rash, dizziness
Adefovir	Elevated LFTs, diarrhea, nausea
Amprenavir	Rash, nausea, headache, vomiting
Delavirdine	Rash, headache, fatigue
Didanosine	Diarrhea, pancreatitis, neuropathy, elevated LFTs
Efavirenz	CNS effects, rash, elevated LFTs
Hydroxyurea	Nausea, headache, stomatitis, white blood cells, platelets, hemoglobin
Indinavir	Nephrolithiasis, elevated bilirubin, nausea, abdominal pain
Lamivudine	Headache, fatigue, nausea
Nelfinavir	Diarrhea, nausea
Nevirapine	Rash, nausea, headache, elevated LFTs
Ritonavir	Nausea, headache, diarrhea, elevated LFTs
Saquinavir	Diarrhea, nausea, elevated LFTs
Stavudine	Neuropathy, elevated LFTs
Zalcitabine	Neuropathy, rash
Zidovudine	Headache, neutropenia, nausea, myalgias

LFT, liver function tests.

▶ Laboratory Data

Obtain an arterial blood gas measurement to aid in investigating pulmonary complaints (Pao_2 <60 or oxygen saturation <90 is suggestive of pneumonitis). A fall in oxygen saturation of greater than 3% with activity is 80% sensitive for PCP. A chest X-ray can be useful in narrowing the differential diagnosis of pulmonary complaints based on appearance, but these findings are often nonspecific. Chest X-rays are read as negative in 15–20% of patients with documented PCP. Obtain blood and urine cultures (remember fungal and mycobacterial studies) as needed to evaluate systemic complaints or for focal complaints related to possible infection. Sputum culture and Gram stain are particularly useful for pulmonary complaints.

A CBC is helpful as a general index to evaluate for infection and for hematologic complications of HIV infection. In the absence of a CD4 count, an absolute lymphocyte count can be helpful. If the total lymphocyte count is less than 1000, then the CD4 is likely less than 200. CMV or MAV usually do not occur unless CD4 is less than 50. CSF should be sent for typical studies such as opening–closing pressures, cell count, glucose, protein, Gram stain, and culture, as well as other studies in selected cases: India ink, viral culture, fungal culture, *Toxoplasma* and cryptococci antigens, and coccidioidomycosis titer.

Evaluation of gastrointestinal complaints should proceed by sending stool for Wright stain, ova and parasite testing, acid-fast stain, and culture. Send standard stool cultures, Thayer–Martin culture, *Chlamydia* culture or immunoassay, and viral culture for HSV if proctocolitis is suspected on clinical examination.

HIV-positive patients should receive a head CT scan prior to lumbar puncture if mental status changes are present. MRI scans are superior to CT scan for detection of cerebral toxoplasmosis and other lesions.

▶ Treatment

Manifestations of HIV infection can range from asymptomatic to life threatening and can affect any organ system. Because of the complexity of opportunistic infections and malignancies occurring in HIV-positive patients, the diagnosis often cannot be made in the emergency department.

▶ Disposition

Disposition depends on the organ system in question. Ensure that the patient is adequately resuscitated. Final diagnoses may require biopsy or complicated studies to obtain a final diagnosis. In general, admit patients if a fever of unknown source or CNS findings are present or in the event of seizure, suspected PCP, hypoxia worse than baseline, intractable diarrhea, disseminated Herpes zoster, marrow suppression, extreme weakness, or inability to care for self or obtain follow-up.

Huang L, Crothers K: HIV-associated opportunistic pneumonias. Respirology 2009;14:474–485 [PMID: 19645867].

Khambaty MM, Hsu SS: Dermatology of the patient with HIV. Emerg Med Clin North Am 2010;28:355–368 [PMID: 20413018].

Rewari BB, Tanwar S: Emergencies in HIV medicine. J Indian Med Assoc 2009;107:317–322 [PMID: 19886387].

Singer EJ, Valdes-Sueiras M, Commins D, Levine A: Neurologic presentations of AIDS. Neurol Clin 2010;28:253–275 [PMID: 19932385].

Volberding PA, Deeks SG: Antiretroviral therapy and management of HIV infection. Lancet 2010;376:49–62 [PMID: 20609987].

INFLUENZA AND PANDEMIC FLU

ESSENTIALS OF DIAGNOSIS

- ▶ Fever
- ▶ Cough
- ▶ Sore throat
- ▶ Influenza known to be in community

▶ General Considerations

Influenza, a staple of emergency medicine practice, took a new twist in April 2009 with the emergence of a new strain of Influenza A H1N1. So genetically different from previous strains that many predicted a pandemic, an epidemic of huge geographical proportions. The virus, which originated in Mexico, spread to the United States and nearly 80 other countries worldwide. An outbreak is when there are more cases of an infection than expected in a community or region. An epidemic occurs when a disease spreads rapidly to many people. A pandemic occurs when there is a global disease outbreak. Responding to a pandemic situation is key at both a departmental and community level.

Between 5% and 20% of the population is infected with influenza yearly and over 200,000 hospitalizations are related to influenza. Influenza viruses that infect humans occur in 3 major types: A, B, and C. Of these, types A and B cause the majority of human illness. While both are associated with seasonal epidemics, only influenza A has been responsible for pandemics; namely, the Spanish Flu of 1918, the Asian Flu of 1957, and the Hong Kong Flu of 1968. About 36,000 deaths/y are caused by influenza. Influenza A viruses have surface proteins, hemagglutinin (H), and neuraminidase (N) that classify them. Subtle changes that occur continuously called antigenic drift do not affect disease or transmission. Major changes in the surface proteins in both human and animal viruses are called antigenic shift. When a shift occurs and there is transmission to a human population that lacks immunity, a pandemic may result. While most transmission of the virus is most commonly from respiratory droplets, both inanimate objects, and other bodily fluids can spread disease. The very young, the elderly, pregnant, and the physically and immune impaired are at greatest risk from pandemic influenza.

▶ Clinical Findings

The incubation period is between 1 and 7 days, and individuals with influenza are contagious 1 day before symptoms emerge. The symptoms of fever, cough, sore throat, rhinorrhea, myalgias, and headache are common to influenza. Up to 15% of patients may be afebrile. The CDC defines a person with an influenza-like illness (ILI), to have only the following symptoms: Fever ≥100° F plus cough and/or sore throat. Lower respiratory symptoms may be present also, and importantly pregnant women present more often with shortness of breath then nonpregnant ones. These symptoms coupled with testing or merely an epidemiological link would define a case of influenza. Testing may be done with one of numerous ways and may be strain specific or just identify Influenza A to be accurate.

▶ Laboratory Data

The CDC recommends that most patients with an illness consistent with influenza who reside in an area where influenza viruses are circulating do not require diagnostic influenza testing. Patients who should be considered for influenza diagnostic testing include hospitalized patients with suspected influenza, patients for whom a diagnosis of influenza will help decisions regarding clinical care, infection control, or management of close contacts, and patients who died of an acute illness in which influenza was suspected.

Treatment and Disposition

The decision to treat influenza (see Table 42–20) should be based on the time of presentation but more importantly on risk factors for severe disease. Because of the variable incubation period, the broad scope of influenza-like illnesses, and the safety of antiviral therapies, most should be considered for treatment, when influenza is in the community. It should be started as soon as possible regardless of testing. Those without risk factors for severe disease can be excluded from treatment if deemed to be recovering. The following risk factors put individuals at a greater threat for severe disease:

- Children less than 2 years old
- Adults over 65 years old
- Pregnant women up to 2 weeks postpartum regardless of how the pregnancy ended.
- Asthma
- Neurological and neurodevelopmental conditions
- Chronic lung disease
- Heart disease
- Blood disorders
- Endocrine disorders
- Kidney disorders
- Liver disorders
- Metabolic disorders
- Immune system disease or steroids

Table 42–20. Outpatient Treatment for Influenza—Treatment in 5 Days.

Drug	Dose
Oseltamivir (Tamiflu®)	Adults 75 mg twice b.i.d. Children 3 mg/kg/dose b.i.d.
Zanamivir (Relenza®)	Adults and Children >7 years old 2 inhalations (10 mg) PO b.i.d. Children <7 do not use

- People younger than 19 years of age who are receiving long-term aspirin therapy

Postexposure antiviral prophylaxis is indicated for patients at high risk of complications from influenza (eg, pregnancy) and should be considered for health care workers who were not using appropriate personal protective equipment during close contacts with a confirmed, probable, or suspected case. This chemoprophylaxis is for 10 days.

Admission should be considered if there are resources for those with risk factors, though many may be discharged with careful planning and follow-up.

Departmental and Community Preparedness and Response

The presence of a pandemic, or epidemic presents additional challenges to the emergency physician beyond the individual patient. The department, the prehospital system, and the community all must be managed to optimize emergency care. There are four tasks that need to be considered in both planning for a pandemic and while in the midst. They include increasing bed availability, developing strategies to deal with the potential staffing shortages, developing strategies for dealing with potential critical equipment and pharmaceutical shortages, and, lastly, the implementation of education, training, and communication strategies for their health care workers and the public they serve.

Blachere FM, Lindsley WG, Pearce TA, et al: Measurement of airborne influenza virus in a hospital emergency department. Clin Infect Dis 2009;48:438–440 [PMID: 19133798].

Centers for Disease Control and Prevention (CDC): Update: Novel influenza A (H1N1) virus infections—worldwide, May 6, 2009. MMWR Morb Mortal Wkly Rep 2009;58:453–458 [PMID: 19444146].

Centers for Disease Control and Prevention (CDC). 2009 H1N1 flu. Atlanta, GA, August 20, 2009. http://www.cdc.gov/h1n1flu (last accessed August 19, 2010).

Jamieson DJ, Honein MA, Rasmussen SA, et al: Novel Influenza A (H1N1) Pregnancy Working Group. H1N1 2009 influenza virus infection during pregnancy in the USA. Lancet 2009;374:451–458 [PMID: 19643469].

Taylor JL, Roup BJ, Blythe D, Reed GK, Tate TA, Moore, KA: Pandemic influenza preparedness in Maryland: Improving readiness through a tabletop exercise. Biosecur Bioterror 2005;3:61–69 [PMID: 15853456].

World Health Organization: Pandemic (H1N1) 2009—update 58. Geneva, Switzerland, July 6, 2009. http://www.who.int/csr/don/2009_07_06/en/index.html (last accessed August 19, 2010).

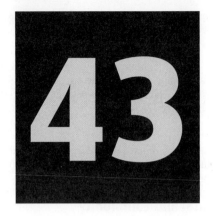

Metabolic & Endocrine Emergencies

Martin R. Huecker, MD
Daniel F. Danzl, MD

Disorders of Glucose Homeostasis
Diabetic Ketoacidosis
Hyperosmolar Hyperglycemic State
Hyperglycemia
Hypoglycemia
Lactic Acidosis
Alcoholic Ketoacidosis

Other Metabolic and Endocrine Abnormalities
Thyroid Disorders
Adrenal Insufficiency and Crisis (Addisonian Crisis)
Pheochromocytoma (Catecholamine Crisis)
Pituitary Apoplexy
Inappropriate Secretion of Antidiuretic Hormone
Diabetes Insipidus

▼ DISORDERS OF GLUCOSE HOMEOSTASIS

Most disorders of carbohydrate metabolism are related to diabetes mellitus (DM) and represent a broad category of emergency conditions. Toxin ingestion, medications, multisystem trauma, head injury, cardiovascular disease, cerebrovascular disease, and infection can mimic or exacerbate these conditions. Clinical appearance may vary dramatically. Patients may present with significant mental status changes or appear well while on the brink of metabolic decompensation.

DIABETIC KETOACIDOSIS

 ESSENTIALS OF DIAGNOSIS

▶ Symptoms and signs include fatigue, tachypnea (Kussmaul's respirations), tachycardia, altered mental status, abdominal pain, vomiting, polyuria, and polydipsia

▶ Arterial pH < 7.3, serum glucose ≥ 250 mg/dL, and serum bicarbonate ≤ 15 mEq/L

▶ General Considerations

Diabetic ketoacidosis (DKA) is the most common acute life-threatening complication of diabetes. It is more commonly seen in type 1 diabetes but may occur in type 2. Patients with type 1 DM have an absolute insulin deficiency. When the production of insulin in the pancreas fails, the decreased glucose utilization creates a relative state of starvation. Counter-regulatory hormones (cortisol, glucagon, catecholamine, and growth hormone) that help maintain blood glucose levels adequate for cellular function during fasting are stimulated. These hormones promote gluconeogenesis and glycogenolysis, increasing glucose levels, and lipolysis, which converts adipose to free fatty acids. Without insulin to allow cellular absorption of glucose, these mechanisms continue to produce glucose. Severe dehydration and electrolyte losses develop as the kidneys filter the highly osmotic glucose. Furthermore, free fatty acids that cannot enter the citric acid cycle without insulin are oxidized into ketones. These accumulate to cause metabolic acidosis, further electrolyte derangement, and exocrine pancreatic dysfunction.

▶ Clinical Findings

A. History

If a diabetes history is elicited or known, ascertain potential precipitating causes of DKA:

- Recent or current infection of any type (most common)
- Injury or trauma
- Acute coronary syndrome or myocardial infarction
- Transient ischemic attack or stroke
- Medications (corticosteroids, thiazides, or sympathomimetics)
- Acute or acute-on-chronic pancreatitis
- Ethanol or drug abuse
- Gastroenteritis or GI bleeding
- Psychosocial factors, such as depression or inability to afford medications, limiting compliance
- Noncompliance with insulin regimen due to psychological or physiological reasons

Although noncompliance or misuse of insulin is a frequent cause of DKA, consideration of other causes of decompensation is imperative. Infection or illness may prompt patients to underdose. Up to 25% of DKA admissions results from new-onset diabetes. Alcoholic ketoacidosis (AKA), starvation, lactic acidosis, renal failure, or ingestions such as salicylates, methanol, ethylene glycol, or paraldehyde should be considered in the differential diagnosis of DKA.

B. Symptoms and Signs

Typical findings include general fatigue and weakness, orthostasis, abdominal pain, and Kussmaul's respirations (rapid deep respirations attempting to compensate for acidosis). A fruity or acetone-like odor is classically described along with historical findings of polyuria, polydipsia, and polyphagia; nausea and vomiting are found in up to 25% of patients. Emesis may have a coffee ground appearance due to hemorrhagic gastritis. Mental status changes ranging from mild confusion to coma may be seen. DKA alone does not cause fever.

C. Laboratory Findings

1. Key findings—Laboratory features include serum glucose ≥ 250 mg/dL, serum ketones or ketonuria, serum bicarbonate ≤ 15 mEq/L, and arterial pH < 7.3. Arterial blood gas (ABG) determination can be limited to patients with an uncertain diagnosis or respiratory concerns. Venous blood is an acceptable alternative. The pH value is usually 0.03 lower than that of arterial blood. This is especially useful for repeated pH determinations. The degree of leukocytosis often correlates with the degree of ketosis.

2. Serum potassium—Because the initial serum potassium is unpredictable, the determination of serum potassium should precede insulin therapy. Acidosis drives potassium out of the cells causing a relatively higher serum potassium level despite total body deficits that may be as much as 3–5 mEq/kg. If serum potassium is initially low, insulin administration will exacerbate the situation by facilitating the cellular entry of potassium. The rapid development of severe hypokalemia may cause symptoms such as fatigue and muscle cramps or lead to a lethal arrhythmia.

3. Serum sodium—Significant diuresis and emesis frequently lower serum sodium. Osmotic shifts from hyperglycemia also dilute the serum and fictitiously lower the reported sodium value. This effect can be corrected by adding 1.8 mEq/L to the serum sodium concentration for each 100 mg/dL above normal.

Sodium deficits may approach 7–10 mEq/kg; however, rapid correction with increasing osmolality may precipitate cerebral edema, especially in children.

4. Serum phosphate—Serum phosphate values may be normal or elevated despite deficits approaching 1 mmol/kg body weight. Routine phosphate repletion does not improve outcome in DKA and is generally not indicated in the emergency department (ED). Severe hypophosphatemia (<1 mg/dL), however, may cause skeletal, cardiac, and respiratory muscle depression. Phosphate should be replaced in this circumstance. This can be done by using potassium phosphate as 1/3 of potassium replacement.

5. Other important laboratory findings—

A. ANION GAP—The anion gap is useful to assess severity of acidosis and to follow progress of therapy. The anion gap is obtained from the formula:

$$\text{Anion Gap} = [Na] - ([Cl] + [HCO_3])$$

Normal values are 8–16.

B. SERUM OSMOLALITY—Serum osmolality values above 340 mOsm/kg usually result in mental status changes. Below this value, other causes for lethargy or coma should be investigated. This value may also be used to diagnose hyperosmolar hyperglycemic state (HHS) and ingestions of ethanol, ethylene glycol, or other alcohols. Effective serum osmolality can be estimated by the formula:

$$\text{Serum osmolality} = 2[Na] + (\text{glucose}/18) + (\text{blood urea nitrogen}/2.8).$$

C. SERUM KETONES—The laboratory determination of serum ketones is not always reliable as a diagnostic test. The primary ketone body formed in DKA initially is β-hydroxybutyrate. However, standard ketone assays measure only acetoacetate. Since insulin is required for the conversion of β-hydroxybutyrate to acetoacetate, these assays may be reassuringly negative even in a severely ill patient. Due to insulin's effect, in most cases serum ketone values will initially increase as the patient improves before resolving.

D. **BLOOD UREA NITROGEN AND CREATININE**—These levels may be elevated because of severe dehydration, acute tubular necrosis, or renal failure. In these circumstances, establish urine output prior to initiating potassium repletion.

E. **AMYLASE/LIPASE**—Levels of both enzymes can be elevated in DKA in the absence of pancreatic pathology.

Treatment

See below.

HYPEROSMOLAR HYPERGLYCEMIC STATE

ESSENTIALS OF DIAGNOSIS

▶ Most symptoms relate to severe dehydration

▶ Absence of acidosis, small or absent serum ketones, and hyperglycemia usually ≥ 600 mg/dL

▶ Kussmaul's respirations and abdominal pain are unusual findings

General Considerations

In contrast to DKA, patients with HHS have sufficient insulin activity to prevent lipolysis and ketogenesis. HHS results from gradual diuresis, resulting in severe dehydration and electrolyte depletion without significant early symptoms. This leads to profound electrolyte deficiencies and eventually mental status changes. In contrast, DKA often manifests symptoms more suddenly over hours to a few days due to acidosis.

HHS is often caused by physiologic stressors such as infection, myocardial infarction, cerebrovascular accident, trauma, decreased access to water, and medication effects or interactions.

Clinical Findings

A. History

Risk factors for HHS include age greater than 65, residence in a chronic care facility or nursing home, change in diabetes regimen, addition of medications that may elevate glucose levels (e.g., corticosteroids, thiazides, anticonvulsants, immunosuppressants, sympathomimetics), recent or current infection, and dementia. Other factors include myocardial infarction, Cushing's syndrome, intracranial hemorrhage, cerebrovascular accident, Down's syndrome, trauma/burns, hemodialysis, and hyperalimentation.

B. Symptoms and Signs

These include polydipsia, polyuria, or polyphagia; generalized weakness; altered mental status (clouded thinking to confusion to lethargy or coma); dry mucous membranes; poor skin turgor; and delayed capillary refill. Since the average fluid deficit is 9 L, tachycardia and orthostatic hypotension are common.

Abdominal pain is not a typical finding in HHS (in contrast to DKA); its presence merits aggressive investigation for a precipitating cause. Acute cholecystitis and appendicitis may be insidious and have an atypical presentation in elderly patients.

C. Laboratory Findings

1. Key laboratory findings—Key findings to diagnose HHS and differentiate it from DKA are as follows:

- HHS typically is associated with a greater fluid deficit (9 L vs. 3–5 L).

- Serum glucose ≥ 600 mg/dL.

- Urine or serum ketones are small or absent (a small amount of ketone may be detected secondary to starvation).

- Glucosuria is prominent.

- Serum bicarbonate is usually >15 mEq/L.

- pH is usually >7.30, but the patient can have acidemia from lactate, starvation ketosis, or renal insufficiency.

- The anion gap may be variable depending on precipitating cause but is usually ≤10.

- Serum osmolality is 320–380 mOsm/kg.

2. Serum sodium—In the early stages of HHS, serum sodium findings are similar to those in patients with DKA. Urinary losses and fluid shifts out of the cell and into the extracellular compartment create hyponatremia usually 125–130 mg/dL. Correct for hyperglycemia with the addition of 1.8–2.4 mg/dL sodium per 100 mg/dL of glucose.

3. Serum potassium—Serum potassium levels will most commonly be normal or low, unless renal failure is present. Total body deficits are often 4–6 mEq/L, which is as much as 500 mEq total.

4. Blood urea nitrogen and creatinine—Blood urea nitrogen (BUN) is often markedly elevated. Gastrointestinal bleeding may also elevate BUN and is a possible precipitating cause of HHS in elderly patients.

5. Other studies—Ancillary diagnostic testing should also be considered including serial ECGs and cardiac enzymes, cranial and abdominal tomography, and evaluation for gastrointestinal hemorrhage. Bedside ultrasonography may also be useful.

Treatment

Treatment of DKA and HHS is very similar. Continuous monitoring of vital signs, mental status, and laboratory parameters is essential. A flow sheet may be helpful during resuscitation due to the complexity of treatment and need for frequent therapeutic changes.

A. Resuscitation Issues

Standard airway management is indicated. If tracheal intubation is required, avoid succinylcholine unless hyperkalemia is excluded. Hypoxia should trigger an investigation for aspiration, pneumonia, or pulmonary edema. Maintain oxygen saturation above 96% or $Po_2 \geq 70$ mm Hg for all DKA or HHS patients.

B. Fluid Therapy

Fluid therapy is dictated by three parameters: vital signs, corrected serum sodium, and serum glucose. Overall fluid deficits approach 6–10 L in most patients. Large-bore ($\geq$18-gauge) intravenous lines are essential. Central venous access may be indicated. Hypotension should prompt a bolus of 1–2 L of 0.9% NaCl solution to restore blood pressure to at least 90 mm Hg.

Caution: Decreased cardiac systolic function and renal failure complicate crystalloid resuscitation. Reassess patients frequently for adequate urine output and signs of pulmonary edema or congestive heart failure. Invasive hemodynamic monitoring may be indicated in very select cases to facilitate fluid management if cardiogenic shock is present.

Serum electrolytes including potassium, bicarbonate, and sodium should be monitored every hour along with hourly glucose determination. The calculated serum osmolality should not decrease more than ~3 mOsm/kg/h due to increased risk of cerebral edema.

- Usually 1–1.5 L of 0.9% saline is infused over the first hour while initial laboratory values are determined. Subsequent infusion can be decreased to 500 mL/h, then 250–500 mL/h, and then 150–300 mL/h as the hydration status improves. Correct one-half of the fluid deficit over the initial 8 hours, and the other half over the following 24 hours.

If the serum sodium is high normal or high, 0.45% saline is recommended after initial fluid boluses to avoid severe hypernatremia. If serum sodium is low or low normal, 0.9% saline should be continued.

- Once serum glucose reaches approximately 250 mg/dL, 5% dextrose in 0.45% NaCl is the fluid of choice at a rate of 250 mL/h; alternatively, use 5% dextrose in normal saline if the corrected serum sodium remains low.

The clinical relevance of the urine output is unreliable while glucose levels remain high due to osmotic diuresis. Once glucose levels approach normal, urine output may be used to guide therapy; 30–50 cc/h is considered adequate.

Cerebral edema may occur in the following cases: correcting acidosis too rapidly, correcting glucose too rapidly, overaggressive IV fluid resuscitation.

C. Electrolyte Replacement

1. Potassium—Potassium repletion may begin once continuous urine output is confirmed and an initial potassium level is determined. With target levels of 4.0–5.0 mEq/L, the following algorithm is useful:

- If the serum potassium is 3.3 mEq/L or less, withhold insulin therapy and give potassium replacement. Give 40 mEq potassium chloride intravenously or a mixture of two-thirds potassium chloride and one-third potassium phosphate (~5 mmol) if serum phosphate is less than 1 mmol/L. Potassium chloride, 40 mEq, may also be given orally or by nasogastric tube. This method allows for safer administration of larger doses of potassium and is the preferred replacement method if oral dosage is tolerated. Assume a deficit of about 100 mEq potassium for each 1 mEq/L below normal.

- If the serum potassium is 3.3–5.0 mEq/L, give 20–30 mEq potassium chloride in each liter of intravenous fluid.

- If the serum potassium is 5.0 mEq/L or more, hold potassium repletion and recheck the serum potassium in 1 hour. If levels remain significantly elevated (above 6 mEq/L) or ECG changes are noted, a regular insulin bolus of 8–12 units can be given along with other standard treatments for hyperkalemia.

- Magnesium is often deficient due to diuresis, and may worsen vomiting.

D. Insulin Therapy

Intravenous regular insulin is used for initial therapy. Subcutaneous insulin may be absorbed erratically in volume-depleted patients. A continuous infusion of regular insulin at 0.1 units/kg body weight per hour is the treatment of choice. Historically, after the serum potassium determination, a bolus of 0.1–0.15 units/kg body weight of regular insulin was considered (not recommended in pediatric patients). Due to the risk of cerebral edema, one should avoid insulin boluses even in adult patients; continuous infusion of insulin is optimal. If glucose is not decreasing by at least 50–70 mg/dL/h, the insulin dosage should be doubled until this rate of decline is achieved. Decrease insulin infusion by 25–75% if the decline in serum glucose is more than 100 mg/dL/h since this results in rapid shifts in serum osmolality.

Insulin therapy should be delayed if the potassium level is less than 3.3 mEq/L until the potassium level is rising.

E. Sodium Bicarbonate Therapy

Sodium bicarbonate therapy is generally not indicated except for unstable patients with severe acidosis such as an arterial pH < 6.9. Bicarbonate therapy is rarely indicated for HHS patients. The incidence of cerebral edema increases with aggressive bicarbonate use (particularly in children). There is no proven impact on outcome in controlled trials when bicarbonate therapy was used for severe acidosis. However, due to the catastrophic potential of severe acidosis, bicarbonate therapy may be considered in these patients. $NaHCO_3$ (50 mmol) is diluted in 200 mL sterile water and infused at 200 mL/h. This may be repeated every 2 hours until the venous pH is greater than 7.

F. Treatment of Precipitants

Infection is the most common pathological precipitant of DKA and HHS. The patient's entire skin surface should be examined for wounds and cellulitis. A pelvic examination may be indicated to rule out infection. Analysis and cultures of all appropriate body fluids (blood, sputum, urine, cerebrospinal fluid) should be obtained. The empiric administration of broad-spectrum antibiotics should be considered until culture results are available.

G. Disposition

Patients with all but very mild cases of DKA and all patients with HHS should have cardiac monitoring and a higher level of nursing care for at least 24 hours. Whether the patient goes to an intermediate care, telemetry unit, or the intensive care unit is based on severity of the case and response to initial therapy as judged by the treating physician.

Kitabchi AE, Umpierrez GE, Fisher JN, Murphy MB, Stentz FB: Thirty years of personal experience in hyperglycemic crises: diabetic ketoacidosis and hyperglycemic hyperosmolar state. J Clin Endocrinol Metab 2008 May;93(5):1541–1552.

Charfen MA, Ipp E, Kaji AH, Saleh T, Qazi MF, Lewis RJ: Detection of undiagnosed diabetes and prediabetic states in high-risk emergency department patients. Acad Emerg Med 2009 May;16(5):394–402.

Charfen MA, Fernandez-Frackelton M: Diabetic ketoacidosis. Emerg Med Clin North Am 2005;23(3):609 [PMID: 15982537].

Kitabchi AE et al: Hyperglycemic crises in diabetes. Diabetes Care 2004;27(Suppl 1):S94–S102 [PMID: 14693938]. (Review on diagnosis and therapy of DKA and HHS by the foremost authorities in these aspects of endocrinology and diabetes care. Contains helpful therapeutic algorithms.)

HYPERGLYCEMIA

Hyperglycemia in the absence of metabolic decompensation (DKA or HHS) is a common finding in the ED. Patients with either known or undiagnosed diabetes may present with symptoms due to hyperglycemia, complications of untreated diabetes, or numerous unrelated conditions that incidentally have high blood glucose levels.

▶ Clinical Findings

A. History

Age greater than 45, obesity, physical inactivity, and family history are risk factors for insulin resistance. Personal history of gestational diabetes, impaired glucose tolerance, hypertension, dyslipidemia, vascular disease, or polycystic ovary disease also increases risk.

B. Symptoms and Signs

Symptoms of hyperglycemia may include polydipsia, polyuria, polyphagia, weakness, fatigue, headache, blurred vision, dehydration, lightheadedness, or dizziness.

Infections are much more common in poorly controlled diabetics. Superficial skin infections such as cellulitis, furuncles, abscesses, nonhealing wounds, and ulcers are very common complaints. Urinary tract infections and candidal infections, malignant otitis externa, and rhinocerebral mucormycosis all have epidemiologic associations with hyperglycemia.

C. Laboratory Findings

A random serum glucose greater than 200 mg/dL with symptoms of hyperglycemia or metabolic decompensation (DKA or HHS) or a fasting serum glucose greater than 126 mg/dL on repeat occasions is diagnostic of diabetes. Impaired fasting glucose is defined as a fasting plasma glucose of 110–126 mg/dL. Glycosylated hemoglobin, or HbA1C, can facilitate the diagnosis of diabetes, and is becoming more valued as a screening test. Levels of 7% or more are nearly always consistent with diabetes.

Severe hyperglycemia (≥400 mg/dL) may foreshadow impending decompensation. An underlying cause should be sought aggressively such as infection, cardiac ischemia, or myocardial infarction. White blood cell count, blood cultures, and ECG with cardiac enzymes may be helpful. Lack of compliance with antidiabetic regimen or diet should always be exclusionary. In this setting evaluate electrolytes, BUN, creatinine, and serum bicarbonate to screen for metabolic decompensation.

▶ Treatment

If diabetes was previously undiagnosed and insulin deficiency (type 1) cannot be excluded, then the patient should be admitted. Insulin resistance (type 2) is much more common. If hyperglycemia is mild (<250–350 mg/dL) with no signs of decompensation, no specific treatment is required if primary care follow-up is readily available. Newly diagnosed patients should also be counseled on diet and the importance of follow-up. If the serum glucose is greater than 300 mg/dL, treatment is as follows:

A. Fluids

Normal saline 1 L given over 1 hour may be adequate mono-therapy for hyperglycemia.

B. Insulin

Usually 0.1–0.15 units/kg regular insulin, insulin lispro (Humalog), or insulin aspart (NovoLog) can be given subcutaneously or intravenously. Insulin may be rebolused intravenously if glucose does not decline by 50–75 mg/dL in the first hour.

C. Oral Hypoglycemic Agents

Oral hypoglycemic agents are generally not indicated for acute therapy of severe hyperglycemia. Oral agents may, however, be initiated or continued by emergency physicians when follow-up is available.

Metformin inhibits fasting hepatic glucose production and promotes weight loss. It is an attractive option that should only be prescribed if follow-up is possible, since it is the least likely to cause hypoglycemia. Metformin can be safely started at 500 mg orally once per day; the dosage can be increased by 500 mg/d each week until 1000 mg twice a day is reached. It should not be given if serum creatinine levels are above 1.4 mg/dL, due to the risk of developing lactic acidosis. Metformin should also be avoided in the following circumstances: risk of hypoxemia, CHF, hepatic impairment, renal insufficiency, acute infection, age >80 or <17, alcoholic, exposure to contrast in the past 48 hours, or planned exposure to contrast.

Initial treatment with sulfonylurea, thiazolidinediones, and α-glucosidase inhibitors is best withheld until the patient has received diabetes education. If education can be provided along with supplies such as glucometer and test strips, these agents can be started in conjunction with consultation and close follow-up. When adjusting an existing oral agent or insulin dosage, do not increase insulin dosages by more than 10% or sulfonylurea dosage by more than about 20%.

▶ Disposition

Most patients with blood glucose less than 250–350 mg/dL in the absence of metabolic decompensation can be safely discharged with follow-up after a thorough evaluation for underlying illness. Patients with serious underlying precipitants or in whom hyperglycemia is resistant to treatment should be hospitalized.

Henderson WR, Chittock DR, Dhingra VK, Ronco JJ: Hyperglycemia in acutely ill emergency patients—cause or effect? CJEM 2006 Sep;8(5):339–343. Review.

Prince LA, Rodriquez E, Campagna J, Brown L, Fischer D, Grant WD: Hyperglycemia in ED patients with no history of diabetes. Am J Emerg Med. 2008 Jun;26(5):532–536.

HYPOGLYCEMIA

 ESSENTIALS OF DIAGNOSIS

▶ Common symptoms and signs include irritability, diaphoresis, and tachycardia related to increased circulating catecholamines

▶ As hypoglycemia progresses, neuroglycopenic effects range from focal neurologic deficits such as diplopia and paresthesias to coma

▶ Always check the fingerstick blood glucose on every patient presenting with altered mental status or who appears to be acutely ill

▶ Background

Symptoms can include altered mental status, focal neurologic deficits, and coma. Even mild, treated episodes can exacerbate preexisting microvascular disease and lead to cumulative brain damage.

▶ Causes

Hypoglycemia is commonly defined as serum glucose of <50 mg/dL. Less than 30 mg/dL is considered severe hypoglycemia. This most commonly occurs in diabetics on exogenous insulin therapy. Changes in daily activities such as diet, exercise, or dosage changes may result in hypoglycemia. Many other factors, however, may result in hypoglycemia such as infection, endocrine disorders, drugs or alcohol, liver failure, intentional overdose of insulin, tumors or malnutrition in both diabetics and nondiabetics.

Other causes of hypoglycemia include glycogen storage disease (esp von Gierke's), carnitine deficiency, sepsis, Addisonion crisis, beta blocker overdose, pregnancy, salicylate toxicity.

A. Exogenous Insulin

In patients with known diabetes, hypoglycemia may occur as a result of the following:

- Delay in eating after taking insulin, general malnutrition, or inadequate caloric intake due to nausea and vomiting or gastroparesis.

- Increased physical activity.

- Increased physiologic stress resulting from infection or injury.

- Excessive dose of exogenous insulin (**Note:** Remember to check the patient's vision and confirm that he or she can read the syringe appropriately.).

- Variable absorption from injection sites.

- Impaired counter-regulatory hormone axis.

- Excessive insulin release produced by sulfonylurea drugs, especially in the presence of renal insufficiency.

- Alterations in therapeutic regimen, particularly increases in insulin or oral agent dosages or the addition of new oral agents such as thiazolidinediones (also known as glitazones), which may reduce insulin resistance and improve therapeutic action of endogenous or exogenous insulin.

- Intentional hypoglycemia may result from insulin or antihyperglycemic agents such as sulfonylurea that may be taken by, or given to, the patients. C-peptide is naturally secreted along with insulin by the pancreas and is not present in manufactured insulin. A high insulin level without a correspondingly high C-peptide level is diagnostic of exogenous insulin.

B. Pancreatic β-Cell Tumor

Tumor of the insulin-secreting β-cells in the islets of Langerhans may cause refractory hypoglycemia and even coma. C-peptide levels will elevate concurrently with insulin levels.

C. ETOH

Acute or chronic excessive ethanol intake, especially without adequate caloric intake, may cause severe hypoglycemia (especially in children). Chronic abuse reduces NADH-mediated gluconeogenesis and depletes hepatic glycogen production and storage.

Caution: Administer thiamine, 100 mg, to alcoholic patients with hypoglycemia to avoid Wernicke's encephalopathy.

D. Postprandial or Reactive Hypoglycemia

The intake of large amounts of concentrated calories in non-diabetics may produce enough excess insulin to induce mildly symptomatic hypoglycemia. Rarely, hypoglycemia may be severe enough to cause briefly decreased level of consciousness.

▶ Clinical Findings

A. History

Try to obtain a history of diabetes from emergency medical services, family, Medic Alert bracelet, necklace, or wallet card. Emergency medical services or family may also be helpful in disclosing alcohol use, recent caloric intake, alterations of medication regimen, and recent illness or injury.

B. Symptoms and Signs

Most early symptoms and signs are the result of increased catecholamine release: tachycardia, irritability, diaphoresis, paresthesias, hunger, and decreased concentration are common. With more severe or prolonged hypoglycemia, symptoms and signs of neuroglycopenia result in mental status changes including confusion or bizarre behavior, lethargy, or coma; visual disturbances such as blurred vision, diplopia, hallucinations; seizures or seizure-like activity or focal neurologic deficits similar to Todd's paralysis that resolves with glucose administration.

C. Laboratory Findings

The capillary or fingerstick glucose is a rapid screen to determine blood glucose levels. Glucometers become unreliable at readings less than 40 mg/dL. Obtain a sample for laboratory determination.

Search for ancillary causes of hypoglycemia such as infection or sepsis, myocardial infarction, cerebrovascular accident, renal insufficiency or failure, alcohol use, pregnancy, drug use (particularly stimulants), occult trauma, depression (poor caloric intake or insulin or oral agent overdose), and other endocrinopathies (Addison's disease, myxedema, thyrotoxicosis, pituitary insufficiency).

▶ Treatment

A. Emergency Therapeutic Measures

1. Intravenous glucose—If intravenous access is readily obtainable, administer 50 cc of 50% dextrose in water (containing approximately 25 g of glucose, which is enough to resolve most hypoglycemic episodes). *Caution:* Remember to give thiamine, 100 mg intravenously or intramuscularly, to alcoholic patients to prevent Wernicke's encephalopathy. Monitor the patient's mental status and recheck capillary blood glucose 15–30 minutes after glucose administration. Repeat dosages of 50% dextrose or infusion of glucose-containing intravenous fluids (5–10%) may be necessary to maintain adequate blood glucose levels. Neuroglycopenia (altered level of consciousness, seizure-like activity, focal neurologic deficits) may take time to resolve completely. If abnormalities persist longer than 30 minutes after glucose administration and hypoglycemia has not recurred, other causes should be investigated with a cranial CT scan and appropriate laboratory studies.

2. Oral feeding—As soon as the patient regains consciousness (or in an already conscious patient), clear fruit juice (eg, apple, grape; 6 oz ≅ 15 g glucose) is a good choice to maintain glucose levels, a snack or meal is appropriate.

3. Glucagon—If intravenous access is not readily available, 1 mg of glucagon may be given intramuscularly. The response time is typically 10–15 minutes, and nausea and vomiting along with overcorrection of glucose levels are common. Since glucagon can be given intramuscularly, all patients with insulin-treated diabetes (or their families) should carry and be familiar with the use of glucagon emergency kits.

4. Monitoring—Consider the duration of action of the insulin or oral agents taken by the patient. Hourly capillary glucose checks should be taken until glucose levels are stable. Generally the patient should be observed through the peak time of the longest-acting insulin, typically 30 minutes to 1–2 hours after the dose with insulin lispro or insulin aspart, 2–4 hours with regular insulin, or 6–8 hours with NPH. Insulin glargine has no peak activity and does not generally cause hypoglycemia by itself. Patients taking long-acting insulins with peak activity, such as lente or ultralente, or patients taking sulfonylurea oral agents should generally be observed in the hospital.

Disposition

Indications for admission include persistent or recurrent hypoglycemia despite appropriate therapy, hypoglycemia related to an oral agent or long-acting insulin, and unknown cause of hypoglycemia or serious ancillary cause (eg, severe infection, persistent nausea, and vomiting).

Conditions for discharge include well-understood cause of hypoglycemia, easily reversible episode, availability of responsible adult to observe the patient for next 8–12 hours; ability to take oral fluids and food; medical follow-up available within 24–48 hours; and ability to check blood glucose levels.

Advances

With advances in the treatment of insulin-dependent diabetes mellitus, more ED physicians will encounter patients who have insulin pumps. These devices come in various brands. The pump consists of a device worn by the patient, which has a reservoir for fast-acting insulin. Tubing connects the reservoir to a subcutaneous site implanted on the trunk or thigh of the patient. Insulin is administered as a continuous basal rate with the addition of bolus therapy with carbohydrate intake. Although associated with iatrogenic hypoglycemia, insulin pumps help the motivated/educated patient achieve tight glycemic control.

Goh HK, Chew DE, Miranda IG, Tan L, Lim GH: 24-Hour observational ward management of diabetic patients presenting with hypoglycaemia: a prospective observational study. Emerg Med J 2009 Oct;26(10):719–723.

Whitmer RA, Karter AJ, Yaffe K, Quesenberry CP Jr, Selby JV: Hypoglycemic episodes and risk of dementia in older patients with type 2 diabetes mellitus. JAMA 2009 Apr 15;301(15):1565–1572.

Sinert R, Su M, Secko M, Zehtabchi S: The utility of routine laboratory testing in hypoglycaemic emergency department patients. Emerg Med J 2009 Jan;26(1):28–31.

LACTIC ACIDOSIS

General Considerations

Lactic acidosis is a common complication of critical illness. It is defined as serum lactic acid concentration greater than 5 mmol/L and arterial pH less than 7.35. Lactic acid is measured as the L isomer; however, the D isomer is being increasingly noticed due to rates of small bowel resection and gastric bypass surgery. Typically lactic acidosis results from the metabolism of glucose under anaerobic conditions or inadequate breakdown of lactic acid by the liver.

Severe acidosis can lead to impairment of cardiac contractility, increased pulmonary vascular resistance, sensitization of the myocardium to dysrhythmias, hyperkalemia, and inhibition of metabolism at the cellular or molecular level. The mortality rate is high, approaching 40–60%.

Causes

Lactic acidosis may occur in any severe illness with a combination of inadequate tissue oxygenation, tissue perfusion, and lactic acid clearance. Common underlying causes include:

- respiratory, hepatic, renal, or heart failure
- sepsis
- shock
- cancer, especially leukemias
- acute infarction of lung, bowel, or extremities
- severe abdominal or multisystem trauma
- ETOH, methanol, ethylene glycol, or cyanide poisoning
- drugs (cocaine, metformin, isoniazid, NRTI HIV medications).

Clinical Findings

Diagnostic efforts should focus on finding the underlying cause of the lactic acidosis. Treatment of the underlying cause is crucial to recovery.

A. Symptoms and Signs

The clinical presentation varies according to the underlying illness or injury. Symptoms may be minimal initially and then progress to include hyperventilation, generalized weakness, abdominal pain, or hypotension.

B. Laboratory Findings

Laboratory findings include pH less than 7.35 and often less than 7.2; anion gap greater than 15 mEq/L; and lack of explanation of acidosis by other causes—such as salicylates; ETOH, methanol, or ethylene glycol poisoning; or diabetic or alcoholic ketoacidosis. Hyperphosphatemia is a common finding secondary to anaerobic glycolysis or cellular disruption.

Samples collected for lactate should be chilled immediately and centrifuged promptly to avoid continued lactic acid production by red and white blood cells.

Treatment

Basic treatment of lactic acidosis is medical resuscitation for improvement of oxygenation and perfusion of tissues along with treatment of the underlying cause of decompensation.

A. Oxygen

High flow rates are indicated. Consider rapid-sequence intubation, mechanical ventilation, or noninvasive ventilation when indicated by blood gas analysis and overall clinical picture.

B. Fluids

Rapid infusion of 1 L of 0.9% saline is indicated to restore intravascular volume. The patient should be frequently reassessed to avoid volume overload in the setting of acute renal failure or cardiogenic shock and circulatory failure.

C. Pressors

Vasoactive pressors such as epinephrine, norepinephrine, and dopamine may be required to support systemic blood pressure and improve overall perfusion in patients with lactic acidosis. One must remember, however, that these agents can increase vasoconstriction to already-hypoxic tissues and increase the metabolic demands of organs such as the heart. For a more detailed discussion of vasopressors use in shock, see Chapter 11.

D. Sodium Bicarbonate

The use of sodium bicarbonate is one of the most controversial issues in the treatment of metabolic acidosis. The majority of data available suggest that no benefit is seen at pH levels greater than 6.9 in the clinical settings of severe metabolic acidosis resulting from DKA and sepsis. Significant risks of administering bicarbonate include hypernatremia, hyperosmolality, volume overload, paradoxical increase of intracellular acidosis secondary to excess carbon dioxide from bicarbonate metabolism, and cerebral edema. If pH is less than 6.9 and the patient exhibits one or more complications of severe acidosis, administration of sodium bicarbonate can be considered using 2–3 ampules (44 mEq/ampule) diluted in 1 L of 5% dextrose in water infused over 2 hours. Reassess pH after allowing at least 2 hours for equilibration. Some experts do not recommend bicarbonate administration at any pH.

E. Treatment of Underlying Causes

Treatment of the underlying cause is the most effective treatment for lactic acidosis. This may include revascularization therapy or balloon pump support in patients with cardiogenic shock, antibiotics for suspected sepsis with appropriate cultures, amputation or revascularization of ischemic extremities, removal or revascularization of ischemic bowel, hemodialysis for renal failure, or removal of toxic components such as ethylene glycol or methanol.

Thiamine should be considered since thiamine deficiency can result from many insults and can produce substantial lactic acidosis.

▶ Disposition

Since the prognosis is grim, prompt identification and treatment of the underlying cause of lactic acidosis remains the best chance for recovery.

Noritomi DT, Soriano FG, Kellum JA, Cappi SB, Biselli PJ, Libório AB, Park M: Metabolic acidosis in patients with severe sepsis and septic shock: a longitudinal quantitative study. Crit Care Med 2009 Oct;37(10):2733–2739.

Howell MD: Lactate: Finally ready for prime time? Crit Care Med 2009 Oct;37(10):2858-9

Perrone J, Phillips C, Gaieski D: Occult metformin toxicity in three patients with profound lactic acidosis. J Emerg Med 2008 [PMID: 18571361].

ALCOHOLIC KETOACIDOSIS

ESSENTIALS OF DIAGNOSIS

▶ Signs include tachypnea (Kussmaul's respirations are common), tachycardia, abdominal tenderness, poor skin turgor, and delayed capillary refill

▶ In general, serum glucose < 250 mg/dL distinguishes alcoholic ketoacidosis from DKA

▶ General Considerations

Alcoholic ketoacidosis is a complex metabolic condition usually developing in chronic alcoholics, but it can also be seen in binge drinkers. It usually develops 24–48 hours after abstinence. Patients are usually either unable or unwilling to consume calories due to abdominal pain, nausea, vomiting, or secondary conditions such as gastritis, pancreatitis, infection, trauma, ingestion, and hepatic or renal failure. Starvation and volume depletion along with depletion of enzymes required for alcohol metabolism inhibit aerobic metabolism. This promotes lipolysis and the release of counter-regulatory hormones as in DKA. A mixed acid–base disturbance from metabolic acidosis results with coinciding volume depletion alkalosis and respiratory alkalosis.

▶ Clinical Findings

A. History

History usually includes chronic alcohol consumption or a recent binge. In either case there is a history of poor food intake, nausea, vomiting, and abdominal pain prior to presentation.

B. Symptoms and Signs

Symptoms are nonspecific and include nausea, vomiting, and abdominal pain. Patients can also present with hematemesis, tremulousness, shortness of air, and dizziness. Common signs are tachypnea (Kussmaul's respiration), tachycardia, and abdominal tenderness.

C. Differential Diagnosis

Because of its vague symptoms the differential diagnosis is quite broad. Most causes of wide anion gap acidosis can present similar to those in AKA. Ingestions of various alcohols, lactic acidosis, infection, DKA, starvation, and renal failure should be considered.

D. Laboratory Findings

1. Metabolic acidosis with a wide anion gap—Serum pH is often <7.2 with a low bicarbonate value.

2. Plasma or urine ketones—The depletion of nicotinamide adenosine dinucleotide by ethanol metabolism slows the conversion of β-hydroxybutyrate to acetoacetate. Since the most common laboratory assessment of ketones is the nitroprusside test, which detects acetoacetate only, initial ketone values may be low or negative. Therefore, negative ketones do not exclude AKA. With treatment, ketone levels may initially rise as the conversion of β-hydroxybutyrate to acetoacetate occurs. They should then fall as ketoacidosis resolves. Of note, the ratio of β-hydroxybutyrate to acetoacetate is usually 6–10:1 in AKA and 3–4:1 in DKA.

3. Electrolyte disorders—Hyponatremia, hyperkalemia, hypokalemia, hypophosphatemia, hypomagnesemia, and hypocalcemia are all common findings in AKA.

4. Glucose—Glucose levels range from hypoglycemia to moderately elevated (up to 250 mg/dL) in the absence of diabetes. DKA can present with lower serum glucose in diabetics who took exogenous insulin just prior to arrival. This may mimic AKA with ketoacidosis and low blood glucose.

5. ETOH levels—ETOH levels may or may not be elevated at the time of presentation because of the inability to maintain oral intake. Watch for signs of withdrawal which can greatly complicate the situation.

▶ Treatment

A. Thiamine

Thiamine 100 mg IV/IM/PO (often along with folic acid 1 mg and a multivitamin) should be given to all patients suspected of chronic ETOH use because of poor nutrition and the risk of Wernicke's encephalopathy.

B. Glucose

After thiamine administration, give 5% dextrose in 0.9% normal saline at 1 L/h for the first 1–2 hours and then 5% dextrose in 0.45% normal saline at ~250 mL/h.

C. Potassium

Total body potassium is usually low due to poor nutrition and losses due to vomiting. Acidosis, however, will shift potassium out of the cells causing initial serum values to be normal to high. Once urine output is established, 10–20 mEq/L of potassium chloride may be given intravenously. Once vomiting is controlled, replacement can be done orally with up to 40 mEq every 2 hours. Assume a 100-mEq deficit for every 1 mEq/L below the normal value. Check potassium every 2 hours during early course of treatment.

D. Insulin

Insulin is generally not required in the treatment of AKA. It may be required in the treatment of diabetics with combinations of AKA and DKA, or it may be used to treat severe hyperkalemia above 6.0 mEq/L with ECG changes.

E. Magnesium

Consider giving 1–2 g of IV magnesium sulfate empirically with the first liter of fluid since magnesium deficiency is very common in alcoholic patients. This will make myocardium less susceptible to dysrhythmias and help restore calcium homeostasis. In addition, replacement of magnesium may be necessary to treat hypokalemia.

F. Bicarbonate

Since acidosis generally responds well to volume and glucose administration, bicarbonate is rarely indicated. Its use may be justified as therapy of severe hyperkalemia or severe acidosis below pH of 6.9 (which is rarely caused by AKA alone).

G. Phosphate

Phosphate replacement is rarely necessary unless levels are below 1 mg/dL. The oral route is preferred because of safety concerns of rapid IV phosphate infusion.

H. Treatment of Underlying Causes

Since AKA has very nonspecific symptoms and signs, do not assume that all symptoms are caused by the syndrome alone. Pancreatitis, GI bleed, infection, or other ingestions may complicate the presentation.

▶ Disposition

Metabolic disorders tend to correct relatively quickly with proper treatment. Many patients with AKA, however, are extremely unreliable and are unlikely to comply with outpatient treatment. Admission is often advisable, and should be considered in patients who remain symptomatic despite hydration. Prior to discharge, the patient should tolerate PO intake, have stable vital signs, and have no underlying illness as a contributor to the AKA. Remember that ETOH withdrawal is also a common and dangerous coinciding problem that will complicate treatment and recovery.

Yanagawa Y, Sakamoto T, Okada Y: Six cases of sudden cardiac arrest in alcoholic ketoacidosis. Intern Med 2008;47(2): 113–117, Epub Jan 15, 2008.

McGuire LC, Cruickshank AM, Munro PT: Alcoholic ketoacidosis. Emerg Med J 2006;23:417:20 [PMID:16714496] (Review).

▼ OTHER METABOLIC AND ENDOCRINE ABNORMALITIES

THYROID DISORDERS

1. Thyroid Storm

ESSENTIALS OF DIAGNOSIS

▶ Typical stigmata of hyperthyroidism, thyromegaly, ophthalmopathy, tremor, stare, diaphoresis, and agitation

▶ Fever (usually)

▶ Tachycardia (out of proportion to fever) often with associated atrial arrhythmias

▶ Mental status changes ranging from confusion to coma

▶ General Considerations

Thyroid storm is a life-threatening disorder that occurs in 1–2% of patients with thyrotoxicosis. A history of previous thyrotoxic symptoms should be sought such as nervousness, restlessness, heat intolerance, sweating, fatigue, muscle cramps, weight loss, tremor, and lighter or less frequent menstrual periods. Thyroid storm should be suspected with a sudden change in mental status (confusion, agitation, delirium more frequent than lethargy or obtundation) with fever and tachycardia out of proportion to fever, and gastrointestinal, cardiac, or central nervous system (CNS) symptoms. Once suspected, treatment should begin immediately and concurrently with treatment for identifiable or suspected precipitating event. Mortality from thyroid storm is high even with proper treatment.

▶ Causes

Thyroid storm usually occurs when an already thyrotoxic patient (Graves disease, toxic multinodular goiter, and toxic adenoma are most common) suffers a serious concurrent illness, event, or injury. Common factors that may trigger a thyroid storm include infection, surgery, trauma, pregnancy/preeclampsia, stroke, MI, PE, amiodarone use, DKA, ketosis, radioiodine

therapy, drug use (usually stimulants), ETOH, iodine contrast material, or discontinuation of antithyroid medication.

▶ Clinical Findings

The diagnosis of thyroid storm should be made clinically. Often a history of partially treated hyperthyroidism or signs of thyroid disease such as thyromegaly, proptosis, stare, myopathy, or myxedema can be found. The diagnosis should be made in the patient with a probable history of thyroid disease, which rapidly decompensates in the setting of fever, tachycardia, gastrointestinal symptoms, and mental status change. Elevated thyroid hormone levels are common in significant illness, and there is no significant difference in levels in thyroid storm and thyrotoxicosis. Therefore, no test will confirm this diagnosis.

A. Symptoms and Signs

Fever may exceed 40°C (104°F). This may be due to the catabolic state of thyrotoxicosis or secondary to precipitating infection. Appropriate cultures and broad-spectrum antibiotics are indicated.

Cardiac findings usually include a friction rub or systolic flow murmur, and either sinus or supraventricular tachycardia. The rate is often characterized as out of proportion to fever. Mental status changes are also common. Gastrointestinal symptoms include nausea, vomiting, diarrhea, and abdominal pain—can mimic an acute abdomen. Neuromuscular findings such as agitation, tremor, generalized weakness (especially in the proximal muscles), and periodic paralysis are also seen. Dermatologic findings include warm, moist, smooth skin and palmar erythema.

Findings consistent with prior thyroid disease include thyromegaly with or without a bruit, orbitopathy, tremor, stare, hyperreflexia, pretibial myxedema, and other integumentary changes such as coarse hair and thick, dry skin. Death may occur from hypovolemic shock, coma, congestive heart failure, or tachydysrhythmias.

Apathetic hyperthyroidism is important to consider in the elderly population. With advanced age and other comorbid conditions, the classic symptoms and signs of thyroid storm and thyrotoxicosis may be absent.

B. Ancillary Diagnostic Findings

Draw blood samples to test for free T_4, T_3, and TSH (thyroid-stimulating hormone) and serum cortisol levels. A complete blood count, serum electrolytes, glucose, renal and hepatic function tests, and ABG analysis should be performed; obtain cultures of the blood, urine, and possibly sputum; chest X-ray and ECG are indicated to look for precipitating causes or complications. Cranial CT scan is indicated for delirious or comatose patients.

Previous abnormal thyroid function tests may suggest a preexisting thyrotoxicosis. TFTs may be misinterpreted based on levels of thyroid binding globulin. TSH will be markedly low in most patients with thyroid storm or thyrotoxicosis. Free thyroxine (T_4) will be elevated, again similar to thyrotoxicosis. Electrolyte and glucose abnormalities may also be present due to gastrointestinal losses, dehydration, physiologic stress, and fever.

C. Electrocardiographic Findings

The ECG is usually abnormal; common findings are sinus tachycardia, increased QRS interval and P wave voltage, nonspecific ST–T wave changes, and atrial dysrhythmias, usually atrial fibrillation or flutter. Conduction defects, most commonly first-degree AV block and nonspecific intraventricular conduction delay, may occur. Ischemic findings or myocardial infarction may be present, especially in older patients with concurrent illness such as diabetes or hypertension.

▶ Treatment

A. Emergency Measures

Initiate standard resuscitative measures.

Volume replacement is commonly indicated with at least 1 L of normal saline or lactated Ringer's solution in the first hour due to volume depletion from fever. Frequent reassessment is required to prevent fluid overload, especially in patients exhibiting signs of high output cardiac failure (tachycardia, dyspnea, wide pulse pressure). Vasopressors may be required for hypotension not correcting with volume resuscitation. Hypotension, however, may be a sign of another problem such as sepsis or adrenal insufficiency.

Phenobarbital should be considered for sedation since it stimulates the clearance of thyroid hormone by inducing hepatic microsomal enzymes. Fever should be treated aggressively with cool IV fluids, cool mist sprays, cooling blankets, and antipyretics.

Avoid iodinated contrast, amiodarone, NSAIDs, aspirin, pseudoephedrine, and ketamine in these patients.

B. Hormone Synthesis Blockers

Thionamides are the standard first-line agents to treat thyroid storm. Propylthiouracil (PTU) 600–1000 mg first dose and 200–250 mg PO every 4 hours is the drug of choice. Methimazole 40 mg PO initially and then 25 mg every 6 hours can also be used. PTU has the additional benefit of blocking the peripheral conversion of T_4 to the active T_3. Neither of the thionamides are available parenterally and must be given PO, via nasogastric tube, or retention enema.

C. Hormone Release Blockers

Iodine therapy is an adjunct to the thionamides. It should not be given until at least 1–2 hours after PTU or methimazole is administered. Early administration can promote further hormone production, thus worsening hyperthyroidism.

Several forms are available such as potassium iodide (SSKI, 35 mg/drop) 5 drops PO every 6 hours or Lugol's solution 8 drops every 6 hours. Other forms include contrast agents such as sodium ipodate (Oragrafin) or sodium iopanoate (Telepaque), both of which would be 1 g a day or 500 mg twice a day by mouth. If iodine allergy is a concern, lithium carbonate can be given instead at 300 mg every 6–8 hours to maintain levels of 1.0–1.2 mEq/L.

D. Hormone Action Blockers

β-Adrenergic agonists such as propranolol block the peripheral effects of excess thyroid hormone. A typical dose is 0.5–1 mg IV every 10–15 minutes until pulse reduction is achieved and then every 2–3 hours. Caution should be used in patients with bronchospastic disease. Metoprolol can be used at a dose of 50 mg PO every 6 hours. Esmolol with a 250–500 µg/kg IV load and then 50–100 µg/kg/min. Beta blockers are the mainstay for high output cardiac failure. Beta blockers may be especially attractive in cases of atrial fibrillation with rapid ventricular response. Calcium channel blockers have been associated with hypotension, amiodarone is contraindicated, and digoxin is often ineffective.

In very severe cases when thyroid hormone effects are not controlled with the above measures, plasmapheresis, plasma exchange, peritoneal dialysis, or charcoal plasma perfusion may be attempted.

E. Corticosteroids

Corticosteroids inhibit peripheral conversion of T_4 to T_3 and block the release of hormone from the thyroid gland. In addition, they treat the relative adrenal insufficiency that may be present. Intravenous hydrocortisone, 100 mg every 8 hours, is the treatment of choice for concurrent adrenal insufficiency; however, dexamethasone, 0.1 mg/kg intravenously every 8 hours, may be given. The advantage of dexamethasone is that an adrenocorticotropic hormone (ACTH) stimulation test of the adrenocortical axis may still be undertaken by consultants.

▶ Disposition

Hospitalization in an intensive care unit is indicated for all patients with thyroid storm, having a mortality rate of 20% if treated, and uniformly fatal if untreated. Invasive hemodynamic monitoring may be necessary to facilitate fluid management and assess progress of therapy in cases complicated by cardiac failure.

Chong HW, See KC, Phua J: Thyroid storm with multiorgan failure. Thyroid 2010 Mar;20(3):333–336.

Martinez-Diaz GJ, Formaker C, Hsia R: Atrial fibrillation from thyroid storm. J Emerg Med. 2008 Dec 19. [Epub ahead of print] [PMID: 19097726].

Ngo AS, Lung Tan DC: Thyrotoxic heart disease. Resuscitation 2006;70:287.

Ngo SYA, Chew HC: When the storm passes unnoticed: A case series of thyroid storm.Resuscitation 2007;73:485.

2. Myxedema Coma

ESSENTIALS OF DIAGNOSIS

▶ A potentially lethal complication of severe hypothyroidism

▶ Look for typical stigmata: dry skin, delayed reflex relaxation, generalized weakness, edema, or a transverse scar across the low anterior neck

▶ Alteration in mental status (although coma is rare).

▶ Often hypothermic (< 35.5°C[95.9°F])

▶ General Considerations

Myxedema coma is a rare complication of extreme hypothyroidism (most often Hashimoto's thyroiditis). Although it can occur as an initial presentation of hypothyroidism, myxedema coma usually occurs in patients with known hypothyroidism or after surgery or ablative therapy for hyperthyroidism. The incidence mirrors that of hypothyroidism with a 4:1 female predominance. Myxedema coma typically occurs in the winter months after exposure to cold in those 60 years and older.

Other predisposing factors include cerebrovascular accident, CHF exacerbation, anesthesia, GI bleed, cardiac ischemia, surgery, trauma, medications, or infection. The cardinal features are CNS depression with hypothermia and hypothyroidism. Hyporeflexia, generalized swelling, coma, bradycardia, and respiratory depression are also common. Onset is often rapid but can be insidious, especially in the elderly. If untreated, mortality is estimated at up to 60–70%. If recognized and treated appropriately, mortality drops to 15–35%.

▶ Clinical Findings

The presumptive diagnosis of myxedema coma should be made when clinical manifestations of hypothyroidism are accompanied by disturbances of consciousness, hypothermia, hypoventilation, bradycardia, and hypotension.

A. History

Cold intolerance, dry skin, constipation, weight gain, muscle cramps, and general fatigue or weakness are common. Slowing of speech, disorientation, apathy, inappropriate humor (myxedema wit), or psychosis may also occur. Discontinuation of thyroid replacement, previous radioactive iodine treatment, thyroidectomy, or medication administration, such as sedatives, iodides, or amiodarone, is a common historical finding.

B. Symptoms and Signs

These include cold intolerance, dry skin, change in voice, heavier or more frequent menstrual periods, constipation, weight gain, irregular or absent menses, muscle cramps, paresthesias, angina, or seizures. Neurologic complaints such as generalized weakness, slow speech, disorientation, apathy, ataxia, inappropriate humor (myxedema wit), or psychosis are also seen. As hypothyroidism worsens, neurologic symptoms progress to lethargy, disorientation, and coma. Seizures may also occur.

Hypothermia is found in approximately 80% of patients with myxedema coma. Hypoventilation is due to decreased respiratory drive and generalized muscle weakness. Hypotension may be present along with gastrointestinal ileus or urinary retention.

Physical findings including bradycardia; generalized puffiness; periorbital edema; ptosis; cutaneous myxedema; coarse, dry, yellow skin; macroglossia; delayed relaxation phase of deep tendon reflexes; thyroidectomy scar or a goiter; or coarse, sparse hair may be the only clues of this condition in a comatose patient.

C. Laboratory Findings

Blood glucose should be assessed initially. Thyroid studies are rarely available on an emergency basis. They typically reveal a low serum free T_4 and T_3. The TSH is usually high in primary hypothyroidism; however, it may be low in secondary and tertiary hypothyroidism. The distinction between hypothyroidism and myxedema coma cannot be made based on TFTs alone.

Blood and urine cultures should be obtained. Arterial blood gases may reveal hypoxemia, hypercapnia, and a respiratory or mixed acidosis. Hyponatremia and hypoglycemia may be potential contributors to CNS depression. Serum creatinine kinase may be elevated. Myocardial pathology or rhabdomyolysis must be excluded as causes. Anemia and hyperlipidemia are common.

D. Imaging

Chest radiography may show an enlarged heart (from a pericardial effusion) or other precipitating cause for the myxedema coma, such as pneumonia. Bedside ultrasonography can confirm a pericardial effusion.

E. Electrocardiographic Findings

The ECG may show bradycardia, low voltage of the QRS complex in all leads, flattening or inversion of the T waves, and conduction abnormalities.

▶ Treatment

A. General and Supportive Measures

1. Stabilization—Patients with myxedema coma will need mechanical ventilation if hypoxemia and hypoventilation are found. Otherwise, supplemental oxygen is indicated. Obtain venous access and blood samples for free T_4, free T_3, TSH, cortisol, CBC, renal and hepatic function tests, arterial blood gases, cultures, and electrolytes and glucose levels.

2. Fluid replacement—Isotonic crystalloid solution (normal saline or lactated Ringer's) should be given for hypotension. Avoid hypotonic solutions because hyponatremia may be present. Watch for the unmasking of congestive heart failure. Treat severe hyponatremia (≤120 mEq/L) with careful administration of 3% saline if mental status is depressed. Thyroid replacement therapy and corticosteroids along with restriction of free water will generally correct mild hyponatremia.

3. Treatment for hypothermia—Active rewarming methods are contraindicated due to the risk of cardiovascular collapse. Passive methods of rewarming such as blankets are preferred.

4. Other therapies—Avoid unnecessary medications that may further depress mental status. Empiric antibiotics are indicated initially in critically ill patients. Hypoglycemia and other electrolyte abnormalities can be treated in the usual manner. Vasopressors are not likely to be effective because of a reduced adrenergic receptor response and may provoke dysrhythmias, especially during intravenous thyroid replacement therapy.

5. Treatment of precipitating causes—Any precipitating cause for myxedema coma must be addressed. Recovery from myxedema coma is slow since reversal of severe metabolic abnormalities is required.

B. Specific Therapy

Levothyroxine (T$_4$) is most often recommended for replacement therapy. This form, however, depends on conversion to the active T$_3$ form that may be inhibited by severe illness. Liothyronine (T$_3$) does not require conversion and can also be given, but higher doses have been associated with increased mortality. Combinations of both are also given as a more physiologic replacement. Some of the protocols are as follows:

- Levothyroxine (T$_4$) alone may be considered in geriatric patients or those with cardiac disease. Use an intravenous loading dose of 200–500 µg over the first hour and then 50–100 µg/d, or oral dosing at 50–100 µg/d when tolerated.

- Liothyronine (T$_3$) alone may be used in young, healthy patients. Give a loading dose of 5–20 µg IV or PO and then 5–10 µg/8 h until improvement.

- Levothyroxine (T$_4$) at 200–250 µg bolus and 50 µg PO daily and liothyronine (T$_3$) 10 µg IV or PO load and 10 µg every 8 hours. Maintenance doses are appropriate when the patient is clinically stable.

All three methods may precipitate a cardiac event such as angina, dysrhythmia, or infarction. Lower dosing regimens are recommended in those at increased risk for cardiac events. All patients receiving intravenous thyroid hormone replacement should have continuous cardiac monitoring. Corticosteroids are also recommended since there is a 5–10% incidence of concurrent adrenal insufficiency. In

this situation, thyroid replacement before corticosteroid replacement can cause further deterioration. Therefore, early corticosteroid replacement is indicated. This can be given as intravenous hydrocortisone 100 mg every 8 hours. This is the preferred replacement method due to its action as both a glucocorticoid and a mineralocorticoid. Acutely however, dexamethasone 2–4 mg IV every 6 hours is often used since it will not alter a cosyntropin stimulation test. This will allow consultants to evaluate the need for chronic replacement once the patient has stabilized.

▶ Disposition

Hospitalization in an intensive care unit is indicated for all patients with myxedema coma.

Benyon J, Akhtar S, Kearney T: Predictors of outcome in myxoedema coma. Crit Care 2008;12(1):111, Epub Jan 23, 2008 [PMID: 18254932].

Kwaku MP, Burman KD: Myxedema coma. J Intensive Care Med 2007 Jul–Aug;22(4):224–231 [PMID: 17712058]. Review.

ADRENAL INSUFFICIENCY AND CRISIS (ADDISONIAN CRISIS)

 ESSENTIALS OF DIAGNOSIS

▶ Consider addisonian crisis in patients with hypotension refractory to intravenous fluids or in acutely ill patients with typical stigmata of chronic glucocorticoid use such as moon facies and buffalo hump

▶ Common symptoms include orthostasis, weight loss, anorexia, lethargy, abdominal cramps, nausea, vomiting, diarrhea, and mental depression

▶ Classic electrolyte abnormalities include hyponatremia associated with hyperkalemia

▶ General Considerations

The adrenal glands produce three different groups of hormones: glucocorticoids, mineralocorticoids, and androgenic hormones. These hormones help the body adjust to metabolic stress. Failure results in a chronic disease state while sudden onset or stress may induce a life-threatening emergency resulting in cardiovascular instability, loss of glucose homeostasis, and extracellular fluid and electrolyte imbalance and shock.

▶ Classification

A. Primary Adrenocortical Insufficiency

Primary adrenocortical insufficiency (Addison's disease) results from primary destruction or inhibition of the adrenal glands. There are several known causes such as autoimmune insults (most common), infection (tuberculosis is most common worldwide while AIDS is most common in the United States), systemic inflammatory response, congenital, trauma, hemorrhage, metastatic carcinoma, and medications.

Bilateral adrenal hemorrhage may occur due to infections such as *Neisseria meningitidis* or pneumococcal septicemia (Waterhouse–Friderichsen syndrome). Patients with coagulopathy, thromboembolic disease, or those taking anticoagulants are also at increased risk.

B. Secondary Adrenocortical Insufficiency

Secondary adrenocortical insufficiency results from pathology of the hypothalamus and pituitary. Corticotropin-releasing hormone and ACTH release are impaired, causing dysfunction along the hypothalamus–pituitary–adrenal axis. Chronic steroid use resulting in ACTH suppression and adrenal hypoplasia is the most common cause of adrenocortical insufficiency. A primary pituitary or hypothalamic mass must also be considered. Traumatic brain injury is becoming a more common cause of secondary or tertiary insufficiency, occurring from 1 day to 6 months after trauma.

▶ Clinical Findings

A. Symptoms and Signs

The most common presentation of adrenal crisis is shock, often refractory to fluids and vasopressors. Adrenal insufficiency presents with symptoms such as fatigue, anorexia, generalized aches, and abdominal pain, which are common with low cortisol levels, while hypotension, hyponatremia, hyperkalemia, metabolic acidosis, and orthostasis are seen with low aldosterone production. ACTH is cleaved with melanocyte-stimulating hormone (MSH), which upregulates melanocytes and causes hyperpigmentation of the axillae and other skin folds in primary adrenal insufficiency. Low androgen levels cause decreased body hair. Amenorrhea develops commonly in women.

B. Laboratory Findings

Mineralocorticoid deficiency causes a classic hyponatremia and hyperkalemia. The finding of the two together in symptomatic patients should suggest the diagnosis of primary adrenal insufficiency.

Other findings may include anemia of chronic disease, elevated BUN, hypoglycemia, hypocalcemia, lymphocytosis, and eosinophilia. Hyperkalemia is typically not seen in secondary adrenal insufficiency because aldosterone production is usually preserved.

C. Imaging

Calcification of the adrenals may be present as a result of tuberculosis, histoplasmosis, or other disseminated fungal disease. Cranial magnetic resonance imaging (MRI) is usually the test of choice for secondary adrenal insufficiency to reveal sellar and hypothalamic–pituitary tumors, and abdominal CT is the test of choice in primary adrenal insufficiency to image the adrenal glands. Enlarged adrenal glands suggest tuberculosis, fungal disease, cancer, hemorrhage, or AIDS. Small adrenal glands suggest autoimmune disease, chronic infection, exogenous corticosteroids, or chronic vascular abnormalities.

D. Electrocardiographic Findings

The ECG may reveal low voltage in all leads and changes characteristic of electrolyte abnormalities such as hyperkalemia with peaked T waves, prolongation of QRS interval, and loss of P waves in severe cases.

▶ Diagnosis

Draw blood for serum cortisol level. A serum cortisol exceeding 20 µg/dL at any time of the day makes the diagnosis of adrenal insufficiency unlikely. A level less than 3 µg/dL is confirmatory. Ideally the blood is drawn when the patient is under duress.

An ACTH stimulation test, however, is the study of choice. After the initial serum cortisol is drawn, 250 µg of synthetic ACTH (cosyntropin) is given. Serum cortisol levels are drawn 30 and 60 minutes later. Failure of the adrenals to produce cortisol to levels of 25–30 µg/dL or an increase of less than 9 µg/dL suggests primary adrenal insufficiency. Administration of hydrocortisone will alter the results of this test. Dexamethasone is an alternative that will not interfere with the diagnosis. This should not, however, be allowed to cause a delay in treatment. A random cortisol sample in an unstable patient should be helpful in making the diagnosis.

▶ Treatment

A. General and Supportive Measures

After standard stabilization, draw blood to test for CBC, electrolytes, glucose, renal and hepatic functions, and random serum cortisol. ACTH stimulation test may be done later by a consultant.

Monitor fluid intake and urine output. Monitor potassium levels carefully. Even though potassium levels may be high initially, total body deficits often exist. Replace fluid volume and correct electrolyte abnormalities as appropriate.

B. Specific Therapy

Hydrocortisone, 100 mg intravenously every 8 hours, is the mainstay for treating adrenal insufficiency. Alternatively, dexamethasone, 0.1 mg/kg every 8 hours, may be used without disruption of diagnostic testing, although it supports only glucocorticoid function. Once diagnostic testing has been done, hydrocortisone is the drug of choice because it has both glucocorticoid and mineralocorticoid functions. Once patients are stable, the dose may be tapered gradually over 1–2 weeks.

Patients receiving less than 50 mg/d of hydrocortisone will likely need mineralocorticoid support as well. Fludrocortisone, 0.05–0.2 mg/d, is the drug of choice. Fludrocortisone therapy is necessary as transition to oral therapy begins.

Disposition

Admission is indicated if an addisonian crisis is suspected or confirmed. Intensive care unit admission is warranted for hemodynamically unstable patients. Adrenal insufficiency will require close follow-up and instructions on stress dosing of adrenal supplementation.

Taub YR, Wolford RW: Adrenal insufficiency and other adrenal oncologic emergencies. Emerg Med Clin North Am 2009 May;27(2):271–282.

Bornstein SR: Predisposing factors for adrenal insufficiency. N Engl J Med 2009 May 28;360(22):2328–2339. Review

PHEOCHROMOCYTOMA (CATECHOLAMINE CRISIS)

 ESSENTIALS OF DIAGNOSIS

► Symptoms of catecholamine crisis are headache, palpitations, flushing, ordiaphoresis associated with hypertension

► Symptoms associated with pheochromocytoma are often intermittent (with asymptomatic periods in between episodes), whereas those of a monoamine oxidase inhibitor (MAOI) crisis or of sympathomimetic intoxication are not

General Considerations

A catecholamine crisis is typically caused by one of three entities: (1) a pheochromocytoma, (2) a monoamine oxidase inhibitor (MAOI) crisis, or (3) intoxication from cocaine or other similar sympathomimetics. Occasionally, a catecholamine crisis may also be induced by sudden cessation of clonidine therapy. Catecholamines bind to α-1 and β-receptors and in excess may cause various symptoms and signs such as headache, palpitations, diaphoresis, and often severe hypertension. A thorough history will usually lead to the cause of catecholamine crisis, except in the case of pheochromocytoma, which often remains elusive since the symptoms are nonspecific and often intermittent.

Clinical Findings

A. Symptoms and Signs

Classic manifestations include hypertension, headache, diaphoresis, pallor, palpitations, nervousness, apprehension, nausea, vomiting, and abdominal pain. Labile hypertension is the hallmark of a pheochromocytoma. Severe hypertension ($\geq$120 mm Hg diastolic) often prompts the clinician to include catecholamine crisis in the differential diagnosis. It is frequently intermittent, however, and may not always be present at the time of examination. Only half of these patients will have sustained hypertension.

Complications that occur late in the course of the disease may be dramatic and often obscure the diagnosis. Abdominal or chest pain, aortic dissection, encephalopathy, cardiomyopathy, pulmonary edema, fever, and anion gap metabolic acidosis are often distracting presentations.

Neurocutaneous syndromes such as neurofibromatosis, von Hippel–Lindau disease, ataxia-telangiectasia, tuberous sclerosis, and Sturge–Weber syndrome are sometimes associated with pheochromocytoma. Cutaneous findings (ie, café-au-lait spots, telangiectasias) may provide clues to the diagnosis.

Mucosal neuromas and a marfanoid appearance suggest multiple endocrine neoplasia type IIB. Other findings include weight loss, heat intolerance, hyperglycemia, and tachycardia.

B. Laboratory Findings and Special Tests

The diagnosis of pheochromocytoma is made along two pathways. First, a biochemical diagnosis must be made. Second, the tumor must be defined by radiologic studies for possible surgical excision.

The initial traditional biochemical test of choice is a 24-hour urine collection for metanephrines and catecholamines. Challenging this tradition, some endocrinologists have advocated plasma fractionated metanephrines as the initial screening test based on high sensitivity of the test (96–100%) and ease of obtaining the specimen. Because of the intermittent nature of secretion, however, 24-hour urine evaluations often produce more consistent results and greater sensitivity (fewer false positives that lead to expensive radiographic testing and sometimes surgery) than with plasma fractionated metanephrine testing.

After positive biochemical tests, localization of the tumor is performed by CT scan, MRI, or isotope scanning with metaiodobenzylguanidine (MUGA). Ninety percent of pheochromocytomas arise from the adrenal glands, however, 10% are found in extra-adrenal sites.

C. Cardiac Effects of a Catecholamine Crisis

In addition to tachydysrhythmias, a prolonged QT interval, which can predispose the patient to lethal arrhythmias, may be present on the ECG. Findings of cardiac ischemia and coronary artery disease also complicate the diagnostic picture. Many of these findings resolve after tumor removal.

▶ Treatment

A. General and Supportive Measures

Obtain blood for routine studies (CBC, serum electrolytes, glucose, hepatic and renal function). Replace volume deficits, and correct electrolyte abnormalities. Avoid drugs or procedures that may exacerbate a catecholamine crisis. Obtain a serum metanephrine specimen or begin 24-hour urine collection for fractionated catecholamines, metanephrine, and vanillylmandelic acid (VMA).

B. Specific Therapy

1. Phentolamine—α-Adrenergic blockade with phentolamine is the traditional cornerstone of acute therapy for pheochromocytoma. The dose is 1–2 mg intravenously every 5 minutes. *Caution:* Higher initial doses may cause sudden severe hypotension. If no response is seen, increase the dose to 5 mg intravenously every 5 minutes until adequate blood pressure control occurs. Orthostatic hypotension is a common side effect and can be managed by ensuring adequate hydration and keeping the patient recumbent.

2. Nitroprusside—Intravenous sodium nitroprusside has classically been the treatment for hypertensive crisis associated with pheochromocytoma. It is still recommended in presentations with a clinical picture of congestive heart failure or myocardial infarction. Newer agents such as nicardipine, labetalol, and fenoldopam are now commonly recommended due to risks of cyanide toxicity with prolonged therapy associated with nitroprusside.

3. Fenoldopam—Fenoldopam, a dopamine-1 receptor agonist, is an alternative to nitroprusside. An intravenous infusion beginning at 0.1 µg/kg/min vasodilates the renal, splanchnic, and coronary circulation. Improved renal blood flow, lack of a toxic metabolite, and a short half-life of 7–9 minutes are its major advantages.

4. Calcium channel blockers—Calcium channel blockers such as nicardipine are commonly used in the treatment of hypertension associated with pheochromocytoma. Both oral and intravenous administrations are very effective in controlling fluctuating pressures. They are also helpful in preventing coronary vasospasm precipitated by catecholamine release.

5. β-Blockers—β-Adrenergic blockade is contraindicated until sufficient α-blockade is initiated due to unopposed α-stimulation, which can precipitate a hypertensive crisis. β-Blockers are usually reserved for patients with severe tachydysrhythmias. Esmolol 50–200 µg/kg/min after a 500 µg/kg loading dose can be used. A mixed α–β-receptor antagonist such as labetalol has a slightly decreased risk of unopposed alpha effects. However, α-blockade is still required since hypertensive crisis has been reported. Labetalol may be given in 10–20 mg intravenous boluses every 10 minutes until the desired blood pressure is achieved with maintenance intravenous infusion of 0.5–2.0 mg/min.

6. Benzodiazepines—Benzodiazepines may also be useful in blunting the body's sympathetic response to excess catecholamines. Lorazepam, 1–2 mg intravenously, and diazepam, 5–10 mg intravenously, are common starting doses. Administer these drugs judiciously to avoid oversedation and hypotension, particularly if the patient is volume depleted.

▶ Disposition

Hospitalization in an intensive care unit is indicated in all patients with pheochromocytoma.

Mitchell L, Bellis F. Phaeochromocytoma—"the great mimic": an unusual presentation. Emerg Med J 2007 Sep;24(9):672–673.

Guerrero MA, Schreinemakers JM, Vriens MR, Suh I, Hwang J, Shen WT, Gosnell J, Clark OH, Duh QY: Clinical spectrum of pheochromocytoma. J Am Coll Surg 2009 Dec;209(6):727–732.

Sawka AM, Jaeschke R, Singh RJ, Young WF: A comparison of biochemical tests for pheochromocytoma: measurement of fractionated plasma metanephrines compared with the combination of 24 hour urinary metanephrines and catecholamines. J Clin Endocrinol Metab 2003 Feb;88:553–558 [PMID: 12574179].

PITUITARY APOPLEXY

ESSENTIALS OF DIAGNOSIS

▶ Rare event with variable presentation

▶ Patients often have a sudden onset of headache

▶ Neurologic deficits including hemiparesis; cranial nerve defects including ophthalmoplegia and bitemporal hemianopsia

▶ General Considerations

Pituitary apoplexy is an infarction or hemorrhage of the pituitary gland. This often occurs in the setting of a preexisting pituitary tumor such as an adenoma. The symptoms seen in pituitary apoplexy result from (1) leakage of blood and necrotic material into the subarachnoid space, (2) development of a rapidly expanding hemorrhagic intrasellar mass lesion compressing the optic chiasm, cavernous sinuses, cranial nerves, and adjacent structures (hypothalamus and internal carotid arteries), and (3) acute hypopituitarism.

Risk factors for pituitary apoplexy include head trauma, irradiation, estrogen, anticoagulation use, DKA, hypertension, diuretics, and use of bromocriptine. Sheehan's syndrome most commonly occurs in the postpartum period, causing hemorrhage and vasospastic necrosis of the pituitary.

▶ Clinical Findings

A. Symptoms and Signs

The diagnosis is challenging, because pituitary apoplexy is a rare disease with variable presentation. Onset is usually acute and dramatic; however, it can rarely be insidious. A headache, often described as a severe sudden-onset retro-orbital or bifrontal, is nearly always present. It is also associated with nausea and vomiting and symptoms of meningeal irritation due to blood in the subarachnoid space. Fever may also be present due to blood or disruption of hypothalamic structures. Neurologic symptoms that are most commonly associated with pituitary apoplexy are ophthalmologic symptoms, including decreased visual acuity, visual field defects, classically bitemporal hemianopia, and opthalmoplegia, due to encroachment of cranial nerves III, IV, and VI. Compression of the internal carotid artery or decreased blood flow from increased intracranial pressure or vascular spasm can lead to mental status changes or stroke-like symptoms caused by hemispheric ischemia. Blood in the subarachnoid space can also cause seizures.

Pituitary hypofunction is seen on presentation in most patients. A history of pituitary hormone dysfunction may be helpful in the diagnosis. Although several hormone deficiencies are often present, adrenal insufficiency is the most life-threatening complication and requires immediate attention. Respiratory failure may also occur from hypothalamic compression or increased intracranial pressure.

B. Laboratory Findings

Global pituitary function should be assessed by thyroid function tests, cortisol levels, growth hormone levels, and prolactin levels. A basic metabolic panel may reveal hyper- or hyponatremia. Cerebrospinal fluid may be xanthochromic or grossly bloody, with an elevated opening pressure.

C. Imaging

MRI is the imaging study of choice for diagnosis of pituitary apoplexy. MRI is superior to cranial CT because it allows differentiation of hemorrhagic and necrotic tissues, as well as abnormalities of the surrounding areas; MRI is up to 50% more sensitive for the detection of pituitary apoplexy than CT. However, these patients are often unstable, which may prohibit the use of MRI. CT is a reasonable alternative in unstable patients and will detect most abnormalities in unstable patients.

▶ Treatment

After initial resuscitation, hydrocortisone 100 mg intravenously should be given to all patients suspected of having pituitary apoplexy to treat frequently concurrent and potentially lethal acute adrenal insufficiency.

Definitive treatment for pituitary apoplexy is usually neurosurgical decompression. Indications for immediate surgery are decreasing consciousness, progressive vision loss, or increasing extraocular motor palsy indicating cavernous sinus compression.

▶ Disposition

Immediate neurosurgical consultation is indicated. Surgery is the definitive treatment, but not every patient will require an operation. Some patients recover without sequelae with conservative management alone.

van der Eerden AW, Twickler MT, Sweep FC, Beems T, Hendricks HT, Hermus AR, Vos PE: Should anterior pituitary function be tested during follow-up of all patients presenting at the emergency department because of traumatic brain injury? Eur J Endocrinol 2010 Jan;162(1):19–28, Epub Sep 25, 2009.

Nawar RN, AbdelMannan D, Selman WR, Arafah BM: Pituitary tumor apoplexy: a review. J Intensive Care Med 2008 Mar–Apr;23(2):75–90. Review.

Espinosa PS, Choudry B, Wilbourn R, Espinosa PH, Vaishnav AG: Pituitary apoplexy: a neurological emergency case report. J Ky Med Assoc 2007 Nov;105(11):538–540.

Agha A, Phillips J, Thompson CJ: Hypopituitarism following traumatic brain injury (TBI). Br J Neurosurg 2007 Apr;21(2): 210–216. Review.

INAPPROPRIATE SECRETION OF ANTIDIURETIC HORMONE

 ESSENTIALS OF DIAGNOSIS

▶ Hyponatremia in the setting of a reduced plasma osmolality, persistent urinary secretion of sodium (>20 mEq/L), and urine osmolality that is inappropriately high for the degree of hyponatremia and hypo-osmolality found

▶ Mental status changes ranging from mild to severe dependent on the degree of hyponatremia and the rate of decline

▶ General Considerations

Arginine vasopressin (AVP), also known as antidiuretic hormone (ADH), is secreted from the posterior pituitary in response primarily to hyperosmolality and decreased circulating volume. AVP acts on the collecting ducts in the nephrons to allow water reabsorption. Inappropriate secretion of antidiuretic hormone (SIADH) is a state of pathological hormone excess in the presence of hyponatremia and hypoosmolality. Classic diagnostic criteria include (1) euvolemic hyponatremia and low plasma osmolality, (2) failure of the kidney to dilute the urine in the presence of reduced serum osmolality (urine osmolality is frequently

Table 43–1. Causes of SIADH.

Tumors
    Small cell carcinoma of the lung
    Pancreatic carcinoma
    Thymoma
    Hodgkin disease
    Neuroblastoma
CNS disorder
    Stroke
    Hemorrhage
    Infection
    Trauma
Drugs
    Antidepressants
    Antipsychotics
    Anticonvulsants
    Sulfonylureas
    ACE inhibitors
    Narcotics
    MDMA (Ecstasy)
    Antineoplastic agents
Pulmonary disorders
    Tuberculosis
    Pneumonia
    Abscess
    Bronchiectasis
    Mechanical ventilation

>300 mOsm/kg), (3) continued sodium excretion (usually >20 mEq/L) despite hyponatremia, and (4) absence of other conditions such as hypothyroidism, adrenal insufficiency, congestive heart failure, cirrhosis, or renal disease, which can cause hyponatremia.

► Causes

Numerous diseases and drugs can cause SIADH. See Table 43–1.

The elderly are at higher risk for SIADH because several physiologic effects of aging contribute to its pathogenesis, including an increased ADH response to osmotic stimulation, declining renal function, and decreased renin, angiotensin, and aldosterone production.

► Clinical Findings

A. Symptoms and Signs

The clinical presentation of SIADH depends on the level of hyponatremia and water intoxication:

- In mild cases (serum sodium ≥ 120 mEq/L), patients are usually asymptomatic.
- When serum sodium reaches 105–120 mEq/L, patients begin to experience neurologic manifestations such

as anorexia, nausea, vomiting, personality changes, depressed tendon reflexes, and muscle weakness.

- With severe hyponatremia (≤105 mEq/L), coma, seizures, delirium, cranial nerve palsies, hypothermia, and altered patterns of respiration (Cheyne–Stokes) may be evident.

Because SIADH can be caused by various pathologic conditions, patients will also present with symptoms or signs of their underlying disease (eg, malignancy, CNS or pulmonary disease). Edema and other signs of volume overload are highly unusual even with severe hyponatremia and water intoxication. Signs of volume overload indicate an alternative diagnosis.

B. Laboratory Findings

Hyponatremia along with reduced plasma osmolality, persistent urinary secretion of sodium (>20 mEq/L), and urine osmolality that is inappropriately high for the degree of hyponatremia and hypo-osmolality is found.

► Treatment

A. General and Supportive Measures

Draw blood for measurement of serum sodium and other electrolytes, creatinine, BUN, osmolality, cortisol levels, and thyroid function studies (TSH and free T_4). Send urine for urinalysis and measurement of urinary osmolality, electrolytes, and specific gravity.

Measure serum and urine electrolytes and osmolality every 1–2 hours during the acute phase if receiving 3% NaCl, and then 1–4 times daily until the patient's condition has stabilized. Assess the patient for evidence of renal, hepatic, or cardiac dysfunction. Obtain a history of drugs and medications used by the patient. Imaging may be indicated for evaluation of causes of SIADH, and evaluate for cancer, CNS disease, or pulmonary disease.

B. Specific Therapy

Fluid restriction is the treatment of choice for the correction of euvolemic (SIADH) or hypervolemic (CHF, cirrhosis) hyponatremia.

1. Mild SIADH (serum sodium ≥ 120 mEq/L)—Restrict fluids to 800–1000 mL per 24 hours.

2. Moderate SIADH (serum sodium 105–120 mEq/L)— Restrict fluids to 500 mL per 24 hour.

3. Severe SIADH (serum sodium < 105 mEq/L or at any level if the patient develops neurologic complications such as coma or seizures)—This is a medical emergency. Treatment is as follows:

- Administer hypertonic saline, 3% solution, at 1–2 mL/ kg/h for the first 3–4 hours.
- Use intravenous furosemide, 1 mg/kg, to counteract volume overload.

- Monitor sodium and potassium every 1–2 hours and adjust fluids and replace as needed.

- Correct to a serum sodium level of 125 mEq/L or until CNS involvement resolves, and then resume fluid restriction therapy as described previously.

Serum sodium correction should average 0.5–2 mEq/L/h and no more than 10 mEq/L in the first 24 hours. Faster rates of sodium correction and longer duration of hyponatremia increase the risk for central pontine myelinolysis. Symptoms of quadripareis and bulbar palsy are seen. Once central pontine myelinolysis occurs as a complication, there is no proven treatment.

Disposition

Responsible patients with mild SIADH without any neurologic symptoms may be managed on an outpatient basis with fluid restriction and close follow-up. Patients with more severe symptoms of SIADH and those who may not follow treatment recommendations should be hospitalized. Patients receiving hypertonic saline should be admitted to the intensive care unit.

Lien YH, Shapiro JI: Hyponatremia: clinical diagnosis and management. Am J Med 2007 Aug;120(8):653–658. Review.

Decaux G: Is asymptomatic hyponatremia really asymptomatic? Am J Med 2006 Jul;119(7 Suppl 1):S79–S82. Review.

Gross P: Treatment of hyponatremia. Intern Med 2008; 47(10):885-91, Epub May 15, 2008. Review.

DIABETES INSIPIDUS

ESSENTIALS OF DIAGNOSIS

▶ Symptoms and signs include lethargy, altered mental status, irritability, hyperreflexia, and spasticity

▶ Urine osmolality of <150 mOsm/kg in the setting of serum hypertonicity and polyuria is generally diagnostic of diabetes insipidus

General Considerations

Patients with diabetes insipidus have an abnormal excretion of large amounts of hypotonic urine. Urine volumes often reach over 3–4 L a day. Most patients will have an intact thirst mechanism and thus may present with only polydipsia and polyuria. Fluid intake >3.5 L/d occurs in an attempt to maintain adequate hydration. If water intake does not keep up with urinary losses, extracellular volume depletion and hypernatremia soon develop.

Causes

Diabetes insipidus occurs in two basic forms. Central diabetes insipidus results from inadequate secretion of AVP (arginine vasopressin or antidiuretic hormone) and nephrogenic diabetes insipidus results from decreased responsiveness of the kidneys to vasopressin.

Central diabetes insipidus may be caused by trauma, neurosurgery, neoplasm, granulomatous infiltration, or autoimmune destruction of cells. Nephrogenic diabetes insipidus is often congenital; however, acquired forms are seen especially in the elderly. Severe forms are more likely to result from renal disease, drug-induced damage to the kidneys (most commonly lithium or demeclocycline), or electrolyte disturbances such as hypokalemia or hypercalcemia.

Clinical Findings

A. Symptoms and Signs

1. ADH deficiency/resistance—Profound polydipsia and polyuria may be present. Polyuria may lead to associated nocturia, incontinence, or enuresis. Urine osmolality is typically less than 300 mOsm/kg.

2. Hypernatremia and hyperosmolality—Hypernatremia and hyperosmolality may be absent in an awake patient with unrestricted availability of hypotonic fluids. If this supply is restricted for any reason, however, hypernatremia and intracellular dehydration will occur. The organ most susceptible to these effects is the brain, resulting in lethargy, altered mental status, irritability, hyperreflexia, and spasticity. Acute changes result in a more symptomatic presentation. Gradual changes can result in adaptation and few symptoms.

Intracranial hemorrhage may occur as the brain shrinks and mechanical tension is placed on dural veins and venous sinuses. Patients with marked volume deficits typically have hypotension, tachypnea, tachycardia, and decreased level of consciousness. Visual field defects and anterior pituitary insufficiency may be present when diabetes insipidus is caused by intracranial neoplasm.

B. Laboratory Findings

A urine osmolality of less than 150 mOsm/kg or specific gravity less than 1.005 in the setting of hypertonicity and polyuria is diagnostic of diabetes insipidus. A trial of 1 µg DDAVP (1-deamino-8-D-arginine vasopressin; exogenous vasopressin) subcutaneously or IV will distinguish central from nephrogenic diabetes insipidus. Urine osmolality will increase and volume will decrease with DDAVP administration in central but not nephrogenic diabetes insipidus.

Hypernatremia and hyperosmolality are found in uncompensated patients. Serum sodium may be greater than 160 mEq/L in severe cases, and prerenal azotemia is common in these patients. Specific gravity and osmolality of urine are low in proportion to serum osmolality. Glycosuria is another cause of polyuria.

If the diagnosis is unclear, a water deprivation test can be performed under controlled conditions by a consultant.

C. Imaging

CT scanning may help exclude some CNS lesions; however in select cases, urgent MRI of the brain is indicated to search for a mass, or hemorrhage, in the region of the hypothalamus or pituitary gland.

▶ Treatment

A. General and Supportive Measures

Provide supplemental oxygen as needed. Draw blood samples for measurement of electrolytes, osmolality, glucose, calcium, and serum cortisol levels and for renal and thyroid function tests. Measure plasma ADH; if very low, this may be diagnostic.

Obtain urine specimens for routine urinalysis and specific gravity and osmolality measurements. Monitor volume status, body weight, fluid intake, and urine output and specific gravity.

B. Volume and Electrolyte Deficits

Water administration whether orally, by nasogastric tube, or intravenously is the treatment for hypernatremia. Whenever possible, the oral or nasogastric route is preferred because water absorption and the decline in serum sodium concentrations are more gradual.

Awake patients will often maintain equilibrium when given free access to water. In patients with altered mental status, the onset of hypernatremia can be catastrophic. The free water deficit should be corrected and fluid balance maintained. The free water deficit can be calculated by the following equation:

$$\text{Free water deficit} = 0.6 \times \text{Premorbid body weight (in kg)} \\ \times [1 - (140/\text{plasma sodium in mmol/L})]$$

Hypotonic saline (0.45% normal saline) or 5% dextrose in water may be given. The latter is given to patients who show severe signs of neurologic compromise from hypernatremia. Avoid iatrogenic hyperglycemia when using dextrose-containing solutions; it may cause an osmotic diuresis and worsen the hypernatremia.

Replace half the free water deficit within the first 12–24 hours. When serum sodium decreases to less than 150 mEq/L, 0.45% or 0.9% saline should be used. Decreasing the serum sodium greater than 1–2 mEq/L/h can cause fluid shifts back into the intracellular compartment causing cerebral edema. Neurologic deterioration after hydration therapy should raise serious concern and prompt action. Idiogenic osmoles found in chronic hypernatremia are thought to cause decompensation; therefore, levels should be corrected over 48 hours.

C. Specific Therapy

Desmopressin acetate or DDAVP is a synthetic vasopressin analogue. A dose of 1–2 μg every 12–24 hours subcutaneously or intravenously or 5–20 μg every 12 hours intranasally is the drug of choice when treating central diabetes insipidus. It is preferred over other vasopressin preparations because it has a longer half-life and has almost no pressor effect.

Nephrogenic diabetes insipidus is more difficult to treat. Thiazide diuretics and sodium restriction are the mainstays of treatment.

▶ Disposition

Patients with diabetes insipidus should be hospitalized for definitive diagnosis and initiation of treatment. Patients who are severely hypernatremic or who present in hypovolemic shock merit intensive care unit admission for at least the first 24 hours of treatment.

Mavrakis AN, Tritos NA: Diabetes insipidus with deficient thirst: report of a patient and review of the literature. Am J Kidney Dis 2008 May;51(5):851–859, Epub Mar 3, 2008. Review.

Loh JA, Verbalis JG: Disorders of water and salt metabolism associated with pituitary disease. Endocrinol Metab Clin North Am 2008 Mar;37(1):213–234, x. Review

Schrier RW: The sea within us: disorders of body water homeostasis. Curr Opin Investig Drugs 2007 Apr;8(4):304–311. Review.

Jane JA Jr, Vance ML, Laws ER: Neurogenic diabetes insipidus. Pituitary 2006;9(4):327–329. Review.

Fluid, Electrolyte, & Acid–Base Emergencies

James E. Morris, MD, MPH

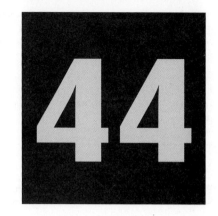

▼ DIAGNOSIS OF FLUID AND ELECTROLYTE DISORDERS

The diagnosis of fluid and electrolyte disorders is complicated by the often-nonspecific symptoms and physical examination findings, which patients suffering from these disorders manifest. A thorough understanding of the homeostatic mechanisms that control fluid and electrolyte balance is essential to the accurate assessment and treatment of the wide variety of pathologies the emergency physician may encounter.

Approximately 60% of an adult male's body weight is composed of water (less in women and the elderly), of which ⅔ is intracellular and ⅓ is extracellular. Of the extracellular volume, ¾ is in the interstitial compartment and ¼ within the vasculature. Osmolality is maintained within a narrow range (285–295 mOsm) and is the same across all fluid compartments; it may be estimated using serum sodium, glucose, and blood urea nitrogen (BUN) values (see Appendix).

Shifts in volume, osmolality, and electrolyte concentrations can occur independently of each other and typically manifest in profoundly different ways. The severity of symptoms is usually contingent on how rapidly the shifts occur. Changes in volume are most readily apparent on the cardiovascular physical examination. Signs and symptoms attributable to changes in osmolality are primarily neurological, resulting from brain dehydration (in hyperosmolar states) or brain edema (in hypoosmolar states). Electrolyte changes are more variable and exert their effect primarily on cell membrane potential with resultant cardiac, neurologic, and musculoskeletal dysfunction. See Table 44–1 for a list of serum electrolytes and normal values.

Table 44–1. Normal Serum Electrolyte Concentrations.

Sodium (Na⁺)	136-146 mEq/L
Potassium (K⁺)	3.5-5 mEq/L
Chloride (Cl⁻)	96-106 mEq/L
Bicarbonate (HCO₃⁻)	24-28 mEq/L
Calcium (Ca²⁺)	8.5-105 mg/dL (4.2-5.2 mEq/L)
Magnesium (Mg²⁺)	1.8-3 mg/dL (1.5-2.5 mEq/L)
Phosphate (PO₄³⁻)	3-4.5 mg/dL (1-1.5 mmol/L)

▼ MANAGEMENT OF SPECIFIC DISORDERS

DISORDERS OF SERUM SODIUM CONCENTRATION

HYPONATREMIA

ESSENTIALS OF DIAGNOSIS

▶ Hyponatremia reflects a relative inability to excrete free water

▶ Symptoms relate to the rate of change

▶ Measure urine osmolality and sodium

▶ Review medications and assess thyroid and adrenal function

▶ Initial treatment is guided by the severity of symptoms and the patient's volume status

▶ General Considerations

Hyponatremia is defined as a serum sodium below 136 mEq/L and is associated with a number of different drugs and disease processes. Hyponatremia may be hyper-, hypo-, or isotonic. Isotonic hyponatremia is the result of laboratory artifact due to a decreased water component of plasma such as may be seen in hyperlipidemia and hyperproteinemia. Newer ion-specific methods of laboratory analysis have essentially eliminated this as a cause of hyponatremia. Hypertonic hyponatremia results from the presence of solutes that do not freely cross cell membranes, such as mannitol and glucose (in the absence of insulin), and represents a hyperosmolar state. With prolonged hyperglycemia, moderation of the hyponatremia or even hypernatremia may result as an osmotic diuresis develops.

Most hyponatremia is hypotonic, representing an excess of total body water relative to total body sodium (which may be low, normal, or even high). In the absence of renal failure, increased levels of arginine vasopressin (AVP), from drugs, paraneoplastic syndromes, or other endocrine abnormalities,

or rarely excess free water intake prevent the kidneys from excreting sufficient free water. Hypotonic hyponatremia can be associated with normal, increased, or decreased volume, and knowledge of the patient's urine sodium concentration and osmolality is invaluable in determining the underlying etiology (Figure 44–1).

▶ Clinical Findings

Symptoms are rare with sodium above 125 mEq/L and when present reflect worsening cerebral edema, ranging from headache, nausea, vomiting, and mental status changes, culminating in seizures, coma, brain-stem herniation, and death. More severe symptoms are associated with a more rapid decrease in serum sodium. The clinician should correlate the measured serum sodium with the patient's presentation to eliminate spurious hyponatremia, such as that produced by a sample contaminated with a hypotonic infusion. In hyperglycemic states, every 100 mg/dL of glucose decreases the measured serum sodium value by 1.5–1.7 mEq/L, and the clinician should calculate the actual serum sodium accordingly.

▶ Treatment

The urgency of treatment is dictated by the severity of symptoms and how abruptly the hyponatremia is thought to have developed. Correction of hyponatremia is controversial, but in acutely symptomatic patients even a 5% increase may be physiologically significant. In the presence of severe hyponatremia (sodium < 120 mEq/L and symptoms to include mental status changes, seizure, or coma), an infusion of 3% hypertonic saline solution (513 mEq/L) should be considered (see Appendix for formulas). The rate of rise of 1 mEq/L/h should be targeted for the first 3–4 hours or until symptoms resolve; otherwise, the rate of correction should not exceed 0.5 mEq/L/h. Simultaneous use of furosemide to limit expansion of the extracellular-fluid volume may be required. A new class of AVP receptor antagonists (the "vaptans") has been approved for the treatment of euvolemic and hypovolemic hyponatremia, but experience with these agents in the ED is lacking. Resolution of symptoms, particularly in the elderly, may lag behind correction of the serum sodium, and frequent monitoring is important to avoid overcorrection.

Consideration should be given to thyroid and adrenal insufficiency, and replacement hormones given after appropriate laboratory samples have been obtained if indicated, and potassium replacement instituted if needed. Patients who do not require urgent treatment may be treated with fluid restriction and observation. Profoundly hypovolemic patients may be treated initially with fluid resuscitation using isotonic saline to prevent cardiovascular compromise. Emergency dialysis should be considered for patients with renal failure, volume overload, and severe hyponatremia.

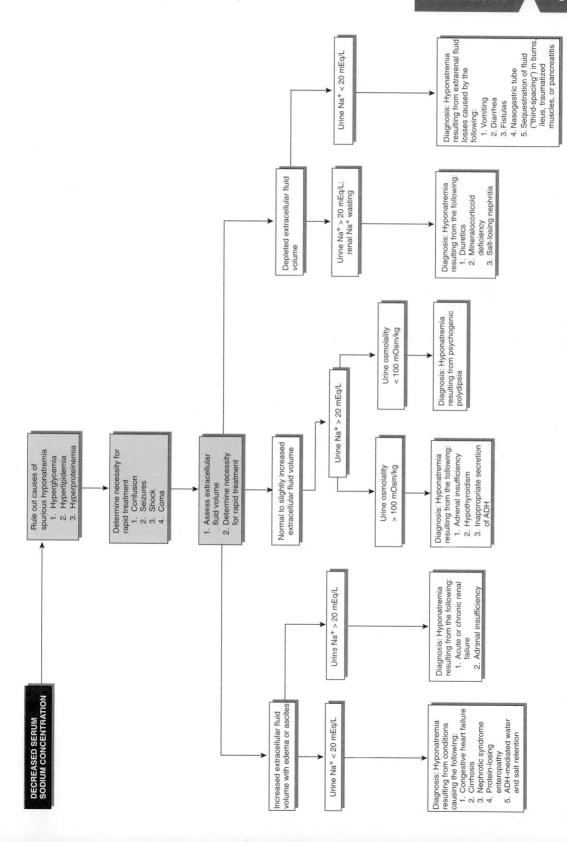

▲ **Figure 44–1.** Evaluation of hyponatremia.

Osmotic demyelination, the most feared consequence of too rapid correction, is rare at a rate of correction below 10–12 mEq/L/d. Alcoholics, hypokalemic patients, burn victims, and women taking thiazide diuretics are more at risk for this consequence. Symptoms of osmotic demyelination include dysarthria, dysphagia, spastic paresis, coma, and occasionally seizures. These symptoms may be delayed for 2–6 days after correction of the serum sodium and imaging by CT may be negative up to 4 weeks. Rapid reinduction of hyponatremia may be beneficial when this disorder is suspected.

Disposition

All patients with clinically significant hyponatremia should be hospitalized. ICU placement should be considered for those with severe mental status changes or seizures.

HYPERNATREMIA

ESSENTIALS OF DIAGNOSIS

▶ Hypernatremia may result from the loss of pure water or hypotonic fluid, or rarely from salt gain

▶ Symptoms are primarily neurologic and those related to severe hypovolemia

▶ Measure urine osmolality and sodium concentration

▶ Use isotonic saline to treat volume deficits on an emergency basis, followed by hypotonic solutions to gradually replace free water deficits

General Considerations

Hypernatremia is defined as a serum sodium above 146 mEq/L, and unlike hyponatremia, it always represents a hyperosmolar state with cellular dehydration. It represents a relative excess of sodium to free water and may result from net water loss, either pure water or hypotonic fluid loss or sodium loading, usually accidental or iatrogenic (Table 44–2). Hypernatremia in outpatients is more common at the extremes of age or in debilitated patients. Although present in only 1% of hospitalized patients, it has a mortality approaching 60%. As with hyponatremia, the severity of symptoms is related to the rate at which they develop.

Clinical Findings

Symptoms from hypernatremia reflect CNS dysfunction and are more prominent with large or rapid changes in serum sodium. Infants with hypernatremia may have muscle weakness, restlessness, a high-pitched cry, lethargy, and coma.

Table 44–2. Causes of Hypernatremia.

Net water loss
  Pure water
    Hypodipsia
    Unreplaced insensible losses
    Neurogenic diabetes insipidus
    Nephrogenic diabetes insipidus (congenital or acquired)
  Hypotonic fluid
    Renal losses
      Loop diuretics
      Osmotic diuresis
      Postobstructive diuresis
      Intrinsic renal disease
  Nonrenal losses
      Vomiting
      NG suctioning
      Diarrhea
      Enterocutaneous fistula
      Burns
      Excessive sweating
Hypertonic sodium gain
    Hypertonic sodium bicarbonate infusion
    Hypertonic feeding preparations
    Ingestion of sodium chloride (emetics, enemas)
    Hypertonic sodium chloride infusion
    Hypertonic dialysis
    Primary hyperaldosteronism
    Cushing syndrome

Elderly patients typically have few or no symptoms until the sodium is over 160 mEq/L. Loss of thirst and progressive decrease in level of consciousness are associated with worsening hypernatremia, but seizures are rare in the absence of aggressive rehydration. When sodium changes occur rapidly, traction on the cerebral vasculature from brain shrinkage may result in tearing with subarachnoid, intraparenchymal, and subdural bleeding. Patients may be clinically hyper-, hypo-, or euvolemic. Skin turgor may be normal despite intravascular volume depletion.

Evaluation of urine osmolality and sodium concentration is necessary to determine the underlying cause, particularly in hypovolemic patients. Hypovolemia with a urine sodium concentration less than 20 mEq/L is consistent with extrarenal losses. Urine osmolality over 400 mOsm/L represents intact renal free water conservation, while dilute urine (less than 250 mOsm/L) is associated with diabetes insipidus (see Chapter 41).

Treatment

In cases of circulatory compromise, volume deficits should be treated initially with isotonic saline. Otherwise, only hypotonic solutions should be used. In hypernatremia that has developed over a period of hours, rapid correction

(~1 mEq/L/h) does not increase the risk of convulsions or brain damage. When the rate of development is unknown, a rate of correction no greater than 0.5 mEq/L/h, or approximately 10 mEq per day, is recommended to avoid cerebral edema (see Appendix).

▶ Disposition

Hospitalization is recommended for all symptomatic patients and patients with a sodium greater than 150 mEq/L. Patients with mild hypernatremia, an intact thirst mechanism, and close follow-up may be discharged home.

DISORDERS OF SERUM POTASSIUM CONCENTRATION

Over 98% of the body's potassium is intracellular, making it the predominant intracellular electrolyte. Because of this, it is often difficult to make extrapolations regarding total potassium stores from serum potassium concentrations. Potassium is sensitive to changes in serum pH caused by the accumulation of mineral acids. Intracellular acidosis promotes the extrusion of potassium with resultant hyperkalemia. In addition to aldosterone, circulating hormones such as insulin and catecholamines also affect the movement of potassium between the serum and intracellular compartments. Symptoms related to changes in serum potassium are related to changes in cell membrane potential, affecting primarily the heart and muscles.

HYPOKALEMIA

ESSENTIALS OF DIAGNOSIS

- ▶ Usually associated with diuretic therapy
- ▶ Symptoms are primarily neuromuscular and cardiac
- ▶ Assess acid–base status
- ▶ Replace potassium orally whenever possible; IV potassium may be given with caution in severe cases with appropriate monitoring

▶ General Considerations

Hypokalemia, defined as a serum potassium below 3.5 mEq/L, is the most common electrolyte disturbance and may represent decreased total body stores of potassium or a shift of potassium into cells. A decrease in total body potassium is most often secondary to diuretic therapy but may also be from increased GI or renal losses, or, in the setting of alcoholism or malnutrition, decreased intake (see Table 44–3). Concurrent digitalis therapy exacerbates the cardiac effects

Table 44–3. Causes of Hypokalemia.

Poor intake
Increased loss
Increased sweating
Gastrointestinal
Vomiting
NG suctioning
Diarrhea (laxatives, VIPoma, villous adenoma, malabsorption)
Jejunoileal bypass
Enteric fistulas
Renal
Diuresis
Liddle syndrome
Bartter syndrome
Gitelman syndrome
Fanconi syndrome
Type I distal renal tubular acidosis
Type II proximal rental tubular acidosis
Diabetic ketoacidosis
Medications (aminoglycosides, amphotericin, cisplatin, etc.)
Cushing syndrome
Primary hyperaldosteronism
Magnesium depletion
Transcellular shifts
Metabolic alkalosis
Respiratory alkalosis
Familial periodic paralysis
Thyrotoxicosis
Hypothermia
Drug induced (insulin, β_2-agonists)

of hypokalemia. Potassium deficiency commonly coexists with other electrolyte abnormalities, particularly magnesium, and may remain refractory to therapy until the other abnormalities are corrected.

▶ Clinical Findings

Symptoms of hypokalemia range from mild weakness, ileus, and rhabdomyolysis to paralysis and lethal arrhythmias (see Table 44–4). The severity of symptoms is often related to how quickly the decrease in serum potassium develops.

Table 44–4. Signs and Symptoms of Hypokalemia.

Generalized weakness
Paralytic ileus
Cardiac arrhythmias
Atrial tachycardia
AV dissociation
Ventricular tachycardia
Ventricular fibrillation
Rhabdomyolysis

Table 44–5. EKG Changes Associated with Hypokalemia.

Decreased T-wave amplitude
T-wave inversion
ST-segment depression
Prominent U wave
Prolongation of QT interval
Ventricular tachycardia
Torsades de pointes

Obtaining a venous pH may be helpful in determining initial treatment. EKG changes are present in over 80% of people with a potassium below 2.7 and may progress rapidly from decreased T wave amplitude to torsades de pointes (see Table 44–5).

▶ **Treatment**

On average, a decrease of 0.3 mEq/L in serum potassium is associated with a 100 mEq deficit in total body stores. Oral replacement using potassium chloride (20–40 mEq every 4 hours) is the preferred method for patients with mild symptoms who are able to tolerate oral intake. Higher doses should be avoided because of the risk of esophageal and gastric irritation or perforation in the presence of strictures. Potassium phosphate preparations may be used for patients with known phosphate deficiency, and potassium bicarbonate may be helpful in patients with severe metabolic acidosis.

For more severe symptoms and in patients with a serum potassium below 2.5, IV replacement is indicated. The concentration of potassium in IV solutions should not exceed 60 mEq/L (20 mEq/L if infusing through a peripheral line). More concentrated solutions are associated with greater pain at the infusion site and sclerosis of the veins. An IV infusion of 20 mEq/h is expected to produce an increase in the serum potassium of 0.25 mEq/h. In rare instances such as acute myocardial infarction with significant ventricular ectopy or in patients with paralysis of the respiratory muscles, rates of infusion as high as 40–100 mEq/h or more concentrated solutions may be indicated. Potassium should not be given in dextrose-containing solutions, as this may stimulate insulin release and result in worsening hypokalemia. All patients receiving IV potassium should have continuous cardiac monitoring, and it should never be given as a "push" because of the risk of precipitating life-threatening hyperkalemia.

▶ **Disposition**

All patients with a serum potassium below 2.5 mEq/L should be hospitalized in a monitored setting. Patients with less severe hypokalemia may be discharged with oral replacement therapy and close follow-up.

HYPERKALEMIA

 ESSENTIALS OF DIAGNOSIS

▶ Hyperkalemia is a true emergency

▶ Suspect hyperkalemia in patients with renal failure, diabetes, or those taking potassium supplements

▶ Symptoms are primarily neuromuscular and cardiac

▶ EKG findings may progress rapidly from peaked T waves to ventricular fibrillation

▶ Beware of spurious hyperkalemia

▶ Treatment stabilizes cardiac membranes, shifts potassium into cells, and removes potassium from the body

▶ **General Considerations**

Hyperkalemia, defined as a serum potassium greater than 5.0 mEq/L, is more rare but more immediately life threatening than hypokalemia. It may rarely result from increased potassium intake but more commonly results from decreased renal excretion or transmembrane shift of intracellular potassium (see Table 44–6). Drugs that interfere with the renin-angiotensin-aldosterone system, such as ACE inhibitors or spironolactone, may result in hyperkalemia, as may drugs such as trimethoprim and triamterene that block secretion of potassium in the distal collecting duct. Digitalis

Table 44–6. Causes of Hyperkalemia.

Increased potassium input (potassium supplements, penicillin G potassium, PRBCs)
Reduced secretion
Renal failure
Medications
Type IV renal tubular acidosis
Hyperkalemic type I distal renal tubular acidosis
Addison disease
Increased release
Hemolysis
Rhabdomyolysis
Tumor lysis syndrome
Transcellular shifts
Acidosis
Exercise
Insulin deficiency
Medications
β-Blockers
Digitalis
Succinylcholine

toxicity may result in hyperkalemia through inhibition of the distal-collecting duct Na^+/K^+ ATP-ase.

Pseudohyperkalemia is frequently encountered and should be suspected when patients with normal renal function and no other evident precipitating cause for true hyperkalemia present with marked elevation in measured serum potassium. Hemolysis, thrombocytosis, marked leukocytosis, prolonged tourniquet time, and long delays between obtaining the lab specimen and analysis may result in release of intracellular potassium within the specimen; analysis of plasma potassium through a specimen collected in a heparinized tube may help differentiate true versus pseudohyperkalemia, with a difference of greater than 0.3 mEq/L suggestive of pseudohyperkalemia.

▶ Clinical Findings

Symptoms attributable to hyperkalemia are nonspecific and include muscular weakness, fatigue, paresthesias, palpitations, and cardiac arrhythmias. EKG changes may progress rapidly from peaked T waves to QRS widening and ventricular

Table 44–7. EKG Changes Associated with Hyperkalemia.

Large-amplitude T waves
"Peaked" T waves
PR interval prolongation
Decreased P-wave amplitude
QRS widening
AV nodal block with escape beats
Sine-wave pattern
Ventricular fibrillation
Asystole

fibrillation (see Table 44–7 and Figure 44–2); however, the presence of EKG changes poorly sensitive for a serum potassium over 6.0 mEq/L and may be absent in up to 80% of patients with significant hyperkalemia. Hyperkalemia is commonly associated with metabolic acidosis, and a venous blood gas may be helpful in guiding treatment. Evaluation of renal function and serum electrolytes is helpful in identifying contributing causes.

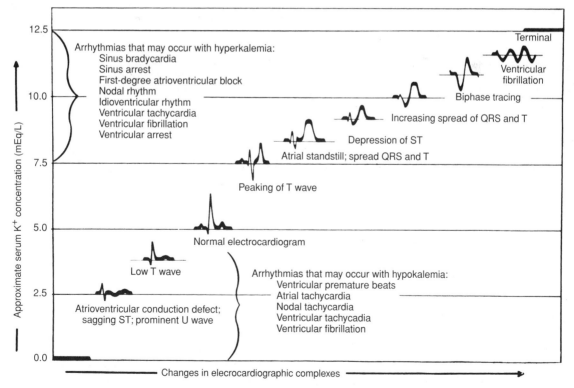

▲ **Figure 44–2.** Correlation between serum potassium concentration and EKG findings. The correlation is approximate and depends on serum pH and concentrations of other ions (particularly calcium and magnesium). (Reproduced, with permission, from Schroeder SA [ed.]: Current Medical Diagnosis & Treatment 1992. Appleton & Lange, Norwalk, CT, 1992.)

▶ Treatment

Emergency treatment of hyperkalemia is warranted for true hyperkalemia exceeding 6.0 mEq/L or in the presence of any EKG changes consistent with hyperkalemia. The goals of therapy are aimed at stabilizing membrane potential, moving potassium intracellularly, and eliminating potassium from the body. Caution should be exercised in patients with conditions such as diabetic ketoacidosis (DKA), in which total body potassium may actually be low and concurrent correction of the acid–base disorder with overly aggressive therapy for hyperkalemia may result in hypokalemia.

A. Membrane Stabilization

Patients with EKG changes or potassium over 7.0 should receive IV calcium, which directly antagonizes the effect of potassium on cardiac membrane potential. Both calcium gluconate and calcium chloride are available as 10% solutions, although calcium chloride contains three times as much available calcium and is more irritating if it extravasates and may worsen acidosis. For these reasons, calcium gluconate is preferred; 10 mL may be given IV over 2–5 minutes and repeated in 10 minutes if there is no effect on the EKG. Effects may be seen within 1–3 minutes and last 30–60 minutes. In patients with hyperkalemia associated with digoxin toxicity, calcium administration should be avoided since calcium potentiates the myocardial toxicity of digoxin. Hypertonic saline may be used in hyperkalemic patients with significant hyponatremia as well.

B. Intracellular Shift

Ten units of regular insulin may be given IV along with 50 mL of D50 (to avoid precipitating hypoglycemia, if necessary) to promote cellular uptake of potassium, with onset within 20 minutes and peak effect between 30 and 60 minutes. Ten to twenty milligrams of nebulized albuterol (or 0.5 mg IV) may also be used, with a slightly delayed onset and peak effect compared to insulin. Infusion of sodium bicarbonate alone has a variable effect and should not be used as monotherapy (particularly in dialysis patients), but it has been shown to potentiate the potassium-lowering effects of insulin and β-agonist therapy.

C. Potassium Elimination

Direct elimination of potassium from the body by methods other than dialysis is the slowest method of reducing serum potassium and should not be used alone in the presence of significant hyperkalemia. Sodium polystyrene sulfonate may be given orally or as an enema in a dose of 25–50 g. The use of sorbitol as a laxative has been associated with intestinal necrosis and perforation, particularly in postoperative patients, and other laxatives may be preferable. Patients with intact renal function may benefit from therapy with potassium-losing diuretics. Dialysis should be considered in patients with renal failure or unstable patients, following institution of the above measures.

▶ Disposition

All patients with hyperkalemia requiring treatment should be admitted to a monitored setting.

DISORDERS OF SERUM CALCIUM CONCENTRATION

Calcium is required for a large number of physiologic processes ranging from nerve conduction to blood coagulation. Calcium is commonly reported in mg/dL, which may be converted to mmol by dividing by 4 or to mEq by dividing by 2. Ninety-eight percent of calcium is bound to bone, and the regulation of extracellular calcium concentrations within the narrow range of 8.5–10.5 mg/dL is complex. Calcitonin, parathyroid hormone (PTH), vitamin D, phosphate, and calcium itself interact through a number of interlocking feedback loops to exert effects on the renal tubules, intestine, and bones.

Serum calcium is approximately 40% protein bound and 10% complexed with organic anions, leaving only 50% ionized. This is the physiologically active portion of serum calcium, which is highly sensitive to changes in pH. Rapid changes in pH may result in symptomatic hypo- or hypercalcemia even with normal serum calcium. As the serum pH increases, more calcium is bound, leaving a lower fraction available for use. Conversely, acidemia increases the amount of calcium available, with a change of 0.1 in pH roughly corresponding to a change in ionized calcium of 0.05 mmol/dL. Also, 1 mg/dL of albumin binds 0.8 mg/dL (0.2 mmol/dL) of calcium, which may be used to estimate expected changes in serum calcium in the setting of hypoalbuminemia; however, there is wide variability, and direct measurement of ionized calcium is preferable to calculation whenever hypo- or hypercalcemia is suspected.

HYPOCALCEMIA

ESSENTIALS OF DIAGNOSIS

- ▶ Occurs often in critically ill patients, although rarely life-threatening in itself
- ▶ Usually asymptomatic until severe
- ▶ Neuromuscular and respiratory symptoms predominate
- ▶ Often associated with disorders of magnesium and phosphate
- ▶ Always check serum phosphate before replacing calcium IV
- ▶ Use caution in giving IV calcium to patients taking digoxin

General Considerations

Hypocalcemia is defined as an ionized calcium less than 1.1 mmol/L, although symptoms are uncommon until the ionized calcium falls below 0.7 mmol/L. Patients with low serum calcium may have a normal ionized calcium. Hypocalcemia may develop gradually from decreased intake or absorption and is commonly associated with decreased PTH and vitamin D levels. It may also be seen with "hungry bone" syndrome, which results after parathyroidectomy for hyperparathyroidism. Hyperphosphatemia and hypomagnesemia commonly coexist with hypocalcemia. More acute changes in calcium may result from shifts in serum pH and the increased concentration of organic anions, such as citrate in the case of massive transfusion or fatty acids in acute pancreatitis. Up to 50% of critically ill patients, particularly those in sepsis, will have hypocalcemia.

Clinical Findings

Symptoms of acute hypocalcemia are primarily neuromuscular, including circumoral numbness, paresthesias, and carpopedal spasm, progressing to tetany, laryngospasm, and seizures (see Table 44–8). Skeletal muscle fasciculations, Chvostek's and Trousseau's signs, and hyperreflexia may be evident on physical examination. Hypocalcemia that develops more slowly may manifest primarily with weakness, irritability, and neuropsychiatric symptoms. Prolongation of the QTc interval without changes in morphology or other intervals is the most common EKG finding in hypocalcemia. Torsades de pointes with hypocalcemia is less common than with hypokalemia or hypomagnesemia.

Evaluation of the patient with hypocalcemia should include measurement of other serum electrolytes (particularly magnesium, phosphate, and potassium), renal function, serum albumin, and a venous or arterial blood gas to evaluate the patient's acid–base status.

Table 44–8. Signs and Symptoms of Hypocalcemia.

Muscle weakness
Myalgias
Cramps
Paresthesias in the hands and feet
Circumoral numbness
Dysphagia
Biliary and intestinal colic
Carpopedal spasms
Trousseau's and Chvostek's signs
Hyperreflexia
Laryngospasm
Bronchospasm
Seizures

Treatment

Asymptomatic hypocalcemia rarely progresses to a life-threatening condition. Even mild symptoms due to hypocalcemia warrant further evaluation and treatment, however, because of the potential for significant compromise should the hypocalcemia worsen. Initial treatment is with IV calcium gluconate, which should be given slowly to avoid serious cardiac dysfunction (20 mL over 10–20 minutes, followed by infusion of 0.5–1.5 mg/kg/h of elemental calcium in dextrose or saline over 4–6 hours). Slower rates should be used in patients on digoxin. In the setting of hypomagnesemia, symptoms may remain refractory until the serum magnesium is also corrected. Hypocalcemia with markedly elevated phosphate (over 6 mg/dL) should not be treated with supplemental calcium to avoid the risk of metastatic calcification; initial treatment should focus on eliminating phosphate (see the Hyperphosphatemia section later in this chapter). Patients with mild or asymptomatic hypocalcemia may be treated with oral supplementation.

Disposition

Patients with acute or symptomatic hypocalcemia should be admitted to a monitored setting. Patients with chronic, asymptomatic hypocalcemia may be discharged with oral calcium supplements and followed up on an outpatient basis.

HYPERCALCEMIA

ESSENTIALS OF DIAGNOSIS

► Usually caused by malignancy or hyperparathyroidism
► Symptoms are primarily neuromuscular and renal
► Volume replacement/expansion is primary therapy
► Treatment promotes calcium excretion, inhibits osteoclast activity, and decreases calcium absorption

General Considerations

Hypercalcemia is defined as a serum calcium over 11 mg/dL. As with most electrolyte disorders, the rate at which the hypercalcemia develops is an important determinant of the severity of symptoms. Although a number of different conditions may result in hypercalcemia, most symptomatic cases result from hyperparathyroidism or malignancy (see Table 44–9). Milk-alkali syndrome due to the use of calcium carbonate supplements for osteoporosis, dyspepsia, or hyperphosphatemia associated with chronic renal failure is an emerging cause of hypercalcemia. Rarely, hyperalbuminemia (such as from dehydration) or paraproteinemia may

Table 44-9. Causes of Hypercalcemia.

Hyperparathyroidism
Increased PTH-related protein in NSCLC, RCC, prostate ca., multiple
   myeloma
Milk-alkali syndrome
Thiazide diuretics
Granulomatous diseases (sarcoidosis, TB, leprosy, coccidiomycosis, etc.)
Vitamin D intoxication
Increased bone resorption
   Immobilization
   Paget disease
   Hyperthyroidism
   Theophylline toxicity
   Skeletal metastases

elevate the measured serum calcium value, and measurement of the ionized calcium will be beneficial. Similarly, hypoalbuminemia may partially mask an elevated ionized calcium and result in symptomatic hypercalcemia even at "normal" serum calcium values.

▶ Clinical Findings

Most symptoms of hypercalcemia are mild and nonspecific, including fatigue, abdominal pain, anorexia, weakness, depression, vomiting, and constipation. Severe hypercalcemia may cause acute pancreatitis, and peptic ulcer disease secondary to prolonged hypercalcemia is also common. With ionized calcium concentrations above 3.0 mmol/L, cognitive dysfunction becomes more prominent, and above 4.0 mmol/L psychosis, stupor, and coma are expected. Although a shortened QTc interval may be seen on EKG, hemodynamically significant arrhythmias are rare.

▶ Treatment

Treatment should be initiated for all patients with clinically significant symptoms. Moderate to severe hypercalcemia (ionized calcium greater than 3 mmol/L) warrants emergency treatment, even if asymptomatic. Specific therapy may be instituted if a precipitating cause is identified; however, general measures aimed at reducing serum calcium levels should be initiated at the same time. Modes of therapy for hypercalcemia consist of promoting calcium excretion, stabilizing or increasing deposition of calcium in the bones, and decreasing dietary uptake. Patients with renal insufficiency or those in whom the previous measures are ineffective may benefit from dialysis.

A. Promoting Calcium Excretion

Most patients with severe hypercalcemia are profoundly volume depleted from hypercalcemia-induced nephrogenic diabetes insipidus, and initial therapy should focus on replacing volume deficits with isotonic saline until the patient is clinically euvolemic. This will help induce calciuresis by increasing the glomerular filtration rate. After extracellular volume status is normalized, a loop diuretic may be used to promote further urinary excretion of calcium. Thiazide diuretics promote calcium resorption and should be avoided.

B. Bone Calcium Stabilization

Bisphosphonates such as pamidronate or zoledronate inhibit osteoclast activity and indirectly stimulate osteoblasts, promoting the deposition of calcium. Their maximum effect is delayed 2–4 days but lasts up to 4 weeks, and both are well tolerated when given as IV infusion. Pamidronate may be given as 60–90 mg in 500 mL isotonic saline over 1–2 hours. Zoledronate (4 mg) may be given IV over 15 minutes and is more effective than pamidronate at reducing serum calcium. Calcitonin (4 IU/kg given SQ or IM every 12 hours) may be used in conjunction with bisphosphonates and has an additive effect, although tachyphylaxis often develops within 2–3 days and it is only effective in 60–70% of patients. It works more rapidly than the bisphosphonates and should be reserved for more severe cases of hypercalcemia. Because of the potential for severe toxicity and the development of second-generation bisphosphonates, the use of mithramycin is not recommended.

C. Decreasing Absorption

Corticosteroids (hydrocortisone 200–300 mg/d IV or prednisone 20–40 mg/d PO) are effective at reducing vitamin D-mediated absorption of calcium from the GI tract and are particularly valuable in hypercalcemia associated with lymphoma and granulomatous diseases. Onset of action is within 3–5 days.

▶ Disposition

Patients with significant symptoms should be hospitalized and consideration given to hospitalization for all patients with an ionized calcium above 3.0 mmol/L regardless of symptoms. Less severe cases may be discharged with close follow-up.

DISORDERS OF SERUM PHOSPHORUS CONCENTRATION

Phosphate is present primarily in bone and skeletal muscle, with less than 1% of total body phosphate present in plasma. In addition to being essential to bone mineralization, it is also important in a large number of cellular functions, particularly energy metabolism. Approximately 15% of serum phosphate is protein bound, and serum levels may not reflect total body stores because of intracellular shift.

HYPOPHOSPHATEMIA

ESSENTIALS OF DIAGNOSIS

▶ Hypophosphatemia is often asymptomatic unless severe and commonly occurs along with disorders of calcium, magnesium, and potassium

▶ Assess acid–base status

▶ Oral replacement is preferred and should be initiated even in asymptomatic patients

▶ IV replacement may be used cautiously in severely symptomatic patients, with frequent monitoring of other electrolytes

General Considerations

Hypophosphatemia is defined as a serum phosphate below 2 mg/dL. It is typically asymptomatic unless it develops rapidly and may result from any combination of decreased intestinal absorption, increased urinary excretion, or intracellular shift (see Table 44–10). Acute respiratory alkalosis and glucose ingestion with insulin release are associated with intracellular shift. Effects on mineralization are seen more

Table 44–10. Causes of Hypophosphatemia.

Decreased absorption
  Decreased intake
  Chronic antacid use
  Vitamin D deficiency
  Diarrhea
Renal losses
  Osmotic diuresis
  Acetazolamide use
  Metabolic or respiratory acidosis
  Hyperparathyroidism
  Glucocorticoid therapy
  Oncogenic osteomalacia
  Renal tubular dysfunction
Transcellular shifts
  Respiratory alkalosis
  Refeeding syndrome
Carbohydrate infusion
Rapid cellular uptake
  Hungry bone syndrome
  EPO therapy
  Blast crisis
Medication/hormone effect
  Insulin
  Calcitonin
  Glucagon
  β-Adrenergic agents

chronically, with phosphate-dependent energy pathways and 2,3-DPG formation impaired acutely.

Clinical Findings

Clinical findings in hypophosphatemia are nonspecific, reflecting the wide range of organs affected. Rhabdomyolysis, seizures, obtundation, coma, depressed cardiac contractility, ileus, dysarthria, and respiratory failure secondary to diaphragmatic weakness have been reported. With severe hypophosphatemia (below 0.5 mg/dL), hemolysis and impaired white blood cell and platelet function may occur.

Treatment

Phosphate replacement is indicated in patients with decreased serum phosphate regardless of symptoms. Oral supplementation is safe and preferred in almost all cases. Milk contains 1 mg of phosphate per milliliter, or oral formulations containing sodium or potassium phosphate are available. For severe symptomatic hypophosphatemia, IV infusion of sodium or potassium phosphate at a rate not to exceed 2.5 mg/kg over 6 hours may be initiated. Frequent monitoring of serum calcium, phosphate, potassium, and magnesium should be undertaken to avoid metastatic calcification from too rapid correction.

Disposition

Hospitalization is advised for all patients with a serum phosphate below 2.0 mg/dL. Patients not hospitalized should have prompt outpatient follow-up.

HYPERPHOSPHATEMIA

ESSENTIALS OF DIAGNOSIS

▶ Hyperphosphatemia is often associated with renal disease or hypoparathyroidism

▶ Increased phosphate may be a manifestation of tumor lysis or rhabdomyolysis

▶ Initial treatment consists of volume expansion and using insulin and glucose to shift phosphate into cells

General Considerations

Hyperphosphatemia is defined as a serum phosphate greater than 5 mg/dL (7 mg/dL in children and the elderly due to increased bone turnover in these age groups). It most commonly results from renal failure but may also be seen with hypoparathyroidism, exogenous loading of phosphate or vitamin D, tumor lysis syndrome, rhabdomyolysis, and acidosis. Pseudohyperphosphatemia may result from hyperglobulinemia, hypertriglyceridemia, hyperbilirubinemia, and hemolysis.

▶ Clinical Findings

Acutely, symptoms from hyperphosphatemia itself are rare and commonly referable to hypocalcemia and hyperkalemia. Chronic hyperphosphatemia may result in metastatic calcification, hyperparathyroidism, and renal dystrophy.

▶ Treatment

Acute hyperphosphatemia should be treated aggressively. In patients with normal renal function, volume expansion using isotonic saline coupled with acetazolamide (15 mg/kg, 500 mg in an average adult) will promote phosphate excretion but requires careful monitoring to avoid lowering serum calcium as well. IV insulin and glucose may also be used as with hyperkalemia to move phosphate into the cells. Dialysis is indicated in patients with renal failure. For hyperphosphatemia that has developed chronically, the primary focus of treatment is reducing intestinal absorption by decreasing protein intake and using phosphate-binding antacids. In patients with renal failure, calcium-containing salts are preferred to reduce the risk of aluminum toxicity.

▶ Disposition

Admission is more commonly indicated by the precipitating cause rather than strictly by hyperphosphatemia itself.

DISORDERS OF SERUM MAGNESIUM CONCENTRATION

Magnesium is primarily an intracellular cation and is important in enzymatic regulation, muscle contractility, and synaptic transmission within the nervous system. Serum concentrations are regulated primarily by the kidney. Because most intracellular magnesium is bound, concentrations are tightly regulated even in the face of large variations in extracellular concentration.

HYPOMAGNESEMIA

ESSENTIALS OF DIAGNOSIS

- ▶ Frequently associated with disorders of calcium, potassium, and phosphate
- ▶ Common in malnourished patients and those with renal disease
- ▶ Symptoms are primarily neuromuscular and similar to those seen with hypocalcemia
- ▶ Oral replacement is preferred except in severe symptomatic cases

Table 44–11. Causes of Hypomagnesemia.

Decreased intake (malnutrition, alcoholism)
GI losses
NG suctioning
Diarrhea
Malabsorption
Acute pancreatitis
Fistula
Primary intestinal hypomagnesemia
Renal losses
Alcohol
Diuresis (osmotic, diuretics, postobstructive)
Correction of chronic acidosis
Hypercalcemia with hypercalciuria
Hypocalcemia with phosphate depletion (hungry bone syndrome)
Hyperaldosteronism
Nephrotoxic drugs
Theophylline and β-agonists
Primary renal magnesium wasting

▶ General Considerations

Hypomagnesemia is defined as a serum magnesium concentration below 1.5 mEq/L and is very common, occurring in 12% of hospitalized patients and almost 2/3 of patients admitted to the ICU. Symptoms are rare until serum concentrations fall below 1 mEq/L. It may result from a number of conditions that produce decreased intake, decreased GI absorption, or increased GI or renal loss (see Table 44–11). Hypokalemia and hypocalcemia frequently occur along with hypomagnesemia, as does metabolic alkalosis.

▶ Clinical Findings

Clinical manifestations of hypomagnesemia are nonspecific and may be attributable to concurrent hypocalcemia or hypokalemia. Neurologic irritability with tremor, clonus, hyperreflexia, and tetany may occur with serum concentrations below 0.8 mEq/L, ultimately progressing to confusion and convulsions. Although there is no set of EKG findings consistently associated with decreased magnesium, both ventricular and supraventricular dysrhythmias appear to be potentiated. Prolongation of the QTc interval may occur secondary to coexistent hypokalemia or hypocalcemia.

▶ Treatment

Correction of other electrolyte abnormalities, particularly calcium and potassium, may be necessary in addition to replacing magnesium. Oral replacement is preferred in patients with mild symptoms and may be accomplished with either magnesium oxide or magnesium gluconate. Parenteral therapy is indicated for patients with symptomatic hypomagnesemia and tetany or seizures, or in the presence of arrhythmias. A typical regimen is 2 g of magnesium sulfate in a 20% solution infused over 20 minutes followed by 1 g IV every 6 hours. Too rapid administration of magnesium may result in apnea secondary to transient paralysis of the respiratory muscles from hypermagnesemia. This may be reversed by the administration of calcium gluconate. In patients with renal failure, doses of magnesium should be reduced by half.

▶ Disposition

Patients with symptomatic hypomagnesemia require admission. Asymptomatic patients may require admission for comorbid illnesses or may otherwise be discharged home with close follow-up.

HYPERMAGNESEMIA

ESSENTIALS OF DIAGNOSIS

- ▶ Symptoms are rare until magnesium levels are severely elevated
- ▶ Usually secondary to renal failure or excess magnesium intake
- ▶ Calcium gluconate can be used to reverse respiratory paralysis until forced diuresis or dialysis lowers serum magnesium levels

▶ General Considerations

Hypermagnesemia is defined as a serum magnesium concentration over 3 mEq/L. It is rare, and typically results from excess ingestion of magnesium-containing antacids or laxatives. Patients with renal failure, bowel disorders, those requiring parenteral hyperalimentation, and the elderly are most at risk.

▶ Clinical Findings

Hypermagnesemia is frequently asymptomatic until magnesium levels are severely elevated. With progressive elevation of the magnesium concentration, patients may experience nausea, vomiting, hypotension, confusion, muscle weakness, lethargy, loss of deep tendon reflexes, coma, and death secondary to respiratory paralysis. EKG changes include bradycardia, AV block, lengthening of the PR interval, QRS widening, and decreased P wave voltage with peaking of the T waves.

▶ Treatment

Calcium gluconate may be used as a temporizing measure in cases of impending respiratory paralysis. Patients with

normal renal function should undergo forced diuresis with isotonic saline and furosemide to promote renal excretion. Dialysis is indicated for severe hypermagnesemia and renal insufficiency.

▶ Disposition

All patients with hypermagnesemia require admission.

Adler SM, Verbalis JG: Disorders of body water homeostasis in critical illness. Endocrinol Metab Clin North Am 2006;35:873–894[PMID: 17127152].

Greenlee M, Wingo CS, McDonough AA, Youn JH, Kone BC: Narrative review: evolving concepts in potassium homeostasis and hypokalemia. Ann Intern Med 2009;150:619–625 [PMID: 19414841].

Kacprowicz RF, Lloyd JD: Electrolyte complications of malignancy. Emerg Med Clin North Am 2009;27:257–269 [PMID: 19447310].

Lin M, Liu SJ, Lim IT: Disorders of water imbalance. Emerg Med Clin North Am 2005;23:749–770 [PMID: 15982544].

Loh JA, Verbalis JG: Disorders of water and salt metabolism associated with pituitary disease. Endocrinal Metab Clin North Am 2008;37:213–234 [PMID: 18226738].

Moe SM: Disorders involving calcium, phosphorous, and magnesium. Prim Care 2008;35:215–237 [PMID: 18486714].

Montague BT, Ouellette JR, Buller GK: Retrospective review of the frequency of ECG changes in hyperkalemia. Clin J Am Soc Nephrol 2008;3:324–330 [PMID: 18235147].

Schaefer TJ, Wolford RW: Disorders of potassium. Emerg Med Clin North Am 2005;23:723–747 [PMID: 15982543].

Sood MM, Sood AR, Richardson R: Emergency management and commonly encountered outpatient scenarios in patients with hyperkalemia. Mayo Clin Proc 2007;82:1553–1561 [PMID: 18053465].

Wald DA: ECG manifestations of selected metabolic and endocrine disorders. Emerg Med Clin North Am 2006;24:145–157 [PMID: 16308117].

Weisberg LS: Management of severe hyperkalemia. Crit Care Med 2008;36:3246–3251 [PMID: 18936701].

▼ ACID–BASE DISORDERS

Emergency physicians frequently encounter critically ill patients with acid–base disorders, and an accurate understanding of the underlying physiology behind these derangements and the body's attempt to compensate for them is essential to appropriately manage these patients.

DEFINITIONS

Hydrogen ion concentration is typically not expressed directly but rather in terms of pH. Normal blood pH ranges from 7.36 to 7.44, with deviations above this range referred to as alkalemia and deviations below referred to as acidemia. Changes in [H$^+$] may result from changes in volatile (P_{CO_2}) or nonvolatile (sulfuric, lactic, etc.) acids. An acidosis is any

Table 44–12. Primary Disorders and Compensatory Responses.

Disorder	Primary Abnormality	Compensation	pH	P_{CO_2} (mm Hg)	Bicarbonate (mEq/L)
Respiratory acidosis	Increased P_{CO_2}	Increased [HCO_3^-]	<7.35	>45	>24
Respiratory alkalosis	Decreased P_{CO_2}	Decreased [HCO_3^-]	>7.45	<35	<24
Metabolic acidosis	Decreased [HCO_3^-]	Decreased P_{CO_2}	<7.35	<40	<22
Metabolic alkalosis	Increased [HCO_3^-]	Increased P_{CO_2}	>7.45	>40	>28

condition that increases the amount of acid in the blood and may be further characterized as respiratory (increased volatile acid) or metabolic (increased nonvolatile acid). Similarly, an alkalosis reduces the amount of acid in the blood and may also be characterized as respiratory or metabolic.

Several different buffer systems exist to help maintain a serum pH close to 7.4. The most important extracellular buffer system is the bicarbonate–carbonic anhydrase system, which converts CO_2 from cellular metabolism to carbonic acid that subsequently dissociates into H^+ and bicarbonate.

An isolated metabolic or respiratory process results in a primary acid–base disorder, and multiple processes result in a mixed acid–base disorder. Metabolic processes affect bicarbonate concentration, and respiratory processes affect P_{CO_2}. As the serum pH is shifted away from the normal range by a primary acid–base disorder, compensatory processes begin that attempt to restore a normal pH. A metabolic acidosis or alkalosis is compensated by changes in ventilation and a respiratory acidosis or alkalosis is compensated by adjusting renal acid excretion. These compensatory mechanisms will shift blood pH toward normal. In primary acid–base disorders, the underlying disorder will be evident from examination of the pH, P_{CO_2}, and serum bicarbonate (see Table 44–12).

Respiratory compensation for primary metabolic disorders begins within minutes as chemoreceptors sense the change in extracellular pH and signal the respiratory center to change minute ventilation. In a primary metabolic acidosis, the acidemia stimulates an increase in minute ventilation and subsequent decrease in P_{CO_2}; conversely, a metabolic alkalosis results in hypoventilation and increased P_{CO_2}. Renal compensation for primary respiratory disorders does not begin in earnest until after 6–12 hours of sustained acidemia or alkalemia. In a primary respiratory acidosis, the kidneys increase bicarbonate synthesis, excrete more protons, and reclaim more bicarbonate from the proximal tubule. Alkalemia promotes the retention of H^+ and increased bicarbonate excretion. Compensatory mechanisms may take several days to reach maximal effect, and with the exception of compensation for chronic respiratory alkalosis never restore the pH to normal. The timing and limits of compensation are detailed in Table 44–13. A normal pH in the setting of an acid–base disturbance should alert the clinician to the presence of a mixed acid–base disorder.

EVALUATION OF ACID–BASE DISORDERS

The patient's history and physical examination often provide important clues to the presence and etiology of acid–base disorders and are particularly valuable in the case of mixed disorders. Beyond the history and physical examination, initial assessment of acid–base disorders requires an

Table 44–13. Degree and Limits of Compensation.

Primary Disorder	Secondary Response	Time	Limit
Metabolic acidosis	Decreased P_{CO_2} of 1 mm Hg for each 1 mEq/L decrease in [HCO_3^-]	24 h	P_{CO_2} of 10 mm Hg
Metabolic alkalosis	Increased P_{CO_2} of 0.7 mm Hg for each 1 mEq/L increase in [HCO_3^-]	24–36 h	P_{CO_2} of 55 mm Hg
Respiratory acidosis			
Acute	Increased [HCO_3^-] of 1 mEq/L for every 10 mm Hg in P_{CO_2}	5–10 min	[HCO_3^-] of 30 mEq/L
Chronic	Increased [HCO_3^-] of 3.5 mEq/L for every 10 mm Hg in P_{CO_2}	72–96 h	[HCO_3^-] of 45 mEq/L
Respiratory acidosis			
Acute	Decreased [HCO_3^-] of 2 mEq/L for every 10 mm Hg in P_{CO_2}	5–10 min	[HCO_3^-] of 18 mEq/L
Chronic	Decreased [HCO_3^-] of 5 mEq/L for every 10 mm Hg in P_{CO_2}	48–72 h	[HCO_3^-] of 14 mEq/L

electrolyte panel and blood gas. Values obtained via venous blood gas sampling (with the exception of Po_2) are quite similar to those obtained via arterial sampling; pH is typically 0.01–0.03 lower, Pco_2 is 6 mm Hg higher, and bicarbonate is 2 mEq/L higher in venous samples when compared to arterial samples. "Arterialization" of the venous blood specimen by warming the hand at 45°C for 10 minutes eliminates even these differences. Because of the decreased pain and morbidity associated with venous sampling, use of venous blood should be considered when oxygenation is not a concern.

The first step in analyzing the laboratory data in acid–base disorders is to ensure the internal consistency of that data using the Henderson-Hasselbalch equation (see Appendix). Following this, an anion gap should be calculated by adding the serum $[Cl^-]$ and $[HCO_3^-]$ and subtracting this sum from the serum $[Na^+]$. The anion gap represents the negative charge from unmeasured serum proteins and averages 10–12 mEq/L. The delta anion gap is the difference between the calculated anion gap and a normal anion gap, and when compared with the change in bicarbonate can be an important clue to the presence of a mixed disorder.

To determine the primary disorder, first examine the bicarbonate. Increased bicarbonate reflects either a primary metabolic alkalosis or metabolic compensation for a primary respiratory acidosis. Examination of the pH will then reveal the primary disorder: an elevated pH indicates a primary metabolic alkalosis, and a decreased pH indicates a primary respiratory acidosis. Decreased bicarbonate may result from a primary metabolic acidosis or as metabolic compensation for a respiratory alkalosis; decreased pH indicates a metabolic acidosis and increased pH indicates a respiratory alkalosis. Normal pH in the presence of either increased or decreased bicarbonate indicates a mixed disorder. In primary disorders, Pco_2 and bicarbonate should deviate in the same direction, while in mixed disorders they deviate in opposite directions. Depending on the clinical setting, examination of serum and urine osmolality and urine electrolytes may be warranted to fully characterize the nature of the disorder.

CLINICAL ACID–BASE DISORDERS

1. Respiratory Acidosis

ESSENTIALS OF DIAGNOSIS

▶ Impairment in alveolar ventilation results in hypercapnia

▶ Alteration in consciousness may result

▶ Treatment is aimed at improving ventilation by treating the underlying disorder

Table 44–14. Causes of Respiratory Acidosis.

Acute
  Respiratory center depression
    Narcotic/sedative overdose
    Cardiac arrest
  Paralysis of respiratory muscles
    Anticholinesterases, anesthetics
    Cerebral, brain stem, or high spinal cord infarct
    Primary neuromuscular diseases: Guillain-Barré, myasthenia gravis, amyotrophic lateral sclerosis, poliomyelitis, botulism, tetanus
    Myopathy of respiratory muscles: muscular dystrophy, hypokalemic myopathy, electrolyte imbalance (decreased phosphorus, magnesium), familial periodic paralysis
    Primary hypoventilation
    Diaphragmatic paralysis
  Airway obstruction
    Upper: laryngeal edema/spasm, tracheal edema/stenosis, obstructive sleep apnea
    Lower: mechanical (foreign body, aspirated fluid, neoplasm, bronchospasm)
  Pulmonic/musculoskeletal abnormalities
    Pneumonia, pulmonary edema, acute respiratory disease syndrome, restrictive lung disease, pulmonary embolism
    Pneumothorax, hemothorax, chest wall trauma, flail chest smoke inhalation iatrogenic (mechanical ventilation)
Chronic
  Chronic airway disease (chronic obstructive pulmonary disease, emphysema)
  Extreme kyphoscoliosis
  Extreme obesity (Pickwickian syndrome)

▶ General Considerations

Respiratory acidosis is defined as an elevated Pco_2 (>45 mm Hg) and a decrease in serum pH below 7.36. Any condition that results in alveolar hypoventilation may cause respiratory acidosis (see Table 44–14).

▶ Clinical Findings

The hallmark of respiratory acidosis is an alteration in level of consciousness. The characteristic features of hypercapnia range from fatigue, irritability, headache, confusion, stupor, and obtundation to coma and are dependent on the severity and chronicity of the hypercapnia. A Pco_2 of 70 may result in coma when secondary to an acute respiratory acidosis, while a person with chronic respiratory acidosis may tolerate Pco_2 levels higher than this without a decrease in mental status.

▶ Physiology

A. Acute Respiratory Acidosis

Acutely, the increased protons resulting from a respiratory acidosis are buffered by intracellular proteins. This results in a rise in $[HCO_3^-]$ of 1 mEq/L for every 10 mm Hg increase in P_{CO_2} up to a maximum $[HCO_3^-]$ of 30 mEq/L and a decrease in pH of 0.08. This compensation is complete within minutes and no further compensation is possible until renal excretion of acid begins, which may take 72–96 hours.

B. Chronic Respiratory Acidosis

Chronic respiratory acidosis commonly results from COPD and extreme obesity. Renal compensation reaches a steady state after 3–4 days and involves the excretion of chloride in addition to acid, with retention of bicarbonate. An increase in the P_{CO_2} of 10 mm Hg is expected to result in an increase in $[HCO_3^-]$ of 3.5 mEq/L (to a maximum of 45 mEq/L) and a decrease in pH of 0.03.

▶ Treatment and Disposition

Treatment consists primarily of reversing and stabilizing the underlying process that generated the respiratory acidosis. Bronchodilators, reversal of opioids, and support of ventilation using either BiPAP or intubation may be warranted depending on the clinical picture. Care should be taken not to decrease the P_{CO_2} too rapidly in the setting of chronic respiratory acidosis, as the shift in pH may result in electrolyte abnormalities with dysrhythmias or seizure. Patients with acute respiratory acidosis requiring therapy should be admitted. Admission for patients with chronic respiratory acidosis is more commonly warranted by other findings such as hypoxemia.

2. Respiratory Alkalosis

ESSENTIALS OF DIAGNOSIS

▶ Hypocapnia may be generated by many common causes

▶ Chronic respiratory alkalosis may be completely compensated

▶ Treat the underlying cause

▶ General Considerations

Respiratory alkalosis is defined as a P_{CO_2} below 35 mm Hg with an increase in serum pH above 7.44. Acutely, respiratory alkalosis is most commonly caused by hyperventilation secondary to other causes (see Table 44–15). These causes may reduce P_{CO_2} to 25–35 mm Hg, with further decreases resulting from concurrent metabolic acidosis or hypoxia.

Table 44–15. Causes of Respiratory Alkalosis.

Early shock
Early sepsis
Trauma
Fear
Anxiety
Pulmonary disease
CHF
Asthma
Pneumonia
Pulmonary embolism
CNS infection
CVA
Pregnancy
Liver disease
Hyperthyroidism
Acute salicylate ingestion

▶ Clinical Findings

The clinical findings of respiratory alkalosis vary depending on the severity and acuity of the process. Acutely, symptoms attributable to hypocalcemia (such as circumoral and digital paresthesia and carpopedal spasm) may occur from the rapid shift in pH. More severe hypocapnia may result in cerebral vasoconstriction with lightheadedness, dizziness, confusion, and altered consciousness. Chronically, respiratory alkalosis may result in hypophosphatemia and a lowered seizure threshold.

▶ Physiology
A. Acute Respiratory Alkalosis

Compensation for acute hypocapnia begins within minutes and involves the movement of protons from the intracellular to the extracellular space. For every decrease in P_{CO_2} of 10 mm Hg, $[HCO_3^-]$ should decrease by 2.5 mEq/L and pH should increase by 0.08.

B. Chronic Respiratory Alkalosis

Renal compensation for chronic respiratory alkalosis results in decreased proton excretion and the retention of chloride for bicarbonate. Chronically, a decrease in P_{CO_2} of 10 mm Hg will result in a decrease in $[HCO_3^-]$ of 5 mEq/L. With prolonged hypocapnia (2 weeks or more), pH may be normal.

▶ Treatment and Disposition

Treatment for respiratory alkalosis focuses on treating the underlying disorder, with disposition based on the precipitating cause rather than the alkalosis itself.

3. Metabolic Acidosis

ESSENTIALS OF DIAGNOSIS

▶ Commonly divided into anion gap and nongap causes

▶ Cardiovascular effects are most immediately life-threatening

▶ Calculate the anion gap and delta gaps

▶ Use Winter's formula to identify respiratory compensation

▶ Treat the underlying cause

▶ General Considerations

Metabolic acidosis occurs due to an imbalance between the plasma concentration of H^+ and HCO_3^- and is defined as a decrease in $[HCO_3^-]$ to below 22 with a decrease in pH below 7.36. It may result from overproduction of organic acids (most commonly lactate or ketones), loss of bicarbonate through intestinal or renal wasting, or the inability to excrete acids from normal metabolism or toxin ingestion.

▶ Clinical Findings

Metabolic acidosis results in a variety of impairments regardless of the underlying etiology (see Table 44–16). The

Table 44–16. Effects of Metabolic Acidosis.

Cardiovascular
  Decreased contractility
  Decreased renal and hepatic blood flow
  Decreased fibrillation threshold
  Decreased cardiac responsiveness to catecholamines
  Tachycardia
Neurologic
  Obtundation
  Coma
  Increased cerebral blood flow
Respiratory
  Increased minute ventilation
  Dyspnea
  Respiratory muscle fatigue
Metabolic
  Inhibition of anaerobic metabolism
  Hyperkalemia
  Hyperphosphatemia
  Increased metabolic rate
  Increased protein catabolism

anion gap is commonly used to help determine the etiology; however, the anion gap can be misleading in patients with low albumin and in the rare patients with an anion gap acidosis who are euvolemic. Winter's formula can be used to predict the P_{CO_2} expected for the measured serum bicarbonate to determine if appropriate respiratory compensation is in place ($P_{CO_2} = 1.5 \times [HCO_3^-] + 8 \pm 2$).

A. Increased Anion Gap

An elevated anion gap is synonymous with the presence of a metabolic acidosis and implies an overproduction of acids or a decrease in acid clearance by the kidney. The accumulation of acidic anions that are not measured by routine laboratory testing lowers the serum bicarbonate via buffering, thus generating an increased anion gap. An increased anion gap is associated with the following conditions:

·   ketoacidosis

·   diabetic

·   alcoholic

·   starvation

·   renal failure

·   lactic acidosis

·   exogenous toxins metabolized to lactate—cyanide, carbon monoxide, ibuprofen, INH, iron, strychnine, toluene

·   exogenous toxins metabolized to acids—aspirin, methanol, ethylene glycol, paraldehyde.

B. Nongap Acidosis

A metabolic acidosis with a normal anion gap is generated by the loss of bicarbonate with a reciprocal increase in chloride concentration, giving it its alternate name of hyperchloremic acidosis. The serum potassium concentration can be used to divide hyperchloremic acidosis into hypo- and hyperkalemic forms. Causes associated with hypokalemia include diarrhea, small bowel or pancreatic fistula, ureteral diversion, ileal loop, type 1 renal tubular acidosis (RTA), and the use of carbonic anhydrase inhibitors. Normal and hyperkalemic causes include type 4 RTA, early renal failure, hydronephrosis, tubulointerstitial renal disease, and hypoaldosteronism. Nongap acidosis may also result from rapid hydration with normal saline.

Calculation of the urinary anion gap can help identify the source of a nongap acidosis. The urinary anion gap is calculated by adding $[Na^+]$ and $[K^+]$ and subtracting $[Cl^-]$ and is used to determine urine ammonium excretion, which is difficult to measure directly. A positive value indicates that the renal ammonium production is impaired, pointing toward a renal source for the acidosis. A negative value is consistent with GI losses.

Table 44-17. Causes of Metabolic Alkalosis.

Saline Responsive (Urine [Cl] <10 mEq/L)	Saline Resistant (Urine [Cl] >20 mEq/L)	Other Causes
Gastrointestinal: vomiting, nasogastric suction, Cl diarrhea, villous adenoma Diuretic therapy Cystic fibrosis Posthypercapnia Alkali syndrome	Mineralocorticoid excess: primary aldosteronism Secondary causes: congestive heart failure, cirrhosis, Bartter syndrome, licorice, renin tumor, tobacco Cushing syndrome, severe K⁺ depletion Congenital adrenal hyperplasia	Refeeding alkalosis Massive blood transfusion Hypercalcemia (bone metastases)

Physiology

The body buffers an acute metabolic acidosis by using intracellular and extracellular proteins, increasing H^+ elimination by the kidney, and stimulating the respiratory drive. Respiratory compensation for a metabolic acidosis involves hyperventilation, and may take 12–24 hours to be fully effective. Under ordinary circumstances, a Pco_2 of 10 mm Hg is the lower limit of compensation, with Pco_2 falling by 1.0–1.3 for every 1 mEq/L decrease in $[HCO_3^-]$.

Treatment

Treatment of metabolic acidosis requires treatment of the underlying cause. In many cases, reversing the underlying causes (e.g., DKA) and replacing volume will allow for the metabolism of organic acids back to bicarbonate or for the kidneys to regenerate bicarbonate. Maintaining adequate tissue perfusion and oxygenation is essential to avoid worsening the acidosis. The use of alkalinizing agents is controversial, as multiple studies have failed to demonstrate benefit from sodium bicarbonate administration and it could theoretically impair oxygen unloading in the tissues as well as result in increased CO_2 formation, thereby worsening the acidosis. In severe cases (dysrhythmias, catecholamine insensitivity, hemodynamic instability), sodium bicarbonate may be used to raise the pH to 7.1 at a dose of 0.5 mEq/L/kg. Disposition depends on the severity of the underlying disorder, although nongap acidosis is rarely life threatening.

4. Metabolic Alkalosis

ESSENTIALS OF DIAGNOSIS

- ► Commonly results from vomiting or volume depletion secondary to diuretics
- ► Evaluate urine chloride concentration to help guide therapy

General Considerations

Metabolic alkalosis is defined as a primary elevation of serum $[HCO_3^-]$ above 28 mEq/L with an elevation in pH above 7.44. A primary metabolic alkalosis results from the loss of acid or, more rarely, the gain of base. Gastric losses via vomiting or NG suctioning and diuretic use are common causes of metabolic alkalosis, with the resultant volume contraction maintaining the alkalosis. Various other medical conditions can result in a metabolic alkalosis, and determination of the urine chloride can help guide therapy (see Table 44–17).

Clinical Findings

Metabolic alkalosis produces hypokalemia, hypocalcemia, and hypomagnesemia. With severe alkalosis, signs of hypocalcemia may predominate. Decreased cerebral blood flow may result in lethargy and confusion, ultimately progressing to coma and seizures. A history of gastric losses or diuretic use may be obtained and signs of volume contraction on physical examination may be evident. Hypertension should raise the suspicion of primary aldosteronism. Patients with chronic hypercapnia may experience a metabolic alkalosis following correction of the hypercapnia.

Physiology

Respiratory compensation for a metabolic alkalosis consists of hypoventilation. For every increase of 1 mEq/L in the $[HCO_3^-]$, Pco_2 will rise by 0.7 mm Hg and pH increase by 0.015. Pco_2 typically will not increase above 55 mm Hg because of the hypoxemia that ensues at that level of ventilation.

Treatment

Urine chloride concentration should be measured to guide initial therapy. Patients with a urine $[Cl^-]$ below 10 mEq/L are characterized as chloride responsive and should be treated with volume expansion using normal saline. Patients with a urine $[Cl^-]$ above 20 mEq/L may be chloride resistant; a urine $[Cl^-]$ above 40 mEq/L always indicates that sufficient volume expansion has occurred. Potassium replacement (up to 100–500 mEq) may be needed to correct the alkalosis in certain settings. Acetazolamide may be used in posthypercapnic metabolic alkalosis if volume status is normal. Disposition depends on the severity of the precipitating cause.

5. Mixed Acid–Base Disorders

ESSENTIALS OF DIAGNOSIS

▶ Up to three disorders can coexist

▶ Analyze the data in a stepwise fashion

▶ Calculate delta gaps and determine if appropriate compensation exists

▶ Metabolic acidosis and respiratory alkalosis commonly coexist

▶ General Considerations

Respiratory acidosis and respiratory alkalosis can never coexist, but any other combination of processes is possible. Consider a mixed disorder whenever the degree of compensation is inadequate, or if an acid–base disorder causes no shift in pH (except in chronic respiratory alkalosis), or if the clinical picture is not consistent with a primary process.

▶ Combined Metabolic Acidosis and Respiratory Acidosis

This is an ominous combination and is found in patients in cardiopulmonary arrest. Once a metabolic acidosis has been identified, determine if the P_{CO_2} is appropriate; if it is higher than expected, a superimposed respiratory acidosis exists. In chronic respiratory acidosis, $[HCO_3^-]$ should increase by 3.5 mEq/L for every increase of 10 mm Hg in P_{CO_2}. A smaller increase in $[HCO_3^-]$ implies incomplete compensation or a superimposed metabolic acidosis.

▶ Combined Metabolic Alkalosis and Respiratory Alkalosis

This mixed disorder is commonly encountered and may result from congestive heart failure, early sepsis, liver disease, or salicylate ingestion. It is identified by a respiratory compensation that is greater than expected for the degree of metabolic acidosis. In patients with chronic respiratory alkalosis, $[HCO_3^-]$ should be decreased by 5 mEq/L for every 10 mm Hg decrease in P_{CO_2}. A greater decrease in $[HCO_3^-]$ implies a superimposed metabolic acidosis.

▶ Combined Metabolic Alkalosis and Respiratory Acidosis

This mixed disorder may occur in patients with chronic respiratory acidosis who develop a metabolic alkalosis from diuretic use. Appropriate compensation for a metabolic alkalosis is an increase in P_{CO_2} of 0.7 mm Hg for each 1 mEq/L increase in $[HCO_3^-]$. A greater increase in P_{CO_2} implies a superimposed respiratory acidosis. For patients with chronic respiratory acidosis, $[HCO_3^-]$ should increase by 3.5 mEq/L for each increase in P_{CO_2} of 10 mm Hg. Greater increases in $[HCO_3^-]$ imply a superimposed metabolic alkalosis.

▶ Combined Metabolic Alkalosis and Respiratory Alkalosis

This mixed disorder may result in patients with hepatic failure who are taking diuretics and in patients who require mechanical ventilation and are taking diuretics or undergoing NG suctioning. An increase in P_{CO_2} of less than 0.7 mm Hg for each 1 mEq/L increase in $[HCO_3^-]$ implies a superimposed respiratory alkalosis. In chronic respiratory alkalosis, $[HCO_3^-]$ should be decreased by 5 mEq/L for every 10 mm Hg decrease in P_{CO_2}, with smaller decreases indicating a superimposed metabolic alkalosis.

▶ Use of Delta Gaps to Identify Mixed Disorders

The use of the delta anion gap and delta bicarbonate can help identify mixed acid–base disorders that would not otherwise be readily apparent, including those with a normal pH. The delta anion gap is derived by subtracting 10 from the calculated anion gap. The delta bicarbonate is derived by subtracting the measured $[HCO_3^-]$ from 24. For most commonly encountered anion gap acidoses, there will be a 1:1 relationship between the delta anion gap and the delta bicarbonate. When the delta bicarbonate exceeds the delta anion gap, a mixed anion gap and nongap acidosis is likely. When the delta bicarbonate is below the delta anion gap, a mixed anion gap acidosis with a metabolic alkalosis is likely (see Table 44–18).

Casaletto JJ: Differential diagnosis of metabolic acidosis. Emerg Med Clin North Am 2005;23:771–787 [PMID: 15982545].

Kaplan LJ, Frangos S: Clinical review: Acid-base abnormalities in the intensive care unit. Crit Care 2005;9:198–203 [PMID: 15774078].

Kellum JA: Disorders of acid-base balance. Crit Care Med 2007;35:2630–2636 [PMID: 17893626].

Kellum JA: Determinants of plasma acid-base balance. Crit Care Clin 2005;21:329–346 [PMID: 15781166].

Table 44–18. Use of the Delta Gaps to Detect Mixed Disorders.

Blood Chemistry	Normal	Anion Gap Acidosis	Anion Gap and Nongap Acidosis	Metabolic Alkalosis	Anion Gap Acidosis and Metabolic Alkalosis
Sodium	140	140	140	140	140
Chloride	106	106	114	94	94
Bicarbonate	24	14	6	34	20
Delta bicarbonate		10	18	10	4
Anion gap	10	20	20	12	26
Delta anion gap		10	10	2	16
pH	7.40	7.29	7.10	7.50	7.38
P_{CO_2}	40	30	20	45	35

▼ APPENDIX

▶ Osmolality

Serum osmolality can be estimated using the following formula:

$$P_{osm} = 2 \times [Na^+]_{serum} + [glucose]/18 + [BUN]/2.8$$
$$+ [ethanol]/4.6.$$

Osmolality is expressed in mOsm/L, sodium concentration is expressed in mEq/L, and glucose, BUN, and ethanol are expressed in mg/dL. A normal serum osmolal gap (measured osmolality minus calculated) is less than 10 mOsm/L. A widened osmolal gap may be seen in any condition that increases the amount of unmeasured osmoles in the blood, such as methanol or ethylene glycol ingestion or in DKA.

▶ Electrolyte Replacement

In treating hyponatremia and hypernatremia, many different formulas that are available to help the clinician estimate total free water deficit or absolute sodium excess or deficiency.

Table 44–19. Total Body Water in Liters as Fraction of Body Weight.

Children	0.6
Adult male	0.6
Adult female	0.5
Elderly male	0.5
Elderly female	0.45

However, the use of the Adrogue–Madias equation offers a simple and reliable method for estimating the effect of infusion of 1 L of infusate on serum sodium.

$$\text{Change in serum } [Na^+] = (\text{infusate } Na^+ - \text{serum } Na^+)/$$
$$(\text{total body water} + 1).$$

Total body water may be estimated by multiplying the patient's weight by the appropriate value in Table 44–19 to obtain a value in liters. Sodium concentrations of common infusate solutions are provided in Table 44–20.

For example, in a 70-kg adult male who is symptomatically hyponatremic with a serum sodium of 120 mEq/L and who is clinically euvolemic, it may be desirable to increase the serum sodium by 2 mEq/L over 2 hours using 3% NaCl. In this case, 1 L of infusate would be expected to have the following effect on serum sodium:

$$(513 - 120)/(42 + 1) = 9.14.$$

Table 44–20. Sodium Concentrations of Common IV Solutions.

Infusate	mEq/L
5% dextrose in water	0
0.2% NaCl in 5% dextrose in water	34
0.45% NaCl in water	77
Ringer's lactate	130
0.9% NaCl in water	154
3% NaCl in water	513
5% NaCl in water	855

Thus, 1 L should raise the patient's serum sodium by approximately 9 mEq/L. Giving the patient 222 mL total, or 111 mL/h for 2 hours, should result in an increase in the patient's serum sodium of 2 mEq/L.

▶ Henderson–Hasselbalch Equation

Internal consistency of the acid–base data acquired from a blood gas can be ascertained by using the Henderson–Hasselbalch equation. For any given set of values, the following equation should be true:

$$pH = 6.1 + \log\left\{\left[HCO_3^-\right] / \left(0.03 \times P_{CO_2}\right)\right\}.$$

Alternatively, the Henderson equation can be used to estimate [H+] directly and does not require the use of logarithms:

$$\left[H^+\right] = 24 \times \left(P_{CO_2} / \left[HCO_3^-\right]\right).$$

Over normal values of pH, [H+] can be estimated by starting at a [H+] of 40 nmol/L for a pH of 7.40, and adjusting the [H+] by 10 for every change in pH of 0.1. Other systems of describing physiologic acid–base balance, such as the standard base error and Stewart method, have been described and are more consistent with the known physical chemistry. However, for most clinical purposes the Henderson–Hasselbalch method is sufficient.

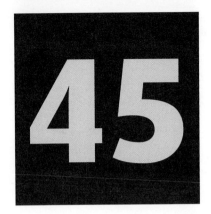

Burns & Smoke Inhalation

Dorian Drigalla, MD, FACEP
Jennifer Gemmill, MD[1]

IMMEDIATE MANAGEMENT OF LIFE-THREATENING PROBLEMS

ESSENTIALS OF DIAGNOSIS

▶ The ABC's
▶ Begin fluid resuscitation
▶ Obtain diagnostic information

See Figure 45–1.

▶ Establish an Adequate Airway

When any patient enters the Emergency Department, the first steps to care involve evaluation of the ABC's—especially in burn patients. Severe burns to the lower face and neck may be associated with upper airway and laryngeal edema that cause airway obstruction. Inhalation of superheated air or steam in a confined space may also cause significant upper airway edema. Full-thickness chest wall burns, especially if they are circumferential, may limit chest wall movement and cause respiratory failure, requiring escharotomy on an emergency basis. Consider early endotracheal intubation in all patients with such injuries and in patients with stridor, hoarseness, or hypoxia.

Airway obstruction may progress rapidly in these patients. When the burn size exceeds 60% total body surface area, early endotracheal intubation should be considered as these patients often deteriorate rapidly. If facial or airway involvement is noted, intubation is advisable. If endotracheal intubation is not successful, cricothyrotomy or tracheostomy may be necessary.

▶ Support Ventilation and Oxygenation

Give oxygen by nasal cannula or face mask. If smoke inhalation may have occurred, give 100% oxygen by tight-fitting reservoir face mask or endotracheal tube. Monitor oxygen saturation by pulse oximetry, but be aware that pulse oximetry readings will be falsely elevated in patients with elevated carboxyhemoglobin levels. Simply subtract the measured carboxyhemoglobin level from the pulse oximetry value to determine the true oxygen saturation. Noninvasive co-oximetry is emerging as a useful tool to monitor the carboxyhemoglobin level in the ED.

[1]This chapter is a revision of the chapter by David A. Fritz, MD, FACEP, from 6th edition.

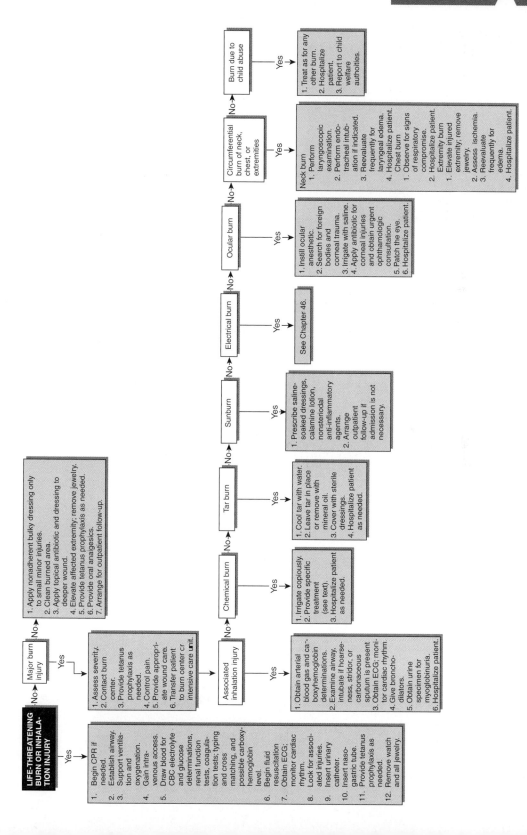

▲ **Figure 45–1.** Management of life-threatening burn or inhalation injury.

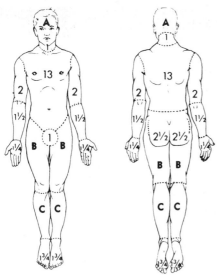

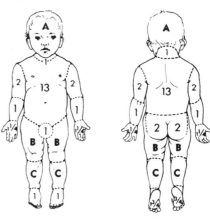

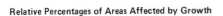

	Age		
Area	10	15	Adult
A = half of head	5½	4½	3½
B = half of one thigh	4¼	4½	4¾
C = half of one leg	3	3¼	3½

Relative Percentages of Areas Affected by Growth

	Age		
Area	0	1	5
A = half of head	9½	8½	6½
B = half of one thigh	2¾	3¼	4
C = half of one leg	2½	2½	2¾

Relative Percentages of Areas Affected by Growth

▲ **Figure 45–2.** Burn size may be estimated using age-adjusted burn chart. (Reproduced, with permission, from Way LW, ed. *Current Surgical Diagnosis and Treatment*, 11th ed. New York, NY: McGraw-Hill; 2003.)

▶ Begin Fluid Resuscitation

Patients with deep burns covering more than 15% of body surface area require intravenous fluid resuscitation. Insert one or two large-bore (≥16-gauge) peripheral intravenous catheters, preferably inserted through unaffected skin, or a central venous catheter if peripheral lines cannot be established. Calculation of the percent of body surface burned can be performed using an age-adjusted burn chart displayed in Figure 45–2. Additionally, the "Rule of Nines" can be used to estimate total burned body surface area, with each of the following representing 9%: head, anterior chest, anterior abdomen, each arm, anterior of each leg, and posterior of each leg. The back and buttocks represent 18%, while the groin and each palm represent 1%. Adjustment of the rule of nines for children changes 9% to 5%, with the head encompassing 20% of the total.

Burns are associated with the loss of large volumes of intravascular fluid, electrolytes, and protein through capillaries with increased permeability. Loss begins soon after injury and is maximal during the first 6–8 hours. Currently there is no universal consensus regarding fluid resuscitation and several formulas may be used as guidelines (Table 45–1).

Studies comparing colloid to crystalloid solutions for resuscitation have not shown an increased benefit with colloids. Most burn centers today use only crystalloid for the first 18–24 hours, utilizing either the Parkland or modified Brook formula. These formulas should be individualized for each patient on the basis of the patient's response to therapy, as well as the accepting physician's preference if the patient is to be transferred to a burn center. Additional variables

Table 45–1. Formulas for Fluid Resuscitation in Burn Patients.

Formula	Day 1[a]
	Crystalloid
Parkland (Baxter)	4 mL crystalloid × TBSA% × weight in kg
Modified Brooke	Using Lactated Ringers: *Adult*: 2 mL/kg × TBSA% burned *Child*: 3 mL/kg × TBSA% burned

[a]One-half of the calculated volume is given in the first 8 hours; the remainder is given over the next 16 hours.

including body temperature, blood alcohol level, and inhalational injury may also affect the volume of fluid resuscitation required. In general, infusion rates should be adjusted to maintain urine output at 0.5–1.0 mL/kg/h for adults and 1.0 mL/kg/h for children under 10 kg.

In the case of extensive burns over a significant body surface area, noninvasive blood pressure monitoring may be impossible due to interference of tissue edema with cuff readings. For these patients, a radial or femoral arterial catheter should be placed to accurately monitor blood pressure during resuscitation.

▶ Diagnostic Studies

Arterial blood gas analysis is helpful if respiratory involvement is present. In addition, for assistance in overall patient management and resuscitation, submit blood for carboxyhemoglobin level, complete blood count, and electrolytes and urine for myoglobin. Obtain chest X-ray and electrocardiogram (ECG) and consider obtaining cardiac enzymes in the patient with suspected carbon monoxide poisoning.

▶ Evaluate for Possible Associated Injuries

Burn patients frequently have other injuries in addition to the burn. Patients who have been burned in motor vehicle accidents or explosions should be evaluated as described in Chapter 12. Consider cervical spine and other traumatic injuries in patients who may have jumped or fallen from a burning building or been burned in a motor vehicle crash.

▶ Insert a Urinary Catheter

An indwelling urinary catheter is the most important monitoring device in burn patients to monitor urinary output and to obtain urine for urinalysis (including myoglobin determination if the patient has sustained an electrical burn). Patients with full-thickness burns of the penile glans or shaft may require suprapubic cystostomy.

▶ Insert a Nasogastric Tube

Patients with deep burns covering more than 20% of their body surface will develop an ileus. Inserting a nasogastric tube will decrease the risk of emesis and possible aspiration.

Alvarado R, Chung KK, Cancio LC et al: Burn resuscitation. Burns 2009;35:4–14 [PMID: 18539396].

Benicke M, Perbix W, Knam F et al: New multifactorial burn resuscitation formula offers superior predictive reliability in comparison to established algorithms. Burns 2009;35:30–35 [PMID: 18945549].

eMedicine: Resuscitation and Early Management Burns. http://emedicine.medscape.com/article/1277360-overview Birmingham, AL, 2009 [Last Accessed on February 4, 2011].

Latenser BA: Critical care of the burn patient: the first 48 hours. Crit Care Med 2009;37:2819–2826 [PMID: 19707133].

FURTHER EVALUATION OF THE BURN PATIENT

ESSENTIALS OF DIAGNOSIS

▶ Evaluate for severity of injury
▶ Provide wound care
▶ Transfer to the appropriate facility

▶ Determine the Severity of Injury

Once initial resuscitation efforts have begun, additional information is often required to determine the disposition of the burn patient. Ask the patient, witnesses, and family about the mechanism of injury (eg, explosion, spilled liquid, house fire) and about the possible presence of combustibles known to be toxic. Find out whether the patient was burned in an open or enclosed space; the latter increases the risk of inhalation injury and should prompt consideration of early intubation. Also ask about underlying medical problems, tetanus immunization status, and medication allergies.

An accurate estimate of the severity of injury is crucial in determining the need for hospital admission or referral to a burn center and in guiding initial fluid resuscitation and establishing a prognosis. In general, patients with minor burns may be managed as outpatients, patients with moderate uncomplicated burns should be hospitalized, and patients with major burns should be transferred to a burn center. Even in the absence of major burn criteria, if the hospital does not have facilities or expertise in caring for burn patients, victims with moderate or major burns should be referred to a burn center. The following factors are used to determine burn severity.

A. Burn Size

Accurate measurement of the burned area, expressed as a percentage of body surface area, should be performed in all burn patients. Burn size may be quickly estimated by using an age-adjusted surface area chart (see Figure 45–2) or by using the "rule of nines" as mentioned earlier in this chapter. The size of scattered small burns can be estimated by comparing them with the size of the patient's hand, which constitutes about 1.25% of body surface area. The extent of all burns should be recorded on a drawing (front and back views) on the patient's chart.

B. Burn Depth

Burns are typically described as first, second, third, or fourth degree. A more useful description, based on the wound's

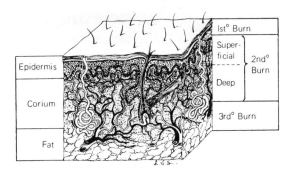

▲ **Figure 45–3.** Layers of the skin, showing depth of first-, second-, and third-degree burns. ((Reproduced, with permission, from Way LW, ed. *Current Surgical Diagnosis and Treatment*, 11th ed. New York, NY: McGraw-Hill; 2003.)

ability to heal, is partial thickness (heals spontaneously) and full thickness (requires skin grafting). Deep partial-thickness burns usually require grafting to expedite healing and decrease contractures and hypertrophic scar. Figure 45–3 shows the level of skin involved with each type of burn. Table 45–2 outlines the physical findings usually associated with each type of burn. The depth of burn should be recorded accurately on a drawing (front and back views) on the patient's chart.

Several principles must be kept in mind when considering burn depth. First, because it is difficult to distinguish deep partial-thickness burns from full-thickness burns, these burns should be assumed to be full-thickness injuries and should be treated accordingly. Second, burn wounds change over 48–72 hours, and what may appear to be superficial injury on initial examination may progress to a deeper-level injury, especially if the patient has poor perfusion or the wound becomes desiccated or infected.

C. Burn Site

Burns in the following areas are considered major injuries:

1. Hands and feet—Deep burns of the hands or feet cause scarring and may produce permanent disability.

2. Face—Partial- or full-thickness facial burns may cause severe scarring, with profound physical and emotional impact. They are also often associated with inhalation injury and compromised airway.

3. Eyes—Burns of the eyes may cause corneal scarring and eyelid dysfunction that may ultimately lead to blindness. *Note*: Patients with possible eye burns should be examined as quickly as possible, preferably in the emergency department, because massive periorbital edema often develops and hinders later examination. Further discussion of eye injury is detailed later in this chapter.

4. Ears—Deep burns of the ears predispose to development of pressure deformity and infection. Examine the tympanic membrane in patients with external ear injuries caused by hot liquids or chemicals. Burns associated with electrical injury, including lightning strikes, also require examination of the tympanic membrane. A high incidence of rupture occurs with this mechanism of injury.

5. Perineum—Burns of the perineum are difficult to manage on an outpatient basis and are more susceptible to infection than are other types of burns.

D. Presence of Circumferential Burns

Any deep circumferential burn is a potential major injury. Circumferential deep burns of the neck may cause lymphatic and venous obstruction that leads to laryngeal edema and airway obstruction. Circumferential burns of the extremities may restrict blood flow, causing an increase in tissue pressure and ischemia. Circumferential chest wall injuries may impede chest wall movement and lead to respiratory failure.

Table 45–2. Characteristics of Burn Depth.

	Depth of Burn	Color and Appearance	Skin Texture	Capillary Refill	Pain/Pinprick	Healing
1st degree	Superficial epidermis	Red	Normal	Yes	Yes	5–10 days; no scar
2nd degree	Superficial partial thickness	Red; may be blistered	Edematous	Yes	Yes	10–21 days; no or minimal scar
	Deep partial thickness	Pink to white	Thick	Possibly	Possibly	25–60 days; dense scar
3rd degree	Full thickness	White, black, or brown	Leathery	No	No	No spontaneous healing
4th degree	Involves underlying subcutaneous tissue, tendon, or bone	Variable	Variable	No	No	No spontaneous healing

E. Inhalation Injury

Inhalation injury signifies a major burn. Signs and symptoms suggestive of inhalational injury include burns sustained in a confined space, singed nasal nares, soot around the nares, carbonaceous sputum, hoarseness, stridor, respiratory distress, and a carboxyhemoglobin level >10%. Diagnosis and management of inhalation injuries are discussed below.

F. Electrical Injury

Damage from electrical injury may be extensive, even though the outward signs of injury are minimal. Cardiac arrhythmias and renal failure from myoglobinuria are possible complications. Electrical currents as little as 100 milliamps can cause ventricular fibrillation. All electrical injuries should be considered major injuries.

G. Age of the Patient

The mortality rate from burn injury is increased in very young or very old patients; these are also the age groups in which burns most commonly occur. Burns in a child younger than 5 years or in an adult older than 55 years are more likely to be serious than are burns in other age groups.

H. Associated Injuries

Burns may occur in patients with other injuries, such as fractures or internal injuries due to vehicular accidents, falls, or explosions. The associated injuries often place the patient at increased risk of serious complications or death, even though the burns themselves are small.

I. Major Underlying Medical Problems

Major pre-existing medical problems in a burn patient are associated with an increased rate of serious complications and death. Any pre-existing condition that prevents normal healing puts a patient with even minor burns at risk for complication. Patients with a history of myocardial infarction, angina, significant pulmonary disease, diabetes mellitus, or renal failure are considered poor-risk patients even if their burns are not serious. Burned patients with a history of alcohol or other drug abuse are also at higher risk for complications following burn injury.

▶ Control Pain

Oral, subcutaneous, or intramuscular administration of narcotic analgesics may provide adequate pain relief for outpatients; however, in patients with moderate or major burn injuries an intravenous opiate such as morphine should be carefully titrated to control pain. Ventilator support may be required in some patients to permit adequate pain control. Recent studies evaluating pain control in burn patients have shown that large amounts of opiates increase the fluid requirements for adequate resuscitation. Fluid volumes should be monitored and adjusted accordingly.

▶ Provide Appropriate Wound Care

Gently remove clothing, dirt, and other foreign material adhering to the burn; irrigation with sterile saline (at room temperature) may be helpful. Do not scrub wounds or use harsh detergents or chemical disinfectants (eg, benzalkonium chloride, povidone–iodine). Little or no debridement of moderate or major wounds should be performed in the emergency department. Redundant skin from ruptured blisters of minor superficial partial-thickness burns may be removed. The wounds of patients with moderate or major burns, especially those who will be transferred to a burn facility, should not be treated with topical ointments or complex dressings in the emergency department, because these will have to be removed for evaluation upon arrival at the receiving facility. A simple nonadherent dressing such as petrolatum-impregnated gauze or sterile saline-soaked dressings should be applied instead. Administer tetanus prophylaxis if indicated. Direct communication with the accepting physician at the burn center can provide specific and individualized instructions for wound care prior to transfer.

▶ Transfer the Patient to a Burn Center

All major burns and many moderate burn injuries are best treated in a burn center, which has the personnel, equipment, and expertise needed to treat major burns effectively. When a patient with a serious burn is first evaluated, the closest burn center should be contacted immediately, so that recommendations for care can be obtained and plans made for transfer, if indicated. If transfer can be carried out quickly, escharotomy may be performed at the receiving facility in patients with circumferential burns of the extremities, chest, or neck and who do not have signs of respiratory compromise or tissue ischemia. Fluid resuscitation and all other supportive measures should be continued during transport, and the patient should be kept warm. See Table 45–3 for treatment and transfer criteria.

▼ OUTPATIENT MANAGEMENT OF MINOR BURNS

▶ General Considerations

Burns that meet the criteria for outpatient management may be treated initially in the emergency department, after which arrangements should be made for close follow-up on an outpatient basis.

▶ Treatment

First-degree burns (erythema only) are best treated with application of nonadherent dressings (eg, petrolatum-impregnated gauze). Clean deeper burns by gently irrigating them with sterile normal saline solution. Studies have shown faster healing of burn wounds by leaving blisters intact, so minimal debridement should be performed. Open blisters

Table 45–3. Summary of American Burn Association Classification of Burn Severity.

	Mild	Moderate	Major
Criteria	<10% TBSA in adults <5% TBSA in children or elderly No 3rd degree burns	10–20% TBSA superficial burns in adults 5–10% TBSA superficial burns in children or elderly No 3rd degree burns Suspected inhalation injury Circumferential burn Concomitant medical problems	>20% TBSA partial thickness burns in adults >10% TBSA partial thickness burns in children or the elderly 3rd degree burns in any age group High voltage burns, including lightening Burns that involve the face, hands, feet, genitalia, perineum, or major joints Chemical burns Inhalation injury Concomitant trauma Inability to provided appropriate care at current facility
Disposition	Outpatient Management	Hospital Admission	Referral to Burn Center

can be unroofed with removal of nonadherent epidermal fragments. Wounds may be covered with a topical antibiotic such as silver sulfadiazine cream or triple antibiotic ointment and wrapped in a bulky dressing. Instruct the patient to keep the wound clean and to change dressings and apply topical antibiotic cream twice a day at home. A nonadherent, semipermeable, polyurethane dressing (eg, Epi-Lock), which is left in place for 5–7 days, may be an acceptable alternative for some patients. Such dressings should be covered with roll gauze, which is changed daily. Have the patient elevate affected extremities to minimize development of edema. All patients should receive tetanus prophylaxis. Prophylactic systemic antibiotics are not indicated. Control pain with oral opiate analgesics or a combination of NSAIDs and opiates.

▶ Disposition

Patients should be seen on an outpatient basis in 1–2 days. Ruptured blisters or dead tissue may be debrided at that time. Promptly treat any minor infection with oral antistaphylococcal drugs (eg, dicloxacillin, 250–500 mg orally four times a day, children <40 kg, 25–50 mg/kg/d orally divided into four equal doses; or a first-generation cephalosporin such as cephalexin, 250–500 mg orally four times a day, children, 25–50 mg/kg/d orally divided into two or four equal doses). Patients who develop infections (fever, extensive cellulitis , lymphadenitis), poor-risk patients (diabetics), and unreliable patients must be hospitalized for administration of parenteral antibiotics and continued wound care.

American Burn Association: Guidelines for the operation of burn centers. http://www.ameriburn.org/Chapter14.pdf Chicago, IL, 2006 [Last Accessed on March 19, 2010].

Brebbia J, Singer AJ, Soroff HH: Management of local burn wounds in the ED. Am J Emerg Med 2007;25:666–671 [PMID: 17606093].

Fish, RM, Geddes, LA: Conduction of electrical current to and through the human body: a review. Eplasty 2009; 9:e44 (Last Accessed on March 19, 2010) [PMID: 19907637].

Wibbenmeyer L, Sevier A, Liao J: The impact of opioid administration on resuscitation volumes in thermally injured patients. J Burn Care Res 2010;31:48–56 [PMID: 20061837].

▼ SMOKE INHALATION INJURY

See Figure 45–1.

 ESSENTIALS OF DIAGNOSIS

- ▶ Look for evidence of thermal injury (airway edema)
- ▶ Consider signs of chemical injury to lung parenchyma
- ▶ Evaluate for carbon monoxide toxicity

THERMAL INJURY

▶ Mechanism

Patients who have been trapped in a fire in a confined space inhale superheated gases and may have thermal injury to the mouth, oropharynx, and larynx. Direct flame injury of the face and neck may also occur and are associated with development of marked upper airway edema and possible airway obstruction. Because of the efficient thermal exchange system of the upper airway, direct thermal injury to the lower respiratory tract is unusual. Rarely, exposure to water or steam in the heated gas mixture may produce thermal damage in the lower trachea and bronchi.

Clinical Findings

Upper airway thermal injury should be suspected in any patient exposed to a fire occurring in a confined location and in patients with obvious neck or facial burns. Soot around the nares, carbonaceous sputum, singed nasal vibrissae, and burned facial hairs are also indicators of thermal injury to the upper airway. Patients may complain of dyspnea; there may be stridor, drooling, or dysphonia. A lack of these findings does not exclude injury. Thermal injury to cutaneous tissues leads to widespread generalized edema which can involve the airway. The diagnosis is confirmed by visualization of the larynx by direct or video-laryngoscopy, or by flexible fiberoptic scope.

CHEMICAL INJURY

Mechanism

Chemical injury to the airways and lung parenchyma may be caused by noxious products from combustion of flammable materials (Table 45–4). Some of these products are directly toxic to the airways and lung parenchyma. Only the most commonly produced toxins are discussed below.

1. Acrolein—Acrolein is a highly reactive aldehyde that results from combustion of wood and petroleum products. It rapidly reacts with lung and airway tissues, causing injury by protein denaturation. Prolonged inhalation or exposure to high concentrations (>150 parts per million) for short periods of time (minutes) can be fatal. Lesser exposure causes pulmonary edema due to alveolar capillary leakage, bronchorrhea and bronchospasm (which may be severe), and ventilation -perfusion disturbances that cause hypoxemia that may persist even after the person is no longer exposed to smoke. Acrolein also causes conjunctivitis and ocular tearing at low concentrations.

Table 45–4. Common Toxic Products of Combustion.

Material Burned	Toxic Product
Wood, paper, cotton	Acrolein, acetaldehyde, formaldehyde, acetic acid, formic acid, nitrogen dioxide, carbon monoxide
Polyvinyl chloride	Hydrochloric acid, phosgene, chlorine
Polyurethane	Hydrocyanic acid, isocyanates (eg, toluene diisocyanate), carbon monoxide
Petroleum products	Acrolein, acetic acid, formic acid
Agricultural wastes, automobile exhaust	Nitrogen dioxide and other oxides of nitrogen; acetic acid; formic acid; carbon monoxide

2. Hydrochloric acid—Hydrochloric acid is one of the main products of combustion of polyvinyl chloride, a material commonly found in the structural components of houses and high-rise buildings as well as in furnishings and plastics. Hydrolysis occurs when hydrochloric acid comes in contact with the mucosa of the upper airway and tracheobronchial tree, causing protein denaturation and cell death. Even limited exposure may cause marked ocular irritation and tearing, although individuals with repeated or prolonged exposure may become desensitized to this effect. More severe exposure is associated with dyspnea, chest pain, and irritation of mucous membranes. Onset of pulmonary edema may be delayed for 2–12 hours after exposure, and the patient may appear asymptomatic in the interim. Toxic levels of hydrochloric acid gas may persist for as long as 1 hour after a fire has been extinguished. Patients exposed to products of combustion of polyvinyl chloride may also demonstrate premature ventricular contractions and may be at risk for development of lethal cardiac arrhythmias.

3. Toluene diisocyanate—Toluene diisocyanate is a product of combustion of polyurethane, a synthetic material found in almost all homes and offices, where it is used in seat cushions, mattresses, and carpet backing. Toluene diisocyanate is also found in insulation material. Toluene diisocyanate may cause severe bronchospasm, especially in persons with underlying obstructive lung disease, and it is also an ocular irritant.

4. Nitrogen dioxide—Nitrogen dioxide is produced in fires involving automobiles or agricultural wastes. It is an uncommon though important toxin, because even brief exposures to high concentrations may cause severe bronchospasm, laryngospasm, and pulmonary edema. If the patient survives, late development of bronchiolitis fibrosa obliterans and chronic interstitial lung disease may occur.

5. Other noxious products—Particulate matter in smoke may stimulate irritant receptors in the large airways and cause bronchoconstriction.

Clinical Findings

Chemical injury to the airways and lung parenchyma is difficult to diagnose in the emergency department. Wheezes, rales, rhonchi, and voice changes may be noted or initially absent in these patients. Direct laryngoscopy or flexible fiberoptic bronchoscopy may reveal mucosal friability and edema of the airways. Fiberoptic bronchoscopy is the burn center standard but is limited to upper airway evaluation. Initially the chest X-ray is often normal and serves as a baseline; noncardiogenic pulmonary edema may develop hours after exposure. Xenon lung scans, pulmonary function tests, and nitrogen washout studies have all been used to document the extent of pulmonary involvement but are not commonly available in the ED.

SYSTEMIC CHEMICAL POISONING

▶ Mechanism

1. Carbon monoxide—(See Chapter 47) The most widely recognized and most common complication of smoke inhalation is carbon monoxide poisoning. Carbon monoxide is a product of incomplete combustion and is produced in varying amounts in all fires. Carbon monoxide binds to hemoglobin with an affinity that is 260 times greater than that of oxygen, forming carboxyhemoglobin. The presence of even small amounts of carboxyhemoglobin drastically alters the affinity of the remaining unbound hemoglobin. Thus, even small concentrations of carbon monoxide may markedly reduce the binding of oxygen to hemoglobin, and the carbon monoxide that is bound is not easily displaced by oxygen. The presence of carboxyhemoglobin shifts the oxy-hemoglobin dissociation curve to the left, making it more difficult for hemoglobin to release bound oxygen to the tissues. The net result is tissue hypoxia and lactic acidosis due to cellular anaerobic metabolism. Carbon monoxide also inhibits mitochondrial function. Brain damage due to excitatory amino acids, inflammation, and oxidative stress may occur. In high concentrations, carbon monoxide is also bound to myoglobin, and may lead to rhabdomyolysis with myoglobinuria and renal failure. The half-life of carboxyhemoglobin is about 4–5 hours, which can be reduced to 60 minutes by administration of 100% oxygen.

2. Cyanide—(See Chapter 47) Reports have documented the presence of cyanide in the smoke of residential fires. Because of the difficulties in measuring cyanide levels in patients and because of the difficulty in recognizing smoke-related cyanide poisoning, the clinical relevance of cyanide poisoning in smoke inhalation is uncertain. Because there are risks associated with traditional treatments of cyanide poisoning—which involves the production of methemoglobin by infusion of sodium nitrite—in a patient who also demonstrates carboxyhemoglobinemia, this empiric therapy for cyanide poisoning is not recommended. More recent evaluation of newer cyanide antidotes continues to develop. Sodium thiosulfate and hydroxocobalamin have potential as empiric treatments in suspected cyanide poisoning.

▶ Clinical Findings

1. Carbon monoxide—Systemic chemical poisoning due to carbon monoxide should be suspected in every victim of fire and may be confirmed by measuring the serum carboxy-hemoglobin level. The often-described cherry-red skin color is not a frequent or reliable finding in patients with carbon monoxide poisoning. Similarly, arterial blood gas measurements are not reliable determinants of carbon monoxide poisoning, because PaO_2 and the calculated percentage of oxygen saturation of hemoglobin (the value

that is routinely reported by clinical laboratories) are not affected by carboxyhemoglobin. The oxygen saturation measured by pulse oximetry does not distinguish oxyhemoglobin from carboxyhemoglobin. Hence, the actual saturation is obtained by subtracting the percent of carboxyhemoglobin from the measured saturation obtained from the pulse oximeter.

Typical nonexposed, nonsmoking individuals may have serum carboxyhemoglobin levels of up to 1%; smokers usually have levels of 4–6%. Levels above 10% signify significant exposure and may be associated with symptoms as outlined in Chapter 47. Patients may be asymptomatic when carboxyhemoglobin levels are below 10–15%. Levels higher than 50–60% are associated with a high incidence of coma and seizures, and levels higher than 70% are frequently fatal. Myocardial ischemia or infarction and cardiac arrhythmias occur frequently, especially in patients with underlying atherosclerotic heart disease. Some patients who initially appear to have recovered may experience delayed onset of a neurologic syndrome characterized by dementia, ataxia, and other sensory and motor abnormalities. This syndrome may be due to infarcts in the globus pallidus. Loss of consciousness may be transitory.

2. Cyanide—Sustained loss of consciousness, dilated pupils, seizures, and hypotension are findings that are more likely in cyanide poisoning. Tachypnea may be followed by central apnea. Lactate levels correlate strongly with toxin levels.

▶ Treatment

For the critically ill patient, proceed as outlined earlier in this chapter. If there are signs of thermal injury to the airway, endotracheal intubation is indicated. In patients with major burns (particularly greater than 40–60% total body surface area), even if the airway is patent initially, edema frequently occurs minutes or hours later. Prophylactic intubation prevents a subsequent difficult intubation or surgical airway.

Obtain arterial blood gas and carboxyhemoglobin determinations in all patients with possible smoke inhalation. While waiting for the results, give 100% oxygen by tight-fitting reservoir mask or, if indicated, by endotracheal tube. Avoid alkalosis and hypothermia, which decrease the dissociation of carbon monoxide from hemoglobin. Indications for hyperbaric oxygen therapy have been described as a carboxyhemoglobin level greater than 25%, neurologic symptoms, seizures, pregnancy, or depressed consciousness. The efficacy of hyperbaric oxygen in clinical management remains unproved and its use cannot be mandated. Although therapy shortens the half-life of carboxyhemoglobin to roughly 20 minutes, the hazards and the length of time involved in transporting a critically ill patient to the nearest hyperbaric oxygen facility and the limited resuscitative environment of the chamber may outweigh the benefits of treatment. Hyperbaric oxygenation may be useful in the severely poisoned patient who fails to respond to therapy with 100% oxygen. If carboxyhemoglobin levels are under 2% and if oxygenation is adequate, the inspired oxygen content can be decreased. In stable patients with suspected thermal or chemical injury of the airway, evaluate mucosa injury using direct laryngoscopy.

Obtain an ECG, and monitor cardiac rhythm. Carbon monoxide poisoning is associated with myocardial ischemia and cardiac arrhythmias. Obtain a chest X-ray to look for signs of lung injury if smoke inhalation has occurred and to serve as a baseline for further changes. Give inhaled and parenteral bronchodilators to patients with clinical evidence of bronchospasm. Obtain a urine specimen for assessment of myoglobinuria. No evidence supports the use of prophylactic antibiotics or systemic corticosteroids in the treatment of inhalation injuries.

▶ Disposition

Because victims of smoke inhalation may develop late respiratory failure, these patients should be hospitalized for 24 hours for observation. All patients with carboxyhemoglobin levels higher than 25% should be hospitalized. Patients who present to the emergency department with respiratory compromise or respiratory failure should be hospitalized in an intensive care unit.

Cancio LC: Airway management and smoke inhalation injury in the burn patient. Clin Plast Surg 2009;36:555–567 [PMID: 19793551].

Hall AH, Dart R, Bogdan G: Sodium thiosulfate or hydroxocobalamin for the empiric treatment of cyanide poisoning? Ann Emerg Med 2007;49:806–813 [PMID: 17098327].

Mlcak RP, Suman OE, Herndon DN: Respiratory management of inhalation injury. Burns 2007;33:2–13 [PMID: 17223484].

Smollin CG: Toxicology: pearls and pitfalls in the use of antidotes. Emerg Med Clin North Am 2010;28:149–161 [PMID: 19945604].

Wolf SJ, Lavonas EJ, Sloan EP: Clinical policy: critical issues in the management of adult patients presenting to the emergency department with acute carbon monoxide poisoning. Ann Emerg Med 2009;51:138–152 [PMID: 18206551].

▼ EMERGENCY TREATMENT OF SPECIFIC TYPES OF BURNS

CHEMICAL BURNS

▶ General Considerations

Most chemical burns result from exposure of the skin to strong acids or alkalis. Other chemicals that may cause skin damage include phosphorus and phenol. Because full development of chemical burns is slower than that of other types, the size of chemical burns is usually underestimated during initial evaluation.

▶ Clinical Findings

Definitive diagnosis of chemical burns depends on the history. The physician should try to ascertain both the type of the chemical involved and its concentration. Physical examination of a patient unable to give a history may aid in diagnosis. Alkali burns are frequently full-thickness injuries, appear pale, and feel leathery and slippery. Acid burns are usually partial-thickness injuries and are accompanied by erythema and erosion. Skin is stained black by hydrochloric acid, yellow by nitric acid, and brown by sulfuric acid.

▶ Treatment

The mainstay of treatment of any chemical burn is copious irrigation with large amounts of tap water. To be most effective, treatment should be started immediately after exposure, preferably before arrival in the emergency department.

Remove any contaminated clothing while preventing personnel exposure. Do not attempt to neutralize the burn with weak reciprocal chemicals (acids for alkali burns or alkali for acid burns), because the heat generated from the chemical reaction may cause severe thermal injury. Occasionally the leathery skin of an alkali burn may make it difficult to completely wash away the alkali, and injury may continue; further irrigation and emergency excision of burned tissue by a surgeon experienced in this procedure may be indicated. Typical cutaneous burn care including pain control and fluid replacement should follow. After copious irrigation *with water,* the following treatment for specific types of chemical burns may be used:

A. Hydrofluoric Acid

Hydrofluoric acid dissociates into its component ions, and acts more like an alkali—penetrating the tissue to cause liquefaction necrosis. Insoluble salts may also form and further damage tissues. Cover burns with calcium gluconate (2.5%) gel prepared by mixing 3.5 g of calcium gluconate powder in 150 cc of water-soluble lubricant (eg K-Y jelly), secured by an occlusive cover. Remove and rinse the gel after 15 minutes and repeat the process until pain relief is achieved. In fingertip burns, the fluoride ion often penetrates under the nail bed and matrix, so that it is usually wise to remove the nail or make a large wedge. For persistent pain or more severe burns, the treatment of choice is subcutaneous and intradermal injections of calcium gluconate (10%), 0.5 mL/cm^2 of burned area by a 30-gauge needle. Larger volumes should not be used, especially in the fingers, because further damage may occur from compartment pressure or the intrinsic toxicity of calcium. Calcium chloride should not be used as it may cause further damage. For extremely severe burns, some physicians recommend intra-arterial perfusion of calcium.

B. Phenol

After copious high-pressure irrigation with water, enhance the removal of phenol by applying polyethylene glycol, which increases the solubility of phenol. Caution is advised with this practice to avoid spreading the area of exposed phenol. Follow with additional water irrigation.

C. Phosphorus

Phosphorus, a potent oxidizing agent found in certain types of ammunition, ignites and melts on air contact and often leaves embedded deposits on the skin. Thermal and chemical burns can be present simultaneously. Immersion in cool water is recommended, followed by attempts to remove embedded material. Hypocalcemia and hyperphosphatemia may result after systemic absorption. Telemetry monitoring is necessary in the case of electrolyte derangement until corrected, as bradycardia or other arrhythmias may occur. Previous recommendations were to apply a solution of copper sulfate to inactivate the phosphorus and aid in its removal. However, systemic toxicity including hemolysis, renal and cardiovascular failure from copper absorption may occur and this practice is no longer recommended. The copper is not an antidote or inactivating agent, but turns phosphorous particulate black to aid in removal. A Wood's lamp may be used alternatively to illuminate the particles and aid in their removal.

Fluid resuscitation in the patient with large chemical burns is the same as that for patients with similar-size thermal burns. Because the size of chemical burns may be underestimated initially, reevaluate the patient after 24–48 hours.

▶ Disposition

The choice between hospitalization and outpatient management of chemical burns should be made using the same criteria as for thermal burns. Noting that the full extent of skin injury may not be readily apparent during an initial emergency department evaluation, inpatient observation is frequently recommended for chemical burns.

TAR BURNS

▶ General Considerations

Road or paving tar may be heated to 135–149°C for application, and roofing tar is heated to 232–260°C. The hands, arms, head, and neck are the most commonly burned areas.

▶ Treatment

Cool the tar immediately with water, which often separates the tar from the skin. If the tar continues to adhere, either leave it in place or apply one of the commercially available cream- or oil-based solvents specially made for this purpose. Shur-Clens®, triple-antibiotic ointment, and mineral oil are among the many reported options to attempt separation. Do not use hydrocarbon solvents, such as paint thinner or gasoline, because they may further injure burned skin. Cover the wound with sterile dressings. When dressings are changed after 6–24 hours, much of the tar will have separated and will be removed with the dressings. Initial stabilization of the patient with large tar burns should follow the procedures outlined for thermal burns.

▶ Disposition

The criteria for admission or transfer to a burn center for patients with tar burns are the same as for patients with thermal burns.

SUNBURN

▶ General Considerations

Most sunburns are first-degree (erythema) or superficial partial-thickness (blisters) burns. Skin changes from sunburn are maximal about 12–24 hours after exposure. Patients usually present to the emergency department for pain relief. Occasionally a patient with extensive superficial partial-thickness burns will require fluid resuscitation and parenteral analgesics for pain control.

▶ Clinical Findings

Diagnosis is based on a history of exposure to the sun (or to ultraviolet light in tanning beds) and physical findings of erythema and blistering.

▶ Treatment

Sunburn can be difficult to treat. Saline-soaked dressings or calamine lotion may provide some relief from pain and itching. Ibuprofen and other nonsteroidal anti-inflammatory agents work by blocking the production of prostaglandins that are thought to be important mediators of pain in sunburned skin. Oral and topical corticosteroids have not been shown to significantly improve symptoms or decrease healing time. Patients with extensive partial-thickness sunburn should receive treatment according to the guidelines described for other thermal burns.

▶ Disposition

Almost all patients with sunburn may receive treatment on an outpatient basis. If there are large blisters, the patient should be seen again in 2–3 days to make sure that secondary infection has not developed. Patients should be advised to avoid prolonged ultraviolet light exposure to the sun in the future and to use a sunscreen (eg, over-the-counter preparations containing PABA [*p*-aminobenzoic acid] or dioxybenzone) before exposure. Patients requiring fluid resuscitation or parenteral analgesics should be hospitalized.

ELECTRICAL BURNS

See Chapter 46.

OCULAR BURNS

See also Chapter 31.

ESSENTIALS OF DIAGNOSIS

- ▶ High level of suspicion in patients with facial burns
- ▶ Evaluate for foreign bodies
- ▶ Examine eyes with fluorescein

▶ General Considerations

Patients with thermal facial burns may also have burns to the eyelid and the eye itself. Chemical burns constitute one of the most common work-related injuries seen in U.S. emergency departments. Both types of burns may be associated with the development of massive periorbital edema that makes delayed examination difficult. Injury of the cornea or anterior chamber may occur and lead to permanent vision loss. It is therefore important that patients with suspected ocular burns be examined promptly, preferably in the emergency department.

▶ Clinical Findings

Instill tetracaine, 0.5%, or proparacaine, 0.5%, in the conjunctival sac to decrease pain during examination. Systemic analgesia should also be provided when needed. Retract and evert the eyelids to look for foreign bodies. Remove particulates and contact lenses to prevent injury to the cornea due to pressure from edematous lids. Assess visual acuity. Corneal abrasions and thermal injury may be detected by instilling fluorescein in the conjunctival sac and examining the eye using the blue light on an ophthalmoscope or, if the patient's condition permits, a slit lamp. Most ocular burns cause uveitis, and cell and flare in the anterior chamber are apparent. Cycloplegics are indicated to prevent synechiae. Phenylephrine is contraindicated.

▶ Treatment

Irrigate any suspected chemical burn of the eye with large amounts (at least 2 L) of sterile normal saline using a Morgan lens. Tap water and Ringers Lactate are sufficient alternatives. Restoration of physiologic pH is paramount, and irrigation should continue to this end. Treat corneal abrasions and thermal injuries by instilling an ophthalmic antibiotic in the conjunctival sac. Alkali burns cause liquefaction necrosis rapidly, may require larger amounts of irrigating fluid, and require emergency ophthalmologic consultation. 1% calcium gluconate drops should be considered for hydrofluoric acid exposure, but only used after discussion with an ophthalmologist.

▶ Disposition

Burns of the eyes are major injuries. Obtain urgent ophthalmologic consultation.

CIRCUMFERENTIAL BURNS OF NECK, CHEST, AND EXTREMITIES

▶ General Considerations

Circumferential deep burns of the neck may cause lymphatic and venous obstruction leading to laryngeal edema and airway obstruction. Circumferential chest wall injuries may impede chest wall movement and lead to respiratory failure. Circumferential burns of the extremities may restrict blood flow, causing increased tissue pressure with resultant ischemia. Scarring can also restrict range of motion and affect fine motor function.

▶ Clinical Findings

Patients with deep circumferential neck wounds should undergo direct visualization of the larynx by laryngoscopy. Because laryngeal edema may develop hours after initial examination, frequent reevaluation may be necessary.

Monitor patients with circumferential chest wounds for signs of respiratory compromise (tachypnea, dyspnea, deteriorating arterial blood gas levels); measurement of forced vital capacity or peak airway pressure may be useful.

Carefully examine the extremity distal to the wound in patients with circumferential burns of the extremities. Look for evidence of ischemia (diminished pulses, poor capillary refill, anesthesia); loss of vibratory sense is an early sign. If available, a Doppler ultrasound device is useful to assess distal blood flow. Because edema continues to develop during the first 6–8 hours after burn injury of the extremities, frequent reevaluation is important.

▶ Treatment

Patients with deep circumferential burns of the neck are candidates for early endotracheal intubation. Elevate the injured limb(s) of patients with circumferential wounds of the extremities in order to minimize development of edema. Remove rings or other jewelry that could act as a tourniquet when edema develops. If evidence of distal ischemia develops, escharotomy is indicated. Ideally this should be performed in a burn center by a surgeon experienced in this procedure. Occasionally escharotomy must be performed in the emergency department before the patient is transported to a burn center for definitive care. Sterilize the overlying skin and make medial and lateral incisions through the eschar using a No. 20 scalpel or electrocautery. Incise deeply enough to cut entirely through the burned skin and release the constricting eschar, being careful to avoid neurovascular structures (typically this occurs at the level of the subcutaneous fat). No anesthesia should be required as full-thickness burns are insensate. Blood loss is seldom significant but can be controlled by cautery or suture if necessary.

Patients with a circumferential chest wall burn may require escharotomy in the emergency department. Using sterile technique, incise the eschar along the anterior axillary line bilaterally to the costal margins, and then join these incisions with incisions along the costal margins and just below the clavicles. This releases a segment of chest wall eschar that can move with respiratory excursion.

▶ Disposition

All patients with deep circumferential burns of the neck, extremities, or chest wall should be hospitalized, preferably in a burn center.

BURNS DUE TO CHILD ABUSE

ESSENTIALS OF DIAGNOSIS

▶ High index of suspicion
▶ Discrepancy between the history and physical findings

▶ General Considerations

Burns represent 8–14% of child abuse injuries seen in the United States; about 15% of abused children have been intentionally burned at some time.

▶ Clinical Findings

Suspect child abuse if there is a delay in seeking medical care, if there is a history of other injuries, or if there is a discrepancy between the history and the physical findings. The injuries most commonly encountered in the emergency department are burns of the buttocks and perineum caused by scalding immersion in hot water in children who are being toilet-trained and cigarette burns in children of any age.

▶ Treatment and Disposition

The treatment of burns in children is the same as that of a burn of comparable size in any other patient, but if there is any suspicion that the injury was due to abuse, *the child must be hospitalized and the attending physician informed of the emergency physician's suspicions.* By law, suspected child abuse must be reported to the appropriate child welfare authorities. Obtain consultation with appropriate personnel as soon as possible (eg, social worker, nurse, psychologist, pediatrician).

Dissanaike S, Wishnew J, Rahimi M et al: Burns as child abuse: risk factors and legal issues in west Texas and eastern New Mexico. J Burn Care Res 2010;31:176–183 [PMID: 20061853].

Frank M, Schmucker U, Nowotny T et al: Not all that glistens is gold: civilian white phosphorus burn injuries. Am J Emerg Med 2008;26:974 [PMID: 18926385].

Faurschou A, Wulf HC: Topical corticosteroids in the treatment of acute sunburn: a randomized, double-blind clinical trial. Arch Dermatol 2008;144:620–624 [PMID: 18490588].

Orgill DP, Piccolo N: Escharotomy and decompressive therapies in burns. J Burn Care Res 2009;30:759–768 [PMID: 19692906].

Robinett DA, Shelton B, Dyer KS: Special considerations in hazardous materials burns. J Emerg Med 2010;39:544–553 [PMID: 18403172].

Salzman M, O'Malley RN: Updates on the evaluation and management of caustic exposures. Emerg Med Clin North Am 2007;25:459–476 [PMID: 17482028].

Spector J, Fernandez WG: Chemical, thermal, and biological ocular exposures. Emerg Med Clin North Am 2008;26:125–136 [PMID:18249260].

Disorders Due to Physical & Environmental Agents

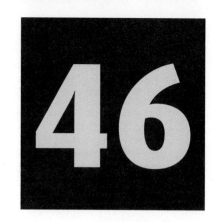

Rebecca C. Bowers, MD, FACEP

M. Virginia Mustain, MD[1]

EMERGENCY TREATMENT OF DISORDERS DUE TO COLD

Individuals vary considerably in their response to environmental cold. Factors that increase the possibility of injury due to cold include poor general physical condition, nonacclimatization, childhood or advanced age, systemic illness, and the use of alcohol and other sedative drugs. High wind velocity (wind-chill factor) and moisture may markedly increase the propensity for cold injury at low temperatures.

SYSTEMIC HYPOTHERMIA

 ESSENTIALS OF DIAGNOSIS

► Signs and symptoms depend on degree of hypothermia

► Rewarming methods include passive external, active external, and active internal rewarming

General Considerations

A. Healthy Persons

Accidental hypothermia occurs when an external cold challenge overwhelms an individual's capacity to produce or

[1]This chapter is a revision of the chapter by Shannon Waters, MD, from the 5th edition.

conserve heat. Hypothermia may occur in otherwise healthy individuals during occupational or recreational exposure to cold or as a result of accidents or other misfortunes. Alcohol and drug abuse is a common predisposing cause.

B. Persons with Predisposing Factors

Systemic hypothermia may follow exposure to even slightly lowered temperatures when preexisting altered homeostasis exists as a result of debility or disease. Accidental hypothermia is more likely to occur in elderly or inactive people and those with cardiovascular, dermatologic, or cerebrovascular disease; mental retardation; myxedema; hypopituitarism; or alcoholism. The use of sedative–hypnotic or antidepressant drugs may be a contributing factor.

▶ Clinical Findings

Because lowered body temperature is the sole finding in some patients brought to the emergency department, the diagnosis often depends on awareness of the possibility of hypothermia.

A. Temperature

In the hypothermic patient, oral and axillary temperatures are not accurate. Instead, rectal probes should be used. The temperature varies widely in hypothermia, and accurate monitoring is essential.

B. Symptoms and Signs

Hypothermia is classified as mild when core body temperature is between 34°C (93.2°F) and 36°C (96.8°F). Patients will exhibit tachycardia, tachypnea, and shivering. Hypothermia is moderate between 30°C (86°F) and 34°C. Loss of the shivering reflex and mild alterations in level of consciousness occur. Bradycardia and atrial fibrillation may start to appear. Hypothermia becomes severe below temperatures of 30°C. Patients may appear dead at this stage with fixed, dilated pupils, loss of other reflexes, and coma.

Ventricular fibrillation and asystole may occur spontaneously at core temperatures below 28°C (82.4°F). *Note*: For this reason, a hypothermic patient should not be considered dead until all reasonable resuscitative measures have failed. No one is dead until he or she is "warm and dead."

C. Laboratory Findings

Several laboratory findings are unique to hypothermia. Hypoglycemia, hypomagnesemia, and hypophosphatemia are common, particularly in alcoholics. Hyperglycemia may be seen as a result of hemorrhagic pancreatitis in patients with prolonged exposure to the cold. Sodium and potassium levels may be elevated or depressed. Arterial blood gas samples drawn at cold temperatures are generally analyzed at 37°C (98.6°F), which causes lowering of pH and elevation of PO_2 and PCO_2 readings. However, clinical therapy is based on the uncorrected determinations recorded at 37°C. The ECG tracing may show

prolongation of any conduction interval. Osborne or J wave, may appear below 32°C (89.6°F) (Figure 46–1).

D. Complications

Metabolic acidosis, pneumonia, pancreatitis, renal failure, sepsis, and ventricular fibrillation may occur. Death due to systemic hypothermia usually results from cardiac arrest associated with ventricular fibrillation, which may occur during rewarming.

E. Underlying Conditions

Obtain a brief history from witnesses or relatives of a patient with hypothermia, and perform a general physical and laboratory examination to detect underlying conditions that might predispose to hypothermia.

Examination should include an evaluation of renal function (uremia), thyroid function (myxedema), and adrenal function (Addison disease). If sepsis is a diagnostic possibility, obtain appropriate cultures.

▶ Treatment

Bundle the victim of suspected hypothermia in dry, warm blankets at the scene of discovery, and transport the person to the nearest hospital as soon as possible. Remove any wet garments. *Note*: Transport should be as gentle as possible because of the risk of cardiac arrhythmias due to increased myocardial irritability.

A. Cardiopulmonary Resuscitation

Adequacy of ventilation and circulation must be ensured by careful clinical observation, continuous ECG monitoring, and serial determinations of arterial blood gases. If cardiac arrest occurs, start cardiopulmonary resuscitation (CPR) (Chapter 9). If the victim has any detectable pulse or breathing, no matter how slow, do not initiate CPR; unnecessary brisk closed chest compression may induce ventricular fibrillation. Because of the protective effects of hypothermia, bradycardia and hypotension are generally well tolerated.

1. Establish an airway—Intubation of the unprotected airway and frequent suctioning may be required.

2. Breathing—Depression of the respiratory center in hypothermia causes hypoxemia or hypercapnia, requiring controlled ventilation and supplemental oxygen. Avoid hyperventilation, because a rapid fall in PCO_2 may trigger ventricular fibrillation.

3. Circulation—Check for a pulse for at least 1 minute. If a pulse is present, do not attempt to correct arrhythmia with drugs or cardioversion. This will be unsuccessful most of the time and may precipitate ventricular fibrillation. Begin the rewarming process (see below). If the patient is pulseless, begin CPR. Attempts at defibrillation are usually unsuccessful at temperatures below 30°C (86°F). If ventricular tachycardia/ fibrillation is present, attempt a shock at 360 J. If there is no success, continue CPR. At temperatures less than 30°C,

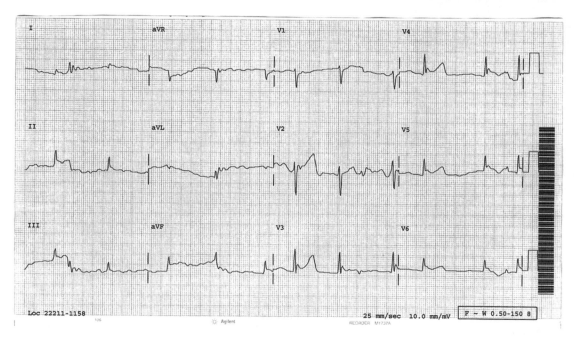

▲ **Figure 46–1.** Hypothermia. The patient is in atrial fibrillation with a slow ventricular response. The QRS complexes are narrow, and there is an additional positive slurred deflection, the J wave (Osborne wave), just prior to the ST segment.

withhold further defibrillation and intravenous medications. Begin aggressive rewarming in conjunction with basic CPR. If temperature is 30°C or greater, then continue with ACLS protocol but space intravenous medications longer than standard (decreased metabolism may induce toxicity of drugs).

4. Correct fluid, electrolyte, and glucose abnormalities—
Give thiamine (100 mg intravenously), naloxone (2.0 mg intravenously), and dextrose (25 g intravenously) to all patients with altered mental status who are thought to be hypothermic. Volume expansion with warmed fluid generally helps the rewarming process. Avoid lactated Ringer's solution because the lactate is not metabolized efficiently by a cold liver.

B. Treatment of Underlying Conditions

Treat underlying and predisposing conditions as necessary (eg, heart disease, hypoglycemia, malnutrition, adrenocortical insufficiency [hydrocortisone, 200 mg intravenously], hypothyroidism [levothyroxine, 400 micrograms intravenously, plus hydrocortisone, 100 mg intravenously]).

C. Rewarming

Rewarming is essential but potentially harmful, because peripheral vasodilatation may divert blood flow from internal organs to the skin and shunt cooled blood to the central circulation, causing a brief drop in core tempera-

ture. *Note*: Rapid rewarming may be hazardous, because hypothermic patients are particularly vulnerable to lethal cardiac arrhythmias. Core rewarming should be undertaken only if hypothermia is severe and the patient shows cardiovascular instability (eg, cardiac arrest and ventricular fibrillation).

1. Mild hypothermia (core temperature ≥34°C [93.2°F])—
Passive rewarming to prevent further heat loss is sufficient for most patients with mild hypothermia, because their thermoregulatory mechanism is intact, and many of these patients are able to generate heat by shivering. Most patients should be wrapped in dry, heated blankets and carefully monitored. Ambient air temperature can be warmed with radiant heat sources. Patients with mild hypothermia who are otherwise healthy usually respond well to heated blankets and the administration of heated (45°C [113°F]) intravenous solutions. Patients must be carefully monitored when using any of these rewarming methods.

2. Moderate to severe hypothermia (core temperature <34°C)—
Moderate to severe hypothermia often requires additional rewarming measures, because thermoregulation is altered or absent. Individualized supportive care is mandatory, because active rewarming is hazardous. As mentioned previously, active core rewarming is necessary only for patients with cardiovascular instability.

A. ACTIVE EXTERNAL REWARMING METHODS—Heated blankets, forced-air blankets (Bair Hugger), or warm baths have been used, with a rate of rewarming of about 1–3°C/h. Because it is easier to monitor the patient and to carry out diagnostic and therapeutic procedures when heated blankets rather than warm baths are used for active rewarming, heated baths are not widely recommended. There is some potential risk with active external rewarming, because marked vasodilation may occur. Combining active external rewarming with active core rewarming may prevent the resultant hypotension and the core temperature after-drop, which are sometimes seen during rewarming. If active external rewarming is used, the patient should be carefully monitored and supported hemodynamically. The application of commercial heat packs directly to hypothermic skin may cause serious burns.

B. ACTIVE INTERNAL (CORE) REWARMING METHODS—Internal rewarming is suggested for patients with profound hypothermia of long duration in which there is suspected underlying debilitation, for patients with complications of cardiovascular or respiratory insufficiency, and for patients in cardiac arrest.

Repeated peritoneal dialysis may be performed using warm (45°C [113°F]) potassium-free dialysate solution or normal saline. The usual exchange rate is 6 L/h, which can increase the core temperature 1–3°C/h.

Warm fluids (crystalloid solutions) administered by gastrointestinal, colonic, or bladder lavage may be employed. Placement of a nasogastric tube is less invasive but may run the risk of stimulating ventricular dysrhythmias owing to the irritability of the hypothermic heart.

Administration of heated intravenous fluids contributes only 17 kcal/h, which accounts for an increase in body temperature of less than 1/3°C/L. Microwave rewarming of crystalloid solutions to 40–42°C (104–107.6°F) may be safely accomplished in about 2–3 minutes. This technique causes some hemolysis of erythrocytes, and if blood products are used they should be administered through a high-flow countercurrent fluid infuser or reconstituted with warmed normal saline.

Heated humidified oxygen, either via a tight-fitting mask or by endotracheal tube, will raise the core temperature 1 or 1.5–2°C/h, respectively.

Thoracic cavity lavage may achieve rapid rewarming with the added advantage of warming the heart more quickly. Insert two thoracostomy tubes, and continuously infuse fluid warmed to 41°C (105.8°F) through one tube and drain it through the other.

Extracorporeal blood rewarming methods are the gold standard for rewarming in the setting of severe cardiorespiratory compromise/arrest. This may be accomplished via cardiopulmonary bypass or hemodialysis. These methods of course are limited to the institutions that have the abilities to perform these functions.

D. Antimicrobials

Patients with severe hypothermia—especially those who are comatose—are at high risk for development of aspiration pneumonia; subsequent pulmonary, urinary tract, or intraperitoneal infections; and sepsis. Many hypothermic alcoholic, debilitated, or elderly patients will have an underlying infection, and the cause should be aggressively sought and treatment initiated.

If sepsis suspected, administer broad-spectrum antibiotics. Prophylactic antimicrobial drugs are unnecessary if infection is unlikely.

E. Complications of Rewarming

Observe the patient for signs of metabolic acidosis, cardiac arrhythmias, acute respiratory distress syndrome, pancreatitis, ischemic bowel, pneumonia, myoglobinuria with renal failure, or clotting abnormalities.

▶ Disposition

Hospitalize all patients who present with core temperatures below 34°C (93.2°F), especially if the sensorium is altered. Patients with coexisting illness and core temperatures under 35°C (95°F) should be hospitalized. The mortality rates in hypothermia are variable and depend on the cause of hypothermia and the patient's underlying condition.

COLD INJURY OF THE EXTREMITIES

ESSENTIALS OF DIAGNOSIS

▶ Tissue injury or death is caused by ischemia and thrombosis in capillaries or by formation of ice in the tissues
▶ Treatment of frostbite or chilblains depends on the severity of the skin injury and includes rewarming by both passive and active measures

In healthy individuals, exposure of the extremities to cold produces immediate localized vasoconstriction followed by reflex generalized vasoconstriction. When skin temperature falls to 25°C (77°F), tissue metabolism is slowed, but the relative demand for oxygen exceeds the supply from diminished circulation; thus, the area becomes cyanotic. At 15°C (59°F), tissue metabolism is markedly decreased and the dissociation of oxyhemoglobin is reduced, which may give the skin a pink, well-oxygenated appearance. Tissue damage occurs at this temperature. Tissue death may be caused either by ischemia and thrombosis in capillaries or by actual freezing. Frostbite is tissue freezing caused by formation of ice crystals in tissue. Frostbite occurs when skin temperature drops to 10–4°C (14–24.8 °F). The body's "hunting reaction," serves to protect the extremity from cold injury by alternating vasoconstriction with vasodilation in 5–10 minute cycles. This occurs with exposure to progressively colder temperatures. The incidence of frostbite depends on factors such as wind, moisture, mobility, venous stasis, trauma, malnutrition, and occlusive arterial disease.

1. Chilblains (Pernio)

▶ Clinical Findings

Chilblains, occurs with exposure to nonfreezing temperatures and is more common in children and women as well as people with any form of peripheral vascular disease. Chilblains are red or violaceous, painful skin lesions common on the ears, nose, hands, and feet. Lymphocytic vasculitis is common. Chilblains may be associated with edema or blistering and are subsequently aggravated by excessive warmth. With continued exposure, ulcerative or hemorrhagic lesions may appear and progress to scarring, fibrosis, and atrophy.

▶ Treatment and Disposition

Treatment of chilblains is mainly supportive. Elevate the affected part on pillows or sheepskin, and allow it to warm gradually at room temperature.

Do not rub or massage injured tissues or apply ice or heat. Protect the area from trauma and secondary infection. Refer the patient to a primary-care physician or clinic for follow-up. Nicardipine and steroids may also have a role in treatment.

2. Frostbite

▶ Clinical Findings

A. Classification

Frostbite is injury of the tissues due to freezing. The classification of injury is applied after rewarming, because the extent of injury is difficult to predict initially. Demarcation is not complete for up to 3–5 weeks.

1. First degree—Freezing without blistering; peeling is occasionally present.

2. Second degree—Freezing with clear blistering.

3. Third degree—Freezing with death of skin, hemorrhagic blisters, and subcutaneous involvement.

4. Fourth degree—Freezing with full-thickness involvement (including bone); ultimate loss or deformity of body part.

B. Symptoms and Signs

Frostbitten tissue appears white or blue–white, is firm or hard (frozen), cool to the touch, and generally insensitive. Skin loses sensation at around 10°C. Because cold injury produces anesthesia, many symptoms are not apparent until rewarming begins or the part is closely inspected. In patients with mild frostbite, the symptoms are numbness, paresthesias, pruritus, and lack of fine motor control. With increas-

ing severity, decreased range of motion, blister formation, and prominent swelling are noted. Thawing unmasks local tenderness and throbbing pain. The tissue becomes discolored, loses its elasticity, and becomes immobile. Profound edema, hemorrhagic blisters, necrosis, and gangrene may occur. Long-term sequel includes cold sensitivity, loss of sensation, and hyperhidrosis.

▶ Treatment

A. Systemic Hypothermia

Treat moderate to severe associated systemic hypothermia before managing frostbite.

B. Rewarming

1. Superficial frostbite—Rewarm extremities affected by superficial frostbite (frostnip) by removing wet clothing and applying constant warmth, which can be accomplished by exerting gentle pressure with a warm hand.

2. Full-thickness frostbite—Rapid rewarming is the most important aspect of management. It should not be attempted, however, if the potential for refreezing exists. Rewarming should be performed with a water bath or whirlpool containing an antimicrobial agent such as iodine or chlorhexidine. Water temperature of 40–42°C (104–107.6°F) is necessary. However, The State of Alaska Cold-injury Guidelines recommend a lower temperature of 37–39°C (98.6–102.2°F). This temperature causes less pain for the patient and only slightly prolongs rewarming. Rewarming should continue until a red-purple color appears and the skin becomes pliable. Recommended rewarming time is anywhere from 15 inutes up to 1 hour.

C. Resuscitation

Unless concomitant hypothermia exists, intravenous hydration is not usually necessary. Severe cases of frostbite have led to subsequent rhabdomyolysis with renal failure, which then requires aggressive hydration. Intravenous narcotics are almost always necessary secondary to the severe pain associated with rewarming.

D. Protection of the Injured Part

In the prehospital setting, padding, splinting, and avoidance of rewarming are all that is necessary. Once in the secure hospital setting and after rewarming has been achieved, avoidance of further trauma is important. Affected body parts should be elevated and padded, uncovered or loosely dressed, and left at room temperature. Debride clear blisters because prostaglandins and thromboxane are present in the exudate. Leave hemorrhagic blisters intact. Administer antitetanus prophylaxis. Apply aloe vera cream every 6 hours. Administer ibuprofen, 400–600 mg every 8–12 hours for 72 hours.

E. Anti-infective Measures

Infection prevention is important after rewarming. Maintain a sterile environment. Protect skin blebs from physical contact. Whirlpool therapy at temperatures of 32–38°C (89.6–100.4°F) twice daily for 30 minutes for a period of 3 or more weeks helps to cleanse the skin and debride superficial dead tissue. Penicillin prophylaxis is recommended in most cases.

F. Adjunctive Therapies

1. Anticoagulation—Consistent benefit from anticoagulation has not been demonstrated.

2. Vasodilators—Have been used with some success.

3. Thrombolysis—Small clinical studies with tissue plasminogen activator have demonstrated success in humans, but the results of larger, multicenter trials are needed.

4. Surgery—Amputation or debridement should not be considered until it is definitely established that tissues are dead. Although rare, the development of a compartment syndrome necessitates fasciotomy. The line of demarcation between injured and normal tissue may not appear until 6–12 weeks after injury; mummification of the injured extremity may require the same length of time. Technetium-99 pyrophosphate and MRI scanning accurately predicts the level of ultimate amputation. Regional sympathectomy performed 24–48 hours after injury has reportedly ameliorated the early sequel of frostbite, including a reduction in edema and decreased subsequent tissue loss. Appropriate clinical studies have yet to be performed to support the use of this therapy.

5. Hyperbaric oxygen—Disagreement still exists as to effectiveness of HBO therapy. Recent studies in humans have yielded good results.

▶ Disposition

Hospitalize all patients with second- or third-degree frostbite and patients with extensive areas of first-degree frostbite.

3. Immersion Syndrome (Immersion Foot; Trench Foot)

ESSENTIALS OF DIAGNOSIS

▶ Caused by prolonged immersion in cold water

▶ Alternating vasospasm and vasodilatation results in initial cold and anesthetic feet followed by blistering and ulceration

▶ Treatment includes rewarming and wound care

▶ Clinical Findings

Immersion foot (or hand) is caused by prolonged immersion in cool or cold water or mud that causes alternating arterial vasospasm and vasodilatation. The affected parts are first cold and anesthetic. Hyperemia follows after 24–48 hours, and the parts become warm, with intense burning and tingling pain. Blistering, swelling, redness, ecchymoses, and ulceration are noted. The posthyperemic phase occurs after 2–6 weeks and causes the limbs to become cyanotic, with increased sensitivity to cold. Complications include lymphangitis, cellulitis, thrombophlebitis, and wet gangrene.

▶ Prevention

Changing out of wet socks and shoes as soon as possible is paramount to the prevention of immersion syndrome. In the military, individuals at risk for immersion foot apply silicone ointment to the bottoms of their feet twice daily as a preventive measure.

▶ Treatment and Disposition

Treatment is best started during or before the stage of reactive hyperemia.

Immediate treatment consists of protecting the extremities from trauma and secondary infection. Rewarm the injured areas gradually by exposing them to air (not to ice or extreme heat). Do not soak or massage the skin. The patient should remain at bed rest until all ulcers have healed. Keep the affected parts elevated to aid in removal of edema fluid, and protect pressure sites (eg, heels) with pillows or booties lined with cotton batting. Give antimicrobials only if infection occurs.

Hospitalize all patients with immersion syndrome.

Bilgic S et al: Treating frostbite. Can Fam Physician 2008;54(3): 361–363 [PMID:18337529].

Imray C et al: Cold damage to the extremities: frostbite and non-freezing cold injuries. Postgrad Med J 2009;85:481–488.

Kuklang K: Protection of feet in cold exposure. Ind Health 2009;47(3):242–253 [PMID: 19531910].

Mohr W et al: Cold injury. Hand Clin 2009;25(4):481–496 [PMID: 19801122].

▼ EMERGENCY TREATMENT OF DISORDERS DUE TO HEAT

The five main disorders due to environmental heat stress are (1) heat edema, (2) heat syncope, (3) heat cramps, (4) heat exhaustion, and (5) heat stroke.

The body maintains temperature homeostasis via four main mechanisms: (1) conduction, (2) convection, (3) radiation, and (4) evaporation. When the body is unable to adequately regulate body temperature using these methods, heat illness occurs.

The extremely young and old, obese, and those with chronic physical and mental impairments have the highest risk of heat illness. The fully heat acclimatized and athletic, healthy individuals are also at risk, however, given the right environmental conditions, if they are impaired by drugs or alcohol, or if they are denied access to hydration and nutrition.

HEAT EDEMA

ESSENTIALS OF DIAGNOSIS

► Swelling of feet and ankles due to vasodilatation and venous stasis
► Treatment is elevation of the limbs

Nonacclimatized individuals, particularly the elderly, may develop swelling of the feet and ankles that is generally associated with periods of prolonged sitting or standing. The edema is not complicated by manifestations of congestive heart failure or lymphatic disease. The cause of heat edema is muscular and cutaneous vasodilation combined with venous stasis. Interstitial fluid then accumulates in the lower extremities. Because the problem is self-limited, treatment involves use of support hose and simple elevation of the lower limbs. Diuretics are not indicated.

HEAT SYNCOPE

ESSENTIALS OF DIAGNOSIS

► Caused by peripheral pooling of the intravascular volume
► Patient responds promptly to rest, cooling, and rehydration

Simple fainting may occur suddenly after exertion in the heat. Cutaneous and muscular vasodilation redistributes intravascular volume to the periphery of the body. Volume loss and prolonged standing (pooling in the lower extremities) also contribute to the development of inadequate central venous return and insufficient cerebral perfusion. The patient's skin is cool and moist, the pulse is weak, and transient hypotension occurs. In general, core temperature is normal or mildly elevated. The patient usually responds promptly to rest in a recumbent position, cooling, and oral rehydration. Evaluate elderly people who experience syncopal episodes for hypoglycemia, arrhythmias, and fixed myocardial or cerebrovascular lesions.

HEAT CRAMPS

ESSENTIALS OF DIAGNOSIS

► Spasms of the voluntary muscles of the abdomen and extremities
► Caused by salt depletion
► Treatment consists of fluid and salt replacement

▶ Clinical Findings

Heat cramps are due primarily to salt depletion and manifested by painful spasms of the voluntary muscles of the abdomen and extremities. The skin may be moist or dry, and cool or warm. Muscle fasciculations may be present. The core temperature is normal or only slightly elevated. Laboratory studies (rarely indicated) may reveal hemoconcentration and low serum sodium levels, although this is variable, and normal serum sodium levels are frequently noted. Hypokalemia occurs occasionally.

▶ Treatment and Disposition

Treatment includes oral fluid and salt replacement with 0.1–0.2% salt solution (¼–½ teaspoon table salt in one cup water) or, in severe cases, intravenous normal saline solution. Give supplementary potassium as dictated by measured serum levels. Replace glucose if needed. An alternative therapy for mild symptoms is a commercial electrolyte solution (eg, Gatorade). Place the patient in a cool place, and massage sore muscles gently.

The patient should rest for 1–3 days, depending on the severity of the attack. Hospitalization is usually not required.

HEAT EXHAUSTION

ESSENTIALS OF DIAGNOSIS

► Caused by either primary water loss or primary sodium loss due to prolonged heat exposure
► Rapidly leads to heat stroke
► Symptoms of dehydration are present, but central nervous system symptoms are not seen
► Treatment includes rehydration and cooling

▶ General Considerations

Heat exhaustion is a systemic reaction to prolonged heat exposure (hours to days) and is due to sodium depletion, dehydration, accumulation of metabolites, or a combination of these factors. It is a premonitory syndrome that rapidly evolves to heat stroke. Central nervous system symptoms are generally not present, and the core body temperature is usually less than 40°C (104°F).

Clinical Findings

Two types of heat exhaustion have been described: hypernatremic (primary water loss) and hyponatremic (primary sodium loss). Heat exhaustion from primary water loss occurs when an individual in a hot environment is denied access to water. Heat exhaustion from primary salt loss occurs when an individual in a hot environment sweats excessive amounts and replaces fluid losses with pure water. It differs from heat cramps in that systemic symptoms are present. Pure forms of either type are rare, and most cases have a mixed salt and water depletion. The signs and symptoms of heat exhaustion are nonspecific and include headache, nausea, vomiting, malaise, muscle cramps, and dizziness. Dehydration is manifested by tachycardia, hypotension, and diaphoresis. In a hypernatremic patient, the water deficit can be calculated by a formula if the current serum sodium and patient's weight and age are known.

Measurement of serum electrolytes and renal function is advisable in most patients, because serum sodium concentration may be markedly low in patients with heat exhaustion. Myoglobinuria indicates subclinical rhabdomyolysis.

Treatment and Disposition

Initial treatment includes placing the patient in a cool place and giving adequate cool water and salted (<200 mOsm/L) fruit drinks or salt tablets according to the estimated amount of water and salt depletion. If the patient is unable to drink fluids, give normal saline or lactated Ringer's supplementation intravenously in accordance with clinical and laboratory findings. If marked hyponatremia with water intoxication is present, administration of intravenous hypertonic saline may be required (Chapter 43).

Hospitalize patients with moderate to severe symptoms and those who are elderly or have comorbid illnesses.

HEAT STROKE

ESSENTIALS OF DIAGNOSIS

▶ Extremely high body temperatures causing altered mental status and multiorgan dysfunction
▶ Rhabdomyolysis and severe hepatic damage occur
▶ Treatment is rapid reduction in body temperature

General Considerations

Heat stroke is caused characterized by dysfunction of the heat regulating mechanism, with altered mental status (ranging from confusion to coma) and elevated core body temperature in excess of 41°C (105.8°F). Sweating is variable. The extremely high body temperature rapidly causes widespread damage to body tissues, with significant rhabdomyolysis and multiorgan dysfunction. Illness and death result from destruction of cerebral, cardiovascular, hepatic, and renal tissue.

Heat stroke usually follows excessive exposure to heat and/or strenuous physical activity under exceptionally hot environmental conditions, although it may develop in elderly, infirm, or otherwise susceptible individuals in the absence of unusual exposure to heat. Cardiovascular disease, diabetes, cystic fibrosis, alcoholism, obesity, recent febrile illness, and debility are predisposing factors. Anesthetics, paralyzing agents, diuretics, sedatives, antidepressants, and anticholinergic drugs may also be contributing factors.

Clinical Findings

A. Symptoms and Signs

Premonitory findings include headache, dizziness, nausea, diarrhea, and visual disturbances. Most patients have profound central nervous system dysfunction including seizures, delirium, and coma. The skin is hot, flushed, and usually dry (although sweating may be present). Prior to cardiovascular collapse, the pulse may be strong and rapid due to an increase in cardiac output with no change in stroke volume. Blood pressure is initially elevated or unchanged, and hypotension is a late finding that signals circulatory collapse. Hyperventilation may cause initial respiratory alkalosis, which is generally followed by metabolic acidosis. Stigmata of coagulopathy may be present and include hematuria, hematemesis, bruising, petechiae, and oozing at sites of venipuncture. Core body temperatures as high as 46°C (114.8°F) have been reported in some patients who have achieved full recovery.

B. Laboratory Findings

Laboratory findings include hemoconcentration, decreased blood coagulation, and evidence of disseminated intravascular coagulation. Hypoprothrombinemia, hypofibrinogenemia, or thrombocytopenia may be present. The white blood cell count is routinely elevated. Hypophosphatemia and hypokalemia sometimes occur. Hyperkalemia is associated with acute renal failure due to rhabdomyolysis. The patient has scantly concentrated urine ("machine oil urine") containing protein, tubular casts, and myoglobin. A consistent finding in patients with heatstroke is severe hepatic injury. Serum transaminase levels rise to tens of thousands, although complete recovery usually ensues if treatment is initiated quickly.

Treatment

Act quickly to prevent further damage. The most critical objectives of treatment are rapid cooling and cardiovascular support.

A. Airway and Ventilation

Maintain an adequate airway and ventilation; monitor arterial blood gas levels. Give supplemental oxygen, 6–10 L/min, by mask or nasal cannula.

B. Temperature Reduction

Reduce body temperature promptly. As a first-aid measure, place the patient in a shady, cool place and remove his or her clothing. Sprinkle the patient's entire body with water, and cool by fanning. Alcohol sponge baths are contraindicated and can result in alcohol toxicity. If the victim is near a cold stream, it may be helpful to immerse the patient in the water to facilitate cooling.

In the emergency department, place the patient on a cooling blanket, and place ice packs on the axilla, posterior neck, and inguinal areas (do not apply ice directly to the skin). Water should be sprayed on the patient with a fan blowing on him or her to maximize evaporative cooling. If the temperature cannot be rapidly lowered, or if the victim is unresponsive and the initial core temperature exceeds 42°C (107.6°F), begin peritoneal lavage with cold potassium-free dialysate, 2 L every 10–15 minutes. If a patient requires dialysis, then extracorporeal blood cooling is possible during dialysis. This is also possible via cardiopulmonary bypass, which is a rarely used but extremely effective option. When the rectal temperature drops to 39°C (102.2°F), discontinue active measures to lower temperature to avoid hypothermia, but continue temperature monitoring. Hyperthermia may recur due to thermoregulatory instability, and additional cooling may be required.

Benzodiazepines may be given as needed to control shivering. Because the hypothalamic set point is not elevated as it is in fever, aspirin and acetaminophen have not been found to be helpful. They may even worsen coagulopathy and liver damage.

C. Maintenance of Urine Output

Maintain adequate urinary output (30–50 mL/h). Insert an indwelling urinary catheter to monitor urine output. If myoglobinuria is present, rehydrate the patient with isotonic saline, alkalinize the urine with intravenous administration of bicarbonate, and consider the use of mannitol, 0.25 g/kg intravenously, to promote diuresis. Maintain blood pressure and urine output with intravenous infusion of crystalloid solutions and inotropic agents as necessary (monitoring of central venous pressure or pulmonary capillary wedge pressure may be required). α-Adrenergic drugs are con-

traindicated because they produce vasoconstriction and decrease heat exchange. Dobutamine may be preferable to dopamine as an inotropic agent, because it does not have the α-adrenergic renal effects associated with dopamine at rapid rates of infusion.

Disposition

Hospitalize all patients whose core temperature has exceeded 41°C (105.8°F) for treatment of possible complications (disseminated intravascular coagulation, renal failure, hepatic failure, rhabdomyolysis, cardiac arrhythmias, myocardial infarction, and coma).

With early diagnosis and proper care, 80–90% of previously healthy patients should survive. Extreme hyperpyrexia (rectal temperature >42°C [107.6°F]), persistent coma after cooling, markedly elevated alanine aminotransferase (serum glutamic pyruvic transaminase) and aspartate aminotransferase (serum glutamic oxalacetic transaminase) levels, and hyperkalemia associated with extensive rhabdomyolysis are unfavorable prognostic signs.

Bouchama A et al: Cooling and hemodynamic management in heatstroke: practical recommendations. Critical Care 2007;11(3):R54 [PMID: 17498312].

Crandall C et al: Cardiovascular function in the heat stressed human. Acta Physiol (Oxf) 2010;Epub [PMID: 20345414].

Schlader Z et al: Exercise and heat stress: performance, fatigue, and exhaustion: a hot topic. Br J Sports Med 2009;Epub 20 [PMID: 19846428].

EMERGENCY TREATMENT OF ELECTRICAL INJURIES

LIGHTNING INJURIES

ESSENTIALS OF DIAGNOSIS

▶ Lightning injuries can result not only in burns but also in multiorgan dysfunction

▶ Respiratory arrest is the most common cause of death; ventricular fibrillation and asystole are also seen in severe cases

▶ Management is the same as that for a person with blunt trauma

General Considerations

The United States National Weather Service estimates approximately 60–100 deaths in the United States and 24,000 deaths worldwide due to lightening strikes annually. A reported 30% mortality and 70% morbidity is noted. Epidemiology centers in the mountainous states and the southeastern United States. Strike events cluster in the summer months and in the mid-afternoon, with 84% of victims being male. Injuries are caused by a direct strike, splash (ie, from trees, buildings, and fences), step voltage (spreading on ground), upward leaders, and blunt trauma from concussive shockwaves.

▶ Clinical Findings

Suspect lightning injury in a person found dazed, unconscious, or injured in the vicinity of a thunderstorm. Certain pathognomonic clinical signs help to establish the diagnosis. Victims may appear initially pulseless with mottled extremities due to autonomic dystrophies and sometimes cardiac standstill. Triage of lightning strike victims differs from other multiple casualty scenarios in that the dead appearing are addressed first.

A. Burns

Lightning contact with the body is instantaneous; a flashover phenomenon may channel most of the current along the outside of the body (over the skin) rather than through the victim, as occurs in other types of electrical injury.

1. Linear burns—Linear burns are first- and second-degree burns that begin at the head and neck and course in a branching pattern down the chest and legs. They tend to follow areas with a heavy concentration of sweat.

2. Punctate burns—Punctate burns are clusters of discrete, circular, partial- or full-thickness burns that form starburst patterns on the skin.

3. Feathering burns—Feathering burns are not true burns but rather cutaneous imprints from electron showers that track through the skin. They create a fernlike pattern with delicate branching. These patterns are also called ferning, keraunographic markings, and Lichtenberg flowers or figures.

4. Thermal burns—Thermal burns from clothing or heated metal are typical second- and third-degree burns. Cranial burns (direct or indirect head strike) and leg burns (ground current) are associated with increased death rates.

B. Altered Mental Status

Victims of lightning strikes are usually amnestic and may be disoriented, combative, or comatose.

C. Cardiac Arrest

Cardiopulmonary standstill may be induced by the massive DC countershock of the lightning strike and is the leading cause of mortality. Asystole is more common in lightning strikes as opposed to fibrillation in electrical shock injury. Spontaneous resumption of normal cardiac function is the rule if cardiac standstill is not complicated by simultaneous respiratory

arrest (brain-stem shock or contusion). Cardiac necrosis may develop with evolving ECG changes and QT prolongation.

D. Neurologic Injuries

Central nervous system injuries include traumatic brain and spinal cord injury, coagulation parenchymal injuries, seizure, and anoxic brain injury. Autonomic dystrophies occur. In addition, epidural and subdural hematomas (due to associated falls), subarachnoid hemorrhage, loss of consciousness, and peripheral neurovascular instability are common. Anterograde amnesia and confusion are noted in most patients. Paraplegia and quadriplegia have also been described. Chronic effects include paralysis, chronic pain, and neuropsychologic disorders.

E. Musculoskeletal Injuries

Victims of lightning strikes are frequently thrown to the ground by tetanic muscle contractions, or they may be injured by falls from heights. Fractures of the spine, ribs, and extremities may occur. Intrathoracic and intra-abdominal injuries result from blunt trauma.

F. Eye and Ear Injuries

Eye injuries associated with lightning strikes include cataracts, corneal abrasions, hyphema, uveitis, vitreous hemorrhage, and iridocyclitis. *Note*: Dilated pupils should never be the sole criterion for termination of resuscitative efforts, because they may merely reflect transient autonomic sympathetic discharge or parasympathetic inhibition. Temporary sensorineural hearing loss with or without rupture of the tympanic membrane may result from acoustic and shock wave barotrauma.

▶ Treatment
A. Maintain the Airway, and Begin Cardiopulmonary Resuscitation

CPR should be instituted immediately. Blown pupils are not a reliable indicator of death as cranial nerve palsy is common. Transport and evacuation should not be delayed; prolonged CPR is only anecdotally successful.

B. Anticipate Traumatic Injury

Managing the lightning strike victim is analogous to the blunt trauma evaluation. Particular attention to hypothermia, skeletal and spinal fracture, and thoracoabdominal injury is necessary. Indicated studies include appropriate radiographs, ECG, and laboratory tests including CK, cardiac enzymes, electrolytes, urinalysis with myoglobin, lactate, and hemogram. CT of the head is indicated in altered and loss of consciousness.

C. Begin Burn Therapy and Fluid Replacement

Management of burn wounds follows standard procedures (Chapter 45). Administration of intravenous fluids should be adjusted according to blood pressure readings and urine output. Rhabdomyolysis is rare, and alkalization of the urine and administration of mannitol are not necessary unless myoglobinuria is present. Overhydration may result in cerebral edema. Tetanus should be updated appropriately (Chapter 30).

Disposition

Prolonged cardiac monitoring and serial cardiac enzymes are required only if the patient has a history of cardiac arrest, loss of consciousness, cardiac arrhythmia, abnormal ECG, or if admission is considered for other reasons (burns, trauma). Record results of visual acuity and hearing tests to establish baseline measurement. If the victim has experienced cardiopulmonary arrest and resuscitation efforts have been successful (resumption of spontaneous cardiac activity), allow a minimum of 12–24 hours before weaning the patient from the ventilator to see if spontaneous respiratory activity resumes. If electroencephalographic abnormalities are present, they may clear over 24–72 hours.

ELECTRIC SHOCK AND BURNS

ESSENTIALS OF DIAGNOSIS

- ▶ Direct current is less dangerous than alternating current (AC)
- ▶ AC (most house current) can cause ventricular fibrillation and respiratory arrest
- ▶ Burns can result from the electrical current and, although they may look mild, can indicate significant internal damage
- ▶ Treatment includes CPR, wound care, and possibly fasciotomy

General Considerations

Electric shock is the response to current flow through the body. Voltage is the pressure behind the current flow. Electrical injuries are the cause of around 1000 deaths in the United States each year. Young men and children are the most commonly injured. The severity of electrical injury is influenced by the type of current as well as the amount of voltage involved.

Alternating current (A/C) refers to an alternating/changing voltage. AC causes tetanic muscle contractions that may lead to inability of the victim to separate from the source, prolonging contact. This may ultimately lead to increased electrical injury to the heart causing fatal arrhythmias.

Direct current refers to unidirectional flow caused by change in voltage difference. For example a utility worker may receive a lethal shock if electric current passes from a high voltage power line in contact with a metal object while the worker is also touching the object. The worker is "grounded" at what is considered 0V (earth). The metal object between the power line and the high voltage wire (7200V) completed the circuit and allowed current to flow from the line to the ground, through the worker.

Tissues of the body differ in resistance to electricity. Skin serves as a protective mechanism at low voltage (<500V). At higher voltage, protective resistance of skin is reduced, generally resulting in more significant injury to internal structures. The protective resistance of skin is decreased with moisture and breaks in the skin. Low resistance pathways include muscular and vascular systems leading to cardiac and vascular damage as well as compartment syndromes.

Clinical Findings

A. Electric Shock

Electric shock may produce momentary or prolonged loss of consciousness. Ventricular fibrillation is the most serious immediate arrhythmia, although ectopic beats, sinus tachycardia or bradycardia, atrial fibrillation, and asystole occur. Seizures, deafness, blindness, aphasia, and neuropathy can also result from electric shock. Multiple orthopedic injuries may be seen, including posterior shoulder dislocations and femoral neck fractures.

After recovery from mild to moderate electric shock, muscular pain, fatigue, headache, and generalized or focal nervous irritability occur. Physical signs vary according to the sites of action of the current.

B. Electrical Burns

Small direct electrical burns may hide significant internal organ burns. Extensive skin necrosis and sloughing may not become evident for several days. With internal organ injury, third spacing of fluid is marked. Rhabdomyolosis may also occur.

Treatment

A. Electric Shock

Free the victim from the current at once. This may be done in many ways, but the rescuer must be protected. Turn off the power, sever the wire with a dry wooden-handled ax, make a proper ground to divert the current, or drag the victim carefully away using dry clothing, a leather belt, rubber, or other dry nonconductive materials. Check cardiac and ventilatory function. If the patient is apneic or pulseless, begin artificial ventilation or CPR (Chapter 9).

B. Electrical Burns

Treat tissue burns conservatively. The direction and extent of tissue injury may not be apparent for 7–10 days. Treat circulatory shock, if present, with intravenous infusion of crystalloid solutions. Serum CK-MB isoenzyme levels may be falsely elevated immediately after high-voltage electrical injuries and should not be considered a reliable indicator of myocardial damage. Monitor cardiac rhythm to detect rhythm disturbances in unconscious victims, those who have presented with cardiac arrhythmias, or those with an abnormal ECG. If myoglobinuria is present, monitor arterial blood pH at regular intervals to detect acidosis, which requires intravenous bicarbonate therapy to alkalinize the urine and maintain blood pH above 7.45. Consider intravenous mannitol, 2.5 g initially, to promote moderate diuresis in patients whom have inadequate urine output inspite of aggressive hydration with intravenous isotonic solutions.

Assess the need for fasciotomy by measurement of intracompartmental tissue pressures. In children who have bitten electrical cords, be alert for delayed (up to 3 weeks) erosion of the labial artery, which can manifest as significant bleeding.

▶ Disposition

Hospitalize patients who have lost consciousness or experienced cardiac or respiratory arrest, as well as those with ischemic chest pain, myoglobinuria, or significant burn wounds. Cardiac/ICU monitoring may be unnecessary for those without extensive injury, ECG changes, or those without cardiac history. Continued monitoring is not necessary for patients, including children, who are asymptomatic with no initial ECG changes and no increased risk factors for arrhythmias if injury is due to low voltage (220–240 V) source.

Bailey B et al: Cardiac monitoring of high risk patients after electrical injury: a prospective multicentre study. Emerg Med J 2007;5:348–352 [PMID: 17452703].

Fish RM: Conduction of electrical current to and through the human body: a review. Eplasty 2009;9:407–421 [PMID: 19907637].

Primavesi R: A shocking episode: care of electrical injuries. Can Fam Physician 2009;7:707–709 [PMID: 19602655].

EMERGENCY TREATMENT OF RADIATION INJURIES

RADIATION INJURIES

ESSENTIALS OF DIAGNOSIS

▶ Radiation exposure can cause damage to multiple organ systems

▶ Organ system damage depends on the dose of radiation delivered

▶ General Considerations

The effects of radiation have been observed in the clinical use of X-rays and radioactive agents, after occupational or accidental exposure, and following the use of atomic weapons or radiologic dispersion device or "dirty bomb." The harm depends on the quantity of radiation delivered to the body, the type of radiation (X-rays, neutrons, gamma rays, or alpha or beta particles), the site of exposure, and the duration of exposure. Clinical signs and symptoms relate directly to amount received. In radiation terminology, a rad is the unit of absorbed dose and a rem is the unit of dose of any radiation to body tissue in terms of its estimated biologic effect. The gray (Gy) is a unit of measurement for the dose of ionizing radiation equal to 1 J/kg of tissue. One gray is equal to 100 rad.

▶ Clinical Findings

A. Localized Radiation Exposure

Irradiation causes delayed erythema, epilation, destruction of fingernails, or epidermolysis, depending on the dose. Symptoms develop 1–3 weeks postexposure.

B. Injury to Internal Organs

1. Hematopoietic tissues—Injury to bone marrow may cause a decrease in production of blood elements. Lymphocytes are most sensitive, polymorphonuclear neutrophils next most sensitive, and erythrocytes least sensitive. Damage to blood-forming organs may vary from transient depression of one or more blood elements to pancytopenia. The degree of lymphocyte depression within the first 24–48 hours can be used to estimate the dose received.

2. Cardiovascular system—Pericarditis with effusion or constrictive pericarditis may occur many months after exposure to ionizing radiation. Myocarditis is less common than pericarditis. Smaller vessels (capillaries and arterioles) are more readily damaged than larger blood vessels. If injury is mild, recovery of function occurs.

3. Gonads—In males, small single doses of radiation (2–3 Gy; 200–300 rads) cause transient aspermatogenesis, and larger doses (6–8 Gy; 600–800 rads) may cause sterility. In females, single doses of 2 Gy (200 rads) may produce sterility. Moderate to heavy irradiation of the embryo in utero results in injury to the fetus or causes embryonic death and abortion.

4. Respiratory tract—High or repeated moderate doses of radiation may cause delayed pneumonitis (weeks or months).

5. Mouth, pharynx, esophagus, and stomach—Mucositis with edema and painful swallowing of food may occur within hours to days after exposure to radiation. The salivary glands are relatively radioresistant. Gastric secretion may be temporarily (occasionally permanently) inhibited by moderately high doses of radiation.

6. Intestines—Loss of mucosa with ulceration and inflammation may follow moderately large doses of radiation leading to massive fluid losses via bloody diarrhea and vomiting.

7. Viscera and endocrine glands—Hepatitis and nephritis may be delayed complications of therapeutic irradiation. Normal thyroid, pituitary, pancreas, adrenals, and bladder are relatively resistant to low to moderate doses of radiation.

8. Nervous system—High doses of radiation may damage the brain and spinal cord by impairing their blood supply. Peripheral and autonomic nerves are highly resistant to radiation.

C. Systemic Reaction (Acute Radiation Sickness)

Symptoms vary with type and amount of exposure. Each phase will be shortened for increasing dosages. The prodromal phase consists of incapacitating vomiting and malaise. Time to onset of vomiting is an excellent screening tool to determine amount of radiation received. An asymptomatic latent phase then follows. A third phase then occurs with dose-dependent symptoms and findings. Bone marrow suppression may occur as early as 24 hours. A gastrointestinal syndrome involving massive fluid losses and bloody diarrhea will begin a few days to a week after exposure to higher doses. The neurovascular syndrome will occur with extremely high doses within a few hours to 1–3 days. This syndrome includes seizures, coma, and eventual death.

1. Mild acute radiation sickness (ARS)—Exposure consists of 1–2 Gy. There is a prodrome of vomiting 2 hours or more postexposure. Patient otherwise feels well. At 30 days or more, there will be a slight decrease in lymphocyte count and platelets. Patient will feel mild malaise and weakness. Lethality is 0%.

2. Moderate ARS—Exposure consists of 2–4 Gy. There is prodrome of vomiting approximately 1–2 hours postexposure. There may be a mild headache with slight increase in body temperature. At 3–4 weeks, there will be a more significant decline in lymphocyte and platelet counts. Patient will manifest fever, infection, bleeding, and weakness. Lethality is 0–50%.

3. Severe ARS—Exposure consists of 4–6 Gy. There is prodrome of vomiting less than 1 hour and bloody but mild diarrhea in 3–8 hours. Patient will have moderate headache. At 1–3 weeks, there will be significant decline in lymphocyte and platelet counts. High fever, infection, bleeding, and epilation will begin. Lethality is 20–70%.

4. Very Severe ARS—Exposure consists of 6–8 Gy. Prodromal vomiting begins at less than 30 minutes. Massive bloody diarrhea, severe headache, and confusion being at approximately 3 hours. In less than 1 week, extreme decline in lymphocyte and platelet counts occur with high fever, infection, massive vomiting, diarrhea, and disorientation. Lethality is 50–100%.

5. Lethal ARS—Exposure consists of more than 8 Gy. Vomiting is immediate. Massive diarrhea, coma, and seizures ensure within 1–2 hours. In less than 3 days, lymphocyte count becomes 0.0–0.1 g/L with platelets counts less than 20,000. Patient remains comatose with seizure, bleeding, and infections. Lethality is 100%.

▶ Treatment

A. Decontamination

Decontamination in most instances will occur prior to arrival at a medical facility. If it does not, simple removal of clothing with placement in marked containers will achieve 90% reduction in contamination. Bare skin and hair should be washed thoroughly with soap and water and the effluent secured for disposal. Radioactive particles will not cause acute injury to medical personnel and should not interfere with emergency management. Wounds should be gently irrigated, debrided, and then covered. Foreign bodies should be removed on an emergency basis. After decontamination, a Geiger counter should be passed over patient to determine effectiveness.

B. Local Treatment

Treatment consists of pain control and prevention of infection. Once the extent of injury is determined, grafting or amputation may be necessary.

C. Systemic Treatment

Resuscitation and stabilization of medical and surgical issues should always occur first. After this is accomplished, minimization or prevention of internal contamination should occur. Finally external decontamination should be performed. Treatment of patients with ARS is largely supportive. Massive fluid resuscitation, antiemetics, and blood products may be needed. There are specific medical treatments for radiation, though their effectiveness and safety are still under investigation: (1) colony-stimulating factors have been recommended for healthy victims with exposures >3 Gy and for injured patients >2 Gy; (2) bone marrow transplants have been successfully used in large-dose irradiation cases with subsequent marrow failure; (3) potassium iodine is used orally with radioiodine exposure to prevent thyroid uptake; (4) Prussian blue taken orally increases excretion of cesium and thallium; and (5) Ca^- and Zn^- DTPA given intravenously chelate plutonium, americium, and curium with subsequent excretion in the urine.

▶ Disposition

All patients with signs or symptoms of radiation exposure must be hospitalized. Advice may be obtained from the Radiation Emergency Assistance Center/Training Site (REAC/TS) in Oak Ridge, TN ([865] 576–3131). The 24-hour emergency network telephone number is (865) 481–1000.

Armed Forces Radiobiology Research Institute, Military Medical Operations Office: Military Manual of Medical Management of Radiological Casualties. Available at: www.afrri.usuhs.mil/www/outreach/pdf/radiologicalhandbooksp99-2.pdf

Koenig K et al: Medical treatment of radiologic casualties: current concepts. Ann Emerg Med 2005;45:643–652 [PMID: 15940101] (Review of pathophysiology, and treatment of radiation injury).

Mettler F et al: Major radiation exposure—what to expect and how to respond. N Engl J Med 2002;346:1554–1561 [PMID: 12015396] (Mechanisms of exposure and how to treat).

▼ EMERGENCY TREATMENT OF NEAR-DROWNING VICTIMS

▶ General Considerations

According to the World Health Organization, 409,272 people died from drowning in the year 2000, following only traffic accidents in worldwide mortality. Drowning affects children disproportionately, with residential pools and shallow water drowning (in toilets and buckets comprising as much as 17% in certain populations). Young males suffer an increased rate of mortality as well. Comorbidities leading to drowning include intoxication, trauma (especially in shallow water and high-speed injuries), seizures, arrhythmia, coronary artery disease, hypoglycemia, and hypothermia. Aspiration invariably seems to be present, "dry" drownings probably occur with preaspiration cardiac arrest, or post-event fluid shifts of the aspirate across the alveoli into the circulation. Pulmonary edema and electrolyte abnormalities occur in fresh and saltwater drowning. Decompression illness (DCI) necessitates consideration in scenarios of diving accidents.

▶ Clinical Findings

The victim of near-drowning may present with a wide range of clinical manifestations. Spontaneous return of consciousness often occurs, as does response to brief CPR, both being predictors of good outcome. Vomiting is common. Patients with more severe near-drowning may develop ARDS, hypoxic encephalopathy, or cardiac arrest. A few patients may be deceptively asymptomatic during the recovery period, only to deteriorate as a result of acute respiratory failure in the ensuing 6–24 hours. Reported complications include unique pneumonias such as leptospirosis due to brackish water aspiration, leading to bacterial seeding and brain abscesses.

A. Symptoms and Signs

The patient may be unconscious, semiconscious, or awake and apprehensive. Cyanosis, trismus, apnea, tachypnea, and wheezing may be present. A pink froth from the mouth and nose indicates pulmonary edema. Cardiovascular manifestations may include tachycardia, arrhythmias, hypotension, shock, and cardiac arrest. Decerebrate or decorticate posturing may be noted in the comatose patient.

B. Laboratory Findings

Metabolic and respiratory acidosis may coexist. Sodium, potassium, calcium, and magnesium electrolyte disturbances are found. Renal failure and rhabdomyolysis may also evolve.

C. X-ray Findings

Initial chest X-rays may show aspiration of fluid; late findings may betray fulminant pulmonary edema or ARDS. Routine chest X-rays are indicated to evaluate for pneumonitis before discharging even in apparent mild cases.

▶ Treatment

Before effective CPR can be accomplished, extract the victim from the water in the prone position. Potential for circulatory collapse exists, with sudden removal of surrounding water pressure in the upright position. Prompt initial resuscitation is best predictor of long-term morbidity. The Heimlich maneuver should not be performed unless there is an airway obstruction. Cervical spine immobilization should be maintained in shallow water, surfing, or trauma victims.

A. Open Airway and Maintain Ventilation

Open the airway, and ventilate the patient with early intubation for airway protection as necessary. Give oxygen in high concentrations; positive end-expiratory pressure ventilation is used to maintain Pao_2 with frequent blood gas measurements. Ventilation is preferred with 6 mL/kg tidal volumes and Fio_2 of 0.6 to avoid barotrauma and oxygen toxicity. Effort is made to maintain normocapnea and normoglycemia.

B. Establish Circulation

Check for a carotid or femoral pulse. Institution of CPR should begin immediately if pulseless; hypothermic vasoconstriction may mask a shallow pulse. Chest compressions and defibrillation in hypothermia may precipitate arrhythmia. Central venous access and monitoring aid in fluid resuscitation.

C. Treat Hypothermia

Monitor core temperature rectally. Rewarming patients with forced air heating is effective in temperatures as low as 26°C. Hypothermia with cardiac arrest is an indication for extracorporeal rewarming and cardiopulmonary bypass. Complete recovery has been reported after prolonged resuscitative efforts, even when victims have had dilated, fixed pupils. This is particularly true of infants and children, in whom the brain is protected by hypothermia. Recovery is unpredictable; therefore, resuscitation efforts should be attempted in most cases. In adults, mild hypothermia in near-drowning-associated coma, with goal temperature of 33°C for 12 hours, has been shown to be of some benefit, though mortality was increased in a series of therapeutic hypothermia in children.

▶ Disposition

Near-drowning victims who are initially asymptomatic must be monitored for respiratory distress that develops typically within 6 hours. If the patient has a normal physical examination and respiratory effort, a presentation of Glasgow Coma Scale score of 15, and a room air oxygen saturation of 95% or better with a normal chest X-ray, they may be safely discharged home after 6–8 hours.

Harries M: Near drowning. Br Med J 2003;6(327):1336–1338 [PMID: 14656846] (Review, with rescue and treatment considerations).

Moon RE: Drowning and near drowning. Emerg Med 2002;14(4):377–386 [PMID: 12534480] (Review, pathogenesis and treatment of drowning).

EMERGENCY TREATMENT OF DISORDERS DUE TO ATMOSPHERIC PRESSURE CHANGES

DECOMPRESSION ILLNESS (CAISSON DISEASE, "BENDS")

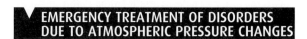

ESSENTIALS OF DIAGNOSIS

▶ Caused by release of nitrogen bubbles from plasma and tissues during ascent

▶ Type1—joint pain; Type2—cardiorespiratory or neurologic involvement

▶ Treatment is immediate recompression in a hyperbaric chamber

▶ General Considerations

The popular sport of scuba diving has exposed a large number of variably trained individuals to the hazards of decompression illness (DCI). DCI occurs in recreational, commercial, and military endeavors involving diving, but also with barometric changes seen in un-pressurized flight. Divers using conventional diving gear (scuba [self-contained underwater breathing apparatus]) breathe oxygen-containing gas mixtures that are at the same pressure as that of the surrounding water. Boyles law dictates that volumes of gas are dependent relative to varying pressures ($P_1V_1 = P_2V_2$). Ambient pressure at 1 atm (sea level) is 760 mm Hg and increases 1 atm for every 33 ft of seawater depth. Boyles law accounts for the barotrauma seen in rapid descent and ascent involving the pulmonary, ENT, gastrointestinal, and other organ systems. Lung squeeze, a descent phenomenon, occurs as total lung volume decreases to less than the residual volume, causing alveolar hemorrhage, pulmonary edema, and hypoxia. On unequalized ascent, pulmonary over-pressurization syndromes arise, leading to pneumothorax, pneumomediastinum, and systemic arterial gas embolism, addressed in the following section. Dalton's gas law integrates the independent partial pressures of various gases in solution adding to total pressure ($P_{total} = PN_2 + Po_2 + Pco_2$). Henry's law shows that gas equilibriation across permeable membranes relates to the partial pressure and concentration of each gas. Dalton's and Henry's laws explain, how during rapid ascent, external pressure decreases, dissolved gases (predominantly nitrogen) escape from solution as gas bubbles, causing endothelial inflammation and problematic mass effects in musculoskeletal, cerebral, and cardiac systems. These effects are known as "the bends." Analogous processes occur in rapid ascend to altitudes above 2000 m (6600 ft) in unpressurized aircraft.

▶ Clinical Findings

Type 1 DCI, or the minor symptom complex, includes deep, aching pain in the large joints and extremities otherwise known as "the bends." The elbow and shoulder are most commonly affected. Cutaneous marmorata is a pathognomic rash involving gas bubbles in small cutaneous vessels.

Type 2 DCI involves any cardiorespiratory or neurologic symptoms, including generalized fatigue. Typical neurologic findings are ataxia, spinal paralysis, vertigo, visual or speech disturbance, and cognitive deficits. Spinal cord emboli can occur in scuba divers, while the upright position in high-altitude flight predisposes to cerebral gas emboli. Chest pain and shortness of breath occur with involvement of pulmonary and cardiac circulation.

▶ Treatment

A. Early Measures

Give oxygen, 100%, by mask for at least 2 hours. Give mild analgesics and crystalloid intravenous fluids to maintain hydration.

B. Recompression

Prompt recompression therapy is indicated in any symptomatic DCI. Resultant chronic symptoms may be altered even by delayed treatment. Persistent symptoms are treated with recompression until resolved or plateau is reached.

Navy dive tables for types I and II illnesses are available for the recompression treatment course. Physicians should know the location of the nearest hyperbaric chamber. In the United States, 24-hour clinical advice may be obtained rapidly by telephoning the National Diving Alert Network (DAN) at Duke University [919] 684–9111.

C. Complications

Further measures may be necessary to relieve some of the complications associated with the bends (eg, shock, spinal cord injury, bladder paralysis, hemoconcentration, and disseminated intravascular coagulation).

▶ Disposition

Transport the patient immediately to the nearest recompression center (hyperbaric chamber) for evaluation and treatment. A patient who is transported to a hyperbaric chamber by aircraft should not be exposed to a cabin altitude higher than 300 m (1000 ft). Commercial flight after DCI should be avoided until resolved or for 1 week. *Caution:* Never attempt recompression in the water.

ARTERIAL GAS EMBOLISM

ESSENTIALS OF DIAGNOSIS

- ▶ Increased pressure in the lungs causing air to escape from alveoli
- ▶ Results in air in the interstitial space or in the pulmonary venous circulation
- ▶ Can result in pneumothorax or occlusion of the coronary and cerebrovascular systems
- ▶ Treatment is immediate recompression in a hyperbaric chamber

▶ General Considerations

In arterial gas embolism, gas bubbles precipitate from solution and cause problematic mass effects in the circulation. Gas bubbles form in the relatively low pressure venous circulation. Entry into the systemic left-sided circulation occurs through arteriovenous connections, commonly a patent foramen ovale. Dramatic presentations will betray arterial gas embolisms. If symptoms occur more than 10 minutes after surfacing, large air embolism is less likely. Many victims of arterial gas embolism die immediately upon surfacing. If air bubbles enter the cerebral circula-

tion, the victim becomes unconscious or has a seizure during ascent or immediately upon surfacing. Presentation is stroke-like, with blindness, confusion, or symptoms based on anatomic distribution.

A. Central Circulation

Cerebral embolism is analogous to stroke presentations. If the bubbles have entered the coronary arteries, the person presents with symptoms similar to those of acute myocardial infarction, with chest pain, arrhythmias, and collapse. Complete, sudden circulatory collapse occurs with occlusion of the central circulation. Pulmonary artery or cardiac chamber obstruction has been described as "the chokes."

B. Pneumothorax

Signs of pneumothorax or mediastinal emphysema develop more slowly and are not as life-threatening; signs include shortness of breath, hyper-resonance of the chest to percussion, and decreased breath sounds on the affected side. Subcutaneous crepitus that may extend into the neck occurs.

▶ Treatment
A. Early Measures

Give oxygen, 100%, by mask. Position the victim supine on the left side to prevent aspiration. Chest tube insertion is indicated for symptomatic pneumothorax. Maintain urine output at 1–2 mL/kg/h with intravenous fluids.

B. Recompression

Immediate recompression is the only effective treatment; the patient should be transported to a hyperbaric chamber immediately (see Decompression Sickness section earlier in this chapter).

▶ Disposition

Transport the patient immediately to the nearest recompression center (hyperbaric chamber) for evaluation and treatment.

HIGH-ALTITUDE SICKNESS (MOUNTAIN SICKNESS)
▶ General Considerations

High-altitude illnesses are a spectrum of diseases that affect unacclimatized people in the relative hypoxia of altitude. The effects can be seen in high rates of ascent of passengers in unpressurized aircraft as low as 1500 m (4921 ft), to the extremely high altitudes of 5500–8850 m (18,000–29,035 ft) reached by expedition trekkers and climbers. Rapid ascent, a history of altitude illness, physical exertion, obesity, and a myriad of comorbid diagnosis predispose individuals to the effects of altitude. Physical fitness is not itself a protective factor. Hypoxic ventilatory response is the key in acclimatization, with eventual adjustment to the respiratory alkalosis with a metabolic compensation.

1. Acute Mountain Sickness

ESSENTIALS OF DIAGNOSIS

- ▶ Headache with a myriad of related symptoms
- ▶ Treatment is descent, oxygen, and antiemetics
- ▶ If descent is not possible, dexamethasone or acetazolamide can be used to aid acclimatization

▶ Clinical Findings

Acute mountain sickness (AMS) is defined as headache at altitude and one of the following: anorexia, nausea, vomiting, fatigue, weakness, dizziness, lightheadedness, or insomnia. AMS is self-limited, but may progress to the more severe manifestations of high-altitude cerebral edema (HACE) or high-altitude pulmonary edema (HAPE). Onset ranges from 1 hour to 3 days.

▶ Treatment

Treat mild cases with rest, allowing physiologic acclimatization before further ascent. NSAIDs and antiemetics may be useful. Avoid alcohol and narcotics/sedatives that may decrease the ventilatory response, especially while sleeping. Moderate cases can be treated with acetazolamide to speed acclimatization, and dexamethazone 4–6 mg PO Q6 hours. Descents of 1000–3000 ft may alleviate symptoms, the definitive treatment for progressive symptoms. Simulated descents of 1000–2000 ft can be achieved with portable pressurized chambers (Gamow bag), when available and rapid descent is not possible in remote settings. Acetazolamide 125–250 mg PO b.i.d. has been shown effective in AMS prophylaxis, starting 1 day prior to ascent, continuing to day 4. Treatment doses are the same; the pediatric acetazolamide dose is 2.5 mg/kg. Avoid acetazolamide in those with sulfonamide/sulfite allergy. Dexamethazone 2–4 mg every 6 hours is also effective. Graded ascents of 600 m per day with rests should allow sufficient acclimatization, preventing AMS.

▶ Disposition

If symptoms persist, descent is the definitive therapy.

2. Acute High-Altitude Pulmonary Edema

ESSENTIALS OF DIAGNOSIS

- ▶ Noncardiogenic pulmonary edema due to rapid ascent above 2400m(8000 ft)
- ▶ Cough and dyspnea on exertion lead to pink, frothy sputum and respiratory distress
- ▶ Chest X-ray findings show patchy infiltrates but normal heart size
- ▶ Treatment is rapid descent, continuous positive pressure ventilation, oxygen, and nifedipine

▶ Clinical Findings

HAPE carries the greatest mortality of the altitude illnesses. Reported as low as 2400 m (8000 ft), a noncardiogenic pulmonary edema arises after hypoxic vasoconstriction and elevated right heart pressures. Risk for HAPE includes AMS, rapid ascent, congenital absence of one pulmonary artery, and brief sojourn at high altitude by persons acclimatized to living at low altitudes.

A. Symptoms and Signs

HAPE diagnosis can be made when two from each of the following are present: symptoms—dyspnea at rest, cough, weakness, decreased performance, and chest tightness; signs—crackles, wheezing, central cyanosis, tachypnea, and tachycardia. Rapid progression may occur to florid pulmonary edema and death.

B. Laboratory Findings

Brain natriuretic peptide levels may differentiate cardiogenic pulmonary edema and HAPE. Secondary signs of inflammation may be seen, with elevated hematocrit. Echocardiogram and/or pulmonary artery wedge pressures may be useful in further differentiating disease.

C. X-ray Findings

Findings on chest X-ray are variable. In mild disease, patchy infiltrates in a solitary lung field (commonly the right middle lobe) are noted. The infiltrates rarely coalesce and generally do not involve the base of the lungs. The central pulmonary arteries are dilated, but the cardiac shadow is of normal size. In severe illness, infiltrates are more generalized, but no left atrial enlargement or Kerley B lines are noted. Unilateral pulmonary edema is consistent with unilateral atresia of the pulmonary artery.

▶ Treatment

Early recognition of the disease is crucial. Persistent dry cough and dyspnea in a person who has recently arrived at high altitude should be considered high-altitude pulmonary edema until proven otherwise. Treatment centers on rest and descent. Exertion and cold stress should be avoided. Oxygen is administered by facemask at 4–6 L/min until symptoms are improved, then 2–4 L/min if supplies need to be conserved. Oxygen is continued for 72 hours even after descent from altitude in severe cases. Remotely, the portable Gamow bag can be used with oxygen, with ventilation of CO_2 intermittently. Continuous positive-airway pressure will improve oxygenation during evacuation of patients when available. Nifedipine may be given sublingually, then 20–30 mg PO in sustained release b.i.d. β-Agonist may also be useful, acetazolamide may hasten acclimatization but will not alter HAPE, and there is no role for dexamethazone.

▶ Prevention

Preventive measures include (1) education of prospective mountaineers about the possibility of serious pulmonary edema, (2) gradual ascent to permit acclimatization, and (3) rest and avoidance of strenuous exercise for 1–2 days after arrival at high altitudes. Medical attention should be sought promptly if respiratory symptoms develop.

Patients with a history of high-altitude pulmonary edema have a 60% chance of the illness recurring with repeat ascents. Prophylaxis with nifedipine, 20–30 mg of the extended release form every 12–24 hours, is helpful.

Mountaineering parties climbing at 2400 m (8000 ft) or higher should carry a supply of oxygen and equipment sufficient for several days if hospital facilities are not available.

People with symptomatic cardiac or pulmonary disease should avoid high altitudes. Detection of a heart murmur and recurrent episodes of high-altitude pulmonary edema should prompt investigation for a previously existing valvular, shunt, or pulmonary hypertension problem.

▶ Disposition

Hospitalization is generally recommended if symptoms persist for more than a few hours after return to lower altitudes. Hospitalization in mild cases at altitude has been done with supportive therapy and oxygen if descent is undesirable. Commercial airline flight and further physical exertion both should be avoided until oxygen is no longer needed.

3. High-Altitude Cerebral Edema

ESSENTIALS OF DIAGNOSIS

▶ Cerebral edema due to rapid ascent to altitudes above 2400 m (8000 ft)

▶ Signs and symptoms include headache, ataxia, papilledema, and global encephalopathy

▶ Treatment is immediate descent, oxygen, and dexamethasone

▶ Clinical Findings

HACE is an end-stage manifestation in the continuum of mountain sickness. It may occur with or without HAPE. Manifestations are principally neurological, with hypoxic failure of cerebral vascular autoregulation. Truncal ataxia and behavior changes may be the first indication of progression to HACE. Symptoms include those of AMS, and may include confusion, apathy, agitation, and focal neurologic signs including cranial nerve palsy, obtundation, and coma. MRI findings show cerebral edema, with death resultant from brainstem herniation. Retinal hemorrhages and papilledema may be seen.

▶ Treatment

Early recognition and intervention is crucial. Because the symptoms of early high-altitude cerebral edema are similar to those of AMS, anyone with headache and fatigue at high altitude must be watched closely for signs of deterioration.

Oxygen should be administered to maintain saturations more than 90%. HACE is an indication for immediate descent/evacuation to preferably an altitude of 1500 m (4000 ft), or at least down 1000 m (3281 ft). Portable hyperbaric chambers may be used if descent is impossible. Dexamethazone, 8 mg and then 4 mg every 6 hours, is indicated. Acetazolamide may be useful, dosed up to 750 mg per day divided b.i.d. When using nifedipine and acetazolamide, monitor closely for hypotension, as cerebral perfusion pressures must be maintained in HACE.

▶ Disposition

Hospitalization is generally recommended if symptoms persist for more than a few hours after return to lower altitudes.

Davies A et al: Determinants of summiting success and acute mountain sickness on Mt. Kilimanjaro. Wilderness Environ Med 2009;20(4):311–317 [PMID: 20030437].

Lynch J et al: Diving medicine: a review of current evidence. J Am Board Fam Med 2009;22(4):399–407 [PMID: 19587254].

Maa E: Hypobaric hypoxic cerebral insults: the neurological consequences of going higher. Neuro Rehabil 2010;26(1):73–84 [PMID: 20130356].

Schoene R: Illnesses at high altitude. Chest 2008;134(2):402–416 [PMID: 18682459].

Stream J: Update on high-altitude pulmonary edema: pathology, prevention, and treatment. Wilderness Environ Med 2008;19(3):293–303 [PMID: 19099331].

Wilson M et al: The cerebral effects of ascent to high altitudes. Lancet Neurol 2009;8(7):604–605 [PMID 19161909].

EMERGENCY TREATMENT OF DISORDERS DUE TO VENOMOUS ANIMALS

SNAKE BITES

ESSENTIALS OF DIAGNOSIS

▶ Venomous bites can result from either pit vipers or elapids

▶ Pit viper envenomation results in symptoms related to cytolysis, whereas elapid bites can result in neurotoxic symptoms

▶ Antivenom is available for both pit viper and elapid bites and should be administered for symptomatic envenomations

General Considerations

Morbidity and mortality from snake envenomation is a significant problem worldwide. Recent estimates put the global number of snake envenomations at around 421,000 annually with an estimated 20,000 deaths. This number is probably higher given very poor tracking of health statistics in underdeveloped countries and rural areas. Only about one out of every four venomous snakebites actually produces venom, with the rest being dry bites. Death from snakebite in the United States is very rare given the low lethality of venom from indigenous species as well as ready access to medical care and antivenin. Two families of venomous snakes exist in the United States. These families are Elapidae or the coral snake and the family Viperidae subfamily Crotalidae or the rattlesnake, water moccasin, and copperhead.

Snake venom is a complex mixture of proteolytic enzymes and toxic proteins. In general, crotalid venom is mainly cytolytic, whereas elapid venom is mainly neurotoxic.

Clinical Findings

The predominantly cytolytic venom of crotalids can cause edema, hemorrhage, and necrosis around the bite site as well as distant from the site in severe envenomations. Systemic signs and symptoms consist of hemolysis, thrombocytopenia, coagulopathy, vomiting, and, rarely, respiratory failure with cardiovascular instability or collapse.

The predominately neurotoxic venom of elapids and the Mojave rattlesnake may produce few or no early local signs of envenomation, but neurologic symptoms (paresthesias, blurred vision, dysphagia, hypersalivation, ptosis, and respiratory depression) may appear after a delay of 12–24 hours.

Treatment

1. Emergency First-Aid Measures

Many of the most well-known first-aid measures are no longer recommended. Cryotherapy, tourniquets, and incision and suction have not been shown to be helpful and, in many cases, cause more harm. The best management is to transport the patient to the nearest hospital. Immobilize the bitten part as if it were a fracture. Keep the patient on strict bed rest, if possible. If the patient has a severe envenomation with progression of symptoms, emergency medical service providers may place a constriction band over the site of the bite. A constriction band is a broad, flat band exerting 20 mm Hg of pressure that still permits one or two fingers under the band. However, if the patient is stable, application of a constriction band is not recommended, even if transport time is long. If a constriction band or suction device has been placed prior to the arrival of emergency medical services, it should be left in place for transport. Suction devices have been shown to cause injury themselves, however, and can be removed if no liquid is being extracted. It is very helpful to hospital providers if the progression of any swelling and ecchymosis can be outlined and timed.

2. Hospital Measures

Assess the patient's respiratory and cardiovascular status. Determine whether airway management or cardiovascular resuscitation with crystalloid or vasopressors is needed.

Obtain intravenous access. Assess bite site for local progression. Determine species of snake if possible. Check complete blood count, electrolytes, coagulation profile, and urine myoglobin. Type and crossmatch blood.

Crotalidae polyvalent immune Fab, also known as CroFab, is now the antivenin of choice for North American crotalidenvenomations. CroFab should be administered per the manufacturer's recommendations. It should be noted that CroFab is only approved for use in rattlesnake envenomation but has been successfully used and shown to be safe for use in copperhead envenomation as well. The severity of envenomation should be determined based on the progression of local soft tissue damage as well the presence of systemic side effects. Please see (Table 46–1) for dosing guidelines and goals of treatment. Antivenin must be reconstituted and then administered slowly intravenously as a test dose for 10 minutes. If no signs or symptoms of anaphylaxis occur, then the infusion rate may be increased to be complete in 1 hour. Although the incidence of severe allergic reaction to CroFab should be much less than that to the previous horse serum antivenin, there are reports of it occurring. Treatment, if reaction occurs, should be halting of infusion and administration of steroids, epinephrine and diphenhydramine. CroFab should continue to be administered until initial control of the progression of envenomation is achieved. The manufacturer recommends a scheduled maintenance dosing at 6, 12, and 18 hours after

Table 46–1. Indications and Dosages of Crotalidae Polyvalent Immune Fab (FabAV).

Symptoms	Dosing	Goal
None	No FabAV required.	
Local progression, systemic symptoms, or clinically significant coagulopathy	The patient should be given enough vials to achieve the goal; this generally ranges from 3 to 12 vials, although up to 25 vials have been used	Achieve control of local progression, resolution of systemic symptoms, or reversal of the coagulopathy
Stabilization of signs and symptoms and no progression of signs and symptoms after FabAV given	Administer two vials at 6, 12, and 18 hours	Prevent recurrence

initial control is achieved for rattlesnake envenomations to prevent recurrence of venom effects. No evidence exists to suggest this is necessary for other crotalid envenomations. CroFab is being used in the pediatric population and recent small studies have shown both safety and efficacy in this age group. The same amount of antivenin is used in children but it must be reconstituted in smaller volumes to avoid fluid overload.

For coral snake (Eastern or Texas variety) bites, give five vials of Eastern coral snake antivenin.

Tetanus immunization should be updated for all patients and antibiotics administered only if clinical evidence of infection is present.

Myonecrosis after snake envenomation is thought to be due to local venom effect, not from increased compartment pressures. Fasciotomy for increased compartment pressures does not tend to improve outcome. Fasciotomy should be withheld until several vials of antivenin have failed to reverse effects.

▶ Disposition

Place patients requiring antivenin in the ICU for monitoring. Asymptomatic patients with no local progression and normal laboratory values may be discharged after 8 hours with close wound follow-up.

Goto CS, Feng SY: Crotalidae polyvalent immune Fab for the treatment of pediatric crotaline envenomation. Pediatr Emerg Care 2009:25(4):27309. [PMID 19369845]

Johnson PN, McGoodwin L, Banner W: Utilisation of Crotalidae polyvalent immune Fab(ovine) for Viperidae envenomations in children. Emerg Med J 2008;25(12):793–798. [PMID 19033492]

Kasturiratne A, Wickremasinghe AR, de Silva N, et al: The global burden of snakebite: a literature analysis and modeling based on regional estimates and envenoming and deaths. PLoS Medicine 2008;5(11):e218. [PMID: 18986210]

Lavonas EJ, Schaeffer TH, Kokko J, et al: Crotaline Fab antivenom appears to be effective in cases of severe North American pit viper envenomation: an integrative review. BMC Emerg Med 2009; June 22;9:13. [PMID 19545426]

BEES AND WASP STINGS

 ESSENTIALS OF DIAGNOSIS

▶ Most people who experience a Hymenoptera envenomation have only a painful and urticarial lesion at the site of the sting; more severe reactions can occur and result in anaphylaxis and multiorgan dysfunction

▶ Oral pain control, tetanus prophylaxis, and diphenhydramine are generally the only treatment needed; in severe reactions, airway management, vasopressors, and even dialysis may be needed

▶ General Considerations

Bees, wasps, and ants are members of the order Hymenoptera. In the United States, domesticated honey bees, feral bumblebees, paper wasps, yellow jackets, and fire ants are the most common attackers, although the aggressive, swarming Africanized bees have been present in the United States since the early 1990s. The venom causes hemolysis and destruction of platelets and leukocytes. It is also capable of destroying vascular endothelium and necrosing skeletal muscle.

▶ Clinical Findings

Patients with Hymenoptera envenomation can present with a wide array of signs and symptoms. The most common effect of a sting is a small pruritic and urticarial-type lesion that also causes pain. Ten percent of people have a large local reaction greater than 5 cm in diameter. These reactions may last longer than the smaller lesions. Less than 1% of patients experience a systemic reaction. Some have a milder reaction with only nausea, vomiting, and diarrhea as well as pruritic urticarial lesions distant from the sting site. Rarely a victim will experience anaphylaxis. Persons who experience multiple stings or who are taking β-adrenergic blocking drugs may experience more severe reactions. Immediate and delayed toxic reactions may occur with envenomation by 50 or more stings.

These reactions include hemolysis and rhabdomyolysis with subsequent renal failure, thrombocytopenia, disseminated intravascular coagulopathy, and liver dysfunction.

► Treatment

Remove stings or fragments by scraping, not with forceps. Apply topical ice packs. Oral pain control, diphenhydramine, and tetanus prophylaxis are usually all that is necessary for small or large local reaction. Mild systemic reactions may require intravenous diphenhydramine as well as intravenous corticosteroids and a short period of monitoring to allow early intervention for progression to anaphylaxis. Anaphylaxis requires intubation, intravenous access, aggressive fluid resuscitation, aerosolized β-agonists for bronchospasm, subcutaneous or intravenous epinephrine, and possibly pressor agents. Toxic reactions will require the above measures with possible blood products, dialysis, and extensive hospital care.

► Disposition

Patients with local reactions may be discharged home. Patients with severe systemic reactions require admission. The Phoenix Poison Control Center recommends mandatory 24-hour admission for children, the elderly, and patients with underlying medical problems or if 50 or more stings are sustained. Otherwise, young healthy individuals with massive envenomation require 6 hours of monitoring with initial and discharge laboratory evaluations of renal and liver function, coagulation studies, and red blood cell count; if no abnormalities are found, patients may be discharged home. Studies of sensitized individuals have found that the vast majority never experience escalating symptoms with future stings; many have less severe reactions. Victims with less severe systemic reactions should undergo immunotherapy and carry an emergency epinephrine pen.

BLACK WIDOW SPIDER BITES

ESSENTIALS OF DIAGNOSIS

▶ Symptoms of envenomation include severe pain in the bitten extremity and muscle spasms of the abdomen and trunk

▶ Abdominal muscle spasms can mimic a surgical abdomen

▶ Severe hypertension and tachycardia can occur

▶ Treatment includes narcotic analgesics and antivenom in the seriously ill

► Clinical Findings

The female black widow spider (*Latrodectus mactans*) is shiny black, with a red hourglass marking on its abdomen. Only the female is dangerous. This spider is common in California and other parts of the United States. Other *Latrodectus* sp. may be found in other countries. The venom is a neurotoxin that results in presynaptic neurotransmitter release. The bite itself is minor and often unnoticed at first. Characteristic symptoms of envenomation occur within 10–60 minutes, including severe pain in the bitten extremity and muscle spasms of the abdomen and trunk. Diffuse paresthesias are noted as well as muscle fasciculation, piloerection, and diaphoresis. Headache, nausea and vomiting, hyperactive deep tendon reflexes, and ptosis may be noted. Victims are in agonizing pain; the rigidity of abdominal muscles may mimic a surgical emergency. Severe hypertension and tachycardia may occur. Deaths are rare; at greatest risk are small infants or older patients with preexisting cardiovascular disease. Symptoms peak at 2–3 hours after the bite and may last up to 3–7 days.

► Treatment

Most patients respond to narcotic analgesics. Calcium gluconate has not been found to be very effective for pain control in most recent studies. Local applications of ice should be used judiciously, along with immobilization and loose compression dressing. Antivenom should be reserved for use in seriously ill infants and older patients and should be preceded by horse serum sensitivity testing. One vial of antivenom is sufficient for most patients; give one ampule (2.5 mL) in 10–50 mL of normal saline by slow intravenous infusion. There is a high rate of allergic reaction and one case of fatal anaphylaxis with antivenom administration.

► Disposition

All patients who have been bitten by a black widow spider should be observed for 12–24 hours, because hypertension and muscle spasm commonly recur. Hospitalization is necessary for all patients under age 14 years, those older than age 65 years, those with a history of hypertension, and those who present with severe symptoms.

BROWN RECLUSE SPIDER BITES

ESSENTIALS OF DIAGNOSIS

▶ The venom of the brown recluse spider is cytotoxic and causes local tissue destruction

▶ The bite progresses from an initial pustule to a bull's eye like lesion to a larger crater like ulcer (severe cases)

▶ Most bites require only tetanus prophylaxis and local wound care; more symptomatic patients may require aggressive wound care including excision

Clinical Findings

The brown recluse spider (*Loxosceles reclusa;* other *Loxosceles* sp.) has a dark, violin-shaped area on its back. It is found in old wood piles, attics, closets, and clothes piles and prefers dark, undisturbed places. The venom, which contains sphingomyelinase D, is chiefly cytotoxic, causing local tissue destruction by destroying endothelial cells; it also has a hemolytic component, which on rare occasions may cause massive hemolysis. The enzyme may also disrupt nerve impulses, thus causing skin anesthesia at the bite site.

The bite initially seems mild and often goes unnoticed. Pain at the site begins 1–4 hours later, and an erythematous area with a central pustule or hemorrhagic vesicle may be seen. The typical bull's eye lesion is created when the red blister is encircled by a pale, irregularly shaped, ischemic halo, which in turn is surrounded by extravasated blood. The pustule may gradually grow to form a craterlike lesion over 3–4 days, with associated lymphadenopathy and low-grade fever. Healing is slow, and large lesions may occasionally require skin grafting. Rarely, ulcerating skin lesions may appear years after a bite. A generalized systemic reaction termed loxoscelism may occur 24–48 hours after the bite, with fever, malaise, arthralgias, rash, and hemolysis. Rare fatalities have occurred in small children, who have shown massive intravascular hemolysis, accompanied by hemoglobinuria, jaundice, hypotension, renal failure, pulmonary edema, and disseminated intravascular coagulation. There appears to be little correlation between the development of a systemic reaction and the severity of the skin lesion.

The bites of many other insects may be mistaken for brown recluse spider bites and lead to unnecessary treatment. One helpful clue (although not absolutely reliable) is that spiders tend to bite only once, whereas other insects leave multiple bites.

Treatment

Because of the progressive necrosis associated with many brown recluse bites, early surgical excision is not recommended. Excision of a necrotic area should occur only after the area has stabilized. Many recent studies have failed to show any significant benefit to corticosteroid therapy. Dapsone has historically been a popular treatment for recluse bites. Its use, however, has come into question given the lack of convincing animal and human studies showing any effectiveness in reducing pain and dermonecrosis. Hyperbaric oxygen therapy and wound coverage with nitroglycerin patches have failed to produce consistent effective reduction in progression of the necrosis. Loxosceles antivenom is commercially available although not in the United States. Its use in other countries has shown improvement in wound healing and helped in treatment of systemic loxoscelism. A new ELISA assay has been developed for detection of brown recluse venom and shows promise for diagnosing this arachnid's bite in dermonecrotic skin lesions when a spider was never identified. Many brown recluse spider bites are minor and heal without specific treatment other than tetanus prophylaxis (Chapter 30) and local wound care.

Disposition

Most brown recluse spider bites can be treated on an outpatient basis. Patients with large or infected wounds or those who have signs of a systemic reaction should be hospitalized.

SCORPION STINGS

ESSENTIALS OF DIAGNOSIS

▶ Most bites produce only local reactions including a painful sting site with or without erythema

▶ The bite of the *Centruroides exilicauda* scorpion can produce severe systemic symptoms including extreme restlessness, diaphoresis, seizures, and hypertension

▶ Severe reactions should be treated in the ICU with neuroleptics, antihypertensives, and atropine; antivenin is available for treatment failures

General Considerations

Most scorpions are relatively harmless, producing only local envenomation reactions. However, *C. exilicauda/ sculpturatus* may produce severe systemic toxicity.

This arthropod is small and yellowish, has a small tubercle (telson) at the base of its stinger, and is 2.5–7.5 cm (1–3 in) long. It is found mostly in the southwestern United States (Arizona, New Mexico, Texas, and along the Colorado River) but may rarely be transported in freight to distant states. Related arthropods are found in many other parts of the world.

The venom of *C. exilicauda* contains a neurotoxin that may produce severe systemic symptoms. Other North American scorpion stings generally produce only local reactions.

Clinical Findings

The initial sting is intensely painful with little or no erythema or swelling. Light percussion of the wound causes intense pain. Although pain and paresthesias generally resolve within 4 hours, local symptoms may persist for several days. Systemic envenomation initially causes a cholinergic-like toxidrome with typical SLUDGE syndrome. Shortly after, massive norepinephrine release is triggered causing hypertension, tachycardia, hyperpyrexia, and pulmonary edema with possible myocardial infarction. Central nervous system effects generally consist of confusion, restlessness, and dystonic reactions.

Treatment

Periodic applications of ice may relieve local pain; avoid intense cooling. Immobilize the affected part. Do not apply a tourniquet.

Most children recover with supportive care alone but should be observed in an ICU. Strong depressants or tranquilizers do not appear to shorten the duration of symptoms and may produce respiratory depression; specifically, opiate analgesics seem to potentiate the toxicity of the venom. Diazepam or phenobarbital may be used to control seizures; sympatholytic antihypertensive agents may be required to control hypertension. Goat serum antivenom is available in Arizona (Arizona Poison and Drug Information Center [800] 222–1222 or [602] 495–6360) but has not been approved by the FDA and therefore is prohibited from transport outside Arizona. It is effective only for stings from *C. exilicauda* and is not of benefit for stings from scorpions from South America, Asia, or the Middle East. It seems to abate local pain and paresthesias but does not appear to be very helpful with treatment of systemic effects unless administered within about 1 hour of envenomation.

Golden D: Stinging insect allergy. Am Fam Physician 2003;67:2541–2546 [PMID: 12825843] (Review of pathophysiology, management, and disposition of insect stings).

Gomez H et al: A new assay for the detection of Loxosceles species (brown recluse) spider venom. Ann Emerg Med 2002;39:608–624 [PMID: 11973553] 469–474 (Study showing usefulness of new test for presence of brown recluse venom in wounds).

Hogan C et al: Loxoscelism: old obstacles, new directions. Ann Emerg Med 2004;44:469–474 [PMID: 15573037] (New treatments for brown recluse envenomations).

Isbister G et al: Antivenom treatment in arachnidism. J Toxicol Clin Toxicol 2003;41:291 [PMID: 12807312] (Pharmacology of arachnid antivenoms).

Saucier J: Arachnid envenomation. Emerg Med Clin North Am 2004;22:405–422 [PMID: 15163574] (Review of types of arachnid envenomations and their treatments).

▼ HAZARDOUS MARINE LIFE

Many ocean-dwelling animals are potentially harmful to humans because of their ability to traumatize, envenom, or otherwise poison their victims with bites or stings. Most human injuries result from envenomation.

1. Stingrays

ESSENTIALS OF DIAGNOSIS

▶ Envenomation occurs when the tail of the stingray releases venom into its victim

▶ The sting causes intense local pain as well as nausea and vomiting, weakness, tachycardia, and muscle cramps

▶ Removal of spines and irrigation with hot water are the mainstays of treatment

▶ General Considerations

Stingrays are the fish most commonly responsible for human envenomations; at least 2000 stings occur annually in the United States. Stingrays are usually encountered in the waters off coastal regions, where they lie partially submerged in the sand. When disturbed, they splash upward with a muscular tail, which carries 1–4 venomous stingers. Injury due to stingrays therefore involves both a traumatic wound (which can be quite severe) and envenomation. The most common sites of injury are the lower extremities, followed by the upper extremities, abdomen, and chest. Wound necrosis is not uncommon.

▶ Clinical Findings

The sting is followed by immediate intense local pain and moderate swelling with bleeding. The pain radiates centrally and can be so severe that it causes disorientation. Systemic symptoms occur within 30 minutes of the sting and include nausea and vomiting, weakness, diaphoresis, vertigo, tachycardia, and muscle cramps. If envenomation has been severe, syncope, paralysis, hypotension, cardiac arrhythmias, and death may occur.

▶ Treatment

1. Irrigate the Wound

Irrigate the wound with whatever dilutent is at hand (preferably sterile saline or water). Remove any obvious pieces of foreign matter. Immediate basic first aid is necessary to help prevent eventual necrosis, ulceration, and infection.

2. Anesthetize the Wound

Soak the wound in hot water to tolerance (45–50°C [113–122°F]) for 30–60 minutes. Stingray venom is heat labile and may be denatured in hot water. If heat fails to relieve the pain, infiltrate the wound with lidocaine, 1–2% without epinephrine, or perform regional nerve block. Do not apply ice to the wound.

3. Explore the Wound

Wound exploration and an X-ray should be performed so that all tissue fragments may be removed. Close the wound loosely around drains, or pack it open.

4. Give Antibiotics

Administer standard tetanus prophylaxis (Chapter 30), and consider starting treatment with trimethoprim/sulfamethoxazole (160 and 800 mg, respectively, twice a day), ciprofloxacin (500 mg twice a day), or tetracycline (500 mg four times a day) for 7 days.

5. Surgical Debridement

If necrosis develops, early surgical debridement is recommended. Serial debridement may be necessary to stop any progression.

6. Hyperbaric Oxygen

Hyperbaric oxygen has been used successfully in the setting of myonecrosis when serial debridement is required. If used, it should be instituted immediately after debridement takes place.

▶ Disposition

Any patient with significant envenomation from a stingray sting should be observed for 4–6 hours for appearance of systemic side effects. Patients who are discharged should have close outpatient follow-up for wound care.

2. Sea Snakes

ESSENTIALS OF DIAGNOSIS

▶ The initial bite is painless, but limb and respiratory paralysis as well as myolysis can occur with envenomation

▶ Treatment is the same as for land snake envenomation and includes sea snake antivenom if paralysis or myolysis is present

▶ General Considerations

Sea snakes are present in all oceans except the Atlantic and are very similar to terrestrial snakes except for the shape of their tail. Although 90% of sea snake bites are dry, the venom is highly toxic to the nervous system and can cause significant myolysis. The sea snake is not aggressive, and some type of provocation is necessary to be bitten.

▶ Clinical Findings

The initial bite is relatively painless, but with significant envenomation comes rapid limb and respiratory muscle paralysis, ptosis, ophthalmoplegia, and myolysis. Renal failure can occur if myolysis is severe. The hemolysis and coagulopathy associated with U.S. snake bites is not seen.

▶ Treatment

The same basic first-aid principles used for terrestrial envenomation still apply. Monitor respiratory status and prepare for intubation. Screen for signs of myolysis with CK, urine myoglobin, and renal function panel. Signs should be present

by 6 hours. If paralysis or myolysis is present, administer sea snake antivenom. Between one and three ampules should be given initially, although more may be necessary. Tiger snake antivenom may be used if sea snake antivenom is not available. Polyvalent snake antivenom is the third-line choice.

3. Jellyfish

ESSENTIALS OF DIAGNOSIS

▶ Jellyfish envenomations are associated with extreme pain both locally and distant from the sting site

▶ Extensive skin changes may be seen shortly after envenomation

▶ Systemic signs and symptoms include nausea and vomiting, autonomic changes, and paralysis

▶ Death is usually caused by respiratory paralysis or drowning secondary to limb paralysis

▶ General Considerations

There are three types of jellyfish that cause the vast majority of the morbidity and mortality associated with jellyfish envenomation of humans: box jellyfish, Irukandji jellyfish, and Portuguese man-o-war. Jellyfish envenomates by touching prey or unsuspecting bathers with long tentacles containing hundreds of stinging cells called nematocysts. The jellyfish sting can cause a wide array of symptoms ranging from skin irritation to death.

▶ Clinical Findings

Most jellyfish stings cause only a localized inflammatory skin reaction and require only symptomatic care. A few jellyfish, however, can cause severe systemic envenomation syndromes.

1. Box Jellyfish

Severe incapacitating localized pain occurs immediately with the development of wide, erythematous bands on the skin. Confusion progressing to unconsciousness as well as respiratory failure and cardiac arrest can occur within 5 minutes. Death is rare and usually occurs in children. Fatalities are due to the cardiotoxic portion of this complex venom. If the patient lives, skin changes occur over the next few hours with the development of blistering and necrosis that may cause permanent scarring.

2. Irukandji Jellyfish

The initial sting is hardly felt. Approximately 30 minutes later, the Irukandji syndrome begins. Unbearable pain generally begins in the sacral area and rapidly progresses to the rest of the body. The pain is always present but worsens in waves. Other symptoms include profuse diaphoresis, restlessness, headache, nausea and vomiting, severe hypertension, and tachycardia. Later complications include pulmonary edema, transient cardiomyopathy, and left ventricular dysfunction.

3. Portuguese Man-o-War

Portuguese man-o-war stings are very painful and leave a "string of beads" appearance. Shortly afterward, an Irukandji-like syndrome can occur, which consists of nausea and vomiting, and muscle cramps, particularly in the abdomen and chest. Pain may be so severe in the chest as to cause hypoxia. Death can occur.

▶ Treatment

1. Box Jellyfish

Due to the rapidity of possible fatality, basic life support on the scene and advanced cardiac life support once in medical hands must be a priority. Vinegar application to the sting sites will inactivate venom. Compression bandages should be applied next. An antivenom exists and should be used immediately to prevent death from severe envenomations, although most victims survive without its use. The antivenom is useful in controlling pain and possibly with preventing scarring. Intramuscular injection above the sting sites should be performed with three ampules. Intravenous pain control is always necessary in all but the most trivial stings.

2. Irukandji Jellyfish

Initial first aid is not usually necessary. The role of vinegar is uncertain because it is not known whether vinegar inactivates the nematocysts. Intravenous pain medication will be needed. Control of blood pressure with an α-adrenergic blocking agent will also be necessary. Monitoring for early signs of heart failure with echocardiography within the first 24 hours is recommended. Respiratory and cardiovascular support may ultimately be needed. Development of an antivenom is under way.

3. Portuguese Man-o-War

First aid consists of removing tentacles. Vinegar is not indicated. Rinsing with seawater, not fresh water, is the treatment of choice. Cold packs and intravenous pain medicine will ease pain. Rarely, respiratory support may be needed.

▶ Disposition

Victims of envenomation should be monitored for 6–8 hours for systemic effects. The elderly or the very young should be monitored for 24 hours.

4. Scorpion Fish

ESSENTIALS OF DIAGNOSIS

► Extreme pain at sting site

► Wound sites commonly become ischemic or secondarily infected

► Systemic signs and symptoms include neurologic changes, respiratory failure, and autonomic dysfunction

▶ General Considerations

Scorpion fish are divided into three groups on the basis of appearance and structure of the venom organ: zebra fish, scorpion fish, and stonefish. The venom apparatus consists of 12 or 13 dorsal spines, 3 anal spines, and 3 pelvic spines, all of which can be erected upon stimulation. The venom can be highly toxic (stonefish) and contains chemical fractions analogous to those contained in stingray venom.

▶ Clinical Findings

Scorpion fish stings vary in intensity depending on the species. Most cause immediate pain, with central radiation of discomfort. Local ischemia at the wound site progresses over days to marked swelling, erythema, and cellulitis. Prolonged indolent wound infections sometimes result. Systemic symptoms occur within the first few hours and include vomiting, weakness, diarrhea, delirium, seizures, paresthesias, fever, arthritis, hypertension, cardiac arrhythmias, respiratory failure, hypotension, and death. The portion of the toxin that is responsible for death causes severe vasodilatation.

▶ Treatment

Manage systemic symptoms and dysfunctions supportively. An antivenom is available in Australia for management of stings by the Indo-Pacific stonefish. For scorpion fish stings occurring in coastal waters surrounding the United States, institute the regimen as described next.

1. Provide Pain Relief

Immerse the wound in hot water to tolerance (45–50°C [113–122°F]) for 30–60 minutes. If heat fails to relieve the pain, infiltrate the wound with lidocaine, 1–2% without epinephrine; or perform regional nerve block. Pain from a stonefish sting may be so severe that it causes delirium requiring parenteral narcotic analgesics for relief.

2. Manage the Wound

Debride and explore the wound, and remove all foreign material. If there is a chance that a spine may have entered a joint, these procedures should be performed in the operating room, and the surgeon should use magnifying loupes to explore the joint. Do not suture wounds tightly; allow adequate drainage.

3. Give Antibiotics

Administer standard tetanus prophylaxis (Chapter 30), and consider starting treatment with trimethoprim/sulfamethoxazole (160 and 800 mg, respectively, twice a day), ciprofloxacin (500 mg twice a day), or tetracycline (500 mg four times a day) for 7 days.

▶ Disposition

Patients who have sustained significant envenomation from a scorpion fish sting should be observed for 4–6 hours for development of systemic symptoms. All patients should be seen frequently on an outpatient basis for wound care after discharged.

Australian Venomous Research Unit at the University of Melbourne: Australian CSL Antivenom Handbook. Available at: www.wch.sa.gov.au/paedm/clintox/cslb index.html.

Currie B: Marine antivenoms. J Toxicol Clin Toxicol 2003;41:301 [PMID: 12807313] (Method of action venom and indication for use of antivenom).

Nomura J et al: A randomized paired comparison trial of cutaneous treatments for acute jellyfish (Carybdea alata) stings. Am J Emerg Med 2002;20:624–626 [PMID: 12442242] (Comparison of vinegar, hot water, and meat tenderizer as treatment for pain of jellyfish stings).

Perkins R et al: Poisoning, envenomation, and trauma from marine creatures. Am Fam Physician 2004;69:885 [PMID: 14989575] (Basic treatment of various marine animal encounters).

EMERGENCY TREATMENT OF INGESTION OF POISONOUS FISH

ESSENTIALS OF DIAGNOSIS

▶ Consider toxic marine ingestion with gastroenteritis, neurologic symptoms, and respiratory compromise

---

Toxic marine poisoning is a worldwide phenomenon involving complex interactions between microbial flora, more than 300 species of fish and shellfish, and regional environmental conditions that may precipitate sometimes epidemic illness. Though varied, the toxins involved are largely heat and gastric acid stable. Treatment is generally supportive and symptomatic. Large ingestions and rapidly progressive symptoms may benefit from activated charcoal, aggressive fluid support, and early airway interventions. Bradycardias generally respond well to atropine. Diagnoses are made by history, epidemiologic, and physical findings.

1. Ciguatera Toxin Poisoning

▶ General Considerations

Ciguatera fish poisoning is caused by tropical and semi-tropical marine coral reef fish whose tissues accumulate toxins from the dinoflagellate, *Gambierdiscus toxicus*. The toxins are multiplied in a food-chain phenomenon in which humans are the final consumer. Ciguaterra, worldwide, is the most common nonbacterial food poisoning. The toxin targets voltage-gated sodium channels; pacific ciguatera toxin has been shown to be ten times as potent as Caribbean isolates with differing regional presentations and severity.

The toxin is ingested by small herbivorous fishes, which are eaten by larger carnivorous fishes. Larger and older fishes are more toxic in ciguatera-endemic areas. The most frequently implicated fishes in the United States include barracuda, jack, snapper, and grouper.

▶ Clinical Findings

Symptom onset ranges from 1–48 hours. First arise perioral parasthesias and mild gastroenteritis or abdominal pain. Symptoms then progress at a rate related to dose, and include parasthesias, pruritis, Lhermitte's phenomenon, myalgias, ataxia, hypotension, and bradycardia. Pathognomonic for ciguatera intoxication is cold allodynia, a sensation of heat–cold reversal. Progressive neurologic symptoms may occur, rarely including respiratory depression and coma. There is a sensitization phenomenon, with subsequent episodes being more pronounced. Untreated, the gastroenteritis usually resolves in 24–48 hours, whereas the neurologic symptoms may become chronic.

▶ Treatment and Disposition

Treat persistent myocardial failure with judicious administration of calcium gluconate, 1–2 g intravenously over 24 hours; the rationale is that the toxin occupies calcium receptor sites that affect the permeability to sodium of the pores in neural and myocardial membranes. Admit patients with cardiovascular symptoms for observation. Antiemetics may be used for gastroenteritis. A double-blinded study recently has shown mannitol to offer no benefit over normal saline administration. Gabapentin has been used recently for chronic neuropathies in anecdotal reports.

2. Scombroid Poisoning

General Considerations

Scombroid poisoning is caused by ingestion of contaminated or unrefrigerated fish with high levels of vasoactive amines. Any dark fleshed species, such as tuna or mackerel, containing high levels of histidine, can produce toxin by endogenous microbial flora. Case reports have included improperly handled canned tuna. Histamine is the dominant toxic product, and urocanic acid, the other one, is a heat and acid stable direct mast cell degranulator. A pseudoallergic reaction develops. Histamine levels higher than 20–50 mg per 100 mL are noted in toxic fish.

Clinical Findings

Symptoms arise within 15–90 minutes of ingestion and last 8–12 hours. Gastrointestinal symptoms are less pronounced. Findings relate to histamine, including flushing, rash, facial swelling, edema, nausea and vomiting, palpitations, respiratory distress, and shock.

Treatment and Disposition

Treatment is directed at reversing the effects of histamine. Histamine 1 and 2 receptor blockade is indicated using diphenhydramine, cimetidine, or ranitidine. Promethazine may be helpful for uncontrolled emesis. If the reaction is severe, give epinephrine, 0.3–0.5 mL of 1:1000 solution subcutaneously. Admit patients with serious illness for observation.

3. Puffer Fish (Tetrodotoxin) Poisoning

General Considerations

Tetrodotoxin is one of the most potent nonprotein poisons found in nature, effective in the nanomolar range on neuronal sodium channels. The poison is found in puffer fish and is the commonest cause of lethal marine poisoning. Historically, cases have centered in Japan with ingestion of the delicacy "Fugu," made by licensed sushi chefs. The toxin accumulates in the skin and liver of the fish.

Clinical Findings

The onset of symptoms can be as rapid as 10 minutes or can be delayed for up to 5 hours. Early symptoms are sensory and include perioral and distal extremity parasthesias. Dizzyness,

muscle weakness, ataxia, hypersalivation, dysrythmia, paralysis, respiratory failure, and coma may evolve rapidly. Sixty percent of victims die, most within the first 6 hours.

Treatment

Early recognition of airway compromise is essential, with anticipating the need for ventilatory support. Sedative and amnestics are necessary as the patient may be conscious. Significantly symptomatic patients should be admitted to an ICU; minimal symptoms require monitoring for 8–24 hours dependent on organ system affected.

4. Paralytic Shellfish Poisoning

Paralytic, diarrhetic, and neurotoxic shellfish poisoning involve the accumulation of toxins in shellfish during phytoplanktonic blooms, largely of dinoflagellate species. Distinction must be made between bacterial and viral shellfish-born infections. Presentation varies geographically and upon the toxin ingested. Symptoms are largely neurologic, including parasthesias, drowsiness, amnesia, respiratory depression, and coma with flaccid paralysis. Gastroenteritis may be an isolated symptom in diarrhetic shellfish poisoning. Symptoms usually resolve in 2–3 days with adequate supportive care.

Treatment

With evidence of dysphagia, obtundation, or progressive paralysis, early airway intervention and endotracheal intubation is indicated. Large ingestions are treated with 50–100 g of activated charcoal. Hypotension is addressed with crystalloid administration. Severe intoxications may lead to arrhythmia; bradycardia responds to atropine, and temporary pacing may be needed for heart block.

Disposition

Patients with respiratory difficulties, cardiovascular symptoms, or paralysis should be hospitalized in an ICU. Patients with symptoms of a minor intoxication, which may be limited to paresthesias and mild dysphagia, should be observed in the emergency department or ICU for at least 8 hours to detect deterioration.

Isbister GK: Neurotoxic marine poisoning. Lancet Neurol 2005;4(4):219–228 [PMID: 15778101] (Review of marine ingestion poisonings).

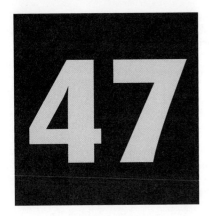

Poisoning

David L. Morgan, MD
Douglas J. Borys, PharmD

IMMEDIATE MANAGEMENT OF LIFE-THREATENING CONDITIONS

Victims of Poisoning with Coma, Seizures, or Marked Obtundation

A. Keep Airway Open

Establish and maintain an adequate airway and ventilation. Begin supplemental oxygen, 12 L/min, by nonrebreathing mask. If the patient has no gag reflex, intubate for airway protection, to facilitate oxygenation and to remove airway secretions. Continuously monitor oxygen saturation.

B. Obtain Arterial Blood Gas and pH Measurements

Obtain arterial blood for blood gas and pH measurements to determine adequacy of ventilation and perfusion.

C. Gain Intravenous Access

Insert a large-bore (≥18-gauge) peripheral or central intravenous catheter, and draw blood for complete blood count, serum electrolyte and blood glucose measurements, and tests of renal and hepatic function.

D. Treat Coma Promptly

Give glucose, 50 mL of a 50% solution (25 g of glucose) intravenously over 3–4 minutes, if a normal blood glucose cannot be determined immediately. If the patient's response is weak or if narcotic overdose is suspected, as indicated by pinpoint pupils and shallow respirations, give repeated doses of naloxone 2 mg every 1–2 minutes up to a total dosage of 10–20 mg. *Note*: The duration of action of naloxone (2–3 hours) is shorter than that of many of the narcotics it reverses. Patients responding to naloxone must be observed for at least 3 hours after the last dose.

If alcoholism or malnutrition is suspected, give thiamine, 100 mg intramuscularly or in intravenous solution with or prior to glucose administration.

E. Maintain Circulation

Maintain circulation, and treat shock by restoring intravascular volume with intravenous infusion of crystal-loid solutions. *Caution*: Fluid overload and pulmonary edema may occur with overly vigorous hydration. Some medications (salicylates) put patients at higher risk for pulmonary edema. If administration of more than 20–30 mL/kg of crystalloid solution and usual doses of dopamine (ie, 5–15 μg/kg/min intravenously) fail to restore blood pressure, insert a central venous catheter and arterial pressure catheter to obtain pressure readings and help guide further therapy with fluids or pressor agents.

F. Treat Seizures

If the patient is experiencing seizures, give diazepam, 0.1–0.2 mg/kg, or lorazepam, 0.05 mg/kg, intravenously. If this is not effective, within a few minutes, repeat the dose. If the seizures continue, administer phenobarbital, 20 mg/kg, intravenously over 20 minutes. Phenytoin is ineffective for stopping seizures caused by most poisonings.

G. Start Electrocardiographic Monitoring

Start cardiac monitoring. Obtain a 12-lead electrocardiogram (ECG) and note especially the rate; rhythm; presence of arrhythmias; and PR, QRS, and QT intervals. If overdose of tricyclic antidepressants is suspected, obtain serial ECGs.

H. Perform Gastric Decontamination

Place a nasogastric or orogastric tube for the administration of activated charcoal. Activated charcoal may be premixed with a 70% solution of sorbitol. Activated charcoal, 1 g/kg, should be given to anyone who may have ingested a toxic substance within 1 hour prior to arrival (see section on decontamination below).

I. Search for Associated Illness

Look for other causes of coma or seizures. In particular, look for (1) head trauma (focal neurologic deficits or asymmetric seizures), (2) other trauma causing hemorrhage or shock, (3) infection (generalized or central nervous system), (4) metabolic disorders (hyponatremia, hypoglycemia, hyperglycemia), (5) hypothermia (use a rectal thermometer that can measure temperatures lower than 32°C [89.6°F]), or (6) hyperthermia.

▼ FURTHER MANAGEMENT OF VICTIMS OF POISONING

For assistance in identifying drugs and poisons and access to expert toxicologic consultation call your local poison center at 1-800-222-1222. Refer to http://www.aapcc.com for other local poison center listings. Experts at the poison center can (1) provide immediate assistance in selecting appropriate laboratory or toxicity tests and (2) in recommending preferred methods of gut decontamination, patient specific care recommendations, or the use of antidotes, and (3) advise on patient disposition.

▶ Obtain Brief History

Obtain as much information as possible from paramedics, bystanders, police, family, and friends. Ask about recent use of drugs or medications, and find out whether any empty pill bottles, medications, or drug paraphernalia were found at the scene. If several patients present with similar symptoms of poisoning, consider carbon monoxide poisoning, food poisoning, or other toxins that can affect multiple victims simultaneously including chemical and bioterrorism. Correlate the history with physical findings and results of laboratory tests, but do not be misled by the history. What the patient or friends say was ingested may differ from what was actually swallowed, especially in suicide attempts.

▶ Decontaminate as Soon as Possible

A. Inhaled Poisons

Remove the patient from the source of poison to fresh air and give oxygen by mask. Inhalation of a water aerosol may help to dilute inhaled irritants in the nasopharynx. Check for hoarseness and singed nasal hairs (eg, after smoke inhalation) and be alert for delayed development of upper airway obstruction or pulmonary edema.

B. Contaminated Eyes

Wash the eyes immediately with copious amounts of plain water or normal saline; *do not* use neutralizing solutions. Hang a bottle containing 500–1000 mL of normal saline above the patient, and dribble the solution slowly into the corner of the injured eye through the intravenous tubing.

If the contaminating material was acidic or basic, tears may be checked with pH paper after the eyes have been washed to make sure that all toxic material has been removed. A careful eye examination is indicated following irrigation.

C. Contaminated Skin

Wash the skin immediately with plenty of water and dilute soap solution. Discard contaminated clothes in a marked plastic bag. Certain toxins, such as organophosphates, are well absorbed through the skin and are difficult to remove. Remove all particulate matter prior to irrigation. Health-care providers should take measures to avoid direct exposure with skin or clothes in an effort to prevent secondary contamination.

Hydrofluoric acid burns are particularly penetrating and corrosive. Following irrigation prompt application of

10% calcium gluconate gel to exposed areas is warranted. A secondary option is immersion of the burn into quaternary ammonium salt solution. Subcutaneous injection of calcium gluconate deep to the burn (0.5 mL of 10% solution per square centimeter of burn area)or intra-arterial calcium may be helpful. Monitor calcium levels closely. Contact a poison control center for additional recommendations. A plastic surgeon (or hand surgeon) should be consulted for injuries involving the fingers.

D. Ingested Poisons

The traditional approach has been to remove ingested toxins by emesis or gastric lavage, followed by activated charcoal and catharsis. However, recent evidence suggests that gastric emptying may have limited efficiency, especially if initiated more than 1 hour after the ingestion, and may delay the administration of charcoal. Activated charcoal is the preferred method of gastric decontamination, particularly in patients who have taken a rapid-acting medication.

1. Ipecac—Induced emesis is no longer recommended.

2. Gastric lavage—Use gastric lavage in patients with suspected serious poisonings, who have a decreased level of consciousness, and who present to the emergency department within 1 hour of ingestion. Unless a patient is intubated, gastric lavage is contraindicated if airway protective reflexes are absent.

Gastric lavage is performed with a large-bore (at least 36F for adults) orogastric or nasogastric tube. (Pill fragments cannot be removed through standard-sized nasogastric tubes.) Use tap water or saline at body temperature in 250-mL increments, and continue lavage until fluid returns clear or free of pill fragments.

3. Activated charcoal—Activated charcoal, 50–100 g as a slurry, can be given if a patient has ingested a potentially toxic amount of most poisons. The administration of activated charcoal is contraindicated in those patients unable to protect their airway. Activated charcoal may be administered by nasogastric or orogastric tube following intubation for patients who do not have an intact airway. For oral administration, charcoal can be made more palatable by adding a small amount of cherry, licorice, or chocolate flavoring just before administration. Mixing the charcoal with 1 mL/kg of 70% sorbitol improves taste and also provides cathartic action. A cathartic should be limited to a single dose of activated charcoal in order to minimize diarrhea and dehydration. The effectiveness of activated charcoal decreases with time, and it will be ineffective for most substances if given more than 1 or 2 hours after the ingestion. Charcoal has great adsorptive properties and can bind most poisons (exceptions include caustics, hydrocarbons, alcohols, iron, lithium, lead, and potassium). If the ingested dose of poison is known, give at least 10 times that weight of charcoal, in divided doses if necessary.

4. Whole bowel irrigation—Indications for whole bowel irrigation include large ingestion of sustained release products, large ingestion of chemicals not absorbed by charcoal (such as lithium), and ingestion of foreign bodies or drug-filled packets. This technique utilizes a balanced electrolyte polyethylene glycol solution (Colyte, GoLYTELY) to flush out the entire intestinal tract. It is given by nasogastric tube, 1–2 L/h (400–500 mL/min in children), until the rectal effluent is clear (3–5 hours or more).

▶ Perform Complete Physical Examination

Look for characteristic physical signs of various kinds of poisoning while immediate treatment measures are being started. Physical signs associated with specific poisons are listed in Tables 47–1 and 47–2.

▶ Order Other Laboratory and X-ray Studies as Needed

Appropriate laboratory evaluation of the patient is determined, in part, by the patient's clinical condition.

A. Blood Tests

Obtain arterial blood gas to determine adequacy of ventilation and circulation. Draw blood for measurement of serum electrolytes, blood urea nitrogen, blood glucose, and serum osmolality. Calculate anion and osmolar gaps (Tables 47–3 and 47–4).

B. Electrocardiogram

Obtain an ECG and look for widened QRS complexes or QT intervals, atrioventricular block, ventricular tachyarrhythmias, or evidence of ischemia (Table 47–5).

C. Radiography

Obtain a chest X-ray to examine for pulmonary edema (caused by opioids, barbiturates, salicylates, ethchlorvynol, or corrosive chemicals) or infiltrates (due to aspiration of gastric contents, inhalation of certain metal fumes, or hydrocarbon aspiration). Obtain an abdominal X-ray to look for radiopaque pills or toxins (Table 47–6).

D. Urine Laboratory Studies

Obtain urine for toxicologic screening and routine analysis. Calcium oxalate crystals may be present with ethylene glycol poisoning. Occult blood in the urine may be indicative of myoglobinuria or hemolysis. Phenylpyruvic acid (eg, Phenistix) may be positive for phenothiazine or salicylate overdose in an alkaline urine.

E. Toxicologic Laboratory Studies

Qualitative determination of the presence of drugs in the urine rarely provides information that alters therapy and

Table 47–1. Physical Findings Associated with Various Types Poisons.

Altered vital signs
  Hypertension: amphetamines, phencyclidine, phenyl propanolamine, anticholinergics, cocaine, nicotine
  Hypotension: sedative–hypnotics, narcotics, antihypertensives, theophylline, clonidine, β-blockers, tricyclic antidepressants
  Hyperthermia: salicylates, amphetamines, cocaine, phencyclidine, anticholinergics, seizures due to any cause
  Hypothermia: narcotics, barbiturates, ethanol, other sedative–hypnotics, clonidine, phenothiazines
  Hyperpnea: salicylates or other agents causing metabolic acidosis
Ocular signs
  Miosis (pinpoint pupils): narcotics, clonidine, organophosphates, phenothiazines, severe sedative–hypnotic overdose, pilocarpine
  Mydriasis (dilated pupils): anticholinergics, amphetamines, cocaine, LSD, glutethimide
  Nystagmus: phenytoin, phencyclidine (especially vertical nystagmus), alcohol, many sedative–hypnotics
  Ophthalmoplegia: botulism, sedative–hypnotics
  Oculogyric crisis: haloperidol, other antipsychotics
  Optic neuritis methanol
Breath odors
  Smoke: fire-associated toxins (see section on inhalants)
  Garlic arsenic, arsine gas, organophosphates
  Bitter almond or silver polish; cyanide
  Wintergreen: methyl salicylate
  Pear-like: chloral hydrate
  Rotten eggs: hydrogen sulfide
  Acetone: diabetic ketoacidosis, isopropanol
  Typical odors of ethanol, ammonia, tobacco, disinfectants, camphor, glue, paraldehyde
Skin signs
  Cyanosis: ergotamine, agents causing hypoxemia, hypotension, or methemoglobinemia
  Flushed, red: carbon monoxide (rare), cyanide (rare), anticholinergics, boric acid
  Acneiform rash: bromides, chlorinated aromatic hydrocarbons
  Bullae: nonspecific for sedative–hypnotic overdose, carbon monoxide, and other causes of coma
Altered muscle tone
  Increased: amphetamines, phencyclidine, antipsychotics
  Flaccid: sedative–hypnotics, narcotics, clonidine
  Fasciculations: organophosphates, lithium
  Rigidity: haloperidol, phencyclidine, strychnine
  Dystonic posturing: antipsychotics, phencyclidine
  Tremor: lithium, nicotine, or stimulant overdose; alcohol or sedative–hypnotic withdrawal
  Asterixis (flapping tremor): agents causing hepatic encephalopathy
  Seizures: tricyclic antidepressants, theophylline, amphetamines, cocaine, phencyclidine, phenothiazines isoniazid, lindane, other chlorinated
    hydrocarbons and pesticides

is seldom helpful in the emergency department. Results of toxicologic studies may be useful in later confirmation of the diagnosis. It is more cost effective to save serum and urine samples in the laboratory and analyze them later only if necessary. For a few types of medication poisoning (eg, lithium, acetaminophen, digoxin), the blood or serum drug concentration may be valuable in determining the need for specific therapy. These specific drugs and their antidotes are discussed later in this chapter.

▶ Accelerate Elimination of Poisons

A. Toxicokinetics

The rational management of drug overdose requires an understanding of the absorption, distribution, and elimination of the toxin. Most published kinetic parameters have

been determined at normal doses, whereas pharmacokinetics in victims of large doses is often more complex.

Dissolution and absorption of toxin or gastric-emptying time may be altered in poisoned patients, so that the peak effects may be delayed (as occurs with anticholinergics). The gastrointestinal tract may be injured, allowing increased absorption of certain materials (eg, iron). If the finite capacity of the liver to metabolize a drug is exceeded, an increased amount of the drug may be delivered to the systemic circulation. If the concentration of the toxin in the bloodstream increases dramatically, protein binding may be saturated (eg, in salicylate poisoning), so that the fraction of free toxin increases. Circulatory insufficiency, hypothermia, and electrolyte and acid–base imbalance influence the metabolism and excretion of ingested drugs. Any of these factors may drastically alter normal kinetics and confuse calculations.

Table 47-2. Toxidromes.

Toxidrome	Representative Agent(s)	Most Common Findings	Additional Signs and Symptoms	Potential Interventions
Opioid	Heroin Morphine	CNS depression, miosis, respiratory depression	Hypothermia, bradycardia. Death may result from respiratory arrest, pulmonary edema	Ventilation or naloxone
Sympathomimetic	Cocaine Amphetamine	Psychomotor agitation, mydriasis, diaphoresis, tachycardia, hypertension, hyperthermia	Seizures, rhabdomyolysis, myocardial infarction. Death may result from seizures, cardiac arrest, hyperthermia	Cooling, sedation with benzodiazepines, hydration
Cholinergic	Organophosphate insecticides Carbamate insecticides	Salivation, lacrimation, diaphoresis, nausea, vomiting, urination, defecation, muscle fasciculations, weakness, bronchorrhea	Bradycardia, miosis/mydriasis, seizures, respiratory failure, paralysis Death may result from respiratory arrest 2° to paralysis and/or bronchorrhea, seizures	Airway protection and ventilation, atropine, pralidoxime
Anticholinergic	Scopolamine Atropine	Altered mental status, mydriasis, dry/flushed skin, urinary retention, decreased bowel sounds, hyperthermia, dry mucous membranes	Seizures, dysrhythmias, rhabdomyolysis. Death may result from hyperthermia and dysrhythmias	Physostigmine (if appropriate) sedation with benzodiazepines, cooling supportive management
Salicylates	Aspirin Oil of wintergreen	Altered mental status, respiratory alkalosis, metabolic acidosis, tinnitus hyperpnea, tachycardia, diaphoresis, nausea, vomiting	Low-grade fever, ketonuria. Death may result from pulmonary edema, cardiorespiratory arrest	MDAC, alkalinization of the urine with potassium repletion, hemodialysis, hydration
Hypoglycemia	Sulfonylureas Insulin	Altered mental status, diaphoresis, tachycardia, hypertension	Paralysis, slurring of speech, bizarre behavior, seizures. Death may result from seizures, altered behavior	Glucose, containing solution intravenously, and oral feedings if able, frequent capillary blood for glucose measurement
Serotonin syndrome	Meperidine/dextromethorphan + MAOI, SSRI + TCA, SSRI/TCA/MAOI + amphetamine, SSRI overdose	Altered mental status, increased muscle tone, hyperreflexia, hyperthermia	"Wet dog shakes" (intermittent whole body tremor). Death may result from hyperthermia.	Cooling, sedation with benzodiazepines, supportive management, theoretical benefit—cyproheptadine

CNS, central nervous system; MDAC, multidose activated charcoal; MAOI, monoamine oxidase inhibitor; SSRI, selective serotonin reuptake inhibitor; TCA, tricyclic antidepressant. Reproduced, with permission, from Tintinalli JE, Kelen GD, Stapczynski S: *Emergency Medicine: A Comprehensive Study Guide*, 5th edn. McGraw-Hill, 2000.

Table 47–3. Drugs Causing Metabolic Acidosis Associated with an Elevated Anion Gap.[a]

Direct causes of acidosis
Alcohols: methanol, ethanol, ethylene glycol
Salicylates
Paraldehyde
Phenformin
Indirect causes of acidosis
Seizures (eg, isoniazid)
Hypotension (eg, barbiturates)
Hypoxemia (eg, carbon monoxide, cyanide)

[a]Anion gap $(Na^+ + K^+) - (HCO_3^- + Cl^-) = 12–16$ mEq/L.

Despite these limitations, pharmacokinetic principles may be useful in the management of drug overdose. Some terms commonly used in toxicology are defined below.

1. Half-life—The half-life of a toxin is the time required to eliminate one half of the toxin from the body. This parameter is most meaningful for the many drugs (eg, barbiturates, theophylline) that exhibit first-order kinetics, in which a fixed percentage of the toxin is removed per unit of time. Other drugs (eg, alcohol) have zero-order kinetics, in which a fixed amount of toxin is removed per unit of time. In an overdose, pathways of elimination are often saturated, and first-order kinetic elimination is replaced by zero-order (fixed amount) elimination.

2. Volume of distribution—The volume of distribution (V_d) is the volume into which the toxin is distributed after absorption. If a drug is sequestered outside the blood and is highly tissue bound, it will have a large volume of distribution. Table 47–7 gives the volumes of distribution for several common drugs.

3. Clearance—Clearance is the volume of plasma that can be cleared of toxin per unit of time. Clearance includes both renal and metabolic components, and the proportion that each contributes to total clearance is important. For

Table 47–5. Electrocardiographic Manifestations of Poisoning.

Sign	Examples of Causes
Prolonged QT interval	Hypocalcemia (ethylene glycol) Tricyclic antidepressants Type I antiarrhythmic agents
Prolonged QRS interval	Phenothiazines (selected) Tricyclic antidepressants Type I antiarrhythmic agents
Atrioventricular block	β-Adrenergic blockers Calcium channel blockingagents Digitalis glycosides Tricyclic antidepressants Type I antiarrhythmic agents
Ventricular tachyarrhythmias	Amphetamines, cocaine Digitalis glycosides Theophylline Tricyclic antidepressants Type I antiarrhythmic agents
Ischemic pattern or current of injury	Cellular, asphyxiants (cyanide, carbon monoxide) Hypoxemia (pneumonia) Hypotension

example, a toxin may be 95% metabolized and 5% renally excreted, in which case doubling the renal clearance of the toxin will not significantly enhance its total elimination from the body.

Knowledge of these parameters is helpful when measures to increase drug elimination (eg, forced alkaline diuresis, hemodialysis, or hemoperfusion) are under consideration. For example, toxins with large volumes of distribution are present in only minute quantities in plasma and are not effectively removed by dialysis or diuresis. Measures to enhance elimination of drugs with rapid intrinsic clearance rates will not contribute significantly to the overall elimination rate.

Table 47–4. Calculation of the Osmolar Gap in Toxicology.

The osmolar gap (Δ Osm) is determined by subtracting the calculated serum osmolality from the measured serum osmolality. Calculated osmolality:
$$Osm = 2(Na^+) + \frac{Glucose}{18} + \frac{BUN}{2.8}$$
Osmolar gap:
$$\Delta Osm = \text{measured Osm} - \text{Calculated Osm}$$

Note: Most laboratories use the freezing point method for calculating osmolality. If the vaporization point method is used, alcohols are driven off and their contribution to osmolality is lost.

Table 47–6. Drugs and Toxins that may be Radiopaque.[a]

Chloral hydrate Heavy metals (iron, arsenic) Iodide Psychotropics (phenothiazines, tricyclic antidepressants) Sodium Enteric-coated tablets	Mnemonic is CHIPS

[a]*Caution*: Recent studies suggest that these drugs are *not* routinely visible on X-ray. If tablets have dissolved, false-negative X-ray results may occur. Abdominal X-rays are therefore useful only if positive findings are seen.

Table 47–7. Volumes of Distribution for Some Common Drugs.

Drugs with Large Volumes of Distribution		Drugs with Small Volumes of Distribution	
Chlorpromazine	10–20 L/kg	Acetaminophen	0.8 L/kg
Haloperidol	20–30 L/kg	Digitoxin	0.5 L/kg
Amitriptyline	>40 L/kg	Ethanol	0.6 L/kg
Imipramine	10–20L/kg	Isoniazid	0.6 L/kg
Digoxin	6–10 L/kg	Lithium	1.1 L/kg
Meperidine	4 L/kg	Phenytoin	0.6 L/kg
Methadone	5 L/kg	Salicylate	0.2 L/kg
		Theophylline	0.5 L/kg

Table 47–8. Indications for Hemodialysis or Hemoperfusion in the Management of Poisoned Patients Unresponsive to Antidotal or Supportive Therapy.

Indicated immediately if intoxication is significant
 Methanol (HD)
 Ethylene glycol (HD)
 Lithium (HD)
 Paraquat (HP)
 Salicylate (HD)
 Theophylline (HP preferred over HD)
Indicated if supportive measures are unsuccessful or if prolonged coma is expected
 Phenobarbital (HP preferred over HD)
 Ethchlorvynol (HP)
 Digitoxin (HP)
 Tricyclic antidepressants (HP)
Not indicated
 Digoxin
 Benzodiazepines (diazepam, chlordiazepoxide)
 Glutethimide
 Narcotics
 Short-acting barbiturates
 Amphetamines, phencyclidine, cocaine
 Quinidine, procainamide
 Chlorpromazine, haloperidol, and other antipsychotics

HD, hemodialysis; HP, hemoperfusion.

B. Methods to Enhance Drug Elimination

The decision to use a specific therapy to improve drug elimination should be based on a rational understanding of the drug's properties and the patient's clinical condition. Most patients respond satisfactorily to appropriate supportive care. The risks, time, and expense involved in hemodialysis or hemoperfusion must be weighed against the possible benefits. In some patients, the severe potential toxicity of the poison warrants immediate hemodialysis (Table 47–8). With other poisons, dialysis is of no theoretic or proved benefit. Poison control center staff may be helpful in identifying those patients who may benefit from enhanced drug elimination.

1. Diuresis and pH manipulations—Because many toxins are weak acids or bases, they can be ionized in solutions of varying pH. In the ionized state, they are less likely to cross cell membranes, and their reabsorption to the renal tubular epithelium is decreased. The clinical significance of these measures depends on the contribution of renal elimination to total body clearance. It is also important to consider the possible adverse effects of overhydration, alkalemia, or acidemia. Most studies have failed to show a significant improvement in the outcome of poisoning by either forced diuresis or by the production of acidemia or alkalemia.

 However, weak acids such as salicylate and phenobarbital are more fully ionized in basic solutions, so that alkalizing the urine may serve to trap them in the tubular lumen, thus increasing excretion of the drug in the urine. Urine acidification is no longer recommended for any poisoning because it may promote myoglobinuric renal failure in patients with rhabdomyolysis.

2. Hemodialysis—During hemodialysis, toxin is removed from the blood into a dialysate solution across a semipermeable membrane. The toxin must be relatively water soluble and not highly protein bound. It should have a small volume of distribution and slow rate of intrinsic elimination (ie, a long half-life). Hemodialysis is effective in removing methanol, ethylene glycol, salicylates, and lithium, among other drugs (see Table 47–8). It is also of value in correcting pH and electrolyte imbalances, especially in anuric patients.

3. Peritoneal dialysis—This method is much less efficient than hemodialysis in removing most drugs.

4. Hemoperfusion—In hemoperfusion, blood is pumped through a column of adsorbent material (charcoal or resin) and returned to the patient's circulation. Vascular access similar to that for hemodialysis is required. The kinetic conditions required are the same as in hemodialysis; that is, the drug should have a small volume of distribution and a slow rate of intrinsic clearance. Hemoperfusion has the advantage that the drug or toxin is in direct contact with the adsorbent material; therefore, high molecular weight, poor water solubility, and even plasma protein binding are not limiting factors as they are in hemodialysis. Hemoperfusion is commonly associated with thrombocytopenia. Hemoperfusion will not correct pH or electrolyte imbalances.

5. Repeated doses of activated charcoal—Repeated doses of charcoal given orally or via gastric tube (20–30 g every 3–4 hours without a cathartic) may enhance elimination of some drugs and toxins from the bloodstream by interrupting enterohepatic or enteroenteric recirculation of the toxic. Drugs for which this may be useful are quinine, aminophylline, phenobarbital, nadolol, carbamazepine, and dapsone.

6. Lipid Emulsion—Recently, successful case reports have been documented in humans with the use of lipid infusion in significant local anesthetic toxicity. A 20% lipid infusion has been used to resuscitate a patients from cardiac arrest following the use of anesthetics. Some have postulated that this treatment could be used for many other fat soluble medication poisonings such as calcium channel blockers.

C. Antidotes

Table 47–9 sets forth several common useful antidotes. Their indications and dosages are discussed below in the sections on specific toxins. The half-life of the antidote relative to that of the toxin must be considered. Most important, antidotes should not be used indiscriminately and without regard for the patient's clinical condition. They may have serious adverse effects and in some cases may be more toxic than the poison. *Note*: Always treat the specific symptoms manifested by the patient, not those known to be associated with a certain poison or by history alone.

Table 47–9. Some Poisons for Which There are Specific Antidotes.

Poison	Specific Antidote
Acetaminophen	Acetylcysteine
Anticholinergics	Physostigmine
Anticholinesterases (organophosphates, carbamates, physostigmine)	Atropine Pralidoxime (2-PAM)
Benzodiazepines	Flumazenil
β-Blockers	Glucagon
Calcium channel blockers	Calcium
Carbon monoxide	100% Oxygen
Cyanide	Sodium nitrite
	Sodium thiosulfate Vitamin B_{12} (not yet approved for use in the United States)
Digoxin	Digoxin-specific antibodies
Heavy metals	Chelating agents
Isoniazid	Pyridoxine (vitamin B_6)
Methanol, ethylene glycol	Ethanol, folate, 4-methyl pyrazole (not approved for use in the United States)
Narcotics	Naloxone
Tricyclic antidepressants	Sodium bicarbonate

MANAGEMENT OF CONDITIONS ASSOCIATED WITH POISONING

▶ Airway Management

It is essential to protect the lungs from aspiration and maintain adequate ventilation and oxygenation.

A. Patients in Coma or with Markedly Depressed Gag Reflex

In the patient with a depressed gag reflex, gastric lavage and administration of activated charcoal may result in significant aspiration. Endotracheal intubation should always be performed in these patients, especially before gastric lavage. Charcoal should be administered through an orogastric or nasogastric tube.

B. Awake Patient with Normal Gag Reflex

Activated charcoal may be administered and gastric lavage may be performed without special precautions.

C. Lethargic Patient

The lethargic patient with fluctuating mental status and a variable gag reflex poses a more difficult problem in management. If the gag reflex is intact, cautious gastric lavage may be performed with the patient in the left lateral decubitus position and with the head of the bed or stretcher tilted down at an angle of 10–20°. *Note*: If there is any doubt about the patient's ability to protect the airway with a gag or cough reflex, charcoal administration and gastric lavage must be preceded by intubation with a cuffed endotracheal tube.

If intubation is not immediately performed, it is critical to monitor the status of the airway closely and to position the patient so as to preserve aspiration. An initially responsive patient may rapidly become more obtunded. Significant swelling and upper airway obstruction may be late developments after thermal, chemical, or caustic burns.

▶ Seizures

A. General Management

Management of drug-induced seizures is generally the same as that for seizures due to other causes, that is, protection of the airway; use of anticonvulsants; and correction of acidosis, hypoxemia, electrolyte abnormalities, and hyperthermia. Seizures unrelated to poisoning may also occur as a result of intracranial bleeding from trauma, hypoglycemia, or hyponatremia. Seizures caused by poisoning are rarely focal, nor are they associated with asymmetric neurologic findings. Meningitis may mimic metabolic or toxic encephalopathy and must be ruled out by lumbar puncture.

B. Specific Therapy

In certain types of poisoning, refractory seizures may require specific therapy:

1. Seizures occurring as a result of theophylline, lithium, or salicylate overdose usually require hemodialysis or hemoperfusion to accelerate removal of the drug.

2. In isoniazid poisoning with seizures refractory to diazepam, administer pyridoxine, 5 g (or 1 g per gram of isoniazid ingested) intravenously.

3. Seizures due to organophosphate poisoning may respond to atropine and pralidoxime. (See Organophosphates & Other Cholinesterase Inhibitors section, below.)

4. Seizures due to anticholinergics that are refractory to conventional therapy may respond to physostig-mine, 0.5–2 mg slow IV push.

▶ Hypotension

Hypotension is a common associated condition in victims of poisoning. The mechanism of hypotension may be direct cardiac depression, peripheral vasodilation, or fluid defects or shifts that result in hypovolemia. Concurrent hypothermia may aggravate hypotension. Be alert for possible concurrent trauma with occult internal bleeding or concurrent infection with septic shock.

In the absence of associated pulmonary edema, a fluid challenge should be given with intravenous boluses of 1 L of normal saline. A central venous or pulmonary artery catheter may need to be inserted to monitor fluid needs and response to therapy in cases of refractory hypotension. Monitoring of urine output with an in-dwelling catheter is recommended. If hypotension and hypoperfusion are severe and unresponsive to administration of fluids and temperature correction, vasopressors may be of benefit.

▶ Thermodysregulation

A. Hyperthermia

1. Causes—Many drugs cause hyperthermia, either by direct toxic effects on temperature-regulating mechanisms or through associated hyperactivity or seizures.

A. SALICYLATES—Salicylate intoxication causes hyperthermia by uncoupling of oxidative phosphorylation, resulting in inefficient (and therefore heat generating) production of ATP.

B. PHENOTHIAZINES—Phenothiazines inhibit the autoregulatory ability of the central nervous system, leading to environmentally induced hypothermia or hyperthermia.

C. SEIZURES OR HYPERACTIVITY—Hyperthermia may result from seizures or extreme hyperactivity (particularly if the patient has to be forcibly restrained) following poisoning by phencyclidine (PCP), cocaine, or amphetamines.

D. ANTICHOLINERGIC PROPERTIES—The anticholinergic properties of many drugs (eg, antihistamines, tricyclic antidepressants) can aggravate hyperthermia by inhibiting sweating.

2. Treatment—For dangerous core temperatures above 41°C (105.8°F), cool the patient rapidly by sponge bathing with evaporation accelerated by fanning and ice packs; treat seizures. Muscular hyperactivity is most effectively treated with benzodiazepines or neuromuscular paralysis and assisted ventilation.

B. Hypothermia

Hypothermia may be caused by certain drugs, exposure to cold, hypoglycemia, sepsis, or hypothyroidism. The diagnosis may be missed if a rectal thermometer capable of reading temperatures in the range of 24–32°C (75.2–89.6°F) is not used.

For severe hypothermia, rapidly restore normal body temperature with warm intravenous fluids, warm gastric or peritoneal lavage, or ventilation with warmed, humidified air. Slow passive rewarming by external means is usually sufficient in milder cases.

▶ Delayed Severe Toxicity

Initial evaluation may fail to reveal the seriousness of poisoning with some drugs. Severe, potentially preventable hepatic damage may occur after acetaminophen overdose unless the physician determines acetaminophen levels and administers the antidote N-acetylcysteine, when appropriate, early in treatment. Other poisons with characteristically delayed severe toxicity are listed in Table 47–10.

The development of sustained-release preparations has increased the chances of nearly normal results on initial evaluation. The possibility that a sustained-release preparation has been used must be considered in theophylline or salicylate poisoning, because with these drugs, serum or blood concentrations are used to evaluate the severity of intoxication. Under these circumstances, it is prudent to observe the patient longer and obtain a second blood-level reading before deciding on further treatment and disposition.

American Academy of Clinical Toxicology; European Association of Poisons Centres and Clinical Toxicologists: Position statement: Single-dose activated charcoal. J Toxicol Clin Toxicol 2005;43:61–87 [PMID: 15822758].

Heard K: Gastrointestinal decontamination. Med Clin North Am 2005;89:1067–1078 [PMID: 16227054].

Eddleston M, Juszczak E, Buckley NA et al: Multiple-dose activated charcoal in acute self-poisoning: a randomized controlled trial. Lancet 2008;371:579–587 [PMID: 18280328].

Jamaty C, Bailey B, Larocque A et al: Lipid emulsioins in the treatment of acute poisoning: a systemic review of human and animal studies. Clin Toxicol (Phila) 2010;48:1–27 [PMID: 20095812].

Table 47-10. Selected Examples of Poisons with Delayed Severe Toxicity.

Poison	Delayed Effect
Acetaminophen	Hepatic necrosis
Amanita mushrooms	Hepatic necrosis
Carbon tetrachloride	Hepatic and renal damage
Methanol	Blindness
Paraquat	Pulmonary fibrosis
Super-warfarins	Bleeding
Thallium	Peripheral neuropathy, hair loss
Ethylene glycol	Renal failure

EMERGENCY TREATMENT OF SPECIFIC POISONINGS

ACETAMINOPHEN

ESSENTIALS OF DIAGNOSIS

▶ Patient may be asymptomatic early after acute ingestion or present with anorexia, nausea, and right upper quadrant pain

▶ Draw 4-hour postingestion levels, and use the nomogram (Figure 47-1) to predict severity following acute ingestion

  – Chronic toxicity should be assessed through clinical examination, an acetaminophen level, and liver function tests

  – N-Acetylcysteine (NAC) therapy is antidote if indicated

▶ General Considerations

Acetaminophen is a widely used ingredient in numerous over-the-counter and prescription preparations. One of the products of the normal metabolism of acetaminophen is hepatotoxic; at toxic levels, it saturates the glutathione detoxification system in the liver and accumulates, causing delayed hepatic injury (24–72 hours after ingestion). The toxic dose of acetaminophen is considered to be over 150 mg/kg in children and seven gin adults.

▶ Clinical Findings

Caution: Shortly after ingestion of acetaminophen, there may be no symptoms or only anorexia, vomiting, or nausea;

hepatic necrosis may not become clinically apparent until 24–48 hours later, when nausea, vomiting, abdominal pain, jaundice, and markedly elevated results on liver function tests may appear. Hepatic failure may follow.

▶ Treatment

A. General Management

Provide intensive supportive care and gastrointestinal decontamination as described previously. Administer activated charcoal regardless of the possibility that *N*-acetylcysteine may be administered.

B. Estimation of Severity

Obtain a 4-hour postingestion acetaminophen serum concentration measurement, and use the Rumack-Matthew nomogram (see Figure 47–1) to predict the range of severity. If the 4-hour level is over 150 µg/mL, begin treatment with *N*-acetylcysteine. Because acetaminophen and salicylate are often ingested simultaneously, a measurement of serum salicylate concentration should also be obtained immediately. The nomogram is not helpful in determining the need for

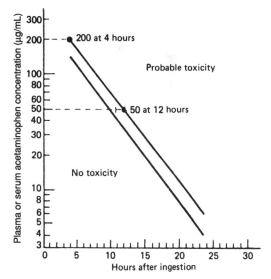

▲ **Figure 47–1.** Nomogram for prediction of acetaminophen hepatotoxicity following acute overdosage. The upper line defines serum acetaminophen concentrations known to be associated with hepatotoxicity. The lower line defines serum levels 25% below those expected to cause hepatotoxicity. To give a margin for error, the lower line should be used as a guide to treatment. (Modified and reproduced, with permission, from Rumack BM, Matthew M: Acetaminophen poisoning and toxicity. Pediatrics 1975;55:871.)

N-acetylcysteine for sustained-release product or chronic ingestions. If a sustained-released product has been ingested, two serum acetaminophen levels should be obtained 4–6 hours apart and treatment given if either level is above the possible toxicity line. For chronic toxicity or for those patients who present after 24 hours postingestion, treatment is based on clinical effects, liver function tests, and the acetaminophen level.

C. *N*-Acetylcysteine Therapy

N-acetylcysteine substitutes for glutathione and binds the toxic metabolite of acetaminophen, thus inactivating and detoxifying it. It is available in both oral and intravenous dosage forms. Both the oral and intravenous routes have been demonstrated in multiple studies to be effective. Give 140 mg/kg orally of a 10 or 20% solution diluted to 5% with citrus juice or soda. Follow with 70 mg/kg orally every 4 hours for 72 hours. If the patient vomits a dose within 1 hour, it should be repeated; slow drip by nasogastric tube and administration of an antiemetic (eg, metoclopramide, 10–20 mg intravenously) may be helpful. Intravenous *N*-acetylcysteine dosing is 150 mg/kg in 200 mL of 5% dextrose for over 15 minutes. Maintenance dosing is 50 mg/kg in 500 mL of 5% dextrose over 4 hours followed by 100 mg/kg in 1-L 5% dextrose infused over 16 hours. Anaphylactoid reactions have been reported with the use of intravenous *N*-acetylcysteine.

To be effective, *N*-acetylcysteine must be given within 12–16 hours of ingestion of acetaminophen and preferably within 8 hours. Do not delay treatment if a serum acetaminophen level is not readily available and a toxic dose may have been taken. Treat with *N*-acetylcysteine empirically and reevaluate treatment after the acetaminophen level has returned. *N*-Acetylcysteine can also be safely given in pregnancy.

▶ Disposition

Use serum concentration of acetaminophen as a guide to the severity of poisoning, and hospitalize all patients requiring acetylcysteine therapy and those with evidence of hepatotoxicity.

Wolf SJ, Heard K, Sloan EP, Jagoda AS; American College of Emergency Physicians: Clinical policy: critical issues in the management of patients presenting to the emergency department with acetaminophen overdose. Ann Emerg Med 2007;50:292–313 [PMID: 17709050].

Dart RC, Erdman AR, Olson KR et al: Acetaminophen poisoning: an evidence-based consensus guideline for out-of-hospital management. Clin Toxicol (Phila) 2006;44:1–18 [PMID: 16496488].

Rowden AK, Norvell J, Eldridge DL, Kirk MA: Updates on acetaminophen toxicity. Med Clin North Am 2005;89:1145–1159 [PMID: 16227058].

AMPHETAMINES AND OTHER RELATED STIMULANTS

ESSENTIALS OF DIAGNOSIS

▶ All drugs in this class are central nervous system stimulants

▶ Predominant symptom is sympathetic hyperactivity

▶ Treatment is supportive; no specific antidote is available

▶ General Considerations

Amphetamines and other stimulants are easily abused because of their wide availability, primarily through street sales. Illicitly obtained stimulants frequently contain methamphetamine and may also contain PCP.

All of these drugs are central nervous system stimulants and cause sympathetic hyperactivity. Some may produce significant vasoconstriction causing hypertension. Most of these drugs have short half-lives and their peak effect and toxicity occur within 30 minutes after intravenous or intramuscular administration and 2–3 hours after oral ingestion. As a result, serum drug level measurements are of little value, and measures to enhance elimination generally do not alter the outcome.

▶ Clinical Findings

Significant amphetamine poisoning is always accompanied by symptoms. Euphoria, mydriasis, and restlessness progress in severe cases to toxic psychosis and seizures. Hypertension can be severe and associated with palpitations or arrhythmias. Seizures and hyperthermia may produce rhabdomyolysis and myoglobinuria.

▶ Treatment

A. General Management

Provide intensive supportive care and gastrointestinal decontamination as described previously. For severe agitation or psychotic behavior, diazepam (5–10 mg in adults and 0.1–0.2 mg/kg in children) or lorazepam (2–4 mg in adults and 0.05–0.1 mg/kg in children) intravenously may be helpful; repeat every 5–10 minutes until sedation has been achieved.

B. Treatment of Seizures

Treat seizures with diazepam (5–10 mg in adults and 0.1–0.2 mg/kg in children) or lorazepam (2–4 mg in adults and 0.05–0.1 mg/kg in children) intravenously. May repeat every 5–10 minutes until seizures have ended. If seizures continue, administer phenobarbital (20 mg/kg intravenously over 20 minutes).

C. Treatment of Hypertension

Hypertension is generally transient and, unless severe, does not require treatment. Often the hypertension responds to benzodiazepine administration, but in severe cases (eg, diastolic blood pressure > 120 mm Hg, encephalopathy), intravenous nitroprusside, 0.5–1.0 μg/kg/min, is effective and easily titratable. Phentolamine, 0.1 mg/kg slowly intravenously, is an alternative drug.

D. Treatment of Arrhythmias

Tachycardia and ventricular tachyarrhythmias rarely require treatment but may respond to administration of propranolol, 0.05–0.1 mg/kg intravenously.

E. Other Measures

Monitor temperature and start cooling measures if hyperthermia occurs. Check the urine for myoglobin. Acidification of the urine is not recommended.

If chest pain is present, perform an ECG and check for cardiac enzymes, and consider hospitalization to rule out myocardial ischemia or infarction. Patients with seizures may require computed tomography (CT) scanning to rule out intracranial hemorrhage.

▶ Disposition

Hospitalize patients with complications (psychotic behavior, hypertension, hyperthermia, chest pain, and arrhythmias) or those with prolonged symptoms.

Greene SL, Kerr F, Braitberg G: Review article: amphetamines and related drugs of abuse. Emerg Med Australas 2008;20:391–402 [PMID: 18973636].

Scharman EJ, Erdman AR, Cobaugh DJ et al: Methylphenidate poisoning: an evidence-based consensus guideline for out-of-hospital management. Clin Toxicol (Phila) 2007;45:737–752 [PMID: 18058301].

ANTICHOLINERGICS

ESSENTIALS OF DIAGNOSIS

▶ Ingestion produces many symptoms prompting the phrase "blind as a bat, hot as Hades, red as a beet, dry as a bone, and mad as a hatter"

▶ Treatment is primarily supportive, although physostigmine can be used in life-threatening situations

▶ General Considerations

Atropine, scopolamine, belladonna, many antihistamines, tricyclic antidepressants, and many plants (eg, jimsonweed [*Datura stramonium*], nightshade, *Amanita muscaria* mushrooms) have anticholinergic effects.

▶ Clinical Findings

These drugs block cholinergic receptors both centrally and peripherally. Ingestion of a significant amount of an anticholinergic drug can produce many clinical effects. The popular phrase "blind as a bat, hot as Hades, red as a beet, dry as a bone, mad as a hatter" describes many of the manifestations of anticholinergic toxicity. Other signs and symptoms include tachycardia, gastrointestinal ileus, urinary retention, seizures, delirium, and hallucinations.

▶ Treatment

Provide intensive supportive care and gastrointestinal decontamination as described previously. Most patients can be managed with supportive measures alone, including sedation with benzodiazepines, cooling, and bladder emptying. If a patient develops life-threatening complications of anticholinergic toxicity (hemodynamically significant tachycardia, hyperthermia, or seizures resistant to benzodiazepines) that is refractory to conventional therapy, physostigmine, 1–2 mg intravenously over 2 minutes, can be given. Physostigmine works within minutes and the duration of effect is 30–60 minutes. It has been associated with severe complications, including bradycardia, heart block, and seizures. Atropine should be readily available if the antidote is used, and ECG monitoring is necessary. Physostigmine is contraindicated in patients with an overdose of tricyclic antidepressants.

▶ Disposition

Hospitalize patients who have incapacitating signs or symptoms of anticholinergic poisoning.

Scharman EJ, Erdman AR, Wax PM et al: Diphenhydramine and dimenhydrinate poisoning: an evidence-based consensus guideline for out-of-hospital management. Clin Toxicol (Phila) 2006;44:205–233 [PMID: 16749537].

Krenzelok EP: Aspects of Datura poisoning and treatment. Clin Toxicol (Phila) 2010;48:104–110 [PMID: 20229618].

ANTIDEPRESSANTS

ESSENTIALS OF DIAGNOSIS

▶ Average toxic dose is 5 mg/kg

▶ Anticholinergic symptoms range from mydriasis, agitation, and tachycardia to seizures and coma

▶ Cardiovascular manifestations are often life-threatening and include QRS widening, profound hypotension, atrioventricular blocks, and ventricular arrhythmias

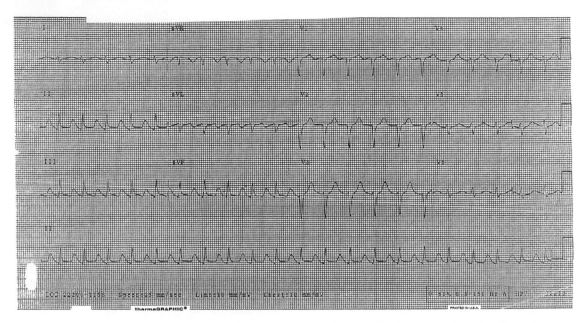

▲ **Figure 47–2.** Supraventricular tachycardia with prolonged QT_c and terminal right axis resulting from tricyclic antidepressant overdose.

▶ General Considerations

Major tricyclic antidepressants include amitriptyline (Elavil, many others), imipramine (Tofranil, many others), and doxepin (Adapin, Sinequan). Maprotiline (Ludiomil) is a tetracyclic antidepressant with similar properties.

The tricyclic antidepressants are analogs of phenothiazines, with complex effects, including anticholinergic, α-adrenergic-receptor blocking, and quinidine-like activity on the heart. They are well absorbed and highly tissue bound, with volumes of distribution of 10–40 L/kg. These drugs are eliminated primarily by metabolism in the liver, and the half-lives are 10–30 hours. The average toxic dose is more than 5 mg/kg, with severe poisoning occurring at doses of 10–20 mg/kg.

Other antidepressants include the selective serotonin reuptake inhibitors (SSRI): fluoxetine, paroxetine, sertraline, citralopram and escitralapam. Other antidresssants include serotonin/norepinephrine reuptake inhibitors (SNRI) (venlafaxine and duloxetine), buproprion (norepinephrine and dopamine reuptake inhibitor) and the antidepressant sedative trazodone.

▶ Clinical Findings

The hallmark of tricyclic antidepressant toxicity is the rapid onset of life-threatening clinical effects. Many symptoms are the result of the anticholinergic activity of these drugs, for example, mydriasis, dry mouth, tachycardia, agitation, and hallucinations. The onset of coma may be rapid, even precipitous. Twitching and myoclonic jerking have been noted, and seizures occur frequently and may be difficult to treat.

Cardiovascular manifestations are the most dramatic and life-threatening (Figure 47–2). Quinidine-like slowing of conduction is reflected by widening of the QRS complex (>100 ms) and prolonged QT and PR intervals. Varying degrees of atrioventricular block and ventricular tachycardia are common. Atypical (torsades de pointes) ventricular tachycardia may occur. Profound hypotension resulting from decreased contractility and vasodilatation may occur and is a frequent cause of death. Hypoxemia and acidosis aggravate the cardiovascular toxicity of tricyclic antidepressants.

Diagnosis is generally based on history, relevant physical findings, widened QRS complexes, and prolonged QT intervals (3 Cs: **c**ardiac abnormalities, **c**onvulsions, and **c**oma). The diagnosis may be confirmed by qualitative or quantitative tests for these drugs in the blood or urine. Plasma concentrations are rarely available and often lack sensitivity in detecting active metabolites. Prolongation of the QRS complex or the terminal axis in lead aVR is a better predictor of severity of poisoning than is the drug concentration.

Some cyclic antidepressants (amoxapine) and antipsychotics (loxapine) can cause seizures and coma without associated cardiovascular toxicity or electrocardiographic changes.

The SSRIs in combination with other serotonergic drugs, or when taken alone, may lead to the development of some degree of serotonin syndrome. Ingestion of the SNRI antidepressants as well as buproprion, may cause seizures.

Treatment

A. General Management

Provide intensive supportive care and gastrointestinal decontamination as described previously. Do not induce emesis because of the well-established risk of seizures and coma. Administer activated charcoal if the patient has ingested a toxic amount and is seen within 1 hour. Consider multidose charcoal for symptomatic patients.

B. Cardiac Monitoring

Constant monitoring of the ECG for at least 6 hours is mandatory. Progressive widening of the QRS complex indicates worsening toxicity.

C. Treatment of Seizures

Treat seizures with diazepam or phenobarbital. Do not use physostigmine to treat seizures, because it may cause seizures and other complications.

D. Treatment of Arrhythmias

Sinus tachycardia is benign and usually does not require treatment. Physostigmine and propranolol may aggravate conduction abnormalities and should not be used.

Ventricular arrhythmias and conduction defects may respond to sodium bicarbonate, 50–100 mEq (1–2 mEq/kg) as an intravenous bolus. It is not clear whether the improvement is merely a result of correction of acidosis, a result of transient hypernatremia, or a result of a shift in the protein binding of the drug with alkalosis. Lidocaine, 1–2 mg/kg as an intravenous bolus, is frequently effective. Quinidine-like drugs (eg, quinidine, procainamide, and disopyramide) are contraindicated, because they worsen cardiotoxicity.

E. Treatment of Hypotension

Treat hypotension initially with intravenous infusion of sodium bicarbonate, 50–100 mEq (1–2 mEq/kg), and crystalloid solutions. If the patient fails to respond after 1–2 L have been infused, further therapy should be guided by measurement of pulmonary artery wedge pressures and cardiac output. Norepinephrine and epinephrine have been found to be more effective than dopamine in refractory hypotension.

F. Other Measures

Hemodialysis and hemoperfusion have no role in tricyclic antidepressant poisoning.

Disposition

Hospitalize all symptomatic patients with overdose of tricyclic antidepressants. Use serial ECGs along with the patient's clinical appearance to predict impending toxicity. Observe asymptomatic patients for a minimum of 6–8 hours, taking repeated measurements of the vital signs and QRS interval.

Flanagan RJ: Fatal toxicity of drugs used in psychiatry. Hum Psychopharmcol 2008;23:43–51 [PMID: 18098225].

Howell C, Wilson AD, Waring WS: Cardiovascular toxicity due to venlafaxine poisoning in adults: a review of 235 consecutive cases. Br J Clin Pharmacol 2007;64:192–197 [PMID: 17298480].

Nelson LS, Erdman AR, Booze LL et al: Selective serotonin reuptake inhibitor poisoning: an evidence-based consensus guideline for out-of-hospital management. Clin Toxicol (Phila) 2007;45:315–332 [PMID: 17486478].

Woolf AD, Erdman AR, Nelson LS et al: Tricyclic antidepressant poisoning: an evidence-based consensus guideline for out-of-hospital management. Clin Toxicol (Phila) 2007;45:203–233 [PMID: 17453872].

β-ADRENERGIC BLOCKING AGENTS

 ESSENTIALS OF DIAGNOSIS

► Ingestion of a large amount of β-blockers primarily affects the cardiac system

► Symptoms of ingestion include hypotension, bradycardia, and bronchoconstriction

► Glucagon can be used to treat hypotension if fluids are unsuccessful; glucagon can also be used to treat arrhythmias, but cardiac pacing may be required in severe cases

General Considerations

β-Adrenergic blocking agents are widely used in clinical medicine to treat hypertension, arrhythmias, angina pectoris, migraine headache, and thyrotoxicosis. β-Blockers act by competing with catecholamines for a finite number of β_1 and β_2 receptor sites. The β_1-receptors are responsible for increasing the force and rate of cardiac contraction. The β_2-receptors mediate vasodilatation; bronchial smooth muscle dilation; and a number of metabolic effects, including glycogenolysis. Excessive β-blockade can therefore cause hypoglycemia, bradycardia, bronchoconstriction, and hypoglycemia.

Clinical Findings

The main features of massive β-blocker overdose are hypotension and bradycardia. Pulmonary edema or bronchospasm may also occur, especially in patients with preexisting congestive heart failure or asthma. Hypoglycemia and hyperkalemia are sometimes seen. Convulsions are common with propranolol and other agents (eg, oxprenolol) with high lipid solubility and marked membrane-depressant effects. The ECG may show sinus bradycardia, atrioventricular blocks, or a prolonged QRS interval. In rare cases, ventricular tachyarrhythmias may occur, especially with sotalol overdose. Death is usually due to profound myocardial depression, with advanced atrioventricular block or asystole. Plasma levels of β-blockers are not clinically useful and are not routinely available.

▶ Treatment

A. General Management

General management of overdose, including airway protection, treatment of hypoglycemia, and gastrointestinal decontamination, should be undertaken as outlined earlier. Give multidose activated charcoal and initiate whole bowel irrigation in a patient who may have ingested a toxic amount of a sustained-release preparation.

B. Treatment of Hypotension

Treat hypotension initially with fluids. If this is unsuccessful, use glucagon, 5–10 mg (100–150 μg/kg) as an intravenous bolus, followed by an infusion of 2–5 mg/h. Glucagon increases intracellular cyclic AMP by a mechanism different from that of β-receptors.

C. Treatment of Arrhythmias

Advanced atrioventricular block or bradycardia resulting in hypotension can also be treated initially with glucagon, 100–150 μg/kg intravenously. If arrhythmia continues, atropine, 0.01–0.03 mg/kg intravenously, or isoproterenol, 0.05–0.3 μg/kg/min by intravenous infusion, may also be used. If these are unsuccessful, cardiac pacing may be necessary. The heart may not respond to attempts at pacing, even with high currents.

D. Other Measures

Because of the relatively large volume of distribution and extensive protein binding, dialysis is not likely to be of value for propranolol overdose. Less lipophilic agents (eg, atenolol, nadolol) have much smaller volumes of distribution and may be eliminated by dialysis or hemoperfusion, but they are less likely to cause profound toxicity.

▶ Disposition

Patients should remain under observation for at least 6–8 hours after ingestion. Patients with significant β-blocker intoxication (eg, profound bradycardia, conduction abnormalities, hypotension, and shock) should be hospitalized. Patients ingesting sustained-release products should be observed for 12–24 hours.

Kerns W: Management of beta-adrenergic blocker and calcium channel antagonist toxicity. Emerg Med Clin North Am 2007;25:309–331 [PMID: 17482022].

CALCIUM CHANNEL BLOCKING AGENTS

 ESSENTIALS OF DIAGNOSIS

- ▶ Ingestion of a large amount of calcium channel blockers can cause hypotension, bradycardia, and central nervous system depression
- ▶ Treatment is primarily supportive, although both calcium and glucagon can be used to treat hypotension and bradycardia

▶ General Considerations

Calcium channel blockers are being used with increasing frequency for supraventricular tachycardia, hypertension, rate control in atrial fibrillation or atrial flutter, angina, and vasospasm. These agents block the slow calcium channels and have the following cardiovascular effects: They depress sinus node activity, slow atrioventricular nodal conduction, cause coronary and peripheral vasodilatation, and depress myocardial contractility. Verapamil and diltiazem have the most marked myocardial effects and are especially dangerous in patients with sinus or atrioventricular nodal disease, Wolff–Parkinson–White syndrome, on digitalis therapy or in patients receiving β-blockers, quinidine, disopyramide, or other myocardial depressant drugs. Nifedipine is especially dangerous in patients receiving nitrates or β-blockers and in patients with obstructive valvular heart disease. Nifedipine is more likely than verapamil or diltiazem to be associated with increased heart rate and vasodilatation. Calcium channel blockers may also block insulin release, resulting in hyperglycemia.

▶ Clinical Findings

The main manifestations of calcium channel blocker overdose are hypotension, bradycardia, and drowsiness. Bradydysrhythmias result from sinoatrial and atrioventricular nodal conduction dissociation. If the ingestion is that of a sustained-release preparation, toxicity and symptoms may be delayed for 6–8 hours. With regular-release preparations, toxicity is generally seen in 2–3 hours. Hyperkalemia and seizures, which are sometimes observed in overdoses of β-blockers, are not prominent in overdoses of calcium channel blockers. The ECG shows evidence of bradyarrhythmia with atrioventricular block. Death results from severe myocardial depression leading to asystole.

▶ Treatment

A. General Management

General management includes airway protection and gastrointestinal decontamination. Give multidose activated charcoal and initiate whole bowel irrigation in a patient who may have ingested sustained-release preparations.

B. Cardiac Care

Constant cardiac monitoring is essential. Appropriate pharmacologic management in seriously ill patients may require placement of central intravenous lines. Leg elevation, Trendelenburg positioning, and fluid management may be required. Advanced atrioventricular block and bradycardia resulting in hypotension may be treated initially with atropine, 0.01–0.03 mg/kg intravenously. Cardiac pacing may be required.

C. Hypotension

In hypotensive patients not responding to the therapy outlined above, calcium solutions have sometimes been successful. Administer 10% calcium chloride, 10–20 mL for adults (10–30 mg/kg for children) intravenously, or 10% calcium gluconate, 10–20 mL for adults (0.2–0.4 mL/kg for children), followed by repeated boluses or continuous intravenous infusion as necessary. Calcium administration improves the blood pressure more than the heart rate. As in β-blocker overdose, glucagon may improve both heart rate and blood pressure. An initial bolus of 2–5 mg intravenously may be given and followed by up to a total of 10 mg if no response is seen. If glucagon improves the patient's hemodynamics, then an infusion should be started. Isoproterenol, epinephrine, phenylephrine, or amrinone may be required for severe, unresponsive hypotension.

▶ Disposition

Asymptomatic patients should be observed for at least 8–10 hours. Patients with significant calcium channel blocker overdose should be hospitalized for monitoring and observation.

Lheureux PE, Zahir S, Gris M, Derrey AS, Penaloza A: Bench-to-bedside review: hyperinsulinaemia/euglycaemia therapy in the management of overdose of calcium-channel blockers. Crit Care 2006;10:212 [PMID: 16732893].

Arroyo AM, Kao LW: Calcium channel blocker toxicity. Pediatr Emerg Care 2009;25:532–538 [PMID: 19687715].

CARBON MONOXIDE

ESSENTIALS OF DIAGNOSIS

▶ Carbon monoxide is a colorless and odorless gas that binds with great affinity to hemoglobin

▶ Severe tissue hypoxia results

▶ Carbon monoxide levels correlate with severity of symptoms and should be used to guide treatment

▶ Treatment is with 100% oxygen; hyperbaric oxygen can also be used in certain circumstances

▶ General Considerations

Carbon monoxide, a colorless, odorless, and tasteless gas, is produced by incomplete combustion of organic materials and is found in engine exhaust, kerosene heaters, burning charcoal briquettes, and from fireplaces. Any fire may also produce large quantities of carbon monoxide.

Carbon monoxide binds to hemoglobin with an affinity about 200 times greater than that of oxygen. The resulting carboxyhemoglobin complex cannot transport oxygen, causing tissue hypoxia that can lead to death or permanent neurologic damage if untreated. Hemoglobin saturation and blood oxygen content are dangerously low despite adequate (or elevated) arterial Po_2 levels. Carbon monoxide also disrupts cellar respiration by binding to cytochrome oxidase.

▶ Clinical Findings

The severity of symptoms usually correlates with carboxyhemoglobin levels (Table 47–11). The carboxyhemoglobin level can be obtained from either venous or arterial blood. The earliest reliable diagnostic symptom is headache. Usually, Po_2

Table 47–11. Clinical findings in carbon monoxide poisoning.

Estimated Carbon Monoxide Concentration (Parts Per Million)	Carboxyhemoglobin (% of Total Hemoglobin)	Symptoms
Less than 35 ppm (cigarette smoking)	5	None, or mild headache
0.005% (50 ppm)	10	Slight headache, dyspnea on vigorous exertion
0.01% (100 ppm)	20	Throbbing headache, dyspnea with moderate exertion
0.02% (200 ppm)	30	Severe headache, irritability, fatigue, dimness of vision
0.03–0.05% (300–500 ppm)	40–50	Headache, tachycardia, confusion, lethargy, collapse
0.08–0.12% (800–1200 ppm)	60–70	Coma, convulsions
0.19% (1900 ppm)	80	Rapidly fatal

is normal, although metabolic acidosis due to tissue hypoxia may be present. Using oxygen saturation calculated from Po_2 (based on assumption of normal hemoglobin) or measured by pulse oximetry will provide an incorrect estimate of oxygen-carrying capacity. Blood may be cherry-red, but the patient rarely appears pink. The ECG may show ischemia or infarction in a person with coronary disease. Delayed central nervous system effects such as Parkinsonism, memory loss, and personality changes can occur after recovery.

Treatment

Note: Act quickly. Delay in treatment may worsen neurologic damage.

A. General Management

Move the patient to fresh air immediately. Administer 100% oxygen by nonrebreathing face mask or endotracheal tube, *not* by nasal cannula or loose-fitting face mask. Oxygen competes with carbon monoxide for hemoglobin-binding sites. The half-life of carboxyhemoglobin in a person breathing room air is 5–6 hours; in 100% oxygen, it is only 1 hour. Hyperbaric 100% oxygen lowers the carboxyhemoglobin level even more rapidly (23 minutes), but it is seldom readily available and no studies have demonstrated a reduction in post carbon monoxide poisoning neurologic deficits in patients receiving hyperbaric oxygen versus 100% oxygen. Consider hyperbaric oxygen for patients with major symptoms of carbon monoxide intoxication such as loss of consciousness or myocardial ischemia or if the patient is pregnant.

B. Blood Tests

Obtain arterial blood for measurement of carboxyhemoglobin content and arterial blood gases.

C. Chest X-Ray

If carbon monoxide poisoning is associated with smoke inhalation, obtain a chest X-ray and consider hospitalization and monitoring for development of noncardiogenic pulmonary edema.

D. Other Measures

The use of corticosteroids and mannitol for cerebral edema has been recommended, but their value in preventing late neurologic sequelae remains unproved.

Disposition

All patients with significant carbon monoxide poisoning (ie, with chest pain or other evidence of cardiac ischemia, neurologic signs, or carboxyhemoglobin concentrations above 25%) and pregnant patients must be hospitalized and given oxygen.

Juurlink DN, Buckley NA, Stanbrook MB et al: Hyperbaric oxygen for carbon monoxide poisoning. Cochrane Database Syst Rev 2005:CD002041 [PMID: 15674890].

Weaver LK: Clinical Practice: carbon monoxide poisoning. New Eng J Med 2009;360:1217–1225 [PMID: 19297574].

CARDIAC GLYCOSIDES

ESSENTIALS OF DIAGNOSIS

► These cardiotoxic drugs result in rhythm and conduction disturbances in the heart and occasionally severe hyperkalemia

► Digoxin levels in combination with serum potassium are indicative of the degree of poisoning in the acute overdose

► Patients with severe arrhythmias or hyperkalemia may benefit from digitalis antibodies to reverse toxicity

General Considerations

Digoxin; digitoxin; and several plant digitalis derivatives including oleander, foxglove, and lily of the valley are the sources of digitalis and the cardiac glycosides. They are used therapeutically primarily for their ability to slow conduction through the atrioventricular node in disease states such as atrial fibrillation. They also increase the force of myocardial contractility and enhance automaticity. These therapeutic effects also mediate the severity of toxicity.

Digoxin has a large volume of distribution (6–10 L/kg) and a half-life of about 40 hours; for the most part, it is excreted unchanged in the urine. Digitoxin, by contrast, has a small volume of distribution, is highly protein bound, and undergoes extensive enterohepatic recirculation; its half-life is 7 days. In the elderly, the half-life may be increased owing to decreased creatinine clearance.

Clinical Findings

Blurred vision, color vision disturbance (especially with green or yellow vision), and neurologic symptoms may occur in a patient with chronic toxicity. The most serious toxic effects are those that cause rhythm and conduction disturbances in the heart, for example, third-degree atrioventricular block, bradycardia, ventricular ectopy, bidirectional ventricular tachycardia, and paroxysmal atrial tachycardia with atrioventricular block. In patients with chronic atrial fibrillation, digitalis toxicity may cause nonparoxysmal junctional tachycardia, which is characterized by a regular rhythm with narrow QRS complexes and a heart rate of 90–120 beats/min. Although hypokalemia may aggravate digitalis toxicity in the patient receiving chronic therapy, acute ingestion of an overdose is often associated with hyperkalemia. The plasma potassium level in digoxin overdose is indicative of the degree of poisoning of the Na^+-K^+-ATPase pump; if the potassium is elevated, the toxicity is severe. Therapeutic serum levels of digoxin are 0.5–2 ng/mL; for digitoxin, they are 18–22 ng/mL.

▶ Treatment

A. General Management

Provide intensive supportive care and gastrointestinal decontamination as described previously. Gastric lavage may worsen bradycardia by enhancing vagal tone.

B. Electrolyte Abnormalities

If hypokalemia is present, replace potassium. For severe hyperkalemia, measures to reduce the potassium level may be necessary in order to reduce the cardiotoxic effects of digitalis. Because the total body potassium is not high, potassium-binding resins (ie, Kayexalate) should not be used. Other measures such as insulin, glucose, and sodium bicarbonate can be attempted in addition to specific antidotal therapy. Avoid the use of calcium, which may potentiate the cardiac toxicity of digitalis. Magnesium replacement may be beneficial.

C. Arrhythmias

For symptomatic bradycardia or second- or third-degree atrioventricular block, atropine, 0.5–1.0 mg intravenously, repeated every 5 minutes if there is no response, may be helpful. The total dose should not exceed 2 mg. A transcutaneous pacemaker may be used.

For ventricular ectopic beats, both lidocaine and phenytoin are effective, although lidocaine is easier to use. Give 1 mg/kg as an intravenous bolus, followed by 1–4 mg/min by continuous infusion. Phenytoin and the new prodrug fosphenytoin are also effective at suppressing atrial and ventricular ectopy.

Avoid direct current countershock, because it may cause serious conduction and rhythm disturbances including asystole or ventricular fibrillation in patients with digitalis toxicity. If countershock is unavoidable, use the lowest voltage that is effective.

D. Drug Removal

Dialysis or hemoperfusion is of no value for digoxin because of its large volume of distribution. Digitoxin may be effectively removed by hemoperfusion and by repeated doses of activated charcoal or cholestyramine, which interrupt enterohepatic recirculation.

E. Digitalis Antibodies

The treatment of choice for cardiac glycoside toxicity is digitalis-specific Fab fragments. Digitalis-specific Fab fragment antibodies are extremely effective and are indicated for patients with serious arrhythmias or severe hyperkalemia. Each vial binds 0.6 mg of digoxin. Toxicity usually is reversed within 5–10 minutes, and the digoxin–antibody complex is excreted in the urine. After administration of the Fab fragment antibodies (Table 47–12), serum digoxin levels are elevated owing to cross-reaction of the complex in the assay. When the ingested amount is unknown, 5–10 vials may be given initially.

▶ Disposition

All patients with digitalis and other cardiac glycoside poisoning require hospitalization in a cardiac-monitored unit for observation and treatment. Onset of cardiac toxicity may be delayed for 6–12 hours after acute ingestion.

Bauman JL, Didomenico RJ, Galanter WL: Mechanisms, manifestations, and management of digoxin toxicity in the modern era. Am J Cardiovasc Drugs 2006;6:77–86 [PMID: 16555861].

Table 47–12. Digoxin Immune Fab Dosing.

To calculate the body load of digoxin:
Dose ingested (if known) $\times$ 0.8
Or

$$\frac{\text{Serum digoxin concentration (ng/ml)} \times 5.6 \text{ L/kg } (V_D) \times \text{wt (kg)}}{1000}$$

$$\text{Digibind dose (number of vials)} = \frac{\text{Body load (mg)}}{0.5 \text{ mg/vial}}$$

$$\textit{Quick estimation}: \text{Number of vials} = \frac{\text{Serum digoxin concentration} \times \text{wt (kg)}}{1000}$$

CAUSTICS AND CORROSIVES

ESSENTIALS OF DIAGNOSIS

- ▶ Includes both acids and alkalis
- ▶ Ingestion can result in coagulative (acids) or liquefactive (alkalis) necrosis of tissue
- ▶ Treatment is supportive and includes dilution of the material with water, milk, or normal saline
- ▶ Endoscopy is recommended to assess degree of damage in symptomatic patients

▶ General Considerations

Corrosive agents include strong agents, alkalis (caustics), oxidizing agents, and other chemicals. They are commonly used in household cleaners (Table 47–13).

A. Acids

Toilet bowl cleaners, bleaches, battery acid, soldering flux (zinc chloride), and many industrial sources contain acids.

B. Alkalis

Lye (drain cleaners, reagent tablets used to detect glucose in urine [Clinitest, many others]), ammonia, and industrial-grade detergents contain caustic alkalis. The mechanism of toxicity is tissue destruction resulting from coagulative (acids) and liquefactive (alkali) necrosis and heat injury during neutralization of the chemical by water in body tissues. Most household bleaches and detergents are dilute and do not cause severe corrosive burns. Concentrated alkalis are

common in the household, especially in granular form or strongly concentrated liquids (pH > 12.5), and these cause severe tissue damage. Corrosive burns may lead to airway or intestinal edema and obstruction, mucosal perforation, and (later) stricture formation.

▶ Clinical Findings

Symptoms are almost always present with significant ingestion and include mouth and throat pain, dysphagia, drooling, and substernal or abdominal pain. However, significant gastric or esophageal burns may be present without oral lesions. Skin and eye burns may also occur.

▶ Treatment

A. General Management

Dilute the corrosive material with water, normal saline, or milk (8 ounces for adults, 4 ounces for children). *Do not* give neutralizers, because they may increase the heat of hydration and worsen subsequent tissue destruction. *Do not* induce vomiting, because this may produce further tissue damage. Activated charcoal is contraindicated because it can interfere with endoscopy.

B. Endoscopy

Diagnostic endoscopy should be performed in any symptomatic patient with or without oral burns. Endoscopy may not be necessary in asymptomatic patients.

C. Pharmacologic Treatment

No studies support the efficacy of corticosteroids in preventing stricture formation, and they are no longer recommended. Esophageal or gastric perforation is a contraindication to their use. Antibiotics are indicated for suspected perforation or infection.

▶ Disposition

Hospitalize all patients known to have ingested or inhaled (aspirated) caustic or corrosive agents with a potential for tissue damage. Skin burns may be managed on an outpatient basis if they are of mild to moderate severity. Eye injuries should be copiously irrigated and evaluated by an ophthalmologist.

Table 47–13. Common Corrosive Agents.

Type	Examples	Injury
Concentrated alkali	Clinitest tablets Drain cleaners Ammonia Lye Oven cleaners Denture cleaners	Penetrating liquefaction necrosis
Concentrated acids	Pool disinfectants Toilet bowl cleaners	Coagulation necrosis
Weaker cleaning agents	Cationic detergents (dishwasher detergents) Household bleach	Superficial burns and irritation; deep burns (rare)

Bauman JL, Didomenico RJ, Galanter WL: Mechanisms, manifestations, and management of digoxin toxicity in the modern era. Am J Cardiovasc Drugs 2006;6:77–86 [PMID: 16555861].

Salzman M, O'Malley RN: Updates on the evaluation and management of caustic exposures. Emerg Med Clin North Am 2007;25:459–476 [PMID: 17482028].

COCAINE AND LOCAL ANESTHETICS

ESSENTIALS OF DIAGNOSIS

▶ Overdose of local anesthetics causes initial central nervous system excitement and seizures, followed by central nervous system depression

▶ Cocaine intoxication causes sympathetic hyperactivity and can result in severe hypertension, hyperthermia, myocardial ischemia, and even aortic dissection

▶ Treatment is supportive and should address any resulting cardiac or central nervous system symptoms

▶ General Considerations

Cocaine is a natural extract from coca leaves. It is a local anesthetic that also has sympathomimetic effects. Overdoses of all local anesthetics are manifested by initial excitement and seizures, followed by central nervous system depression. Peak effects occur rapidly, usually in less than 1 hour.

A. Cocaine

All significant overdoses are associated with symptoms. Intravenous injection of cocaine and inhalation (smoking) of freebase, or crack, cocaine may result in very high levels. Cocaine causes euphoria, excitement, and restlessness; toxic psychosis, seizures, hypertension, tachycardia, dysrhythmias, and hyperthermia are common. Chest pain, myocardial ischemia and infarction, and aortic dissection have occurred. Blood cocaine and metabolite concentrations vary widely and do not predict the development of clinical findings.

B. Local Anesthetics

Common local anesthetics such as lidocaine, mepiva-caine, and procaine have no toxic effects in usual doses. With excessive doses, they cause tremors, anxiety, and restlessness, followed by seizures and then cardiorespira-tory depression. Toxic doses for these drugs vary and depend on the route and duration of administration. Maximum recommended doses for infiltration anesthesia in adults are lidocaine, 4.5 mg/kg; bupivacaine, 2 mg/kg; and procaine, 7 mg/kg. Larger doses may be tolerated if epinephrine has been included in the preparation.

▶ Treatment

A. General Management

Provide intensive supportive care and gastrointestinal decontamination as described previously.

B. Treatment of Cocaine Overdose

Treat manifestations of sympathetic hyperactivity in the same way as for amphetamine overdose. Because effects peak rapidly, measures to enhance elimination of the drug from the body are unnecessary. The exception is those patients who ingest packets of cocaine to avoid arrest. If a patient is thought to have ingested packets of cocaine (body packers), whole bowel irrigation should be instituted immediately to hasten removal of the packets.

Patients with chest pain suggestive of ischemia should be evaluated with a 12-lead ECG and considered for admission to rule out myocardial infarction. Myocardial infarction may be present even with a normal ECG. Patients with a new onset of seizures may need CT scanning to rule out intracranial hemorrhage.

C. Treatment of Overdose with Common Local Anesthetics

Treatment consists of supportive measures with particular attention to respiratory depression and hypotension. Seizures are usually brief and easily treatable with benzodiazepines and usually do not require other anticonvulsant therapy. Recently, successful case reports have been documented in humans with the use of lipid infusion in significant local anesthetic toxicity. A 20% lipid infusion has been used to resuscitate a patients from cardiac arrest following the use of anesthetics.

▶ Disposition

Hospitalize patients with cocaine or local anesthetic poisoning manifested by multiple seizures, hyperthermia, ischemic chest pain, or severe hypertension.

Karch SB: Cocaine cardiovascular toxicity. South Med J 2005;98:794–799 [PMID: 16144174].

CYANIDE

ESSENTIALS OF DIAGNOSIS

▶ Cyanide acts as a cellular asphyxiant that inhibits the use of oxygen by the body's tissues

▶ Symptom onset is rapid and ultimately results in hypotension

▶ In mild cases, supportive care including 100% oxygen is adequate

▶ If poisoning is severe, a cyanide antidote kit of sodium nitrite, amyl nitrite, and sodium thiosulfate should be used

▶ Cyanide levels are not readily available and should not be used to determine treatment

▶ All patients with cyanide intoxication should be hospitalized

General Considerations

Fumigants, hydrocyanic acid gas used in industry, and burning plastics and fabrics are sources of cyanide. Sodium nitroprusside used to treat severe hypertension undergoes a biotransformation to methemoglobin and cyanide and can be a source of poisoning. Cyanide poisoning has also resulted from metabolism of ingested acetonitrile in an artificial nail-removing solution.

Cyanide is a rapidly absorbed cellular asphyxiant that inhibits the cytochrome oxidase system for oxygen utilization in cells. The inability of the body's tissues to use oxygen leads to anaerobic metabolism and a profound metabolic acidosis. Death may occur within minutes after a dose of 200 mg. In fatal poisoning, blood levels usually exceed 1–2 mg/mL. Cyanide gas is much more toxic than salt forms because of its rapid absorption, and its effects are usually immediate.

Clinical Findings

Significant poisoning is associated with rapidly developing symptoms, including headache, nausea and vomiting, anxiety, confusion, and collapse. Initial hypertension and tachycardia progress to hypotension, bradycardia, and apnea. The smell of bitter almonds is present occasionally. The skin may appear pink. The measured oxygen saturation of venous blood may be elevated as a result of failure of oxygen uptake by the tissues.

Treatment

Note: Act quickly. To be successful, treatment must be started within 5–10 minutes in cases of severe poisoning. In witnessed cases of cyanide poisoning, begin therapy without waiting for symptoms.

A. General Management

Supportive care only, including 100% oxygen, may be given to asymptomatic patients as well as those with mild to moderate symptoms. Close observation is needed because the antidote may need to be administered if the patient deteriorates. If activated charcoal is available, administer it at once. Although its binding affinity for cyanide is low, it can adsorb a lethal dose.

B. Antidote Administration

Every emergency department should have a prepackaged cyanide antidote kit containing sodium nitrite, 300 mg in 10-mL ampules (2); sodium thiosulfate, 12.5 g in 50-mL ampules (2); amyl nitrite inhalant, 0.3 mL (12 Aspirols); and syringes and stomach tube (Table 47–14).

Table 47–14. Prepackaged Cyanide Antidote Kit.[a]

Antidote	How Supplied	Dose
Amyl nitrite	0.3 mL (aspirol inhalant)	Break 1–2 aspirols under patient's nose Sodium nitrite
Sodium nitrite	3 g/dL (300 mg in 10 mL [vials])	300 mg intravenously
Sodium thiosulfate	25 g/dL (12.5 g in 50 mL [vials])	500 mg intravenously

[a]In the United States, manufactured by Taylor Pharmaceuticals.

1. Nitrites—Nitrites produce methemoglobin, which binds free cyanide.

1. Break a capsule of amyl nitrite under the patient's nose for deep inhalation while starting an intravenous infusion of sodium nitrite and thiosulfate. A new ampule should be used every 3 minutes until intravenous medication has begun.

2. Give sodium nitrite, 300 mg (10-mL ampule) intravenously for adults; for children, 0.12–0.33 mL/kg up to 10 mL with a normal hemoglobin concentration (for alternate dosing in a child with abnormal hemoglobin, consult Poisindex). *Caution:* Do not over treat; fatal methemoglobinemia has resulted from overzealous use of nitrites. After initial therapy, guide subsequent treatment by monitoring symptoms and signs. The goal of nitrite therapy is a methemoglobin level of 25–30%.

2. Thiosulfate—Sodium thiosulfate is a cofactor in the rhodanese enzyme conversion of cyanide to thiocyanate, which is less toxic and readily excreted. Give thiosulfate, 50 mL of a 25% solution to adults and 1.65 mL/kg of a 25% solution to children, intravenously.

C. Vitamin B$_{12A}$

Vitamin B$_{12A}$ (hydroxocobalamin) has been successfully used in Europe. Hydroxocobalamin reverses cyanide toxicity by combining with cyanide to form cyanocobalamin (Vitamin B$_{12A}$). The usual dose is 50 mg/kg; a single dose of 5 g is usually sufficient.

Disposition

All patients with suspected or documented cyanide poisoning should be hospitalized.

Hall AH, Saiers J, Baud F: Which cyanide antidote? Crit Rev Toxicol 2009;39:541–552 [PMID: 19650716].

DRUG-INDUCED METHEMOGLOBINEMIA

ESSENTIALS OF DIAGNOSIS

▶ Methemoglobin cannot bind oxygen or carbon dioxide

▶ Symptoms correlate with the degree of methemoglobinemia and can include asymptomatic cyanosis, dyspnea, and severe central nervous system depression

▶ Treatment includes methylene blue, which can reduce methemoglobin levels in less than 1 hour

General Considerations

Hemoglobin becomes methemoglobin when iron is oxidized from the ferrous to the ferric form. Methemoglobin is dark chocolate like in color and can no longer bind to oxygen or carbon dioxide. Conversion of hemoglobin to methemoglobin decreases both delivery of oxygen to the tissues and removal of carbon dioxide, and tissue hypoxia may result.

Methemoglobin is produced endogenously in small quantities and is reduced by methemoglobin reductase; normally, less than 1–2% of hemoglobin is methemoglobin. Methemoglobinemia is caused by various oxidant drugs and poisons, including nitrites, some well water, nitrous gases, chloroquine and primaquine, phenazopyridine, sulfonamides, sulfones, aniline dye derivatives, phenacetin, dapsone, local anesthetics, and nitrobenzenes.

Clinical Findings

Symptoms correlate with the degree of methemoglobinemia. At concentrations of 1.5 g/dL (about 10% of the total hemoglobin), patients may seek care for cyanosis without any shortness of breath. When the level of methemoglobin exceeds 15% of total hemoglobin, blood appears chocolate brown when it is dripped onto filter paper. The exact concentration of methemoglobin in the blood may be determined spectrophotometrically. However, the Po_2 and calculated oxyhemoglobin on routine test of arterial blood gases are falsely normal, and the measured saturation by pulse oximetry is unreliable.

Conversion of up to 25% of normal hemoglobin to methemoglobin is usually not associated with clinical findings other than peripheral and perioral cyanosis, although anxiety, headache, weakness, and lightheadedness can develop. At conversion levels of 35–40%, patients experience lassitude, fatigue, and dyspnea. At conversion levels exceeding 60%, coma and death may occur as a result of severe central nervous system depression. Anemia, acidosis, respiratory compromise (eg, chronic obstructive pulmonary disease), and cardiac disease may make patients more symptomatic than expected for a given methemoglobin level.

▶ Treatment

A. General Management

Provide intensive supportive care and gastrointestinal decontamination as described previously.

B. Oxygen

Oxygen per se does not affect the methemoglobin level, but it should be given to improve tissue oxygenation pending the start of specific therapy. Give oxygen, 5–10 L/min by mask; in comatose or severely acidotic patients, give 100% oxygen by rebreathing mask or endotracheal tube. Continue oxygen therapy for 1–2 hours after giving methylene blue (see below). Always give oxygen if the percentage of methemoglobin is higher than 40% or if the patient has severe symptoms.

C. Methylene Blue

Methylene blue is a specific antidote for methemoglobinemia. The dose is 1–2 mg/kg, or 0.1 mL/kg of a 1% solution, given intravenously over 5 minutes. The dose may be repeated at 1 mL/kg once after 1 hour, but the amount specified should not be exceeded, because an overdose of methylene blue can also cause methemoglobinemia. Methylene blue should reduce methemoglobin levels significantly in less than 1 hour. Patients with glucose-6-phosphate dehydrogenase deficiency may not respond to methylene blue and may experience hemolysis. Exchange transfusions may be required in these patients. *Note*: Methylene blue is contraindicated in patients with methemoglobinemia associated with nitrite treatment of cyanide poisoning because it may cause release of cyanide, resulting in toxic concentrations.

D. Removal of Source

Discontinue the offending drug or chemical.

▶ Disposition

Symptomatic patients with methemoglobinemia should be hospitalized for treatment. Some agents (eg, dapsone) may produce prolonged or recurrent methemoglobinemia over several days.

Guay J: Methemoglobinemia related to local anesthetics: a summary of 242 episodes. Anesth Analg 2009;108:837–845 [PMID: 19224791].

ETHANOL AND OTHER ALCOHOLS

ESSENTIALS OF DIAGNOSIS

▶ Ethanol, methanol, ethylene glycol, and isopropanol are all central nervous system depressants. Levels of all alcohols should be obtained, although the level may not predict the severity of the intoxication

▶ Treatment of ethanol intoxication is supportive and includes glucose and thiamine

▶ Treatment of methanol and ethylene glycol ingestions includes either fomepizole or an ethanol drip to inhibit the formation of toxic metabolites

▶ Treatment of isopropanol ingestion is supportive and may include dialysis if the level is greater than 400 mg/dL

▶ General Considerations

Methanol, ethylene glycol, and even isopropanol have been used as cheap substitutes for ethanol, although this practice is less common now than formerly. These alcohols may also be ingested accidentally or in suicide attempts. All are capable of causing intoxication similar to that produced by ethanol, and all can widen the osmolar gap (see Table 47–4). Additional toxic effects and death can occur as a result of the metabolism of ethylene glycol and methanol.

1. Ethanol

Ethanol is a central nervous system depressant. It is metabolized by alcohol dehydrogenase (in most cases by fixed-rate, zero-order kinetics) at a rate of about 7–10 g/h, resulting in a decrease in blood alcohol concentration of 20–30 mg/dL/h. The rate of elimination among individuals varies, as does tolerance. In the United States, legal impairment for purposes of driving is generally defined as blood (or breath) ethanol concentrations above 80–100 mg/dL; coma usually occurs with levels exceeding 300 mg/dL, except in chronic ethanol abusers who have developed tolerance.

▶ Clinical Findings

Symptoms of alcohol intoxication include ataxia, dysarthria, depressed sensorium, and nystagmus. The breath may smell of alcohol, but this finding is neither sensitive nor specific. Alcohol intoxication is frequently seen with trauma and can contribute significantly to morbidity and mortality. Coma and respiratory depression with subsequent pulmonary aspiration due to intoxication are also common causes of illness and death. Laboratory diagnosis may be aided by direct determination of the blood ethanol concentration

or by its estimation from the calculated osmolar gap (see Table 47–4).

▶ Treatment

A. General Management

Provide intensive supportive care and gastrointestinal decontamination as described previously. Supportive care is the primary mode of therapy. Special care should be taken to prevent aspiration.

B. Thiamine and Glucose

Give thiamine and glucose as needed. Give thiamine, 100 mg intramuscularly or intravenously, to prevent Wernicke's syndrome. Check for hypoglycemia, because ethanol inhibits gluconeogenesis, and give glucose, 50 mL of a 50% solution (25 g of glucose) intravenously over 3–4 minutes, if needed.

C. Other Measures

Diagnose and correct disorders such as hypovolemia, hypothermia, infection, trauma, or gastrointestinal tract bleeding. Do not use fructose therapy or forced diuresis.

▶ Disposition

Hospitalize patients with ethanol poisoning if ethanol intoxication has caused abnormalities that would by themselves require hospitalization (eg, obtundation, seizures, and refractory hypoglycemia).

2. Methanol

Methanol is a highly toxic alcohol found in a variety of commercial products, including paint stripper, antifreeze, automobile windshield washer fluid, and solid alcohols (Sterno Canned Heat, and many others). It is metabolized by alcohol dehydrogenase to formaldehyde and formic acid. An osmolar gap and profound metabolic acidosis with an anion gap result. Optic neuritis (caused by formate) that results in blindness has been described after overdose. Early diagnosis is essential, because permanent blindness or death may result if methanol intoxication is left untreated.

▶ Clinical Findings

The major clinical effect of methanol before it is metabolized is central nervous system depression. As the methanol is metabolized to formic acid (this may be delayed 6–18 hours if ethanol has also been ingested), visual disturbances invariably occur (blurred vision or hazy and snow-like patterns), along with hyperemia of the optic disk, headache, dizziness, and breathlessness. In severe toxicity, seizures and coma may occur.

Examination shows variable degrees of central nervous system dysfunction (agitation and intoxication to coma). Pupillary dysfunction has been shown to be a strong predictor of mortality. The retinas may appear suffused and bright red. Early after ingestion, the only finding may be inebriation with an elevated osmolar gap. Later, severe metabolic acidosis occurs.

▶ Treatment

If serious intoxication is suspected, begin therapy even before receiving the results of blood methanol concentration determination.

A. General Management

Provide intensive supportive care and gastrointestinal decontamination as described previously. The main objective of treatment is to limit the accumulation of formate by blocking the metabolism of methanol by alcohol dehydrogenase. Two drugs have been shown to be effective, fomepizole (Antizol) and ethanol.

1. Fomepizole—Fomepizole is the treatment of choice. It is approved by the FDA for the treatment of ethylene glycol and methanol poisoning. Fomepizole, like ethanol, inhibits alcohol dehydrogenase and the formation of toxic metabolites. Give a loading dose of 15 mg/kg intravenously, followed by 10 mg/kg every 12 hours for 48 hours. After 48 hours the dose is increased to 15 mg/kg every 12 hours until the level of methanol is undetectable or both symptoms and acidosis resolve and the level is less than 20 mg/dL. Fomepizole has several advantages over ethanol infusion, including ease of dosing, lack of central nervous system depression, and no requirement for constant serum monitoring because of its reliable therapeutic concentration. Ethanol infusion can also be used if fomepizole is unavailable.

2. Ethanol—In the absence of fomepizole ethanol may be used. Ethanol is metabolized in preference to methanol by alcohol dehydrogenase, thus blocking further metabolism of methanol. The loading dose of ethanol for an average 70-kg adult is 0.7 g/kg (2 mL/kg of 100-proof [50%] ethanol orally; or 7 mL/kg of 10% ethanol intravenously). Maintain continuous infusion of 0.07–0.1 g/kg/h to keep blood concentration of ethanol between 100 and 200 mg/dL. These levels are sufficient to produce clinically evident intoxication. Ethanol may be given intravenously or orally, but intravenous solutions must be at concentrations of 10% or less to prevent hypertonicity of the solution. Monitor and maintain adequate ventilation during the infusion of ethanol.

B. Other Measures

Correct metabolic acidosis with sodium bicarbonate; keep the pH at 7.2 or higher. Because folate deficiency increases the toxicity of methanol (in animals), folate replacement may be helpful. It can be given as a 50-mg intravenous dose every 4 hours for five doses, then once a day.

C. Hemodialysis

Hemodialysis is indicated for methanol blood concentrations higher than 50 mg/dL and in patients with severe acidosis, high formate levels, seizures, optic changes, or mental status changes; it should be started as soon as possible. The ethanol infusion must be adjusted to replace ethanol lost in dialysis (increase ethanol to 0.15–0.2 g/kg/h). Fomepizole is also dialyzed, and dosing should be increased to every 4 hours during dialysis.

▶ Disposition

Hospitalize all patients with suspected or documented methanol poisoning. If the osmolar gap and anion gap are both normal 1 hour after suspected ingestion, serious intoxication is unlikely.

3. Ethylene Glycol

Ethylene glycol is a common ingredient of deicers and antifreeze products. It is sweet tasting, and some preparations are attractively colored. Following ingestion, it is metabolized by alcohol dehydrogenase to glycolate and ultimately to oxalate, which precipitates with calcium to form calcium oxalate crystals. Symptoms may occur within 30 minutes or after a delay of several hours. Severe toxicity has resulted from the inhalation of ethylene glycol containing carburetor cleaner.

▶ Clinical Findings

The clinical course of ethylene glycol intoxication can be divided into three phases. The first phase occurs less than 1 hour after ingestion and is characterized by central nervous system depression. The second phase affects the cardiopulmonary system, and heart failure or pulmonary edema can occur approximately 12 hours after ingestion. The final phase occurs 24–72 hours after ingestion and is characterized by renal tubule necrosis, flank pain, hematuria, and renal failure. Visual symptoms are usually not present, and the ocular fundi appear normal (as distinguished from their appearance in methanol poisoning). An osmolar gap is present, and after metabolism to toxic products, a severe acidosis usually occurs, and crystals of calcium oxalate may be seen in the urine. The urine may be fluorescent under an ultraviolet lamp owing to the fluorescence often added to commercial antifreeze products.

▶ Treatment

Fomepizole is the treatment of choice, although ethanol can be used if fomepizole is unavailable. The dosing is the same as in methanol poisoning. Hemodialysis is now indicated only in patients with severe acidosis or abnormal renal function; the ethylene glycol level by itself does not determine the need for dialysis.

▶ Disposition

Hospitalize all patients with suspected or documented ethylene glycol intoxication.

4. Isopropanol

Isopropanol is a common ingredient in many household products, especially rubbing alcohol. It causes intoxication with central nervous system and cardiac depression; blood concentrations of 150 mg/dL are frequently associated with deep coma. It is metabolized by alcohol dehydrogenase to acetone, although most of the clinical effects of isopropanol intoxication are due to the parent compound. Both the alcohol and acetone cause an elevated osmolar gap, but acidosis is rare. The odor and acetonemia without acidosis is characteristic of isopropanol intoxication.

▶ Treatment

Treatment is primarily supportive and similar to that for ethanol intoxication. Hemodialysis is indicated for patients with an isopropanol level greater than 400 mg/dL and significant central nervous system depression.

▶ Disposition

Hospitalize patients with isopropanol intoxication who have significant signs (eg, stupor, coma, or hypotension).

Brent J: Fomepizole for ethylene glycol and methanol poisoning. N Engl J Med. 2009;360:2216–2223 [PMID: 19458366].

HYDROCARBONS

ESSENTIALS OF DIAGNOSIS

▶ Choking, gagging, or gasping following ingestion

▶ Hypoxia

▶ Delayed (4–6 hours) physical findings

▶ Infiltrates on chest X-ray (chemical pneumonitis)

▶ General Considerations

Hydrocarbons—a large group of compounds that includes petroleum distillates—exert various toxic effects. They are classified by two characteristics: viscosity (lowviscosity products are more likely to cause chemical aspiration pneumonia) and their potential for systemic toxicity (central nervous system or cardiac toxicity). These properties are summarized in Table 47–15.

The major complication following ingestion of petroleum distillates is aspiration pneumonitis, which may occur with poisoning caused by any of the lowviscosity compounds. Most cases of poisoning are accidental, and exposure is rarely more than a taste (5–10 mL). As little as 1–2 mL of low-viscosity compounds may produce severe chemical pneumonitis if aspirated into the tracheobronchial tree.

A coincidental or intentional inhalation of hydrocarbon vapors may produce irritation, nausea, and headache. Exposure to volatile vapors in an enclosed area may result in hypoxia owing to displacement of oxygen from the atmosphere. Inhalation of aromatic (eg, toluene) or halogenated (eg, freon and trichloroethylene) hydrocarbon solvents may cause euphoria, confusion, hallucinations, coma, and cardiac arrhythmias. Chronic exposure to toluene may cause myopathy, hypokalemia, renal tubular acidosis, and neuropathy.

▶ Clinical Findings

Symptoms suggesting aspiration are choking, coughing, or gasping immediately following ingestion of a toxic compound. Physical signs of aspiration are often present but may be delayed for up to 4–6 hours. For example, chest X-ray may reveal infiltrates before physical signs appear. Systemic signs of toxicity include narcosis, delirium, and for certain compounds, seizures. Some of these effects may result from hypoxemia due to pneumonitis. Hydrocarbons may sensitize the myocardium to the arrhythmogenic effects of endogenous catecholamines.

▶ Treatment

Gastric decontamination is controversial. Activated charcoal does not absorb hydrocarbons very well. Gastric lavage should be considered in hydrocarbon ingestion for substances that cause significant systemic toxicity. These include camphor, halogenated hydrocarbons, and aromatic hydrocarbons. The risk of aspiration may outweigh the benefit of decreasing toxicity with gastric lavage. Perform endotracheal intubation to protect the airway before performing gastric lavage.

A. High-Viscosity Lubricants

No treatment is required.

B. Low-Viscosity Compounds with No Known Systemic Toxicity

If there are unequivocal signs of aspiration pneumonitis, protect the airway if necessary to prevent further aspiration, and give oxygen. If the patient is asymptomatic and has no history of coughing or choking after ingestion, aspiration is unlikely. Do not induce emesis or perform gastric lavage, because it may increase the risk of aspiration. Observe the patient closely for 4–6 hours to detect signs of possible aspiration. Obtain a chest X-ray even in asymptomatic patients.

Table 47–15. Clinical Features of Hydrocarbon Poisoning.

Type	Examples	Risk of Pneumonia	Risk of Systemic Toxicity	Treatment
High-viscosity	Vaseline, motor oil, gasoline	Low	Low	None
Low-viscosity, nontoxic	Furniture polish, mineral spirits, kerosene, lighter fluid	High	Low	Observe for pneumonia. *Do not* induce emesis
Low-viscosity, unknown systemic toxicity	Turpentine, pine oil	High	Variable	Observe for pneumonia. *Do not* induce emesis if less than 1-2 mL/kg was ingested
Low-viscosity, known systemic toxicity	CHAMP: **C**amphor, **H**alogenated or **A**romatic hydrocarbons (benzene, toluene), **M**etals, **P**esticides	High	High	Gastric aspiration followed by activated charcoal

C. Low-Viscosity Compounds with Unknown or Unproved Toxicity

It is unclear whether these compounds have inherent systemic toxic effects apart from chemical pneumonitis, and controversy exists regarding the use of lavage to clear a compound of this group from the body. Evaluate the patient, and give treatment for possible pulmonary aspiration, as described above.

D. Low-Viscosity Compounds with Known Systemic Toxicity

Consider gastric emptying for ingestions of more than 30 mL of hydrocarbons with systemic toxicity, intentional overdoses, and mixed overdoses with other toxins. In the absence of the above scenarios, avoid gastric emptying. Activated charcoal should also be initiated under the same pretenses. Activated charcoal is especially useful if the toxin (eg, camphor) is known to produce coma or seizures abruptly. If lethargy, coma, or seizures are present, intubate the patient with a cuffed endotracheal tube and perform gastric lavage. Evaluate the patient for possible pulmonary aspiration.

▶ Disposition

Hospitalize patients who have ingested low-viscosity petroleum distillates if symptoms or signs of systemic toxicity (lethargy and seizures) or pneumonitis (coughing, choking, and abnormal findings on chest X-ray) are present. Because delayed onset of pulmonary complications may occur after hydrocarbon poisoning, it is prudent to observe patients for 4–6 hours before discharging them from the emergency department.

Lin CY et al: Toxicity and metabolism of methylnaphthalenes: comparison with naphthalene and 1-nitronaphthalene. Toxicology 2009:16;260:16–27 [PMID: 19464565].

Manoguerra AS, Erdman AR, Wax PM et al: Camphor Poisoning: an evidence-based practice guideline for out of hospital management. Clin Toxicol (Phila) 2006;44(4):357–370 [PMID: 16809137].

INHALANTS (TOXIC GASES AND VAPORS)

ESSENTIALS OF DIAGNOSIS

▶ Hypoxia

▶ Irritation of upper airway and conjunctiva

▶ Chemical pneumonitis and pulmonary edema

▶ General Considerations

Many toxic inhalants (eg, carbon monoxide and phosgene) are produced by combustion of household or industrial products in accidental fires or as byproducts of work activity (eg, welding). Many toxic chemicals exist in gaseous form (eg, chlorine, arsine) and exposure occurs during an accidental spill or leak. Toxic gases can be classified as (1) simple asphyxiants, (2) chemical asphyxi-ants and systemic poisons, and (3) irritants or corrosives (Table 47–16).

A. Simple Asphyxiants

Methane, propane, and inert gases cause toxicity by lowering the ambient oxygen concentration.

B. Chemical Asphyxiants and Systemic Poisons

Examples include carbon monoxide, cyanide, and hydrogen sulfide. These substances possess intrinsic systemic toxicity manifested after absorption into the circulation.

C. Irritants or Corrosives

These substances cause cellular destruction and inflammation when they come in contact with the tracheobronchial tree, usually by producing acids or alkali upon contact with moisture. Gases that are highly water soluble (eg, chlorine and ammonia) cause immediate irritation, mainly of the

Table 47–16. Clinical Features of Toxic Gases and Fumes.

Class of Toxin	Toxin	Source	Clinical Features	Treatment
Simple asphyxiants	Propane Methane Carbon dioxide Inert gases (nitrogen, argon)	Cooking gas Cooking gas All fires Industry (especially welding)	All displace normal air and lower F_{IO_2}. Symptoms of hypoxemia, without airway irritation	Remove patient from source; give oxygen
Chemical asphyxiants	Carbon monoxide	Fires	Forms carboxyhemoglobin; inhibits oxygen transport. Headache is earliest symptom	100% oxygen
	Hydrocyanic acid	Industry; burning plastics, furniture, fabrics	Highly toxic cellular asphyxiant (see section on cyanide).	Use cyanide antidote (Table 47–14)
	Hydrogen sulfide	Liquid manure pits, decaying organic materials	Highly toxic cellular asphyxiant similar to cyanide; sudden collapses; ability to smell characteristic odor of rotten eggs is rapidly fatigued	Use sodium nitrite as for cyanide (makes sulmethemoglobin). *Do not* use thiosulfate
Irritants: High solubility in water	Chlorine gas Hydrochloric acid Ammonia	Industry; swimming pool chemical; bleach mixed with acid at home Industry, burning fabrics	Early onset of lacrimation, sore throat, stridor, tracheobronchitis; with heavy exposure, may progress to pulmonary edema in 2–6 h	Humidified oxygen; bronchodilators; airway management
Low solubility in water	Nitrogen dioxide Ozone Phosgene	Burning cellulose; fabrics. Grain silos (acid red gas) Inert gas arc welding industry Burning of chlorinated organic material	Has sweet "electric" smell. Delayed onset (12–24 h) of tracheobronchitis, pneumonitis, and pulmonary edema. Late chronic bronchitis	Oxygen; observation for 24–48 h; steroids (controversial)
Allergenic	Toluene diisocyanate	Manufacture of polyurethanes	Reactive bronchoconstriction; may have long-term effects (chronic obstructive pulmonary disease) in susceptible persons	Bronchodilators.
Metal fumes	Zinc Copper Tin Teflon	Welding (especially galvanized metal welding)	"Metal fumes fever." Chills, fever, myalgias, headache, nonproductive cough, leukocytosis (4–8 h after exposure)	Self-limited (12–24 h)
	Arsine	Burning arsenic-containing ores; electronics industry	Highly toxic. Hemolysis, pulmonary edema, renal failure; chronic arsenic toxicity	Exchange transfusion; use dimercaprol (BAL) for chronic arsenic toxicity only
	Mercury Lead	Industry, welding	See specific metals	

upper airway and conjunctiva, whereas gases that are poorly soluble in water (eg, nitrogen dioxide) may be more deeply inhaled, producing delayed lower airway destruction with chemical pneumonitis and pulmonary edema.

▶ Clinical Findings

Symptoms and signs vary depending on the toxin. In an accidental fire, combinations of all classes of toxic inhalants may be responsible for symptoms of toxicity, for example, a burning sensation in the eyes and mouth, sore throat, brassy cough, dyspnea, and headache. Look for singed nasal hairs, carbonaceous deposits on the nose and face, upper airway swelling or obstruction, wheezing or signs of pulmonary edema, and manifestations of systemic toxicity. Obtain arterial blood gas determinations, carboxyhemoglobin level measurements, and chest X-ray.

▶ Treatment

Remove the patient from the source of toxic gases, and begin supplemental oxygen, 10 L/min, by mask. For victims of smoke inhalation or carbon monoxide poisoning, give 100% oxygen.

Treatment of poisoning caused by chemical asphyxiants and systemic toxins depends on the specific toxin. For cyanide, see previous discussion; for hydrogen sulfide poisoning, use sodium nitrate and hyperbaric oxygen, as outlined in the Cyanide section. Although unproved, nitrite therapy may decrease sulfide toxicity by binding it with methemoglobin. Do not give thiosulfate for hydrogen sulfide intoxication, because the enzyme rhodanese is not involved in elimination of sulfide.

For upper airway irritation, humidified oxygen is often effective. Carefully observe the patient for stridor and other signs of progressive airway obstruction that would require endotracheal intubation. For bronchospasm, give nebulized bronchodilators.

▶ Disposition

Hospitalize for observation and treatment all patients with significant symptoms or signs of poisoning caused by inhalation of toxic gases. Patients exposed briefly to high-solubility irritant gases whose symptoms have resolved can be safely discharged; however, those exposed to low-solubility irritants such as nitrogen oxides or phosgene may experience delayed-onset pulmonary edema or chemical pneumonitis and should be admitted for 16–24 hours' observation.

Yalamanchili C: Acute hydrogen sulfide toxicity due to sewer gas exposure. Am J Emerg Med 2008;26:518.e5–7 [PMID: 18410836].

IRON

ESSENTIALS OF DIAGNOSIS

▶ Signs and symptoms of iron poisoning can vary widely and include all major organ systems

▶ Levels can be obtained and in many cases guide treatment

▶ Chelation therapy is available for iron poisoning

▶ General Considerations

Iron poisoning results primarily from ingestion of mineral supplements containing divalent iron: ferrous sulfate (20% elemental iron), ferrous fumarate (33%), and ferrous gluconate (12%).

Absorption of iron is dose related and may increase dramatically with overdose levels, especially when the corrosive action of iron has damaged the intestinal mucosal barrier. Iron also causes vasodilatation and disruption of cellular electron transport. The elemental iron equivalent should be used when toxic doses are being estimated; an amount higher than 40 mg/kg causes toxicity, and amounts over 60 mg/kg are potentially lethal. Blood concentrations of

iron may assist in the diagnosis of acute toxicity but may be unreliable owing to concurrent absorption of iron and distribution in the tissues. A peak concentration in serum often occurs 4–6 hours after ingestion. Serum concentrations over 500 μg/dL are potentially toxic, and levels over 1000 μg/dL are associated with severe poisoning.

▶ Clinical Findings

Four stages of intoxication are commonly described:

1. Severe nausea and vomiting and abdominal pain occur within 1–4 hours. Hyperglycemia and leukocytosis are common. In severe cases, hemorrhagic gastroenteritis, shock, acidosis, and coma may follow. A plain film of the abdomen may show radiopaque iron tablets.

2. During the next period, which lasts 6–12 hours and sometimes up to 24 hours, the patient may appear relatively well or may even improve. Patients with significant ingestions, however, can still have progressive, silent systemic deterioration.

3. A stage of shock, acidosis, coagulopathy, and hypoglycemia may occur 12–24 hours after ingestion of significant amounts of iron and reflects a severe course and poor outlook. Serum iron concentration at this stage may be deceptively low, because most absorbed iron has been taken up by tissues.

4. The last stage is characterized by hepatic poisoning with possible progression to hepatic injury.

▶ Treatment

A. General Management

Provide intensive supportive care and gastrointestinal decontamination as described previously. For serious or massive ingestion, enhance removal of iron from the gastrointestinal tract with whole bowel irrigation. Activated charcoal is not effective.

B. Chelation Therapy

Intravenous chelation with deferoxamine is the treatment of choice when symptoms of iron poisoning are evident or when the serum iron level is over 500 μg/dL. The iron–deferoxamine complex is excreted in the urine and has a pink color. If urinary output is inadequate, the complexes may be removed with hemodialysis. The deferoxamine intramuscular challenge is no longer recommended, and any patient with a significant ingestion who appears toxic or has a serum iron level greater than 500 mg/dL should receive treatment. The dose of deferoxamine is 10–15 mg/kg until serum iron levels fall to less than 400 μg/dL or until urine no longer has characteristic pink color. Rapid IV administration may cause hypotension.

Observe the patient for several hours when ingestion of significant amounts of iron is suspected, because symptoms in the initial phase may be deceptively mild.

▶ Disposition

Hospitalize all patients with suspected or documented cases of iron poisoning. If patients remain asymptomatic, with a negative abdominal X-ray and no elevation of white blood cell count or blood glucose 6 hours after ingestion, they may be discharged to home care.

Madiwale T, Liebelt E: Iron: not a benign therapeutic drug. Curr Opin Pediatr 2006;18:174–179 [PMID: 16601499].

ISONIAZID

ESSENTIALS OF DIAGNOSIS

- ▶ Seizures, metabolic acidosis, and coma
- ▶ Seizures may be refractory to standard management (benzodiazepines)
- ▶ Estimated acute toxic dose is 80–100 mg/kg

▶ General Considerations

Isoniazid is a common antituberculosis drug often prescribed as a 3–6-month supply. The principal manifestations of isoniazid overdose are seizures, metabolic acidosis, and coma. Seizures may be due to depression of γ-aminobutyric acid levels in the central nervous system. Severe metabolic acidosis accompanies recurrent seizure activity. The estimated acute toxic dose is 80–100 mg/kg, although this range may be lower in patients with preexisting seizure disorders, vitamin B_6 deficiency, or chronic alcoholism.

▶ Clinical Findings

Symptoms occur 30 minutes to 3 hours following ingestion and include nausea and vomiting, slurred speech, dizziness, lethargy progressing to stupor, hyperreflexia, seizures, metabolic acidosis, hyperglycemia, and cardiovascular and respiratory depression. Symptoms and signs occur promptly after significant poisoning.

▶ Treatment

A. General Management

Provide intensive supportive care and gastrointestinal decontamination as described previously.

B. Treatment of Seizures

Treat seizures with lorazepam or diazepam, as described in Chapter 17. If these medications are not effective, continue benzodiazepines and give pyridoxine (vitamin B_6) in doses

equivalent to the amount ingested (gram for gram). If the amount ingested is unknown, start with 5 g (0.1 g/kg) intravenously given over 3–5 minutes, and repeat every 10–15 minutes until seizures are controlled. If the intravenous form of pyridoxine is not available, pyridoxine can be given as a slurry in a similar dose via a nasogastric tube.

C. Enhanced Elimination

Consider hemodialysis for patients unresponsive to conventional therapy.

▶ Disposition

Hospitalize all patients who have ingested more than 80 mg/kg of isoniazid and those who have signs or symptoms suggesting isoniazid poisoning.

Menzies D, Long R, Trajman A et al: Adverse events with 4 months of rifampin therapy or 9 months of isoniazid therapy for latent tuberculosis infection: a randomized trial. Ann Intern Med 2008;18;149:689–697 [PMID: 19017587].

Forget EJ, Menzies D: Adverse reactions to first-line antituberculosis drugs. Expert Opin Drug Saf 2006;5:231–249. [PMID: 16503745].

LITHIUM

ESSENTIALS OF DIAGNOSIS

- ▶ Apathy, lethargy, tremor, slurred speech, and ataxia
- ▶ In severe overdose, choreoathetosis, seizures, and coma
- ▶ Toxicity often accidental and seen with diuretic therapy and dehydration
- ▶ Lithium levels >2 mEq/L are usually toxic

▶ General Considerations

Lithium is frequently used to treat bipolar disorder and other psychiatric disorders. It is a monovalent cation like sodium and potassium; unlike these cations, however, it has only a small gradient of distribution across cell membranes and cannot maintain membrane potentials. It is rapidly absorbed into extracellular fluid, with an initial volume of distribution of 0.1–0.2 L/kg. Its distribution into selected tissues then occurs slowly over several hours. Its final volume of distribution is about 1 L/kg. It is excreted unchanged in the urine and actively reabsorbed, with a half-life of approximately 22 hours (with normal renal function). Sodium and water depletion lead to marked increases in the reabsorption of lithium and to elevation of blood concentrations of lithium.

▶ Clinical Findings

Symptoms of lithium overdose include apathy, lethargy, tremor, slurred speech, ataxia, and fasciculations, which may progress in severe overdose to choreoathetosis, seizures, coma, and death. Persistent neurologic sequelae may occur. Toxicity is frequently accidental and occurs secondary to chronic sodium depletion, diuretic therapy, and dehydration. In these cases, the serum lithium level is a more reliable index to the severity of overdose, because adequate time has passed for distribution into the central nervous system. In such circumstances, blood concentrations of lithium greater than 2 mEq/L are usually associated with toxicity.

In acute overdose, in contrast, initially elevated serum lithium concentrations may be misleading, because distribution into tissues occurs over several hours. For example, an initial toxic level of 4 mEq/L may easily fall to 1 mEq/L with final distribution. Thus, in acute overdose, repeated measurements of serum lithium levels and assessment of mental status (eg, every 4 hours) are more helpful than a single assessment in evaluating toxicity.

▶ Treatment

A. General Management and Prevention of Absorption

Provide intensive supportive care. Whole bowel irrigation is an effective means of increasing lithium removal. Activated charcoal does not adsorb lithium.

B. Enhanced Elimination

The treatment of choice for serious intoxication is hemodialysis. Specific indications for hemodialysis have not been well defined by careful studies, but dialysis should be considered for any patient with obtundation, seizures, or coma. Dialysis is the only route of elimination in patients with renal failure. Hemoperfusion is not effective.

Because lithium is reabsorbed in the kidney when sodium and fluids are depleted, sodium levels should be followed closely. Administration of intravenous saline may prevent reabsorption of lithium. Normal urine flow rates are adequate.

C. Prevention of Accidental Toxicity

To prevent chronic (accidental) toxicity, frequent assessment of fluid and sodium balance and lithium levels is recommended for patients taking lithium.

▶ Disposition

Hospitalize all patients with serum lithium concentrations above 2–3 mEq/L and those who show objective signs of lithium intoxication.

Waring WS: Management of lithium toxicity. Toxicol Rev 2006;25:221–230 [PMID: 17288494].

OPIATES

ESSENTIALS OF DIAGNOSIS

▶ Sedation, hypotension, bradycardia, hypothermia, and respiratory depression

▶ Diagnosis is confirmed if patient regains consciousness after naloxone

▶ General Considerations

Codeine, heroin, hydrocodone, oxycodone, and other opiates with varying potencies and durations of action are found in a wide range of prescription analgesic preparations. Some opiates, such as dextromethorphan, are found in nonprescription drugs.

The opiates act on central nervous system receptors and cause sedation, hypotension, bradycardia, hypothermia and respiratory depression. Most opiates have a half-life of 3–6 hours; the major exceptions are methadone (15–20 hours) and propoxyphene (12–15 hours).

▶ Clinical Findings

Consider opiate intoxication in any comatose or lethargic patient, especially when the clinical findings listed above are present. Pinpoint pupils are a typical sign, although in mixed overdoses, pupils may be in middle position. Signs of parenteral drug abuse may or may not be apparent. Pulmonary edema may occur. The diagnosis is confirmed if toxic concentrations of opiates are found in blood or urine or if the patient regains consciousness after administration of naloxone.

▶ Treatment

A. General Management

Provide intensive supportive care and gastrointestinal decontamination as described previously. Maintain adequate airway and ventilation.

B. Naloxone or Nalmefene

1. Naloxone—Give naloxone (a specific narcotic antagonist) to all patients with suspected opiate overdose. Start with 0.4–2 mg intravenously. Repeat 2 mg every 2–3 minutes three or four times if no response occurs and narcotic overdose is suspected. Some authorities recommend up to 10–20 mg to treat suspected narcotic overdose. Naloxone may also be administered intramuscularly or intranasal. Because naloxone has a half-life of 1 hour and effects lasting only 2–3 hours (shorter than many opiates), its effects may wear off before those of the narcotic, permitting the patient to lapse into coma again. If relapse occurs after the first response to naloxone, a naloxone continuous infusion may be started, using approximately two-thirds of the dose required to initially awaken the patient given over each hour.

2. Nalmefene—Another option in the busy emergency department is a long-acting opioid antagonist such as nalmefene. Nalmefene (2 mg) has been shown to last for as long as 8 hours, thereby reducing the need for any drips or repeated doses of naloxone. Naloxone is still the preferred initial antidote for comatose patients when the cause is uncertain because it will produce a shorter period of withdrawal in the chronically opioid-dependent patient.

C. Prevention of Narcotic Withdrawal Symptom

Watch carefully for withdrawal symptoms caused by naloxone or nalmefene. Chronic narcotic abusers who have developed tolerance to opiates may develop acute narcotic withdrawal when these agents are given. Although this syndrome is not life-threatening, it is a management problem in the emergency department if the patient becomes combative or uncooperative or signs out of the hospital before adequate treatment can be given. Careful titration of the naloxone dose may help to prevent narcotic withdrawal syndrome.

▶ Disposition

Hospitalize and observe all patients thought or known to have ingested significant amounts of opiates and those who relapse after the initial response to naloxone. Patients with heroin overdose who respond to naloxone may be safely discharged if they are asymptomatic 3 hours after the last dose.

Merlin MA, Saybolt M, Kapitanyan R et al: Intranasal naloxone delivery is an alternative to intravenous naloxone for opioid overdoses. Am J Emerg Med 2010;28:296–303 [PMID: 20223386].

Aquina CT, Marques-Baptista A, Bridgeman P, Merlin MA: OxyContin abuse and overdose. Postgrad Med 2009;121: 163–167 [PMID: 19332974].

ORGANOPHOSPHATES AND OTHER CHOLINESTERASE INHIBITORS

ESSENTIALS OF DIAGNOSIS

- ▶ Toxicity and potency vary widely
- ▶ DUMBELS (**d**iarrhea; **u**rination; **m**iosis; **b**ronchorrhea; **e**xcitation with muscle fasciculation, **e**mesis; **l**acrimation; and **s**alivation, **s**eizures). Death is usually from respiratory depression
- ▶ Diagnosis usually confirmed with low plasma or red blood cell cholinesterase level

▶ General Considerations

Cholinesterase inhibitors are found in a variety of insecticides (organophosphates and carbamates) available for home and commercial use (eg, crop sprays, bug bombs, and flea collars). Some chemical warfare agents (nerve gases) are also cholinesterase inhibitors.

These compounds inhibit acetylcholinesterase and therefore allow accumulation of acetylcholine at muscarinic and nicotinic receptors in nerve endings. Organophosphates bind irreversibly with the enzyme, whereas carbamates are considered reversible inhibitors. All are rapidly absorbed from the skin, gastrointestinal tract, and respiratory tract. Toxicity and potency vary widely. Workers chronically exposed to organophosphates and infants with underdeveloped cholinesterase activity are at greater risk for intoxication.

▶ Clinical Findings

Miosis, excessive salivation, bronchospasm, hyperactive bowel sounds, and lethargy typically occur shortly after exposure. Either bradycardia (muscarinic effect) or tachycardia (nicotinic effect) may be observed. QT-interval prolongation and pleomorphic ventricular tachyarrhythmias are a late consequence of poisoning. Symptoms of toxicity are easily remembered with the mnemonic DUMBELS. (**d**iarrhea; **u**rination; **m**iosis; **b**ronchorrhea; **e**mesis, **e**xcitation with muscle fasciculation; **l**acrimation; and **s**alivation).

Measurement of the plasma or red blood cell cholinesterase level is helpful in confirming acute toxicity; cholinesterase levels become low soon after exposure.

▶ Treatment

A. General Management

Provide intensive supportive care and gastrointestinal decontamination as described previously. Careful management of the airway is important, because significant bronchial secretions, bronchospasm, and hypoventilation may occur. Position the patient so as to avoid aspiration, and provide suction and oxygen as required. Early recognition of respiratory distress and subsequent intubation may decrease the mortality among these patients. Remove and isolate the patient's clothing, and carefully wash the skin with soap and water. Medical personnel should be careful to avoid cross-contamination.

B. Pharmacologic Treatment

Atropine is a symptomatic treatment for muscarinic signs (salivation, bronchorrhea, bronchospasm, and sweating). Large doses may be required. Start with 1–2 mg intravenously (0.5 mg in children), followed by repeated doses of 2–4 mg every 5–10 minutes until signs of atropinization occur (ie, flushing, mydriasis, drying of secretions, and tachycardia). The use of up to 50 mg in 24 hours is not unusual.

Pralidoxime (Protopam, 2-PAM) competitively inhibits binding of organophosphates to acetylcholinesterase and should be given to all patients with significant intoxication. It is not required for carbamate poisoning, because carbamate toxicity is transient. The dose is 1–2 g (25–50 mg/kg in children) in saline intravenously over 5–10 minutes. Continuous pralidoxime infusion has also been shown to improve the outcome in organophosphate poisoning. Adequate renal function is a prerequisite for use of pralidoxime, because it is excreted in the urine.

Other experimental treatments include magnesium, fresh frozen plasma and hemoperfusion.

C. Neurologic Sequel

Patients who receive prompt treatment usually recover from acute toxicity. However, two neurologic sequelae of severe intoxication—organophosphate-induced delayed neuropathy and intermediate syndrome—may occur after significant exposure.

▶ Disposition

Hospitalize all patients with clinical effects of organophosphate poisoning. Carbamate poisoning is usually transient, and patients who recover rapidly may be discharged.

Eddleston M, Buckley NA, Eyer P, Dawson AH: Management of acute organophosphorus pesticide poisoning. Lancet 2008;371:597–607 [PMID: 17706760].

Peter JV, Moran JL, Graham PL: Advances in the management of organophosphate poisoning. Expert Opin Pharmacother 2007;8:1451–1464 [PMID: 17661728].

PHENCYCLIDINE

ESSENTIALS OF DIAGNOSIS

▶ Rapid onset of action

▶ Vertical and horizontal nystagmus are common

▶ Symptomsmayfluctuate, unpredictably, fromsevere agitation to quiet stupor

▶ Hyperthermia and rhabdomyolysis may lead to myoglobinuria and renal failure

▶ General Considerations

Phencyclidine is a common adulterant of marijuana, amphetamines, and street hallucinogens. PCP is also called angel dust, crystal, supergrass, ozone, whack, rocket fuel, and peace pill by its users. It may be smoked, snorted, ingested, or injected.

PCP is a sympathomimetic, hallucinogenic, dissociative anesthetic agent originally used in veterinary practice. It has a rapid onset of action when smoked or snorted, causing euphoria and hallucinations. Serious overdose does not usually occur with smoking, because users can titrate the dose to achieve the desired effect. Ingestion of 20–25 mg of PCP can cause severe intoxication. PCP has a large volume of distribution (2–4 L/kg) and a half-life of several hours to days.

▶ Clinical Findings

Symptoms typically fluctuate, with patients alternating unpredictably from severe agitation to quiet stupor. Bizarre, paranoid behavior and extreme violence may occur unexpectedly. Both vertical and horizontal nystagmus is common. The pupils may be large or small. Hypertension, tachycardia, and hyperthermia are common. Marked muscle rigidity, dystonias, and seizures may occur. Hyperthermia and rhabdomyolysis resulting in myoglobinuria and renal failure are a major cause of subsequent illness. The diagnosis is made primarily on clinical grounds but may be confirmed by demonstrating PCP in urine or gastric aspirate. Serum PCP concentrations are not of value in emergency management.

▶ Treatment

A. General Management

Provide intensive supportive care and gastrointestinal decontamination as described previously. Most instances of PCP intoxication are mild and self-limited, and patients need no specific treatment other than to be in a quiet and supportive environment.

B. Treatment of Moderate to Severe Poisoning

Diazepam, 2–5 mg intravenously every 10 minutes until sedation is achieved, is effective in controlling moderate agitation or anxiety.

C. Treatment of Rhabdomyolysis or Myoglobinuria

If the patient has rhabdomyolysis or myoglobinuria, maintain urine output with intravenous fluids and mannitol.

▶ Disposition

Hospitalize patients who have moderate to severe PCP poisoning, particularly if hyperthermia, severe muscular rigidity, or evidence of rhabdomyolysis is an accompanying manifestation.

Moeller KE: Urine drug screening: practical guide for clinicians. Mayo Clin Proc 2008;83:66–76 [PMID: 18174009].

PHENOTHIAZINES AND ATYPICAL ANTIPSYCHOTICS

ESSENTIALS OF DIAGNOSIS

▶ Extrapyramidal side effects (eg, dystonia, orofacial spasms)

▶ Sedation, miosis, and hypotension are common

▶ Coma, seizures, and ventricular arrhythmias may occur with large doses

▶ General Considerations

Antipsychotic drugs include chlorpromazine (Thorazine, many others), prochlorperazine (Compazine), haloperidol (Haldol, others), and many other phenothiazines and butyrophenones. More recent antipsychotics do not have the same adverse effects of these older medications and are called "atypical." These include aripiprazole, quetiapine, risperidone, olanzapine, and ziprasidone.

The mechanism of toxicity of the antipsychotics is complex. Antiadrenergic properties cause sedation and hypotension, anticholinergic effects are manifested by dry mouth and tachycardia, and antidopaminergic properties may produce extrapyramidal side effects (most commonly seen with haloperidol). The contribution of each of these effects in drug overdose depends on the specific drug and on the individual patient. Most of these compounds have large volumes of distribution (10–30 L/kg) and long half-lives (12–30 hours); dialysis is not effective.

▶ Clinical Findings

With acute overdose, sedation, miosis, and hypotension are common. Coma and seizures may occur with very large ingestions. Prolongation of the QT interval and ventricular arrhythmias may occur. Disruption of the temperature-regulating mechanism may lead to hyperthermia or hypothermia. Extrapyramidal side effects may occur even at therapeutic doses and include dystonic posturing, spasm of orofacial muscles, cogwheel rigidity, and spasticity. Clinical effects following atypical antipsychotic overdose include sedation, anticholinergic effects, QT prolongation and rarely extrapyramidal effects.

▶ Treatment

A. General Management

Provide intensive supportive care and gastrointestinal decontamination as described previously. Treat hypotension with intravenous crystalloid solution; if a vasopressor is needed, norepinephrine is preferable.

B. Treatment of Extrapyramidal Reactions

Diphenhydramine (Benadryl, many others), 0.5–1 mg/kg intravenously slowly, or benztropine (Cogentin), 1–2 mg intramuscularly for adults, is recommended for extrapyramidal reactions. Relapse may occur; dispense oral anticholinergics for 2–3 days.

C. Treatment of Atypical Antipsychotic Overdose

Patients who overdose on atypical antipsychotics present in a manner similar to patients who overdose on the high-potency antipsychotics and should be managed similarly including close cardiac monitoring.

▶ Disposition

Hospitalize patients with clinically significant poisoning due to antipsychotics. In the acute period, close cardiac monitoring for arrhythmias and hypotension is warranted. Indications of significant poisoning include (1) rapidly worsening clinical findings and (2) obtundation. Patients with extrapyramidal reactions who respond to anticholinergic therapy may be discharged.

Tan HH, Hoppe J, Heard K: A systemic review of cardiocascular effects after atypical antipsychotic medication overdose. Am J Emerg Med 2009;27:607–616 [PMID: 19497468].

Isbister GK, Balit CR, Kilham HA: Antipsychotic poisoning in young children: a systemic review. Drug Saf 2005;28:1029–1044 [PMID: 16231955].

POISONOUS MUSHROOMS

ESSENTIALS OF DIAGNOSIS

▶ Delayed onset of symptoms (gastrointestinal irritation) of 6–12 hours suggests a toxic mushroom ingestion

▶ Mushrooms containing amatoxin may produce fatal hepatic necrosis

▶ General Considerations

Of the over 5000 varieties of mushrooms found in the United States, about 100 can be toxic. Most poisonous mushrooms act as gastrointestinal irritants. Table 47–17 lists several types of poisonous mushrooms, symptoms, and treatment. The most significant are *Amanita phalloides* and other mushrooms containing amatoxin, which may produce fatal hepatic necrosis.

Assistance with identification of specimens can often be obtained from a university biology department or mycology society. The regional poison control centers may also

Table 47-17. Mushrooms: Symptoms, Toxicity, and Treatment.

Symptoms	Mushrooms	Toxicity	Treatment
Gastrointestinal symptoms Onset < 2 h	*Chlorophyllum molybdites* *Omphalotus illudens* *Cantharellus cibarius* *Amanita caesarea*	Nausea, vomiting, diarrhea (occasional bloody). Initial: Nausea, vomiting, diarrhea	IV hydration Antiemetics IV hydration, glucose, monitor, AST, ALT, PT, PTT, bilirubin, BUN, creatinine
Onset 6–24 h	*Gyromitro esculenta*: fall season *Amanita phalloides, Amanita verna,* and *Amanita virosa*: spring season	Day 2: Rise in AST, ALT; day 3: hepatic failure	For *Amanita*: activated charcoal Penicillin G, 300,000–1,000,000 U/kg/d Silymarin, 20–40 mg/kg/d. Consider cimetidine, 4–10 g/d
Muscarinic (SLUDGE) syndrome Onset < 30 min	*Inocybe* *Clitocybe*	Salivation, lacrimation, diarrhea, gastrointestinal distress, emesis	Hyperbaric oxygen Supportive atropine, 0.01 mg/kg, repeated as needed for severe secretions.
CNS excitement Onset < 30 min	*Amanita muscaria* *Amanita pantherina*	Intoxication, dizziness, ataxia, visual disturbances, seizures, tachycardia, hypertension, warm dry skin, dry mouth, mydriasis (anticholinergic effects)	Supportive sedation with phenobarbital, 30 mg IV, or diazepam, 2–5 mg IV, as needed for adults
Hallucinations Onset < 30 min	*Psilocybe* *Gymnopilus*	Visual hallucinations, ataxia	Supportive sedation with phenobarbital, 0.5 mg/kg, or, for adults, 30–60 mg IV, or diazepam, 0.1 mg/kg or 5 mg IV, for adults
Disulfiram 2–72 h after mushroom, and < 30 min after alcohol	*Coprinus*	Headache, flushing, tachycardia, hyperventilation, shortness of breath, palpitations	Supportive IV hydration. Propranolol for supraventricular tachycardia. Norepinephrine for refractory hypotension

ALT, alanine amino transferase; AST, aspartate amino transferase; BUN, blood urea nitrogen; CNS, central nervous system; PT, prothrombin time; PTT, partial thromboplastin time; SLUDGE syndrome, salivation, lacrimation, urination, defecation, gastrointestinal hypermotility, and emesis.

Reproduced, with permission, from Tintinalli JE, Keten GD, Stapczynski S: *Emergency Medicine: A Comprehensive Study Guide*, 5th edn. McGraw-Hill, 2000.

help with identification. However, because accurate identification of mushrooms is difficult without an experienced mycologist and impractical because many types of mushrooms are often ingested at one time, the best approach to mushroom ingestion is to assume that the most toxic types have been consumed. Delayed onset (6–12 hours) of gastrointestinal symptoms suggests amatoxin or monomethylhydrazine poisoning.

▶ Treatment

Provide intensive supportive care and gastrointestinal decontamination as described previously. Unintentional pediatric ingestion of unknown "little brown mushrooms" rarely requires treatment or admission. If poisoning with amatoxin is suspected, perform gastric decontamination in the emergency department. Activated charcoal should be administered every 2–4 hours. Hospitalize the patient for observation and obtain baseline hepatic and renal function measurements. A variety of potential antidotes have been recommended, including corticosteroids, penicillin

G, thioctic acid, silymarin, and *N*-Acetylcysteine. Currently silymarin (Legalon, Madaus Inc.) is in phase III clinical trial. More important than specific antidotes is supportive care, including aggressive fluid replacement for massive gastroenteritis, supplemental glucose, and supportive treatment for hepatic encephalopathy. Early charcoal hemoperfusion or dialysis may be beneficial. Liver transplant has been successful in several patients with massive hepatic necrosis. Table 47–17 describes specific treatment for various kinds of mushroom poisoning.

▶ Disposition

Hospitalize patients thought or known to have ingested mushrooms known to cause serious poisoning (see Table 47–17).

Saller R, Brignoli R, Melzer J, Meier R: An updated systemic review with meta-analysis for the clinical evidence of silymarin. Forsch Komplementmed 2008;15:9–20 [PMID: 18334810].

POISONOUS PLANTS

ESSENTIALS OF DIAGNOSIS

▶ Identification of plant is often difficult but essential to diagnosis of toxicity

▶ Symptoms are dependent on the plant toxin ingested (eg, cyanide, cardiac glycosides, anticholinergics)

▶ General Considerations

Several hundred species of plants in the United States contain toxic compounds. Tables 47–18 and 47–19 give examples of nontoxic and toxic plants. Details about identification, mechanism of toxicity, and treatment are best obtained from a local poison control center. If the identity of a plant is unknown, it is helpful to send a sample to a local nursery or university botanist.

Treat the specific symptoms manifested by the patient, not those thought to be associated with the type of poisonous plant believed to have been ingested. Many similar species of plants have widely varying potencies and combinations of toxins; the plant's age, the soil conditions, and other factors influence the severity of toxic symptoms.

▶ Classes of Toxins

Some of the more common plant toxins are described below. The list is not complete.

A. Oxalates

Insoluble calcium oxalate crystals in the leaves and stems of some plants irritate the mucous membranes and can cause edema of the mouth, throat, and tongue. In rare severe reactions, drooling, dysphagia, and airway obstruction may

Table 47–18. Some Nontoxic Plants.

African violet (*Saintpaulia ionantha*)
Baby tears (*Helxine soleirolii*)
Bridal veil (*Genista monosperma pendula*)
Coleus species
Fuchsia species
Gardenia (*Gardenia radicans*)
Jade plant (*Crassula argentea*)
Piggyback *Begonia* (*Begonia hispida* var. *cucullifera*)
Piggyback plant (*Tolmiea menziesii*)
Rubber plant (*Ficus elastica "Decora"*)
Spider plant (*Chlorophytum comosum*)
Swedish ivy (*Plectranthus australis*)
Wandering Jew (*Tradescantia albiflora, T. fluminensis, Zebrina pendula*)
Zebra plant (*Calathea zebrina*)

Table 47–19. Some Poisonous Plants.[a]

Plant Name	Type of Toxin
Azalea (*Rhododendron* species)	Andromedotoxin (nicotine-like and cardiotoxic)
Black nightshade (*Solanum nigrum*)	Solanine
Caladium	Oxalates
Castor bean (*Ricinus communis*)	Toxalbumin (ricin)
Deadly nightshade (*Atropa belladonna*)	Anticholinergic
Delphinium	Nicotine-like
Dumb cane (*Dieffenbachia*)	Oxalates
Elderberry (*Sambucus*)	Cyanogenic (ripe berries nontoxic)
Foxglove (*Digitalis purpurea*)	Cardiac glycosides
Hydrangea	Cyanogenic
Jequirity bean, rosary bean (*Abrus precatorius*)	Toxalbumin (a lectin)
Jerusalem cherry (*Solanum pseudocapsicum*)	Solanine
Jimsonweed (*Datura stramonium*)	Anticholinergic
Lantana	Anticholinergic
Lily of the valley (*Convallaria majalis*)	Cardiac glycosides
Lobelia	Nicotine-like
Mistletoe (*Viscum album, Phoradendron flavescens*)	Tyramine (hypertension; gastroenteritis)
Mountain laurel (*Kalmia latifolia*)	Andromedotoxin (nicotine-like and cardiotoxic)
Oleander (*Nerium oleander*)	Cardiac glycosides
Philodendron	Oxalates
Pits (of cherry, apricot, peach)	Cyanogenic (amygdalin)
Poison hemlock (*Conium maculatum*)	Nicotine-like
Poinsettia (*Euphorbia pulcherrima*)	Oxalate-like
Tobacco (*Nicotiana tabacum*)	Nicotine
Water hemlock (*Cicuta maculata*)	Cicutoxin (seizures)
Yew (*Taxus* species)	Taxine (gastroenteritis, cardiac toxicity)

[a]This short list is for illustrative purposes only. Consult other sources (eg, regional poison control center) for information on specific plants.

occur. Renal failure may occur if sufficient amounts of oxalates are absorbed.

B. Amygdalin and Cyanogenic Glycosides

Cyanide is produced by the gastrointestinal hydrolysis of chewed-up fruit pits or seeds (*Prunus* species: cherry, apricot, peach) or leaves and stems (*Hydrangea*, elder-berry). Severe poisoning is uncommon. See Cyanide section for symptoms and therapy.

C. Cardiac Glycosides

Digitalis and similar compounds are present in varying amounts in certain plants. Serious clinically effects after consumption of only one oleander leaf, or oleander tea, have been reported (see Cardiac Glycosides section).

C. Anticholinergics

The typical anticholinergic syndrome of dry mouth, tachycardia, delirium, urinary retention, and mydriasis is seen. Most poisonings are mild, and supportive treatment is sufficient. Abuse of anticholinergic plants has been frequently reported. (see Anticholinergics section).

D. Nicotine-Like Toxins

These toxins include nicotine and aconitine. Symptoms include nausea and vomiting, salivation, diarrhea, restlessness, and seizures. Mydriasis may also occur. Following an initial phase of excitement, respiratory depression and hypotension may occur.

E. Solanine

Solanine produces gastrointestinal symptoms similar to those of nicotine. In addition, plants containing solanine often have significant amounts of atropinic alkaloids, so that the net effect is unpredictable. Onset of symptoms may be delayed several hours.

F. Toxalbumins

These highly toxic compounds (eg, abrin, ricin, and phallin) can cause acute gastroenteritis, dehydration, and shock. Convulsions, hemolysis, and renal and hepatic injury can also occur. Oral and esophageal irritation or burns may be seen.

▶ Treatment

In general, observation is recommended after ingestion of plants with known potentially serious toxic effects and activated charcoal may be beneficial in such cases. Begin specific treatment as indicated for the specific toxins involved.

▶ Disposition

Disposition depends on the plant ingested and the symptoms experienced.

Schep LJ, Slaughter RJ, Becket G, Beasley DM: Poisoning due to water hemlock. Clin Toxicol 2009;47:270–278 [PMID: 19514873].

Froberg B, Ibrahim D, Furbee RB: Plant poisoning. Emerg Med Clin North Am 2007;25:375–433 [PMID: 17482026].

SALICYLATES

ESSENTIALS OF DIAGNOSIS

▶ Toxicity generally occurs at levels >150 mg/kg

▶ Early manifestations include nausea, vomiting, and hyperventilation

▶ Initial respiratory alkalosis is often followed by a severe metabolic acidosis, creating a mixed acid-base status

▶ Hypoglycemia is prominent in children

▶ General Considerations

Salicylates are present in numerous prescription and non-prescription medications, for example, analgesics, bismuth subsalicylate (Pepto-Bismol, many others), or oil of wintergreen (methyl salicylate).

The mechanism of toxicity with salicylate poisoning is complex and includes direct central nervous system stimulation, uncoupling of oxidative phosphorylation, inhibition of Krebs cycle enzymes, and interference with hemostatic mechanisms. The volume of distribution is dose dependent and usually small; with significant ingestion, however, the drug is redistributed into the central nervous system. Because salicylate is a weak acid, acidemia increases its penetration of the central nervous system. The half-life may increase from 2 to 20 hours at overdose levels as a result of saturation of liver metabolism. The elimination of salicylate is increased in alkaline urine. The minimum acute toxic dose is 150 mg/kg, with severe toxicity occurring at doses over 300–500 mg/kg. However, many cases of toxicity are a result of prolonged excessive treatment of minor illnesses (subacute or accidental overdose). The chronically ill and the elderly are at greater risk for subacute toxicity because of relative hypoalbuminemia and renal insufficiency.

▶ Clinical Findings

Early manifestations of overdose include nausea and vomiting, tinnitus, listlessness, and hyperventilation. Loss of fluid and electrolytes is common. Initial respiratory alkalosis is followed by severe metabolic acidosis, hypokalemia, and hypoglycemia. Seizures, hyperpyrexia, and coma occur as toxicity becomes more severe. Measurement of the blood salicylate concentration is essential for effective management, although it is not as reliable an indicator of the severity of illness if subacute toxicity is present. In cases of acute salicylate ingestion the prognosis and patient management should not be based solely on an aspirin level. Consider the patient's clinical presentation, age, aspirin level, and acid–base status in making treatment decisions. In the presence of acidosis, toxicity occurs with considerably lower levels. Salicylate determinations should be repeated every 4–5 hours. Repeated measurements are especially important for ingestion of sustained-release or enteric-coated preparations, which are absorbed slowly and may result in delayed peak levels.

With subacute (accidental) toxicity, severity of poisoning does not correlate well with serum salicylate concentration, but levels above 30 mg/dL (300 mg/L) are significant. Patients with subacute toxicity are frequently very young or very old and they usually present with dehydration, obtundation, and acidosis. The diagnosis is often missed while the physician concentrates on the more prominent secondary complications. Cerebral and pulmonary edema and death are more common in patients with subacute toxicity.

▶ Treatment

A. General Management

Provide intensive supportive care and gastrointestinal decontamination as described previously. After acute overdose, give adequate charcoal to bind ingested salicylate. Multidose activated charcoal may be beneficial. For enteric-coated aspirin, toxicologists recommend multidose activated charcoal and possibly even whole bowel irrigation if the salicylate level is rising.

B. Correction of Acid–Base Status

Correct dehydration, hypoglycemia, hypokalemia, and acidosis. Fluid resuscitation is imperative. For significant dehydration, start with 20 mL/kg of an intravenous crystalloid solution given over 1–2 hours, and then give 3–5 mL/kg/h to maintain the urine output at 2–3 mL/kg/h. To correct acidosis and promote excretion of salicylate in the urine, give sodium bicarbonate, 1 mEq/kg/h. Concurrent correction of potassium deficit is mandatory. Urine pH should be maintained at 7–7.5. Alkalization of the urine is often unsuccessful in critically ill patients (especially the elderly), and it may aggravate pulmonary and cerebral edema.

C. Enhanced Elimination

Hemodialysis is recommended for critically ill patients with persistent seizures, acidosis that fails to respond to treatment, or cerebral or pulmonary edema. Although high salicylate concentrations (eg, > 120 mg/dL [1200 mg/L] at 6 hours) generally represent severe toxicity, hemodialysis should be based on the patient's complications and not the drug level. Hemodialysis is efficient in removing salicylate

and can help to correct pH and electrolyte abnormalities. Consider early hemodialysis in ill patients with subacute overdose. Although there are no proved guidelines, elderly patients with serum salicylate levels over 60 mg/dL, and those with significant neurologic toxicity, should probably receive immediate hemodialysis. If the patient is hemodynamically unstable or hemodialysis is unavailable, continuous hemodiafiltration has been reported to be a viable alternative.

D. Other Measures

Obtain measurements of serum salicylate every 4–6 hours to monitor adequacy of treatment. If evidence of salicylate-induced hypoprothrombinemia is present, give vitamin K, 10 mg intramuscularly.

Rehydration, control of hyperthermia, and rapid correction of acidemia are essential. Give glucose, and replace potassium deficits.

▶ Disposition

Hospitalize all patients with known or suspected severe salicylate poisoning.

Pearlman BL, Gambhir R: Salicylate intoxication: a clinical review. Postgrad Med 2009;121;162–168 [PMID: 19641282].

SEDATIVE–HYPNOTICS

ESSENTIALS OF DIAGNOSIS

▶ Symptoms include nystagmus, atonia, lethargy, somnolence, respiratory depression, hypotension, and hypothermia

▶ Sedative–hypnotics such as γ-hydroxybutyric acid may be associated with symptoms ranging from respiratory depression and coma to seizure-like activity with aggressive behavior

▶ General Considerations

Sedative–hypnotics include a broad range of drugs used to treat anxiety or insomnia. Included are benzodiazepines, zolpidem, and a variety of medications for insomnia. They can induce tolerance and can cause a withdrawal syndrome similar to that associated with ethanol withdrawal (except for the time of onset and duration). These agents are found singly and in various drug combinations. Of note, one sedative–hypnotic, γ-hydroxybutyric acid (GHB), has become a common drug of abuse. Effects range from respiratory depression, apnea, and coma to seizure-like activity along with aggressive behavior.

Absorption, distribution, and elimination of sedative–hypnotics vary. In general, the mechanism of toxicity of these drugs is central nervous system depression similar to that caused by ethanol.

▶ Clinical Findings

Clinical manifestations of overdose include nystagmus, ophthalmoplegia, ataxia, dysarthria, lethargy, somnolence, respiratory depression, hypotension, and hypothermia. With the onset of deep coma, oculocephalic reflexes are lost and the pupils become nonreactive to light. The initial electroencephalogram may be flat, although the patient may subsequently recover completely. Serum drug levels may be misleading because levels of intoxication and rates of elimination vary enormously from person to person, depending on prior drug use and the patient's physical state.

▶ Treatment

A. General Management

Provide intensive supportive care and gastrointestinal decontamination as described previously. Treat shock and hypotension with an initial bolus of 200–1000 mL of intravenous crystalloid solution (Chapter 9). Restore the patient's core temperature to normal levels, because hypothermia will worsen hypotension. Monitoring the pulmonary capillary wedge pressure is helpful in avoiding fluid overload and determining the need for pressor agents. Vasopressors should be used only if adequate fluid replacement is ineffective (as determined by pulmonary capillary wedge pressure measurements).

B. Enhanced Elimination

Reserve hemodialysis or hemoperfusion for patients who remain hypotensive or otherwise unstable despite aggressive supportive care. These measures successfully remove only a few sedative–hypnotics (eg, phenobarbital, meprobamate, and ethchlorvynol).

C. Other Measures

The benzodiazepine antagonist flumazenil (Romazicon) should be used with extreme caution, if at all. The dose is 0.2 mg intravenously slowly repeated every 5–10 minutes as needed, up to a maximum 3–5 mg. Effects wear off in 1–3 hours, and repeated sedation is common. Contraindications include known seizure disorder, coingestion of drugs known to cause seizures, benzodiazepine addiction, and tricyclic antidepressant overdose. General supportive care usually suffices.

▶ Disposition

Hospitalize patients with sedative–hypnotic drug poisoning resulting in depression of vital reflexes (eg, respiration and gag reflex).

Charlson F, Degenhardt L, McLaren J, Hall W, Lynskey M: A systematic review of research examining benzodiazepine-related mortality. Pharmacoepidemiol Drug Saf 2009;18:93–103 [PMID: 19125401].

THEOPHYLLINE AND METHYLXANTHINES

ESSENTIALS OF DIAGNOSIS

▶ Minimum acute toxic dose is 10 mg/kg
▶ Mild symptoms include nausea and vomiting, tremor, anxiety, and abdominal cramping
▶ Severe symptoms include arrhythmias and seizures

▶ General Considerations

Theophylline, caffeine, and other methylxanthines cause bronchodilatation; gastric, central nervous system, and cardiac stimulation; and vasodilatation. The half-life is 4–8 hours and is shortened in chronic smokers and prolonged in patients with congestive heart failure or cirrhosis. In acute overdose, the half-life may be markedly prolonged (up to 50 hours).

The minimum acute toxic dose is over 10 mg/kg, or 700 mg, in the average adult. Because drug metabolism varies markedly depending on the patient's clinical status, careful monitoring of patients receiving therapeutic doses is necessary to avoid iatrogenic toxicity.

▶ Clinical Findings

Mild symptoms of toxicity are nausea and vomiting, abdominal cramps, tremor, and anxiety. Arrhythmias and seizures occur with more serious intoxication. Seizures are often refractory to treatment with standard anticonvulsants. The characteristics of acute single overdose differ from those of chronic, subacute overmedication. Acute overdose is characterized by hypotension, tachycardia, and hypokalemia. Seizures and serious arrhythmias are common with levels over 100 mg/L but rare with levels under 90 mg/L. By contrast, chronic intoxication more commonly results in seizures and arrhythmias with much lower serum levels (ie, 20–70 mg/L). Hypotension and hypokalemia are uncommon. The elderly are at highest risk for fatal outcome.

Sustained-release theophylline preparations are now commonly used, so that after acute overdose, early blood concentrations of the drug may be low and gastrointestinal symptoms absent. Obtain serial blood levels until the theophylline level begins to fall.

▶ Treatment

A. General Management

Provide intensive supportive care and gastrointestinal decontamination as described previously.

B. Gastrointestinal Decontamination

Consider activated charcoal if a significant dose has been ingested within 1 hour of arrival at the emergency department. Administer multidose activated charcoal and consider whole bowel irrigation for sustained-release preparations.

C. Treatment of Seizures

Seizures are usually difficult to control with standard drugs. Start with diazepam, 0.1–0.2 mg/kg as an intravenous bolus, followed by phenobarbital, 15 mg/kg intravenously over 20–30 minutes. Perform hemoperfusion immediately if seizures are not controlled.

D. Treatment of Hypotension

Treat hypotension with intravenous fluids. Propranolol, 0.02–0.05 mg/kg, or esmolol, 25–50 μg/kg/min, intravenously, may reverse hypotension associated with tachycardia, both of which are mediated by excessive β-adrenergic stimulation.

E. Treatment of Arrhythmias

Ventricular tachyarrhythmias and rapid atrial fibrillation may be controlled with propranolol or esmolol intravenously or with standard antiarrhythmics.

F. Enhanced Elimination

Charcoal hemoperfusion, hemofiltration, or hemodialysis is the treatment of choice for severe poisoning. Hemoperfusion is the treatment of choice for severe poisoning (intractable seizures, acute overdose with serum level over 80–100 mg/L, and hemodynamic instability). Repeated doses of activated charcoal may be effective at lowering theophylline levels, obviating extracorporeal treatment.

▶ Disposition

Hospitalize patients with significant theophylline poisoning (serum concentrations above 30 μg/mL or signs or symptoms of toxicity).

Dhar R, Stout CW, Link MS et al: Cardiovascular toxicities of performance-enhancing substances in sports. Mayo Clin Proc 2005;80:1307–1315 [PMID: 16212144].

WARFARIN AND OTHER ANTICOAGULANTS

ESSENTIALS OF DIAGNOSIS

▶ A single overdose with warfarin usually does not cause significant bleeding

▶ May see ecchymosis, hematuria, melena, epistaxis, gingival bleeding, hematoma, and hematemesis

▶ Life-threatening cardiac tamponade and intracranial hemorrhage may occur

▶ General Considerations

Dicumarol and other natural anticoagulants are found in sweet clover. Warfarin and other synthetic coumarin-like anticoagulants are used therapeutically and as rodenticides.

Warfarin and other coumarin-like compounds inhibit blood clotting by interfering with the synthesis of vitamin K dependent clotting factors (II, VII, IX, X). Only the synthesis of new factors is affected, and the anticoagulation effect is delayed until currently circulating factors have degraded. Thus, effects may be seen within 8–12 hours after ingestion because factor II has only a 6-hour half-life, but peak effects are usually not observed until 1–2 days after ingestion because of the longer half-lives (24–60 hours) of the other clotting factors.

The potency and pharmacokinetics of the different coumarin anticoagulants vary. Warfarin is highly bound to albumin and has a half-life of 35 hours. It is metabolized by the liver. Multiple drug interactions are known to increase or decrease the anticoagulation effect (Table 47–20).

A single overdose with warfarin does not usually cause significant bleeding, because the half-life of warfarin is shorter than that of some of the clotting factors. Chronic warfarin administration carries a greater risk of excessive anticoagulation and bleeding. However, some extremely potent and long-acting anticoagulants, also known as super-warfarins (brodifacoum, indanediones), may produce severe bleeding disturbance for several weeks to months.

▶ Clinical Findings

Excessive anticoagulation may result in ecchymoses, hematuria, uterine bleeding, melena, epistaxis, gingival bleeding, hemoptysis, or hematemesis. Hematomas may result in compression neuropathy or compartment syndrome. Life-threatening cardiac tamponade and intracranial hemorrhage have been reported. Such complications can be prevented if the international normalized ratio (INR) is carefully monitored and kept within the desired therapeutic range, if interacting drugs are avoided, and if antidotal therapy is begun promptly when necessary.

Table 47–20. Interactions of Warfarin and Oral Anticoagulants with Selected Drugs.

Increased Anticoagulation Effect	Decreased Anticoagulation Effect
Allopurinol	Barbiturates
Chloral hydrate	Carbamazepine
Cimetidine	Cholestyramine
Disulfiram	Glutethimide
Indomethacin	Oral contraceptives
Quinidine	Antibiotics (rifampin)
Salicylates	
Sulfonamides	
Antibiotics (erythromycin)	

▶ Treatment

A. General Management

Provide intensive supportive care and gastrointestinal decontamination as described previously. Treatment is rarely required for acute single overdose of warfarin, because the dose involved (eg, from typical rodenticide) is small, and any anticoagulation effect is usually brief and mild. However, caution and careful follow-up are indicated after ingestion of the super-warfarins. Obtain a baseline prothrombin time and repeat the measurement after 24 and 48 hours. Children who ingest a rodenticide rarely require treatment.

B. Treatment of Major Hemorrhage

For major hemorrhage (eg, intracranial hemorrhage, aortic dissection, and shock), control bleeding with fluid resuscitation and withhold further doses of warfarin. Vitamin K, 5–10 mg intravenously, should be given along with fresh-frozen plasma, 15 mL/kg, or prothrombin complex concentrates. For patients with asymptomatic prolongation of the INR (>10), give vitamin K, 2–5 mg orally, without fresh-frozen plasma. Recheck the INR in 6–12 hours. If the INR is between 6 and 10, give vitamin K, 2 mg, orally without fresh-frozen plasma and recheck the INR in 12–24 hours. In all the above cases, vitamin K should be given intravenously or orally, not intramuscularly, because of the risk of erratic absorption and hematoma formation.

▶ Disposition

Hospitalize all patients with significantly prolonged prothrombin times, evidence of bleeding, or history of ingestion of massive amounts of anticoagulants. Patients who have documented anticoagulant effect after ingestion of the super-warfarin rodenticides will need close follow-up and repeated vitamin K dosing for up to several weeks.

Watt BE, Proudfoot AT, Bradberry SM, Vale JA: Anticoagulant rodenticides. Toxicol Rev 2005;24:259–269 [PMID: 16499407].

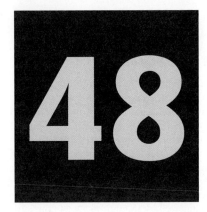

48

Dermatologic Emergencies

Kavon Azadi, MD
Boyd Burns, DO, FACEP, FAAEM[1]

IMMEDIATE RECOGNITION AND MANAGEMENT OF LIFE-THREATENING PROBLEMS

To some, emergency medicine and dermatology may seem to be two of the most unrelated specialties in medicine, and in our daily practice dermatologic complaints most likely respresent a small percentage of our normal daily census but the emergency physician will encounter many patients presenting with dermatologic complaints. The astute clinician will realize that, although rare, some of these problems can be life-threatening. Some patients may even require emergency airway protection and vigorous resuscitation. This chapter reviews those special situations and discusses common and uncommon dermatologic complaints.

▶ Initial Evaluation

The initial evaluation begins with the primary survey and vital signs. Always focus special attention on airway, breathing, and circulation (the ABCs). Note any abnormal vital signs and oxygen saturation, and be alert to subtle changes in mental status or behavior that may indicate impending airway or cardiovascular collapse. The ABCs apply to all clinical situations, and a thorough history and examination are often the most helpful tools in arriving at any diagnosis. The dermatologic examination must be performed on a disrobed patient. Inspect all areas of the skin and mucosal surfaces before addressing specific lesions.

▶ History

Parallel to the assessment of the ABCs is a thorough history that includes potential recent exposures to foods, medications, plants, insects, and the like that may have triggered the condition. An ample history, addressing the patient's allergies, medications, medical and surgical history, last meal, and

[1]This chapter is a revision of the chapter by: Ben H. Chlapek, DO, FACEP, FACOEP from the 6th edition.

events leading up to the presentation may provide information necessary to begin appropriate management.

ANGIOEDEMA AND URTICARIA

1. Angioedema

 ESSENTIALS OF DIAGNOSIS

▶ Swelling of face, lips, tongue
▶ May lead to airway compromise

▶ General Considerations

Angioedema forms in the deeper dermal and subcutaneous tissues of the distal extremities, tongue, lips, mouth, face, and neck. Particularly dangerous is the involvement of the mouth, tongue, and lower airway, which can lead to severe airway compromise. Angioedema is believed to be a similar to urticaria, which is present in half of the cases, but a deeper reaction. Two subtypes exist, the rare hereditary form and the acquired form. The autosomal dominant hereditary variant is usually due to C1-esterase deficiency or defect with 75% of patients with hereditary angioedema (HAE) having their first episode before 16 years of age. The acquired form is most commonly secondary to angiotensin-converting enzyme (ACE) inhibitors and has increased in prevalence because of widespread usage of these drugs. Patients who have been using ACE inhibitors for months or years can still develop angioedema from these agents.

▶ Treatment

Emergency airway protection is mandated if airway compromise is impending or present. Treat shock if present. Discontinue any implicated medications or substances. Supply oxygen to maintain oxygen saturation at greater than 90%. In severe angioedema with airway compromise, administer epinephrine 0.1–0.5 mg (1:1000 solution) subcutaneously or preferably intramuscularly. This may be repeated every 5–10 minutes. Give an H_1 antihistamines such as diphenhydramine HCl, 1–2 mg/kg, or in adults, 25–50 mg parenterally. Consider an H_2 antihistamine such as ranitidine 50 mg intravenously. Methylprednisolone sodium succinate, 125 mg intravenously, may be repeated every 6 hours. Life-threatening HAE attacks may not respond well to epinephrine in normal dosages, antihistamines, or steroids. In these cases, airway protection is mandatory and fresh frozen plasma should be considered as it contains C1 inhibitor.

▶ Disposition

Admit patients to an ICU if airway compromise is present; otherwise, they may need observation in a non-ICU hospital bed or in the emergency department. If a patient is thought to have experienced a reaction to a medication, instruct the patient to discontinue that medication and contact his or her primary-care physician to discuss an alternative medication.

2. Urticaria

 ESSENTIALS OF DIAGNOSIS

▶ Localized areas of dermal edema
▶ Intense itching

▶ General Considerations

Urticaria (hives) may be either acute or chronic and may appear in any age group. The condition represents one end of a continuum, ranging from urticaria to anaphylactic shock. Because various medications and foods are most often implicated as causes, take a thorough history of possible exposures. The lesions themselves represent localized areas of edema in the dermis. They appear as intensely pruritic, sharply demarcated raised circular or annular areas with either an erythematous or a blanched base and border. Their appearance may wax and wane, and individual lesions often resolve within an hour. With anaphylaxis (see Chapter 9), there may be an initial decrescendo of the presenting symptoms with early interventions. A late-phase response may occur hours later with a more severe presentation than the initial symptom complex.

▶ Treatment

If airway compromise is not present, patients can be given H_1-receptor blockers (see diphenhydramine dosing, above), steroids, and even epinephrine. H_2-receptor blockers, such as ranitidine, may also be added. If airway compromise is present, treat on an emergency basis as for angioedema.

▶ Disposition

Disposition is the same as for angioedema (see above). Remember the sometimes biphasic nature of anaphylactic reactions. Instruct patients to avoid any potentially responsible agents. Give any patient with a history of anaphylaxis a prescription for an autoinjector epinephrine device and instruct the patient on its proper use prior to discharge.

Hoover T, Lippmann M, Grouzmann E, Marceau F, Herscu P: Angiotensin converting enzyme inhibitor induced angio-oedema: a review of the pathophysiology and risk factors. Clin Exp Allergy 2010;40:50–61 [PMID: 19659669].

Kaplan AP, Greaves MW: Angioedema. J Am Acad Dermatol 2005;53:373–388 [PMID: 16112343].

Levy JH, Freiberger DJ, Roback J: Hereditary angioedema: current and emerging treatment options. Anesth Analg 2010;110:1271–1280 [PMID: 20418292].

STEVENS–JOHNSON SYNDROME AND TOXIC EPIDERMAL NECROLYSIS

ESSENTIALS OF DIAGNOSIS

▶ Epidermal detachment
▶ Drug-induced or postviral illness
▶ Patients may be critically ill

▶ General Considerations

A disorder of epidermal detachment was initially reported in 1922 when Stevens and Johnson published a description of two children with fever, erosive stomatitis, severe conjunctivitis, and a disseminated cutaneous eruption. It is now known to be a drug-induced state or one that follows a viral illness. Stevens–Johnson syndrome (SJS) and toxic epidermal necrolysis (TEN) are now thought to represent ends of a spectrum of reactions involving detachment of the epidermis. Both conditions share inciting factors and mucosal involvement. The range of disorders has been classified into three categories: SJS, involving less than 10% of body surface area (BSA); transitional cases, involving 10–30% of BSA; and TEN, with greater than 30% of BSA with detached epidermis. Mortality rates for SJS are approximately 5%; rates are much higher (30%) with TEN. Death is most commonly from sepsis secondary to infections from *Staphylococcus aureus* and *Pseudomonas aeruginosa*.

▶ Clinical Findings

With a few exceptions, SJS/TEN results from drug exposure. The main culprits are sulfonamide antibiotics. Others on the list include aromatic anticonvulsants, β-lactam antibiotics, NSAIDs, *allopurinol*, tetracyclines, quinolones, and *abacavir*. Over 200 medications have been implicated along with vaccinations, malignancy, HIV and herpes viral infections. Patients with SJS/TEN typically present with 1- to 2-week prodrome of arthralgia, anorexia, fever, pruritus, pharyngitis, and conjunctivitis prior to skin involvement. With re-exposure of a drug, the time to onset to skin involvement is typically 1–3 days. Any mucous membrane site can be involved. Mucous membrane involvement often precedes but may accompany skin lesions. Patients with

SJS/TEN present with severe, intensely painful macules and mucosal ulcerations with a truncal and occasionally facial distribution of target like lesions. The skin lesions begin as macules and are often described as burning. Over time macules coalesce into wide areas of erythema as the eruption expands. As lesions age, the skin becomes necrotic and bullae may form. The Nikolsky sign may be elicited. This refers to easy separation of the upper layers of the epidermis from the lower layers with very minor trauma, such as lateral traction or gentle rubbing on the skin. There may be eroding of the bullae, or the affected skin may slough in large sheets. This may progress over hours to days. The sloughing may involve other organ systems, including the gastrointestinal tract, genitourinary system, and the respiratory tree.

▶ Treatment

Discontinue any potentially inciting medications. This usually requires that all nonessential medications be stopped, because no tests are available to identify the offending agents. Careful correction of electrolyte abnormalities and fluid replacement are critical, because significant fluid losses occur with loss of the protective skin barrier. Airway protection and mechanical ventilation may be necessary if the trachea and upper airway are involved. Sloughing and detachment of mucosa can lead to airway compromise. Antibiosis may be necessary to avoid sepsis-related complications. Pain control is essential. For uveitis, corneal ulceration, and/or vision loss, ophthalmologic consultation is strongly encouraged. Skin biopsy can aid in ruling out other deadly bullous diseases such as pemphigus vulgaris.

▶ Disposition

In severe cases, treatment in a burn center may be necessary. Guard carefully against infection. Avoid steroids because they have not proved beneficial.

Borchers AT, Lee JL, Naguwa SM, Cheema GS, Gershwin ME: Stevens-Johnson syndrome and toxic epidermal necrolysis. Autoimmun Rev 2008;7:598–605 [PMID: 18603022].

Knowles S, Shear NH: Clinical risk management of Stevens-Johnson syndrome/toxic epidermal necrolysis spectrum. Dermatol Ther 2009;22:441–451 [PMID: 19845721].

EXFOLIATION AND ERYTHRODERMA

ESSENTIALS OF DIAGNOSIS

▶ A diffuse, generalized erythema and scaling
▶ Occurs secondary to many disease states

General Considerations

Many cutaneous diseases present with exfoliative erythroderma, or generalized redness and scaling. This condition is associated with a high risk for morbidity and mortality, independent of the inherent risks of the disease process it represents. Most commonly, this condition occurs secondary to psoriasis, atopic dermatitis, Hodgkin's disease, or mycosis fungoides (aka cutaneous T-cell Non-Hodgkin's lymphoma), or reactions to any of a wide range of inciting drugs. The erythrodermic state usually has a slow progression, but an acute onset may occur in patients who have cutaneous dermatoses or severe drug reactions.

Clinical Findings

Clues to the diagnosis may be from the underlying disease, such as psoriatic plaques or characteristic nail changes. Bullous pemphigoid typically exhibits tense bullae in addition to erythroderma. Long-standing erythroderma may be associated with keratoderma, alopecia, and ectropion. Peripheral edema occurs in 50% of patients. Patients with severe drug reactions may appear acutely ill with fever, malaise, and lymphadenopathy. A leukocytosis with eosinophilia, organomegaly, and hepatic or renal impairment may be present. In the most severe cases, high-output cardiac failure may occur. Severe alterations in fluid balance may occur, leading to shock. Sepsis may ensue, and hepatic necrosis may be fatal.

Treatment

Correction of derangements in fluid balance must begin early. Take care with the skin, applying moist dressings to weeping areas. Low-potency topical steroids may be used. Avoid high-potency preparations, because the large surface areas involved could lead to the absorption of large doses of steroids. Treat secondary infections.

Disposition

Hospital admission is often required, preferentially in an ICU, depending on the needs of the patient.

Sehgal VN, Srivastava G: Erythroderma/generalized exfoliative dermatitis in pediatric practice: an overview. Int J Dermatol. 2006;45:831–839 [PMID: 16863521].

STAPHYLOCOCCAL SCALDED SKIN SYNDROME

ESSENTIALS OF DIAGNOSIS

- ▶ Skin appears scalded and blistered
- ▶ Affects primarily children
- ▶ Skin barrier is broken and leads to S. aureus infection

General Considerations

Primarily a disease of children, staphylococcal scalded skin syndrome (SSSS) refers to a series of toxin-induced blistering dermatoses. SSSS lies within a spectrum of blistering skin disorders beginning with localized bullous impetigo. The exfoliative toxins, collectively known as *exfoliatin*, are primarily attributed to S. *aureus*, and page group 2 exotoxin-producing staphylococci are most implicated. Mortality rates are low (2–3%) in children but can reach as high as 60% in adults who have comorbidities or preexisting conditions.

Clinical Findings

The clinical presentation ranges from a milder form with localized eruption of a few fragile fluid-filled bullae surrounded by normal skin, to a more involved state. The more widespread form is often associated with fever, generalized erythema, and poor feeding in infants. Subsequently, large bullae form with a predilection for sites of friction. Erosion can occur in large areas, resulting in open, painful lesions. The Nikolsky sign is present. Unlike in SJS or TEN, mucous membranes are spared in SSSS. This may be a helpful distinguishing factor. The process is thought to result from a break in the protective skin barrier, which leads to S. *aureus* infection. Typical areas involved in the primary infection include the umbilicus in neonates, as well as the nasopharynx, urinary tract, and other sites.

Treatment

Cases of localized eruptions may be treated with oral antibiotics. The widespread form usually requires parenteral antibiotics to cover penicillin-resistant S. *aureus*. Treatment for adults is nafcillin, 1.5 g, or oxacillin, 2 g intravenously every 4 hours. For pediatric patients, treatment is nafcillin or oxacillin, 150 mg/kg/d intravenously in divided doses for 5–7 days. If superinfection is suspected, an aminoglycoside may be needed. Vancomycin or clindamycin should be considered. Rehydration and thermoregulation are essential, as is adequate pain control.

Disposition

Severe cases require treatment in an ICU or burn center. Because the cleavage of the epidermis and exfoliation are extremely superficial, the lesions typically heal with little or no residual scarring.

Kapoor V, Travadi J, Braye S: Staphylococcal scalded skin syndrome in an extremely premature neonate: a case report with a brief review of literature. J Paediatr Child Health 2008;44:374–376 [PMID: 18476932].

▼ **RECOGNITION AND MANAGEMENT OF POTENTIALLY LIFE-THREATENING PROBLEMS**

CELLULITIS AND ERYSIPELAS

ESSENTIALS OF DIAGNOSIS

Cellulitis
▶ Deeper infection
▶ Affects skin and subcutaneous tissues

Erysipelas
▶ Well-demarcated, superficial, erythematous infection
▶ Often affects face and extremities

▶ General Considerations

Cellulitis and erysipelas refer to infections of the subcutaneous tissues. Erysipelas involves the more superficial upper dermis, and cellulitis is deeper, with more extensive involvement of the subcutaneous tissues and fat. Both conditions are acute and related to a breach in the skin's protective barrier function. This can be secondary to fissuring and maceration, burns, venous stasis, malnutrition, lymphedema, or any of a number of other factors. The primary causative agent is group A β-hemolytic streptococcus. Other causes include streptococci B, C, and G and staphylococci infection. Other causative organisms associated with cellulitis include *S. aureus*, *H. influenzae*, *Streptococcus pneumoniae*, and *Pseudomonas*. If untreated, both conditions can lead to devastating complications such as local abscesses and gangrene with severe cellulitis. Facial erysipelas may lead to cavernous sinus thrombosis. Both cellulitis and erysipelas may lead to septicemia.

▶ Clinical Findings

Erysipelas is characterized by well-demarcated, erythematous, indurated plaques. The borders may be palpable. Primary sites include the face, scalp, and lower extremities. Patients are usually in the extremes of age. Cellulitis is usually associated with painful swelling and erythema of the involved area. The borders are usually less well defined, and the affected area is typically warm.

▶ Treatment

Although many cases can be managed on an outpatient basis, patients may have constitutional symptoms, and those with comorbid conditions may be quite ill and require hospitalization. Antibiotics are used empirically to cover streptococci and *S. aureus*. Recommended therapies include penicillin G, 600,000 to 2 million units intravenously every 6 hours, for streptococci; and nafcillin, 1.5–2 g intravenously every 4 hours, for staphylococci. Treat methicillin-resistant cases with vancomycin 1.5–2 g intravenous q day. Patients who appear well and without constitutional symptoms may be given oral therapy. This includes dicloxacillin, 250–500 mg orally four times daily, or erythromycin, 0.25–0.5 g orally four times daily, in the penicillin-allergic patient. If methicillin-resistant staphylococcus is suspected treat with trimethoprim–sulfamethoxazole or minocycline. Simple measures may be helpful in both conditions, including rest, cool compresses, elevation of the affected part, and antibacterial soaks. Debridement is used in secondary abscesses.

Bernard P: Management of common bacterial infections of the skin. Curr Opin Infect Dis 2008;21:122–128 [PMID: 18317033].

Celestin R, Brown J, Kihiczak G, Schwartz RA: Erysipelas: a common potentially dangerous infection. Acta Dermatovenerol Alp Panonica Adriat 2007;16:123–127 [PMID: 17994173].

PEMPHIGUS VULGARIS

ESSENTIALS OF DIAGNOSIS

▶ Blistering of skin and mucous membranes
▶ Usually affects older adults

▶ General Considerations

Pemphigus is one of several autoimmune diseases of the skin that present with blistering. The antibodies attack skin proteins and result in the inability of cells in the epidermis to hold together normally. Blisters form within the superficial epidermis. Although rare, pemphigus can be life threatening. Several subtypes exist, and pemphigus vulgaris is the most common and the most severe. Prior to newer developments in therapy, mortality rates were as high as 50% at 2 years and 100% at 5 years.

▶ Clinical Findings

Pemphigus most often occurs in older adults. The skin and mucous membranes are usually affected, and oral lesions often appear first. All mucous membranes may eventually be affected. As described earlier, the blistering is superficial. This results in fragile, flaccid blisters. The underlying skin may be erythematous. In the oral cavity, the blisters often slough prior to presentation, and the clinician may find only ulcerations. Hoarseness may occur if the lower airway is involved. Oral involvement can be extremely painful, interfering with the patient's ability to tolerate oral intake. The blisters slough easily, and the erosions enlarge by extending their borders. Nikolsky sign is present. These erosions often crust over, but scarring is not usually a problem.

▶ Treatment

Patients may have only isolated lesions, but more commonly there is widespread involvement. Patients may appear ill or toxic. Initial management involves fluid resuscitation, because fluid losses from the blistering are significant. Institute antibiotic therapy if secondary infection is present. Causative organisms are usually streptococci or staphylococci. This chronic disease usually mandates lifelong immunosuppressive therapy. The advent of glucocorticoids has decreased the mortality rates to approximately 5%. Start steroid therapy immediately. The suggested doses are 1–2.5 mg/kg/d of prednisone. Prednisone doses of 60 mg/d are recommended for treating isolated oral lesions. Topical high-potency steroids, such as clobetasol propionate 0.05%, can also be used in mild cases of skin involvement but should not be used on mucous membranes. Other immunosuppressive agents, such as azathioprine, cyclophosphamide, and methotrexate, are usually added to the oral steroid regimen later.

▶ Disposition

Admit patients who appear ill to an ICU for careful management of their fluid balance.

Groves RW: Pemphigus: a brief review. Clin Med 2009;9:371–375 [PMID: 19728517].

▼ RECOGNITION AND MANAGEMENT OF NON-LIFE-THREATENING PROBLEMS

CONTACT DERMATITIS AND *RHUS* DERMATITIS

ESSENTIALS OF DIAGNOSIS

Rhus dermatitis
▶ Intense itching
▶ Erythema with vesicles
▶ Linear distribution
▶ Lesions appear 8–48 hours after exposure to poison ivy, poison oak, or poison sumac

▶ General Considerations

Contact dermatitis refers to a collection of disorders resulting from an inciting environmental agent that has contacted the skin. The usual manifestation is a papulosquamous eruption, but vesicles may also be present.

A classic example is *Rhus* dermatitis, which is induced by plants in the *Rhus* genus (Toxicodendron). These include poison ivy, poison oak, and poison sumac. The culprit agent is the plant oil urushiol, and 50–70% of the U.S. population is sensitive to this substance. Factors affecting the clinical significance of any contact include the extent of exposure, the patient's age and activity level, and the patient's immunocompetence. Poison ivy, poison oak, and poison sumac are native plants of North America, rarely found at elevations above 4000 ft. Their appearance is quite variable, and they do not always exhibit the classic three-leaf morphology. The oil urushiol is widely distributed in almost all parts of the plant. The resultant dermatitis is classically described as a form of delayed hypersensitivity (type IV) reaction.

▶ Clinical Findings

After the first exposure, lesions can erupt within 8–48 hours, and they may persist for up to 3 weeks. The presence of an intensely pruritic, erythematous, papulovesicular eruption after an environmental exposure is highly suggestive of *Rhus* dermatitis. The lesions are usually linear. Transfer of the allergenic urushiol can continue and produce more lesions if it is not completely removed. It must be cleansed from the fingernails, skin, and clothing and from pets. Transfer of the oil, not the vesicles or the vesicular fluid, is responsible for the development of new lesions.

Immediate eruption after exposure is not consistent with *Rhus* dermatitis, because it takes at least 8 hours for the cell-mediated response to develop. The most common sites for eruptions are the face and extremities. The lesions may range from erythematous papules to large bullae. Any of the commonly used rules for estimation of BSA of burns, such as the "rule of nines" or preprinted estimation sheets, may be used to estimate the percentage of BSA involved.

▶ Treatment

The condition is self-limiting, with resolution within 3 weeks if all of the urushiol is removed. The most important therapy is prevention of exposure, but if exposure occurs, the individual should attempt to remove the oil within 10–30 minutes of exposure with warm water and soap remembering to wash under the fingernails to prevent spreading. Many new products have been introduced containing bentoquatam which binds urushiol and prevents absorption.

Treatment can decrease the severity of the symptoms, but it does not shorten the course. Oral antihistamines are effective symptomatic therapy for the intense pruritus. Topical preparations, including calamine, camphor, and cool compresses, are useful measures for comfort. Extreme caution must be used with topical antihistamines, zirconium, and benzocaine. These medications are no longer advocated, secondary to systemic absorption and sensitization. Over-the-counter steroid preparations are typically not helpful, because they contain too little steroid to be of benefit.

The backbone of therapy is usually a moderate-potency topical corticosteroid, such as triamcinolone 0.1% cream or betamethasone 0.1% cream. If the case is more severe or widespread, high-potency preparations such as clobetasol propionate 0.05% may be used. Extreme caution must be used with these creams, because systemic effects can occur secondary to steroid absorption.

Steroid therapy can also be used orally, but to be effective it must begin within 18 hours of exposure. Therapy must be tapered for 2–3 weeks. If the dose is too low or the course is too brief, intense rebound flares will often occur. A single 40-mg intramuscular dose of triamcinolone will typically produce good results in adults. Superinfection of the lesions with staphylococci or streptococci is the most common complication.

▶ Disposition

Outpatient therapy is sufficient in all but the most severe cases, which may require parenteral steroids. Systemic gluco-corticoids, such as prednisone or prednisolone at oral doses starting with 1 mg/kg/d, may be used and continued until the symptoms resolve. If prolonged steroid therapy is required, a gradually tapering dose may be advisable.

Gladman AC: Toxicodendron dermatitis: poison ivy, oak, and sumac. Wilderness Environ Med 2006;17:120–128 [PMID: 16805148].

Nosbaum A, Vocanson M, Rozieres A, Hennino A, Nicolas JF: Allergic and irritant contact dermatitis. Eur J Dermatol 2009;19:325–332 [PMID: 19447733].

IMPETIGO

ESSENTIALS OF DIAGNOSIS

▶ Infection due to Staphylococcus or Streptococcus sp.

▶ Lesions appear honey-crusted

▶ More common in children but may affect all ages

▶ General Considerations

Impetigo is an infection of the skin primarily due to group A streptococci and, less commonly, *S. aureus*. The infection is classified into bullous and nonbullous forms; the nonbullous form comprises approximately 70% of cases.

Young children are the predominant age group affected, but adults are not excluded. A break in the protective skin barrier is the inciting event. Conditions such as chick-enpox, abrasions, and burns are typically associated with impetigo. Predisposing situations include crowded living conditions, poor hygiene, and contact sports.

▶ Clinical Findings

Impetigo is associated with the classic history of the emergence of a small vesicle or pustule. This is often in the context of one of the above-mentioned conditions. The vesicle or pustule develops into the classic honey-crusted lesion. These lesions are usually less than 2 cm in diameter and may be mildly pruritic. The lesions are usually not painful. Although in healthy individuals the lesions will usually heal spontaneously with little scarring, the potential complications can be life-threatening. Complications include septicemia, pneumonia, osteomyelitis, and glomerulonephritis.

▶ Treatment

Correction of predisposing environmental conditions is important. The honey-colored crust must be removed. Cleansing with antibacterial soaps and solutions is helpful. The only topical antibiotic therapy currently indicated for the treatment of localized lesions is mupirocin (Bactroban) ointment. Patients should apply the ointment until the lesions resolve. Scalp and oral lesions typically require oral therapy, as do disseminated cases. Effective oral therapies include cloxacillin, amoxicillin–clavulanate, or clindamycin. Cephalosporins may be used, such as cephalexin, cefaclor, cefadroxil, cefprozil, or cefpodoxime proxetil. Seven days of therapy has been demonstrated as effective. If symptoms persist beyond 7 days, cultures should be taken and further treatment should be based on the results. Treat lesions suspected of being due to *S. aureus* with a β-lactamase-resistant penicillin such as oxacillin or nafcillin.

Epps RE: Impetigo in pediatrics. Cutis 2004;73:25–26 [PMID: 15182164].

HERPES ZOSTER

ESSENTIALS OF DIAGNOSIS

▶ Most cases are very painful

▶ Prodrome of paresthesias may occur

▶ Rash appears as a bandlike distribution of vesicles

▶ Usually has a dermatomal distribution

▶ Usually does not cross the patient's midline

General Considerations

Herpes zoster (HZ), or shingles, is a painful condition that results from reactivation of a latent infection with the varicella zoster virus (VZV). A patient who is naive to the virus develops chickenpox after an initial exposure. After resolution of this primary infection, the VZV remains dormant in the satellite cells of the dorsal root ganglion of the sensory nerves. It remains there for the rest of the patient's life. The triggers of subsequent reactivation in certain patients are not fully understood. Events such as trauma and exposure to ultraviolet radiation have been implicated in provoking eruptions of shingles. The incidence of HZ is increased in the elderly population. This is thought to result from diminishing immune function with increasing age. Although usually a localized process, disseminated HZ can develop in immunocompromised individuals.

Clinical Findings

The diagnosis is primarily clinical. Previous history of chickenpox and the progression of current symptoms are important points in the history.

Three phases of HZ have been described: prodrome, acute, and chronic phases. During the prodrome phase, 80% of patients feel altered sensations in the affected dermatome. These are typically described as pain, burning, or paresthesias. These feelings may be intense and will often be present several days before the appearance of any lesions. This can often make the diagnosis difficult during this phase.

Patients in the acute phase present with the eruption of vesicles, usually in a bandlike pattern, which follows a dermatomal distribution. Only rarely will the lesions cross the midline. The two most common sites are the trunk and face, respectively. The lesions will dry and form a crust within 7–10 days, and they usually resolve within 2–3 weeks.

An unfortunate subset of patients will go on to develop the chronic phase of HZ, known as postherpetic neuralgia (PHN). This is an extremely painful condition, which persists at least 30 days after the eruption resolves. PHN can be quite difficult to treat and is much more likely in the older patient. It may occur in up to 50% of elderly patients with HZ.

Several dangerous complications can develop from HZ, including ophthalmic HZ. This condition occurs when the ophthalmic branch of the trigeminal nerve is involved. Up to half of these patients will have ocular HZ. A clue to the presence of ocular HZ can be involvement of the tip of the patient's nose. Conjunctivitis, uveitis, and ulcerative keratitis can occur as a result of HZ. These serious conditions can lead to blindness if not managed properly. A complete ocular examination and urgent ophthalmologic referral are essential. Other potential complications of HZ include the Ramsay Hunt syndrome (an acute facial paralysis), meningitis, and encephalitis.

Treatment

It is important to educate patients who have HZ. They must understand that they are contagious to those who are not immune to VZV and to those who have not had chickenpox. This infective state lasts until the vesicles have dried and crusted, or approximately 1 week from the onset of the rash. During this time, patients should avoid pregnant women, those who are immunocompromised, and those who have never had chickenpox.

Pain relief is important and usually achieved with short-term combinations of oral analgesics and narcotics. Antiviral drugs are of use in the treatment of HZ, if therapy is started within 72 hours of the eruption of the rash. Oral acyclovir, 800 mg five times daily for 7–10 days, is effective in improving resolution of the rash and decreasing the incidence of PHN. Famciclovir, 500 mg three times a day for 7 days, and valacyclovir, 1 g three times a day for 7 days, are other options with similar efficacy to acyclovir. One study showed valacyclovir as having some superiority in pain control. Antiviral agents have been shown to decrease the severity of PHN but not the incidence.

Studies have shown that steroids do not prevent the development of PHN. Some authors suggest that steroids are beneficial in treating Ramsay Hunt syndrome. Treatment of ocular involvement requires the assistance of an ophthalmologist. Varicella-zoster immunoglobulin and intravenous acyclovir is recommended for immunocompromised individuals.

Gilden D: Varicella zoster virus and central nervous system syndromes. Herpes 2004;11(Suppl 2):89A–94A [PMID: 15319095]

Johnson RW, Whitton TL: Management of herpes zoster (shingles) and postherpetic neuralgia. Expert Opin Pharmacother 2004;5:551–559 [PMID: 15013924].

Liesegang TJ: Herpes zoster virus infection. Curr Opin Ophthalmol 2004;15:531–536 [PMID:15523199].

HERPES SIMPLEX

ESSENTIALS OF DIAGNOSIS

► Vesicles on an erythematous base
► HSV-1: usually oral; HSV-2: usually genital
► Spread by direct contact

General Considerations

Herpes simplex virus (HSV) is a major cause of recurrent orofacial and genital lesions and causes other types of illness as well (eg, keratitis and encephalitis). Infection is spread by direct contact. Primary infection is often the most severe, although it may be asymptomatic. After the primary lesion has healed, the virus remains latent in sensory neurons in ganglion tissue, where it periodically reactivates in response to diverse stimuli.

HSV type 1 (HSV-1) tends to be associated with oral lesions and is spread through contact with saliva from an infected person, whereas HSV type 2 (HSV-2) causes mainly genital lesions and is spread primarily by sexual contact. This is classically taught, but both infections can occur in either location.

▶ Clinical Findings

A. Primary Herpes Simplex Infection

The first clinical attack of HSV infection is usually the most severe. Patients may present with fever, malaise, and arthralgias. Infection is characterized at first by grouped vesicles and later by denudation, erosions, or punctate lesions on a swollen, tender, painful erythematous base. Local pain and regional adenopathy are usually marked. Gingivostomatitis is the most common manifestation of HSV-1 infection; patients with HSV-2 infection usually present with genital lesions (ie, of the vulva, vagina, penis, anus, or perineum). Patients (especially women) with genital herpes may have aseptic meningitis. The primary illness usually disappears in 2–3 weeks but may last as long as 6 weeks.

B. Recurrent HSV Infection

Recurrence of infection is common and may be triggered by fever, exposure to ultraviolet light, friction or trauma associated with sexual intercourse, menstruation, and possibly stress or fatigue. Focal itching, pain, or aching may precede the appearance of vesicles by hours to a few days in some patients. Vesicles usually rupture spontaneously within a few days and heal within a week without scarring. The virus may be recovered as long as lesions are moist; until the area is completely dry and healed, the patient should avoid direct skin-to-skin contact with others.

C. Specific Diagnosis

For either primary or recurrent herpes simplex, especially genital herpes, confirm the diagnosis by culture or antigen detection.

▶ Treatment

A. Primary Infection

Antipyretics or analgesics may help to relieve systemic symptoms. Give oral acyclovir, valacyclovir, or famciclovir to all patients who have primary infection for 7–10 days. Hospitalize severely ill patients for administration of intravenous acyclovir, 10 mg/kg every 8 hours. Give other patients oral acyclovir, 400 mg threetimes daily for 10 days, valacyclovir, 1 g twice a day for 7–10 days, or famciclovir, 250 mg three times daily for 7–10 days.

Antibiotics are not necessary unless local purulence or cultures or Gram-stained smears positive for bacteria suggest concomitant bacterial infection. *Candida* vaginitis occurs frequently in women with primary genital herpes.

B. Recurrent Infection

Patients should not touch or manipulate lesions and should avoid physical contact with others around the area of moist or active lesions. Acyclovir, 400 mg orally three times daily for 5 days, valacyclovir, 500 mg twice daily for 3 days, or famciclovir, 125 mg two times daily for 5 days, will somewhat reduce healing time and the duration of virus shedding if started within a day of lesion onset.

▶ Disposition

Hospitalization is often indicated for patients with primary genital herpes, who may have severe pain, systemic symptoms, and other complications (eg, aseptic meningitis, neuropathic bladder). Hospitalization is also required for patients with large or rapidly progressive lesions, especially if the patient is immunocompromised.

Refer pregnant patients with newly diagnosed genital herpes to an obstetrician. Order a serologic test for syphilis (eg, VDRL) for all patients to rule out the possibility of coexisting syphilis. Consider testing for HIV if risk factors are present.

Aga IE, Hollier LM: Managing genital herpes infections in pregnancy. Womens Health (Lond Engl) 2009;5:165–172 [PMID: 19245354].

Chayavichitsilp P, Buckwalter JV, Krakowski AC, Friedlander SF: Hepers simplex. Pediatr Rev 2009;30:119–129 [PMID: 19339385].

Opstelten W, Neven AK, Eekhof J: Treatment and prevention of herpes labialis. Can Fam Physician 2008;54:1683–1687 [PMID: 19074705].

PSORIASIS

ESSENTIALS OF DIAGNOSIS

▶ Common disorder
▶ Well-circumscribed plaques
▶ Erythematous base with silvery scale
▶ Predilection for extensor surfaces

▶ General Considerations

Psoriasis is a common skin condition affecting up to 2% of the U.S. population. It has been described among all age groups with a similar male-to-female ratio. Onset is usually in the third decade of life. The disease process is well described and understood, but its cause is still unknown. A family history is present in 30% of patients. Psoriasis significantly affects the patient's quality of life. It is chronic, and there is no known cure. The plaque variant of psoriasis, or psoriasis vulgaris, is the most common form.

▶ Clinical Findings

Thorough examination reveals the characteristic erythematous, raised, scaly plaques. These are often described as having a salmon-colored base with tightly adherent silvery scales. They are typically found on the extensor surfaces of major joints, such as elbows and knees. Other sites of predilection include the scalp, ears, and umbilicus. Lesions are often found to be in various stages of plaque formation and healing. Potassium hydroxide preparations can be used to differentiate psoriasis from tinea. Classic nail findings, such as pitting and onycholysis, can also aid in the diagnosis.

▶ Treatment

Many remedies have been tried over the years, but no cure has been found for psoriasis. Therapies often merely decrease scaling and increase the patient's comfort. The use of emollients such as petroleum jelly, Aquaphor healing ointment, or Eucerin cream should be encouraged. Tar preparations and shampoos are well-known effective keratolytics, which decrease scaling. Avoidance of skin trauma is helpful, because the Koebner phenomenon is associated with psoriasis. This phenomenon refers to a flare in symptoms and initiation of plaque formation after local skin trauma, including scratching and even surgical incisions. Judicious use of topical low-potency steroids may be helpful initially. Calcipotriene is a newer preparation that is a topical vitamin D_3 analogue. Applied twice daily, effects are typically seen within 8 weeks. Oral and parenteral steroids play little or no role in the treatment of plaque psoriasis. Their use has been demonstrated as harmful in certain situations, such as the exacerbation of the more serious pustular psoriasis. Topical steroids are helpful in limited disease. Restrict the highest-potency corticosteroids, such as betamethasone, to 2 weeks of BID use. Afterwards, a midpotency corticosteroid should be considered. Narrow-band UVB light exposure three times weekly with or without tar preparations will help clear lesions over weeks, but maintenance may be needed since relapses are frequent.

▶ Disposition

Outpatient therapy is sufficient, except in the most severe cases. Referral should be made to a primary-care physician or a dermatologist for more involved therapies, including topical preparations, ultraviolet phototherapy, and systemic agents such as methotrexate.

Ferrándiz C, Carrascosa JM, Boada A: A new era in the management of psoriasis? The biologics: facts and controversies. Clin Dermatol 2010;28:81–87 [PMID: 20082956].

SCABIES

ESSENTIALS OF DIAGNOSIS

- ► Human parasite
- ► Causes intense itching
- ► Spread by contact
- ► May affect entire households

▶ General Considerations

Scabies have been known to affect the human condition for thousands of years. The culprit organism in scabies is a mite, *Sarcoptes scabiei*. This mite is found in varying stages of development in the epidermis of the infested individual. There it makes tunnels, leaving behind eggs and feces. The mites are obligate parasites of humans and are spread by skin-to-skin contact between persons. This includes both sexual and nonsexual interactions.

▶ Clinical Findings

The diagnosis of scabies is primarily a clinical one, with the usual history of intense pruritus that is especially worse at night. Consider scabies when entire households complain of the onset of pruritus. The classic physical findings are tiny burrows in the web spaces between the fingers, in intertriginous areas, and in flexor creases. Burrows may not always be seen. Only excoriations and impetiginization may be found. The lesions may be difficult to differentiate from atopic dermatitis. In the most extreme cases, heavy mite loads may result and lead to the crusted or Norwegian variant. This is usually limited to individuals with severe disabilities or in immunocompromised states. The diagnosis of scabies is confirmed by microscopic visualization of mites or eggs in skin scrapings.

▶ Treatment

A. Adults

The treatment for adults (except pregnant or lactating women) and older children includes permethrin 5% cream (Elimite). It should be applied after a shower or bath over the entire body from the neck down. It should be left on for 8 hours, after which it should be carefully washed off. A 60-g tube is usually sufficient to treat one to two people. All clothing and bed linens should be laundered in hot water to kill all remaining mites.

Alternative regimens include lindane cream or lotion. Used for many years, it is effective but some strains of lindane-resistant scabies exist. Also, dangerous central nervous system side effects have occurred in the elderly and in immunocompromised patients, or in normal hosts after repeated uses.

Sulfur in petrolatum 6% is another treatment option. It should be applied to the entire body from the neck down for three consecutive nights. Patients should bathe between applications and 24 hours after the final treatment. Although it has no dangerous systemic effects, this remedy has an unpleasant odor. Crotamiton 10% cream may be applied for two consecutive nights and then washed off 24 hours after the last application.

B. Children

The treatment for infants, children younger than 10 years of age, and pregnant or lactating women is permethrin 5% cream, crotamiton 10% cream, or sulfur and petroleum as described above. The lindane preparation should not be used due to potential toxicity.

PEDICULOSIS

ESSENTIALS OF DIAGNOSIS

▶ Lice infestation
▶ Different distributions: head, body, pubic area
▶ Spread by direct contact or sharing of personal items

▶ General Considerations

Pediculosis refers to infestation of the body with lice. Similar to scabies, pediculosis results from a parasite. These organisms feed on the blood of humans. Several variants exist, and the organisms are named in reference to the area of the body they inhabit. These include *Pediculus humanus capitis* (head lice), *P. humanus corporis* (body lice), and *Pediculosis pubis* (pubic lice). Head lice are the most common, with the classic scenario of outbreaks in school children seen in all levels in society. The lice are transmitted by direct contact as well as by sharing of hats, brushes, and other personal items. Body lice predominantly affect adults of lower socioeconomic standing such as the homeless and those in refugee situations. Pubic lice are spread by sexual contact, and they often occur in conjunction with other sexually transmitted diseases.

▶ Clinical Findings

Recognition of the lice as described above is essential in the diagnosis. Pruritus may lead to excoriations that may become secondarily infected. Infestation of head lice is diagnosed by visualizing live lice or nits (eggs) attached to the proximal portion of the hair shaft. Body lice and eggs are found in the clothing of the affected individual, with excoriations over the body. A body louse does not attach to hair but in clothing, coming out to feed on blood. Pubic lice are intensely pruritic,

and the lice themselves may be transferred to other hair-bearing areas of the body. Remember to screen these patients for other sexually transmitted diseases. When pubic lice are found in children, they have often resulted from nonsexual contact; however, abuse should be considered in the differential.

▶ Treatment

For the treatment of pediculosis capitis, corporis, and pubis, permethrin 1% cream rinse can be used. It can be applied to the groin, armpit, or scalp for 10 minutes and then washed off. Lindane 1% shampoo may be used as an alternative regimen. It is applied as above but is left on for 8 hours before washing off. For pediculosis capitis, it may be used as a shampoo, left on for 4 minutes, and then rinsed. Lindane should never be used on pregnant or lactating women, or on children younger than 10 years of age. Clothes should be washed in hot water and dried with high heat. Since Pediculus corporis resides in clothing, discarding or sealing clothing for 2 weeks leads to eradication.

Leone PA: Scabies and pediculosis pubis: an update of treatment regimens and general review. Clin Infect Dis 2007;44: S153–S159 [PMID: 17342668].

CUTANEOUS DERMATOPHYTES/TINEA

ESSENTIALS OF DIAGNOSIS

▶ Superficial fungal infections
▶ Flat, scaly patches

▶ General Considerations

Dermatophytes include a group of fungi that infect the skin. The organisms themselves survive on the dead keratin found in the uppermost layer of the epidermis. The infections are limited to this superficial distribution in immunocompetent individuals. The dermatophytoses are classified by the distribution of the lesions.

▶ Clinical Findings

A. Tinea Corporis

Tinea corporis refers to tinea of the body. Some authors and clinicians include the face in this category, but the American Academy of Dermatology refers to tinea of the face separately as tinea faciei. The most common causative organisms are *Trichophyton rubrum*, *Microsporum canis*, and *Trichophyton mentagrophytes*. Classic ring-worm (tinea circinata) is the most common form of tinea corporis. It usually begins as a flat scaly patch with a raised, palpable border. It enlarges by advancing its border outward, leaving an area of central clearing.

B. Tinea Pedis

Also known as athlete's foot, tinea pedis is a common condition. It affects up to 70% of adults. It is divided into three subtypes. The most prevalent is the interdigital type. It is chronic and occurs with fissuring and maceration between the toes. Moccasin-type tinea pedis has a plantar distribution. The plantar surface is tender and erythematous. It is usually covered with a silvery scale. The third type is the wet, vesicular type.

C. Tinea Cruris

Tinea cruris, commonly called "jock itch," affects the groin area, sparing the genitalia. Men are affected more commonly than women, and the condition has a predilection for summer months.

D. Tinea Versicolor

Tinea versicolor affects a deeper layer of the skin than the previously described tineas. It is caused by the yeast *Malassezia furfur*. It often is associated with multiple hypopigmented macular lesions distributed over the trunk and extremities. Exposure to sunlight accentuates the lesions, because they do not tan normally like the surrounding skin. A fine scale is often present.

▶ Treatment

A. Tinea Corporis

Mild cases of tinea corporis can usually be treated with over-the-counter topical preparations, such as miconazole nitrate or clotrimazole. Prescription agents include ketoconazole 2% cream or econazole nitrate. All topical remedies should be used for 1–2 weeks after resolution of symptoms. Extensive disease or difficult cases may require oral therapy. Agents include griseofulvin, itraconazole, terbinafine, and fluconazole.

B. Tinea Pedis

Most mild cases of tinea pedis can be treated successfully with 1–4 weeks of therapy with an over-the-counter preparation, in conjunction with the use of drying powders. Severe cases may require oral therapy. Drugs such as griseofulvin, fluconazole, and itraconazole are effective. Cases are often recurrent if concomitant nail disease is present.

C. Tinea Cruris

Tinea cruris can often be treated with topical antifungal therapies used for 2–3 weeks (see as for tinea corporis). The area should be kept dry, because moisture and maceration are

problems with this disease. Antifungal powders and loose-fitting clothing are often useful adjuncts. A mild topical corticosteroid may be used cautiously for a short time to help relieve the pruritus, which is often severe. Corticosteroids may be used only for 48–72 hours; longer use is contraindicated. As with tinea corporis, resistant disease may require oral therapy.

D. Tinea Versicolor

Limited tinea versicolor can be treated with topical selenium sulfide 2.5%. Daily application of ketoconazole to the affected areas for 3 days is an alternative regimen. Recurrence of the disease may be prevented with the use of a once-monthly bedtime application of selenium sulfide 2.5%.

Mendez-Tovar LJ: Pathogenesis of dermatophytosis and tinea versicolor. Clin Dermatol 2010;28:185–189 [PMID: 20347661].

PITYRIASIS ROSEA

ESSENTIALS OF DIAGNOSIS

▶ Herald patch is initial lesion
▶ Rash is usually truncal and has a "Christmas tree" distribution
▶ May be pruritic

▶ General Considerations

Pityriasis rosea is a common rash that may easily be confused with tinea corporis. It is a papulosquamous eruption that most commonly affects patients in the second to the fourth decades of life. Pityriasis rosea affects men and women equally. Although its cause is thought to be related to a viral exanthem associated with reactivation of human herpesvirus 7 (HHV-7) and sometimes HHV-6, the exact cause of pityriasis rosea is unknown.

▶ Clinical Findings

The classic progression of the exanthem begins with the appearance of a herald patch. This is an isolated salmon-colored macule usually found on the trunk. It is typically oval shaped and can be as large as 10 cm in diameter. It usually has an erythematous scaling border, and there may be central clearing. The subsequent lesions usually develop within 1–2 weeks, and their distribution has been described as resembling the shape of a Christmas tree. The individual lesions are smaller than the herald patch, are usually of a lighter shade, and have a scaly border.

Treatment

The lesions are self-limiting and usually disappear within 6–8 weeks. The initial lesions regress, and new lesions develop during this time. No effective treatment has been found for pityriasis rosea. If pruritus is present, it may be treated symptomatically with oatmeal baths, antihistamines, or topical hydrocortisone 1% ointment. Patients should be reassured that recurrences are uncommon, occurring in only approximately 3% of cases.

Broccolo F, Drago F, Careddu AM et al: Additional evidence that pityriasis rosea is associated with reactivation of human herpesvirus-6 and -7. J Invest Dermatol 2005;124:1234–1240 [PMID: 15955099].

Stulberg DL, Wolfrey J: Pityriasis rosea. Am Fam Physician 2004;69:87–91 [PMID: 14727822].

MOLLUSCUM CONTAGIOSUM

ESSENTIALS OF DIAGNOSIS

▶ Viral infection
▶ Pearly pink papules with central umbilication

General Considerations

Molluscum contagiosum is a viral infection of the skin. It is associated with multiple lesions, typically papules, spread over the skin. Molluscum contagiosum is present worldwide and is a member of the poxviruses. In normal hosts, it is a self-limited disease and usually resolves within 8 weeks. Recently there has been increased prevalence in the immunocompromised population, especially in patients with HIV. In this population, the disease presentation can be dramatic, with large, widespread lesions and a longer duration.

Clinical Findings

The diagnosis is made by the identification of the lesions. They are typically flesh-colored papules. The lesions may also appear pearly pink. The papules are rounded with a distinctive central umbilication and are firm to palpation. They usually are 1–5 mm in diameter, but in certain situations they may be quite large. The lesions may be distributed anywhere on the body, but they are rarely found on the palms or soles. They are usually found in groups, and usually fewer than 20 lesions are present. Molluscum contagiosum is spread by close contact with infected persons, by contact with contaminated surfaces, or by autoinoculation with scratching or shaving. It can also be spread by sexual contact.

Treatment

Most lesions resolve without treatment in immunocompetent patients. Lesions involving the perineum and genitalia should be treated to avoid spread via sexual contact. If lesions require treatment, the two most commonly used modalities are cryosurgery and curettage. Various topical therapies have had varying levels of success, including lactic acid, podophyllin, cantharidin, and silver nitrate. In pediatric patients, use of a topical anesthetic, such as lidocaine plus prilocaine, should be considered prior to curetting. Instruct patients to avoid contact sports, swimming pools, and other such activities until the lesions have resolved.

Coloe J, Burkhart CN, Morrell DS: Molluscum contagiosum: what's new and true? Pediatr Ann 2009;38:321–325 [PMID: 19588675].

Psychiatric Emergencies

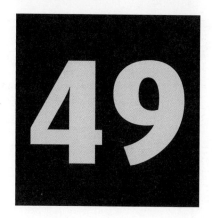

Eric J. Brown, MD, MS
Lori Whelan, MD[1]

▼ INTRODUCTION

Psychiatric emergencies are acute changes in behavior that negatively impact a patient's ability to function in his or her environment. Often such patients are in a state of crisis in which their baseline coping mechanisms have been overwhelmed by real or perceived circumstances. In dealing with such emergencies, the emergency physician faces many challenges and must prioritize his or her clinical efforts toward four main concerns.

First, the physician must ensure his or her own safety and the patient's well-being if violence or agitated behavior

is present. Second, the physician must perform an effective screening assessment, probing for organic causes and completing a psychiatric safety check. The screening assessment ensures that there is no underlying medical cause for the patient's condition, either initially inducing the aberrant behavior or evolving as a consequence of that behavior (eg, malnutrition or dehydration). The screening assessment also involves a psychiatric safety check to explore for suicidal ideation, homicidal ideation, or patients' inability to care for themselves. Third, the physician must ensure that the patient receives appropriate psychological support and medical treatment, even if the treatment needs to be provided without the patient's consent. Lastly, the physician must determine the appropriate disposition for the patient.

The algorithm in Figure 49–1 provides a decision-making guide to the management of psychiatric emergencies. This

---

[1]This chapter is a revision of the chapter by Gregory Hall, MD and Denis J. FitzGerald, MD from the 6th edition.

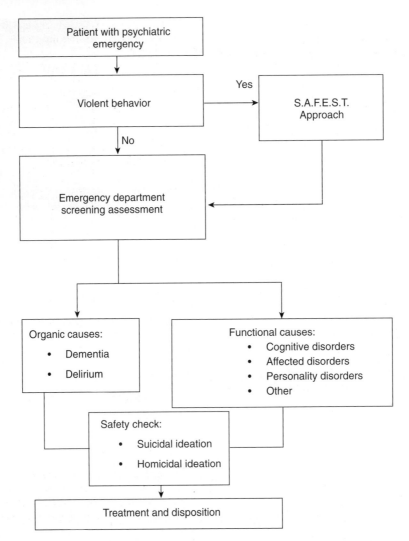

▲ **Figure 49–1.** Decision-making algorithm for psychiatric emergencies.

algorithm reflects the four main priorities in patient care and provides a framework for this chapter.

THE S.A.F.E.S.T. APPROACH TO VIOLENT OR AGITATED PATIENTS

The emergency physician may encounter patient who threatens or exhibits violent behavior toward staff. In these cases, it is important to recognize the early warning signs of impending violence and adopt an approach to management that reduces the likelihood of injury to staff and patient. Early warning signs of impending violence include threatening statements, clenched fists, loud vocalizations, shifting body positions toward a fighting posture, agitated movements,

and striking inanimate objects. If such behavior is detected, adopt the **S.A.F.E.S.T.** approach:

Spacing—Maintain distance from the patient. Allow both the patient and you to have equal access to the door. Do not touch a violent person.

Appearance—Maintain empathetic professional detachment. Use one primary contact person to build rapport. Have security staff available as a show of strength.

Focus—Watch the patient's hands. Watch for potential weapons. Watch for escalating agitation.

Exchange—Delay by calm, continuous talking is crucial to permit de-escalation of the situation. Avoid punitive or judgmental statements. Use good listening skills. Target the current problem or situation in order to find face-saving alternatives for resolution and to elicit the patient's cooperation with treatment.

Stabilization—If necessary, use three stabilization techniques to get control of the situation: physical restraint, sedation, and chemical restraint.

1. **Physical restraint**—Once the situation permits, it is advisable to restrain any violent or agitated person to ensure safety. This activity is best done by trained security personnel who should also search the patient for weapons. Implement documentation that indicates the need for restraints and provides a record of safety checks on the restrained patient.

2. **Sedation**—If agitation persists, sedation is best achieved by administering lorazepam, 1–2 mg intramuscularly or intravenously. Dosing may be repeated to achieve effect while monitoring for side effects including respiratory depression.

3. **Chemical restraint**—Chemical restraint is best achieved with neuroleptics. For patients not responding to sedation, haloperidol 5 mg may be administered intramuscularly. In elderly patients, it is best to start with lower dosing and increase by 1–2-mg increments. Dosing may be repeated every 30 minutes until the patient is in more control. Be alert for the emergence of extrapyramidal symptoms, seizure activity, or neuroleptic malignant syndrome.

Treatment—Once the patient is more manageable, initiate treatment based on the patient's symptoms. The patient may refuse treatment and may need to receive treatment involuntarily in order to ensure his or her safety.

American College of Emergency Physicians: Use of patient restraints. www.acep.org/practres.aspx?id=29836. Dallas, TX, October 2007 [Last Accessed on August 26, 2010].

FitzGerald D: S.A.F.E.S.T. Approach. Tactical Intervention Guided Emergency Response (TIGER) Textbook. 2003.

Rocca P, Villari V, Bogetto F: Managing the aggressive and violent patient in the psychiatric emergency. Prog Neuropsychopharmacol Biol Psychiatry 2006;30:586–598 [PMID: 16571365].

▼ EMERGENCY DEPARTMENT SCREENING ASSESSMENT

TARGETED HISTORY

Focus on precipitating causes and circumstances that brought the patient to the emergency department. It may be necessary to elicit information from multiple sources such as family, friends, or ambulance personnel. Other key topics include previous psychiatric treatment, seizure disorders, polysubstance abuse, and any recent suicidal attempts including possible ingestions.

FOCUSED PHYSICAL EXAMINATION

Perform a thorough physical examination, including neurologic assessment. Complete vital signs are essential. Look for physical clues to the source of an altered mental status, such as evidence of head injury, drug use, or toxidromes. Assess the patient for adverse consequences of his or her behavior such as malnutrition or dehydration.

MENTAL STATUS EXAMINATION

It is important to document the mental status examination in patients presenting with psychiatric emergencies. The mental status assessment should probe for global functioning, thought disorders, mood disorders, and personality disorders.

A. Global Functioning

Assess the patient for general orientation (person, place, time, reason for visit), memory (short and long term), judgment, and concentration.

B. Thought Disorders

Assess the patient for abnormal thought content such as hearing voices, experiencing command hallucinations, or having paranoid thoughts.

C. Mood Disorders

Assess the patient for evidence of depression or mania. Compare the appropriateness of the patient's stated mood with his or her overt affect. Look for clues such as emotional lability or unbalanced emotional extremes.

D. Personality Disorders

Try to assess whether the patient's current behavior is an acute psychiatric event that represents a decompensation in his or her normal functioning or a representative sample of a maladaptive pattern of behavior derived from an underlying socially inappropriate personality matrix.

SCREENING LABORATORY TESTS

The utility of screening tests remains a controversial topic. Recent American College of Emergency Physician (ACEP) guidelines recommend directing laboratory evaluations based on history and physical findings. Routine testing of all patients is very low yield and is not necessary for Emergency Department assessment. Given these recommendations, the following studies may be helpful in the evaluation of patients presenting with psych emergencies if the history and physical suggests an organic cause:

- Electrolyte panel with glucose
- Pulse oximetry
- Toxicology screen (blood and urine)
- Blood ethanol level
- Liver function tests
- Computed tomography (CT) scan of the head
- Electrocardiogram (ECG)
- Thyroid function tests

Lukens TW, Wolf SJ, Edlow JA et al: Clinical Policy: Critical issues in the diagnosis and management of the adult psychiatric patient in the emergency department. Ann Emerg Med 2006;47:79–99 [PMID: 16387222].

DIAGNOSTIC FOCUS: ORGANIC VERSUS FUNCTIONAL CAUSE

The etiology of psychiatric emergencies involves the classic triad of brain, mind, and behavior. Often a patient presents with an alteration in his or her behavior manifested as change in mental state, level of functioning, mood, or personality. The emergency physician must distinguish between those patients needing medical treatment for an organic problem affecting the brain (eg, delirium or dementia) and those individuals who would benefit from psychiatric treatment for a functional problem of the mind (eg, thought disorder, mood disorder, or personality disorder).

Traditional psychiatry involves the diagnosis and treatment of functional entities. The psychiatric *emergency*, however, is an acute, undifferentiated presentation of altered behavior that may result from either functional or organic conditions. In fact, sometimes both types of problems coexist in the same patient. The emergency physician must consider all these possibilities, first ruling out organic conditions before diagnosing functional entities that may require psychiatric care. This is often referred to as "medical clearance".

Many patients present to psychiatric facilities with acute altered behavior. Emergency physicians often provide the first and possibly only medical evaluation the acute psychiatric patient is likely to receive. In addition, psychiatric facilities may not be equipped with either appropriate staff or equipment to provide comprehensive medical evaluation and/or treatment. Emergency department personnel are tasked with excluding a medical etiology for the patient's symptoms. Unfortunately, the term "medical clearance" can imply different things to psychiatric staff and emergency staff. Emergency staff must determine the appropriate evaluation based on a focused history and physical. No agreed upon standard exists and therefore emergency physicians must use patient presentation to determine the appropriate evaluation.

Organic disorders may be very difficult to differentiate from behavioral changes caused by a functional condition. However, some factors may point to an organic cause of the behavioral change. Organic causes often are acute in onset, whereas functional disorders develop over time. Visual hallucinations are much more common with organic syndromes or medical illness than are auditory hallucinations. Age of onset may also be a clue. Patients presenting with functional etiologies are usually younger, typically 12–40 years of age. Exceptions are always possible, but older patients need special consideration when disease is being attributed to functional origin, especially when no history of previous psychiatric disorder is present. Patients with organic disorders generally present with emotional lability, whereas patients with a flat affect usually have functional disease. Finally, any abnormality in vital signs or features of a toxidrome should immediately point to an organic cause.

PSYCHIATRIC SAFETY CHECK

▶ General Considerations

The emergency physician must directly assess for the presence of suicidal or homicidal ideation in all patients presenting with a psychiatric emergency. In general, the patients' ability to care for themselves is a cardinal component of the initial assessment.

▶ Suicidal Patients

The management of suicidal ideation involves recognition of the problem, an assessment of risk, and development of a treatment plan.

A. Recognition of Suicidal Ideation

Patients with suicidal ideation may present with an obvious attempt to cause self-harm. However, suicidal patients may present to the emergency department more indirectly, with suicidal ideation as the underlying cause behind other presentations, such as through an automobile accident. The best screening approach involves general questions about the patient's emotional state. Inappropriate, irrational, or dysphoric answers should prompt further investigation, culminating in direct questions about suicidal intent.

B. Assessment of Risk

Several factors increase the risk of suicide. Patients with prior suicide attempts are at increased risk. Patients who employ violent means are more serious about their intent. Existence of a detailed plan reflects significant commitment to following through with the suicide attempt, particularly when coupled with a depressed emotional state or altered mental status. Poor social support or inadequate coping mechanisms also put patients at increased risk.

C. Treatment

Admit patients who have clear suicidal ideation, unless immediate psychiatric evaluation is an option. The admission may be directly to the psychiatry service or to the medical service with a psychiatry consult. It may be necessary to sign involuntary admission holds on patients who resist efforts to ensure their safety. Patients with suicidal ideation should be monitored closely at all times, ideally with a one-to-one sitter. They should be given emotional support throughout their stay and their environment should be screened for any potential means of suicide.

▶ Homicidal Patients

Patients expressing homicidal intent require special measures to ensure staff safety and the safety of the third party threatened by the patient. The patient's threats should be believed, particularly if he or she has a specific plan. The third party, if specifically named, should be contacted through appropriate authorities to ensure his or her safety. The patient should be closely monitored by security personnel, with restraints, as indicated, in a setting devoid of potential weapons. Acute psychiatric consultation is mandatory.

Doshi A et al: National study of US emergency department visits for attempted suicide and self-inflicted injury, 1997–2001. Ann Emerg Med 2005;46:369.

▼ ORGANIC CAUSES FOR PSYCHIATRIC EMERGENCIES

Patients with acute behavior, mood, or thought disturbances must be medically evaluated for the presence of dementia or delirium. Dementia is a chronic, progressive alteration in memory associated with cognitive decline, agnosia (inability to recognize familiar objects), apraxia (inability to perform tasks), and aphasia (defective language function). Alzheimer's disease is the classic type of dementia. However, infections, such as HIV, and other neurologic conditions, such as stroke, can also cause dementia.

Delirium, by contrast, is an acute disturbance in consciousness. It may also involve cognitive decline, but the patient's level of consciousness is decreased, unlike in dementia. Delirium has a short onset and usually a fluctuating course.

DEMENTIA

Alzheimer's disease is the most common type of dementia. It starts with memory loss affecting recent memory. Long-term memory is usually preserved. As the disease progresses, more cognitive deficits become apparent until the patient is no longer able to function. History and physical examination are the most important contributors to the diagnosis. Magnetic resonance imaging (MRI) is an important adjunct.

Acetylcholinesterase inhibitors (eg, tacrine, donepezil) are used to increase central nervous system (CNS) levels of acetylcholine. This treatment helps to delay the progression of disease in some patients. However, no agent is currently available that can prevent the ultimate progression of Alzheimer's disease.

DELIRIUM

Multiple medical problems can cause a delirious state, which may be confused with psychosis. Drug intoxication or withdrawal; infection; and endocrine, metabolic, neurologic, and cardiopulmonary disturbances are most often implicated.

DRUG INTOXICATION AND WITHDRAWAL

See Chapter 47.

▶ Stimulants

The stimulant drugs such as cocaine and amphetamines, including MDMA (Ectasy), can cause symptoms of behavioral and personality disturbance. These drugs can also induce someone with a compensated psychiatric illness such as schizophrenia to decompensate. Therefore, when evaluating a patient with mental status changes and bizarre behavior, the physician should determine whether stimulant drugs are present. The diagnosis is based on history of substance abuse, characteristic signs, and a positive drug screen.

Cocaine and amphetamines both cause a sympathetic hyperactivity. They cause hypertension, tachycardia, dilated pupils, and diaphoresis. MDMA causes less sympathetic hyperactivity and has more hallucinogenic properties. Psychological manifestations of stimulants include dysphoria, paranoid psychosis, and potentially a delirious state. Stimulants also cause a disinhibition leading to poor impulse control. As a result, patients with acute intoxication are more likely to be violent, homicidal, or suicidal. This property is seen especially in patients taking amphetamines.

Management of patients with acute toxicity is supportive. Benzodiazepines are the treatment of choice for the acutely agitated and violent person taking cocaine or amphetamines.

Withdrawal from stimulants initially involves anxiety, anhedonia, depression, fatigue, and severe craving for the drug of abuse. Withdrawal does not cause a significant risk for death from cardiac or pulmonary disturbances. The withdrawal state may be a risk factor, however, for suicide. Patients receive supportive measures, usually lasting 1–2 weeks until improvement in the anxiety and lethargy is seen. However, the anhedonia and cravings may continue for weeks.

▶ Depressants

Alcohol and benzodiazepines are the classic depressants. The diagnosis is based on clinical findings coupled with a positive drug level. They cause a decrease in sensorium, lethargy, ataxic gait, nystagmus, and respiratory depression. Individuals presenting with symptoms of intoxication and lethargy warrant evaluation for depressant use. These chemicals, however, can inhibit impulse control, and some people have a paradoxical excitation using depressants. Monitoring of airway and breathing status is crucial. Searching for any other cause of the behavior (eg, head injury) is also important.

Alcohol withdrawal is noteworthy due to the continued morbidity and even mortality that occurs from such a widely used substance. Delirium tremens can cause a clinical picture very similar to that of an acute psychotic break. Patients with delirium tremens have stopped drinking for as little as a few hours to days. Patients clinically show signs of sympathetic overload, including hypertension and tachycardia. They are usually diaphoretic and, by definition, tremulous. This delirious state can be differentiated from functional psychosis on the basis of the history, autonomic dysfunction, and visual hallucinations. Treatment is with benzodiazepines. A titrated lorazepam infusion may be needed to decrease the hypertension, tachycardia, and CNS symptoms.

Narcotics

All narcotic substances, such as morphine and heroin, can cause the classic triad of respiratory depression, miosis, and decreased mental status. Diagnosis is based on the clinical picture, positive drug screen, or response to naloxone. Usually the patient abusing narcotics presents with lethargy and not bizarre behavior. However, if these chemicals are mixed with stimulants (eg, cocaine or amphetamines), the result may be any type of delirium that can mimic functional psychosis or mood disorder.

Hallucinogens

Lysergic acid diethylamide (LSD) and phencyclidine (PCP) are the traditional hallucinogenic drugs. LSD is absorbed through the oral mucosa and binds to post-synaptic serotonergic receptors. The patient may report kaleidoscopic hallucinations. However, the drug may also cause violence, suicidal ideation, and bizarre memories or flashbacks.

PCP is a dissociative anesthetic. Patients are awake but exhibit bizarre behavior that can become suddenly violent. Patients may be hypertensive and tachycardic. Patients may also experience a host of behavioral and neurologic changes such as loss of concentration or the presence of illogical speech, nystagmus, or ataxia. Diagnosis is based on the history of use, clinical findings, and drug screen results. Treatment for hallucinogens includes ruling out any other associated acute medical problem and providing supportive care in a calm, quiet environment. Benzodiazepines may be used in acutely agitated patients.

INFECTION

See Chapter 42.

Systemic

Many patients with systemic infections, especially the elderly, present with delirium. Sometimes the delirious state involves behavioral changes. Any elderly patient with acute mental status changes should be evaluated for systemic infection. Diagnosis is based on the clinical picture coupled with the source of infection detected on urinalysis, chest X-ray, or from cultures.

Central Nervous System

Encephalitis is an infectious process that causes inflammation around the brain. The etiology often is viral (eg, herpes). Clinical manifestations usually involve fever and headache. If the infection affects the limbic area of the brain, personality and behavioral changes may occur, including floridly psychotic behavior and aggression. Meningitis, likewise, may cause delirium and altered mental status. Therefore, if an infectious cause is suspected, especially in a patient with fever, the patient should undergo a head CT scan and lumbar puncture. Diagnosis is based on these two tests in the appropriate clinical setting. Treatment is aimed at the underlying infectious or inflammatory process. If infection is suspected, initiate acyclovir and antibiotics as soon as possible.

ENDOCRINE AND METABOLIC DISORDERS

Hepatic Encephalopathy

(See Chapter 37) Patients with stigmata of liver failure routinely present with altered mental status. These patients may be delirious. At times they may be violent or aggressive. In the context of liver failure, an elevated ammonia level may be helpful in narrowing down the differential diagnosis to hepatic encephalopathy. Treatment is usually supportive along with lactulose to enterally eliminate toxins usually cleared by the liver.

Electrolyte Abnormalities

(See Chapter 44) Hypercalcemia and alterations in sodium, either hyponatremia or hypernatremia, are the most common electrolyte causes of altered mental status. Personality and behavioral changes are much less common than lethargy. Seizures, coma, and death are possible if the electrolyte abnormality is not corrected appropriately. Fortunately, the diagnosis is easily made with routine electrolyte panels.

Hypoglycemia

(See Chapter 43) The brain requires glucose to function. A low blood glucose level can mimic any type of CNS event. Patients may present with decreased consciousness or focal neurologic findings similar to a stroke. Blood glucose level should be checked as soon as possible in any patient with behavioral changes. Rapid correction of hypoglycemia can itself cause behavioral changes. Violence and aggression from the rapid correction are usually short in duration. However, if a patient continues to have symptoms after the glucose level has been corrected, further investigation into the cause is warranted.

Thyroid Disease

(See Chapter 43) Hyperthyroidism and hypothyroidism have been implicated in acute behavioral changes mimicking functional disorders. Hyperthyroidism may cause anxiety and tremor. These patients usually present with mild to moderate hypertension and tachycardia along with weight loss and heat intolerance. Patients with hypothyroidism can present with symptoms of fatigue all the way to delirium or coma. Other symptoms include gastrointestinal complaints such as constipation, cold intolerance, weight gain, and menstrual irregularities. Diagnosis can be reliably made based on laboratory levels of thyroid hormones.

NEUROLOGIC DISORDERS

Seizure Disorder

(See Chapter 19) Patients who have had a seizure may present with a normal mental status or may have decreased consciousness from a postictal state. A history of seizure or witnessed seizure activity may guide the workup. Nonconvulsive status epilepticus is much more difficult to determine. These patients may present with decreased consciousness or may be awake and alert. Patients may even have behavioral changes from blank stare to aggression depending on the location of the seizure focus. Nonconvulsive status epilepticus should be considered in patients with behavioral or neurologic changes, especially if a history of epilepsy is present. If necessary, neurologic consultation and an electroencephalogram would be appropriate to confirm the diagnosis.

Cerebral Vascular Accident

(See Chapter 37.) Cerebral vascular accidents (CVAs) are usually associated with focal weakness and a variable level of consciousness. Depending on the area of the brain affected, patients may have significant cognitive deficits. Patients may present with bizarre behavior secondary to aphasia or neglect. Therefore, a CVA should be considered in patients with risk factors for vascular disease or cardioembolic phenomenon. CT scanning and MRI can be helpful in the diagnosis.

Wernicke-Korsakoff Syndrome

Wernicke's encephalopathy, a clinical diagnosis, is due to thiamine deficiency and occurs mostly in alcoholic patients. The main features clinically are ataxia, ophthal-moplegia (either nystagmus or gaze palsy), and mental status changes. The mental status change involves anything from confusion to delirium or even coma. Thus, this entity should be considered in anyone with a history of alcohol abuse, eye changes, and mental status changes. The development of Korsakoff's psychosis can accompany these findings. Altered patients with malnutrition and alcohol abuse should be given thiamine.

CARDIOPULMONARY DISEASE

Diseases of the cardiopulmonary system can cause significant behavioral changes. Myocardial infarction, pulmonary edema, and pulmonary embolism can cause anxiety secondary to pain, shortness of breath, and a possible sense of doom. These disorders may elicit significant fear in patients, which may manifest itself as panic attack or even aggression.

Patients may also be hypoxic or hypotensive, which may cause decreased consciousness and cognitive dysfunction. Diagnosis is based on clinical suspicion coupled with basic cardiac function evaluation (EGG, cardiac enzymes, pulse oximetry, and chest X-ray).

FUNCTIONAL CAUSES FOR PSYCHIATRIC EMERGENCIES

Patients with functional illness present to the emergency department with a disorder of behavior secondary to abnormal thought process, mood, or personality traits. The changes that result in the visit to the emergency department usually occur over a period of weeks. Patients may present with depressed mood, labile affect, paranoid delusions, auditory hallucinations, and psychomotor retardation, or they may be in a manic state. The clinical picture is quite variable, and organic cause for the decompensation should be investigated.

COGNITIVE (THOUGHT) DISORDERS: SCHIZOPHRENIA

Diagnosed clinically, schizophrenia is a common disorder. Most patients with schizophrenia are not institutionalized and routinely present to the emergency department for acute medical care. The visit may be due to medication noncompliance, ineffective medication, or substance abuse. Onset of the disease is usually in the late teens or early adult years. The cause of schizophrenia is not fully understood, but it is heralded by a disturbance in thought process called psychosis. Current medications work on dopamine and serotonin receptors.

Clinical Findings

Patients with schizophrenia present with positive symptoms (delusions, hallucinations, and bizarre behavior) and negative symptoms (withdrawal, blunted affect, catatonia). Organic causes of the behavior must be sought (eg, steroid toxicity, substance abuse or withdrawal, encephalitis, HIV encephalopathy). Common manifestations of disorganized thought include the following:

- Social withdrawal, often with poor personal hygiene
- Preoccupation with inner thoughts and auditory hallucinations, which are often violent, sexual, or religious in nature
- Labile affect, often presenting with flat, emotionless affect but rapidly changing
- Poor ability to focus on a topic, making it difficult to follow the patient in conversation
- Flight of ideas
- Hallucinations, often derogatory to the patient
- Grandiose or persecutory delusions
- Catatonia
- Paranoia

▶ Treatment

Provision of a safe and supportive environment is important, both for the patient and the emergency department staff. Patients with aggression and grossly disruptive or dangerous behavior require antipsychotic agents such as haloperidol, 5–10 mg intramuscularly, often in combination with lorazepam 2–4 mg or midazolam 5–15 mg intramuscularly. Newer atypical antipsychotics such as ziprasidone, 10 mg intramuscularly, are also used for management of acute agitation. Patients who are unable to care for themselves or who pose a high risk of harm to themselves require psychiatric consultation and admission. Often patients present in a withdrawn state (catatonia). These patients are at high risk for dehydration, electrolyte imbalances, and malnutrition. Therefore, along with psychiatric consultation, evaluation for organic disease that results from the functional condition is imperative.

▼ AFFECTIVE (MOOD) DISORDERS

DEPRESSION

Diagnosed based on a constellation of symptoms, depression is the most common mood disorder. Patients have variable presentations ranging from an acute depressive state lasting days after an emotionally taxing event to chronic depression lasting years.

▶ Clinical Findings

Depression is characterized by a change in mood. Patients commonly have intense feelings of sadness, guilt, and hopelessness. Patients are often anhedonic, with no interest in pleasurable activity. These patients may also have psychomotor retardation or agitation with variable sleeping patterns.

Depressed patients are routinely evaluated in the emergency department for complaints of fatigue or decreased appetite, suicidal ideation or attempt, overdose, substance abuse, dehydration, or malnutrition.

Patients with depression may present with delusions or frank psychosis. These patients may or may not have a diagnosis of schizoaffective disorder, which is a disorder of both thought and mood. The delusions are usually persecutory or somatic in nature.

▶ Treatment

Life-threatening medical conditions must be detected and treated. Dehydration, overdose, and illicit drug in-gestion must be medically managed. Many general medical conditions may cause depression and must also be ruled out. Neurodegenerative disorders, stroke, thyroid disorders, epilepsy, metabolic disorders, and infection are just some of the conditions that may involve a depressed state. Once patients are medically stable, those at risk of harming themselves or others must receive psychiatric consultation and be admitted.

MANIC STATES

Mania is another type of mood disorder. Many patients with mania have bipolar affective disorder, alternating between episodes of mania and depression. Mania is diagnosed clinically and is characterized by variable degrees of heightened mood and activity. The symptoms may be mild, characterized by an overly friendly or talkative personality. This condition is called hypomania. Others may present with grandiose delusions, insomnia, and aggressive behavior. Caution must be used in the emergency department when dealing with a manic patient. The disorder can cause unpredictable behavior.

▶ Clinical findings

The predominance of an infectious, inappropriate euphoria coupled with hyperactivity and talkativeness suggests the diagnosis. Mania is also characterized by decreased need to eat or sleep. Patients routinely are awake all hours of the night and may go for extended periods of time without a significant amount of sleep. The disorder is also characterized by flight of ideas, decreased ability to concentrate on a task, inappropriate laughing and joking, increased uninterrupted speech, and grandiose delusions.

Patients with bipolar affective disorder may be rapid cycling. In this state, patients, over hours to days, alternate between severely depressed mood and a state of euphoria. When disorganization of thought process is a prominent feature, a diagnosis of schizoaffective disorder should be considered.

▶ Treatment

Initially, evaluate patients for an organic cause or signs of organic disease resulting from the manic state. Illicit drug use, especially stimulants, may cause a clinical picture of mania. In addition, patients with mania may be dehydrated or have an electrolyte or nutritional disorder secondary to decreased consumption of food and water while in a manic state.

Evaluate patients for toxicity from drugs used to treat mania, such as lithium or antiepileptics. Once patients are medically stable, evaluate them for risk of harming themselves or others. If a patient is found to be at risk, psychiatric consultation and admission are required.

Treat acute hostile behavior as appropriate. Reducing the environmental stimuli in the emergency department is important. Place the patient in a safe and quiet room after ensuring that he or she has no objects that may be used to cause harm. If the patient continues to be agitated, medical management with lorazepam, 1–2 mg intravenously or intramuscularly, or haloperidol, 5–10 mg intramuscularly, is appropriate.

BORDERLINE PERSONALITY DISORDER

Borderline personality disorder presents a special situation in the emergency department. Patients with this disorder regularly present to the emergency department. The diagnosis is clinical, based on patient behavior.

▶ Clinical Findings

Patients with borderline personality disorder are characterized by their volatile interpersonal relationships. They can be very impulsive and have labile affect. Patients are usually very demanding, frequently presenting with suicide threats and other self-destructive behavior. They commonly experience paranoid thoughts and have other comorbid conditions such as substance abuse and affective disorders.

▶ Treatment

Evaluation of the patient for organic illness is the first priority. Treat medical and surgical issues resulting from self-destructive behavior rapidly, and evaluate the patient for continued threat to self or others. If such a threat exists, seek psychiatric consultation for the patient and arrange for admission. Additional techniques for dealing with patients with borderline personality disorder involve contacting the patient's support structure (eg, family, friend, or therapist) and ensuring adequate follow-up. The number of visits to the emergency department is inversely proportional to the amount of social support that the patient receives outside the hospital. Furthermore, emergency department staff should treat the patient's abrasiveness as a symptom of the disorder and avoid an inappropriate response. Addressing the patient's complaints promptly may prevent escalation of symptoms.

OTHER FUNCTIONAL CAUSES

SOMATOFORM DISORDERS AND HYSTERICAL STATES

Patients with somatoform disorders and hysterical states present with different types of physical complaints. Patients perceive the symptoms as real, even though no underlying physical organic cause is found responsible. These disorders must be separated from malingering, which involves deliberate and conscious deception for secondary gain.

1. Conversion Disorder

Conversion disorder is characterized by motor or sensory dysfunction caused by psychological stress with no true physical dysfunction. These symptoms are not intentionally produced and may occur in patients after a traumatic event, especially if a loved one is injured or killed. Conversion disorder may present with motor symptoms, sensory symptoms, or even apparent seizures.

▶ Clinical Findings

The emergency physician must differentiate between somatic symptoms due solely to functional cause and true organic disease exacerbated by psychologic stress. Evaluate patients for disorders such as Guillain–Barre syndrome, botulism poisoning, herpes encephalitis, and CVAs. Obtain a thorough history, including history of psychiatric disease, and conduct a complete physical examination. Pay close attention to any discrepancies in the physical findings. A patient with hysterical blindness can be tested for nystagmus by running a strip of paper with multiple vertical lines on it (eg, EKG paper) in front of the patient's eyes. This procedure will elicit tracking and nystagmus if the patient has vision (optokinetic reflex).

The diagnosis of conversion disorder is strengthened by a fluctuating pattern of disability; a lack of concern about the disability; a pattern that does not follow known anatomic relationships; intact sphincter tone; and, when the complaint is paralysis, presence of the Hoover sign (in which counterpressure with the heel of the unaffected leg is absent when the patient is asked to lift the affected leg).

▶ Treatment

Differentiating a conversion disorder from a true motor or sensory disorder is imperative. If the diagnosis is difficult, an elaborate workup may be initiated. If the diagnosis of conversion disorder is made, psychiatric consultation and counseling are appropriate.

2. Somatization Disorder

Somatization disorder is characterized by four or more different pain complaints along with at least two gastrointestinal complaints, a sexual complaint, and a neurologic complaint. Patients usually have a history of multiple surgeries, numerous emergency department visits, multiple medications, multiple reported allergies, and no relief from intractable chronic pain. The emergency physician must rule out significant organic disease and at the same time avoid elaborate workups. Evaluating available medical records and contacting the patient's other physicians or counselors is imperative.

3. Hypochondria

Hypochondriasis is an anxious and inappropriate preoccupation with physical signs and symptoms. Patients live in fear that they have a serious medical condition. Evaluation of the patient based on clinical reasoning is important, followed by reassurance and referral for psychiatric counseling.

PSYCHOGENIC FUGUE

▶ Clinical Findings

Psychogenic fugue is the dissociative state most commonly encountered in the emergency department. The disorder is diagnosed clinically and characterized by the sudden loss of memory. It usually begins abruptly after a psychologically catastrophic event, such as the loss of a close family member. Patients are usually in good health and able to communicate, but they are unable to answer personal questions, for example, regarding their name and address. Patients may travel long distances without recall and are often found in bus or train stations. Recovery of memory can occur within a few hours or take several weeks. Afterward, the patient often has amnesia for the period of dissociation.

▶ Treatment

The emergency physician must rule out organic disorders. Alcohol abuse is the most common cause of blackouts, which may mimic psychogenic fugue. Malingering must also be considered, especially if the patient is confronted with legal problems. Once other etiologies have been ruled out, it is important to reassure the patient that the disorder is not permanent. Social support is important to help the patient emotionally cope until the problem resolves.

Alderfer BS, Allen MH: Treatment of agitation in bipolar disorder across the life cycle. J Clin Psychiatry 2003;64:3–9 [PMID: 12672259].

Bethell J, Rhodes AE: Adolescent depression and emergency department use: the roles of suicidality and deliberate self-harm. Curr Psychiatry Rep 2008;10:53–59 [PMID: 18269895].

Broderick KB, Lerner EB, McCourt JD, Fraser E, Salerno K: Emergency physician practices and requirements regarding the medical screening examination of psychiatric patients. Acad Emerg Med 2002;9:88 [PMID: 11772676].

Lukens TW, Wolf SJ, Edlow JA et al: Clinical Policy: Critical issues in the diagnosis and management of the adult psychiatric patient in the emergency department. Ann Emerg Med 2006;47:79–99 [PMID: 16387222].

Marco CA, Vaughan J: Emergency management of agitation in schizophrenia. Am J Emerg Med 2005;23:767–776 [PMID: 16182986].

Oyama O, Paltoo C, Greengold J: Somatoform disorders. Am Fam Physician 2007;76:1333–1338 [PMID: 18019877].

Piechniczek-Buczek J: Psychiatric emergencies in the elderly population. Emerg Med Clin North Am 2006;24:467–490 [PMID: 16584967].

Sood TR, Mcstay CM: Evaluation of the psychiatric patient. Emerg Med Clin North Am 2009;27:669–683 [PMID: 19932400].

Thomas P, Alptekin K, Gheorghe M, Mauri M, Olivares JM, Riedel M: Management of patients presenting with acute psychotic episodes of schizophrenia. CNS Drugs 2009;23:193–212 [PMID: 19320529].

Zaheer J, Links PS, Liu E: Assessment and emergency management of suicidality in personality disorders. Psychiatr Clin North Am 2008;31:527–543 [PMID: 18638651].

▼ PSYCHOPHARMACOTHERAPY

Psychiatric medications have changed significantly in recent years. Emergency physicians commonly encounter patients who are taking these drugs. An understanding of their indications, side effects, and potential toxicities is essential.

ANTIPSYCHOTICS (NEUROLEPTICS)

TYPICAL ANTIPSYCHOTICS

Typical antipsychotics include both high-potency and low-potency agents. High-potency antipsychotic agents such as haloperidol are used to treat agitation, violence, and acute psychosis in the emergency department. The high-potency agents are associated with less sedation, hypotension, and anticholinergic effects than are the low-potency agents such as chlorpromazine or thioridazine. However, the high-potency agents are associated with a higher incidence of dystonic reactions and extrapyramidal side effects (EPS).

The usual dose of haloperidol for agitation in a patient without evidence of other toxic overdose is 5–10 mg intramuscularly. These agents may be used in combination with minor tranquilizers such as benzodiazepines, but prolonged sedation is a risk. Studies have shown that combination of haloperidol and benzodiazepines are more effective than either agent alone. Effects should start within 20–30 minutes and peak at 1–2 hours. One comparison of two major benzodiazepines showed significantly shorter time to sedation with midazolam 5 mg intramuscularly (18.3 minutes) compared to lorazepam 2 mg intramuscularly (32.2 minutes).

Like its closely related cousin droperidol, haloperidol has the potential to cause a prolonged QTc. In 2007, the Food and Drug Administration placed warning on use of intravenous haloperidol citing literature concerns for cardiac dysrhythmias and torsades de pointes. Currently, use of haloperidol via intravenous administration is not recommended by the Food and Drug Administration. It may also lower seizure threshold. These factors should be considered before use, particularly in patients with overdose or toxin exposure.

An overdose of typical antipsychotics should be treated with supportive care. Dyskinesias are treated with diphenhydramine, 25–50 mg intravenously or intramuscularly, or benztropine, 1–2 mg intravenously or intramuscularly.

ATYPICAL ANTIPSYCHOTICS

The atypical antipsychotic medications (eg, risperidone, clozapine, quetiapine, olanzapine, ziprasidone) demonstrate equivalent efficacy in treating schizophrenia as do typical agents. These agents have a lower side-effect profile than typical antipsychotics, with less likelihood of EPS and tardive dyskinesia. However, the atypical agents have also been associated with significant weight gain in patients.

Atypical antipsychotics are often promoted as more favorable alternatives to typical agents, however considerations must be made. While atypical agents have been shown to be more effective in exacerbations of chronic psychiatric disorders, they have not been fully evaluated in respect to acute undifferentiated psychosis. In addition, the typical agents, including haloperidol, have advantages of decades of research and lower cost. Therefore many considerations must be made to determine whether typical or atypical agents are best for the individual patient.

While these agents are relatively safe, toxic effects can include CNS effects, respiratory depression, hypotension, and anticholinergic symptoms. Prolongation of the QTc and dysrhythmias happen infrequently. Of note, elderly individuals with dementia taking atypical agents for behavioral disorders have been found at increased risk for death. Treatment for intentional overdose is largely supportive, paying attention to airway, breathing, and cardiac monitoring.

Some of the agents have more specific side effects. Clozapine, the drug of choice for treatment-resistant schizophrenia, has a higher risk of seizures, myocarditis, and agranulocytosis. Therefore, a complete blood count should be routinely obtained in patients taking this medication. Ziprasidone has a higher risk of associated cardiac arrhythmia related to prolongation of the QTc interval. Appropriate caution should be exercised if using this agent in the acute setting.

NEUROLEPTIC MALIGNANT SYNDROME

▶ Diagnosis

Neuroleptic malignant syndrome (NMS) is an uncommon and potentially fatal reaction usually due to antipsychotic medications. The condition is characterized by hypertension, tachycardia, hyperthermia, and muscle rigidity. It may also occur in cases of acute delirium. Consider NMS in any patient who is known to have a psychiatric condition and who is taking neuroleptic medications.

▶ Treatment

Treatment begins with management of airway, breathing, and circulation. Discontinue antipsychotic medication immediately. The patient should be cooled and rehydrated with crystalloid. Initiate muscle relaxation with intravenous benzodiazepines or dantrolene (1 mg/kg). Bromocriptine has also been used to help treat this condition because it is potentially caused by depletion of dopamine in the CNS. Further management includes supportive care and evaluation for rhabdomyolysis.

ANTIDEPRESSANTS

TRICYCLIC ANTIDEPRESSANTS

Developed in the 1960s, the tricyclic antidepressants (eg, imipramine, amitriptyline, nortriptyline) are no longer first-line agents. They are effective but have the potential for serious side effects or death, particularly if taken as an overdose. Multiple side effects include dry mouth, constipation, dizziness, and elevated heart rate. In toxic overdose, rapid administration of sodium bicarbonate can correct lethal cardiac arrhythmia.

MONOAMINE OXIDASE INHIBITORS

Monoamine oxidase inhibitors include phenelzine, tranylcypromine, and isocarboxazid. These agents can be used to treat depression and panic disorder. The potential for serious interaction with tyramine-containing foods (eg, cheeses, wines, and pickles) and other antidepressants has limited the use of this class of medication.

SELECTIVE SEROTONIN REUPTAKE INHIBITORS

Selective serotonin reuptake inhibitors (SSRIs) are now the predominant antidepressant agents. The SSRIs include fluoxetine, sertraline, paroxetine, and fluvoxamine. Metabolized by cytochrome P450 enzymes, SSRIs can inhibit these enzymes, causing altered levels of other medications such as theophylline or warfarin. Side effects may include headache, nausea, sleep disturbance, and nervousness. The serotonin syndrome, marked by tremulousness and delirium, is also a risk. SSRI overdoses usually cause minor symptoms but rarely death. Symptoms of SSRI overdose can include nausea, vomiting, tachycardia, dizziness, and drowsiness. Seizures, coma, and death are possible but rare. Treatment includes supportive measures and observation.

NEWER ANTIDEPRESSANTS

Newer combination agents are increasingly becoming available that combat depression and other disorders such as anxiety and obsessive-compulsive disorder. Newer agents such as venlafaxine (Effexor) and mirtazapine (Remeron), like SSRJs, are relatively safe agents. Common symptoms of overdose include drowsiness and sinus tachycardia. Patients who overdose on these agents usually require only observation and supportive care. However, two exceptions should be noted. Citalopram in doses greater than 600 mg has caused seizures and cardiac conduction abnormalities. A patient who has ingested a large quantity may require monitoring in an intensive care setting. Bupropion, likewise, has been associated with seizures in people with bulimia nervosa and in individuals who overdose on high doses.

ANTIMANIC AGENTS

Mania may be managed pharmacologically with several different regimens. Lithium is the most common agent used for bipolar disorder, but it has a narrow therapeutic-to-toxic window. Lithium can cause complications in the thyroid and kidney in addition to cardiac and neurologic systems. As a result, lithium levels should be checked in any patient on the medication presenting with acute systemic complaints (eg, altered mental status or seizure).

Anticonvulsants, such as valproic acid, are used as alternative mood stabilizers in mania, particularly for rapid-cycling bipolar disorder. Manic patients may ultimately require combination therapy, including the use of antidepressants or antipsychotics, to control their symptoms.

Drugs for depression and bipolar disorder. Treat Guidel Med Lett 2010;8:35–42 [PMID: 20414177].

Foussias G, Remington G: Antipsychotics and schizophrenia: from efficacy and effectiveness to clinical decision-making. Can J Psychiatry 2010;55:117–125 [PMID: 20370961].

Lieberman JA, Stroup TS, McEvoy JP et al: Effectiveness of antipsychotic drugs in patients with chronic schizophrenia. N Engl J Med 2005;353:1209–1223 [PMID: 16172203].

National Institutes of Mental Health: Mental Health Medications. www.nimh.nih.gov/ health/publications/mental-health-medications/index.shtml, Bethesda, MD, 2008 [Last Accessed on August 26, 2010].

Margetić B, Margetić BA: Neuroleptic malignant syndrome and its controversies. Pharmacoepidemiol Drug Saf 2010;19:429–435 [PMID: 20306454].

DISPOSITION

▶ General Considerations

Disposition is critical in patients with psychiatric emergencies. Patients should be admitted to the hospital if they meet any of the following criteria, which constitute a psychiatric crisis:

- Unable to care for self
- Actively suicidal
- Actively homicidal
- Unresolved symptoms with an organic cause

Admit such patients to the psychiatric service or, alternatively, to the general medicine service with a psychiatry consult. Assign patients full-time sitters for their safety.

▶ Involuntary Procedures and Admission

One of the unique aspects of managing patients with psychiatric emergencies is the potential need to initiate involuntary procedures or admission when such patients refuse lifesaving intervention. Generally, patient care is conducted under the auspices of the patient's informed consent. However, care can be rendered without the patient's consent if he or she is not exhibiting a rational pattern of behavior with regard to self-preservation and what reasonable individuals would consider to be consistent with the patient's best interests. In such situations, the physician must act to preserve the patient's life until the situation changes to permit the patient's consensual participation in the care. Patients experiencing an acute psychiatric crisis may therefore need procedures and admission performed for their safety without their consent.

Involuntary procedures may include physical or chemical restraint. Such patients may also require involuntary admission or 72-hour holds to permit psychiatric assessment. In most venues, this type of involuntary care may be authorized by a practicing physician, police officer, or social service worker who has reason to believe that the patient is a safety risk to him or herself or another. This individual must document evidence to support the decision, and it is good practice to seek the independent corroboration of two physicians if available. Under such circumstances, the patient may then receive treatment and be held against his or her will for up to 72 hours until the psychiatry evaluation is completed.

Pediatric Emergencies

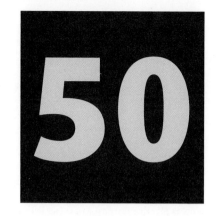

Maria Stephan, MD
Craig Carter, DO
Shah Ashfaq, BS[1]

Cardiovascular Emergencies
  Dehydration
  Shock
  Congestive Heart Failure
  Cardiac Dysrhythmias
Respiratory Distress
  Apnea
  Upper Airway Obstruction
  Lower Airway Disorders
Neurologic Emergencies
  Seizures
  Encephalitis
Infectious Diseases
  Fever
  Meningitis
  Acute Otitis Media
  Pharyngitis
  Cellulitis and Subcutaneous Abscesses

  Periorbital and Orbital Cellulitis
  Urinary Tract Infection
  Gastroenteritis
  Septic Arthritis
  Acute Osteomyelitis
Gastrointestinal Disorders
  Abdominal Pain
  Vomiting
  Gastrointestinal Bleeding
  Foreign Body
Hematological Diseases
  Anemia
  Sickle Cell Disease
  Idiopathic Thrombocytopenic Purpura
Newborn Emergencies
Child Abuse
  Physical Abuse
  Sexual Abuse

▶ General Considerations

A. Epidemiology

Children constitute one of the most diverse and challenging patient populations facing the emergency physician. While comprising almost 30% of emergency department patients, critical illness and injury are present in only approximately 5%. The majority of pediatric emergency visits are evaluated not in pediatric hospitals, but community emergency departments. Early recognition and aggressive management of illnesses and injuries effecting pediatric patients is of utmost importance.

The epidemiology of pediatric emergency medicine changes with the clinical setting. In the prehospital environment, the common presenting complaints are trauma, seizures, respiratory distress, and toxicologic emergencies. In the emergency department, the most common complaints are fever, trauma, injury, respiratory distress, vomiting, diarrhea, or upper respiratory tract infection.

B. Assessment

Assessment of the pediatric patient in the emergency department requires an age-specific approach. A calm, reassuring, and gentle manner on the physician's part will facilitate information collection and encourage patient cooperation in examining and testing.

Knowledge of the child's growth and development often is required for the diagnosis, management, and disposition

[1]This chapter is a revision of the chapter by Eric Yazel, MD, & Sandra Herr, MD from the 6th edition.

Table 50–1. Pediatric Procedural Equipment Sizing.

Age	Weight (Kg)	Endotrachel Tube	Laryngoscope Blade	Chest Tube (F)	Nastrostic Tube (F)	Foley Catheter (F)	Femoral IV
Premie 32 week gestation	2	2.5-3.0	1 straight	8	5	5	3 F, 8 cm
Newborn	3	3.5	1 straight	10	5	8	3 F, 8 cm
1 month	4	3.5	1 straight	10	5	8	3 F, 8 cm
3-5 months	6-7	3.5	1 straight	10-12	5-8	8	3 F, 8 cm
6-11 months	8-10	3.5-4.0	1 straight	10-12	8	8-10	3 F, 8 cm
1 year	10-11	4.0	1 straight	16-20	8-10	8-10	3 F, 8 cm
2-3 years	12-14	4.5	1.5-2 straight	20-24	10	8-10	5 F, 15 cm
4-5 years	15-18	5.0	2 straight or curved	20-28	10-12	10-12	5 F, 15 cm
6-8 years	20-28	5.5-6.0	2 straight or curved	30-32	14-18	10-12	5 F, 15 cm
10-12 years	35-50	6.5-7.0	3 straight or curved	32-38	18	12	5-7 F, 15-20 cm
14 years	60	7.0-7.5	3-4 straight or curved	38-40	18	12	7 F, 20 cm

of the pediatric patient. Severity of acute pediatric illness and injury is often difficult to discern. Recognition of anatomic and physiologic differences remind the examiner of large surface area to weight ratio leading to heat loss and trauma to internal organs may exist with little signs of external injury. Airway differences are important to understand in order to manage respiratory distress and failure. Observational methods of assessment may be more sensitive to illness and injury acuity in children taking into account such variables as quality of cry, reaction to parent stimulation, state variation, skin color, hydration status, and response social overtures such as talking and smiling. Such observations appear to be more predictive of serious illness than anatomic physical examination using standard palpation, percussion, and auscultation techniques.

Assessment and management of the distressed pediatric patient requires appropriately sized equipment. Table 50–1 provides equipment sizes for invasive procedures in children of different age groups.

Vital signs may vary by age (Table 50–2). A rapid formula for estimating normal systolic blood pressure is 80 + (2 × age [in years]). The maximum effective heart rate in

Table 50–2. Age-related Vital Signs.

Age	Mean Weight (kg)	Minimum Systolic Blood Pressure	Normal Heart Rate	Normal Respiratory Rate
Premature	2.5	40	100-170	40-50
Newborn	3	50	90-180	30-50
3 months	6	60	110-180	24-40
6 months	8	70	110-17	24-40
1 year	10	72	90-150	24-40
2 years	13	74	90-150	22-30
4 years	15	78	65-135	20-40
6-8 years	20-28	80-86	60-130	18-24
9-10 years	30-36	90	60-110	16-22
11-14 years	50-60	90	60-110	14-20

Table 50–3. Common Topical Local Anesthetics.

Drug	Components	Applied To	Effect (min)	Cautions
EMLA (Eutectic Mixture of Local Anesthetics)	Lidocaine 2.5% Prilocaine 2.5%	Intact skin	90	Methemoglobinemia Max dose: 5 mglk Lidocaine
Elamax LET	Lidocaine 4% Epinephrine 0.1% Tetracaine 0.5%	Both intact and non intact skin	30	Vasoconstriction Max dose: 5 mglk Lidocaine
TAC	Tetracaine 0.25-0.5% Adrenaline 0.025-0.05% Cocaine 4%-11.8%	Both intact and nonintact skin	15	Vasoconstriction Cocaine toxicity Reapplication Contraindicated Max dose: cocaine 3 mglk
Viscous Lidocaine	Lidocaine 2%	Both intact and and nonintact skin	10	Max dose: 5 mglk Lidocaine

infants is 200 beats/min, in young children 150 beats/min, and in school-aged children 120 beats/min. Respiratory rate decreases with advancing age (Table 50–2). The use of vital signs to assess vital functions in pediatric patients, however, is hazardous. Appropriate-sized measuring equipment is imperative, techniques must be applied carefully, and interpretation must be age-related. Furthermore, even accurately obtained, age-adjusted vital signs may be insensitive and are often affected by fever, pain, and ambient features of the emergency department environment. Instead, other measures of cardiopulmonary function, such as skin color, temperature, and capillary refill, are often better triage and assessment tools.

C. Concept of the Distressed Family

The emergency department physician must appreciate the intimate relationship of the child to the family. Acute pediatric illness and injury are inextricably part of the family environment and dynamics. The child as well as the entire nuclear and extended family may experience major psychological, emotional, and financial consequences of pediatric emergencies. Effective care requires appropriate consideration of the child within the distressed family, enlistment of parental assistance in evaluation and management, and provision of psychological support.

D. Pain and Sedation

Too often, the inexperienced physician neglects pain control or procedural sedation because of misunderstanding the significance of pain in the young child, unwarranted fear of addicting children to narcotic agents, or ignorance of appropriate agents. When a painful procedure is necessary, an effective approach integrates careful explanation directly to the child and enlistment of parental understanding and assistance. Whenever conscious or deep sedation procedures

are performed, the emergency department physician must ensure patient's safety by strict adherence to the guidelines of monitoring. This includes preparation for any potential airway complications, such as aspiration or apnea. In general, only previously healthy or mildly chronically ill children should be considered candidates for sedation procedures in the emergency department. Sometimes a restraint apparatus will facilitate the procedure.

The guidelines for a variety of clinical situations are given next.

1. Topical anesthetics— (Table 50–3)

A. FOR WOUND REPAIR:—The formulation LET (2% lidocaine, 1:1000 epinephrine, and 2% tetracaine) is easily applied and has a favorable safety profile. It is available as gel or solution. The onset of action is approximately 30 minutes; thus it should be applied early in the laceration evaluation process. TAC (tetracaine, adrenaline, and cocaine) is occasionally used as well; however caution should be used as seizures have been reported secondarily to systemic cocaine absorption. Any anesthetic containing epinephrine (such as LET or TAC) should be avoided on end-arterial structures, such as the ears, nose, digits, or penis. (See Table 50–3.)

B. FOR IV LINE PLACEMENT, BLOOD DRAWS:—Eutectic mixture of local anesthetics (EMLA) or Elamax 4%, ethyl chloride spray preparations, J-tip lidocaine applicators have been advocated for local analgesic use on intact skin.

2. Sedation and analgesia for painful procedures—

There are numerous agents (Table 50–4) which are useful in sedation and pain management in the pediatric patient. Familiarity with several of these is useful for the emergency physician, allowing tailoring of the most appropriate agent to the clinical situation. The most commonly used agents are discussed next.

Table 50–4. Pediatric Sedation and Analgesia.

Agent	Route	Pediatric Dose	Onset	Duration	Comments
Commonly Used Sedative/Analgesic Agents					
Sedation					
Propofol	IV	1 mg/kg bolus: followed by 0.5 mg/kg every 3-5 min	30-45 s	<15 min	Max dose 4.5 mg/kg Contraindicated in egg, soy allergies No analgesia
Ketamine	IM IV PO	3-5 mg/kg 0.5-2 mg/kg 0.5 mg/kg	5-10 min 1 min 30-45 min	0.5-1.5 h 15 min-1 h 2 h	Laryngospasm occurs in 2% Vomiting in up to 20% May use atropine or glycopyrrolate to decrease secretions Contraindicated in patients with increased intraocular or intracranial pressure
Midazolam	IV 1 m PO Nasal	0.05-0.1 mg/kg 0.1-0.2 mg/kg 0.5 mg/kg 0.2-0.5 mg/kg	2-3 min 10-20 min 15-30 min 10-15 min	1 h 1-2 h 1-2 h 1 h	
Nitrous Oxide	Inhaled	50-70% Concentration	1-2 min	5 min	Vomiting in up to 10%
Analagesia					
Acetaminophen	PO PR	15 mg/kg 15 mg/kg	20-40 min	4 h	No anti-inflammatory effects Max 1 g Use with caution in hepatic disease
Ibuprofen	PO	10 mg/kg	20-30 min	6h	Beware in ASA allergic Use with caution in renal or hepatic disease
Hydrocodone Morphine	PO 1m IV	0.15-0.2 mg/kg 0.1-0.2 mg/kg 0.05-0.2mg/kg	10-30 min 10-30 min Immediate	4-6 h 3-6 h 2-4 h	Maximum dose 10 mg
Fentanyl	Nasal[a] IV	1.7 mcg/kg of 150 mcg/cc concentration 1-4 mcg/kg	10-20 min Immediate	1 h 0.5-1h	Chest wall rigidity with rapid infusion

[a]Source for this dose and route: Borland M. Ann Emerg Med 2007;49(3):335–340.

A. MIDAZOLAM—Midazolam is a relatively fast acting benzodiazepine providing anxiolysis, sedation, and antegrade amnesia, commonly used in emergency department sedation. It is commonly used in conjunction with a narcotic analgesic such as morphine or fentanyl. Some children will have a paradoxical excitation to midazolam and will experience agitation instead of sedation. There is some evidence that this unpleasant reaction may be reversed with flumazenil. Patients may also respond favorably to additional administration of benzodiazepines.

B. KETAMINE—Ketamine, IM/ may be used for procedural situations involving children of any age, especially burn debridement, foreign body removal, deep wound care, abscess incision and drainage, or orthopedic reductions. Some clinicians recommend adding atropine, 0.01 mg/kg (maximum, 0.5 mg), or glycopyrrolate, 0.005 mg/kg (maximum 0.25 mg),

to avoid hypersalivation, although current literature has not demonstrated a clear benefit. Intravenous administration is better for longer procedures. Ketamine may elevate intracranial and intraocular pressure, induce emesis, and occasionally precipitate laryngospasm. Ketamine use in older children may also cause an adverse behavioral reaction upon emergence from sedation. Some clinicians recommend the concomitant use of midazolam in children over 5 years. Studies, however, have not demonstrated a clear benefit to administering midazolam with ketamine to prevent emergence phenomenon.

C. PROPOFOL—Propofol, 0.5–1.0 mg/kg by slow IV injection over 3–5 minutes, followed by an infusion of up to 0.5 mg/kg over 2–3 minutes with at least 1 minute between infusions. The advantage to this drug is the rapid onset of sedation and quick recovery time. Propofol is easily titrated to appropriate level of sedation. As with other agents, respiratory depression can occur and therefore ability to manage the airway and assist ventilation is extremely important when using this agent. Common uses of propofol include sedation for orthopedic reduction and suturing. Because of the potential for allergic reaction, the drug is contraindicated in patients with egg or soy allergies. Although the clinical significance of the effect is often not apparent, blood pressure frequently drops during propofol infusion. For this reason, most clinicians avoid propofol in patients who have been hypotensive and/or are significantly hypovolemic.

3. Sedation for imaging studies—For individuals requiring imaging studies such as computed tomography (CT) scan or magnetic resonance imaging (MRI), pentobarbital intramuscularly, midazolam, etomidate , methohexital or dexmedetomidine are commonly and safely used with proper monitoring as for any procedural sedation.

4. Precautions—Sedation agents should only be used by those with appropriate training and familiarity with the agents used. Proper precautions should be taken such as constant vital sign and pulse oximetry monitoring. End-tidal CO_2 monitoring is advised to more closely assess the adequacy of a patient's ventilation. Rescue airway equipment and reversal agents such as naloxone, 0.01–0.1 mg/kg IV, and flumazenil, 0.01 mg/kg IV should be readily available.

5. Outpatient analgesia—Outpatient analgesia ordinarily includes a nonsteroidal, anti-inflammatory drug such as ibuprofen, 10 mg/kg every 6–8 hours. This drug can also be used in combination with oral narcotic agents for the treatment of severe pain. Acetaminophen, 10–15 mg/kg every 4–6 hours, can also be used for the treatment of mild pain on an outpatient basis. Narcotics as hydrocodone/acetaminophen combination or codeine/acetaminophen every 4–6 hours may be used for severe pain.

E. Drug and Fluid Administration

All parenterally and orally administered agents should be given strictly on a per-kilogram basis, until maximum adult doses and volumes are reached. Over dosing and over hydration are dangerous errors in emergency pediatrics. Under dosing is also frequent, especially in infants and small children. Initial treatment of dehydration should include isotonic fluids (normal saline or lactated Ringer's). Physicians and nurses should meticulously review drug and fluid orders to ensure that they are age and weight corrected.

Vascular access is often the rate-limiting step in provision of life-saving therapy to critically ill and injured children. The emergency department physician must be familiar with a variety of techniques for access into the cardiopulmonary system.

1. Endotracheal tube—In critically ill, intubated patients, the endotracheal route is an effective conduit for administration of a variety of life-saving drugs, including epinephrine, atropine, lidocaine, naloxone, and diazepam. Epinephrine is by far the most commonly used. When administered through the endotracheal tube, higher doses, up to 10 times the IV dose, must be used to obtain adequate serum concentrations. The pharmacokinetics of endotracheal epinephrine administration may be optimized by delivery of the drug directly into the highly vascular trachea and proximal tracheobronchial tree instead of directly into the endotracheal tube. The preferred technique required is the insertion of a nasogastric tube or a size 5F umbilical catheter past the distal tip of the endotracheal tube with direct instillation of drugs through the tube. Because endotracheal drugs may be more effective if aerosolized, dilute the drug with normal saline to a maximum volume of 0.5–1.0 mL/kg, and then inject rapidly to achieve a partially aerosolized form.

2. IV access—In infants, the scalp is an ideal site for cannulation; use a size 24 gauge IV catheter. In children past the neonatal period, the dorsal veins of the hand, antecubital fossa, or dorsum of the foot are usually accessible with a 24 or 22-gauge IV catheter. The external jugular vein is a large vein, usually easily visualized and readily cannulated with a 20-gauge catheter if the child is properly restrained and the head is held in a dependent position.

3. Intraosseous infusion—(See also Chapter 8.) For patients under age 5 years in extremis and requiring life-saving drug and fluid administration, intraosseous infusion is an alternative method of administration. This method of access is also a viable alternative in older children and adults; however, successful cannulization is more difficult in this population. A short, thick needle with a trocar tip is inserted into the intramedullary space of the bone. The richly vascularized intramedullary space allows for direct entry of drugs into the central circulation through emissary veins. The easiest insertion sites are the medial proximal tibia or the distal midline femur. Intraosseous infusion is a rapid and effective technique of achieving therapeutic serum concentrations of almost all important drugs; moreover, a large fluid volume can be rapidly administered in injured or dehydrated patients. The most common complication of this procedure is osteomyelitis.

F. Death in the Emergency Department

The sudden and unexpected death of an infant or child in the emergency department constitutes one of the most difficult situations in emergency practice. Chaplin and social services should be made available to aid in support to the family. Careful and compassionate dialogue between the physician and parents, and between the physician and emergency department staff, is essential to minimize chaos in the clinical setting and to reduce confusion and anger among bereaved families and department personnel. Provide the parents with a hospital contact should questions arise after their return home. Debriefing for health-care workers may also be appropriate within 48–72 hours to alleviate stress that may impair work performance or cause psychological disability.

CARDIOVASCULAR EMERGENCIES

Evaluation of cardiopulmonary function in children, especially in infants and younger children, requires special techniques. Vital signs are generally insensitive and nonspecific. Blood pressure poorly reflects volume status. In children, hypovolemia triggers compensatory tachycardia and intense peripheral vasoconstriction, which effectively maintains blood pressure until volume loss exceeds about 50% of intravascular volume.

Tachycardia, while sensitive to cardiopulmonary duress, is nonspecific. Normal heart rate also varies with age, and tachycardia is a common response to many types of stress (eg, fever, anxiety, hypoxia, hypovolemia). In children, assessment of volume status should focus primarily on skin signs (temperature, color, capillary refill, turgor) in combination with heart rate. Rate of urine output may be the next best measure of core perfusion. Adequate core blood flow results in 1–2 mL/kg/h of urine production. Therefore, in the unstable child with suspected perfusion abnormalities, a urinary bladder catheter is imperative to monitor output. Also, close monitoring of mental status and interaction with the surrounding environment is important indicators of adequate cardiopulmonary perfusion.

Cardiac rhythm disturbances in children are unusual. The most common disturbance is bradycardia, usually secondary to hypoxia. Properly applied pulse oximetry, at the triage desk or part of an initial clinical assessment, is an easy and useful method for rapid evaluation of oxygen saturation in patients with slow or rapid heart rates. When a primary tachycardia occurs, it is usually supraventricular in origin. In the distressed child, ECG monitoring will assist in evaluating cardiovascular status and in judging response to therapy.

DEHYDRATION

ESSENTIALS OF DIAGNOSIS

► Commonly occurs after severe or prolonged episodes of diarrhea and vomiting
► Significant signs include acute weight loss, listlessness, sunken eyes, dry mucous membranes, poor capillary refill, and tachycardia

▶ General Considerations

Acute dehydration is a common pediatric emergency. Diarrhea and vomiting are the most frequent causes. Other common causes are burn wounds, open wounds, fever or hyperthermia, sweating, inadequate fluid intake, polyuria, and poisoning.

▶ Clinical Findings

The smaller the child, the greater the risk for developing dehydration secondary to the high water body requirement resulting from their surface area/volume ratios. Clinical evaluation of the dehydrated child requires assessment of hydration status. Comparison of presenting weight with recent weights may be useful. Management is dictated by degree of acuity (mild, 3–5% weight loss; moderate, 10%; severe, 15%). Formulate initial treatment on the basis of clinical evaluation of degree of dehydration. Only three clinical signs have been found to be specific for diagnosis of 5% dehydration: prolonged capillary refill time, abnormal skin turgor, and abnormal respiratory pattern. Laboratory assessment of type of dehydration assists the physician in later strategies for specific electrolyte replacement. Serum sodium concentration is the most important laboratory parameter. Serum sodium concentration does not indicate degree of hydration but does provide a useful measure for titrating sodium repletion (ie hyponatremic, isotonatremic, or hypernatremic dehydration).

▶ Treatment

After rapid assessment of degree of dehydration, management must match severity of illness.

A. Oxygen and IV Access

For severely dehydrated patients, provide supplemental oxygen, attach pulse oximeter and cardiac monitor, and establish IV or intraosseous access with one or two secure catheters.

B. Volume Resuscitation

For a severely dehydrated infant or young child, rapidly infuse a balanced isotonic solution (eg, normal saline or lactated Ringer's). Infants and children have limited glycogen stores and are prone to hypoglycemia when stressed; rapid blood glucose analysis (eg, fingerstick blood sugar) should be performed, and glucose should be replaced if less than 60 mg/dL. Administer 5–10 mL/kg 10% dextrose in water for infants and young children and 2–4 mL/kg 25% dextrose in water for older children.

Administer an isotonic fluid bolus of 20 mL/kg, and then repeat boluses of 20 mL/kg until physical signs (heart rate, skin temperature, and capillary refill) indicate improved perfusion. After 60 mL/kg of isotonic fluid have been administered, if vital signs have not normalized, consider administration of albumin. Packed red blood cells, 10–20 mL/kg, should be considered in cases of blood loss from trauma.

Table 50–5. Daily Maintenance Requirements for Fluids and Electrolytes.

Weight	Water Requirement[a]	Sodium Requirement	Potassium Requirement[b]
1–10 kg	100 mL/kg		
11–20 kg	50 mL/kg + 1000 mL	3 mEq/kg	2 mEq/kg
>20 kg	20 mL/kg + 1500 mL		

[a]Assume that the child is normothermic. Fever significantly increases insensible water losses.
[b]Do not exceed 0.25 mEq/kg/h intravenously. Use oral route when possible. Add KCl to intravenous infusion after urination.

C. Other Measures

After stabilizing the patient, slow IV infusion to a maintenance rate (Table 50–5) and devise a therapeutic plan. Insert a urinary bladder catheter if the child has uncertain volume replacement requirements. Send blood for complete blood count (CBC); electrolytes; and glucose, blood urea nitrogen (BUN), and creatinine measurements. Obtain a urinalysis. Blood gas determination is indicated for the child who remains unstable after 60 mL/kg of volume administration.

When laboratory data are available, titrate sodium and water repletion accordingly. For hyponatremic and isonatremic dehydration, replace the calculated volume deficit over 24 hours, giving 50% of the deficit in the first 8 hours and the remaining 50% over the following 16 hours. Ongoing losses and maintenance requirements must also be included. Control fever, because insensible water losses are significantly increased by temperature elevation. Add small amounts of potassium to the ongoing infusion, once urination is observed, and replace calculated potassium deficits over 48 hours. The minimum daily maintenance requirements for water, sodium, and potassium are noted in Table 50–5. For hypernatremic dehydration, divide fluid and electrolyte replacement evenly over 48 hours to avoid rapid osmolal shifts and CNS complications.

D. Oral Rehydration Therapy

Use oral rehydration therapy (ORT) in most dehydrated patients. Children can usually take fluids by mouth. Vomiting does not contraindicate the use of ORT. Unless shock, altered mental status, or severe weakness is present, ORT may be used as part of early emergency department and inpatient management for most dehydrated patients. Other patients not requiring hospitalization can be easily rehydrated using this technique. ORT in the ED has been underutilized in favor of IV fluid therapy. Recently oral ondansetron (dose 0.15 mg/kg/dose) has been shown to reduce vomiting and facilitate successful ORT. The composition of ORT as set by the World Health Organization includes 90 mEq/L of sodium, 20 mEq/L potassium, 30 mEq/L of citrate, and

1–2% glucose concentration. Commercial preparations that provide approximately these constituents include Pedialyte®, Lytren®, and Infalyte®. Other commonly used clear liquids, such as colas, have too few electrolytes (Na, K, Cl), and their high sugar content may contribute to worsening of osmotic diarrhea. If the child can be discharged, prescribe home fluid replacement that is appropriate for the age of the child, the calculated deficit, and ongoing losses.

Freedman S, Thull-Freedman J: Pediatric dehydration assessment and oral rehydration therapy. Ped Emerg Med Rep 2008;13(2):13–28.

SHOCK

ESSENTIALS OF DIAGNOSIS

▶ Altered mental status
▶ Tachypnea, tachycardia
▶ Hypotension is a late sign in children

▶ Clinical Findings

Shock is inadequate oxygen delivery to tissues (See Chapter 11). Most causes of shock in children (eg, gastrointestinal fluid losses, burns, blood loss from acute injury) involve decreased stroke volume usually from hypovolemia (hypovolemic shock). Septic shock, a form of distributive shock, occurs usually in the patient under 2 years of age and must always be considered in the sick-appearing, febrile child. Anaphylactic shock, another form of distributive shock, may develop after bee stings or after in-hospital use of parenteral drugs or contrast agents. Cardiogenic shock is extremely rare in children but may complicate congenital heart disease or toxicologic emergencies. Neurogenic shock occurs in trauma, presenting with hypotension and bradycardia (Table 50–6).

Table 50–6. Management of Shock.

Hypoglycemic		
A.	Hemorrhagic	20 mL/kg NS/LR x 2-3 boluses Transfuse PRBC's as indicated
B.	Nonhemorrhagic	20 mL/kg NS/LR as needed Consider colloid after 3rd bolus
Distributive		
A.	Septic	See algorithm
B.	Anaphylactic	Epinephrine: 1:1000 (IM) 0.01 mg/kg to maximum of 0.5 mg Antihistamines Corticosteroids Albuterol nebulizer Racemic Epi nebulized for stridor
C.	Neurogenic	20 mL/kg NS/LR as needed vasopressors
Cardiogenic		
A.	Secondary to arrhythmia	Treat/manage the arrythymia
B.	Cardiomypoathy/myocarditis/congetive heart failure	5-10 ml/kg NS/LR Vasoactive infusion (doubtamine/milrinone)
Obstructive shock		
A.	Ductal dependent (LV outflow obstruction)	Prostaglandin E, consult cardiology
B.	Tension pneumothorax	Needle decompression, chest tube
C.	Cardiac tamponade	Pericardiocentesis 20 mL/kg NS/LR
D.	Thrombolytics	20 mL/kg NS/LR bolus Anticoagulants

Shock is not hypotension. Successful management includes early recognition of the compensated, normotensive phase of shock. During the compensated phase of hypovolemic shock, vital signs in the supine patient are usually normal, except for mild tachycardia. Skin signs of hypoperfusion are usually evident, and laboratory testing may disclose metabolic acidosis. Intervention is usually successful during this phase. When the hypotensive, de-compensated phase develops in the absence of recognition and effective treatment, irreversible shock and death may result.

▶ Treatment

Rapid clinical assessment should disclose a shock category so that focused treatment can be immediately instituted. Failure to act expeditiously and aggressively is a common error and may significantly increase mortality risk. Figure 50–1 is an algorithm for the treatment of uncompensated shock in neonates and Figure 50–2 is an algorithm for treatment of infants and children with uncompensated shock.

A. General Management

Consider immediate endotracheal intubation. In the ill-appearing child with signs of shock and sepsis or the frankly hypotensive child, intubation should be accomplished either immediately or after the patient fails to respond to first-line resuscitation with oxygen and fluids. After intubation, insert a nasogastric tube.

Apply supplemental oxygen, attach pulse oximeter and cardiac monitor, establish two secure IV catheters, check fingerstick blood glucose, and insert urinary bladder catheter.

B. Volume Resuscitation

Initiate volume resuscitation. Start with 20 cc/kg of isotonic saline administered as rapidly as access will allow. The bolus may be repeated up to two times if no clinical response. If there remains no response after 60 mL/kg, consider colloid or packed red blood cell transfusion or administration of an inotropic agent. When inotropic agents are used, the intravascular volume must be adequate. Inotropic infusions used are dependent on etiology of shock. They can then be titrated at bedside, often using multiple infusions (dopamine, epinephrine, dobutamine), until perfusion is restored. Start with epinephrine at 0.1–1.0 μg/kg/min or dopamine 10–20 μg/kg/min, and then add a second inotropic agent if cardiovascular response does not occur. If physical examination is equivocal for hydration status, a chest X-ray may help: dehydration or overhydration is reflected in the appearance of pulmonary vessels.

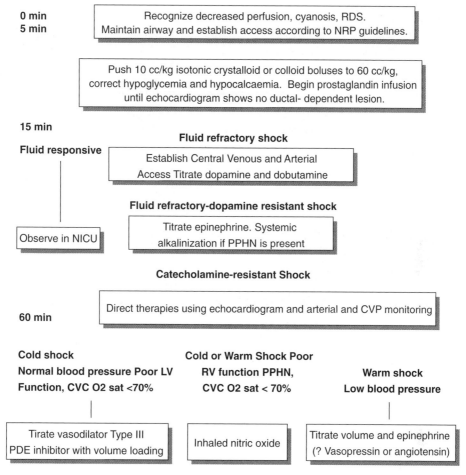

0 min
5 min
Recognize decreased perfusion, cyanosis, RDS.
Maintain airway and establish access according to NRP guidelines.

Push 10 cc/kg isotonic crystalloid or colloid boluses to 60 cc/kg,
correct hypoglycemia and hypocalcaemia. Begin prostaglandin infusion
until echocardiogram shows no ductal- dependent lesion.

15 min

Fluid responsive

Fluid refractory shock

Establish Central Venous and Arterial
Access Titrate dopamine and dobutamine

Fluid refractory-dopamine resistant shock

Observe in NICU

Titrate epinephrine. Systemic
alkalinization if PPHN is present

Catecholamine-resistant Shock

Direct therapies using echocardiogram and arterial and CVP monitoring

60 min

Cold shock
Normal blood pressure Poor LV
Function, CVC O2 sat <70%

Cold or Warm Shock Poor
RV function PPHN,
CVC O2 sat < 70%

Warm shock
Low blood pressure

Tirate vasodilator Type III
PDE inhibitor with volume loading

Inhaled nitric oxide

Titrate volume and epinephrine
(? Vasopressin or angiotensin)

▲ **Figure 50–1.** Recommendations for stepwise management of hemodynamic support in neonates with goals of normal perfusion and perfusion pressure. PDE, phosphodiesterase; PPHN, persistent pulmonary hypertension, $CVCO_2$, central vena cava oxygen saturation. In refractory shock: rule out and correct pericardial effusion, pneumonthorax. Use hydrocortisone for absolute adrenal insufficiency and consider ECMO. (From Carcillo JA, Fields AI et al: Clinical practice parameters for hemodynamic support of pediatric and neonatal patients in septic shock. Crit Care Med 2002;30 (6)1372.)

C. Other Measures

Obtain arterial blood gases, CBC, electrolytes, platelets, coagulation studies, blood, urine, and spinal fluid cultures (if infection is suspected), and urinalysis. A urine drug screen may also be considered. A chest X-ray is also necessary in most cases. Administer broad spectrum antibiotics if infection suspected.

Carcillo JA: Pediatric septic shock and multiple organ failure. Crit Care Clin 2003;19:413 [PMID: 12848313].

Freedman SB, Adler M, Seshadri R et al: Oral ondansetron for gastroenteritis in a pediatric emergency department. N Engl J Med 2006;354:16,1698–1705 [PMID: 16625009].

CONGESTIVE HEART FAILURE

 ESSENTIALS OF DIAGNOSIS

► Sweating during feeding or crying; failure to thrive

► Tachypnea, tachycardia

► Hepatomegaly

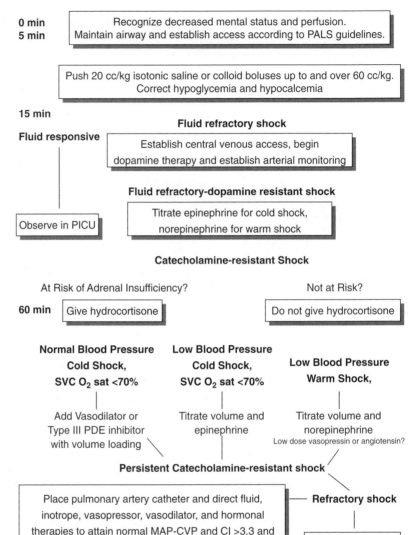

▲ **Figure 50–2.** Recommendations for stepwise management of hemodynamic support in infants and children with goals of normal perfusion and perfusion pressure (mean arterial pressure–central venous pressure [MAP–CVP]). Proceed to next step if shock persists. PALS, pediatric advanced life support; PICU, pediatric intensive care unit; SVC O$_2$, superior vena cava oxygen; PDE, phosphodiesterase; CI, cardiac index; ECMO, extracorporeal membrane oxygenation. (From Carillo JA, Fields AI: American College of Critical Care Medicine Task Force Committee Members: clinical practice parameters for hemodynamic support of pediatric and neonatal patients in septic shock. Crit Care Med 2002;30:1370.)

▶ Clinical Findings

Congestive heart failure (CHF) is unusual in childhood. When it does present, it is usually as a manifestation of congenital heart disease and is seen in the first year of life. Table 50–7 lists the structural conditions causing CHF at different times during infancy. The classic triad of symptoms for pediatric CHF is tachypnea, tachycardia, and hepatomegaly. There may also be a history of poor feeding, sweating or color change with feeding, and poor weight gain. Lower extremity edema and jugular venous distention are less likely in the pediatric population.

▶ Evaluation of the Neonate with Cyanosis

Cyanosis in neonates is usually due to either pulmonary or cardiac disease. A CXR, ECG, and hyperoxia test should be obtained in all neonates with unexplained cyanosis. The hyperoxia test is performed by obtaining an initial ABG from the right radial artery on room air. A second ABG is obtained after 10 minutes of breathing 100% FiO$_2$. In general, the PaO$_2$ will rise on 100% FiO$_2$ to greater than 80 mmHg in neonates with pulmonary disease. In contrast, it will remain unchanged or only slightly increase in those with cyanotic heart disease (Table 50–8).

Table 50–7. Differential Diagnosis of Congestive Heart Failure Based on Age of Presentation.

Age	Spectrum	

1 min
1 h
	Noncardiac origin: anemia,
	  acidosis, hypoxia, hypoglycemia,
	  hypocalcemia, sepsis
		} Acquired

1 day 1 week 2 weeks 1 month	PDA in premature infants HPLV Coarctation Ventricular septal defect	} Congenital
3 months 1 year 10 years	Supraventricular tachycardia Myocarditis Cardiomyopathy Severe anemia Rheumatic fever	} Acquired

Abbreviations: HPLV, hypoplastic left ventricle; PDA, patent ductus arteriosus. (Source Tintinalli. 6th ed. 763.)

▶ Treatment

When CHF has progressed to frank pulmonary edema, the treatment is as follows.

A. General Management

Apply supplemental oxygen as necessary including endotracheal intubation in the severely distressed, hypotensive, or hypoxic patient (pulse oximetry < 85% on 100% oxygen). Apply a pulse oximeter and cardiac monitor. Establish secure IV access. Insert urinary bladder catheter and check fingerstick blood sugar.

B. Pharmacologic Treatment

Pharmacologic treatment can be critically important for patients with left heart obstructive lesions such as hypoplastic left heart syndrome, severe coarctation of the aorta, interrupted aortic arch, and critical valvular aortic stenosis. The newborn is extremely dependent on a patent ductus arteriosus to supply systemic flow. Initial management may require

Table 50–8. Cardiac Lesions Causing Cyanosis in the Infant.

Cyanotic Lesions
Tetrology of fallot
Transposition of great vessels
Tricupid atresia
Total anomalous pulmonary venous return
Triscusid ateriosus
Complete artervioventricular canal
Epstein's anomaly of the tricuspid valve
Single ventricle states

administration of prostaglandin E1 (.05–0.1 μg/kg/min) if a ductal-dependent cardiac lesion is suspected. Apnea is the main side effect of prostaglandin E1; therefore consider intubation prior to transport of a patient during an infusion. In other cases, first-line pharmacologic management is furosemide, 1 mg/kg IV.

C. Other Measures

Obtain chest X-ray, ECG, CBC, and serum electrolytes, with additional studies if indicated. Consider digoxin in refractory cases. Occasionally, patients with severe pulmonary edema unresponsive to initial therapy require dopamine, dobutamine, or both.

Costello J, Almodovar M: Emergency care for infant and children with acute cardiac disease. Clin Ped Emerg Med 2007;8:145–155.

Yee L: Cardiac emergencies in the first year of life. Emerg Med Clin North Am 2007;25:981–1008 [PMID: 17950133].

CARDIAC DYSRHYTHMIAS

▶ Clinical Findings

Dysrhythmias are relatively rare in the pediatric population, with the most common being sinus tachycardia, supraventricular tachycardia, and bradycardia. Atrial flutter may be present in patients having undergone cardiac shunting surgeries (ie Fontan procedure) These can present a diagnostic challenge to the emergency physician as vague and nonspecific symptoms may be the rule. Evaluation of dysrhythmias includes a rapid cardiopulmonary assessment and ECG interpretation using a systematic approach and comparison with age-specific norms.

▶ Treatment

See Table 50–9.

A. General Management

Apply supplemental oxygen; attach pulse oximeter and cardiac monitor. Establish a secure IV line. Obtain an ECG.

B. Cardioversion

Unstable patients with tachydysrhythmias require immediate electrical cardioversion or defibrillation. Unsynchronized mode is recommended for ventricular fibrillation and pulseless ventricular tachycardia, synchronized for the remaining rhythms. Exact energy levels are dictated by the nature of the dysrhythmia (see Table 50–9).

Ensure that paddles are held firmly against chest wall and a good conductive agent is employed. If standard 4.5-cm pediatric paddles are unavailable for sternoapical placement, use adult paddles in an anteroposterior configuration.

Table 50–9. Treatment of Common Pediatric Dysrhythmias.

Rhythm	Rate/min	QRS	Initial Treatment	Drug Therapy
Narrow complex tachycardia's				
1. Sinus tachycardia	100-250	<0.10	Oxygen, fluids, warmth, calm manner	Treatment of primary condition
2. Atrail flutter	300-500	<0.10	If unstable, synchronized electrical DC cardioversion 0.5-1 J/kg If unaffected, increase to 2 J/Kg. Sedate if possible If stable see Drug Therapy	Digoxin 10 mcg/k Procainamide 15 mg/kg IV over 30-60 min Amiodarone 5 mg/kg over 20-60 min (max 300 mg)
3. Atrail fibrillation	Ventricle response 60-90 irregularly Irregular	<0.10	See atrail flutter May need anticoagulation pretreatment	See atrail flutter Consider cardiology consult
4. Supraventricular Wolf-Parkinson-White	120-300	<0.10	If stable try vagal maneuvers If unstable: synchronized cardioversion at 0.51-1 J/kg	Adenosine 0.1 mg/k rapid IV push max 6 mg single first dose if unaffective repeat at 0.2 mg/kg (max 12 mg)
Wide complex tachycardias				
1. Ventricular tachycardic	150-260	>0.10	If unstable with a pulse, synchronized cardioversion 0.5 J/kg If pulseless, treat like ventricular fibrillation	Amiodorone5 mg/k over 20-60 min or Procainamide 15 mg/kg over 30-60min Do not administer procainamide and amiodarone together or Lidocaine 1 mg/kg IV bolus
2. Wolff- Parkinson White	150-300	>0.10	As for ventricular tachycardia	As for ventricular tachycardia
Ventricular fibrillation	300-500	Variable	DC defibrillation 2 J/kg if unaffected, double to 4 J/kg	Epinephrine (1:10,000) 0.1 ml/k Amiodarone 5 mg/kg or Lidocaine 1mg/kg bolus
Torsades de points	300-500	Variable		Magnesium sulfate: 25-50 mg/kg (max 2 grams)
Bradycardia				
1. Sinus	Age-related	<0.10	Oxygen, airway management stimulation	Epinephrine (1:10,000) 0.1 ml/kg Atropine 0.02 mg/kg (minimum 0.1 mg) If vagal in nature Pacing
2. AV-V block	Age-related	Variable	Oxygen if unstable transcutaneous pacing	as for sinus brady cardia

Pretreat conscious patients requiring cardioversion with light sedation, and be prepared to perform endotracheal intubation and full cardiopulmonary resuscitation if necessary.

Samsin R, Atkins D: Tachyarrhythmias and defibrillation. Ped clin North Am 2008;55:887–907 [PMID: 18675025].

O'Connor M, Mc Daniel N, Brady W: Pediatric dysrrthymias. Am J Emerg Med 2008;26:348–358 [PMID: 18358948].

▼ RESPIRATORY DISTRESS

In children, normal ventilation and oxygenation occurs with minimal visible effort. Evaluation of respiratory function includes assessment of rate, work of breathing, skin and mucous membranes color, and mental status. Respiratory rate alone is an insensitive means of evaluating for respiratory distress. Rates vary greatly with age, anxiety, excitement, or fever, and interobserver reproducibility is often poor. Tachypnea may be an early manifestation of respiratory distress, or it may result from respiratory compensation for metabolic acidosis caused by shock, diabetic ketoacidosis, inborn errors of metabolism, salicylism, or chronic renal insufficiency. A slow respiratory rate may indicate impending respiratory failure.

Observation alone will usually disclose distress or increased work of breathing. Increased work of breathing is also evidenced by nasal flaring and by suprasternal, intercostal, and subcostal retractions. Retractions become more pronounced cephalad to caudad with increasing hypoxia. Grunting is produced by premature glottic closure and usually represents alveolar collapse and loss of lung volume, which develops in patients with pulmonary edema, pneumonia, or atelectasis. Auscultation will provide further differentiation of disease possibilities. Wheezing, rales, or decreased breath sounds may be present. Cyanosis, when present, represents severe distress and is best seen on mucous membranes of the mouth and nail beds. Peripheral cyanosis is more likely due to circulatory failure than a primary pulmonary source. Finally, mental status changes may be a clue to gas exchange abnormalities. Hypoxic patients are restless and agitated; hypercapnic patients are drowsy or even comatose.

Rapid evaluation of respiratory function is imperative in all distressed pediatric patients. Respiratory failure and respiratory arrest due to a wide spectrum of causes (eg, head trauma, coma, poisoning, pneumonia, asthma, foreign body aspiration) are the most common causes of cardiac arrest in childhood. Timely, aggressive intervention in the early stages as well as meticulous respiratory monitoring by means of pulse oximetry and continuous observation will avert preventable adverse patient outcomes. Children with respiratory distress should not be sent for imaging studies without qualified personnel in attendance. Early hospital admission is usually warranted for such patients.

Pulse oximetry should be used liberally in the emergency department setting in order to disclose undetected oxygen desaturation states. Pulse oximetry is noninvasive, simple, and reasonably accurate. Readings may be difficult to obtain in patients with poor perfusion or cold sites of placement. In selected patients, especially those with significant tachypnea or work of breathing, pulse oximetry may underestimate degree of distress, and it provides no indication as to the adequacy of ventilation. In such patients, it may be necessary to obtain arterial blood gas levels to help measure the severity and nature of the ventilation or oxygenation disturbance.

APNEA

▶ General Considerations

Apnea is defined as an unexplained episode of cessation of breathing for 20 seconds or longer, or a shorter respiratory pause associated with bradycardia, cyanosis, pallor, and/or marked hypotonia. Ordinary sleep will sometimes cause breathing irregularities easily confused with apnea. There are two classifications of apnea: central and obstructive. Central apnea is characterized by an absence of respiratory effort secondary to diminished muscular activation. It occurs in newborn infants, most commonly in preterm infants. Infection, metabolic abnormalities, anemia, hypoxia, or CNS injury may be associated with newborn apnea. Obstructive apnea occurs in later infancy and childhood and is related to obstructive upper airway conditions. This results in cessation of airflow despite respiratory effort, as can be seen with chest and abdominal movement. Apnea may be accompanied by color change, marked change in muscle tone (usually limpness), choking or gagging which is frightening to the observer. This is the definition for apparent life-threatening event (ALTE).

▶ Treatment

A. Apnea in Infants

Apnea in infants may be symptomatic of life-threatening illness. Such patients ordinarily require hospital admission for observation and full workup for infections and for CNS, metabolic, and feeding problems. Initial management in the emergency department is discussed here.

1. Oxygenation and ventilation—Place child on supplemental oxygen, and apply pulse oximeter and cardiac monitor or apnea monitor.

2. Volume resuscitation—If evidence of dehydration is present, establish IV access and replete with an isotonic fluid bolus.

3. Laboratory and imaging studies—Obtain blood for CBC with differential, electrolytes, BUN, creatinine, ionized calcium and magnesium, and cultures. Obtain urinalysis and urine cultures as well as toxicology studies. CT of the head should be strongly considered for evaluation of any infant with abnormal mental status, bulging fontanelle, or focal neurological examination. Spinal fluid analysis should also be considered in any lethargic- or toxic-appearing infant.

4. Other measures—Admit for observation and further evaluation on an apnea monitor.

B. Apnea in Children

Obstructive apnea may be serious. Focus evaluation on obstructive upper pharyngeal lesions such as tonsillitis and pharyngitis or laryngomalacia. Chest X-ray and lateral neck films are often necessary. Emergency department evaluation may be insufficient to exclude a serious diagnosis, such as airway masses, and hospital admission may be indicated.

C. ALTE

The evaluation for ALTE is primarily dependent upon the history and physical exam. Currently, in-hospital observation and monitoring remain an accepted treatment, especially in infants less than 48 weeks postconceptional age.

UPPER AIRWAY OBSTRUCTION

ESSENTIALS OF DIAGNOSIS

▶ Inspiratory stridor

▶ Suspect foreign body aspirations if symptoms develop rapidly without associated signs of infection

▶ Anteroposterior and lateral neck X-rays are helpful to differentiate croup from epiglottitis and foreign body

▶ Clinical Findings

Upper airway obstruction is usually readily apparent. Inspiratory stridor is the hallmark. The child is dyspneic and shows signs of respiratory distress, including tachypnea, nasal flaring, and supraclavicular, intercostal, and subcostal retractions. Ventilation and oxygenation abnormalities are sometimes present. If obstruction is severe, hypercapnia will be present, usually along with depressed mental status, cyanosis, and decreased air movement. Arterial blood gases will demonstrate carbon dioxide retention and often hypoxemia. Pulse oximetry will be abnormal in most advanced cases but normal in typical cases (see Figure 50–3).

▶ Differential Diagnosis

In children, the common causes of stridor and upper airway obstruction are croup, epiglottitis, and foreign body aspiration (see Table 50–10). Other less common conditions producing stridor are bacterial tracheitis (usually *Staphylococcus aureus, Streptococcus pneumoniae*, or *Haemophilus influenzae*), retropharyngeal or peritonsillar abscess, trauma, caustic ingestions, neoplasm, or angioneurotic edema.

▶ Treatment

Clear the airway using procedures recommended in Table 50–11 for the patient with complete airway obstruction. Avoid airway clearance maneuvers in the patient with partial airway obstruction as this may result in further progression to a complete obstruction. Allow the child to adopt a position of comfort, usually on a parent's lap. Apply supplemental oxygen, and attach pulse oximeter and cardiac monitor. Avoid procedures or interventions that cause agitation or worsening symptoms.

A. Anaphylaxis

Anaphylaxis is a life-threatening manifestation of immediate hypersensitivity. It is an IgE-mediated reaction that occurs after re-exposure to an antigen. Symptoms develop within 30 minutes of exposure to the inciting agent. Manifestation may be mild, demonstrating urticaria or severe involving

upper airway obstruction resulting from edema of the larynx, epiglottis, and surrounding structures. Hypotension, secondary to profound vasodilatation and seizures may occur.

Management consists of maintenance of airway and oxygenation. Attach a pulse oximeter and cardiac monitor. Initial pharmacologic management consists of administration of epinephrine (1:1000), 0.01 mL/kg (max 0.5 mL) IM. For bronchospasm (wheezing), administer albuterol by metered-dose inhaler (MDI) or nebulizer. For stridor, racemic epinephrine 2.25% solution dosed 0.05 mL/kg (max 0.5 mL) diluted with normal saline to volume of 3 mL for nebulization. For hypotension, administer 20 mL/kg bolus isotonic fluids with the addition of inotropic agents if needed. Other therapies include: H-1 receptor-blocking antihistamines, such as diphenhydramine (1 mg/kg) IV/PO/IM; corticosteroids (1–2 mg/kg methylprednisolone IV, max 125 mg, or oral prednisone 1–2 mg/kg (max 80); H-2 receptor-blocking antihistamines such as cimetidine (5 mg/kg, max 300 mg) or ranitidine (1–2 mg/kg, max 50 mg) work synergistically with H-1 blocking antihistamines. Children with airway involvement should be monitored for 24 hours. Discharge instructions must involve instruction and dispension of epinephrine auto-injector use.

B. Epiglottitis

Epiglottitis has become much less common since the introduction of the *H. influenzae* type B vaccine. The epidemiology has now changed to more commonly involve older children and adolescents, with *Staphylococcus* and *Streptococcus* being the most common etiologic agents. The patient often presents with dysphonia and dysphagia and sits in the sniffing position. The findings on oropharyngeal examination are typically unimpressive. However, the patient may rapidly progress to stridor and complete airway obstruction. In such cases, early airway management is essential, preferably in the operating room. In the meantime, minimize all invasive procedures in order to avert patient agitation and potential precipitous airway obstruction, and ensure that equipment for airway management is readily available. The patient should not be left unattended at any point.

Once the airway is secured, obtain blood and throat cultures and begin antibiotic therapy with second or third generation cephalosporins plus coverage for the treatment of possible methicillin-resistant Staphylococcus with vancomycin.

In a patient with a lower likelihood of epiglottitis, a soft tissue lateral film of the neck may be useful to help demonstrate the swollen epiglottis (Figure 50–4).

C. Bacterial Tracheitis

Bacterial tracheitis is also known as psuedomembranous croup, is characterized by prodromal viral upper respiratory symptoms with low grade fever, cough, and stridor similar to croup. Unlike epiglottis, a cough may be present. Typically, the child is without drooling and may be comfortable lying

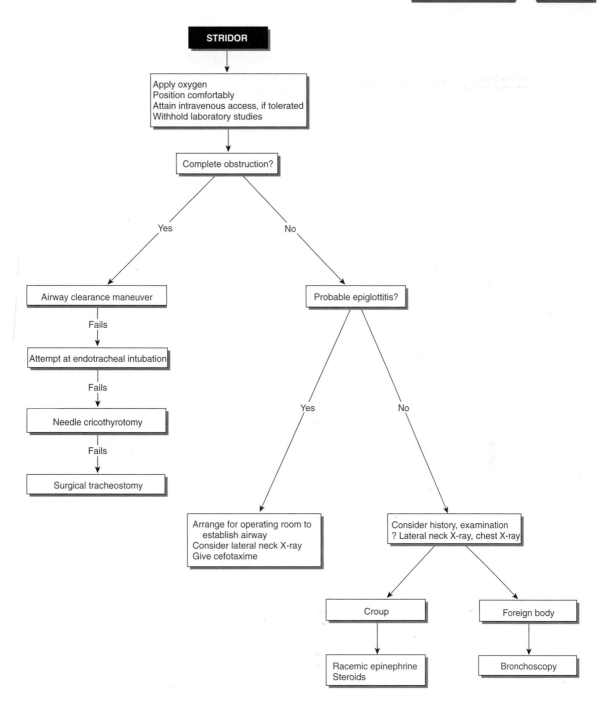

▲ **Figure 50–3.** Treatment algorithm for pediatric stridor.

flat. Routine laboratory data are not indicated. The diagnosis is made endoscopically by visualizing normal supraglottic structures with prominent subglottic edema, ulcerations, and copious purulent secretion. Patients with severe distress are best managed in the operating suite for endoscopic diagnosis and intubation. If emergency department intubation is required, an endotracheal tube smaller that the calculated size for the patient may be necessary. Antibiotic coverage should be initiated with a third generation cephalosporin plus vancomycin.

Table 50–10. Differential Diagnosis of Upper Airway Obstruction.

	Croup	Epiglottitis	Foreign Body
Age	6 months to 3 years	2–5 years	Under 3 years
Cause	Parainfluenza	*Strep. pyogenes, Strep. pneumoniae, Staph. aureus, H. influenzae* (rare)	Foreign body
Season	Fall or winter	Any	Any
Time of day	Night or morning	Any	Daytime
Illness features			
Onset	Slow	Abrupt	Abrupt
Upper respiratory infection	Yes	No	No
Fever	Generally low grade	High	None
Toxic	Mild	Yes	No
Pharyngitis	Possible	Yes	No
Drooling	No	Yes	No
Stridor	Inspiratory + expiratory	Inspiratory	Inspiratory + expiratory
Position	Variable	Sitting	Variable
Hoarseness	Yes	Rare	No
Ancillary tests			
White blood count	Normal	High	Normal
Chest X-ray	Steeple sign	Normal	Hyperinflation
Lateral neck	Normal	Swollen epiglottis, "thumbprint sign"	May show radiopaque body

Table 50–11. Management of Complete Foreign Body Obstruction in Infants and Children.

Status	Infant (up to age 1 year)	Child (1–8 years)
Conscious	Patient unable to ventilate: five back blows with infant in prone, head-down position, then five chest thrusts with infant supine, head-down position Repeat as above until patient becomes unconscious	Patient unable to ventilate: perform Heimlich maneuver—abdominal thrusts above the umbilicus standing behind the victim Continue thrusts until foreign body is expelled or victim becomes unconscious
Unconscious	Open airway, perform tongue–jaw lift If able to visualize foreign body, remove it If no spontaneous respirations, attempt rescue breathing If unsuccessful . . . Reposition airway and try again, then . . . Start cycle again, repeat back blows, chest thrusts, open airway, attempt to ventilate Emergency medical services activation after 1 min If spontaneous respirations resume, place in recovery position	Lower victim to the ground Open airway with tongue–jaw lift Remove any visible foreign body If no spontaneous respirations, attempt to ventilate If unsuccessful . . . Straddle or kneel beside the victim Begin abdominal thrusts with heel of hand positioned above umbilicus and below xiphoid process Open airway and repeat steps until obstruction is relieved

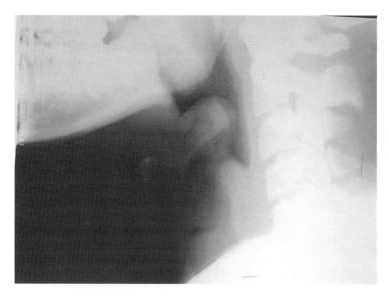

▲ **Figure 50–4.** Lateral soft tissue X-ray of the neck, showing thumbprint sign of epiglottitis.

D. Croup (Laryngotracheobronchitis)

Croup is infection and inflammation of the subglottic airway causing upper airway obstruction. It is characterized by barking cough, hoarseness, and inspiratory stridor. The physician must note that symptoms are typically more severe at night; thus the presentation may not be as impressive in daytime hours. Therapy includes the following:

1. Initial steps—Attach pulse oximeter and cardiac monitor. Keep the child in a position of comfort, usually on the parent's lap. Cool humidified mist, although frequently administered, has not been shown to be effective in improving clinical symptoms in children presenting to the ED.

2. Pharmacologic treatment—Give glucocorticoids to any child who presents with croup symptoms and demonstrates increased work of breathing. Give PO/IM/IV dexamethasone, 0.6 mg/kg (max 10 mg) once. In more severe cases, nebulized epinephrine should be considered. This can provide immediate improvement though reduction in edema and secretions. Dosage for nebulization is 0.5 mL/kg (maximum of 5 mL) of 1:1000 preparation of epinephrine, or racemic epinephrine 2.25% is dosed at 0.05 mL/kg (maximum 0.5 mL) diluted with normal saline to a total volume of 3 mL. In severe croup, consider administration of heliox (a mixture of helium and oxygen). In patients unresponsive to nebulized epinephrine, steroids or heliox, endotracheal intubation and ventilation may be necessary. Using a tube with a diameter smaller than recommended for patient age and size should be used.

For the minimally distressed child, treatment with steroids may be adequate. For patients who receive nebulized epinephrine, caution must be taken because the clinical effects of epinephrine wane after 2 hours. All patients should be monitored during this time period for worsening or return of symptoms. Those who remain without stridor or hypoxia, appear comfortable, and tolerating oral fluids may be discharged with a reliable parent. All others should be hospitalized for observation and further treatment.

E. Foreign Body Aspiration

Foreign body aspiration can have a constellation of physical findings depending on the degree of occlusion of the airway. The presentations can range from a complete obstruction managed by the Heimlich maneuver to a protracted course of wheezing not responsive to bronchodilators. The history can be highly suggestive, with a brief asymptomatic interval followed by severe dyspnea, coughing, and gagging, after the child has handled a small object. In 20% of cases, the object is in the upper airway; in 80% it is in the main-stem or lobar bronchus. Stridor is present if the object is lodged high, at the level of the larynx; wheezing and decreased breath sounds occur if it is lodged below the larynx. Mild tachypnea may be the only clinical sign in some instances. Useful X-ray views include the lateral neck, chest, and bilateral lateral decubitus end-expiratory chest, which may show hyper-inflation in the affected lung.

1. Complete obstruction—If obstruction is complete and airway clearance maneuvers (see Table 50–11) fail, perform laryngoscopy immediately, and attempt to remove the foreign body with Magill forceps under direct visualization. After removal of a foreign body, insert a properly sized endotracheal tube to prevent later inflammatory obstruction.

2. Partial obstruction—In most patients, obstruction is partial. Apply supplemental oxygen, and attach pulse oximeter and cardiac monitor. Allow the patient to assume a position of comfort, usually on parent's lap. Obtain airway and chest X-rays. Maintain constant observation of the patient by nurse or physician. Arrange for rigid bronchoscopy, under general anesthesia, to remove the foreign object.

Shah S Sharieff G: Pediatric respiratory infections. Emerg Med Clin North Am 2007;25:961–979 [PMID: 17950132].

Silverstri J: Apparent life-threatening eents in the young infant and neonate. Clin Ped Emeg Med 2008;9:194–190.

Al-Kindy H et al: Risk factors for extreme events in infants hospitalized for apparent life-threatening events. J Pediatr 2009;154:332–337 [PMID: 1895079].

LOWER AIRWAY DISORDERS

Lower airway disorders are a disparate group of conditions with varying clinical presentations that may affect oxygenation and ventilation. Lower airway disease includes both obstructive conditions and parenchymal or alveolar disease. The clinical hallmarks are dyspnea and tachypnea, often with cough. Wheezing denotes an obstructive process.

In children, the most common causes of lower airway obstruction are bronchiolitis, asthma, and foreign body obstruction. In infants, congenital abnormalities of the airway (tracheal web, cysts, vascular rings, lobar emphysema) must also be considered. Pneumonia is the most frequent pediatric alveolar disorder, although pulmonary edema, pneumonitis, inhalation injury, and cystic fibrosis must also be excluded.

1. Bronchiolitis

▶ Clinical Findings

Bronchiolitis is a clinical syndrome characterized by the acute onset of respiratory symptoms in a child younger than 2 years of age. The typical course consists of an upper respiratory tract infection progressing within 4–6 days to involve the lower respiratory tract with the onset of cough and wheezing. Respiratory syncytial virus (RSV) is the most common underlying viral infection. More than half of the affected children are between 2 and 7 months of age. Clinical signs of respiratory distress are variable. The white blood cell (WBC) count may be slightly elevated or normal. Hyperinflation, patchy infiltrates, and atelectasis may all be seen on chest X-ray.

▶ Treatment

A. General Management

Supportive care is the mainstay of therapy. Ensure hydration, oxygenation, and clearing of secretions with nasal suction. Intubation may be required for respiratory failure. Attach pulse oximeter, apply supplemental oxygen for saturations < 92%.

B. Medical Therapy

There is conflicting evidence as to the efficacy of bronchodilator therapy in bronchiolitis.

If wheezing is present, a trial of nebulized epinephrine or albuterol can be considered. Bronchodilators should be continued only if there is a documented clinical response.

Deep nasal suctioning is helpful. Nebulized 3% hypertonic saline seems to provide a beneficial effect as an adjunct to aid in clearance of thickened secretions. Recent reviews recommend that steroid therapy not be given. Heliox (a mixture of helium and oxygen), high flow nasal oxygen, or nasal continuous positive airway pressure (CPAP) may be trialed prior to intubation for severe or refractory disease.

C. Other Measures

Obtain a chest X-ray and consider a nasopharyngeal swab for RSV viral testing.

▶ Disposition

Infants younger than 2 months of age, former premature infants, any history of apnea or cyanosis, and those with underlying chronic medical conditions or congenital abnormalities should be strongly considered for admission, as well as any patient with persistent tachypnea, hypoxia, or toxic appearance.

Seiden J, Scarfone R Bronchiolitis: An evidence-based approach to management. Clin Ped Emerg Med 2009;10:75–81.

2. Asthma

▶ Clinical Findings

Asthma is one of the most common diseases of childhood and accounts for over 15% of all emergency department visits. It is characterized by bronchial hyperreactivity, airway inflammation, and reversible airway obstruction. The overall prevalence of asthma is increasing. Despite significant efforts in treatment and management, mortality rates have not improved, especially in urban areas.

Pulmonary function tests are also of great importance in assessing the severity of an exacerbation. Peak flow testing is relatively easy to perform and has been shown to be relatively successful even in young children. The patient's baseline value is especially useful, if known; otherwise comparison can be made with the patient's predicted value. Chest X-rays are usually not indicated in afebrile patients with known disease, but may be of assistance when the etiology is unclear. Arterial blood gas is indicated in more severe exacerbations. Close monitoring of PCO_2 should occur as normalization or elevation can indicate impending respiratory failure.

When a patient presents during and asthma exacerbation, important historical information includes recent steroid use, prior intensive care unit admissions, prior intubations secondary to asthma, preceding triggers, medications and frequency of their use, and baseline peak expiratory flow rates (PEFRs).

▶ Treatment

See Figure 50–5.

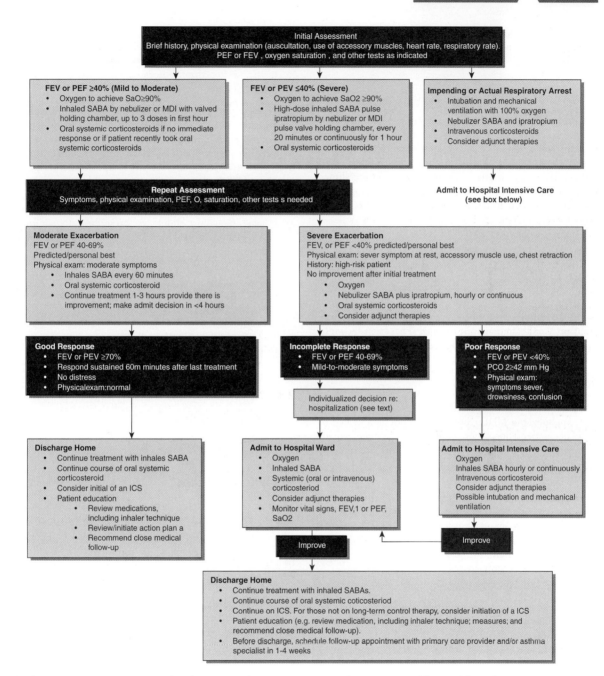

▲ Figure 50–5. Management of asthma exacerbation: emergency department and hospital-based care. Key: FEV1, forced expiratory volume in 1 second: ICS, inhaled corticosteroid; MDI, metered-dose inhaler; $_{PCO_2}$, partial pressure carbon dioxide; PEF peak expiratory flow; SABA, short-acting β2-agonist; SaO_2, oxygen saturation. (Reproduced from National Institutes of Health: National Asthma Education and Prevention Program. Expert Panel 3: guidelines for the diagnosis and management of asthma. August 2007. NIH publication no 07-4051.)

A. General Management

Attach pulse oximeter, provide supplemental oxygen therapy, if required.

B. Pharmacologic Therapy

1. Inhaled β_2-agonists—These are the first-line agents for the treatment of the acute asthma exacerbation, causing the rapid relaxation of bronchial smooth muscle. Albuterol is typically the agent used (0.15 mg/kg; maximum 5 mg). Both metered dose inhaler and nebulizer have been shown to be equally efficacious. Nebulizer is the method of choice in young children who may have difficulty with proper inhaler use.

2. Glucocorticoids—Glucocorticoids are indicated for all children with asthma who present in an acute exacerbation. The initial dose of prednisone is 1–2 mg/kg, with a maximum of 60 mg. Oral and IV routes have been shown to be equivalent.

3. Ipratropium bromide—Ipratropium is used as an adjuvant therapy to β-agonist therapy. It has been shown to decrease ED treatment time and improve pulmonary function testing. Dosing is 250 mcg per nebulized treatment for patients' weights less than 15 kg and 500 mcg for weights greater than 15 kg.

4. Epinephrine or terbutaline—In severe exacerbations where nebulizer or MDI treatments may not be tolerated or rapid decompensation occurs, subcutaneous epinephrine or terbutaline (0.01 mg/kg up to 0.3–0.5 mg) or IV terbutaline (10 μg/kg over 10 minutes followed by infusion of 0.4 μg/kg/min) may be considered.

5. Magnesium—Several conflicting studies exist but data have been shown that magnesium sulfate has improved pulmonary function and reduce hospitalizations in certain subgroups. Dosage is 25–50 mg/kg (maximum of 2.0 g) over 20 minutes. Close monitoring for hypotension is indicated.

C. Adjunctive Treatments

Bi-level positive airway pressure (BiPaP) in treating pediatric status asthmatics is safe and effective with resulting prevention of intubation.

Ketamine intravenous infusions have also been controversial in the management of severe asthma exacerbations. However, infusion at a bolus dose of 0.2 mg/kg followed by an infusion of 0.5 mg/kg was not found beneficial.

D. Intubation

The only absolute indications for intubation in an asthma exacerbation are coma and respiratory arrest. Worsening ventilatory status despite maximized treatment is a relative indication. Clinical judgment must be used on a patient by patient basis. Due to significant difficulty attaining adequate ventilation and oxygenation while avoiding barotraumas, permissive hypercarbia by means of low tidal volumes and a prolonged expiratory phase has been used.

▶ Disposition

There are no absolute guidelines for admission or discharge of a pediatric asthma patient and the decision is highly dependent on response to therapy. Intensive care unit admission is required for patients with an altered level of consciousness, hypotension, or respiratory failure. Hospitalization is highly recommended for patients with poor social situation, history of near-fatal asthma, or inability to tolerate oral medications. If the clinical decision is made to discharge the patient home, an inhaled β_2-agonist should be prescribed. In addition, steroids (eg, prednisone 2 mg/kg/d) should be strongly considered and close follow-up should be arranged.

Allen J, Macias G: The efficacy of ketamine in pediatric emergency department patients who present with acute severe asthma. Ann Emerg Med 2005;46 (1):4350 [PMID: 15988425].

Beers S, Abramo T et al: Bilevel positive airway pressure in the treatment of status asthmaticus in pediatrics. Am J Emerg Med 2007;25:6–9.

Bolte RG: Emergency department management of pediatric asthma. Clin Ped Emerg Med 2004;5:256 [PMID: 17157675].

Busse et al: Expert panel Report 3 (EPR-3): guidelines for the diagnosis and management of asthma- summary 2007. J Allerg Clin Immun 2007;120(5):S94–S138.

3. Pneumonia

▶ Clinical Findings

There is a wide spectrum in presentation of pediatric pneumonia, ranging from the classic fever, productive cough, and tachypnea to nonspecific presentations such as lethargy, vague abdominal pain, and poor feeding. Physical examination may reveal crackles, rhonchi, or dullness to percussion. Often adventitious lung sounds are difficult to discern secondary to the ambient noise level in the emergency department. Chest X-rays show various patterns from lobar consolidation to diffuse interstitial patchy opacities depending on the etiologic agent.

The exact etiologic agent causing pneumonia is not known in a majority of cases. It is typically inferred from factors such as age, season, and clinical characteristics. Table 50–12 summarizes the most common pathogens in each pediatric age bracket. While clinical practice typically involves chest X-rays, blood counts, and cultures, these tests are of limited utility in pathogen identification. However, certain clinical or laboratory features suggest specific causes. Rapid onset of lobar pneumonia is often *Streptococcus pneumoniae*. Empyemas are frequently associated with Streptococcus or Staphylococcus, including methicillin-resistant staph. Nonspecific symptoms with patchy interstitial infiltrates are

Table 50-12. Treatment of Pediatric Pneumonia According to Age and Etiology.

Age	0-4 Weeks	4-8 Weeks	8-12 Weeks	12 Weeks-4 Years	5 Years-Adolescence
Etiology (in order of prevalence)	Group B strep Gram-negative enteric bacteria *L. monocytogenes*	*C. trachomatis* Viruses (RSV, parainfluenza) *Strep. pneumoniae B pertussis* Group B streptococcus Gram-negative enteric *L monocytogenes*	*C. trachomatis* (RSV, parainfluenza) *Strep. pneumoniae B. pertussis*	Viruses (RSV, parainfluenza, influenza, adenovirus, rhinovirus) *Strep. pneumoniae H. influenza* (nontype b) *M. catarrhalis* Group A streptococcus *M. pneumoniae M. tuberculosis*	*M. pneumoniae C. pneumoniae Strep. pneumoniae* Viruses (RSV, parainfluenza, influenza, adenovirus, rhinovirus) *M. tuberculasis*
Treatment outpatient (in order of initial choice)		For pertussis or chlamydia: Erythromycin or other macrolides	For pertussis or chlamydia: Erythromycin or other macrolides Sulfonomides For *Strep. pneumoniae*: see next column	Amoxicillin or amoxicillin–clavulanate or cefuroxime Macrolides	Macrolides or tetracyclines (>8 years) Fluoroquinolones (>16 years)
Treatment inpatient	Neonatal pneumonia or sepsis: Ceftriaxone or cefotaxime plus ampicillin	Neonatal pneumonia or sepsis: Ceftriaxone or cefotaxime plus ampicillin	For *Strep. pneumoniae*: see next column	Penicillin or ampicillin or cefuroxime Cefotaxime or ceftriaxone Clindamycin Vancomycin until alternative susceptible agents identified	Macrolides Cefuroxime plus macrolides Macrolides plus cefotaxime or ceftriaxone or clindamycin Vancomycin

Lichenstein R, Suggs, AH, Campbell J: Pediatric pneumonia. Emerg Med Clin North Am 2003;21:447 [PMID: 12793623].
(Used with permission from Lichenstein R, Suggs AH, Campbell J: Pediatric pneumonia. Emerg Med Clin North Am 2003;21:447 [PMID: 12793623].)

consistent with atypical pneumonias such as *Mycoplasma* or *Chlamydia*. A newborn with staccato cough, eosinophilia, and bilateral diffuse infiltrates on radiograph is likely to have *Chlamydia trachomatis* pneumonia. A paroxysmal cough followed by posttussive emesis combined with a lymphocytosis on peripheral blood smear is suggestive of pertussis.

▶ Treatment

Rapid evaluation of respiratory status, in combination with pulse oximetry and, in more severe cases, arterial blood gas determination, will direct the immediate therapy.

A. General Management

Provide supplemental oxygen, and attach pulse oximeter and cardiac monitor. Evaluate degree of respiratory distress.

B. Laboratory and Imaging Studies

Obtain a chest X-ray (posteroanterior and lateral). Consider CBC with differential, RSV studies, and blood culture. If a pleural effusion is suspected, a lateral decubitus X-ray is useful.

C. Antimicrobial Therapy

Administer antimicrobial therapy based on age and clinical appearance. See Table 50–12 for guidelines.

▶ Disposition

Most cases may be treated on an outpatient basis with close follow-up. Hospitalization is appropriate for any child appearing toxic, dehydrated, hypoxic, or in respiratory distress, any child failing outpatient therapy, and child less than 1 month old, and those with chronic medical conditions or preexisting pulmonary disease. Close follow-up is mandatory for all pediatric pneumonia patients who are discharged.

Chang A et al: Lower respiratory tract infections. Ped Clin N Am 2009;56:1303–1321.

Rafei K, Lichenstein R: Airway infectious disease emergencies. Ped Clin N Am 2006;53:215–242.

Ranganathan S, Sonnappa S: Pneumonia and other respiratory infections. Ped Clin N Am 2009;56:135–156.

▼ NEUROLOGIC EMERGENCIES

Objective neurologic evaluation of the emergency department patient involves recognition of age-appropriate differences in cognitive function. For patients with altered mental status, an objective scale, such as the pediatric Glasgow Coma Scale (Table 50–13) will help reduce interobserver differences in assessment and provide a measure for comparison during serial examinations.

Table 50–13. Pediatric Glasgow Coma Scale[a].

Eye opening response	
Spontaneous	4
To speech	3
To pain	2
None	1
Verbal response: Child (*Infant modification*)[b]	
Oriented (*Coos, babbles*)	5
Confused conversation (*Irritable cry, consolable*)	4
Inappropriate words (*Cries to pain*)	3
Incomprehensible sounds (*Moans to pain*)	2
None	1
Best upper limb motor response: Child (*Infant modification*)[b]	
Obeys commands (*Normal movements*)	6
Localizes pain (*Withdraws to touch*)	5
Withdraws to pain	4
Flexion to pain	3
Extension to pain	2
None	1

[a]The appropriate number from each section is added to total between 3 and 15. A score less than 8 usually indicates CNS depression requiring positive-pressure ventilation.
[b]If no modification is listed, the same response applies for both infants and children.
(Used with permission from *Current Diagnosis and Treatment Pediatrics*, 20th ed. 310.)

SEIZURES

▶ General Considerations

Seizures are common pediatric emergencies in both the prehospital environment and the emergency department. Approximately 5% of all children have had one or more seizures by the age of 16. Epilepsy is a chronic condition of recurrent seizures that develops in only a small percentage of patients who have a single seizure. Most seizures in childhood are single, generalized, tonic-clonic events, lasting a few minutes. Seizures may be generalized or focal. Status epilepticus is defined as continuous seizure activity for 30 minutes or as recurrent seizures without intervening return of consciousness. Status epilepticus may be the first presentation of seizures in childhood.

The causes of seizures and status epilepticus in children are multiple and age-dependent. Children under age 3 years presenting with status epilepticus are most likely to have serious conditions, for example, CNS infections or vascular disorders, anoxia, trauma, intoxications, or metabolic abnormalities. Many of these conditions are treatable. In older children, however, status epilepticus is usually the result of chronic epilepsy with noncompliance for anticonvulsive medications, chronic progressive encephalopathy, or idiopathic encephalopathy. The likelihood of serious underlying disease in a child with status epilepticus is inversely proportional to age.

Febrile seizures are also common in childhood. The peak age is 8–20 months, although they may occur in children from approximately 6 months to 6 years of age. Often, underlying diseases are simply upper respiratory tract infections or gastroenteritis. Febrile seizures may be simple or complex. A simple febrile seizure typically occurs as a generalized self-limited tonic-clonic seizure of several minutes' duration. Complex febrile seizure denotes a seizure with high-risk features, including focal onset, postictal neurologic abnormalities, or duration greater than 15 minutes. Other high-risk features include prior neurologic or developmental abnormalities or a history of epilepsy in the nuclear family. The simple febrile seizure is usually benign and requires no therapy; however, children presenting with high-risk features are a greater risk for recurrent afebrile seizures.

▶ Clinical Findings

Many children will present in the postictal state. In such patients, search for a specific cause. A thorough history is of extreme importance. Information must be obtained about potential precipitating factors such as fever, trauma, ingestions, the patient's medical history, and family history. A detailed description of the event is necessary, including length of event, movements during the event (including eye movements), incontinence, and the presence of a postictal state. Exclude head trauma and alcohol/drug intoxication and hypoglycemia. Consider syncope, hysteria, breath holding, and night terrors as alternative causes. Several drugs are well known to cause seizure activity, including tricyclic antidepressants, sympathomimetics (cocaine, amphetamines), theophylline, isoniazid, phenothiazines, camphor, antihistamines, anticholinergics, and lindane. Physical examination should specifically exclude head trauma, bulging fontanelle, papilledema, meningeal irritation, focal neurologic signs, cutaneous lesions, and systemic disease.

▶ Treatment

A well-organized approach to seizure management minimizes the complications of the acute electrical and metabolic derangements and averts iatrogenic complications. Ensure adequate ventilation and oxygenation in the patient with active seizures, and then address termination of the seizure and reversal of metabolic imbalances. Finally, attempt to establish the cause in order to implement specific therapy.

A. General Management

1. Initial steps—Open the airway, use suction to clear secretions or foreign bodies, and then administer oxygen. Reserve intubation for failure of medical management, or respiratory depression from medication administration.

2. Laboratory studies—Establish IV access, and draw blood for immediate bedside glucose determination and other appropriate laboratory investigations, which may include CBC, glucose, lead, calcium, and magnesium levels; liver and renal function; and electrolytes, ammonia, and pertinent drug levels. Send urine for toxicologic screening. Consider obtaining an arterial blood gas if significant acidosis is suspected.

3. Volume resuscitation—If rapid bedside glucose determination is less than 70 mg/dL, administer 25% dextrose in water, 2 mL/kg per dose slowly. If evidence of dehydration is present, provide lactated Ringer's solution or isotonic normal saline. Otherwise, if the patient is euvolemic, start 5% dextrose in normal saline at maintenance rate for weight.

4. Pharmacologic therapy—If the child is febrile, administer rectal acetaminophen, 15 mg/kg. If fever fails to respond to acetaminophen, ibuprofen may be administered at a dose of 10 mg/kg to infants greater than 6 months of age. Consider pyridoxine (vitamin B_6) if the child could have been exposed to isoniazid in the setting of refractory seizures.

5. Other measures—After a febrile seizure, children who appear toxic or do not return to baseline mental status (after a brief postictal period) should undergo a full septic workup including a lumbar puncture. In addition, a lumbar puncture should be strongly considered in all children less than 1 year of age with seizures associated with fever.

B. Specific Management

If seizures continue after first-line supportive care, consider immediate anticonvulsive therapy (Figure 50–6). Duration of seizure activity may be related to ultimate neurologic outcome, particularly in patients with severe underlying disease. In patients with difficulty obtaining IV access, alternatives include rectal diazepam, 0.5 mg/kg, or intramuscular midazolam 0.2 mg/kg, phenytoin, barbiturates, and benzodiazepines also may be given intraosseously.

For treatment of status epilepticus in neonates use of benzodiazepines (lorazepam, midazolam) and phenobarbital loading at 10–20 mg/kg is recommended. For older infants and children, administer benzodiazepines, then loading with fosphenytoin at 20 mg/kg. Consider use of phenobarbital or levetiracetam as secondary intravenous medicatious for status epilepticus.

Blumstein M, Friedman M: Childhood seizures. Emerg Med Clin N Am 2007;25:1061–1086 [PMID: 17950136].

Freedman SB, Powell EC: Pediatric seizures and their management in the emergency department. Clin Ped Emerg Med 2003;4:195.

1. ABCs
   a. Airway: maintain oral airway; intubation may be necessary.
   b. Breathing: oxygen.
   c. Circulation: assess pulse, blood pressure; support with IV fluids, drugs. Monitor vital signs.
2. Start glucose-containing IV (unless pt on ketogenic diet); evaluate serum glucose; electrolytes, HCO_3^-, CBC, BUN, anticonvulsant levels.
3. May need arterial blood gases, pH.
4. Give 50% glucose if serum glucose low (1–2 mL/kg).
   for infants use D10 at 5mL/kg.
5. Begin IV drug therapy; goal is to control status epilepticus in 20–60 min.
   a. Diazepam, 0.3–0.5 mg/kg over 1–5 min (20 mg max); may repeat in 5–20 min; or, lorazepam, 0.05–0.2 mg/kg (less effective with repeated doses, longer-acting than diazepam).
      [a]Midazolam: IV, 0.1–0.2 mg/kg; intranasally, 0.2 mg/kg.
   b. Phenytoin, 10–20 mg/kg IV (not IM) over 5–20 min; 1000 mg maximum); monitor with blood pressure and ECG. Fosphenytoin may be given more rapidly in the same dosage and can be given IM; order 10–20 mg/kg of "phenytoin equivalent."
   c. Phenobarbital, 5–20 mg/kg (sometimes higher in newborns or refractory status in intubated patients).
6. Correct metabolic perturbations (eg, low-sodium, acidosis).
7. other drug approaches in refractory status:
   a. Repeat phenytoin phenobarbital (10 mg/kg). Monitor blood levels. Support respiration, blood pressure as necessary.
   b. [a]Midazolam drip: 1–5 mcg/kg/min (even to 20 kg/min). Valproate sodium, available as 100 mg/mL for IV use; give 15–30 mg/kg over 5–20 min.
   c. Levetiracetam may be helpful (20–40 mg/kg/dose IV)
   d. Pentobarb coma. Propofol. General anesthetic.
8. Consider underlying causes:
   a. Structural disorders or trauma: MRI or CT scan.
   b. Infection: lumbar puncture, blood culture, antibiotics.
   c. Metabolic disorders: consider lactic acidosis, toxins, and uremia. May need to evaluate medication levels, Toxin screen. Judicious fluid administration.
9. Give maintenance drug (if diazepam only was sufficient to halt status epilepticus): phenytoin (10 mg/kg); phenobarbital (5 mg/kg); daily dose IV (or by mouth) divided every 12 h.

[a]Much supportive data.
BUN, blood urea nitrogen; CBC, complete blood count; CT, computed tomography; ECG, electrocardiogram; IM, intramuscularly; IV, intravenously; MRI, magnetic resonance imaging.

▲ **Figure 50–6.** Management of status epilepticus. (Reproduced, with permission, from Current Diagnosis and Treatment Pediatrics, 20th edition, Chapter 23, page 720.)

Hanhan UA, Fiallos MR, Orlowski JP: Status epilepticus. Pediatr Clin North Am 2001;48:683 [PMID: 11411300].

Reuter D, Brownstein D: Common emergent pediatric neurologic problems. Emerg Clin North Am 2002;20:155 [PMID: 11826632].

ENCEPHALITIS

Encephalitis is an inflammation of the brain parenchyma. Etiologies include postinfectious, viral and arthropod–borne. Acute disseminated encephalomyelitis (ADEM) is an immune-mediated disorder of the central nervous system, also identified as postinfectious.

▶ Clinical Findings

Symptoms range from headache to a severe presentation with seizures, coma or death. Focal neurologic deficits may be seen with Herpes simplex virus infections. ADEM typically appears with abrupt onset of neurologic symptoms 2-3 weeks after the occurrence of a preceding infection or vaccination. CNS white matter demyelination is the pathologic hallmark of this disease.

A. General Management

1. Initial steps—Manage the airway. Intubate if needed for altered mental status.

2. Laboratory studies—Establish IV access, and draw blood for immediate bedside glucose determination and other appropriate laboratory investigations, which may include CBC, glucose, liver and renal function; and electrolytes, ammonia. Send urine for toxicologic screening. Perform lumbar puncture after obtaining a brain CT to ascertain any existing intracranial pathology. Consider emergent MRI to determine if white matter disease is present.

B. Specific Management

Neurologic consultation is appropriate. Current management is the administration of high-dose glucocorticoid therapy with dexamthasone (1 mg/kg) or methylprednisolone (10–30) mg/kg/day.

Management of encephalitis is mainly supportive care. Acyclovir should be initiated if there is a suspicion of viral herpetic encephalitis. In the case of ADEM, intravenous immunoglobulin has been used in combination with high-dose steroids.

Noorbakhsh F, Johnson R et al: Acute disseminated encephalomyelitis: clinical and pathogenesis features. Neurol Clin 2008;26:759–780 [PMID: 18657725].

INFECTIOUS DISEASES

FEVER

Fever is one of the most common presenting complaints in the pediatric patient. Despite the regularity with which it is seen, appropriate management is one of the most difficult dilemmas facing the emergency physician. While a vast majority will have benign infections, a few will have significant bacterial infections that, when untreated, can lead to morbidity or even death. The identification of this subset of patients at increased risk is of extreme importance. Most authorities agree that two primary risk groups for managing fever in young children are (1) those younger than 2 months (fever in infants) and (2) those aged 2–24 months (fever in young children).

1. Fever in Infants

General Considerations

Fever in infants under age 2 months is typically managed by a conservative clinical approach. This is secondary to the fact that younger children are at greater risk of serious infections and the relative immaturity of their immune system leaves them at risk for invasive disease. Numerous studies have shown that identifying patients at increased risk by means of physical examination findings and laboratory results lacks the necessary sensitivity. This leads to a more cautious approach with generous use of laboratory testing. Common organisms causing infection in this age group that should be considered include Group B *Streptococcus*, *Listeria*, *Escherichia coli*, *Strep. pneumoniae*, herpes, and congenital infections such as cytomegalovirus, rubella, and syphilis.

Clinical Findings

Initial evaluation begins with a detailed history, including the length of gestation, any complications, maternal infections during pregnancy including Group B *Streptococcus*, and Herpes simplex status of mother, whether antibiotics were administered, and hospital course after delivery. Examine the patient for general signs and symptoms of sepsis such as grunting, respiratory distress, lethargy, irritability, fever or hypothermia, hypo- or hyperglycemia, apnea, poor feeding, cyanotic spells, petechiae, and unexplained jaundice.

A. Laboratory Findings

The laboratory evaluation of febrile infants under age 2 months often includes the following:

CBC with differential and blood culture—High-risk infants include those with WBC count of <5000 or greater than 15,000 and/or a total band count of 1500 or more, or a band/neutrophil ratio of 0.2.

Lumbar puncture—Lumbar puncture is mandatory for all infants under 1 month of age and should be strongly considered in those aged 1–2 months. There are no conclusive data to support omission of lumbar puncture from routine evaluation in infants 4–8 weeks of age. Nevertheless, for a selected group of older well appearing infants who meet all low risk criteria both clinical and diagnostic, some experienced clinicians will elect to delay or omit the LP, provided follow-up can be arranged and the provider is confident the parents have appropriate skills. Immediate lumbar puncture may be deferred in patients who are hypotensive or have respiratory failure. Spinal fluid studies include Gram stain and culture, glucose and protein, cell count and differential, and antigen testing dependent on local laboratory capabilities.

Urinalysis—Obtain urine dipstick and microscopic analysis. Clues to the diagnosis of UTI include urine nitrate, leukocyte esterase, bacteria, or WBCs. Less than 10 WBCs per high-powered field are considered normal.

Urine culture—Urine culture is the most accurate means to diagnose UTI in infants. A bagged specimen is not adequate because of the high incidence of contamination. Bladder catheterization is the preferred method of obtaining urine.

B. X-ray Findings

Findings of pneumonia may be present on chest X-ray even in infants without cough tachypnea or rales.

Treatment

A. General Management

Management must be conservative. If evaluation discloses a local infection (eg, meningitis, pneumonia, or urinary tract infection [UTI]), hospitalize the infant and promptly institute IV antibiotic therapy. Most clinicians recommend IV coverage with either ampicillin 50–100 mg/kg **or** cefotaxime 50–100 mg/kg, plus gentamycin 2 mg/kg, and acyclovir 20 mg/kg for treatment of neonatal sepsis.

B. Treatment of Fever Without Clear Cause

Emergency department treatment of febrile infants less than 1 month of age without clear evident source of infections after history, physical examination, and diagnostic workup requires admission to the hospital and IV antibiotics until blood, urine, and CSF cultures are negative or reveal a source that can be more specifically treated. The shift in management over the last few years is that febrile infants between 1 and 2 months of age who are well appearing and have a normal sepsis workup can be considered for discharge and close outpatient follow-up. This is a decision that should be made in consultation with the patient's primary physician and be reserved for reliable parents with readily available follow-up access. Reevaluation should occur within 12–24 hours. All other infants should be admitted and managed in a similar fashion to those less than 1 month of age.

2. Fever in Children

▶ General Considerations

Febrile illness is an extremely common presenting complaint for children aged 2–36 months. While careful history and examination can elicit a source in many of these subjects, there is a small risk of occult bacteremia—unsuspected presence of bacteria in the bloodstream. The current prevalence of occult bacteremia among febrile children aged 2–36 months is thought to be between 0.5 and 1%. Less than 1% will later develop serious complications such as septic arthritis, osteomyelitis, meningitis, or sepsis. The widespread use of the *H. influenza* type b (Hib) and 7-valent pneumococcal vaccines have decreased the incidence of occult bacteremia but some risk remains.

▶ Clinical Findings

A thorough history and physical examination is essential in the febrile child aged 2–36 months. A precise fever history should be elucidated including maximum temperature, method of temperature obtainment, timing, antipyretic use, and any associated symptoms. Past medical history, ill contacts, and immunization status should all be included in the routine history. As *Strep. pneumoniae* remains the most common organism isolated in occult bacteremia, history of the pneumococcal vaccine is of importance. Physical examination should include close inspection of the tympanic membranes, oropharynx, auscultatory findings of the lungs, and abdominal and genitourinary examination. UTIs are a common culprit in this age range and must be considered as dysuria, frequency, and urgency are difficult and often impossible symptoms to screen for in this age group

▶ Treatment

A. General Management

A rapid cardiopulmonary survey should be performed. Any patient appearing toxic or in distress should be managed aggressively (see below). Antipyretics should be administered early in the emergency department course to improve the patient's comfort level. However, response to antipyretic medication does not change the likelihood of a child having serious bacterial infections and should not be used for clinical decision making. If a source of infection can be elucidated, it should be addressed.

B. Fever Without an Apparent Source

The management of infants over 3 months of age with fever and no apparent source on physical examination remains controversial. Current clinical guidelines suggest children with fever < 39°C and a nontoxic appearance may be managed on an outpatient basis with antipyretic therapy only. Children > 6 months of age with fever ≥ 39°C and history of three doses of both the pneumococcal and Hib vaccine should be screened with a urinalysis and urine culture and discharged with antipyretic therapy if negative. The rate of bacteremia in these children is determined to be < 1%. Some clinicians advocate that children < 6 months of age and/or less than three doses of the aforementioned vaccines should be screened with a urinalysis and urine culture, CBC and blood culture, and chest X-ray. Others will take a less aggressive approach and trust clinical judgment to determine if an extensive laboratory evaluation is indicated in infants and children with fever. Regardless of the approach employed by the ED physician, febrile infants and children should have follow-up in 12–24 hours for reexamination and to check on any cultures that were obtained.

C. Management of the Child Appearing Seriously Ill

Any child on rapid cardiopulmonary survey appearing seriously ill requires aggressive diagnostic evaluation and prompt institution of parenteral antibiotic therapy within 1 hour of arrival to the emergency department. Obtain cultures of blood, urine, and CSF (if clinical status allows), and begin antibiotics. If physical examination or laboratory evaluation does not disclose a source of infection, use third-generation cephalosporin IV, or piperacillin/tazobactam, + vancomycin. Regardless of whether a source of infection is found, hospitalize seriously ill febrile children for continued antibiotic therapy and observation.

American College of Emergency Physicians: Clinical policy for children younger than three years presenting to the emergency department with fever. Ann Emerg Med 2003;42:530 [PMID: 14520324].

Baker D, Avner J: The febrile infant: what's new? Clin Ped Emerg Med 2008;9:213–220.

Gerdes JS: Diagnosis and management of bacterial infections in the neonate. Pediatr Clin North Am 2004;51:939 [PMID: 15275982].

Mahajan P, Stanley R: Fever in the toddler-aged child: old concerns replaced with new ones. Clin Ped Emerg Med 228; 9:221–227.

Nigrovic LE, Malley R: Evaluation of the febrile child 3 to 36 months old in the era of pneumococcal conjugate vaccine: focus on occult bacteremia. Clin Ped Emerg Med 2004;5:13.

MENINGITIS

 ESSENTIALS OF DIAGNOSIS

▶ Fever, headache, stiff neck, mental status changes, or excessive irritability

▶ CSF Gram stain or culture may be diagnostic for a specific organism

▶ General Considerations

Meningitis is defined as inflammation of the membranes that surround the brain and spinal cord. Potential pathogens include bacteria, viruses, fungi, and parasites. These organisms reach the CNS by either hematogenous spread or by direct extension from a contiguous site. In neonates, pathogens are acquired from nonsterile maternal genital secretions such as Group B-Beta Streptoccus(GBBS) and Herpes Simplex Virus (HSV). In infants and children, many of the organisms that cause meningitis colonize the upper respiratory tract. Direct inoculation can occur from trauma, skull defects with CSF leaks, congenital malformation, or extension from nearby suppurative foci. Bacterial meningitis typically presents acutely as bacterial penetration of the blood–brain barrier elicits an intense inflammatory response. Prompt diagnosis and aggressive treatment is paramount as delays can lead to significant morbidity and possibly death.

▶ Clinical Findings

A. Symptoms and Signs

Manifestations of meningitis depend on the age of the patient. Symptoms may be subtle in infants such as poor feeding, decreased interactiveness, increased crying, and lethargy. Other signs include fever, apnea, seizures, a bulging fontanel, and a rash. Neck stiffness and mental status changes may be apparent in older children. Kernig's and Brudzinski's signs are useful signs of meningeal irritation, but their presence is not specific for meningitis. Headache, focal neurologic deficits, persistent vomiting, and seizures are commonly seen. Petechiae and purpura may be seen with several etiologic agents, but are most common in patients with meningococcal meningitis.

B. Laboratory Findings

1. Lumbar puncture—Lumbar puncture is necessary for the definitive diagnosis of bacterial meningitis. Neuroimaging (Head CT) should occur before lumbar puncture in patients with signs or symptoms of increased intracranial pressure or focal neurologic deficits. This should occur on an emergency basis and antibiotic administration should not be delayed for imaging. Analysis should include Gram stain and culture, cell count and differential, and glucose and protein levels. A herpes PCR can be considered as well as a viral battery panel. Table 50–14 demonstrates typical findings associated with bacterial, viral, fungal, and tubercular meningitis.

2. Other tests—CBC and blood cultures are indicated. A comparison of serum to CSF glucose is often useful. Urinalysis, urine culture, and chest X-ray should be strongly considered. If septic shock is evident, add PT/PTT and a Basic Metabolic Panel.

▶ Treatment

A. General Management

The initial focus of attention remains the primary survey. Assess the airway, including elective intubation if indicated. Apply supplemental oxygen, place the child on a monitor, and perform a rapid cardiovascular assessment.

B. Volume Resuscitation

Assess the child's intravascular volume by means of blood pressure, heart rate, and capillary refill. Hypovolemia can compromise perfusion of the CNS. Aggressive rehydration with isotonic fluid is indicated if signs of hypovolemia are present.

C. Steroid Therapy

The administration of steroids (dexamethasone) in patients with bacterial meningitis is controversial. Studies have shown a benefit in reducing hearing loss in patients with *H. influenzae* meningitis. However, the decrease in *H. influenzae* meningitis due to the advent of the Hib vaccine makes this data less significant. Studies have suggested benefit for pneumococcal meningitis if steroids are given before antibiotics. Further complicating recommendations, steroids may decrease antibiotic penetrating through the blood–brain barrier. Current recommendations support the use of steroids in infants and children with Hib meningitis. For infants and children 6 weeks and older with pneumococcal meningitis, steroids should be considered after weighing risks and benefits. Steroids for neonates with bacterial meningitis are not recommended. The dosing of dexamethasone ranges from 0.6–0.8 mg/kg daily in two or three divided doses for 2 days to 1 mg/kg in four divided doses for 2–4 days.

Table 50–14. Characteristics of Cerebrospinal Fluid in the Normal Child and in Central Nervous System Infections and Inflammatory Conditions.

Condition	Initial Pressure (mm H$_2$O)	Appearance	Cells/μl	Protein (mg/dl)	Glucose (mg/dl)	Other Tests	Comments
Normal	<160	Clear	0–5 lymphocytes, first 3 mo, 1–3 PMNs; neonates, up to 30 lymphocytes, rare RBCs	15–35 (lumbar), 5–15 (ventricular); up to 150 (lumbar) for short time after birth; to 6 mo up to 65	50–80 (two-thirds of blood glucose); may be increased after seizure	CSF-IgG index[a] <0.7[a]; LDH 2–27 U/L	CSF protein in first month may be up to 170 mg/dL in small-for-date or premature infants; no increase in WBCs due to seizure
Bloody tap	Normal or low	Bloody (sometimes with clot)	One additional WBC/700 RBCs; RBCs not crenated	One additional milligram per 800 RBCs[b]	Normal	RBC number should fall between first and third tubes; wait 5 min between tubes	Spin down fluid, supernatant will be clear and colorless[c]
Bacterial meningitis, acute	200–750+	Opalescent to purulent	Up to thousands mostly PMNs; early, few cells	Up to hundreds	Decreased; may be none	Smear and culture mandatory; LDH >24 U/L; lactate, IL-8, INF elevated, correlate with prognosis	Very early, glucose may be normal; PCR meningococci and pneumococci in plasma, CSF may aid diagnosis
Bacterial meningitis, partially treated	Usually increased	Clear or opalescent	Usually increased; PMNs usually predominate	Elevated	Normal or decreased	LDH usually >24 U/L; PCR may still be positive	Smear and culture may be negative if antibiotics have been in use
Tuberculous meningitis	150–750+	Opalescent; fibrin web or pellicle	250–500, mostly lymphocytes; early more PMNs	45–500; parallels cell count; increases over time	Decreased; may be none	Smear for acid-fast organism: CSF culture and inoculation; PCR	Consider AIDS, a common comorbidity of tuberculosis
Fungal meningitis	Increased	Variable; often clear	10–500; early more PMNs then mostly lymphocytes	Elevated and increasing	Decreased	India ink preparations, cryotococcal antigen, PCR, culture, inoculations, immuno-immuno-fluorescence tests	Often superimposed in patients who are debilitated or on immuno-suppressive therapy

(continued)

Table 50-14. Characteristics of Cerebrospinal Fluid in the Normal Child and in Central Nervous System Infections and Inflammatory Conditions. (*Continued*)

Condition	Initial Pressure (mm H$_2$0)	Appearance	Cells/μL	Protein (mg/dL)	Glucose (mg/dL)	Other Tests	Comments
Aseptic meningo-encephalitis (vital meningitis, or parameningeal disease); encephalitis in similar	Normal or slightly increased	Clear unless cell count >300/μl	None to a few hundred, mostly lymphocytes; PMNs predominate early	20–125	Normal; may be low in mumps, herpes, or other viral infections	CSF, stool, blood, throat washings for viral cultures; LDH < 28 U/L; PCR for HSV, CMV, EBV, enterovirus, etc	Acute and convalescent antibody titers for some viruses; in mumps, up to 1000 lymphocytes; serumamylase often elevated; up to 1000 cells present in enteroviral infection
Parainfectious encephalomyelitis (ADEM)	80–450, usually increased	Usually clear	0–50+, mostly lymphocytes; lower numbers, even 0, in MS	15–75	Normal	CSF-IgG index, oligoclonal bands variable; in MS, moderate increase	No organisms; fulminant cases resemble bacterial meningitis
Polyneuritis	Normal and occasionally increased	Early: normal; late: xanthochromic if protein high	Noraml; occasionally slight increase	Early: normal; late: 45–1500	Normal	CSF-IgG index may be increased; oligoclonal bands variable	Try to find cause (viral infections, toxins, lupus, diabetes, etc)
Meningeal carcinomatosis	Often elevated	Clear to opalescent	Cytologic indentification of tumor cells	Often mildly to moderately elevated	Often depressed	Cytology	Seen with leukemia, medulloblastoma, meningeal melanosis, histocytosis X
Brain abscess	Normal or increased	Usually clear	5–500 in 80%; mostly PMNs	Usually slightly increased	Normal; occasionally decreased	Imaging study of brain (MRI)	Cell count related to proximity to meninges; findings as in purulent meningitis if abscess ruptures

[a]CSF-IgG index = (CSF IgG/serum IgG)/ (CSF albumin/serum albumin).

[b]Many studies document pitfalls in using these ratios due to WBC lysis, Clinical judgment and repeat lumbar punctures may be necessary to rule out meningitis in this situation.

[c]CSF WBC (predicated) = CSF RBC × (blood WBC/blood RBC). O:P ratio = (observed CSF WBC)/(predicted CSF WBC). Also, do WBC: RBC ratio. If O:P ratio ≤ 0.01,and WBC: RBC ratio ≤ 1:100, meningitis is absent.

ADEM, acute disseminatd encephalomyelitis; AIDS, acquired immunodeficiency syndrome; CMV, cytomegalovirous; CSF, cerebrospinal fluid; EBV, Epstein-Barr virus; HSV, herpes simplex virus; IL-8, interleukin 8; LDH, lactate dehydrogenase; MRI, magnetic resonance imaging; MS, multiple sclerosis; PCR, polymerase chain reaction; PMN, polymorphonuclear neutrophill; RBC, red blood cell; TNF, tumor necrosis factor; WBC, white blood cell.

(Used with permission from Current Diagnosis and Treatment Pediatrics, 20th ed. 699–700.)

Table 50–15. Common Causes of Meningitis and Empiric Antibiotic Therapy.

Age of Patient	Common Bacterial Causes	Antibiotic	Dose	Other Causes
Preterm to <1 month	Group B streptococcus E. coli Listeria	Ampicillin plus cefotaxime or gentamicin	50 mg/kg, q 6–8 h 50 mg/kg q 8–12 h 2.5 mg/kg q 12 h	Enterovirus Candida albicans
1–3 months	Group B streptococcus E. coli Listeria Strep. pneumoniae N. meningitidis H. influenzae type B (rare)	Vancomycin plus cefotaxime or ceftriaxone	15 mg/kg q 6 h 50 mg/kg q 6 h 100 mg/kg q 24 h	Enterovirus
3 months–6 years	Strep. pneumoniae N. meningitidis H. influenzae type B (rare)	Vancomycin plus cefotaxime or ceftriaxone	15 mg/kg q 6 h 50 mg/kg q 6 h 100 mg/kg q 24 h	Enterovirus Mumps M. tuberculosis
>6 years–adult	Strep. Pneumoniae N. meningitidis	Vancomycin plus cefotaxime or cefriaxone	15 mg/kg q 6 h 50 mg/kg q 6 h 100 mg/kg q 24 h	Enterovirus Mumps M. tuberculosis

D. Antimicrobial Therapy

In critically ill children suspected of having meningitis, administer antibiotics rapidly without delay prior to lumbar puncture. In neonates, during the first month of life, ampicillin with either an aminoglycoside or cefotaxime is typically used as initial empiric therapy. For children older than 1 month, vancomycin plus a third-generation cephalosporin (ceftriaxone or cefotaxime) is recommended as initial therapy (see Table 50–15). Acyclovir should be considered for suspected herpetic CNS infections.

E. Other Measures

Treat seizures aggressively with anticonvulsants. Attempt to maintain euvolemic status. Hyperglycemia and hypoglycemia should be avoided. Electrolytes should be closely monitored and any abnormalities should be corrected.

▶ Disposition

Children with proven or clinically suspected meningitis require prompt hospitalization, ideally in a pediatric intensive care unit.

Chavez-Bueno S, McCracken GH: Bacterial meningitis in children. Pediatr Clin North Am 2005;52:795 [PMID: 15925663].

Schneider JI: Rapid infectious killers. Emerg Med Clin North Am 2004;22:1099 [PMID: 15474784].

Seehusen DA, Reeves MM, Fomin DA: Cerebrospinal fluid analysis. Am Fam Phys 2003;68:1103 [PMID: 14524396].

ACUTE OTITIS MEDIA

 ESSENTIALS OF DIAGNOSIS

▶ Redness and bulging of the tympanic membrane is highly suggestive of otitis media

▶ Loss of tympanic membrane landmarks and decreased mobility are sensitive indicators

▶ General Considerations

Otitis media is one of the most common pediatric infectious diseases and accounts for a large number of emergency department visits. A large majority of pediatric patients will have an episode of otitis media at some point during childhood. Otitis media most commonly occurs during the period of speech and language development in children, making appropriate management essential to assist the child in reaching appropriate developmental milestones.

Impaired eustachian tube function is key in the pathogenesis of otitis media. This often occurs after an upper respiratory infection. Serous fluid accumulates behind the tympanic membrane and often becomes inoculated with organisms from the nasopharynx. In infants and children, Strep. pneumoniae, H. influenzae, and Moraxella catarrhalis are the most common pathogens.

▶ Clinical Findings

The classic symptom complex for otitis media is ear pain and hearing loss. This may occur after antecedent upper respiratory infection or may occur spontaneously. Fever is often associated with this presentation, but may be absent. Younger children typically present with more nonspecific signs, such as poor feeding, decreased activity level, and irritability. Very young infants with otitis media associated with fever are at increased risk for hematogenous spread of disease and must be managed aggressively.

On otoscopic examination, a red bulging tympanic membrane provides an easy diagnosis. The absence of this finding does not rule out otitis media, however. The loss of tympanic membrane landmarks on visual inspection and decreased movement by pneumatic otoscopy often will facilitate the diagnosis.

Most cases of otitis media are self-limited and will resolve with symptomatic treatment only. In recent years, some clinicians have advocated a more watchful waiting approach to decrease the administration of antibiotics, which may not ultimately be necessary for all cases of otitis media. Although rare, complications do occur and include brain abscess, cavernous sinus thrombosis, mastoiditis, as well as progression to meningitis and sepsis. Any focal neurologic signs on physical examination should alert the physician to the potential for these complications. The mastoid area should be inspected carefully for swelling, tenderness, or erythema.

Otitis media is a clinical diagnosis and typically no ancillary tests are needed to assist the diagnosis. Treatment is directed at the most common bacterial pathogens. Further testing is necessary when complications are a clinical concern. CT scan of the head may be indicated when intracranial pathology or mastoiditis is suspected on basis of physical examination.

▶ Treatment

A. Antimicrobial Therapy

While controversy exists, typical clinical practice includes administration of antibiotics at the onset of symptoms, especially in children less than 2 years and those with severe symptoms. Figures 50–7 and 50–8 indicate appropriate antibiotic selection. Typical treatment length is 10 days. If symptoms persist, alternative antibiotic treatment may be necessary. Table 50–16 lists the various antibiotics commonly used to treat otitis media. The "observation option" for treatment entails deferring antibiotic prescription for 48–72 hours. If the child improves clinically in that time frame, no prescription is required. Close follow-up is a necessity for this treatment option.

B. Treatment of Pain and Fever

The pain and fever associated with otitis media may be quite significant and are managed with acetaminophen and ibuprofen. Topical anesthetic agents may also be useful, but cannot be used if perforation has occurred.

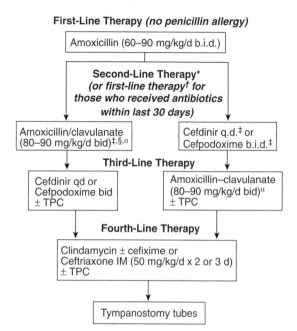

▲ **Figure 50–7.** Antibiotic choices for acute otitis media. TPC, tympanocentesis with culture and susceptibility testing. Recommendations are for children aged 3–36 months with acute otitis media (AOM). †If fully vaccinated with pneumococcal conjugated heptavalent vaccine, cefixime can be used as an alternative second-line antibiotic. Azithromycin (5 days) may be an alternative for the older child with recurrent AOM who has (1) concomitant pneumonia suggestive of atypical pathogens or (2) significant gastroenteritis. ‡Because azithromycin has limited coverage of *H. influenza* (approximately 50%), some experts recommend adding trimethoprim–sulfamethoxazole. §Also AOM with concomitant conjunctivitis. ¶Also AOM with concomitant impetigo. Augmentin ES-600 may be substituted. (Reproduced, with permission, from Block SL, Harrison CJ: *Diagnosis and Management of Acute Otitis Media*, 1st ed. Professional Communications, 2001.)

C. Treatment for Infants Under Age 4 Weeks

Due to the risk of hematogenous spread of infection in this age group, any febrile or ill-appearing neonate should undergo a full sepsis evaluation.

▶ Disposition

A vast majority of children with uncomplicated otitis media can be appropriately discharged home. However, an emergency department presentation of otitis media is an excellent

First-Line Therapy

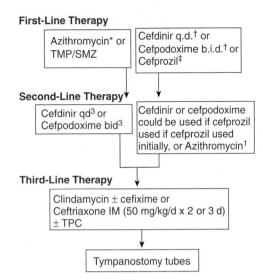

▲ **Figure 50–8.** Antibiotic choices for acute otitis media for the penicillin-allergic child. TMP-SMZ, trimethoprim-sulfamethoxazole; TPC, tympanocentesis with culture and susceptibility testing. *Recommendations are for children aged 3–36 months with acute otitis media (AOM). Because azithromycin has limited coverage of *H. influenza* (approximately 50%), some experts recommend adding TMP-SMZ. †Also AOM with concomitant pneumonia suggestive of atypical pathogens. ‡Also AOM with concomitant conjunctivitis. With concomitant impetigo (*Staph. aureus*). In AOM, coverage of β-lactamase-positive *H. influenza* is 10–25%. (Reproduced, with permission, from Block SL, Harrison CJ: *Diagnosis and Management of Acute Otitis Media*, 1st ed. Professional Communications, 2001.)

time to discuss risk factor modification with parents, including passive tobacco smoke exposure, allergens in the household, and pacifier use.

A reevaluation is necessary in 1–2 days if no improvement in condition occurs and again at the conclusion of antibiotic therapy.

If complications such as cavernous sinus thrombosis, brain abscess, or mastoiditis occur, admission to the hospital and IV antibiotics are indicated.

Eskin B: Should children with otitis media be treated with antibiotics? Ann Emerg Med 2004;44:537 [PMID: 15520716].

Pelton SI: Otitis media: re-evaluation of diagnosis and treatment in the era of antimicrobial resistance, pneumococcal conjugate vaccine, and evolving morbidity. Pediatr Clin North Am 2005;52:711 [PMID: 15925659].

Singh A, Bond B: Does this child have acute otitis media? Ann Emerg Med 2006;47:113 [PMID: 16395779].

Weber SM, Grundfast KM: Modern management of acute otitis media. Pediatr Clin North Am 2003;50:399 [PMID: 12809330].

American Academy of Pediatrics, Subcommittee on Management of Acute Otitis Media. Diagnosis and management of acute otitis media. Pediatrics. 2004;113:1451–1465 [PMID: 15121972].

PHARYNGITIS

▶ General Considerations

Acute pharyngitis is one of the most common illnesses for which children present to the emergency department. There are a wide range of viral and bacterial pathogens which may cause pharyngitis. Group A β-hemolytic streptococcus (GABHS) is the most significant of the bacterial pathogens. Discerning between the more common viral causes and GABHS, for which antibiotic treatment can prevent significant morbidity, is essential. Other important bacterial causes of pharyngitis include *Corynebacterium diphtheriae*, which may present with a gray–white membrane (now rare due to immunization practices), and gonococcal/chlamydial pharyngitis which may be seen in sexual abuse and must be considered in sexually active patients. Pharyngitis by the Epstein-Barr virus (EBV), the causative agent in infectious mononucleosis, can also cause a significant exudative pharyngitis. It can be associated with hepatitis and splenomegaly which should preclude the patient from contact activities.

▶ Clinical Findings

The clinical findings associated with pharyngitis overlap between viral and bacterial causes. Typical presentation includes sore throat, pain on swallowing, and fever. Other symptoms that may be present include headache, nausea, vomiting, abdominal pain, an inflamed swollen uvula, and rash. The associated abdominal pain may be quite significant and distract the physician from the true diagnosis. These may be present in both viral and bacterial causes including GABHS. The four most reliable clinical features for diagnosis of GABHS are tonsillar exudates, tender anterior cervical lymphadenopathy, absence of cough, and temperature of at least 100.4°F.

While the diagnosis of pharyngitis is on a clinical basis, ancillary testing may be considered to determine the necessity of antibiotic therapy. The decision to perform a test should be based upon clinical characteristics that may indicate GABHS or other bacterial cause is likely. Prevalence of GABHS in the community as well as close contacts with known GABHS pharyngitis can be useful in this decision.

The most commonly used ancillary test is the rapid antigen detection test followed by a throat culture. While rapid antigen tests are convenient, the sensitivity remains

Table 50–16. Drugs Used for the Treatment of Acute Otitis Media.

Drug	Dosage	Comments
Amoxicillin (Amoxil)	40–60 mg/kg/d (b.i.d.) × 10 d	Standard dose for children without risk factors >age 24 months
Amoxicillin (Amoxil) high dose	80–90 mg/kg/d (b.i.d.) × 10 d	Indicated for children >age 24 months with any risk factors (daycare attendance, multiple antibiotic courses, or antibiotics use in previous 30 days)
Amoxicillin-clavulanate (Augmentin)	80–90 mg/kg/d of amoxicillin 10 mg/kg/d of clavulanate (b.i.d.-t.i.d.) × 10 d	Alternative to high-dose amoxicillin, gastrointestinal intolerance common
Azithromycin (Zithromax)	10 mg/kg/d × 1 d then 5 mg/kg/d × 4 d	Alternative for penicillin-allergic patients
Cefdinir (Omnicef)	14 mg/kg/d (q.d.) × 10 d	Alternative to high-dose amoxicillin
Cefpodoxime (Vantin)	10 mg/kg/d (q.d.) × 10 d	Alternative to high-dose amoxicillin
Cefprozil (Cefzil)	30 mg/kg/d (b.i.d.) × 10 d	
Ceftriaxone (Rocephin)	50 mg/kg/d IM × 3 d	Documented efficacy in acute otitis media treatment failures from other antibiotics
Cefuroxime axetil (Ceftin)	30 mg/kg/d (b.i.d.) × 10 d	
Clarithromycin (Biaxin)	15 mg/kg/d (b.i.d.) × 10 d	Alternative for penicillin-allergic patients
Clindamycin (Cleocin)	25 mg/kg/d (t.i.d.)	No activity against *H. influenzae* or *M. catarrhalis*
Trimethoprim-sulfamethoxazole (TMP-SMZ; Septra, Bactrim)	8 mg/kg/d IMP 40 mg/kg/d SMZ (b.i.d.) × 10 d	No activity against DRSP, alternative for penicillin-allergic patients

DRSP, drug resistant Strep. pneumoniae.

approximately 80–90%, necessitating the confirmatory throat culture when rapid test is negative. CBC may show an elevated WBC count with pharyngitis, but is nonspecific and does little to guide management. Leukocytosis with predominantly atypical lymphocytes is common with EBV pharyngitis. Screening with the monospot test can be useful but has limited sensitivity. In patients for whom a confirmatory diagnosis is essential, EBV antibody titers should be obtained.

The complications of pharyngitis are classified as suppurative (peritonsillar abscess and retropharyngeal abscess) and nonsuppurative (rheumatic fever and poststreptococcal glomerulonephritis). Peritonsillar abscesses (PTA) occur when pharyngitis progresses to cellulitis followed by abscess formation. Patients may present with drooling, muffled voice, and trismus. It is most commonly seen in adolescents. Retropharyngeal abscesses (RPA) typically occur from suppuration of retropharyngeal lymph nodes from adjacent pharyngitis and present similarly to PTAs. This complication is more commonly seen in toddlers and school-aged children. Imaging may include a plain lateral soft tissue study of the neck to evaluate RPA and to rule out epiglottitis. It is rare that more extensive imaging such as a CT with contrast of the neck would be required. Appropriate diagnosis and treatment of GABHS pharyngitis has led to

a dramatic decrease in the incidence of rheumatic fever. Treatment does not appear to prevent poststreptococcal glomerulonephritis.

▶ **Treatment**

A. Symptomatic Therapy

Symptomatic therapy can be used to decrease the discomfort from an inflamed pharynx, including acetaminophen, NSAIDs, and saltwater gargles in age appropriate patients. In severe cases, dexamethasone can be used to decrease pharyngeal edema.

B. Antimicrobial Therapy

If pharyngitis is determined to be GABHS by rapid antigen test, or is later confirmed by throat culture after negative rapid antigen test, administer antimicrobial therapy immediately. Treatment of patients with a high clinical suspicion of GABHS pharyngitis before test results are available is an option, provided a mechanism is in place to discontinue antibiotics if GABHS infection is not confirmed. Penicillin, which has never shown resistance to GABHS, remains the drug of choice for treatment of GABHS. In patients diagnosed with GABHS and acute otitis media amoxicillin appears to be efficacious.

Penicillin V is administered orally at 250 mg b.i.d. or t.i.d. in children and 250 mg t.i.d. to q.i.d. in adolescents. A 10-day course is recommended. A single intramuscular injection of benzathine penicillin is dosed at 6 million units for children less than 27 kg and for 1.2 million units for all others. For patients allergic to penicillin, erythromycin and possibly cephalosporin drugs are reasonable alternatives.

C. Treatment of Peritonsillar Abscesses and Retropharyngeal Abscesses

The definitive treatment of PTAs and RPAs includes broad-spectrum antibiotics and abscess incision and drainage. Antibiotic choices include penicillin and a β-lactamase inhibitor, carbapenem, or clindamycin. PTAs often require aspiration or incision and drainage, while RPAs are often managed nonoperatively.

► Disposition

Most patients with pharyngitis can be safely discharged with close follow-up. Patients in whom there is suspicion for potential airway difficulty or who are unable to tolerate oral intake with dehydration should be admitted for observation and fluid resuscitation. In noncomplicated cases where the abscess is minimal and easily visualized, bedside drainage of PTAs may occur in the emergency department, with close oto-rhinolaryngology follow-up. The remainder of patients should be hospitalized for IV antibiotics, airway monitoring, intravenous fluid resuscitation, and definitive incision and drainage.

Belleza WG, Kalman S: Otolaryngologic emergencies in the out-patient setting. Med Clin North Am 2006;90:329 [PMID: 16448878].

Bisno AL et al: Practice guidelines for the diagnosis and management of group: a streptococcal pharyngitis. Clin Infect Dis 2002;35:113 [PMID: 1207516].

Gerber MA: Diagnosis and treatment of pharyngitis in children. Pediatr Clin North Am 2005;52:729 [PMID: 15925660].

Whitman JH: Upper respiratory tract infections. Clin Fam Pract 2004;6:1535.

CELLULITIS AND SUBCUTANEOUS ABSCESSES

► General Considerations

Simple superficial cellulitis in the pediatric population is routinely treated for the basic skin flora organisms of streptococcus and staphylococcus aureus. In recent years, however, subcutaneous abscess and cellulitis management have become more common and complex due to the increase of infections caused by community acquired methicillin resistant staphylococcus aureus (CA-MRSA). With the outbreak of CA-MRSA, there has been a sharp increase of emergency department visits for abscess management in the healthy pediatric population nationwide. One study found a sevenfold increase in CA-MRSA from 1999 to 2006. Many emergency departments are seeing over 50–60% of all abscesses in children culture positive for CA-MRSA. CA-MRSA is spread via direct contact with skin surfaces. Increased risk factors associated with the spread of CA-MRSA include: (1) close skin-to-skin contact, (2) open wounds in the skin, (3) crowded living conditions, and (4) poor hygiene.

► Clinical Findings

Classic findings of superficial cellulitis are also hallmark signs of an early abscess infection. These can include redness, swelling, warmth, pain, and tenderness. Unique to abscess formation, the patient will commonly complain of a preceding "spider bite." As the infection worsens, fluctuance will become apparent with a white or yellow center and can spontaneously drain pus. CA-MRSA infections are more commonly found on the buttocks, legs, and thighs. In some cases, CA-MRSA can evolve into bacteremia, empyema, and sepsis. It can also be found in conjunction with "super-infections" with preceding viral or influenza infection.

► Treatment

When treating superficial cellulitis, one must consider anti-microbial therapy with coverage for Streptococcus as well as other basic skin flora organisms. Antibiotic choice can include cephalexin, dicloxicillin, or cefazolin. If an abscess is present, simple incision and drainage is the treatment of choice. Needle aspiration is also an option for draining a small subcutaneous fluid collection. Currently there are mutiple antimicrobial options for out-patient management of CA-MRSA which include: (1)trimethoprim-sulfamethoxazole(TMZ), (2) clindamycin, (3) rifampin (not used in montherapy), and (4) linezolid. Some strains of CA-MRSA have an inducible resistance to clindamycin. If the culture sensitivities show CA-MRSA susceptibility to clindamycin but resistance to erythromycin, the strain could have an inducible resistance to clindamycin. Definitive efficacy can be confirmed with a D-test through the laboratory. The regional rates and types of inducible CA-MRSA resistance should be evaluated to determine the best out-patient antimicrobial choice. Some physicians consider adding a second antimicrobial agent to treat both superficial cellulitis and early CA-MRSA in the patient who has a history of previous infection or exposure to CA-MRSA or if there is significant cellulitis surrounding the abscess.

Severe infections with large abscesses and patient symptoms consistant with systemic bacteremia need emergent surgical consultation for operative incision and drainage as well as IV antimicrobial therapy, usually vancomycin. Supportive and aggressive management of the septic pediatric patient is a necessity with IVF resuscitation, laboratory evaluation including CBC, BMP, blood and urine cultures as well as possible CSF evaluation and inpatient admission.

▶ Disposition

Close follow-up is a necessity for patients that receive abscess incision and drainage to evaluate for resolution of infection as well as any culture results and antimicrobial sensitivities. If CA-MRSA infection becomes a recurring problem, refer the patient to pediatric infectious disease specialist.

Buckingham S, McDougal L, Cathey L et al: Emergence of community-associated methicillin-resistant *Staphylococcus aureus* at a memphis, tennessee children's hospital. Ped Inf Dis J 2004;23(7):619–624 [PMID: 15247599].

Centers for Disease Control and Prevention: Overview of community-associated MRSA. http://www.cdc.gov/ncidod/dhqp/ar_mrsa_ca_clinicians.html#4

Jaggi P, Paule S, Peterson L, Tan T: Characteristics of *Staphylococcus aureus* infections, Chicago Pediatric Hospital, Emerg Infect Dis 2007;13(2). www.cdc.gov/eid

PERIORBITAL AND ORBITAL CELLULITIS

ESSENTIALS OF DIAGNOSIS

- ▶ Erythema and swelling around the eye
- ▶ Pain with limitation of ocular motility and decreased visual acuity differentiates orbital from periorbital cellulitis

▶ General Considerations

Periorbital cellulitis, also commonly referred to as preseptal cellulitis, is an infection anterior to the orbital septum. This is an important distinction as the orbital septum provides a barrier to spread of infection into the orbit and breach of this barrier may provide access to intracranial structures. It is often secondary to eyelid infections, sinusitis, upper respiratory infection, otitis media, or eye trauma. *H. influenzae,* *Staphylococcus* sp., and *Streptococcus* sp. are the most common pathogens. Orbital cellulitis differs in that it is an infection of the contents of the orbit posterior to the septum. It usually results from severe sinusitis and is also typically caused by *Staphylococcus* and *Streptococcus* sp. as well as *H. influenzae.*

▶ Clinical Findings

Patients with periorbital cellulitis present with erythema and edema of the eyelid and surrounding skin and may be associated with chemosis, conjunctivitis, fever, and nasal discharge.

Periorbital cellulitis is often a clinical diagnosis; blood and wound cultures may be of assistance in pathogen identification. In orbital cellulitis, physical examination often demonstrates unilateral proptosis, pain with limitation of ocular motility, decreased visual acuity, or an afferent papillary defect. This can indicate progression past the orbital septum. Orbital cellulitis is evaluated by CT scan of the orbits to determine extent of infection and to evaluate for a periosteal abscess. CBC and blood cultures should also be obtained.

▶ Treatment

Mild periorbital cellulitis is typically treated on an ambulatory basis with dicloxacillin, 25 mg/kg/d divided four times daily, or cephalexin, 25–100 mg/kg/d divided four times daily. For children who do not respond to outpatient therapy, have severe infection, or are ill appearing, use IV ceftriaxone, 100 mg/kg/d divided twice daily, or IV cefuroxime, 100 mg/kg/d divided three times daily. IV antibiotic treatment is indicated for orbital cellulitis (second- or third-generation cephalosporins or ampicillin–sulbactam are appropriate choices).

▶ Disposition

Children with mild periorbital cellulitis can be managed on an outpatient basis with close follow-up. Patients with extensive cellulitis, toxic appearance, or those who do not respond to outpatient management require admission. A nasal decongestant and warm compresses may also be beneficial to patients.

Management of orbital cellulitis should include blood cultures and CBC if the patient is febrile or appears bacteremic. Infants under age 3 months with these symptoms should be worked up as outlined previously. Obtain a CT scan without contrast for all patients suspected of having orbital cellulitis. Mild cases may be managed with daily ceftriaxone injections. More severe cases should receive inpatient IV antibiotics (second or third-generation cephalosporins or ampicillin–sulbactam are appropriate choices). Consultation with ophthalmology is highly advised.

Greenberg MF, Pollard ZF: The red eye in childhood. Pediatr Clin North Am 2003;50:105 [PMID: 12713107].

Naradzay J, Barish RA: Approach to ophthalmologic emergencies. Med Clin North Am 2006;90:305 [PMID: 16448877].

Pasternak A: Opthalmologic infections in primary care. Clin Fam Pract 2004;6:19.

URINARY TRACT INFECTION

▶ General Considerations

Similar to adults, UTIs are relatively common in the pediatric populations. However, the implications of UTIs in pediatric population differ significantly. UTI in the pediatric population may be a hallmark of an anatomic anomaly, such as obstruction or vesicoureteral reflux. Children also have a greater risk of renal scarring after a UTI.

Among children 2 months to 2 years of age with a fever without a source, ~5% are diagnosed with a UTI. Premature infants have greater risk of UTI as well. Males have a higher rate of UTI in the first months of life. From that point forward, the incidence is higher in females than males, and is lowest in circumcised boys. Studies have shown a 5–20% increase risk of UTI in uncircumcised males versus circumcised males under age 2. Recurrence rates are similar between the sexes, but recurrence in males greater than 1 year after primary infection is rare.

In the healthy child, pathogens typically reach the urinary tract as a result of retrograde migration of enteric bacteria colonizing the periurethral area, most commonly *E. coli*. Other common pathogens include *Klebsiella*, *Proteus*, other *Enterobacteria*, *Staphylococcus saprophyticus* (especially in sexually active females), and *Staph. aureus*. In neonates, hematogenous seeding of the urinary tract may occur during sepsis. Infants and children with recurrent infections, abnormal urinary tract anatomy, or frequent urinary instrumentation are at greater risk for *Enterococcus* or *Pseudomonas*.

▶ Clinical Findings

Nonspecific presentations are typical in patients under 2 years of age. Symptoms may include fever, fussiness, vomiting, diarrhea, abdominal pain, or poor feeding. A caretaker may notice foul-smelling or cloudy urine. In this population, fever is often the only presenting symptoms and UTI should be in the differential for any febrile patient without an apparent source. Older children may present with the more classic symptoms of dysuria, urgency, frequency, and suprapubic or low back pain. Incontinence and enuresis should raise suspicion for the presence of UTI as well. In adolescents, the presence of dysuria and other associated symptoms may be a hallmark of sexually transmitted disease (STD) and should be evaluated by the physician.

The key to diagnosis of UTI is the demonstration of bacteria in the urine. Obtaining an appropriate specimen in the pediatric patient is of great importance and may be quite difficult. Urine specimens may be obtained by suprapubic bladder aspiration, urethral catheterization, or midstream clean catch in a toilet-trained child. A urine bag collection technique in a nontoilet-trained child can be considered as a screening tool, however, due to the high rate of contamination, it is only useful if negative for signs of infection. A urine sample collected via urine bag technique should never be sent for a culture. If the urine is positive for infection, further confirmatory testing should be done by one of the other collection techniques listed. Once collected, the urine specimen should be processed as rapidly as possible.

Urine specimens should be sent for culture and microscopy. Culture results are typically not available until at least 12–24 hours from initial processing; thus urinalysis by microscopy is commonly used for a presumptive diagnosis.

The presence of bacteria on urinalysis can be due to infection or contamination, but the presence of greater than 10 WBCs per high-powered field has a relatively high positive predictive value. The presence of nitrites (a by-product of bacterial metabolism) is 98% specific for UTI. Positive leukocyte esterase (produced by activated leukocytes) is 83% sensitive and 78% specific for UTI.

Neonates with UTI on urinalysis or culture should have CBC and blood cultures drawn and CSF studies considered. Blood cultures should also be obtained for any infant or young child with high fever or toxic appearance. Diagnostic imaging tests are seldom indicated in the acute setting.

▶ Treatment

A. Outpatient Treatment

Patients older than 2 months with a nontoxic appearance and ability to tolerate oral intake may be managed on an outpatient basis. Initial therapy should be broad spectrum and cover the most common pathogens. Common oral antibiotics used include TMP-SMX, amoxicillin (although *E. coli* resistance is increasing), nitrofurantoin (unless pyelonephritis is a consideration), or oral cephalosporins. The choice can be further tailored when results of the urine culture are available. Physicians may consider an IV or intramuscular dose of antibiotic, such as ceftriaxone, while the patient is in the emergency department followed by oral antibiotics upon discharge. A 7–10-day course is recommended for uncomplicated UTI and 14 days for complicated infections or suspected concomitant pyelonephritis. For patients requiring inpatient treatment, IV ampicillin with gentamycin or ceftriaxone are commonly administered antibiotics.

B. Inpatient Treatment

Neonates and any additional patients who do not meet criteria for outpatient management should be admitted for IV antibiotics.

C. Evaluation for Urinary Tract Anomalies

Because of the frequency of urinary tract anomalies in children who have UTIs, renal and bladder ultrasound is recommended for all children younger than 2 years with first UTI. It should also be considered in males older than 2 years with UTI and girls with repeated UTIs. Vesicocystourethrogram is also recommended in this subset of population to evaluate for vesicourethral reflux. Imaging is not typically necessary in the emergency department and may be done after admission or on an outpatient basis if the patient meets discharge criteria.

▶ Disposition

Hospital admission for IV antibiotics is indicated for patients younger than 2 months with UTIs, as well as toxic, vomiting or dehydrated patients. Patients with urosepsis, who are immunocompromised, have decreased renal function, or who appear to be failing outpatient management should also be admitted. Nontoxic, febrile, older infants, and children with UTI can receive treatment on an outpatient basis with follow-up at 24–48 hours. Urine cultures results should be evaluated to ensure appropriate antibiotic selection.

Layton KL: Diagnosis and management of pediatric urinary tract infections. Clin Fam Pract 2003;5:367.

Ma JF, Dairiki Shortliffe LM: Urinary tract infection in children: etiology and epidemiology. Urol Clin N Am 2004;31:517 [PMID: 15313061].

Malhotra SM, Kennedy WA: Urinary tract infections in children: treatment. Urol Clin N Am 2004;31:527 [PMID: 15313062].

Shlager TA: Urinary tract infections in infants and children. Infect Dis Clin North Am 2003;17:353 [PMID: 12848474].

Bachur R. Nonresponders: prolonged fever among infants with urinary tract infections. Pediatrics. 2000;105:E59.

Schoen EJ: Circumcision for preventing urinary tract infections in boys: North American View. Arch Dis Child 2005;90:772–773 [PMID: 16040868].

GASTROENTERITIS

▶ General Considerations

Diarrhea is a common reason for bringing a child to medical attention. Dehydration frequently complicates diarrhea in children, particularly young children who experience a greater net fluid and electrolyte loss. Acute diarrhea in children most commonly results from infectious gastroenteritis. Keys to management include identification of children who will benefit from antimicrobial therapy, prevention and treatment of dehydration, and identification of children with diarrhea secondary to other processes (eg, intussusception, hemolytic uremic syndrome). In the United States, rotavirus is the most common cause of acute diarrhea, particularly in winter months.

▶ Clinical Findings

A. Symptoms and Signs

Information regarding the duration of diarrhea, number of stools per day, frequency of urination, presence of tears when crying, and most recent weight of the child are helpful in assessing the risk of dehydration. A history of frequent vomiting, particularly early in the course of the disease, suggests a viral cause. High fever, lack of vomiting, abdominal pain with bowel movements, and the presence of gross blood and mucus in the stool suggest a bacterial cause. A history of recent antibiotic use suggests the possibility of pseudomembranous colitis. A history of recent travel suggests the possibility of a parasitic infection or traveler's diarrhea. Children in daycare are particularly susceptible to infections with *Giardia lamblia*. Inquire about a common outbreak of symptoms in family members that may suggest food poisoning. When more than one family member has symptoms of

nausea, vomiting, or headache, explore the possibility of carbon monoxide poisoning. Assess the child's hydration status, and look for signs of appendicitis or intussusception. Serial abdominal examinations are recommended to rule out surgical conditions. Gastroenteritis is one of the most common diagnoses listed in cases of missed appendicitis.

B. Laboratory Findings

1. Stool culture—A stool culture is the most reliable means of identifying a bacterial cause. It is not cost effective, however, to culture the stool of every child with diarrhea. Obtain cultures from children at highest risk for bacterial disease. Stool cultures for *Shigella*, *Salmonella*, *E. Coli* 0157:H7, and *Campylobacter* should be obtained in the following circumstances:

- If the child presents with obvious symptoms of acute bacterial dysentery (ie, fever, watery stool, fecal leukocytes, and gross blood in the stool).

- If the child has abrupt onset of frequent stools without the initial vomiting common to viral gastroenteritis. Perform methylene blue slide examination for the presence of fecal leukocytes. A positive result (>5 WBCs per high-power field) is a sensitive indicator of a bacterial pathogen. Trophozoites of *G. lamblia* may also be identified.

- If the child has hemoglobinopathies or immunodeficiencies.

2. Peripheral WBC count—While not necessary in most cases, a peripheral WBC count may be helpful, because *Salmonella* and *Shigella* can cause leukocytosis. Some patients with *Shigella* infection may have a low WBC count with a marked shift to the left.

3. Other laboratory tests—If the child appears dehydrated, check serum electrolytes, BUN, creatinine, and fingerstick blood sugar. Blood cultures are also indicated in febrile young infants with bloody diarrhea and any child who appears significantly ill. If the child is in day-care or has a recent history of travel, consider examination of the stool for ova and parasites.

▶ Treatment

A. Rehydration

The use of oral rehydration solutions for children with mild to moderate dehydration and of IV fluids for children with more severe dehydration is critical to prevent severe morbidity and mortality. Breast-feeding infants should continue to breast feed while taking oral rehydration.

B. Antiemetics and Antidiarrheal Agents

Antiemetic and antidiarrheal drugs occasionally worsen symptoms in children with gastroenteritis. Promethazine is contraindicated in children younger than 2 years. Some recent studies have seen improvement with tolerating oral rehydration after dosing a patient with ondansetron and it is frequently used to control vomiting in children with gastroenteritis.

C. Antimicrobial Therapy

Antibiotic therapy is not indicated for a majority of gastroenteritis infections, as most are self-limited. The empiric use of antibiotic therapy can be considered for obvious symptoms of most bacterial dysentery. TMP-SMZ (TMP, 8–12 mg/kg/d, and SMZ, 30–60 mg/kg/d, in divided doses every 12 hours) can be given empirically until culture results are available. Regarding pediatric specific treatment of salmonella, antibiotics are only indicated in patients < 2 months old, in those with sickle cell disease, patients with extra intestinal infection or in those who are immunocompromised.

▶ Disposition

Hospitalize children with moderate to severe dehydration, particularly if vomiting prevents oral rehydration, and young infants with fever and bloody diarrhea. Young infants are at increased risk for *Salmonella* bacteremia.

Instruct parents about the signs of dehydration and the proper use of oral rehydration solutions. Parents should encourage children to continue small but frequent amounts of liquids at home and to resume a low-fat diet as tolerated.

Infants under 6 months of age should be followed up by telephone or be seen in 24 hours. Reevaluate older children if diarrhea persists longer than 3 days. Stable children with bloody diarrhea should be reexamined in 24 hours.

Reeves J, Shannon M, Fleisher G: Ondansetron decreases vomiting associated with acute gastroenteritis. Pediatrics 2002;109;62–68 [PMID: 11927735].

Freedman S, Adler M, Seshadri R, Powell E: Oral ondansetron for gastroenteritis in a Pediatric Emergency Department. N Engl J Med 2006;354:1698–1705 [PMID: 16625009].

SEPTIC ARTHRITIS

ESSENTIALS OF DIAGNOSIS

- ▶ Patients usually febrile
- ▶ Involved joint is tender, swollen, erythematous, with painful range of motion
- ▶ Aspiration with fluid analysis is diagnostic

▶ General Considerations

Septic arthritis is the bacterial invasion of a joint space and the subsequent inflammatory response. The synovium is highly vascular and prone to bacteremic seeding. Contiguous spread and direct inoculation from penetrating trauma may also lead to this condition. Patients with sickle cell disease (SCD) and diabetes mellitus are at increased risk. The knees and hips are the most commonly affected joints.

Most cases of septic arthritis are caused by gram-positive organisms, particularly *Staph. aureus*. GABHS and *Strep. pneumoniae* are also noted causes. Patients with sickle cell anemia are at increased risk for septic arthritis due to *Salmonella* sp. In the neonatal population, *Staph. aureus* remains the most common, but group B *Streptococcus* and gram-negative enteric organisms are also seen. *Neisseria gonorrhoeae* should be considered as a causative agent in sexually active adolescents.

▶ Clinical Findings

A. Symptoms and Signs

Patients typically present with focal findings at the infected joint. Warmth, erythema, swelling, and pain with range of motion are common findings. Systemic symptoms, such as fever and malaise, are often present. Children will usually keep the affected joint in a position that maximizes comfort. Any sudden onset of refusing to move a limb or joint should raise concern for this condition. In neonates and infants, discomfort may be noted during manipulation of the knees and hips during diaper changes. Toxic synovitis can closely mimic septic arthritis. These patients may have similar complaints but in general have a lower-grade temperature, less pain on joint manipulation, and a more indolent course.

B. Laboratory Findings

1. Joint aspiration—Definitive diagnosis is established by joint aspiration. Examine joint fluid for Gram stain and culture, cell count and differential, glucose, and protein. In general, the WBC count for septic arthritis will be over 50,000 (with greater than 75% PMNs) as compared to transient synovitis in which the WBC count in the synovial fluid is usually between 5000 and 15,000 (with less than 25% PMNs). The glucose level is usually low at less than 40 mg/dL in septic arthritis.

2. Blood tests—CBC with differential, C-reactive protein, and erythrocyte sedimentation rate are often elevated in septic arthritis. When normal, these do not rule out septic arthritis, but are helpful when considering other etiologies. Blood cultures should also be obtained.

C. Imaging

X-rays may show a widened joint space in septic arthritis, especially when comparing the hip joint space, and are useful to rule out fractures and other conditions. If septic arthritis is suspected, obtainment of plain films should not delay joint aspiration and treatment. Ultrasound is useful in identifying location and size of effusions, especially in deeper joints such as the hip, and may be used to guide aspiration. Bone scan

Table 50–17. Commonly Encountered Organisms in Septic Arthritis.

Patient/Condition	Expected Organisms	Antibiotic Considerations
Neonates and infants	*Staphylococcus*, gram-negative bacteria, group B *Streptococcus*, *Candida*	Nafcillin[a] plus aminoglycoside or third-generation cephalosporin, ampicillin-sulbactam
Children younger than 5 years	*Staphylococcus*, group A Streptococcuss, pneumococcus, *Hoemophilus influenzae*	Nafcillin[a] plus aminoglycoside or third-generation cephalosporin, ampicillin-sulbactam
Older children and healthy adults	*Staphylococcus*, *Gonococcus*, *streptococcus*	Nafcillin[a] plus third-generation cephalosporin, ampicillin-sulbactam
Involvement of the foot	*Staphylococcus*, *Pseudomonas*	Nafcillin[a] plus ceftazidime or aminoglycoside
Intravenous drug users	*Staphylococcus*, gram-negative bacilli	Nafcillin[a] plus aminoglycoside, ampicillin-sulbactam
Sickle-cell patients	*salmonella*	Ciprofloxacin, ofloxacin, or ceftriaxone

[a]First generation cephalosporins may be substituted for penicillinase-resistant penicillin, Vancomycin should be employed for the treatment of suspected methicillin-resistant Staphylococci.
(Used with permission from Tintinalli JE, Kaplan GD, Stapczynski JS (editors): *Acute Disorders of Joints and Bursae*, 5th ed. Table 278–4.)

and MRI are often helpful diagnostic adjuncts, but are more typically used in the inpatient setting.

▶ Treatment

Antibiotic therapy should be initiated without delay. A list of the typical organisms involved in septic arthritis can be found in Table 50–17. If Gram stain is available, results can be used to guide antibiotic selection. Traditionally, if gram-positive cocci are seen, a penicillinase-resistant penicillin (eg, oxacillin, 150 mg/ kg/d, divided in four doses) has been appropriate. In the current era of increasing community-acquired MRSA, however, vancomycin or clindamycin should be strongly considered. If gram-negative or no organisms are seen on Gram stain, a third-generation cephalosporin, such as cefotaxime or ceftriaxone, should be used. This will also provide coverage for gonorrheal septic arthritis. Neonates are often treated with oxacillin or nafcillin plus cefotaxime or gentamicin. Coverage can be tailored once culture results are available. Despite the early initiation of antibiotics, septic arthritis remains a surgical emergency. Timely orthopedic consultation and drainage are essential. Pain management can be addressed though the use of NSAIDs and narcotic medication as needed.

▶ Disposition

Hospitalize children with suspected septic arthritis for IV antibiotic therapy. Obtain orthopedic consultation to evaluate the need for surgical drainage of the affected joint.

Frank G et al: Musculoskeletal infections in children. Pediatr Clin North Am 2005;52:1083 [PMID: 16009258].

Ross JJ: Septic arthritis. Infect Dis Clin North Am 2005;19:799 [PMID: 16297733].

ACUTE OSTEOMYELITIS

ESSENTIALS OF DIAGNOSIS

▶ Usually warm, tender, swollen area
▶ Initially X-rays tend to be normal

▶ General Considerations

Acute osteomyelitis is a pyogenic infection of bone that occurs in about 1 in 5000 children before the age of 13 years. Although any bone may be involved, in children, the long bones are more frequently infected. Infection usually is the result of seeding, although spread from a contiguous focus or through direct traumatic inoculation can also occur.

Over 90% of cases of acute hematogenous osteomyelitis are caused by *Staph. aureus*. Group A streptococci and *H. influenzae* are less common causes. In neonates, osteomyelitis may also be caused by group B streptococci and gram-negative enteric organisms. Children with SCD are at risk for *Salmonella* and *Strep. pneumoniae* osteomyelitis. Puncture wounds to the plantar surface of the foot may result in *Pseudomonas aeruginosa* osteomyelitis.

▶ Clinical Findings

A. Symptoms and Signs

The clinical hallmarks are fever and well-localized bone tenderness. Chills, malaise, and ill appearance are frequently present. Lower extremity disease will frequently result in a limp. Point tenderness is usually evident on careful examination. There may also be swelling, warmth, redness, and focal induration at the site of infection. The young infant is usually irritable when the affected extremity is touched or moved. Pseudoparalysis is common, and occasionally significant swelling of the extremity will occur.

B. Laboratory Findings

Draw blood for culture, CBC with differential, C-reactive protein, and erythrocyte sedimentation rate. Blood cultures are positive in about 30–50% of patients with osteomyelitis.

C. Imaging

Obtain plain X-rays of the affected extremity. Radiographic changes are usually not evident until 7–10 days after disease onset. However, soft tissue swelling and obliteration of the tissue planes may be the initial radiographic findings. Later findings include periosteal reaction and osteolysis.

After the child has been admitted to the hospital, technetium bone scans or MRI may be helpful. Bone aspiration under CT or ultrasound guidance may reveal the etiologic agent.

▶ Treatment

The mainstay of treatment of acute osteomyelitis is parenteral antibiotics. Because culture results are usually not available when the diagnosis is first made, empiric therapy depends on the patient's age. In children with puncture wound osteomyelitis of the foot, surgical debridement is an important part of therapy and parenteral antibiotics active against *Pseudomonas* should be started.

▶ Disposition

Hospitalize children in whom acute osteomyelitis is suspected.

Kaplan SL: Osteomyelitis in children. Infect Dis Clin North Am 2005;19:787 [PMID: 16297732].

Kothari NA, Pelchovitz DJ, Meyer JS: Imaging of musculoskeletal infections. Radiol Clin North Am 2001;39:653 [PMID: 11549164].

▼ GASTROINTESTINAL DISORDERS

ABDOMINAL PAIN

▶ General Considerations

Abdominal pain and gastrointestinal disturbances are frequently encountered in the care of the pediatric patient. There are a vast number of conditions that appear in the differential diagnosis of abdominal pain and differentiating the benign causes from the true emergencies can be a challenging and extremely difficult task. The causes of abdominal pain vary by the age of the patient (see Table 50–18). Gastroenteritis is the most common medical complaint, appendicitis the most common of a surgical nature.

Abdominal pain occurs via three separate pathways: visceral, parietal, and referred. Visceral pain occurs when stimuli such as tension, stretching, or ischemia affect a viscus, such as the stomach or intestines. Visceral pain fibers are bilateral and enter the spinal cord at multiple levels. Irritation of these fibers causes pain that is dull, poorly localized, and midline in location. Parietal pain results from irritation of the parietal peritoneum. These fibers transmit to the same side and dermatomal level of the site of irritation. This pathway leads to sharp, intense, well-localized pain. Referred pain is similar to parietal pain with the exception that the pain is felt in remote areas supplied by the same dermatome as the site of local irritation.

▶ Clinical Findings

A. Symptoms and Signs

A thorough history is essential; the character of the pain, onset, duration, severity, and location should be elicited. Aggravating and relieving factors, associated symptoms, gynecologic and sexual history, and medical history are also important information.

Rapid cardiopulmonary assessment is the initial step in the physical examination. If the patient appears toxic or has unstable vital signs, aggressive resuscitation should coincide with history and further physical examination. Much can be learned by simple direct observation before manual examination. Is the patient active and playful or lying in bed avoiding any movement? The abdomen should be inspected for distention, masses, or peristaltic waves. Auscultate the abdomen in all quadrants to evaluate the nature of the bowel sounds. If the child is able to indicate the area of maximal tenderness, start with gentle palpation away from the site and move slowly to the area. Percussion should be used to elicit rebound tenderness. Deeper palpation is used to discover masses or organomegaly.

A thorough extra-abdominal examination is indicated. Lower lobe pneumonia can be a cause of referred abdominal pain, as can Streptococcal pharyngitis. Genitourinary examination may reveal a testicular torsion or hair tourniquet. In sexually active females, pelvic examination is indicated. Rectal examination can be helpful in numerous conditions, including retrocecal appendicitis, intussusception, gastrointestinal bleeding, abscess, or impaction. Signs associated with appendicitis such as Rovsing's sign (palpation of left lower quadrant causes pain in right lower quadrant), iliopsoas (reproduction of pain with extension of right hip and flexion of right thigh), and obturator (pain reproduced with rotation of flexed right hip) should be checked and documented. A modified heel tap sign can be performed by having a child stand and jump, then evaluate for right lower

Table 50-18. Common Nontraumatic Causes of Abdominal Pain.[a]

Organ System	Clinical Entity and Demographics	History	Physical Examination and Laboratory Findings	Imaging Studies
Gastrointestinal	Appendicitis peak: 10-1 2 years M:F3:2	Periumbilical pain followed by right lower quadrant pain, anorexia, and emesis	Temperature > 100.5°F, right lower quadrant pain, peritoneal signs (if perforated); often elevated white blood cell count	X-rays: Concave curvature of the spine to the right; fecalith (5-10%) Ultrasound: Pericolic or appendiceal fluid; edema Abdominal CT scan with intravenous contrast: Enlarged appendix or right lower quadrant stranding or fluid
	Meckel diverticulitis Mean: 2 years	Typically painless gastrointestinal bleeding; stool appears bright red or tarry	Anemia, elevated blood urea nitrogen and creatinine	X-rays: Typically normal, possible obstruction or perforation Meckel's scan with technetium 99m recommended
	Intussusception 5-9 months M:F3:2	Paroxysmal crampy abdominal pain followed by periods of calmness, emesis, currant jelly stools	Fever, distension (late), right-sided mass; dehydration, anemia, leukocytosis (late)	X-rays: Obstructive pattern Ultrasound: Intussusception "pseudokidney" and "target" signs Contrast enema: Intussusception and failure of gas or contrast to reflux into the small bowel is diagnostic and often therapeutic
	Pyloric stenosis	Nonbilious projectile vomiting following feeds	Scaphoid abdomen, peristaltic waves, palpable olive; hypochloremic, hypokalemic metabolic acidosis	X-rays: Dilated stomach Ultrasound: Hypertrophied pylorus "bulls-eye" and "sausage" sign
	Malrotation/midgut volvulus < 1 month M:F3:2	Sudden onset of bilious emesis, abdominal pain, and feeding intolerance	Normal (early), tenderness, possible distension, peritonitis (late); dehydration; anemia; leukocytosis (late)	X-rays: Distended stomach, gasless abdomen (high obstruction) Upper gastrointestinal: Abnormal duodenal sweep Lower gastrointestinal: Cecum in the left abdomen or right lower quadrant
	Incarcerated inguinal hernia < 1 year F > M	Irritability; crampy, abdominal pain; nonbilious emesis (early); bilious emesis (late)	Firm, tender groin or scrotal mass; dehydration leukocytosis (late)	X-rays: Obstructive pattern
	Hirschprung disease	Infant unable to pass meconium in 24 h after birth, diarrhea ± emesis, no rectal stool	Asymptomatic (early), lethargy, fever, obtunded, shock (late), abdominal distension, normal or hyperactive bowel sounds	X-rays: Distended bowel loops, abrupt cutoff below pelvic brim; relatively airless rectum Barium enema: Postevacuation films show transition zone
	Constipation	Two or fewer bowel movements per week with excessive straining	Crampy abdominal pain without peritoneal signs; may have abdominal mass	X-rays: Not required; may show large amount of stool in colon or rectum

(continued)

Table 50–18. Common Nontraumatic Causes of Abdominal Pain.[a] (*Continued*)

Organ System	Clinical Entity and Demographics	History	Physical Examination and Laboratory Findings	Imaging Studies
Gynecologic	Ectopic pregnancy	Delayed menses, abdominal pain, vaginal bleeding	Positive urine pregnancy test, lower quadrant pain and tenderness, amenorrhea, adnexal tenderness	*Ultrasound:* Free fluid in pelvis, adnexal mass, gestational sac outside uterus, ectopic fetal heart beat activity
	Salpingitis	Increased vaginal discharge, pelvic pain, symptoms of urethritis	Cervical motion tenderness, adnexal tenderness, possible fever	*Ultrasound:* Free fluid in pelvis, adnexal mass
Pulmonary	Influenza	Signs and symptoms of viral illness	Altered breath sounds, low grade fever	*X-rays:* Viral pattern
	Pneumonia	Dyspnea, cough, ± chest pain	Altered breath sounds, fever; elevated absolute neutrophil count, elevated C-reactive protein	*X-rays:* Infiltrate, possible consolidation
Renal	Cystitis F > M	Urinary frequency, dysuria, nocturia, history of congenital abnormalities	Suprapubic tenderness, pyuria, bacteruria, varying degrees of hematuria	None recommended
	Pyelonephritis F > M	Flank pain, possible frequency or dysuria, nausea and vomiting, history of congenital abnormalities	Flank and occasionally lower quadrant tenderness, fever	*Ultrasound:* May show hydronephrosis in cases of chronic reflux. *Abdominal CT scan with intravenous contrast:* Decreased enhancement, enlargement of kidney

[a]Modified and reproduced, with permission, from Irish MS, Pearl RH, Caty M, Glick P: The approach to common abdominal diagnoses in infants and children. Pediatr Clin North Am 1998;45(4):730.

quadrant discomfort/peritoneal signs upon landing. When considering a pediatric specific abdominal pathology differential, one should include intussusception, Hisrchsprungs Disease, malrotation resulting in a midgut volvulus, streptococcal pharyngitis, lower lobe pneumonia and pain from trauma or abuse.

B. Laboratory Findings

1. Urinalysis—Look for evidence of a UTI. More than five white or red blood cells per high-power field can occasionally be seen in patients with appendicitis.

2. CBC with differential—CBC with differential may be useful in suggesting an infectious cause for abdominal pain. The WBC count is an insensitive and nonspecific test and cannot be used to rule out appendicitis.

3. Other laboratory studies—Electrolytes, BUN, and creatinine measurements should be obtained for children who appear dehydrated after protracted vomiting or diarrhea. Consider lipase and hepatic function tests if biliary disease, pancreatitis, or hepatitis are possible causes. Obtain a pregnancy test in adolescent girls.

C. Imaging

Obtain a chest X-ray for any patient with abdominal pain and respiratory symptoms to evaluate for the presence of a lower lobe infiltrate. Plain film abdominal X-rays are helpful in identification of intestinal obstruction, perforated viscus, constipation, and some types of kidney stones. CT scan of the abdomen is a sensitive test to evaluate for a variety of abdominal pathologies and may be indicated in acute abdominal pain where etiology is unclear. This must be balanced with the risks of radiation exposure, use of contrast agents, and possible need of sedation. Ultrasound may be helpful in diagnosing testicular, gynecologic, and biliary pathology, and it may also show periappendiceal inflammation and intussusception.

▶ Treatment and Disposition

Treatment is directed at the underlying cause. Often repeat physical examinations by the same physician are necessary to elicit the cause. IV fluid hydration may be necessary. Analgesics should be given for patient comfort. Recent studies indicate that appropriate pain management may assist diagnosis by allowing a more thorough examination on a comfortable patient. Any patient with an acute abdomen should remain on nothing-by-mouth status and have an immediate surgery consult. Broad-spectrum antibiotics should be given without delay if a perforated viscus is suspected. Patients with significant abdominal pain but no signs of acute abdomen may be admitted for serial abdominal examinations. In cases of mild abdominal pain with no additional concerning signs or symptoms, or known nonsignificant causes of abdominal pain, outpatient management

is acceptable. Strong precautions should be given upon discharge and follow-up for reexamination should be arranged in 12–24 hours.

D'Agostino JD: Common abdominal emergencies in children. Emerg Med Clin North Am 2002;20:139 [PMID: 11826631].

Halter JM et al: Common gastrointestinal problems and emergencies in neonates and children. Clin Fam Pract 2004;6:731.

Leung AK, Sigalet DL: Acute abdominal pain in children. Am Fam Physician 2003;67:2321 [PMID: 12800960].

McCollough M, Sharieff GQ: Abdominal pain in children. Pediatr Clin North Am 2006;53:107 [PMID: 16487787].

VOMITING

▶ General Considerations

Causes of vomiting in children may be categorized due to direct irritation to the gastrointestinal tract, intestinal or gastric outlet obstruction, effect of a toxin or other noxious stimulus on the CNS, or elevated intracranial pressure.

▶ Clinical Findings

Look for precipitating factors including trauma, medications, feeding techniques, and recent illness. It is helpful to know the nature of the vomitus (eg, bilious, bloody, coffee ground, bright red, or feculent), the relationship to eating and position, and whether projectile vomiting occurs. The absence of passage of stool or gas implies obstruction. Inspect the abdomen for signs of obstruction, and look for evidence of a systemic illness (eg, otitis media, UTI, strep pharyngitis).

A. Vomiting in the Newborn

Infants commonly regurgitate a portion of feedings. Nonforceful regurgitation is usually benign. Forceful vomiting, however, often indicates serious disease. Causes of gastrointestinal obstruction in newborns include:

1. Intestinal atresia—Intestinal obstruction will occur in the first days of life with emesis. Emesis will often be nonbilious in duodenal atresia and bilious of atresia occurs distal to the duodenum. Patients will often have abdominal distention and failure to pass meconium. Diagnosis is made by presenting symptoms and abdominal X-ray. Early surgical intervention is necessary.

2. Meconium ileus—Obstruction due to thick meconium can lead to ileus and perforation if unrecognized. A vast majority of these patients will have cystic fibrosis.

3. Meconium plug syndrome—The distal colon becomes obstructed with a plug of meconium. A barium enema shows the plug and usually relieves the obstruction. This entity is suggestive of Hirschsprung disease.

4. Midgut volvulus—This abdominal emergency typically presents in the first month of life as a result of malrotation during development. Midgut volvulus must be considered in the presence of emesis in this age range. The emesis is classically bilious in nature, but nonbilious emesis may occur in up to 20% of patients. Abdominal X-rays should be performed but a normal pattern does not rule out volvulus. An upper gastrointestinal tract contrast study is the choice for definitive diagnosis. Immediate pediatric surgery consult is essential.

5. Hirschsprung disease—This condition is characterized by aganglionosis of the distal colon. It presents most commonly in the newborn with abdominal distention and bilious vomiting. There is often a delay in passing meconium beyond in the first 24 hours of life. Diagnosis is made by barium enema.

6. Pyloric stenosis—This condition results from thickening of the antral-pyloric muscle resulting in gastric outlet obstruction. Pyloric stenosis usually presents between the third and sixth week of life, with an increased frequency in first born males, with progressive nonbilious vomiting, often described as projectile. The diagnosis can be made on physical examination with the observation of a gastric peristaltic wave, or palpation of an olive-shaped mass in the epigastrium. Diagnosis can be confirmed by ultrasound. Definitive treatment is surgical pyloromyotomy.

B. Vomiting in Infants and Children

A majority of infants and children with emesis have gastroenteritis. More serious causes of vomiting include the following:

- Intussusception—Intussusception is the prolapse of one section of the intestine into the distal adjoining section, often seen between 3 months and 5 years of age. It often presents as gastrointestinal obstruction. The classic triad consists of colicky abdominal pain, vomiting, and bloody mucous stools, and is variably present. On physical examination, an elongated mass in the right upper or right lower quadrant may be present. Rectal examination may reveal either occult blood or bloody, foul-smelling stool, often referred to as "currant jelly" stool. This is often a late finding.

- Duodenal hematoma—Consider if a history of trauma is present, traumatic pancreatitis as well as abuse should be considered.

- Appendicitis—May begin with a history or nausea and vomiting prior to the appearance of right lower quadrant abdominal pain. Associated with anorexia and classically starts with periumbilical pain that progressively localizes to the right lower quadrant.

- Hepatitis—Commonly associated in children with anorexia and vomiting as well as in teenagers and preteen population who have infectious mononucleosis.

- Incarcerated inguinal hernia—Common in children with abdominal pain and vomiting, often will have a palpable firm, indurated groin mass with an increased frequency in premature born males.

- Intracranial pathology—A mass or lesion, hemorrhage, or hydrocephalus can lead to increased intracranial pressure and should be considered as an etiology of vomiting.

► Treatment

Administer fluids if the child is dehydrated or if an obstruction is present. Obtain upright and supine X-rays and if signs of obstruction are present, insert a nasogastric tube for decompression. An air-contrast enema is indicated for both the diagnosis and treatment of intussusception. Perform an upper gastrointestinal series on an emergency basis in the infant with bilious emesis who may have a midgut volvulus. Obtain urinalysis, CBC, platelet count, and electrolyte measurement as indicated by the child's clinical condition. Imaging with ultrasound or CT is dependent on the presumed etiology of the vomiting.

A pediatric surgery consult is essential for any child with an acute abdomen and vomiting, or surgically correctable condition that cannot clinically tolerate outpatient treatment.

Brousseau T, Sharieff GQ: Newborn emergencies: the first 30 days of life. Pediatr Clin North Am 2006;53:69 [PMID: 16487785].

Gosche JR et al: Midgut abnormalities. Surg Clin North Am 2006;86:285 [PMID: 16580924].

Halter JM et al: Common gastrointestinal problems and emergencies in neonates and children. Clin Fam Pract 2004;6:731.

McCollough M, Sharieff GQ: Abdominal pain in children. Pediatr Clin North Am 2006;53:107 [PMID: 16487787].

GASTROINTESTINAL BLEEDING

► General Considerations

Gastrointestinal hemorrhage in children can result from numerous sources. The first step in evaluation is to determine if the bleeding is from an upper or lower source. Patients with hematemesis (vomiting of blood) usually have a lesion proximal to the ligament of Treitz (upper source). Bleeding from sources distal to the ligament of Treitz is referred to as lower gastrointestinal bleeds. The appearance of stool may also indicate the site of bleeding. If stools are dark or black in appearance (melena), this typically indicates a longer transit time for stool, such as upper gastrointestinal, small bowel, or slow right colon bleeding. Patients with bright red blood per rectum (hematochezia) typically have distal colon or rectal lesions. There are exceptions to this as profuse bleeding from an upper gastrointestinal source may lead to hematochezia, while slow transit from a distal colon source may lead to melena.

▶ Clinical Findings

The patient's age and the amount and type of bleeding help determine the most likely etiology. Bleeding in neonates is usually benign and self-limited. Profuse, painless bleeding may indicate Meckel's diverticulum. Bleeding associated with colicky pain may occur with intussusception. Diarrhea associated with bleeding per rectum may indicate bacterial dysentery.

Obtain vital signs to detect cardiovascular compromise. Clinical signs of liver disease may indicate a coagulopathy or esophageal varices as a possible cause of bleeding. Elicit a careful history for nonsteroidal anti-inflammatory drug use or exposure to warfarin containing drugs.

Occasionally what appears to be gastrointestinal hemorrhage is not truly from the gastrointestinal tract. Epistaxis, nasopharyngeal trauma, oral or pharyngeal postoperative bleeding (eg tonsillectomy) and hemoptysis may result in coffee-ground emesis. Some substances may color the emesis or stool red (eg, food colorings, beets, red gelatin, artificial fruit drinks, and antibiotic elixers such as cefdinir). The stool should be routinely checked with a guaiac test for occult blood.

A. Bleeding in the Newborn

1. Maternal blood ingestion—Swallowed maternal blood at delivery or from a bleeding nipple can result in hematemesis or melena in the newborn. These infants usually appear otherwise healthy. An Apt-Downey test can differentiate infant from maternal blood by identifying fetal hemoglobin.

2. Hemorrhagic disease—Newborns with hemorrhagic disease may present with melena or hematochezia. However, other evidence of a generalized bleeding disorder is usually present. Maternal medications such as aspirin or anticoagulants may result in neonatal hemorrhage. Consider vitamin K deficiency if the neonate did not receive an intramuscular injection after birth.

3. Stress ulcers—Stress ulcers can be secondary to sepsis, asphyxia, intracranial pathology, or heart disease. These ulcers may cause significant gastrointestinal bleeding.

4. Other causes—Consider necrotizing enterocolitis, anal fissures, malrotation or midgut volvulus, and Hirschsprung disease with enterocolitis.

B. Upper Gastrointestinal Bleeding in Infants and Children

The most common cause of upper gastrointestinal bleeding is esophagitis or gastric and duodenal ulceration. Esophageal varices are an uncommon cause of bleeding in young children but may develop with severe liver disease. With forceful vomiting, tears of the distal esophagus (Mallory–Weiss syndrome) can occur, causing upper gastrointestinal hemorrhage.

C. Lower Gastrointestinal Bleeding in Infants or Children

1. Anal fissures—Anal fissures are the most common cause of hematochezia in infants. This usually is from constipation and passing a large, firm stool. In pediatric patients with rectal trauma or fissures, one must also consider abuse in the differential diagnosis.

2. Cow's milk sensitivity—Sensitivity to cow's milk protein can result in severe colitis with bloody stools.

3. Intussusception—Always consider intussusception in a child who presents with colicky abdominal pain followed by vomiting. Typically, these children may appear well between episodes of vomiting. Bloody stool helps establish the diagnosis but is often a late finding.

4. Meckel diverticulum—Patients with Meckel diverticulum may present with painless appearance of bright red blood per rectum. Sufficient blood loss may result in cardiovascular compromise. The gastric mucosa within the diverticulum can be identified on technetium scan.

5. Bacterial or viral infection—Fever and diarrhea associated with blood per rectum are usually secondary to an invasive bacterial infection of the colon. Culture stool for *E. Coli*, *Campylobacter*, *Shigella*, and *Salmonella*. Viral pathogens such as rotavirus and Norwalk virus must also be considered as possible causes.

6. Hemolytic uremic syndrome (HUS)—HUS is characterized by acute renal failure with thrombocytopenia, hemolytic anemia, and bloody diarrhea. Children with this syndrome are usually quite ill and require hospitalization and close observation.

7. Intestinal polyps—Intestinal polyps are sometimes found in young children and may result in bright red blood per rectum. A diagnosis can be established by colonoscopy.

8. Henoch-Schonlein Purpura (HSP)—This disorder is characterized by small vessel vasculitis of the skin, gastrointestinal tract, and kidneys. Patients will at times have palpable purpura of the skin, joint swelling and pain, and colicky abdominal pain. Gastrointestinal bleeding may be secondary to submucosal hemorrhage. Abdominal pain and gastrointestinal bleeding may occur before the classical skin findings, complicating the diagnosis. Children with HSP are also at increased risk for intussusception.

9. Inflammatory bowel disease—Patients with inflammatory bowel disease may present with evidence of gastrointestinal bleeding associated with anemia, poor growth, abdominal pain, and diarrhea.

10. Thrombocytopenia—Children can present with low platelets resulting in gastrointestinal bleeding from new onset leukemia or secondary to the side effects of chemotherapy, as well as Idiopathic Thrombocytopenia (ITP)

▶ Treatment

Evaluate cardiovascular status. Obtain IV access and initiate blood volume as indicated by cardiovascular assessment. Send blood for CBC, coagulation studies, and type and crossmatch. Consider stool evaluation for fecal leukocytes, bacterial culture, ova, and parasites.

Place a nasogastric tube to determine if the site of bleeding is in the upper gastrointestinal tract. Lavage with saline (10 mL/kg) until active bleeding stops. Unstable patients are at risk for aspiration and may require intubation.

▶ Disposition

Admit children with acute and persistent upper gastrointestinal bleeding to the hospital for stabilization and endoscopic evaluation. Children with lower gastrointestinal bleeding can be evaluated as outpatients as long as they appear well and are hemodynamically stable with no active bleeding. Patients with abnormal hemodynamics need to be stablized prior to performing diagnostic procedures. Emergency surgical intervention may be necessary to identify the site of bleeding.

Dennehy P: Acute diarrheal disease in children: epidemiology, prevention, and treatment. Infect Dis Clin North Am 2005;19:585 [PMID: 16102650].

Gosche JR et al: Midgut abnormalities. Surg Clin North Am 2006;86:285 [PMID: 16580924].

Halter J, Baesl T, Nicolette L, et al. Common gastrointestinal problems and emergencies in neonates and children. Clin Fam Pract. 2004;6:731–754.

Lin S, Rockey DC: Obscure gastrointestinal bleeding. Gastroenterol Clin North Am 2005;34:679 [PMID: 16303577].

McCullough M, Sharieff GQ: Abdominal pain in children. Pediatr Clin North Am 2006;53:107 [PMID: 16487787].

McCullough M, Sharieff GQ: Abdominal surgical emergencies in infants and young children. Emerg Clin North Am 2003;21:909 [PMID: 14708813].

Moustafa MH et al: "My two-week-old daughter is throwing up blood." Acad Emerg Med 2005;12:775 [PMID: 16079432].

Naik-Mathuria B, Olutoye OO: Foregut abnormalities. Surg Clin N Am 2006;86:261 [PMID: 16580923].

FOREIGN BODY

▶ Esophageal Foreign Bodies

Foreign bodies within the esophagus become lodged at the cervical esophagus, aortic arch, or lower esophageal sphincter. Esophageal obstruction secondary to a foreign body may result in substernal chest pain and increased salivation secondary to inability to swallow. The physical examination is usually normal unless perforation has occurred. X-ray examination of the chest usually will identify the foreign body; in the esophagus it is best seen on an anteroposterior film (Figure 50–9). A radiolucent foreign body (eg, plastic) may not be visible on X-ray.

▶ Gastric and Small Bowel Foreign Bodies

Most foreign bodies, regardless of shape, that successfully pass through the esophagus will navigate the remainder of the gastrointestinal tract without difficulty. The occasional object that is unable to pass through the stomach after a period of 3 days should be removed by endoscopy. Intestinal obstruction may occur if a foreign body becomes lodged in the region of the ileocecal valve. Small disc batteries or "button" batteries need to be removed emergently via upper endoscopy if they have not passed within 24–48 hours. If two or more magnets are ingested, endoscopy or surgical consultation is warranted.

Baliga SK, Hussain D, Sarfraz SL, Hartung RU: Magnetic attraction: dual complications in a single case. J Coll Physicians Surg Pak 2008;18(7):440–441.

Cortes C, Silva C: Accidental ingestion of magnets in children. Report of three cases. Rev Med Chil 2006;134(10):1315–1319.

▼ HEMATOLOGICAL DISEASES

ANEMIA

▶ General Considerations

In children, over 75% of anemias are due to iron deficiency or thalassemia minor, both of which are characterized by microcytosis. The most common cause of anemia in children aged 6 months to 2 years is nutritional iron deficiency. Typically, this results from excessive cow's milk intake. Less commonly iron deficiency anemia will occur secondary to chronic blood loss, usually from the gastrointestinal tract (eg, duodenal ulcers, Meckel diverticulum, and polyps).

Anemias not due to iron deficiency may occur as a result of either of the following two: (1) Decreased erythrocyte production or release from the bone marrow, for example transient erythorblastopenia of childhood (TEC). TEC typically occurs in children aged 1–2 years. Severe anemia and reticulocytopenia spontaneously resolve in 1–2 months. (2) Increased destruction, sequestration, or acute loss of circulating red cells owing to sickle cell disease, autoimmune hemolytic anemia, or hemolytic uremic syndrome, or blood loss due to trauma, surgery, or peptic ulcer disease.

▶ Clinical Findings

A. Symptoms and Signs

With rapid onset of anemia from blood loss or hemolysis, signs of cardiovascular compromise as well as impending cardiac failure may be present. With slow onset of anemia, children typically show pallor and decreased exercise tolerance but no evidence of cardiovascular compromise even with extremely low levels of hemoglobin. Hemolytic anemias

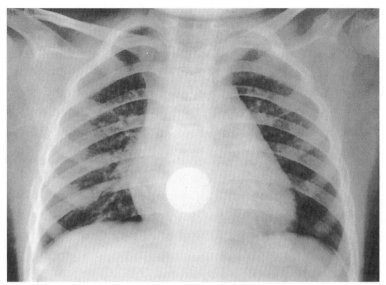

A

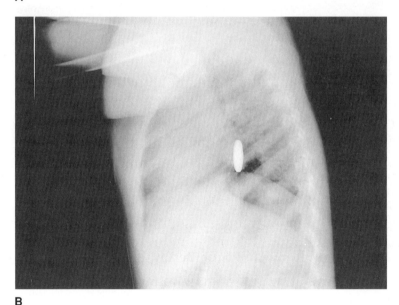

B

▲ **Figure 50–9.** Posteroanterior (A) and lateral (B) chest X-rays, showing esophageal foreign body.

may cause jaundice and splenomegaly. Petechiae may indicate hemolytic uremic syndrome and thrombocytopenia.

B. Laboratory Findings

Laboratory evaluation should include a CBC with hemoglobin, red blood cell indices, WBC, and platelet counts, peripheral smear, and reticulocyte counts. Anemia with microcytosis in a young child strongly suggests iron deficiency. If the stool is negative for occult blood, further tests are not necessary if the child is not severely anemic.

▶ Treatment

A. Iron Therapy

Treat iron deficiency with elemental iron at 3–6 mg/kg/d. Continue iron therapy for 2 months after the anemia is corrected. Restrict cow's milk intake.

If anemia has developed slowly, patients can often tolerate remarkably low hemoglobin levels, even to 4–5 g/dL, without the need for transfusion if other effective therapy is available.

B. Transfusion

Transfuse children who experience a rapid decline in hemoglobin to less than 7 g/dL, particularly if signs of cardiovascular compromise are present.

In patients with gradual onset of anemia who require transfusion, slow transfusion is recommended, because these children are at risk for CHF with rapid transfusion. Consider use of a diuretic to prevent fluid overload.

▶ Disposition

Consult with a hematologist for anemias requiring transfusion, anemias associated with hemolysis, and anemias without obvious cause.

Recheck the hemoglobin level in children receiving iron therapy in 2–4 weeks to document response.

SICKLE CELL DISEASE

▶ General Considerations

SCD is a group of inherited disorders of hemoglobin structure characterized by hemolysis, unpredictable acute complications, and chronic organ damage. SCD is an autosomal recessive genetic disorder that results in an abnormally (sickle) shaped hemoglobin molecule. This leads to hemolysis and intravascular sludging, particularly in times of oxidative stress.

▶ Clinical Findings

A. Symptoms and Signs

Vaso-occlusive events are associated with fever, leukocytosis, joint effusions, and local tenderness. These symptoms may not be apparent at initial presentation but develop gradually during the course of the illness. The location is most often in the long bones or joints. Vasoocclusive events may also occur in the scalp, jaw, abdomen, pelvis, and various other locations. Pain in these areas may mimic numerous other medical conditions.

Splenic sequestration results from an accumulation of sickled red blood cells within the spleen. This can lead to rapid enlargement of the spleen, and precipitous drops in hemoglobin. Progression to shock and death can occur. Over time, sludging of red blood cells in the splenic vasculature leads to infarcts, causing abdominal pain and progressive decrease in splenic function. Any patient with SCD should be managed as if they are asplenic and are vulnerable to overwhelming infection by encapsulated bacteria.

Vaso-occlusive crises affect numerous other organs such as the chest, CNS, and penis. Acute chest syndrome is characterized by an infiltrate on chest X-ray, combined with lower respiratory tract symptoms and/or hypoxemia. This may be an isolated presentation or develop 2–3 days after a pain crisis. Any neurologic symptom more severe than a minor headache requires urgent evaluation, as occlusion of the CNS blood supply may be occurring. Symptoms may be significant (aphasia, hemiparesis) or more subtle (developmental delay, poor school performance). Occlusion of the vascular supply of the penis can lead to priapism (prolonged painful erection of the penis).

B. Laboratory Findings

Obtain a CBC and reticulocyte count. A decrease in hematocrit from baseline may indicate the need for transfusion. The absence of reticulocytosis indicates an aplastic crisis (often due to parvovirus B19 infection) and heralds an abrupt decrease in the hematocrit.

Obtain cultures of blood and urine if fever is present. Obtain electrolyte studies if dehydration is a concern.

If bone pain is associated with high fever, chills, toxicity, and leukocytosis, orthopedic consultation and bone aspiration is indicated to evaluate for osteomyelitis.

C. Imaging

Obtain X-rays of the chest if hypoxemia, cough, tachypnea, or dyspnea is present. Infiltrates may be present in patients with acute chest syndrome.

▶ Treatment

A. General Management

Administer oxygen if the patient is hypoxemic or in respiratory distress. IV fluid hydration is important in reversing the sickling process.

B. Venous Access

Begin an IV line if need for fluids or parenteral pain medications is anticipated. For patients with acute splenic sequestration, give bolus with IV fluids and perform exchange transfusion when available.

C. Antimicrobial Therapy

Due to increased risk for severe infection from encapsulated organisms, febrile SCD patients should be managed aggressively. CBC, blood cultures, urinalysis, urine culture, and chest X-ray should be performed, and CSF studies strongly considered. Empiric antibiotics should be administered while cultures are pending.

D. Pain Management

Effective pain management is essential in sickle cell crises. Patient's self-report is often the most accurate way to assess pain level. Patients may be able to use an objective scale or compare the current episode to prior crises. Even younger patients are often capable of relating the pain management regimen that has worked for them in past episodes. Acetaminophen with or without codeine can be used for mild pain. For severe pain, give IV morphine sulfate, 0.1 mg/kg every 2–4 hours. The patient should be reassessed frequently and medications adjusted according to pain level.

E. Treatment of Acute Chest Syndrome

Treatment of acute chest syndrome includes hospitalization, IV antibiotics, and supplemental oxygen to keep oxygen saturation above 95% on pulse oximetry. Administer IV fluids judiciously to maintain hydration. Over-hydration can lead to pulmonary edema. Frequent chest X-rays are necessary as radiologic appearance often lags behind clinical appearance. If hypoxemia worsens or respiratory distress occurs, exchange transfusion may be required to improve oxygen-carrying capacity and reduce the cardiac workload.

▶ Disposition

Children who can maintain adequate oral fluid intake and whose pain is controlled with oral medication can be managed as outpatients with close follow-up.

Hospitalize children who require continued parenteral therapy for pain, those who cannot maintain adequate oral hydration, or those who have required more than two visits for treatment of the same painful crisis. Any febrile child with SCD should be considered for admission.

Ballas SK: Pain management of sickle cell disease. Hematol Oncol Clin North Am 2005;19:785 [PMID: 16214644].

Freeman L: Sickle cell disease and other hemaglobinopathies: approach to emergency diagnosis and treatment. Emerg Med Pract 2001;3:11.

Johnson CS: The acute chest syndrome. Hematol Oncol Clin North Am 2005;19:857 [PMID: 16214648].

Sadowitz P, Amanullah S, Souid AK: Hematologic emergencies in the pediatric emergency room. Emerg Clin North Am 2002;20:177 [PMID: 11826633].

Section of Hematology/Oncology Committee on Genetics: Health supervision for children with sickle cell disease. Pediatrics 2002;109:526 [PMID: 12612266].

Wanko SO, Telen MJ: Transfusion management in sickle cell disease. Hematol Oncol Clin North Am 2005;19:803 [PMID: 16214645].

IDIOPATHIC THROMBOCYTOPENIC PURPURA

ESSENTIALS OF DIAGNOSIS

▶ Usually children present with petechia, purpura, or spontaneous bleeding involving the mucous membranes

▶ Platelet counts usually less than 100,000

▶ General Considerations

There are three mechanisms by which thrombocytopenia occurs: (1) increased destruction (idiopathic thrombocytopenia purpura [ITP], hemolytic uremic syndrome, or disseminated intravascular coagulopathy), (2) decreased production (aplastic crisis, marrow infiltrating neoplasms), and (3) splenic sequestration (sickle cell disease). ITP is an autoimmune disorder from increased destruction of platelets causing severe isolated thrombocytopenia. It commonly follows a viral illness. It is usually benign and self-limited; approximately 80–90% of cases resolve within 6 months.

▶ Clinical Findings

A. Symptoms and Signs

The clinical presentation is a healthy child who acutely develops petechiae and ecchymoses. Bleeding may occur from mucous membranes and significant epistaxis may occur. Physical examination should not reveal significant lymphadenopathy, hepatosplenomegaly, or joint swelling. These can be signs of other conditions such as leukemia or infectious mononucleosis. Children with platelet counts under 10,000 are at risk for life-threatening complications. Patients who manifest severe headache or altered level of consciousness should be evaluated for intracranial hemorrhage.

B. Laboratory Testing

Obtain a CBC with manual differential, blood smear, and platelet count. Typically the platelet count is less than 100,000 and sometimes less than 20,000.

▶ Treatment

A. General Management

Mild thrombocytopenia can be managed with observation and close follow-up.

B. Drug Therapy

Drug therapy for ITP remains controversial. Platelet levels with which therapy should begin and efficacy in improving thrombocytopenia are debated. Commonly used agents include corticosteroids, IVIG, and platelets. It is currently recommended that if the platelet count is less than 10,000–20,000, or if extensive bleeding is present, consultation with a pediatric hematologist and emergency therapy should be initiated.

C. Emergency Interventions

Emergency intervention is needed for severe gastrointestinal bleeding, hematuria, or intracranial hemorrhage. Whole-blood transfusion may be required for severe anemia. IV corticosteroids should be administered such as methylprednisolone, 10–30 mg/kg/d for 3–5 days (maximum, 1 g over 30 minutes). The optimal dose of IVIG is not known, but 0.25–1.0 g/kg is the usual range used.

D. Platelet Transfusions

Platelet transfusions are indicated for refractory ITP and life-threatening hemorrhage, but the half-life of transfused platelets is brief. Splenectomy may be indicated if medical treatments fail.

▶ Disposition

Hospitalize children with ITP if the platelet count is less than 10,000 or if significant bleeding is present, particularly young children for whom avoidance of traumatic play is difficult.

Advise older children to avoid all contact sports and vigorous playground activities during the acute phase of the disease.

Obtain emergency neurosurgical consultation for any signs of intracranial hemorrhage. Obtain hematologic consultation and a bone marrow examination before corticosteroid therapy is initiated.

Kaplan RN, Bussel JB: Differential diagnosis and management of thrombocytopenia in childhood. Pediatr Clin North Am 2004;51:1109 [PMID: 15275991].

Sadowitz P, Amanullah S, Souid AK: Hematologic emergencies in the pediatric emergency room. Emerg Clin North Am 2002;20:177 [PMID: 11826633].

Tarantino MD, Buchanan GR: The pros and cons of drug therapy for immune thrombocytopenic purpura in children. Hematol Oncol Clin North Am 2004;18:1301 [PMID: 15511617].

▼ NEWBORN EMERGENCIES

▶ Clinical Findings

The need for resuscitation of the newborn infant is based on the primary survey. Immediate attention should be placed on any deficiencies in airway, breathing, or circulation. Secondary survey and Apgar scores (Table 50–19) can be used to further guide the resuscitation efforts. Vital signs should be recorded frequently to monitor the success of resuscitation. Physical examination should establish the degree of maturity of the infant as well as the integrity of the infant's respiratory and cardiovascular functions.

▶ Treatment

A. General Management

The key to treatment in the newborn infant is to be prepared and use an organized team approach. A "code card" posted in the emergency department, or use of the Broselow tape, can help guide drug dosing and choice of equipment sizes.

If time permits, alert the obstetric service and nursery staff prior to the birth of the baby. Electronic fetal monitoring is helpful if time and equipment availability permit.

An overhead radiant warmer should be present and turned on. If one is not available, use heating lamps or warm blankets. Proper equipment should be available and functioning.

At birth, the umbilical cord should be quickly clamped and then cut. Remember to leave 1–3 cm of cord in the event the infant needs an umbical central line. The infant should be placed under the radiant warmer and immediately assessed, and an Apgar score should be assigned (see Table 50–19). The heart rate can be monitored by palpation of the umbilical arterial pulse. The oropharynx can be gently suctioned and the infant stimulated by rubbing its back. The infant should be towel dried. Apgar scores should be assigned at 1 and 5 minutes.

B. Neonatal Resuscitation

Infants who are bradycardic, apneic, or significantly depressed require immediate resuscitative efforts (Figure 50–10).

Epinephrine, atropine, or naloxone can be administered via the endotracheal tube after intubation during resuscitative efforts prior to the establishment of vascular access. When this route is used, double the usual IV dosages of these medications.

Umbilical vein catheterization can also be used for emergency drug administration or volume expansion. Umbilical artery catheterization can be used for frequent arterial blood gas analysis and blood pressure readings.

Continue to reassess the cardiovascular function of the child to guide resuscitative efforts. Be alert to complications particular to the newborn when resuscitation does not result in expected improvement (eg, meconium aspiration, respiratory distress syndrome, shock, maternal substance abuse, pneumothorax, choanal atresia, diaphragmatic hernia, tracheoesophageal fistula, volume/ blood loss). As the Apgar score improves, prepare the infant for transport to the nursery for close monitoring and care as indicated.

▼ CHILD ABUSE

PHYSICAL ABUSE

▶ General Considerations

Each year child protective services find evidence of abuse in almost 1 million children. Over 1700 childhood deaths occur each year as a result of abuse, with over 75% being less than 3 years of age. The initial presentation of an abused

Table 50–19. Evaluation of the Newborn Infant Using the Apgar Score.

	Score		
	0	**1**	**2**
Appearance (color)	Pale or blue	Pink trunk and pale limbs	Pink trunk and limbs
Pulse (heart rate)	Absent	<100	>100
Grimace	Absent	Some response	Crying withdraws
Activity	Absent	some flexion	Extremities well flexed
Respiration	Absent	Weak cry	Active cry

child frequently occurs in the emergency department. This requires the coordination of the emergency medicine practitioner with other community members responsible for the investigation, management, and adjudication of child abuse cases. Risk factors that increase the likelihood of child maltreatment include poverty, substance abuse, single parenthood, young maternal age, social isolation, parental psychiatric illness, and parental history of childhood abuse. While these variables may be present, there is no typical patient or caregiver who is a victim or abuser. The physician's responsibilities are to (1) acknowledge that a problem exists, (2) maintain a high index of suspicion, (3) discuss concerns with the parents in a sensitive and compassionate manner, (4) ensure protection of the child, (5) perform a complete medial evaluation of the injuries or neglect, including documentation and radiologic imaging if indicated, and (6) report suspicions to child protective services.

The history given by the caretaker that is inconsistent with the physical examination of the child may suggest the diagnosis of abuse. Child abuse should be considered when: (1) a child presents with significant injuries and history of trauma is denied or does not explain the injuries identified (2) the history changes over time or from different caregivers (3) a history of self-inflicted trauma is beyond the child's developmental milestones (4) delay in seeking medical attention, (5) multiple injuries in different stages of healing (6) failure to thrive, (7) any injury pathognomonic for child abuse. Current research is being devoted to developing clinical models involving force required to generate various injuries to assist the physician in determining the plausibility of given histories. The history documented should include location, time, and mechanism of injury, as well as all caregivers present at time of injury.

▶ **Clinical Findings**

A. Symptoms and Signs

1. Bruises—Bruises are the most common injury identified in abused children. However, bruising is also ubiquitous in the normal ambulatory child. Factors that may alert the physician to nonaccidental trauma are bruising to infants who are not yet cruising and bruising in an unusual distribution or location, such as the ears, buttocks, chest, or abdomen. Bruises may also demonstrate pattern injuries that demonstrate a specific object that struck the child. It must be remembered that a subtle bruise may be the only external indicator of significant internal trauma. Additionally, severe or even fatal abuse can occur without a single external mark. Any child suspected of being abused needs a full body skin exam.

2. Skeletal trauma—Skeletal injuries are more common in infants and young children but can be seen in all ages. Patterns of fractures that raise suspicion for abuse include fractures in nonambulatory infants, multiple fractures, and fractures of different ages. Specific locations of fractures listed below can also increase clinical suspicion.

A. **Femoral fractures**—Femoral fractures (spiral or transverse) in children under age 3 years are suspicious. Minor falls, less than 30–60 cm, usually do not result in femoral fractures.

B. **Epiphyseal–metaphyseal fractures**—Epiphyseal–metaphyseal fractures in young infants and children are virtually diagnostic of abuse because they usually do not occur with accidental falls. These fractures usually occur as a result of severe pulling, twisting, or shaking of the child's limbs. These activities produce severe acceleration–deceleration forces on the limbs, resulting in metaphyseal chip or "corner" fractures.

C. **Rib fractures**—Rib fractures in infants under the age of 2 years are extremely uncommon because the infant's rib cage is extremely pliant. Multiple, bilateral posterior rib fractures are virtually pathognomonic for abuse and are caused by significant squeezing pressure to the chest.

3. Burns—Burns sustained by infants and toddlers may be accidental, inflicted, or the result of poor supervision and neglect. Inflicted immersion burns often demonstrate clear lines of demarcation where the child was held in scalding water with areas above spared. Accidental immersion burns typically have indistinct borders, varying depths of injury, irregular margins, and splash pattern burns outside the primary burn area. Burns also may be inflicted by cigarettes, irons, or stoves. Care must be taken in examining the burn area to identify pattern injury.

4. Head injuries—Head injuries carry the highest incidence of morbidity and mortality. These injuries can occur by blunt impact or shaking with sudden acceleration–deceleration forces. Head injury is most common in patients under 3 years

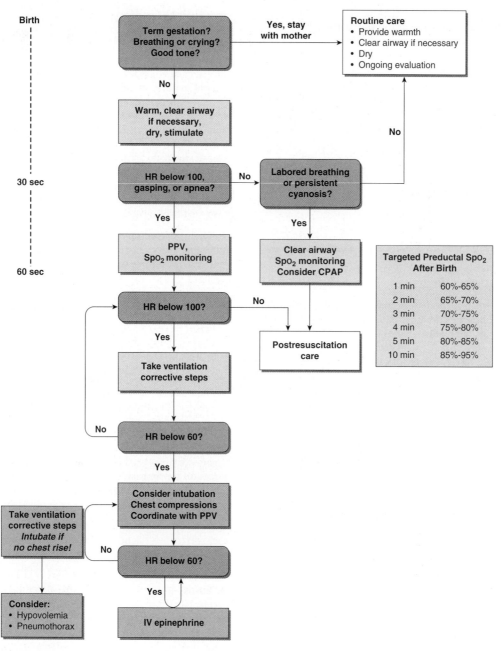

▲ **Figure 50–10.** Algorithmic guide to neonatal resuscitation. Endotracheal intubation may be considered at several steps. The recommended IV dose of epinephrine is 0.01 to 0.03 mg/kg per dose. While access is being obtained, administration of a higher dose (up to 0.1 mg/kg) through the endotracheal tube may be considered, but the safety and efficacy of this practice have not been evaluated. The concentration of epinephrine for either route should be 1:10,000 (0.1 mg/mL). (Reproduced, with permission, from 2010 American Heart Association guidelines for cardiopulmonary resuscitation and emergency cardiovascular care, part 15: Neonatal resuscitation. *Circulation.* 2010;122(Suppl 3): S909–S919. Copyright © 2010 American Heart Association, Inc.)

of age, especially infants. Subdural hematomas can occur with resulting cerebral compression. In addition, these forces can cause direct neuronal injury within the brain. Infants who are severely shaken can present with sudden onset of seizure or coma but have no signs of head trauma. Typically, infants who are severely shaken will have bilateral subdural and inter-hemispheric hemorrhages.

5. Abdominal injuries—Nonaccidental abdominal injury may produce severe injury to the viscera, including intramural hematomas of the small bowel, splenic or hepatic lacerations, traumatic pancreatitis, and renal contusions.

B. Diagnostic Procedures

The following studies should be ordered:

- CBC and coagulation studies
- urinalysis (recommend urine pregnancy for adolescent females)
- abdominal enzymes (lipase, liver functions) should be considered
- a skeletal X-ray series of the skull, ribs, and long bones in any known or suspected cases of abuse in children younger than 3 years (a babygram does not provide satisfactory bone resolution to rule out abuse)
- CT head should be performed in children with abuse related head trauma, neurologic signs and symptoms, and considered in all abuse cases involving children younger than 1 year.

Christian CW: Assessment and evaluation of the physically abused child. Clin Fam Pract 2003;5:21.

Hudson M, Kaplan R: Clinical response to child abuse. Pediatr Clin North Am 2006;53:27 [PMID: 16487783].

Pierce MC et al: Femur fractures resulting from stair falls among children: an injury plausibility model. Pediatrics 2005;115:1712 [PMID: 15930236].

National Clearinghouse on Child Abuse and Neglect Information. Available at: http://www.childwelfare.gov/can/faq.cfm

SEXUAL ABUSE

General Considerations

Sexual abuse is involvement of children and adolescents in sexual activities that they cannot comprehend because of their developmental level, activities to which they are unable to give informed consent, or activities that violate social taboos. Sexual abuse accounts for 7% of all abuse cases reported. These activities may physically injure the child and leave detectable patterns of trauma, but often sexual abuse may involve genital touching or fondling that does not cause detectable injury. Most victims of sexual abuse are female, and the mean age is 7–8 years. Children are usually molested by males who are well known to them, either as family member or trusted friends. Adolescents are more commonly molested by strangers.

Clinical Findings

Various behavioral reactions may ensue following sexual abuse. In preschool and grade school aged children, these can be fear states (eg, fear of adult males), nightmares, precocious sexual behavior, sexual aggression toward other children, crossdressing, school failure, truancy, running away, or depression. Adolescents may demonstrate behavioral problems with drugs, promiscuity, prostitution, running away, sexual aggression toward other children, depression, somatic complaints, or school failure.

Disclosures of sexual abuse are often incomplete and may later be retracted because the perpetrator is typically someone to whom the child feels great allegiance and on whom the child is dependent.

Some children who are sexually abused show signs of abuse, including genital and nongenital trauma as well as the presence of STDs. A STD may be the only indication of molestation. Direct injuries to hymenal tissue are rarely accidental. Hymenal lacerations should always raise the possibility of sexual abuse. Typically straddle injuries do not cause hymenal lacerations. Anal penetration may result in erythema and swelling of the perianal tissue as well as lacerations, abrasions, and bruising.

Children in whom sexual abuse is being considered should be evaluated at a center where health-care providers accustomed to examining sexual abuse victims are located. The goals of the medical evaluation are to (1) treat any medical illness or injuries, (2) provide crisis counseling, (3) provide protection for the child if necessary, and (4) document injuries and collect evidence for use by the legal system.

Approach the child in a compassionate, nonthreatening manner, and ask nonleading questions in an attempt to uncover whether sexual abuse has occurred. The physical examination should be performed immediately if sexual assault has occurred within 72 hours or if the child has signs or symptoms of genital injury or infection. Look for both nongenital and genital injuries. Many examiners employ a colposcope with a camera attachment to provide photographic documentation of genital injuries. A speculum examination in a prepubertal child is indicated only when symptoms of vaginal injury (eg, vaginal bleeding) are present. This is best done under general anesthesia. Laboratory testing for the diagnosis of STDs should be obtained routinely, including wet mount and Gram staining of genital or rectal discharge; genital and rectal cultures for *N. gonorrhoeae* and *Chlamydia trachmatis*; pharyngeal cultures for *N. gonorrhoeae*; culture of lesions suspicious for herpes simplex; and serologic studies for hepatitis B, syphilis, and human immunodeficiency virus, if indicated.

If the sexual assault has occurred within 72 hours of the examination, seminal fluid may be present on or within the child. The proper collection of this evidence is essential. Physicians who examine sexual abuse victims must be fully knowledgeable of the protocol for evidence collection in their locale.

▶ Treatment

A. Treat Physical Injuries

Treat physical injuries as necessary. Inspect vaginal lacerations for possible extension into the abdominal cavity. Significant perineal or vaginal lacerations are best examined under general anesthesia in the operating room.

B. Treat STDs

Because STDs are relatively uncommon in prepubertal victims of sexual abuse, empiric therapy is recommended only if the child has a vaginal or rectal discharge that on Gram staining is suggestive of gonorrhea. Adolescent victims of sexual assault should routinely be given treatment for STDs at the time of examination, because the incidence of STDs in this group is significant. Give empiric treatment for both *Chlamydia* (patients > 8 years doxycycline, 100 mg twice a day for 10 days, Children ≤ 8 years use weight-based erythromycin) and gonorrhea (ceftriaxone, 125 mg intramuscularly).

C. Offer Pregnancy Prevention

After documentation of a negative urine pregnancy test, adolescent girls should be offered prophylaxis against conception with norgestrel (Ovral), two pills at the time of examination and two pills 12 hours later orally.

D. Offer Counseling

Pediatric and adolescent victims of sexual abuse should be offered counseling following the initial evaluation. Many children will require extensive counseling, particularly those who are victims of long-term incestuous relationships.

▶ Disposition

Children and adolescents may be discharged home if their medical condition permits and safety can be ensured. Disposition home should be confirmed by child protective services involved in the case and documented in the medical record. If the child is at risk for further sexual abuse, removal from parental custody and placement in shelter care is indicated.

National Clearinghouse on Child Abuse and Neglect Information. Available at: http://www.childwelfare.gov/can/faq.cfm

INDEX

Page numbers followed by *f* indicate figures; page numbers followed by *t* indicate tables.

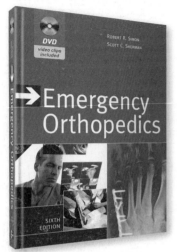
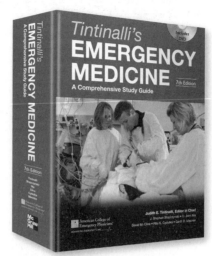
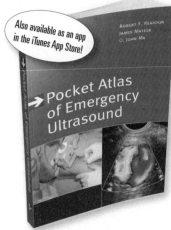
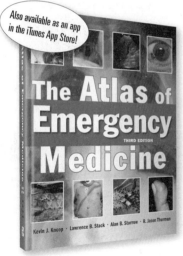
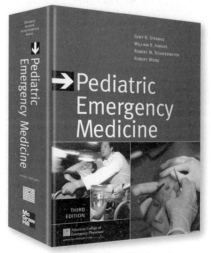
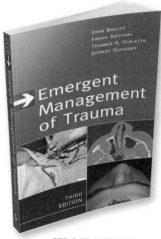
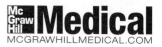